CLINICAL SURGERY

THIRD EDITION

EDITED BY

MICHAEL M HENRY MB FRCS
Formerly Consultant Surgeon, Chelsea and Westminster and Royal Marsden Hospitals;
Formerly Honorary Consultant Surgeon, National Hospital for Neurology and
Elizabeth Garrett Anderson Hospital, London, UK

JEREMY N THOMPSON MA MB MCHIR FRCS
Consultant Surgeon, Chelsea and Westminster and Royal Marsden Hospitals, London, UK

Foreword by
PARVEEN KUMAR & MICHAEL CLARK

Illustrations by Gillian Lee FMAA HonFIMI AMI RMIP
and Louise Perks MIMI RMIP

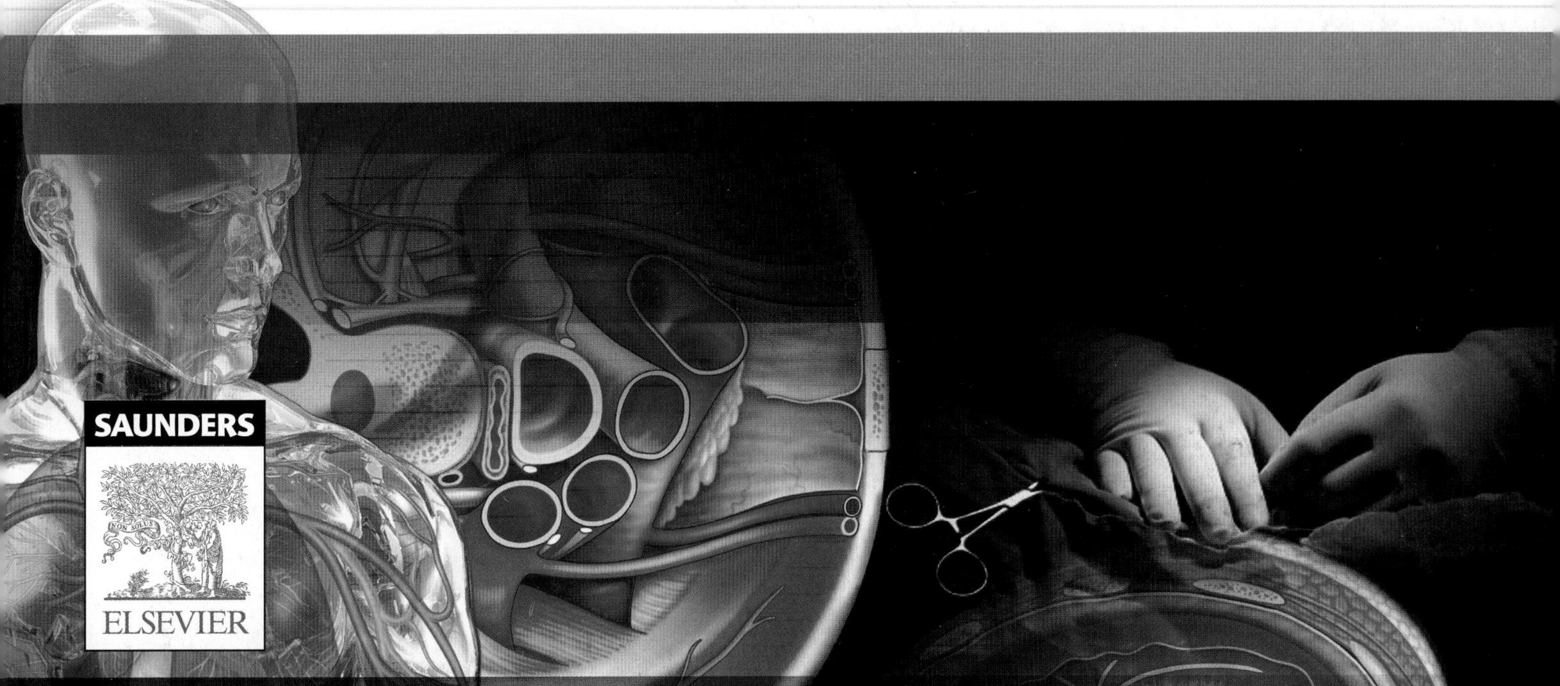

SAUNDERS
ELSEVIER

Edinburgh London New York Oxford Philadelphia St Louis Sydney Toronto 2012

SAUNDERS
ELSEVIER

Third edition 2012
Second edition 2005
First edition 2001

ISBN 978-0-7020-3070-3
International ISBN 978-0-7020-3074-1

British Library Cataloguing in Publication Data
A catalogue record for this book is available from the British Library

Library of Congress Cataloging in Publication Data
A catalog record for this book is available from the Library of Congress

Printed in China

Contents

SECTION 2 REGIONAL SURGERY

SECTION 3 SURGICAL SPECIALTIES

Contributors

Solomon Abramovich MSc FRCS
Consultant Ear, Nose and Throat Surgeon, Department of Otolaryngology, Head and Neck Surgery, Imperial College Healthcare NHS Trust, St Mary's Hospital, London, UK
Ear and nose

Matthew Barry MBBS MS FRCS(Orth)
Consultant Orthopaedic Surgeon, Department of Orthopaedics, The Royal London Hospital, London, UK
Principles of orthopaedics

Duncan Arthur Black BSc(Med Hons) MBChB FRCS(Ed) PhD
Honorary Consultant Vascular Surgeon, Department of Vascular Surgery, St Mary's Hospital, Imperial College Healthcare NHS Trust, London,UK
Venous and lymphatic disorders

Roger C Bloomer MBChB FRCA
Specialist Registrar in Anaesthetics, Imperial School of Anaesthesia, London, UK
The seriously ill and injured patient

Gianluca Bonanomi MD FRCS
Consultant Surgeon, Chelsea and Westminster NHS Foundation Hospital, London;
Honorary Senior Lecturer, Imperial College, London, UK
Bariatric surgery

S Jeremy Booth MBBS FCEM
Consultant in Emergency Medicine, Chelsea and Westminster Hospital, London, UK
Formerly:
Clinical Director of Accident and Emergency Medicine, Chelsea and Westminster Healthcare NHS Trust, London
Honorary Consultant in Accident and Emergency, Royal Brompton and Harefield Hospitals NHS Trust, London
Immediate Past President (Accident and Emergency Section), Royal Society of Medicine
Senior Examiner in Surgery to the University of London
Emergency medicine

Tim Campbell-Smith BSc(Hons) MBBS FRCS (Gen Surg)
Colorectal Fellow, University College London Hospital, London, UK
Anal and related disorders

Nicholas H Cawrse FRCS(Plast)
Specialist Registrar in Plastic Surgery, Abbey Ward, Royal Devon and Exeter Hospital (Wonford), Exeter, UK
Principles of plastic surgery

Simon Clarke BSc(Hons) FRCS(Paed Surg)
Consultant Paediatric Surgeon, Chelsea and Westminister Foundation NHS Trust;
Honorary Senior Lecturer, Imperial College London, London, UK
Principles of paediatric surgery

Simon Anthony Clint BSc MBBS FRCS(Tr & Orth)
Specialist Registrar, Royal National Orthopaedic Hospital, Middlesex, UK
Principles of management of fractures, joint injuries and peripheral nerve injuries

C Richard G Cohen MD FRCS
Consultant Colorectal Surgeon and Honorary Senior Lecturer, University College London Hospital, London, UK
Anal and related disorders

David Corless BSc MD FRCS(Gen)
Consultant General and Upper Gastrointestinal Surgeon, Mid-Cheshire Hospital Foundation Trust, Cheshire and University Hospital, North Staffordshire, Staffordshire, UK
Organisation of surgical services

Lord Ara Darzi PC KBE HonFrEng FMedSci
Professor of Surgery, Division of Surgery, Imperial College London, St Mary's Hospital, London, UK
The operation
Perioperative management and postoperative complications

Michael Dialynas MS FRCS(Ed) FRCS(Gen Surg)
Consultant Vascular Surgeon, King's College Hospital, London, UK
Arterial disease

Daryl Dob BSc(Hons) MBBS FRCA
Consultant Anaesthetist, Maghill Department of Anaesthetics, Chelsea and Westminster Hospital, London, UK
Anaesthesia and pain control

Philip J Drew BSc MD(Hons) MS FRCS (Ed, Eng & Glasg) FRCS(Gen)
Professor and Consultant Breast Surgeon, Royal Cornwall HospitalTrust, Treliske Hospital, Truro, Cornwall, UK
Breast disease

Michael Dusmet MD FMH
Consultant Thoracic Surgeon, Royal Brompton Hospital, London, UK
Chest and lungs

Timothy E E Goodacre MBBS BSc FRCS
Florey Lecturer in Clinical Medicine and Consultant Plastic and Reconstructive Surgeon, Oxford Children's Hospital, Oxford Radcliffe Hospitals, Headington, Oxford, UK
Surgery in the developing world

Seyed Habib Kashi MB ChM FRCS
Consultant Surgeon, University Hospital of Coventry and Warwickshire NHS Trust, Coventry, UK
Organ transplantation

Kevin Haire MBBS FRCA
Consultant Anaesthetist, Maghill Department of Anaesthesia, Chelsea and Westminster Hospital, London, UK
Anaesthesia and pain control

Michael M Henry MB FRCS
Formerly Consultant Surgeon, Chelsea and Westminster and Royal Marsden Hospitals; Formerly Honorary Consultant Surgeon, National Hospital for Neurology and Elizabeth Garrett Anderson Hospital
London, UK
Large bowel, including appendix

Michael J Hershman DHMSA MSc(Hons) MS(Hons) FRCS(Eng, Ed, Glas & I) FICS
Consultant Surgeon, Stafford Hospital, Stafford, UK
Hernia

Andrew L Hine MBBS MRCP FRCR
Consultant Radiologist, Department of Radiology, Central Middlesex Hospital, North-West London Hospitals NHS Trust, London, UK
Investigation of the surgical patient

Michael Philip Jenkins BSc MS FRCS FRCS (Gen Surg) FEBVS
Consultant Vascular Surgeon, Regional Vascular Unit, St Mary's Hospital, Imperial College Healthcare NHS Trust, London, UK
Arterial disease
Venous and lymphatic disorders

Pankaj Kumar MA FRCS(C/Th)
Consultant Cardiac Surgeon, Morriston Hospital, Swansea, UK
Cardiac surgery

Tim P Lawrence BM MRCS
Neurosurgery Registrar, Department of Neurosurgery, The John Radcliffe Hospital, Oxford, UK
Neurosurgery

Jonathan Leonard BSc MD FRCP
Consultant Dermatologist, St Mary's Hospital, Imperial College Healthcare NHS Trust, London, UK
Skin Disorders

Christopher P Macklin BMed BM BS FRCS DM
Consultant General and Colorectal Surgeon
Mid Yorkshire Hospitals NHS Trust, Yorkshire, UK
Reader

Timothy K McCullough MS FRCS
Consultant General and Colorectal Surgeon
Lister Hospital, East and North Hertfordshire NHS Trust, Stevenage, Hertfordshire, UK
Hernia

Satvinder Mudan BSc MBBS MD FRCS
Consultant Surgeon, Royal Marsden Hospital, London, UK
Surgical infection
Liver and biliary tree

Nuala O'Donoghue MBChB MRCPI
Consultant Dermatologist, Salford Royal NHS FoundationTrust, Salford, UK
Skin disorders

Christopher William Ogden MS FRCS Eng(Urol) FEBU
Consultant Urologist, The Royal Marsden Hospital, Urology Unit, London, UK
Urology

Paraskeva Paraskevas PhD FRCS
Consultant Surgeon and Senior Lecturer, Department of Biosurgery and Surgical Technology, St Mary's Hospital, Imperial College Healthcare NHS Trust, London, UK
The operation
Perioperative management and postoperative complications

John Pepper MChir FRCS
Professor of Cardiothoracic Surgery, Department of Surgery, Royal Brompton Hospital, London, UK
Cardiac surgery

Sanjay Purkayastha BSc(Hons) MD MRCS(Eng) MBBS(Hons)
Clinical Lecturer in Surgery, Division of Surgery, Department of Surgery and Cancer, Faculty of Medicine, St Mary's Hospital, Imperial College Healthcare NHS Trust, London, UK
The operation

Warwick Radford ChM FRCSEd(Orth)
Consultant Orthopaedic Surgeon, Chelsea and Westminster Hospital, London, UK
Principles of orthopaedics

Peter Richards FRCS FRCPCH
Consultant Paediatric Neurosurgeon, Department of Neurosurgery, John Radcliffe Hospital, Oxford, UK
Neurosurgery

Peter J Saxby MBChB FRCS(Plast) ChM
Consultant Plastic Surgeon, Department of Plastic Surgery, Royal Devon and Exeter Hospital, Exeter, UK
Principles of plastic surgery

Wilhelm Edmund Schulenburg FRCS FRCOphth
Consultant Ophthalmic Surgeon, The Western Eye Hospital Imperial College Healthcare NHS Trust, London, UK
Ophthalmology in clinical surgery

David Michael Scott-Coombes MS FRCS
Consultant Endocrine Surgeon, University Hospital of Wales, Cardiff, UK
Surgery of the endocrine glands

Philip J Shorvon FRCP FRCR FBIR
Consultant Radiologist, Department of Radiology, Central Middlesex Hospital, North West London Hospitals NHS Trust, London, UK
Investigation of the surgical patient

Dishan Singh MBChB FRCS(Orth)
Consultant Orthopaedic Surgeon, Royal National Orthopaedic Hospital, Middlesex, UK
Principles of management of fractures, joint injuries and peripheral nerve injuries

Neil Soni MBChB FRCA FANZCA FJFICM MD
Consultant in Anaesthesia and Intensive Care, Chelsea and Westminster Hospital NHS Trust, London, UK
The seriously ill and injured patient

Duncan Richard Castell Spalding BSc(Hons) MD FRCS(Eng) FRCS(Gen Surg)
Clinical Senior Lecturer and Honorary HPB Surgeon, Hammersmith Hospital, Imperial College Healthcare NHS Trust, London, UK
The spleen

Allan D Spigelman MBBS MD FRACS FRCS
Clinical Associate Dean and Professor of Surgery, Surgical Professorial Unit, UNSW St Vincent's Hospital Clinical School, Sydney;
Director of Cancer Services, St Vincent's and Mater Health, Sydney;
Director Cancer and Imunology Program, St Vincent's Hospital, Sydney, Australia
Acute abdominal conditions

Nicholas D Stafford MBChB FRCS
Professor of Head and Neck Surgery, Postgraduate Medical Institute, University of Hull, Hull, UK
The neck and upper aerodigestive tract

Jeremy N Thompson MA MB MChir FRCS
Consultant Surgeon, Chelsea and Westminster and Royal Marsden Hospitals, London, UK
Surgery – what it is and what a surgeon does
Wound healing and management
The pancreas
Small bowel disease and intestinal obstruction

Robin C N Williamson MA MD MChir FRCS(Ed) FRCS(Eng)
Consultant Surgeon, Hammersmith Hospital, Imperial College Healthcare NHS Trust, London;
Professor of Surgery, Imperial College London, London, UK
The spleen

Alastair C J Windsor MD FRCS
Consultant Colorectal Surgeon, University College Hospital, London, UK
Anal and related disorders

John Winstanley BDS MD FRCS (Eng, Glas) FDSRCPSG
Consultant Surgeon, Royal Bolton Hospital, Bolton, UK
Breast disease

International Advisory Panel

Foreword

Undergraduate curricula are continually changing to suit the needs of the patient and over the last few years there has been an emphasis on communication skills, clinical skills and patient involvement. However, the basic practise of medicine and surgery remains unchanged and requires a good grounding of knowledge.

Despite the onslaught of the technological age, textbooks still remain an integral part of learning. This textbook has now become well established in the undergraduate curriculum and we are delighted to see this 3rd edition. It builds on the previous editions bringing all aspects of surgery right up-to-date. The book is extremely practical as well as informative. It gives an excellent insight into the life of a surgeon, starting with the training of a surgeon, the organisational aspects of being a surgeon, and the pre- and post-operative care management of the patient. It also touches on the legal and ethical issues which are a necessary part of being a doctor. The remaining chapters take you through the various specialities in a logical fashion providing the knowledge to be able to understand surgical decisions and techniques.

This new edition, once again, has been written to harmonise with our own textbook, *Kumar and Clark's Clinical Medicine*. We hope that these books will be helpful companions through your career in clinical practice.

Parveen J. Kumar
Michael L. Clark

Preface

Clinical Surgery aims to provide a comprehensive textbook of surgical disorders for both an undergraduate and postgraduate readership. The book encompasses a wide range of surgical specialties within a single volume.

The Third Edition has been comprehensively revised and updated in response to comments and suggestions from our readers, authors, Chris Macklin, Parveen Kumar and Michael Clark. An extra chapter on *Bariatric Surgery* has been added.

We believe that these changes have further strengthened *Clinical Surgery*.

Michael M. Henry
Jeremy N. Thompson

Acknowledgements

The Third Edition of Clinical Surgery follows on from the success of the first two editions. We remain grateful to those authors that contributed to the first two editions. In particular we are indebted to several authors who contributed to both the previous editions including: Shaun Appleton, Saswata Banerjee, Rolfe Birch, Reuben Canello, Richard Coombs, David Drake, Omar Faiz, Pierre Guillou, Nagy Habib, Dimitri Hadjiminas, Andrew Leather, Hamish McClure, Jonathan Northway, Michelle Slater, the late Nick Taffinder, Alison Waghorn and Gordon Williams.

We are extremely grateful to all those existing and new authors who contributed to the current edition. We would also like to thank Chris Macklin for his input as reader. We are particularly thankful to Michael Clark and Parveen Kumar who have made helpful contributions to the editorial review of this edition.

Finally we are very grateful for the support and patience of Alan Nicholson, Sally Davies and Pauline Graham at Elsevier during the preparation of the Third Edition.

Michael M. Henry
Jeremy N. Thompson

Abbreviations

A&E accident and emergency
AAA abdominal aortic aneurysm
ABGs arterial blood gases
ABPI ankle:brachial pressure index
ACE angiotensin-converting enzyme
ACL anterior cruciate ligament
ACTH adrenocorticotrophic hormone
ADH antidiuretic hormone
AEE activity energy expenditure
AFP alpha-fetoprotein
AION anterior ischaemic optic neuropathy
APC antigen-presenting cell
APPT accelerated partial thromboplastin time
APUD amine precursor uptake and decarboxylation
ARDS adult respiratory distress syndrome
ARMD age-related macular degeneration
ATLS advanced trauma life support
ATP adenosine triphosphate
AV (1) atrioventricular; (2) arteriovenous
AVM arteriovenous malformation
BMR basal metabolic rate
BMT best medical therapy
BP blood pressure
BPH benign prostatic hyperplasia
BST basic surgical training
CA 19-9 carbohydrate antigen 19-9
CABG coronary artery bypass grafting
CAD coronary artery disease
CCD charge couple device
CCK cholecystokinin
CCST Certificate of Completion of Specialist Training
CDC Centers for Disease Control
CEA (1) carcinoembryonic antigen; (2) carotid endarterectomy
CLI critical limb ischaemia
CNS central nervous system
COPD chronic obstructive pulmonary disease
CPAP continuous positive airways pressure
CPB cardiopulmonary bypass
CPP cerebral perfusion pressure
CQC Care Quality Commission
CSF cerebrospinal fluid
CSSD central sterile supply department
CT computed tomography
CVA cerebrovascular accident
CVP central venous pressure
DCIS ductal carcinoma in situ
DGH district general hospital
DIC disseminated intravascular coagulation
DIT dietary-induced thermogenesis
DMSA dimercaptosuccinic acid
DSA digital subtraction angiography
DTPA diethylene-triamine-penta-acetic acid
DTSI deep-to-superficial incompetence
DVT deep-vein thrombosis
ECF extracellular fluid
ECG electrocardiogram
ECMO extracorporeal membrane oxygenation
EEG electroencephalogram
EGF epidermal growth factor
ELISA enzyme-linked immunosorbent assay
EMG electromyography
ENT ear, nose and throat
ER oestrogen receptor
ERCP endoscopic retrograde cholangiopancreatography
ESR erythrocyte sedimentation rate
FDPs fibrin degradation products
FEV_1 forced expiratory volume in the first second
FFA free fatty acids
FNA fine-needle aspiration
FNAC fine-needle aspiration cytology
FNH focal nodular hyperplasia
FSH follicle-stimulating hormone
FVC forced vital capacity
GA general anaesthetic
GCS Glasgow Coma Score
G-CSF granulocyte colony-stimulating factor
GFR glomerular filtration rate
GI gastrointestinal
GMC General Medical Council
GnRH gonadotrophin-releasing hormone
GORD gastro-oesophageal reflux disease
GTN glyceryl trinitrate
HAART highly active antiretroviral therapy
hATI human anti-tetanus immunoglobulin
hCG human chorionic gonadotrophin
HDU high-dependency unit
HRT hormone replacement therapy
HST higher surgical training
i.m. intramuscular
i.v. intravenous
IABP intra-aortic balloon pump
ICF intracellular fluid
ICP intracranial pressure
ICU intensive care unit
IFN interferon
IL interleukin
INR international normalised ratio
IVN intravenous nutrition
IVU intravenous urogram
JVP jugular venous pressure
L litre
LA local anaesthetic
LAD left anterior descending coronary artery
LATS long-acting thyroid stimulators
LCA left coronary artery
LCIS lobular carcinoma in situ
LDH lactate dehydrogenase
LH luteinising hormone
LHRH luteinising hormone-releasing hormone
LMA laryngeal mask airway

LMWH	low-molecular-weight heparin
LVEDP	left ventricular end-diastolic pressure
MAG3	technetium-99m mercaptoacetyltriglycine
MAP	mean arterial pressure
MCV	mean corpuscular volume
MG	myasthenia gravis
MHC	major histocompatibility complex
MODS	multiple organ dysfunction syndrome
MOSF	multiple organ system failure
MRCP	magnetic resonance cholangiopancreatography
MRI	magnetic resonance imaging
MRSA	methicillin-resistant Staphylococcus aureus
MS	multiple sclerosis
MSU	midstream urine
NHS	National Health Service
NICE	National Institute for Clinical Excellence
NSAID	non-steroidal anti-inflammatory drug
NSCLC	non-small-cell lung cancer
NTN	National Training Number
NVE	native valve endocarditis
NYHA	New York Heart Association
OA	osteoarthritis
OPSI	overwhelming postsplenectomy infection
PABA	p-aminobenzoic acid
PACS	picture archive and communication system
PAD	peripheral arterial disease
PCA	patient-controlled analgesia
PCL	posterior cruciate ligament
PCR	polymerase chain reaction
PCT	Primary Care Trust
PE	pulmonary embolism
PEEP	positive end-expiratory pressure
PEG	percutaneous endoscopic gastrostomy
PET	positron emission tomography
PGA	persistent generalised lymphadenopathy
PiCCO	pulse-induced contour cardiac output
PNO	pneumothorax
PONV	postoperative nausea and vomiting
PPV	positive-pressure ventilation
PR	progesterone receptor
PSP	peak systolic pressure
PTA	percutaneous transluminal angioplasty
PTC	percutaneous transhepatic cholangiography
PTCA	percutaneous transluminal coronary angioplasty
PTH	parathyroid hormone
PUJ	pelviureteric junction
PUO	pyrexia of unknown origin
PVD	posterior vitreous detachment
PVE	prosthetic valve endocarditis
RA	rheumatoid arthritis
RAPD	relative afferent pupillary defect
RAS	renal artery stenosis
RCA	right coronary artery
REE	resting energy expenditure
RP	Raynaud's phenomenon
RSI	repetitive strain injury
RTI	respiratory tract infection
RVF	rectovaginal fistula
SA	sinoatrial
SAC	Specialist Advisory Committee
SCC	small-cell carcinoma
SCFAs	short-chain fatty acids
SCID	severe combined immune deficiency
SIRS	systemic inflammatory response syndrome
SPECT	single-photon emission computed tomography
SpR	Specialist Registrar
TBW	total body water
TEE	total energy expenditure
THI	tissue harmonic imaging
TIA	transient ischaemic attack
TIBC	total iron-binding capacity
TNF	tumour necrosis factor
TNM	tumour–node–metastasis
TPN	total parenteral nutrition
TRH	thyrotrophin-releasing hormone
TRUS	transrectal ultrasound
TSH	thyroid-stimulating hormone
TSSU	theatre sterile supply unit
TUR	transurethral resection
U&E	urea and electrolytes
UGI	upper-gastrointestinal
UICC	International Union against Cancer
UTI	urinary tract infection
VATS	video-assisted thoracic surgery
VIP	vasointestinal peptide
VMA	vanillylmandelic acid
VVF	vesicovaginal fistula
WBC	white blood cell

SECTION 1
GENERAL ISSUES

1 Surgery – what it is and what a surgeon does

THE PROFESSION

Surgery is defined in the *Oxford English Dictionary* as:

The art or practice of treating injuries, deformities and other disorders by manual operation or instrumental appliances.

The surgeon, therefore, attempts to make people better chiefly by the exercise of manual skills in performing 'invasive' procedures. In the development of medicine, surgeons have in consequence tended to be regarded as technicians, in contrast to physicians who have been seen as contemplative, analytical and devoted to the philosophical. However, these distinctions, if they ever existed, between the roles of physicians and surgeons have become increasingly blurred. Invasive procedures are frequently done within medical specialties. For example, a gastroenterologist will remove bile duct stones by endoscopic methods (ERCP) avoiding the need for surgical exploration; an interventional radiologist will deal with a narrowed artery, which would once have been bypassed using a surgical procedure. In addition, surgeons have skills in patient management other than manipulative ones; they look after many patients who might possibly need an operation but in the event do not, e.g. patients with head injuries or acute abdominal pain.

A further stereotype of the surgical personality has been that of a dominant leader. The biographical accounts of pioneer surgeons contain many examples of such men, who, even if they made notable contributions to the advancement of surgery, were often dogmatic in their views and wrong as often as they were right. One early-20th century surgical master (Berkeley Moynihan) remarked that it was necessary for the surgeon to have 'the eye of an eagle, the hand of a lady' and, he added (in that he saw himself as a leader whom all should follow), 'the courage of a lion'. In the development of surgery of 'new territories' of Moynihan's time – the abdomen, the thorax and the head – this was probably true. But inbred dexterity and charismatic leadership have now largely given way to careful training and recognition by surgeons themselves of the limits to both their cognitive and physical skills.

Current medical practice is 'patient centred' and based on multidisciplinary teamwork. The complexity of both modern surgical procedures and perioperative patient care makes a well-functioning team essential. Such teams need a leader (or leaders), but leadership is in general based on discussion and consensus, and should be focused on the individual patient's needs and wishes. Whenever possible, recommendations about patient management are 'evidence-based'. The development of multidisciplinary and multiprofessional teams has changed the surgeon's relationship with other doctors, nurses and healthcare workers. The members of a team share a common interest in a group of disorders. Gastroenterology is a good example: surgeons, physicians (internists in North America), radiologists and pathologists investigate and look after patients with alimentary disease and all gain from joint activities. The same is true in the care of cardiological and neurological patients. For such professional groupings to be effective, joint meetings must take place regularly at which the problems of patients and the results of investigations, such as imaging and pathological findings, are discussed and decisions reached on recommended management. Over the last few years in the United Kingdom, these multidisciplinary team meetings (MDMs or MDTs) have been formally incorporated into the management of patients with cancer and other conditions.

There is also often a place for seeing and managing patients together – for example, the surgeon may meet with a gastroenterologist to discuss patients with inflammatory bowel disease, or with a radiologist to discuss a possible interventional vascular procedure. Patients requiring intensive care need close cooperation between surgeons and intensivists. The same team approach is valid for the broader matters of patient care where the close incorporation of social workers, occupational and other therapists into the decision processes about a patient may simplify return to the community and work after a major operation.

Teamwork has not, however, led to a reduction in accountability – surgeons in particular are subjected to increasing scrutiny, both from within and outside the specialty (see Ch. 2). All treatments, but especially operations, carry the risk of unintended injury to the patient. Such complications of surgery often cause distress to patient and surgeon and may lead to complaint and litigation.

Surgical practice is now more formally regulated by audit, which maintains a running peer-controlled check on the performance of individuals or teams. The introduction of periodic re-certification or revalidation for both individual surgeons and also multidisciplinary teams is increasingly common in Western countries. External inspection and quality control, and the development of national protocols and guidelines, are common features of modern medicine. In England and Wales the Care Quality Commission (CQC) and the National Institute for Health and Clinical Excellence (NICE) undertake such roles.

SURGERY AS AN ASSAULT – PSYCHOLOGICAL EFFECTS

The implied and legal view of surgery as an assault inevitably impinges on the relationship between the practitioner and the patient. The biological effects of a surgical procedure are increasingly well known and discussed in detail throughout this book (Chs 5–8), but there are important psychological matters that have been less studied and sometimes ignored by surgeons. Most patients are relatively ignorant about their body deep to their skin. One study showed, for example, that less than 10% of UK patients could accurately locate the gallbladder or define its function. A proposed attack on a structure or organ may therefore inspire alarm or dismay a patient out of proportion to what the surgeon believes to be appropriate. Irrespective of the organ or area which requires surgical attention, any physical invasion of the body creates fear, and there is a lingering belief that surgery means a close brush with death. The surgeon must understand such fears and attempt to relieve them by careful explanation of the procedure and a frank account of possible complications, including, when appropriate, the risk of death. Surgeons must recognise that certain operations have a particular psychological impact. Mastectomy for breast cancer is a good and obvious example of a severe injury to a woman's body image (Ch. 28). There are also less visible threats such as removal of the womb (hysterectomy) with resultant loss of fertility. The circumstances in which the operation is done are also important. An urgent total colectomy with creation of an ileostomy for toxic megacolon in a young woman (Ch. 25) may be life-saving but she is unlikely to be prepared for the psychosexual consequences. A surgical procedure should always be expected to result in such benefit for the patient that the upside outweighs any downside. For example, in inflammatory bowel disease (Ch. 25), to have to put up with an ileostomy may be preferable to enduring years of frequent loose bowel motions, periodic hospitalisation, the side effects of prolonged medical therapy and the risk of cancer development.

Surgeons must at all times consider the psychological impact of their advice and actions. A caring approach, considerate discussion with patient and their families, and a detailed, honest consent process will help patients overcome these problems.

TRAINING

Surprisingly, training in surgery has differed markedly between regions of the world. However, these cultural differences are beginning to disappear. Increasingly medical students learn basic surgical skills such as venous cannulation and skin suturing in a clinical skills laboratory using simulation techniques whenever possible. For those doctors who wish to pursue a surgical career the training has become more standardised (Fig. 1.1). Currently in Great Britain and Ireland there is a 2–3-year period of core surgical training after the foundation training programmes (Years 1 and 2). This core surgical training should lead to obtaining the MRCS Diploma of the Royal Surgical Colleges of Great Britain and Ireland. Trainees are strongly advised to attend both an Advanced Trauma Life Support (ATLS) course and a Care of the Critically Ill Surgical Patient (CCrISP) course. The MRCS examination consists of two parts: an MCQ test on applied basic sciences and the principles of surgery in general and an OSCE (objective and structured clinical examination) on anatomy, surgical pathology, surgical skills, patient safety, communication skills, applied surgical science and critical care, and clinical skills in history taking and physical examination.

Further training in the UK is the responsibility of the Postgraduate Medical Education and Training Board (PMETB), supported by the individual Surgical Specialist Advisory Committees (SACs). Trainees are appointed as Specialist Registrars (SpRs) to a 4–5-year specialist surgical training programme by competitive interview. On appointment they obtain a specialty National Training Number (NTN) which they keep until completion of training (or expiry of their contract). Trainees are assessed at 6 months and annually thereafter. They must pass these assessments and the Intercollegiate Specialty Examination (FRCS, or 'exit exam') to obtain a Certificate of Completion of Training (CCT). This confers eligibility for the Specialist Register of the General Medical Council (GMC) and to apply for Consultant (Specialist) posts.

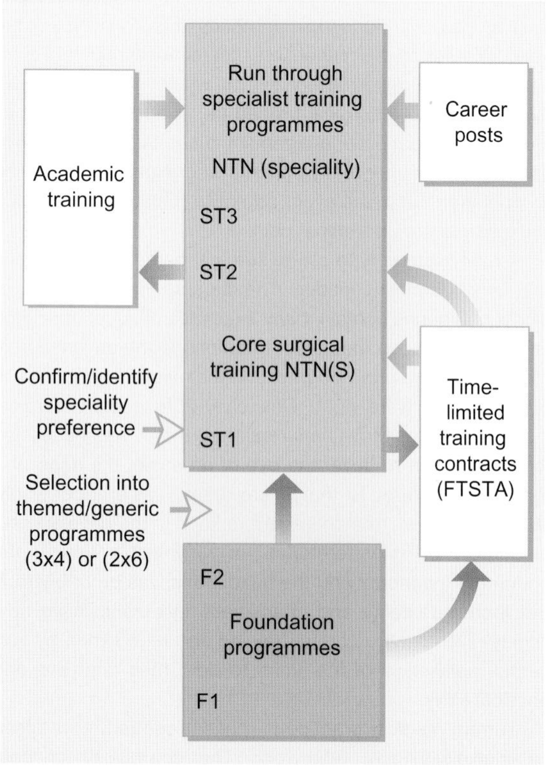

Fig. 1.1 Structure of surgical training (2007).

A further optional component of surgical (and also of most other specialist) training is to spend a period in research. This is commonly undertaken after core surgical training (post-MRCS) or as an additional period of 1–2 years during specialty training. All medicine has become increasingly based on applied science. Hands-on experience of scientific method and the production of new ideas at the scientific frontier may result in a better and more perceptive clinician. How true this is in surgery is uncertain, but the prosecution of research by surgeons is regarded by most as essential to the progress of the discipline, however skill-based it may continue to be. For this to continue requires that some, if not all, surgeons gain formal training in science as applied to their discipline; most also find it exciting.

FURTHER READING

Surgery in general

Douglas C 1975 The houseman's tale. Canongate, Edinburgh. *(A cynical but realistic novel on relatively recent hospital practice, based on the Royal Infirmary of Edinburgh)*

Hger, K, Calne R, Calne R 2000 The illustrated history of surgery, 2nd edn. Routledge, Oxford

Moore F 1995 A miracle and a privilege. National Academy Press, Washington. *(Personal recollections of the growth of surgical biology)*

Mosley M, Hollingham R 2008 Blood and guts: a history of surgery. BBC Books, London

Moynihan, Lord 1967 Selected writings. Pitman Medical, London

Starzl T 1992 The puzzle people – memoirs of a transplant surgeon. University of Pittsburgh Press, Pittsburgh

Professional relationships and training

Department of Health 2009 Reference guide to consent for examination or treatment, 2nd edn. DoH, London

General Medical Council 2006 Good medical practice. General Medical Council, London

General Medical Council 2008 Consent: patients and doctors making decisions together. General Medical Council, London

Intercollegiate Surgical Curriculum Programme: www.iscp.ac.uk

Royal College of Surgeons of England 2008 Good surgical practice

2 Organisation of surgical services

Surgery, like many aspects of medicine, needs to be organised in such a way as to provide a timely and quality service. Similarly, the complexity of all branches of surgery continuously increases and requires the support of a complex infrastructure of an extended surgical team, including the surgical consultant, surgeons in training, other medical professionals such as anaesthetists, nurses and professions allied to medicine such as physiotherapists. An IT and administrative team is also needed to bring the correct patient to the correct clinic and then to the appropriate operating list. As in all systems, errors will occur and safety measures need to be inbuilt.

An operation for an individual is a major life event. Anxiety and fear need to be addressed. All organisational issues need to function well to provide confidence as well as to lead to efficiency. For accountability and simplicity it remains a cornerstone of the UK health system that all patients admitted to hospital are the responsibility of a named consultant. An operation may be a single visit such as a day-case procedure with no or very little follow-up or it may be part of a complex programme of treatment, such as in cancer treatment.

The early part of the 21st century has seen many changes to the provision of surgical services. New 'providers' of surgical care have arrived, albeit still funded in the main by the NHS. Essentially, new providers are private and by definition profit-driven organisations but they still must address all the parameters of quality as the main NHS Trusts. The complexity of the administration of each of these systems interacting has increased. It is controversial to utilise private companies within the NHS and not all professionals approve. This extra provision has probably helped reduce the time people wait for their procedures. As 'waiting times' reduce, quality needs to be ensured.

The fact that additional providers of surgery have arrived is due mainly to the hitherto unprecedented increase in spending the UK Government has allocated to health in the last decade. This has brought the UK in line with the rest of Europe in the proportion of GDP allocated to health. The current economic situation is unlikely to lead to further additional spending. It would therefore be very difficult to predict whether the pace of change in the provision of health care and particularly surgery will continue or falter. Currently, however, the NHS is no longer the sole provider of surgical care but remains the guarantor of care still free at the point of delivery.

Surgery needs to attempt to keep pace with a rapidly changing society and its expectations. Generally, increased broadband availability and instant communications make many NHS carbon-copied handwritten illegible letters obsolete. Investment and advances in IT should improve this and help with accurate data recording and analysis, which should improve patient safety, the effectiveness of care and the experience of the patient.

Likewise, socio-economic changes will work through to affect surgical practice. One of the most obvious is the rise in obesity. Not only does this make most types of surgery considerably more difficult but also it adds significantly to the risks involved and the likelihood of complications. It has also spurred on surgical innovation to help such people with what is called bariatric surgery specifically designed to promote weight loss by reducing the size of the stomach and/or shortening the functional part of the small bowel. Such lifestyle-type surgery remains controversial, particularly in terms of NHS funding.

There are nine surgical specialties, each with its own particular issues but sharing many common organisational issues. They are:

- General surgery, now sub-specialising into breast, vascular, colorectal, upper gastrointestinal, endocrine and transplantation surgery
- Trauma and orthopaedics
- Urology
- ENT
- Oral and maxillofacial
- Paediatric
- Plastic surgery
- Cardiothoracic surgery
- Neurosurgery.

THE SURGICAL TEAM

The surgical consultant needs to lead a clinical team and coordinate the complex pathway to surgery alluded to above. As the complexity of surgery increases, many surgeons may become particularly specialised in a certain area. The majority of routine surgery, however, needs to be delivered with high quality in operating lists optimising the time available. Surgeons of all disciplines in the UK are required to provide emergency care and provide an elective service in their particular specialty. The generality of emergency work and the increasingly specialised elective work is an area which is influencing the organisation of surgical services, particularly in general surgery.

ELECTIVE SURGERY IN THE NEW NHS

In the UK, unlike many areas of Europe and North America, patients are referred for a surgical opinion via their family doctor or general practitioner (GP). In other parts of Europe a problem with the ear, for example, may take a person directly to the relevant ENT specialist. There are advantages in both systems. In the UK it seems likely that the traditional system will continue. Now, however, the GP and patient have a choice of where this opinion may be. The majority of patients have confidence in their local hospital and currently continue to choose to have their surgery there. Patients, however, may choose to have surgery in another NHS hospital, in one of the newer Independent Treatment Centres or via a local Private Hospital Provider. Using a centralised appointment system called 'Choose and Book' a patient can confirm their appointment with a specialist shortly after their GP consultation, utilising appointment times dedicated to this system. The potential choice can be bewildering and difficult for patients to be truly informed about their choices. Needless to say that the concept of more providers of routine surgery is controversial and may destabilise a local Trust, which also has to train future surgeons and provide emergency surgery whilst losing the revenue of its routine work and the routine training cases. Currently, hospitals receive payment for the work done by a 'payment by results' system, whereby the more operations performed the more revenue received. An alternative method of payment is called a 'block payment' system (e.g. Wales) where a service is bought regardless of the number of cases performed. Strategic planning by the Department of Health obviously tries to calculate the need for surgery and provide the funding for it. As the requirements may differ around the country there are about 28 Strategic Health Authorities which manage the local NHS budget and commission (plan and fund) local services. Highly specialised services, for example paediatric cardiac surgery, can only be commissioned nationally. Recently, many Trusts have achieved 'Foundation Trust' status, which gives them some degree of financial autonomy. This may affect the range of services offered. The next few years will hopefully see the stabilisation of the routine provisions of surgical care. Many factors will influence the direction this will take, including the economic climate and the training needs of future surgeons with more stringent control of their working time by means of the European Working Time Directive (EWTD). These features may lead to the separation of emergency surgical care and elective care to improve the efficiency and quality of both. Many Trusts have adopted a 'consultant of the week' system in which one surgeon looks after all the emergency cases and is freed from elective responsibility. This leads to improved continuity of care and is now widely adopted in the UK.

TRAINING

The majority of hospitals in the UK have an important role in training the surgeons of the future. Traditionally there has been an apprenticeship-type component to this training with much of the service being delivered by surgeons in training. Trainees spent long hours in hospital dealing with both the daytime elective work and out of hour's emergencies. This allowed a great deal of experience to be gained but at the expense of many unproductive hours waiting for that same experience. Recent years have seen a progressive and continuous move away from this system. The principal driving force is the EWTD, which the UK government remains committed to and which limits the time a trainee can work each day and each week and will be no more than 48 hours per week. Compulsory periods of rest are built into the system and its goal is safety by avoiding over-tired people making difficult decisions or being required to work long continuous hours. Adhering to the EWTD appears to be reducing the training opportunities for trainees and there are strongly held views that the particular requirements of surgical training cannot be met within the shortened period of training that results. However, it seems unlikely that any move back from the EWTD is planned. There are serious potential consequences for both training and emergency surgery which are probably not yet fully realised and which may influence the organisation and provision of surgical services in the years to come

THE PATIENT'S PATH TO SURGERY

Definitions

- **An elective** patient is an individual with a condition that may require surgical management but in whom the matter is not sufficiently progressive to need immediate treatment.
- **An emergency** patient, by contrast, requires assessment at once, either because of the nature of the problem (e.g. acute injury, fracture, infection or bleeding) or because of the possible rapid progression of a disease (e.g. an acute abdomen such as appendicitis).

An emergency patient may be assessed, treated and stabilised to become an elective patient.

Elective patients

In the UK the majority of patients initially see their GP with their problems. Subsequent assessment by their GP may identify a surgical problem and referral to a consultant for further assessment. Surgeons may also see patients referred from other medical specialists or accident and emergency (A&E) departments. The referring doctor will usually have made an assessment about the urgency of the referral, which guides the surgeon in allocating a clinic appointment. All patients who are referred need to be seen promptly and increased capacity and efficiency may lead to the majority of patients being seen in a sufficiently timely fashion such as to remove the need to classify the referrals by urgency. Currently, however, referrals are divided into those who need to be seen **urgently** (i.e. within 2 weeks) or **routinely**.

Patients with suspected cancer are referred via a fast-tracked system in which the patient is seen and assessed within 2 weeks. Any subsequent tests are also expedited to provide a rapid diagnosis and subsequent treatment.

Additional targets to begin treatment within a timeframe have further influenced streamlining patient assessment with open access and one-stop clinics.

Open access is a system in which primary care physicians can refer their patients directly to a clinical service, e.g. an endoscopy or flexible sigmoidoscopy or some minor surgery. These patients are receiving a test or treatment and are not having a comprehensive assessment.

One-stop clinics provide assessment and sometimes treatment in one visit. Examples where this works well include the assessment of breast lumps where a definitive diagnosis can be achieved in one visit with clinical examination, imaging and pathology, all organised at the same visit so greatly reducing the anxiety of waiting for results. Similarly, rectal bleeding and haemorrhoids can be evaluated and treated in one visit. If more serious problems are encountered, time has also been saved as initial tests have already been done.

Potentially more complex surgical problems require conventional assessment, usually in an out-patient setting.

In such a consultation, a full relevant history is taken and, coupled with clinical examination, will lead to a diagnosis or further investigations. This process may result in the patient being listed for a surgical procedure. The best system also allows for a date to be agreed with the patient at that same appointment. If this is not possible, the patient is added to a waiting list but should be given an idea of the length of time to wait before surgery.

MINOR PROCEDURES

No operation is minor for the patient and the clinician needs to be sensitive to a patient's anxiety even if it is routine.

A considerable proportion of minor surgery is performed in general practice. The range of cases undertaken is increasing as larger 'poly clinics' are built with more facilities (e.g. vasectomy, endoscopy and in some cases hernia repair).

Day-case surgery

A lot of routine general, orthopaedic, ophthalmological and ENT surgery can safely be performed without requiring the patient to stay in hospital overnight. Such day-case surgery requires careful planning and patient selection. It is best performed in dedicated units where the day-case processes are well established. This type of surgery lends itself to protocols, which can be followed safely and efficiently. Preoperative assessment is a key component of this process. The patient is seen, usually by a trained nurse, on a date prior to surgery to assess the patient's fitness for the operation and general anaesthetic if that is required. The protocol will guide the necessity of additional tests such as blood tests and ECG. The procedure is further explained. Explanatory leaflets may be given and consent for procedures can be taken. Clinical and anaesthetic staff, depending on the patient, mix may also support this preoperative assessment.

The range of cases that are suitable for day surgery continues to develop and many laparoscopic cases such as cholecystectomy can be safely performed. Currently over 50% of general surgery may be performed as a day case.

In-patient management

Cases that are not suitable for day surgery require in-patient care. This may involve surgery that would usually be a day case but the patient has other medical problems that require treatment or has no social support to care for him or her.

Generally, however, in-patient surgery usually means more major surgery. These are cases during which a major physiological challenge is created such as blood loss, which requires prolonged observation and management afterwards. Examples would be major cancer surgery or joint replacement.

The other main group of in-patient cases is emergency patients. These patients can range from being constitutionally well with a relatively minor problem such as an abscess which requires drainage to patients needing immediate life-saving surgery due to blood loss in, for example, a patient with multiple injuries or a ruptured aortic aneurysm. Other patients may be critically ill with a surgical emergency such as a perforated intra-abdominal viscus. These patients need the physiological consequences of their illness correcting by resuscitation and then urgent surgery to deal with the cause.

Surgical services in hospitals which receive such diverse emergency cases need an infrastructure which can adapt to cope with these differing cases and the availability of appropriately trained and experienced staff. The sophisticated equipment, medical infrastructure and access to critical care emergency patients need are the same as needed for complex elective cases. Often, however, elective cases and emergency cases may clash in terms of their respective needs. Hospitals may therefore separate the running of elective and emergency services so that the surgical team dealing with the emergency patients have no elective work for that day. They also have a dedicated operating theatre for any surgery required. Consequently, both elective and emergency work may proceed more efficiently. At many hospitals this system is called the 'consultant of the week' system, whereby one team deals with the emergency cases for a week at a time. Patients requiring certain specialist skills will still need to be 'transferred' to the appropriate clinician and so there still needs to be adaptability in the concurrent elective surgical services.

Emergency patients may be referred from their general practitioner, from A&E or from other specialists such as physicians.

Emergency, life-saving surgery is very seldom indicated within the A&E. Most conditions can be stabilised to transfer to a fully equipped operating theatre.

Many A&E departments may have an observation ward. Here cases usually admitted to an in-patient bed may be safely dealt with. Head injuries can be observed. Some minor surgery can be performed: for example, fracture manipulation or abscess drainage.

An increasing number of hospitals now have an **Admissions Unit** where the majority of general surgical patients can be assessed, further tests or investigations arranged and if required the patient can be stabilised and resuscitated before transfer to theatre. Such units work well because the medical team responsible for emergencies have all the cases in one place and the nursing team become skilled in their management.

Acute hospitals which receive and deal with emergency cases in both medical and surgical disciplines require a minimum range of interdependent services such as acute medicine, critical care, anaesthesia, radiology, coronary care and laboratories. They also need to be supported by networked liaison with services which may be on site or in nearby hospitals such as paediatric surgery, cardiothoracic surgery, neurosurgery, ophthalmology, ENT, maxillofacial surgery, urology and obstetrics and gynaecology.

Elective operating lists need to be carefully planned. Operating lists in the UK (but not in all countries) tend to be of a set length of time such that there are two lists per day, one in the morning and one in the afternoon. These are often combined to give a team an 'all day' list, particularly if long or complex operations are planned. The lists therefore need to be planned to be completed in these timeframes. This operating list scheduling may have been compiled by the surgeon or structured by secretarial or administrative staff. Other factors need to be addressed to optimise the safety and efficiency of operating lists:

The patients should be medically and psychologically prepared; this is best facilitated by **preoperative assessment clinics** where it is checked that the correct procedure is planned, and the patient's fitness for surgery is assessed. This may involve further clinical examination and, if needed, further tests such as blood tests (including grouping and saving blood in case a transfusion is required) and an electrocardiogram (ECG) are performed. Patients are instructed where to report on the day of surgery, or the day before if more detailed planning is required, and what to bring with them as well as how long to have fasted prior to surgery. These clinics are held prior to surgery and aim to produce well-prepared patients and avoid the cancellation of operations due to unforeseen problems. Appropriately trained nurses or medical staff may run clinics. Consent may also be taken at these clinics.

Complex cases should be at the start of operating lists to allow time to deal with any unexpected problems. Patients with medical problems such as diabetes should be prioritised on an operating list because of the difficulties managing their insulin. Children should ideally be operated on dedicated paediatric lists with specialist surgeons, anaesthetists, theatre staff and equipment.

The operating suite

Most students remember their first visit to an operating theatre. There is often trepidation and a feeling of 'being in the way'. There are many professionals within an operating theatre and there is an apparent unwritten code of practice and behaviour that at first seems daunting. It is important that when a medical student first attends an operating theatre that he or she is made to feel welcome and is offered explanations of why, for example, certain areas are not touched because they are sterile. By attending theatre regularly these rituals of behaviour soon make sense and students enjoy being part of the team. More importantly, the student sees operations at first hand and gains an added understanding of the medical problem that was treated by surgery. Even if the student does not follow a surgical career, this knowledge will be invaluable in explaining issues to patients.

An operating suite usually comprises several individual operating theatres. They should be easily accessible from the A&E and close to the ITU for obvious reasons. Increasingly, individual theatres are dedicated to one or two specialties. This is because each specialty often requires its own equipment and theatre layout: for example, a laminar flow theatre for orthopaedics where joint replacements are performed and theatres dedicated to minimal access surgery.

Postoperative pathway

After each operation, apart from some minor cases, patients are taken to a recovery area. Patients remain vulnerable just after surgery and require special monitoring and care in this time. Recovery staff have expertise to recognise and manage problems of breathing and ventilation after general anaesthetic and to recognise surgical problems such as bleeding which occasionally necessitates further surgery. Such a recovery facility is part of a theatre complex and patients remain there until they are stable and can be safely returned to the ward for ongoing but usually less intense observation.

More complex or high-risk cases may be transferred directly to a critical care facility (ITU or HDU) to continue medical treatment and observation after surgery such as ventilation. Patients who are in an ITU after surgery may require not only ventilation but also accurate monitoring and support of the other body systems. Patients typically require lines to monitor the central venous pressure (CVP) and arterial pressure (arterial line). Only with the accurate knowledge and monitoring of parameters such as these can the patient's condition be managed well (see Ch. 10).

LEGAL AND ETHICAL ISSUES FOR THE SURGEON

All doctors occupy a privileged position in society in which others may put the ultimate trust of their life in the doctor's hands. The vast majority of doctors only ever act with the best interest of their patients at heart. The nature of medical work and especially surgery requires a supporting legal framework for both patients and doctors

All medical practitioners need to be aware of the legal issues related to their practice. Surgeons may be taken to court by a patient seeking compensation where negligence is deemed to have occurred. Surgeons may also face allegations of negligence through complaints made to the General Medical Council (GMC). This body regulates and advises doctors and protects patients. Most complaints about doctors can be addressed without a prolonged investigation. In potentially more serious cases a court system operates where issues of negligence are investigated and tried. The GMC, thereafter, has the powers to suspend or 'strike a doctor off' the medical register either temporarily or permanently.

The complexity of surgery ceaselessly increases. There are many areas where patients may suffer adverse outcomes or misadventures. Society in general has higher expectations and less tolerance of these perceived failures. Patients are therefore now more likely to complain or take legal action against their doctor, hospital or both.

DUTY

Before describing matters relating to negligence in more detail it would be helpful to outline a doctor's legal duty to his or her patient and how this is interpreted in common law. Duty is the primary legal test. This is a duty of care and a duty to act in the best interest of the patient. By exercising this duty a doctor is striving to prevent disease and promote health, relieve pain and suffering and care for those who may not be cured. Surgeons often have to take very difficult decisions with and on behalf of their patients. For example, whether to proceed with high-risk surgery when potential complications could ensue. Surgeons need to always have in mind that they have a duty of care and not a duty to try to cure and operate on all their patients.

NEGLIGENCE

To prove negligence it must be proved that the doctor had a duty of care, that this duty was breached with the claimant suffering as a consequence and that any resulting damage was due to this breach in care. Any claim for negligence must be brought within 3 years and the burden of proof lies with the claimant.

It would be fair to say that many 'medico-legal' cases can be protracted and very costly. It is hard to see who, apart from solicitors, gains from this. No fault compensation or fixed tariff settlements may be a way forward.

When a professional skill is involved and negligence is alleged, the question that arises is: 'What level of skill and care does the law require?' The evolution of common law has, over the years, provided a number of guidelines of the standards of care expected so as to avoid or counter a charge of negligence.

The first and most general is:

A fair, reasonable and competent degree of skill is brought to the procedure.

This should be dealt with in surgical training and clinical governance. It is any doctors' responsibility to keep up to date and work within their limitations and seek help when needed.

The second guideline relates to circumstances in which there are alternative treatments for a given condition:

Failure to act in a way that a surgeon of ordinary skill would have done.

This is sometimes expressed as the practice accepted as proper by a reasonable body of medical people skilled in that particular area. Interpretation of this point can be difficult, as not infrequently seemingly contradictory views can exist. However, a doctor cannot be judged to be negligent because a contrary view exits.

The third guideline is the causal chain:

A direct causal link justified in terms of logic and medical knowledge must exist between the alleged negligent act and the damage or loss that has been sustained.

Proving such a link can be contentious, especially if the case is complex, and may involve difficult decisions and sometimes multiple procedures. The importance of accurate, legible, contemporaneous notes can never be overestimated in these circumstances.

CONSENT

Patients may give implied consent for such matters as clinical examination, X-ray or blood tests. Explicit or written consent is needed for all invasive and surgical procedures and treatments incurring risk such as chemotherapy.

Consent is not just obtaining a signature on a form prior to an operation. Informed consent is a legal entity. It must be obtained with a clear understanding of all the relevant facts and all consequences. In terms of surgery this means the diagnosis and how certain that is, the prognosis, the proposed operation and any alternative surgical or non-surgical treatments. It should also include details of the likely outcome and risks and side effects. Generally speaking, an adult is presumed to be competent to understand the consent process and give consent for a surgical procedure. Some common problems impair reasoning and could invalidate an informed consent process. Examples may be Alzheimer's, senile dementia and alcohol intoxication. Surgical procedures may be justly indicated where informed consent cannot be taken. Each hospital will have guidelines about consent based on national consent guidelines. In such circumstances the most senior doctor responsible should be integral to this type of decision. In life-saving scenarios with an unconscious patient surgery can take place without consent, provided what is done can be judged to be reasonable (as judged by other doctors).

Consent is ideally taken by the operating surgeon. Doctors in training can very ably take consent provided they have a full understanding of the procedure and its benefits and risks, and are able easily to discuss with the operating surgeon any problem that arises. Likewise, other professionals such as nurses can be trained to take consent.

Patients have rights both in civil and criminal law and these have been reaffirmed and strengthened by the Human

Rights Act of 1998 which became law in 2000 and brought the provisions of the European Convention of Human Rights. If a patient suffers harm in a procedure and consent was not taken or was not adequate, this may be a factor in a claim of negligence. Thus, anything that can be construed as invading the body or mind in any way without consent is unlawful and may attract proceedings for the crime of assault and battery. For such a charge there must also be intent. Such events are extremely rare and fortunately allegations like this are also very rare. It is possible for mischievous and deluded patients to make false allegations possibly in the hope of gain. Having a witness or chaperone is vital when conducting intimate or invasive examinations or procedures.

The following principles must be satisfied for the consent to be valid:

- Consent must be voluntary.
- The patient must have the capacity to give consent.
- The patient must have adequate knowledge to understand what they are consenting to.

The complexity and possible ramifications of many surgical procedures makes taking fully informed consent nearly impossible. In North America the patient is informed of every possible complication, however rare it may be. In English law it is necessary to give sufficient information for patients to make a balanced judgement. To explain every rare potential risk may impart unnecessary anxiety in many cases for which the procedure may be usually straightforward and necessary. A grave risk of adverse complications is judged by the standards of a reputable body of medical practice – a court of law uses peer review by experienced clinicians who form expert opinions after having appraised all the facts of the cases. There is little to guide the clinician about disclosing the risks involved in a particular procedure. Case law gives some guidance and suggests that a risk of 10% should always be disclosed. Surgeons should also take into account the likelihood and seriousness of any risk for the individual patient. It is probably sensible to explain risks which occur at a level of 1% or even more rarely if the consequences are significant.

Additional matters have emerged from the detailed judgements handed down in some leading cases and may be summarised as follows:

- The surgeon must weigh the balance of good and harm before treatment is recommended and is ethically required to provide information which is adequate to enable the patient to reach a balanced judgement.
- The patient is entitled to reject treatment and for that purpose must understand the possibility that harm may result.
- Information about the procedure may both (unduly) confuse and alarm.

Implicit in the above are that:

- The surgeon should take into account the nature and severity of the patient's condition in determining how much to disclose.
- The urgency of the situation (see consent in emergency care below) and the effect of the condition to be treated on the patient's emotional state, must be taken into account.
- A judgement must be made on the patient's intellect and capacity to understand and deal with any information offered.

Surgeons must cultivate and be trained in sensitive interpersonal and communication skills to provide balanced and impartial advice to their patients and not to unduly favour a favourite operation. False hopes should not be raised and undue fears should not be caused. If the patient requires treatment in the ITU, this should be explained and fears helped by an introduction to the unit and the staff preoperatively.

Age of consent

Above the age of 16, statute law (Family Law Reform Act 1969) empowers patients to provide valid consent for their own medical, surgical or dental treatment. For those younger than 16, tradition rather than law has vested consent in parents or guardians. However, in the 1980s a Lord Justice said in a particular case:

Provided the patient … is capable of understanding what is proposed and expressing his or her own wishes, I see no good reason for holding that he or she lacks the mental capacity to express them effectively and to authorise the medical man …

In light of this, the surgeon must make a clinical judgement in those under 16 as to whether:

- There is sufficient capacity in the patient to comprehend the implications of treatment
- It is sensible and proper for an agreement regarding treatment to be entered into directly with the patient, independent of the views of the parents.

Mental illness and capacity

The Mental Capacity Act for England and Wales (2005) has clarified the procedures to be followed when assessing an adult patient's ability to make his or her own decision about treatment and who can make decisions for those who lack such capacity. In general, a patient is assumed to have capacity unless proven otherwise. Just because a decision seems wrong or irrational to the attending doctor does not mean that the patient lacks mental capacity. Support must be given to help a patient make her or his own decision when possible. Anything done for a patient who lacks capacity must be done in their best interests and be least restrictive of their basic rights and freedoms. In certain circumstances an independent mental capacity advocate (IMCA) must be consulted. The act also provides a framework for patients to appoint someone else to make decisions for them if they lose capacity (a Lasting Power of Attorney) and to make advance decisions about treatment.

Unconsciousness

Life-saving treatment to resuscitate and stabilise can be performed without consent.

Jehovah's Witnesses

Surgeons in particular may face the occasion when a patient facing imminent death from haemorrhage refuses a blood transfusion because of religious beliefs. This is a legal right but it is unlikely that any criminal proceedings would be brought against those who administer a blood transfusion to save life. However, that this is an area of difficulty is shown by a successful action by a Jehovah's Witness because of the mental trauma which followed a blood transfusion. Jehovah's Witnesses may also refuse blood transfusion for elective operations. All operations are performed to minimise the need to transfuse blood but many, particularly long and complex procedures, often require blood to be available. Modern equipment to aid vessel sealing help to minimise blood loss and cell-saving suction devices can re-transfuse the patient's own blood. Likewise, in some circumstances, a patient may store their own blood preoperatively.

Undue influence

Children of Jehovah's Witnesses

If there is a threat to life, the surgeon is not entitled to assume that the parent's beliefs are shared by their children. There is a greater duty to act in the best interest of the child protected by the view that the courts do not regard children as capable of forming profound religious beliefs.

In similar circumstances not related to Jehovah's Witnesses, when it can be shown that parental or other influence has caused the patient to withhold consent for life-saving treatment, the courts have taken the view that legal liability shall not attach to those who have acted in good faith.

For those just starting a medical career it may seem daunting to cope with the potential legal manifestations of everyday practise. The risk of inadvertently being entwined in legal matters can be reduced by always acting in good faith and seeking advice and counsel for any doubt. Record keeping and paperwork should be legible and in sufficient detail to reflect all decisions, particularly with such things as consent forms. All doctors in the NHS are protected by indemnity for work carried out within the NHS, provided of course the doctor followed good practise. All doctors should, however, have medical insurance (a necessary condition of employment in most countries). In the UK there are two agencies: the Medical Defence Union and the Medical Protection Society.

DEATH AND BEREAVEMENT

Death comes to us all but in a surgical context may be unexpected and sudden and may be the direct consequence of efforts to try to help the patient. Sensitive and speedy handling of the physical and emotional turmoil and awareness of cultural and social differences in those bereaved are essential.

Terminal care

All clinicians, including surgeons, are responsible in some way for the management of the last stages of life. The common aims are to allay suffering and maintain dignity, both of which require close and sympathetic contact with relatives. Although surgeons may feel the human and honourable need to strive against potential therapeutic defeat, it is not their task to wring the last drop of life out of their patients. For instance in extreme old age the correct management of an abdominal catastrophe may be pain relief rather than major surgery with very little prospect of survival. These are very difficult decisions only experience can make. They are subjective and the reasons why one particular decision was taken should of course be recorded because in different circumstances elderly patients can do very well from surgery. At all times the surgeon should try to follow the wishes of the patient (including living wills), involve the relatives in difficult decisions and seek advice from colleagues if needed.

It is better to anticipate the special needs of the dying in consort with the general practitioner and sometimes religious representative, especially if special care is going to be necessary.

Many hospitals have protocols and pathways for patients who are dying and in need of terminal care. Groups such as Macmillan nurses can be invaluable at these difficult times.

Informing relatives

This task, especially at night, may fall upon the most junior member of the medical team. At other times a senior doctor may be able to answer more questions to alleviate anxiety. Nurses can also play a key role. All questions should be answered honestly and directly. Handling these issues sensitively and with understanding is greatly appreciated by most relatives.

Death certification

Trainee doctors are nearly always those responsible for the recording of death. The death certificate is a legal document and also the basis of national population statistics. It should be completed accurately to avoid subsequent wrangles, anxieties and confusion for relatives. Referral to a coroner (in England, Wales and Northern Ireland) or a procurator fiscal (in Scotland) may be necessary (Box 2.1). Many other countries have similar procedures to observe. A cause of death should be recorded rather than the mode of death (e.g. ruptured aortic aneurysm rather than shock).

Box 2.1 Reasons for referral to the coroner or procurator fiscal

Doctor:
Did not treat the deceased in the final illness
Did not see the deceased in the last 14 days of life

Death in relation to surgical operation:
During the procedure
Before recovery from anaesthesia
Within 24 hours

Circumstances:
Suspected industrial cause of death
Patient in receipt of a war or industrial pension
Accidental death
Suspected or known
- violence
- neglect
- poisoning or administration of drugs

Medical mishap
Death in police custody
After abortion in mother or stillbirth of child
Within 24 hours of admission to hospital

Doubt and complaint:
Doubt as to cause, including sudden or unexplained death
Complaint by relatives

Postmortem examination

Opinions can be divided on the need and benefit of such examinations. Pathologists, in particular, point out that unexpected and instructive information is often discovered. Others, in contrast, often feel that functional causes such as adult respiratory distress syndrome and multi-organ system failure are apparent during life and are not well reflected in postmortem examinations. If a death certificate cannot be issued, the death must be reported to the coroner. In other circumstances where a death certificate can be issued and a postmortem would be of value to discover more about the cause of death, the consent of the relatives must be requested.

3 Emergency medicine

The primary purpose of an Emergency Department (ED) is to diagnose and treat acute life-threatening injury and illness. Of necessity, such departments need always to be open – 24 hours a day – and adequately staffed. Inevitably, therefore, they also deal with large numbers of patients who do not strictly fall into the category of having a life-threatening illness.

Emergency medicine is a rapidly expanding specialty in the UK, and all EDs now have much improved consultant supervision when compared with a decade ago. It is regrettable that some Foundation Year 2 doctors only spend 4 months in the ED; this is a vital part of their training and it is important that they get as much out of their period in the ED as possible.

Because of the ready availability of the ED, all manner of patients pass through its doors. These include the lonely, people who abuse drugs, society's misfits, and those who find conventional access to healthcare difficult. It is important that every medical student and trainee doctor sees these patients, because they have much to instruct us about the nature of humanity.

Surgical workload

Only about 1% of patients who attend an ED have suffered multiple trauma. There is currently a trend to concentrate these patients into specifically designed trauma centres; however, it will still be the case that most EDs will receive multiple injured patients. A few more, although not many, come with surgical conditions which require urgent intervention: a leaking aneurysm of the abdominal aorta, a perforated abdominal viscus or a femoral artery blocked by an embolus. There is a much commoner third group of surgical patients: those who suffer from minor surgical conditions such as abscesses, paronychias and perianal haematomas.

Given this wide range of presentation, it is important for patients to be prioritized – a process known as 'triage' (from the French word meaning 'to sort').

LIFE-SAVING PROCEDURES IN THE EMERGENCY DEPARTMENT

A number of surgical conditions demand immediate intervention if the patient's life is to be saved. These are usually related to trauma – advanced trauma life support (ATLS) guidelines should be followed in the management of all trauma patients.

AIRWAY

Never forget to call for help if it is apparent that the patient has a problem with their airway. A duty anaesthetist should be asked to attend urgently if there is an airway problem. It is a good principle for the inexperienced trainee doctor to call for help at an early stage *before* he or she gets out of depth, rather than afterwards. It is no shame, and is indeed commendable, to ask for senior and more experienced help when the situation demands. Never let one's own pride get in the way of asking for assistance, it is a sign of maturity, *not* weakness, to ask for senior help when the situation demands it.

In all accident victims and in anyone who is unconscious, say after a head injury, care of the airway is paramount; for example, it is quite wrong to waste time dealing with a dislocated ankle if the patient is unable to breathe because of an obstructed glottis. Always deal with the airway first (Emergency Box 3.1).

The common objects which obstruct the airway are the tongue, food and dentures. The most useful instrument to have to hand is a wide-bore (Yankers) sucker. The first action to be undertaken in dealing with an unconscious patient or an accident victim is to check that the upper airway – mouth to larynx – is patent, to suck out any food and to remove dentures if these are present.

It is important to bear in mind that, in trauma cases, the cervical spine must be protected by means of a stiff-neck

Emergency Box 3.1

Management of airway obstruction

- Protect cervical spine in trauma patients
- Remove any foreign bodies, e.g. food, dentures
- Displace tongue forwards by chin lift or jaw thrust
- Insert oropharyngeal or nasopharyngeal airway if possible
- Perform cricothyroidotomy if obstruction not relieved.

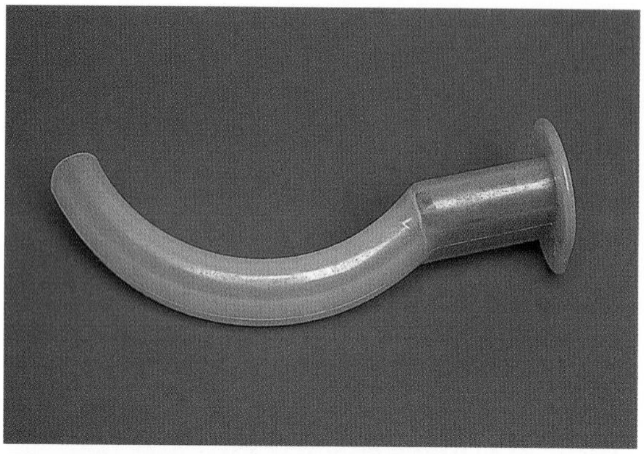

Fig. 3.1 Oropharyngeal airway (Guedel).

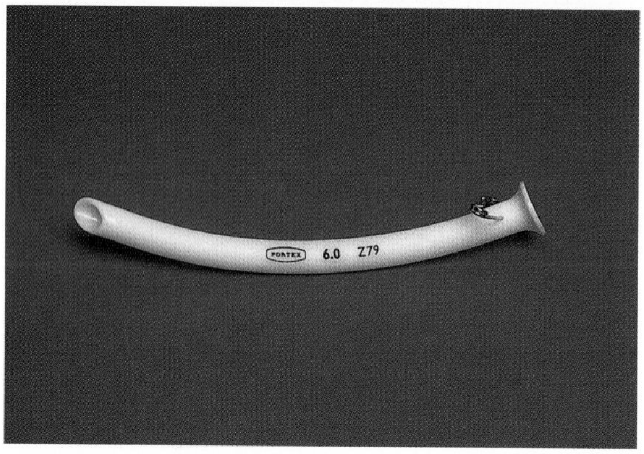

Fig. 3.2 Nasopharyngeal tube for airway maintenance.

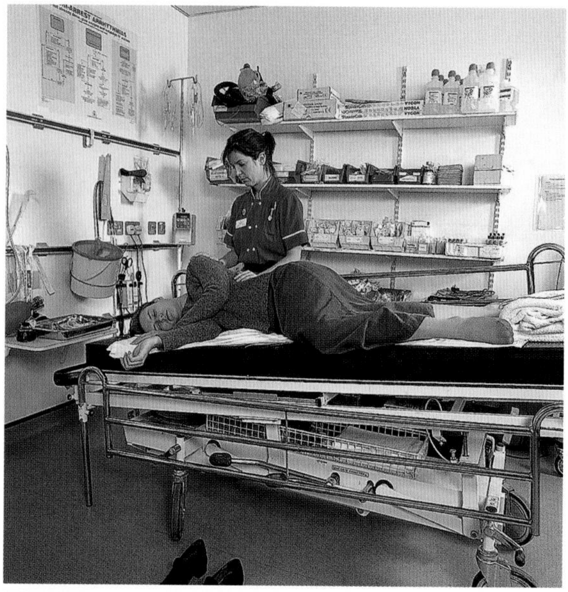

Fig. 3.3 The semi-prone position for the unconscious patient.

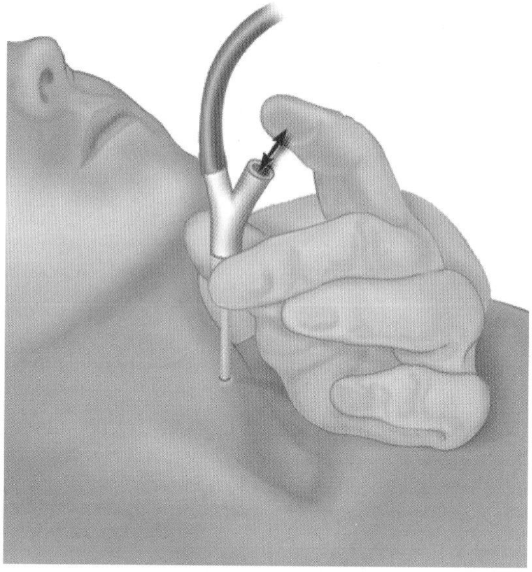

Fig. 3.4 Technique of jet insufflation. Carefully palpate for the cricothyroid membrane before insertion of the cannula.

cervical collar, and the spine must be kept 'in line' until spinal trauma has been excluded.

Because the tongue has its main muscular attachment to the posterior aspect of the body of the mandible, drawing the jaw forward automatically brings the tongue with it. Therefore, obstruction caused by the tongue falling back can be dealt with by either of two simple measures: chin lift or jaw thrust. An oropharyngeal airway (Fig. 3.1) helps to keep the tongue forward. Alternatively, a nasopharyngeal tube can be inserted along the floor of the nose (Fig. 3.2). It is important to insert a safety pin at the nasal end to prevent the tube disappearing down the back of the patient's throat. Whenever it is feasible, the unconscious patient should be kept semi-prone (Fig. 3.3).

When there is an immediate need for a definitive airway, endotracheal intubation should be performed by an appropriately experienced doctor with in-line stabilisation of the cervical spine. If the trachea cannot be intubated, then this is an indication for creating a surgical airway; an example of where this might be the case is severe maxillofacial trauma. A cricothyroidotomy is the method used to establish a surgical airway. An incision is made directly over the cricothyroid membrane (Ch. 11) and an endotracheal tube is inserted into the upper trachea. Alternatively, the less experienced operator should pass a wide-bore intravenous trocar and cannula through the cricothyroid membrane and then remove the trocar. The stem of a Y-shaped connector is then attached to the cannula and one of the limbs of the Y is connected to an oxygen supply; insufflation of the lungs is achieved by intermittent obstruction of the remaining vent (Fig. 3.4). This procedure, although crude, can buy very valuable time for more definitive management, usually by orotracheal intubation or tracheostomy (Ch. 14).

BREATHING (VENTILATION)

Oxygenation of the tissues cannot be achieved, even if the airway is patent, if there is either absence of respiratory activity or impairment of cardiac output. There are four such conditions commonly encountered in the ED:

- tension pneumothorax
- haemothorax
- flail chest
- acute cardiac tamponade.

Tension pneumothorax

Aetiology

There are two causes:

- closed trauma in which a fractured rib penetrates the lung
- rupture of an emphysematous bulla.

Pathophysiology

More air passes out through a hole in the lung during inspiration than is returned on expiration, and in the most acute examples there is one-way traffic only. With each inspiration the volume of intrapleural air increases, the intrapleural pressure rises and, in consequence, the lung collapses and the mediastinum is displaced towards the opposite side. The compressed lung causes a right-to-left shunt with cyanosis; the displaced mediastinum kinks the superior and, more importantly, the inferior vena cava, so reducing venous return and resulting in death from abolition of cardiac output.

Clinical features

History

There may be a story of closed injury or of previous emphysema, and a conscious patient may complain of progressive dyspnoea.

Physical findings

There will be gasping attempts to breathe and, in the very final stages, cyanosis. There may be distended neck veins. Local physical signs on the affected side are:

- decreased chest wall movement
- a hyperresonant percussion note
- absent breath sounds.

In addition, although these are of late occurrence and difficult to detect, there will be:

- displacement of the trachea in the suprasternal notch away from the affected side
- movement of the apex beat – laterally in a right and medially in a left pneumothorax.

Management

A chest X-ray should not be done until urgent relief has been achieved by the insertion of a wide-bore needle through the second intercostal space in the midclavicular line (see Ch. 11). Formal chest drainage with an underwater seal can then be undertaken (Ch. 11) once deterioration of the patient has been averted.

Haemothorax

Aetiology

The cause is usually trauma to the chest as the result of either penetration (knife or projectile) or blunt injury which is usually severe, such as a fall from a height or a crush by a vehicle.

Pathophysiology

The usual cause of a haemothorax is rupture of one or more intercostal arteries. The intercostal vessels are segmental in nature and come directly off the thoracic aorta; hence, haemorrhage is often brisk. Bleeding can also come from torn bronchial arteries or veins when the substance of the lung is itself lacerated.

Loss of blood can be severe and is combined with compression of the lung on the affected side to produce a right-to-left shunt.

Haemothorax may also be caused by an acute transection of the aorta as a result of a sudden deceleration injury.

Clinical features

Symptoms

In addition to a history of a physical injury, there may be chest pain and dyspnoea.

Physical findings

There will usually be general features of hypovolaemia and occasionally cyanosis. Local signs are:

- bruising of the chest wall
- evidence of fractured ribs, including subcutaneous emphysema
- imprinting – a mark left on the skin by the object responsible for the injury, such as a tyre mark or other evidence of cause
- an entry wound, perhaps with, in a projectile injury, a complementary exit wound
- dull percussion note on the affected side
- absent or reduced breath sounds also on the affected side.

Investigation

Provided there is not urgency to restore ventilation, a chest X-ray often shows shadowing on the affected side with a fluid interface with the lung. If there is also a pneumothorax, an erect film reveals a horizontal fluid level.

Management

Treatment is different from that of a tension pneumothorax; a needle is inadequate for drainage. A wide-bore chest drain must be inserted and positioned so that it lies in the dependent part of the chest cavity. However, large-calibre intravenous lines and intravenous fluid resuscitation must be instituted so that blood volume is restored as the chest cavity is being decompressed.

Drainage and re-expansion of the lung are frequently followed by cessation of the bleeding. However, if the rate of blood loss is greater than 200 mL/h, or if 1500 mL is drained immediately, then it is likely that an urgent thoracotomy is indicated, and a thoracic surgical team needs to be urgently contacted.

Flail chest

Aetiology

Trauma is the only cause and, once again, may be open or closed – usually the latter.

Pathophysiology

The injury is always serious and very frequently associated with an underlying contusion of the lung. The chest wall injury is a fracture of one rib (but usually more) at both the anterior and posterior ends. Thus a segment of chest wall moves independently in a paradoxical manner – inwards on inspiration and outwards on expiration. The size of the involved segment determines the degree of reduction in respiratory efficiency, which is made worse by any lung contusion which causes a right-to-left shunt.

Clinical features

Symptoms

The symptoms are those of hypoxia and respiratory distress.

Physical findings

The physical findings are:

- dyspnoea
- paradoxical respiration in the involved segment of chest wall.

Diagnosis

Early recognition can be surprisingly difficult, particularly when breathing is shallow, but is important in that the whole thrust of management is to avoid tissue hypoxia. The majority of those with a flail chest that is causing respiratory insufficiency require positive-pressure ventilation, which can be established in the ED by intubation of the trachea and either hand or mechanical ventilation. The procedure must be continued until the flail segment has stabilised, which may take several weeks. Surgical fixation of the chest wall is only occasionally indicated.

CIRCULATION

Acute cardiac tamponade

Aetiology and pathophysiology

Blood accumulates within the pericardial sac and compresses the heart so that cardiac output is decreased. The source is a leak from the heart either because of a penetrating injury, such as a knife wound, or from blunt trauma. The outcome is a low cardiac output which will eventually cause death; venous return is reduced, so that there are features of right heart failure.

Clinical features

History

Penetrating or blunt trauma is usually obvious. The victim becomes progressively ill from low cardiac output, with confusion and eventually unconsciousness.

Physical findings

Apart from an external injury in penetrating trauma, physical findings may be few. Dilated neck veins are universal, and loss of a palpable apex beat may be suggestive but this may be difficult to evaluate. Heart sounds are quiet and arterial blood pressure low. Pulsus paradoxus is characteristic (decrease in systolic pressure by >10 mmHg on inspiration) but not always present.

Management

Unless there is prompt relief, continuing hypoxia and death result. Tamponade caused by a stab wound requires immediate thoracotomy, if necessary at the place where injury occurred or in the ED. The thorax is entered via the left fifth rib space, the bulging pericardial sac is incised longitudinally avoiding the phrenic nerve, the blood is evacuated, and a finger is placed over the myocardial wound to arrest further bleeding while preparations are made to close the wound with simple sutures. This dramatic management results in survival of at least a quarter of victims. For those untrained in thoracotomy, time may be bought by performing needle pericardiocentesis.

IMAGING IN THE TRAUMA PATIENT

Any imaging must be related to the clinical state of the patient and, in particular, a competent clinical individual should accompany the patient during the procedure.

There are three standard radiological views which, in trauma, should be taken:

- chest X-ray
- anteroposterior pelvis
- cervical spine X-rays, which now form part of the secondary patient survey.

Chest X-ray

An upright (Ch. 4) chest X-ray should be obtained in any patient who has sustained trauma to the trunk – chest or abdomen. There are numerous possible abnormalities, but commonly missed diagnoses include:

- pneumothorax (see above); it is important to check that lung markings go right out to the periphery of the lung field
- ruptured diaphragm
- traumatic aortic dissection (Ch 29), which often reveals itself as a widened mediastinum.

Pelvis

A *diastasis* (abnormal widening) at the symphysis pubis (Fig. 3.5) may indicate damage to the urethra (Ch. 33), which can be confirmed by urethrography. This is easily performed in the resuscitation room by inserting a urinary balloon catheter (Ch. 11) and securing it in the meatal fossa by gently inflating the balloon and instilling contrast medium under gentle pressure.

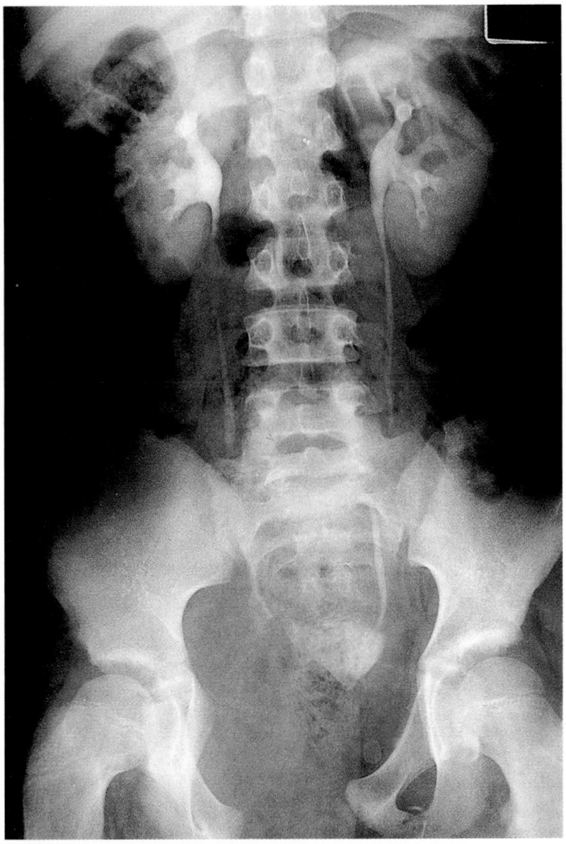

Fig. 3.5 Abnormal widening of the pubic symphysis with an associated rupture of the urethra and high-riding bladder.

Concurrent with or subsequent to the information derived from these basic imaging techniques, other methods may be indicated.

Cervical spine

A cross-table cervical spine X-ray which shows all seven cervical vertebrae and the cervicothoracic junction is mandatory to avoid the possibility of a missed diagnosis of a cervical spine injury. Unrecognised, this may lead on to damage to the spinal cord. Such views are facilitated if the patient's shoulders are pulled down (Fig. 3.6). If the cervical spine cannot be completely imaged, then a swimmer's view can be obtained, where one arm is extended over the patient's head, the X-ray tube is brought into the axilla, and a plate is placed on the opposite side and then exposed. There are four lines on a lateral cervical spine X-ray:

- prevertebral
- the anterior aspect of the vertebral bodies
- the posterior aspect of the vertebral bodies
- the spinous processes.

All of these must be smooth curves. A feature which is commonly missed in interpreting these X-rays is a haematoma deep to the prevertebral fascia which clearly shows as a soft tissue swelling. Odontoid peg fractures are also commonly missed, and it is important to check that the distance between the posterior aspect of the body of the first cervical vertebra and the anterior aspect of the odontoid peg is no greater than 3 mm.

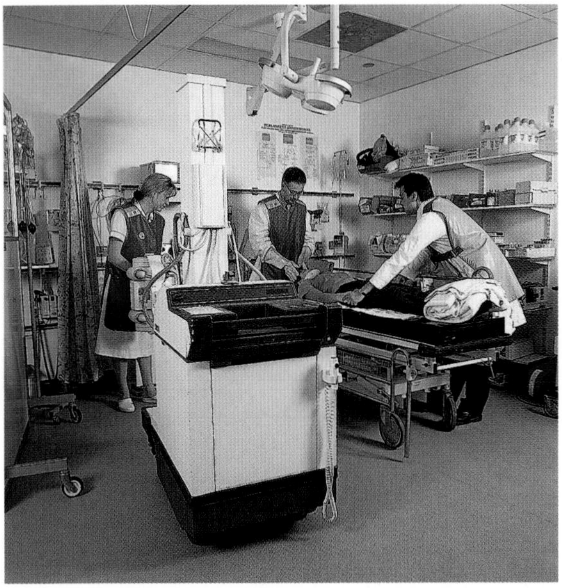

Fig. 3.6 Method of obtaining a cross-table X-ray of the cervical spine.

Ultrasound

Ultrasound images can be obtained on small, portable machines that can easily be used in the resuscitation room. This can be very useful in cases of abdominal trauma. The Focused Assessment with Sonography for Trauma (FAST scan) is a rapid, bedside, ultrasound examination performed to identify intra-peritoneal haemorrhage or pericardial tamponade. FAST examines four areas for free fluid:

- Perihepatic and hepato-renal space
- Perisplenic
- Pelvis
- Pericardium.

Computed tomography (CT)

This technique has transformed radiological practice, particularly in neurotrauma (Ch. 31). Spiral CT makes imaging more rapid than was previously the case and an increasing number of EDs have a CT scanner for the rapid assessment of trauma cases and selected patients with acute abdominal or chest disease. CT scanning has helped greatly in the acute management of these patients.

URGENT SURGICAL CONDITIONS WHICH CAUSE HYPOVOLAEMIC SHOCK

Management of hypovolaemic shock is summarised in Emergency Box 3.2.

Emergency Box 3.2

Management of hypovolaemic shock

- Arrest external blood loss by pressure/elevation
- Insert two 14 G cannulae and take blood samples for full blood count, biochemistry, clotting studies and urgent cross match
- Administer 0.9% saline 1–2 L as fast as possible, followed by plasma substitutes and blood (O-negative universal donor, type specific or fully cross matched as time permits)
- Monitor pulse, blood pressure, tissue oxygenation (by pulse oximetry) and urine output (catheterisation required)
- Assess/investigate and treat cause of blood loss.

The commonest causes of non-traumatic massive blood loss are:

- ruptured abdominal aortic aneurysm (Ch. 29)
- ectopic pregnancy
- gastrointestinal haemorrhage (usually from the upper GI tract) (Ch. 23).

In civilian ED practice in the UK, the common traumatic causes are:

- ruptured spleen
- rupture of other intra-abdominal viscera such as the liver and tearing of the mesenteric vessels
- long bone fractures – a single femoral shaft fracture leads to the loss of 1.5 L of blood, which is 30% of the total blood volume
- pelvic fractures – several litres of blood may be lost and the patient may rapidly die from hypovolaemia. Hence, if a pelvic fracture is suspected clinically, very urgent resuscitation is required and the haemorrhage can often be abated by applying an external fixator to the pelvis in the resuscitation room.

Ectopic pregnancy

This condition should be considered in any woman who presents to the ED with acute abdominal pain and who may, even as a remote possibility, be pregnant. A denial of recent sexual intercourse is not a guarantee that the patient is not pregnant.

Clinical features

History

There is frequently (90%) a short history of lower abdominal pain followed by more generalised and constant pain which may also be felt in the shoulder if blood tracks up the paracolic gutters to the undersurface of the diaphragm. Dysuria is also common. Vaginal bleeding is absent in 25%.

Physical findings

General features of bleeding are often apparent – pallor, circulatory collapse and air hunger may be present together with abdominal tenderness and rigidity, initially most marked in the lower abdomen. Cervical excitation also causes pain.

Management

In any patient in which an ectopic pregnancy is likely, two large intravenous cannulae should be inserted even if the circulation is apparently stable; in such circumstances it may be possible to confirm the diagnosis by obtaining a positive pregnancy test. A patient with signs of hypovolaemia should go immediately to the operating room for surgery, preferably by a gynaecologist who may be able to save the affected fallopian tube.

SURGICAL CONDITIONS COMMONLY SEEN IN THE ED

Soft-tissue abscesses

These represent a very considerable component of the surgical work of an ED. An abscess is defined simply as a collection of pus, and the pain of an abscess is caused by the build-up of pressure in the inflamed soft tissues. It is true to say that the smaller the abscess, the greater the pain and, because an abscess may appear small, this is not a reason to underestimate the distress caused.

An abscess in the finger (e.g. a pulp space abscess) is much more painful than, say, an abscess on the scrotum, because in the former there are strong fibres which connect the pulp of the fingertip to the periosteum of the distal phalanx, and also pressure rises in a confined space. Thus there is little opportunity for the abscess to expand and the tension in the affected area is high.

Diagnosis

This is usually straightforward. The symptoms are of inflammation, the signs of which are heat, redness, tenderness, swelling and loss of function of the affected part. In addition there is often fluctuation.

Management

Once an abscess has been diagnosed, the correct treatment is incision and drainage rather than recourse to antibiotics, although these may be administered to deal with the possibility of spread when a surgical procedure is undertaken, or any associated cellulitis.

Before incision is performed, an appropriate method of anaesthesia needs to be established. For pulp space abscesses and those beside the fingernail (paronychia), ring block regional anaesthesia is suitable. A solution of 1% lidocaine (lignocaine) is introduced on either side of the base of the digit to anaesthetise the digital nerve. It takes 5 or 10 minutes for the anaesthetic to take effect; then an incision is made over the chosen point where the abscess is at its most prominent. In all abscesses, it is a cardinal error to make the incision too small.

There are some abscesses which are better dealt with under general anaesthesia, e.g. in the breast, the axilla or the ischiorectal fossa.

There is now a school of thought that maintains that after drainage and the use of appropriate antibiotics, the drainage site can be closed primarily. There is certainly a case for this, but caution should be observed unless drainage and excision of dead tissue are indubitably complete.

Traumatic haematoma

There are two small haematomas (which cause severe pain) that can easily be dealt with in an ED: subungual and perianal.

Subungual haematoma

This usually occurs when the extremities of either a finger or a toe have been damaged. Blood oozes out beneath the affected nail and, because there is initially little room for expansion, the pain soon becomes severe and requires urgent release. The old-fashioned method of trephine, in which the red hot end of a paper clip is pushed down on the nail in order to bore a hole and allow the escape of blood, is very effective, but ring block anaesthesia should be used.

Perianal haematoma

See Chapter 26.

'Minor' wounds

Relatively simple lacerations to the skin and underlying tissues are common in the ED, but a wound should never be regarded as minor. It is imperative that the basic principles of wound management are observed (Ch. 8). Chemoprophylaxis is required for all animal (including human) bites.

Tetanus prophylaxis

In dealing with a laceration in the ED, consideration should always be given to whether or not the patient is immune to the effects of *Clostridium tetani* (Ch. 9). Tetanus is rare in developed countries but is a major cause of mortality in developing communities. The very low rates of tetanus in the UK are attributable to an effective immunisation programme and good standards of hygiene. However, previous and often repeated immunisations, as took place during the 1940s, have produced a population which is now ageing and in whom resistance to *C. tetani* may be on the decline.

Tetanus-prone wounds are wounds including burns:

- sustained more than 6 hours before surgical treatment
- with a significant degree of devitalised tissue
- resulting from a puncture injury
- which have come into contact with soil or manure, and
- where there is associated clinical evidence of sepsis, foreign body or a compound fracture.

In a patient who has sustained such a wound, and who has received a full five dose course of tetanus vaccine at the recommended intervals, or who is up to date with their tetanus immunisation schedule, then no further doses of vaccine are recommended since within the incubation period of tetanus vaccine given at the time of the tetanus-prone injury may not boost immunity early enough to give additional protection. However, if the risk of tetanus is especially high, e.g. the wound is contaminated with stable manure, then human tetanus immunoglobulin should be given to provide immediate additional protection. If the patient's immunisation schedule is not up to date, or if their status is unknown, a reinforcing dose of Td/IPV (this is tetanus, diphtheria, and inactivated polio vaccine) should be given provided there are no contraindications. Further doses should be given as required to complete the recommended five dose schedule. In this situation immunoglobulin should be given for any injury which is defined as a tetanus-prone wound.

The preventative dose of human tetanus immunoglobulin is 250 IU, intramuscular in most case, except if more than 24 hours have elapsed since the injury, or if there is a risk of heavy contamination or following burns, when the dose is 500 IU.

For all other wounds if the patient is not up to date with his/her tetanus immunisation a reinforcing dose of Td/IPV should be given (or a course of immunisation started).

Antibiotic prophylaxis

There are some wounds which, by definition, will be heavily contaminated by bacteria, e.g. agricultural injuries and human and animal bites. These should not be primarily sutured (see below) but should be thoroughly washed out with normal saline, left open and prophylactic antibiotics (Ch. 9) prescribed.

Initial examination

Examination must include that part of the body distal to the wound to ensure that nerves, blood vessels and tendons have not been damaged. For example, in a laceration to the hand caused by a broken glass, all the fingers must be carefully examined to ensure that nerve and tendon function is intact. It is inadequate merely to ask the patient to make a fist – each finger must be examined, and flexor digitorum profundus and flexor digitorum superficialis tendons must have their integrity established.

The possibility that there might be a foreign body should always be considered.

Management

The principles of excision and suture are outlined in Chapter 8. Lacerations over the pretibial (shin) area should not be sutured because the skin is already quite tight and additional tension easily results in ischaemia of the wound edges. The correct management is for the wound edges to be approximated only, often by means of sterile adhesive plastic strips (Steristrips; see also Ch. 6) and a light dressing applied. These wounds usually heal well, although they can take many months to do so.

Head injury

Definitive management is considered in Chapter 31. Initial decision-making and management in the ED are vital to subsequent success.

Every year, 3 per 1000 000 of the population are admitted to hospital with head injuries; they make up approximately 20% of acute surgical admissions. The majority are admitted under the care of general surgeons and therefore it behoves those in training to have a thorough working knowledge of their initial management and to be able to detect warning signs of deterioration. They must be fully conversant with the in-house arrangements for the procedures to be undertaken with such patients and must also know the lines of referral to their local neurosurgical unit.

History and progress

For every victim of a head injury, the following clinical matters must be recorded, if necessary with the help of witnesses and family:

- time of injury
- time seen by the examining doctor
- mechanism of injury
- evidence of loss of consciousness
- period of amnesia both before (retrograde) and after sustaining the injury and whether the patient now has a continuous memory of events
- any visual disturbance
- vomiting
- headache
- fits
- an alcohol and drug history (if possible).

Clinical features

Physical findings

Urgent findings are:

- presence of blood behind the eardrum (haemotympanum)
- cerebrospinal fluid coming from the nose or ears, often blood-stained (rhinorrhoea and otorrhoea)
- pupillary signs, including inequality between the two sides and dilatation, particularly if unresponsive to light.

The first two findings are an indication of a fracture of the base of the skull.

The pupillary signs are possible indications of compression of the ocular motor (third cranial) nerve against the edge of the tentorial hiatus from critically raised intracranial pressure, perhaps because of an expanding supratentorial extradural haematoma.

Level of consciousness

This is recorded against the Glasgow Coma Scale (GCS) scoring system (see Ch. 31). The initial and subsequent estimates must be, together with the time, recorded in the notes both as individual scores and as a total.

Urgent management

Any patient known or suspected to have a head injury is dealt with according to the protocols laid down by the advanced trauma life support (ATLS) system (Emergency Box 3.3). As in every other circumstance of injury, the airway is of overriding importance – however severe the injury to the head, the airway always comes first in an attempt to ensure survival.

As is also emphasised above, arterial hypotension in the presence of a head injury should not be presumed to be caused by damage to the head. Although scalp lacerations can bleed profusely, intracranial bleeding of itself does not produce hypotensive shock; the systemic response to raised intracranial pressure caused by an expanding intracranial haematoma is usually bradycardia with later hypertension. Therefore, other causes for hypotension should be sought. An algorithm for the investigation of head injuries has been produced by NICE (Fig 3.7).

For further discussion on management of head injuries, see Chapter 31.

Emergency Box 3.3

Advanced trauma life support (ATLS)

A – airway maintenance with cervical spine control
B – breathing and ventilation with supplemental oxygen as required
C – circulation with haemorrhage control
D – disability – neurological status
E – exposure – completely undress patient.

SOME APHORISMS IN ED MEDICINE

Always introduce yourself to the patient

In the ED, patients are nearly always frightened and in pain. When there is time and a pressing state of emergency does not exist, an early rapport is established by introducing yourself to the patient. The patient will forgive most things related, for example, to delay if you are perceived as being a kind and caring doctor. By contrast, forgiveness is uncommon for one who is seen to be offhand. Being kind does not require any special training and is therapy needed by every patient you meet.

Do not be distracted by the spectacular

Spectacular injuries are not uncommonly seen in a busy ED. It is easy to become distracted by a patient with bilateral fractured femurs with the bone ends clearly visible, but concentration on the local injury may divert attention from a need to attend to the airway or to make sure that there is a channel for fluid replacement. The injury that is spectacular is not necessarily the one that should be attended to first.

Clinical notes are a medicolegal document, and legible, timed and signed records should be taken in every instance

This good professional practice is easy to forget in the hurly-burly of an ED. However, these records are a legal document (see Ch. 2) and may later have to be made available to the patient or legal advisors, not necessarily because legal action is being taken but perhaps because an insurance claim is pending (sometimes years after the accident) which can only be dealt with properly if clear notes were taken initially. Further, if, at a later date, malpractice (Ch. 2) is alleged, comprehensive and legible clinical notes are a necessary part of the defence; by contrast, absence of a record or its incomplete nature makes defence difficult.

The diagnosis of a fracture is clinical, not radiological

A normal X-ray should not lead to a false sense of security that a fracture is absent. A classical example of this is after

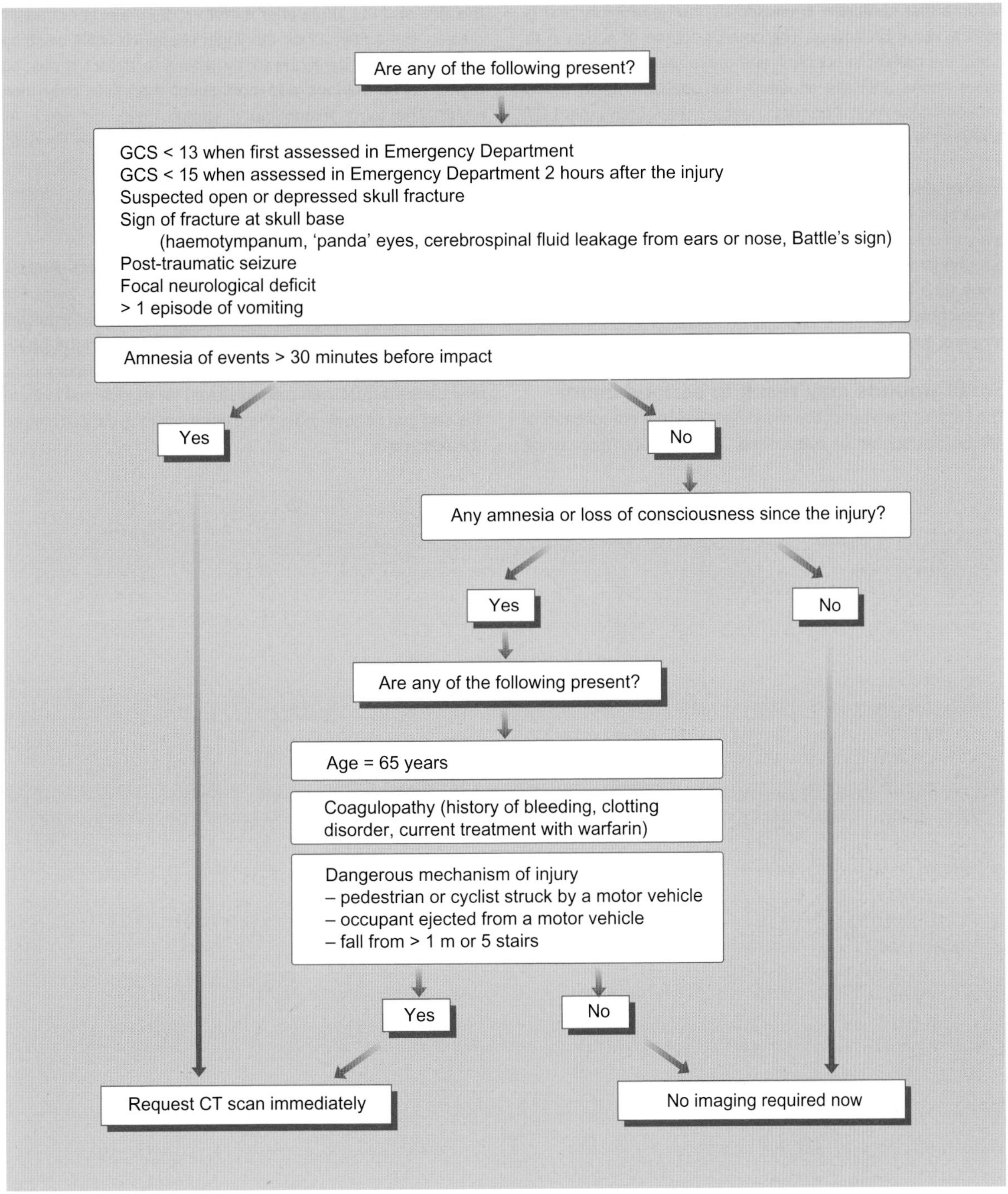

Fig. 3.7 Investigation for clinically important brain injury. (Adapted from CG 56 Head injury: triage, assessment, investigation and early management of head injury in infants, children and adults, London: NICE, 2007. Available from www.nice.org.uk/CG56 Reproduced with permission. Note: this guidance is current at the time of going to press. All NICE guidance is subject to review.)

a fall onto the outstretched hand (Ch. 35) when there is a fracture of the head of the radius or of the scaphoid. Similarly, an elderly lady who has fallen on her hip and is complaining of local pain could have a fracture that is impacted and permits walking (Ch. 35), even if the initial X-ray looks normal – never make a diagnosis of a bruised hip; admission to hospital is the best course.

Consider carefully the diagnosis of drunkenness

It is often unsatisfactory and sometimes very dangerous for both the patient and the medical attendant to make a diagnosis of alcohol intoxication in the ED. Other conditions such as head injury and hypoglycaemia must be excluded. If the patient has sustained a head injury, then it is prudent to assume that confusion is caused by the head injury and is not the result of alcohol. The correct course of action is to admit the patient to hospital, and make regular neurological observations until the situation has declared itself. If the patient's neurological condition deteriorates, then urgent CT scanning is indicated with appropriate airway management.

Never diagnose hysteria

It has been known for a patient to be labelled 'hysterical' after a minor chest injury; the patient is then given a paper bag to breathe into and put into a cubicle, only to be found dead some time later from a tension pneumothorax. A diagnosis of psychological problems in ED should only be made after physical causes have been properly excluded.

Small wounds may result in serious injury

The smaller the wound, the more likely it is that complications will be discounted or overlooked. A compound fracture of the tibia and the fibula after a motorcycle crash is not easily missed, but a tiny cut on the finger sustained while washing the dishes may be followed by failure to detect a divided digital nerve. Serious and permanent morbidity may then result. The term 'minor injury' should never be used. All injuries have a potential for morbidity and should be dealt with in this light.

If there is abdominal pain, examine the chest (and vice versa)

Chest problems often cause abdominal pain, and similarly abdominal conditions may cause referred chest pain. For example myocardial infarction not infrequently presents with epigastric pain, and pleural involvement in lower lobe pneumonia can cause referred pain to the abdomen. Biliary colic may cause retrosternal pain mistaken for myocardial ischaemia and gas or fluid under the diaphragm may cause referred shoulder pain.

4 Investigation of the surgical patient

Decision-making in the surgical patient is not often based on clinical findings alone. More frequently, investigations are undertaken to support or refute a clinical suspicion. Any investigation increases the cost of healthcare and often carries a risk both to the patient and to healthcare workers (e.g. exposure to X-rays). In consequence, investigations should only be undertaken if they are thought to contribute significantly to patient management (see also Ch. 7). It has now become customary to grade investigations by their degree of invasiveness (Ch. 1). There is not an agreed scale to define this, but the amount of compromise of the body surface and the likelihood of complications (both morbidity and mortality) are a rough guide; for example, a venepuncture is regarded as less invasive than an arterial puncture.

Objectives

There are three objectives to carrying out investigations:

- to establish a diagnosis, which includes the determination of the extent of the pathological process and the planning for its surgical correction
- to assess system physiological impairment (e.g. pulmonary or cardiac) and therefore the possible risk which is present if surgical treatment is needed
- to screen for disorders that are common but without symptoms; however, this is only worthwhile if their presence results in a change in management (e.g. previously undiagnosed hypertension, diabetes mellitus or coronary artery disease in those who require operations for vascular disorders).

There is an additional meaning of the word 'screen'. It can be, and often is, a synonym for a group of tests designed to detect a specific abnormality, such as in clotting (see below). The surgical student should understand the difference between the two senses.

Efficacy

A given investigation (just as with any clinical or laboratory observation) has a given degree of association with an underlying disease or disorder. This degree is a measure of the probability that, in a run of patients with disease X, the investigation will be positive in a given fraction of those who actually have X. For example, in patients with perforated peptic ulcer (Ch. 18), an upright chest X-ray reveals gas under the diaphragm in 60 out of 100 consecutive patients – a probability of 0.6. Observations of this kind can be incorporated into mathematical formulae using Bayes' theorem (see 'Further reading') to calculate the likelihood that a given set of observations (which include clinical findings and investigations) implies the presence of a particular disease/disorder.

Sensitivity, specificity, positive and negative predictive values

Sensitivity describes the ability of the clinical test to identify patients with a particular abnormality, even though it may also select patients who do not actually have the condition. It is calculated as:

$$\frac{\text{true positives}}{\text{true positives} + \text{false negatives}}$$

Specificity describes the ability of the test to identify the healthy individuals who do not have that particular abnormality, even though it may miss some patients who have the condition. It is calculated as:

$$\frac{\text{true negatives}}{\text{true negatives} + \text{false positives}}$$

Positive predictive value describes the probability that an individual who tested positive actually has the abnormality. It is calculated as:

$$\frac{\text{true positives}}{\text{true positives} + \text{false positives}}$$

Negative predictive value describes the probability that an individual who tested negative actually does not have the abnormality. It is calculated as:

$$\frac{\text{true negatives}}{\text{true negatives} + \text{false negatives}}$$

False negatives are those patients who truly have the condition but were not detected by the clinical test, and *false positives* are those who, on subsequent analysis, turn out not to have the condition under study but had a positive test.

The ideal investigation is one whose sensitivity and specificity approach unity. In practice, however, there is a trade-off between the two ratios – the greater the sensitivity, the less the specificity, and vice versa. This matter is particularly important in screening for early disease.

HAEMATOLOGICAL INVESTIGATIONS

Full blood count

The diagnostic use of full blood count in surgical patients is less common than in assessment and screening, e.g. to ensure that the patient has a haemoglobin level sufficient for oxygen carriage during anaesthesia (see Ch. 6) and a platelet count which ensures adequate haemostasis. Nevertheless, the full blood count is the commonest haematological investigation ordered in surgical patients (Table 4.1).

In diagnosis, the mean corpuscular volume (MCV) helps to identify the cause of anaemia, because chronic occult bleeding produces a low MCV (microcytic anaemia), whereas acute haemorrhage is associated with a normal value but a low haemoglobin level. A high MCV may be encountered in chronic alcoholism and vitamin B_{12} or folate deficiency (e.g. in patients with a previous total gastrectomy without vitamin B_{12} replacement, Crohn's disease [Ch. 24] of the terminal ileum or previous resection of this part of the gut). High haemoglobin and red blood cell counts are commonly the result of severe dehydration and compensation for chronic respiratory failure. Occasionally they direct attention to the possibility of polycythaemia vera, a myeloproliferative disorder in which there is not only excessive production of normal erythrocytes but also increased production of leucocytes and platelets.

Table 4.1 Full blood count

Component	Normal value
Haemoglobin	
–Male	12.5–16.5 g/dL
–Female	11.5–15.5 g/dL
Haematocrit	
–Male	0.42–0.53
–Female	0.39–0.45
Red blood cell count	
–Male	$4.4–6.5 \times 10^{12}$/L
–Female	$3.9–5.6 \times 10^{12}$/L
White blood cell count	$4–11 \times 10^9$/L
Platelet count	$150–400 \times 10^9$/L
Mean corpuscular volume (MCV)	80–98 fL
Mean corpuscular haemoglobin (MCH)	27–32 pg

White cell count

A raised white cell count with neutrophilia may be indicative of the presence of bacterial infection or necrotic tissue (Ch. 9). A severe septic response, however, may be associated with an abnormally low count. Eosinophilia may be a manifestation of parasitic infestation or allergic reaction, and a high lymphocyte count can indicate the possibility of viral infection. Low white cell counts follow cytotoxic chemotherapy. Patients with HIV infection may have low numbers of lymphocytes.

Platelets

Thrombocytopenia may be the result of a drug reaction (e.g. heparin), hypersplenism, an autoimmune process (idiopathic thrombocytopenic purpura), leukaemias or excessive consumption (disseminated intravascular coagulation). Thrombocytosis is seen in chronic sepsis and after splenectomy (Ch. 21) or haemorrhage.

Coagulation

In certain surgical patients, disorders of the clotting mechanism are more common. A coagulation screen should be obtained in:

- obstructive jaundice in which absence of vitamin K absorption leads to lack of prothrombin synthesis (Ch. 20)
- patients on anticoagulants
- patients who have undergone significant haemorrhage, e.g. during operation or after trauma
- patients who appear, during operation, to have coagulation defects, i.e. those with unexpectedly heavy bleeding.

Coagulopathies are not common but can occur in the course of other serious illness that may require surgical management.

Disseminated intravascular coagulation (DIC)

This condition is usually part of another severe illness or widespread malignancy and is characterised by activation, within the intravascular compartment, of both the coagulation and the fibrinolytic cascades. Clotting factors are consumed at a higher rate than they are replaced. The results are:

- depletion of clotting factors, and coagulopathy characterised by high prothrombin time and a low platelet count and fibrinogen levels
- increased circulating products of fibrin degradation (FDPs).

The cause of the syndrome is probably the activation of the vascular endothelium in capillary beds, which assumes a pro-coagulant state and initiates the coagulation cascade. Many bacterial products such as endotoxin and cytokines (e.g. tumour necrosis factor, interleukin-1) are capable of inducing a pro-coagulant state in endothelial cells.

BIOCHEMICAL TESTS

Table 4.2 lists the most commonly used biochemical tests.

Blood levels

Previously well patients who are not taking medication can undergo minor surgery without any biochemical studies other than routine urinalysis for the presence of glucose (see below). Levels in the blood are, however, important screening tests for many surgical patients: those with a cardiovascular disorder, on diuretic treatment or with known diabetes mellitus should always have their blood levels of sodium and potassium determined before an anaesthetic. Potassium changes (usually hypokalaemia) make patients vulnerable to cardiac arrhythmias; correction is necessary and usually easy. Elevated serum urea concentration is common with dehydration or renal insufficiency, whereas serum creatinine concentration is a more reliable marker of renal disease and is usually not affected by moderate dehydration. Elevation usually signifies the loss of 50% of renal function. Creatinine clearance (calculated from 24-hour urinary and serum creatinine values) is an accurate measure of glomerular filtration rate (GFR) and should be done in those who are to undergo major vascular reconstructions (e.g. aortic aneurysm repair), when it may reveal impaired renal function.

Table 4.2 Commonly used biochemical tests

	Normal value
Sodium	135–146 mmol/L
Potassium	3.5–5.5 mmol/L
Urea	2.6–6.7 mmol/L
Creatinine	60–120 mmol/L
Calcium	2.2–2.6 mmol/L
Glucose	3.9–5.6 mmol/L
Urate	0.18–0.42 mmol/L
Total protein	62–80 g/L
Albumin	35–50 g/L
Bilirubin	<17 mmol/L
Alkaline phosphatase	25–120 U/L
Aspartate aminotransferase	10–40 U/L
Alanine aminotransferase	5–30 U/L
Lactate dehydrogenase	40–195 U/L
Creatine phosphokinase	24–195 U/L
C-reactive protein	<5 mg/L

Postoperative abnormalities in serum electrolyte concentrations are very common, chiefly because, in many surgical circumstances, the gastrointestinal tract cannot be used for the administration of maintenance fluids and electrolytes. In addition, postoperative requirements may be difficult to calculate when losses are complicated – fistulae, nasogastric suction and fluid sequestration into either the intestine or large inflamed areas. Although sepsis and inappropriate antidiuretic hormone (ADH) secretion can cause a low serum sodium concentration (hyponatraemia), the commonest cause of this is water overload. If the patient is dependent on parenteral fluid therapy, the levels of electrolyte and urea in the blood should be measured daily.

Changes in serum potassium concentration are particularly likely in patients with an unusually high urine output (low potassium – hypokalaemia) or pathologically low output (raised potassium – hyperkalaemia). Prompt correction of the underlying cause is mandatory. Renal blood flow may be reduced during and after prolonged hypotension caused by uncorrected loss of blood volume or in patients with systemic sepsis. Postoperative elevations of urea and/or creatinine concentration are often the consequence of this. Serial measurements of urea concentration may provide an early warning of the development of renal failure.

Other blood levels, such as calcium and enzyme concentrations, are dealt with under the heading of the disorders or disturbances which cause their change.

Urinalysis

Testing of the urine has been greatly simplified by the use of dipstick and other prepackaged tests. Relevant findings in surgical patients are:

- glucose as an indicator of diabetes and the need for further preoperative investigation
- nitrites – particularly in acute undiagnosed abdominal pain; a positive test should lead to microscopy for the presence of leucocytes and bacteria indicative of a urinary tract infection
- blood (haematuria) suggests disease of the urinary tract, but the test is likely to give a false-positive result in a woman who is menstruating
- bilirubin – see Chapter 20
- human beta-chorionic gonadotrophin – pregnancy.

Twenty-four hour collections of urine are sometimes diagnostically valuable.

Microbiological investigation

Routine preoperative testing is indicated in the following circumstances:

- multiple antibiotic screening for carriage of resistant bacteria (e.g. MRSA – see Ch. 10)
- urinary infection in patients undergoing urological operations
- hepatitis virus infection (B and C) in patients from high-risk areas.

Tumour markers

See Chapter 12.

IMAGING

Surgery is a discipline based largely on anatomy and the function of anatomically discrete organs. With the increase in minimally invasive approaches to surgery, precise pre-operative localisation of disease processes is becoming more important. In consequence it is highly dependent on techniques which can give insight into the position and activity of organs and systems. Until the 1970s, this was achieved largely by the use of X-rays. However, although most hospitals still have organisations which are usually known as X-ray or radiology departments, many other techniques of imaging are now practised both in these departments and elsewhere. For this reason, 'departments of imaging' would now be the more appropriate phrase.

Imaging now has a central role in the management of patients, and image guidance is widely used for both diagnosis and treatment. Therapeutic procedures carried out utilising an imaging technique are called interventional, although they are no more – and are usually less – invasive than surgical techniques.

In addition, some methods and their physical basis (ultrasound, radioisotope imaging and functional MRI) overlap with studies of organ function.

Requests for imaging

Because there are so many different ways of performing all types of imaging and also many specific contraindications and complications, it is essential that adequate clinical information is given when requests are made. This ensures not only that the test is carried out in the optimal way to answer the question posed but also that any action is avoided that may be, at best, inappropriate and, at worst, dangerous. The term 'an order' is therefore clearly inappropriate for an imaging request.

It is also important that whoever makes the request is aware of what is involved, the contraindications and the possible hazards. If the surgical team is in any doubt, then a discussion with the imaging department is mandatory.

Finally, to make intelligent decisions on requests, it is also essential that the team has a general understanding of the physical basis of the various forms of imaging – their capabilities and limitations.

There are currently many different types of imaging, some of which interact with each other:

- radiological – plain X-rays (including tomography), contrast studies and computed tomography (CT)
- ultrasonography
- magnetic resonance imaging (MRI)
- isotope scanning.

All have a place in surgical diagnosis, and they are discussed separately below.

RADIOLOGICAL IMAGING

Physical basis

X-rays and gamma rays (γ-rays) are part of the spectrum of electromagnetic radiation (Fig. 4.1); both have short wavelengths and are therefore of high frequency. All electromagnetic waves travel through space at approximately 3×10^8 metres per second and are identified either as fluctuations of electrical and magnetic fields (waves) or as the effect of discrete photons (particles) on sensitive receptors. Their short wavelength and high frequency are associated with a large photon energy. To produce X-rays, electrons which have been accelerated to a high velocity by a potential difference (known as the peak kilovoltage, kVp) across a vacuum tube strike a suitable target such as tungsten or molybdenum. On impact, the electrons lose energy which, for the most part, is dissipated as heat. However, a small proportion is converted into X-rays, and the target can be arranged so that these pass through tissues. The higher the kilovoltage, the greater is the penetration but the smaller the differential absorption by tissues, and hence the lower is the inherent contrast produced in the receptor device on the far side of the structure towards which the X-rays are directed.

Interaction of X-rays with matter

In the energy range of diagnostic (as distinct from therapeutic) X-rays, three interactions occur:

- **coherent scattering.** In this interaction the incident photon undergoes a change of direction without a change in wavelength. Only a small proportion of the radiation interacts in this way.
- **photoelectric effect.** The photon is completely absorbed by an atom, with ejection of an electron and ionisation; the so-called characteristic radiation of a fixed and typical wavelength is released. This occurs more commonly with low-energy X-rays.
- **Compton scattering.** A photon strikes an outer shell electron of an atom, ejects it and leaves an ionised

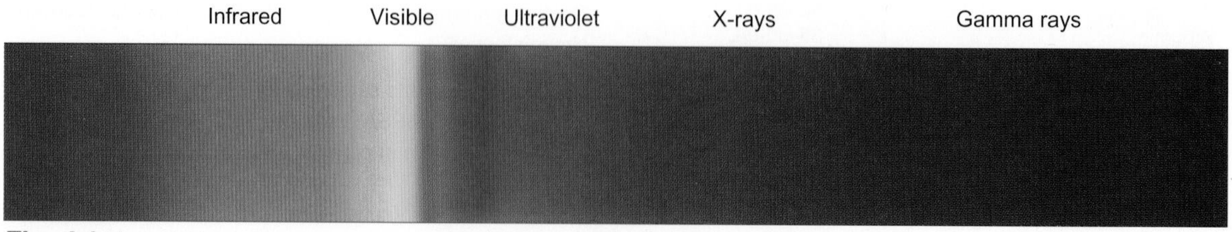

Fig. 4.1 The position of X-rays and gamma rays on the electromagnetic spectrum.

atom; the incident photon is deflected but retains some of its energy. Compton scattering accounts for most of the scattered radiation encountered in diagnostic radiology.

Detection: plain films

The original method of detection was by the effect that the beam of X-rays emerging from the patient had on a photographic plate – the less absorption there is by body tissues, the greater the electrochemical conversion on the plate and the darker the image. The X-rays alone can form a spatial image, but this requires a higher radiation dose than does the commonly used practice of having a fluorescent plate in contact with an X-ray film, which amplifies the effect of the X-rays and reduces the overall dose (at the cost of a slight reduction in spatial resolution). Film is rapidly being replaced by 'computed radiography – CR' and 'direct radiography – DR'. Both these technologies allow input of these X-ray images into digital networks (picture archive and communication systems or PACS), and these networks can incorporate all digital imaging. Conventional film can also be 'scanned' to form a digital image to be stored on PACS. In CR a photostimulable phosphor image plate replaces the film. The phosphor image is 'developed' by a red laser light creating energy release in the form of light, which in turn is captured as a digital image by highly specialised monitors. The plate can then be 'wiped clean' by fluorescent light and reused. With DR, the plate itself is dispensed with and the digital image formed directly by the X-ray equipment. This is a developing field; similar to CR but in-built phosphor plate technology can be used or X-ray photons can generate a flow of electrons in a dielectric plate and the image formed by an electrode collection plate.

Detection: fluoroscopy

Image amplification using image intensifiers, colloquially known as screening, or 'real-time' imaging, has been available for many years. Initially this was by a fluorescent screen in a darkened room during face-to-face encounters between radiologists and their patients. However, more complex methods are now routine which subject the raw output after tissue passage to recognition by photon detectors and amplification by photoelectronic techniques. These can include digital methods that allow storage in a form which is available for subsequent manipulation by computer (see also 'Digital subtraction' below). As with all digital images these real-time images can be stored, replayed from storage and modified (post-processed) to aid in interpretation by highlighting areas of interest and increasing their contrast.

Safety

The photoelectric and Compton effects cause ionisation which leads to breaking of chemical bonds with, importantly, damage to DNA. Large amounts of X-rays produce so-called non-stochastic (which roughly means non-random) or deterministic (consequent on a known biological effect of given frequency) effects: cell death, bone marrow suppression, cataract formation and hair loss. However, all of these occur at levels in excess of those used in diagnostic radiology. Stochastic (chance) effects, however, can also occur and include the induction of malignancy (including that of the bone marrow) and genetic mutations in germ cells (Table 4.3). Some tissues are more radiosensitive than others: in particular the ovaries, testes, thyroid and bone marrow. There is often a long (up to 30 years) latent period before these effects become evident clinically. In consequence, any X-ray examination is not without risk, however small that may be. The higher the dose, the greater the risk, although this has to be placed in context with life's other hazards (Table 4.4). Radiology departments have a duty to comply with the 'ALARA principle' – keeping radiation doses 'as low as reasonably achievable'. In any proposed X-ray examination there is a duty to weigh up the risk of irradiation against the benefit that may ensue. There is no such thing as a routine X-ray or one performed out of interest only. It is also important to be particularly cautious before performing X-ray examinations in:

- infants and children
- pregnant women
- patients who have been much exposed to X-rays in the past.

Proposed examinations in all such patients must be discussed with radiologists. In addition, X-rays which expose especially sensitive structures, such as the gonads, thyroid and bone marrow, should be kept to a minimum.

Plain X-ray films

These are images taken without any modification by the clinician or radiologist. Because the beam is differentially absorbed as it passes through the body, a two-dimensional

Table 4.3 Typical risks from X-ray examinations (per million)

	Hereditary effect		Effect on fetus	
Irradiation examination	Paternal	Maternal	Childhood cancer	Mental retardation
Lumbar spine	0.2	16	200	1560
Abdomen	2	11	170	1300
Pelvis	24	6.3	100	740
IVU	23	19	220	1610
Barium meal	0.8	9.4	220	1620
Barium enema	5.4	26	960	7200

IVU, intravenous urogram
From Plaut (1993).

Table 4.4 Effective dose equivalent of X-ray examinations, and the comparative risk

Examination (millisieverts[a])	Effective dose equivalent
Chest X-ray	0.02
Mammography	0.4
Abdomen X-ray	0.7
CT chest	7
CT chest for pulmonary embolus (CT-PE)	15
CT abdomen	8
CT pelvis	6
CT lumbar spine	6
CT neck	3
Myocardial perfusion imaging	15.6
Coronary angiography	7
Relative contribution to deaths in the UK	
Smoking 10 cigarettes/day	1 in 200
Influenza (all ages)	1 in 5000
Road traffic accidents	1 in 8000
Radiation dose equivalent of 10 millisieverts	1 in 10 000
Accident at work	1 in 43 500
Being hit by lightning	1 in 10 million

[a]The sievert is the SI unit of dose equivalent, which is a compound measurement derived from absorbed dose, the type of radiation and other modifying factors; it has replaced other measures such as the rem and the roentgen.
From Fazel et al, New England Medical Journal 2009, 361: 849-857.

impression of a three-dimensional structure is created on the output device.

Tomography

This is an X-ray technique that allows imaging of a defined section of the body. There are two types:

- analogue – using plain films
- digital – using computation as in computed tomography (CT) (also known as computed axial tomography or CAT).

Plain film tomography

In this technique, images are produced using an X-ray source and film combination that move with each other, so that only a single plane (slice) of interest is unaffected by the movement and all other planes are blurred out. It is now not commonly used except as part of intravenous urography.

Computed tomography

This technique uses a rotating X-ray beam to acquire tomographic slices, the information being detected by multiple receptors. By mathematical processing of the output (rendered possible by the high speed of the digital computer) an attenuation value is assigned to each small volume (voxel) of tissue that the beam has traversed. By combining these, a digital picture of the slice of the body at which the beam is directed is assembled and this can be further converted into grey scale values to be displayed on a screen. By altering the centring point and the range of units ascribed to each grey scale point, images which demonstrate soft tissue, bone or air-containing structures to the best advantage can be produced (Fig. 4.2). The most recent scanners use slip ring techniques to allow the continuous transfer of data while the X-ray beam is rotated, thus acquiring data in a spiral pattern as the patient is moved slowly through the scanning aperture. Original 'spiral' CT scanners used a single beam, but multislice scanners now have simultaneous multiple parallel beams, with rows of detectors working also in parallel, resulting in multiple spirals being imaged in one movement of the table (Fig. 4.3): 64-slice scanners are now widely installed and 256- and 320-slice scanners are available. Images can be obtained in a short space of time over quite large sections of the body, e.g. the whole chest while the patient stops breathing, in just a few seconds. Because of the design principles outlined above and also the practical constraints of positioning the patient, most CT scans are performed in the axial plane – hence the original name, computed axial tomography (CAT). Two-dimensional reformatting of axially acquired data into any plane (Fig. 4.4a) and three-dimensional reconstruction (Fig. 4.4b) are also possible, although this had until recently resulted in some loss of quality of the image. However, in that multislice detector CT (MDCT) produces volume rather than axial data, loss of quality has now become less of an issue. With very thin slices (narrow collimation –0.625 mm is now commonly used) possible with MDCT, any plane of reconstruction can be utilised with minimal loss of resolution, but sometimes with some cost in terms of radiation exposure. Reconstruction is of particular use to the surgeon who wishes to judge the relationship of structures to each other.

Volume data sets have also allowed improvement in advanced 3D processing tools such as 'virtual colonoscopy' where the computer produces images that resemble those obtained from within lumens by endoscopy. This eliminates the potential complications of endoscopy (see Box 4.1). Complex 3D reconstructions from the volume data sets can be made quickly on modern workstations. Angiographic reconstruction of 3D data sets is now used in place of conventional angiography except when detailed views of small vessels are required.

Radiological cross-sectional studies of this kind have revolutionised imaging and are now supplemented by similar techniques using ultrasound and MRI, both of which are considered later in this chapter.

Contrast studies

It is a common practice to enhance contrast in an X-ray, including CT, usually by the use of radio-dense substances which outline organs or areas of interest. In the biliary, vascular and urinary tracts, iodine-containing compounds are used, and in the gastrointestinal tract both iodine-containing compounds and barium sulphate. These materials are known collectively as contrast media or agents, although this is sometimes shortened to 'contrast' (used as a noun). The term 'dye' is often applied but it is incorrect and should be avoided. Although contrast media are usually substances containing atoms of high atomic number that strongly absorb X-irradiation (positive media), fat-containing

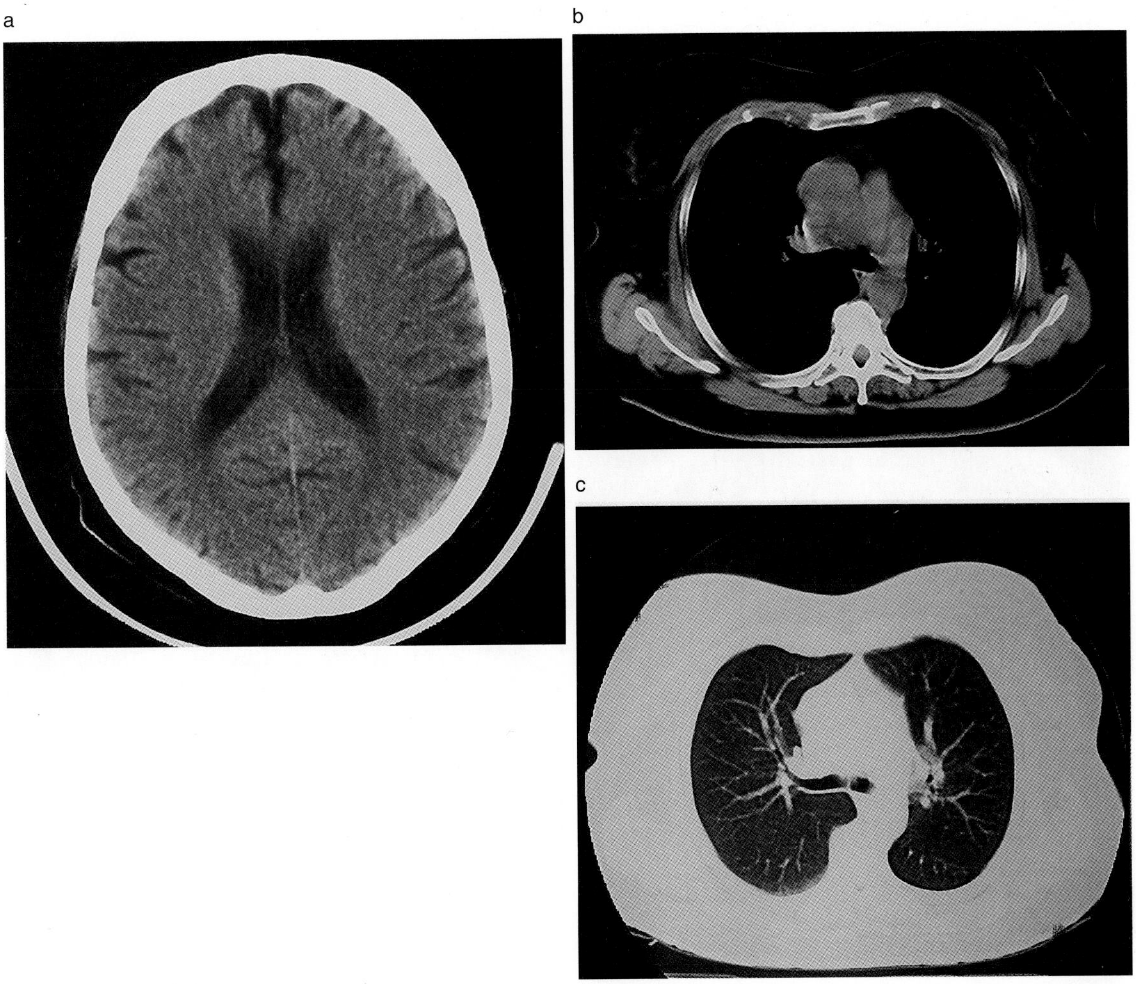

Fig. 4.2 (a) Axial image of brain at the level of the lateral ventricles. The CSF, ventricles and sulci are of low density (black) and the cerebral substance – cortex and medulla – are of intermediate density (grey). The bone is high density (white). (b) Axial CT image of the chest with the grey scale set to show soft tissues of the mediastinum and chest wall. The lungs are not shown, because of the position and width of the grey scale. (c) The same CT image as (b) with the grey scale set to show the lungs. Note that the mediastinum and chest wall are poorly seen with this grey-scale setting as the soft tissue, fatty tissue and bone are all represented by 'white' on the scan.

and gas-containing (negative media) contrasts are occasionally employed, and in the GI tract double contrast with barium sulphate and gas is commonly utilised. Many examples of the use of contrast media are found in other chapters of this book, such as the gastroenterological and urinary tracts (Chs 18 and 33), the cardiovascular system (Chs 17 and 29 and the neurological system (Ch. 31).

As indicated above, plain films are relatively insensitive in distinguishing minor changes in radio-density (as opposed to photon detectors used in computed tomography and in digital subtraction). Enhancement can be achieved by:

- opacifying the organ or tissue by adding an agent to the blood which perfuses it, e.g. the brain in computed axial tomography
- specifically outlining blood vessels so as to demonstrate these either directly on a record such as a film or after removal of the tissue background by digital subtraction (see below); both a normal vascular supply and unusual circulations such as that to a tumour (neovascularisation) can be demonstrated. The technique is also used in the direct study of blood vessels (angiography, see Ch. 29)
- administration of a contrast agent that is selectively concentrated by the organ as part of its function, e.g. uptake and concentration of contrast medium by the kidney for urography (see Ch. 33).

When the uptake and distribution of intravascular contrast agents is studied sequentially by ordinary X-ray exposures or CT, the investigation is often called 'dynamic' and can give useful information on patterns of blood flow in normal and diseased tissues (Fig. 4.5).

Intravascular contrast media

The objective is to deliver large amounts of substances containing atoms of high atomic number into the vascular system. The molecules must be:

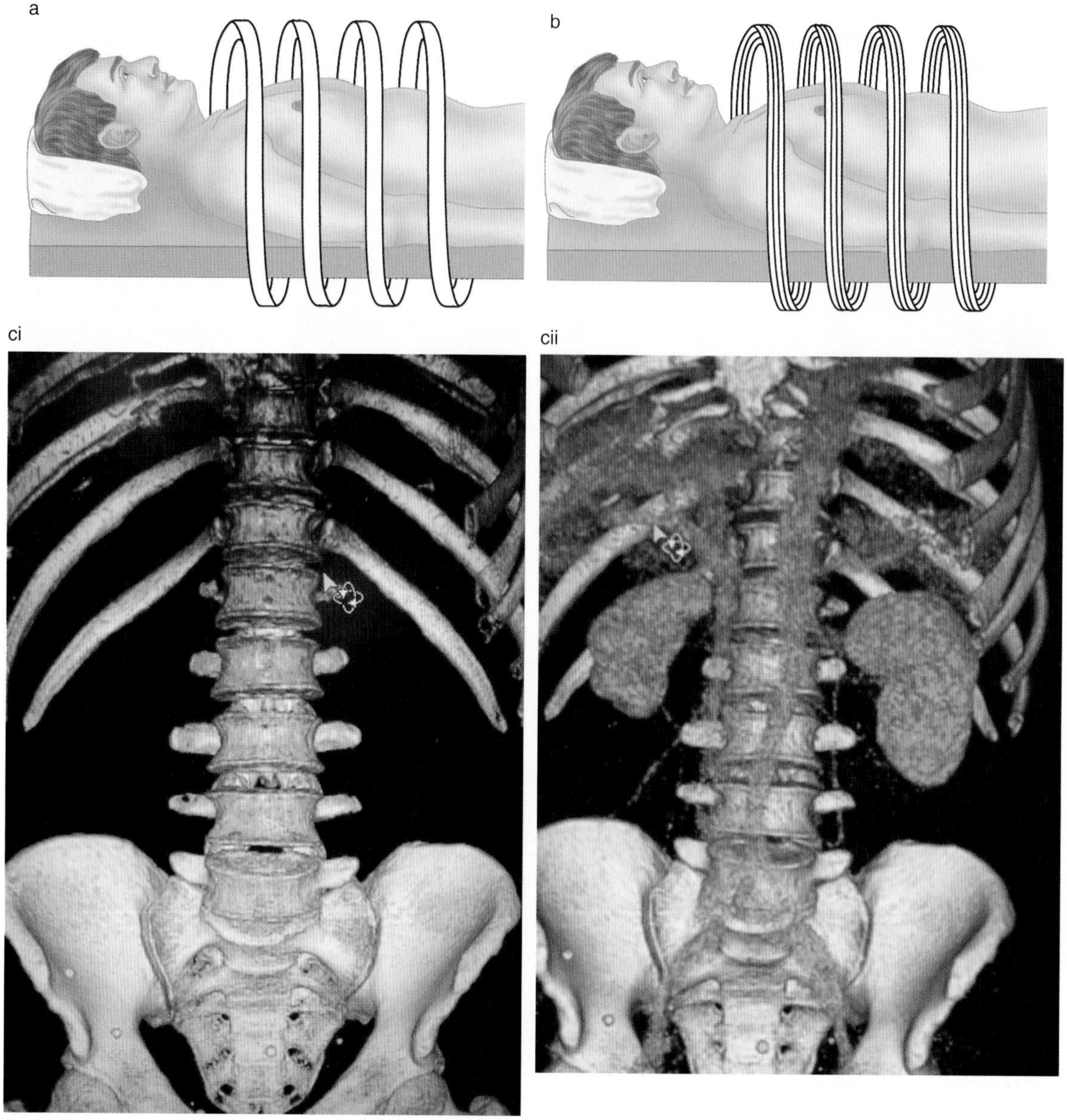

Fig. 4.3 (a) Diagrammatic representation of a single-slice spiral scanner in acquisition of data. The spiral is more stretched out (increased pitch) and thicker (greater collimation) than in real practice. Normally the pitch is less than 2 (when the gap between the rings of the spiral is equal to the width or collimation) but greater or equal to 1 (when the rings of the spiral are contiguous but do not overlap), (b) The same scan with a four-slice scanner. The original width of the beam is now taken up by four separate beams, all a quarter of the original width. The multislice scanner can cover the same length of scan with thinner collimation, or utilise the same collimation to image a greater length of the subject in the same time, or a combination of both of these; (c) a series of 3D images all produced from a single data set acquired in a normal single scan. These images are produced quickly on modern workstations with a few mouse clicks in a matter of seconds. (ci) demonstrates the bones, (cii) the kidneys and the aorta are added, (ciii) the abdominal wall musculature is shown, (civ) the skin surface is shown and (cv) is a work station display of a virtual colonoscopy study in the same patient.

ciii

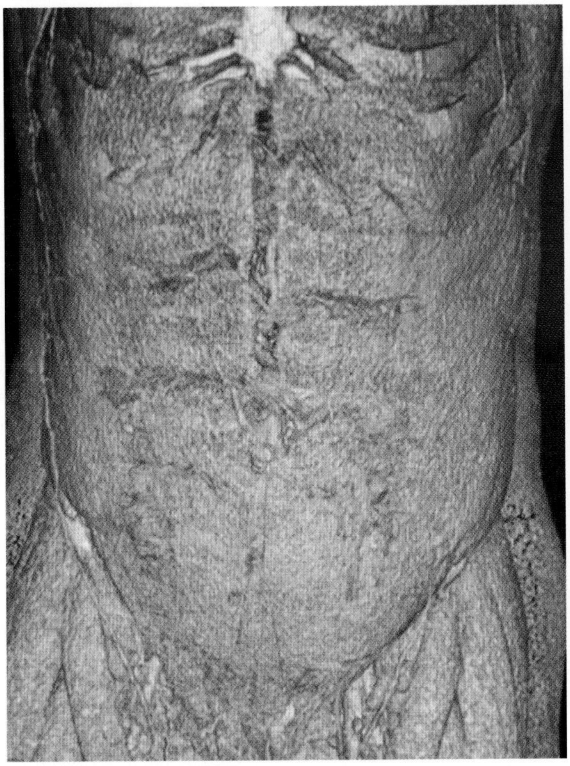

civ

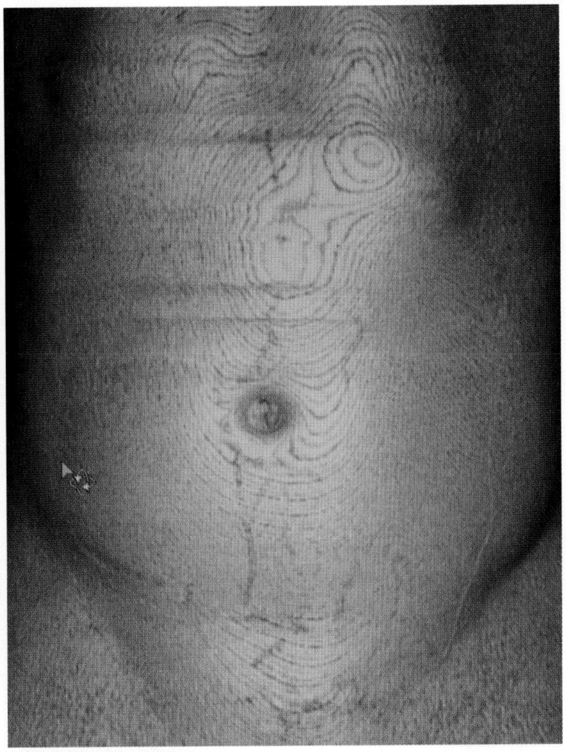

cv

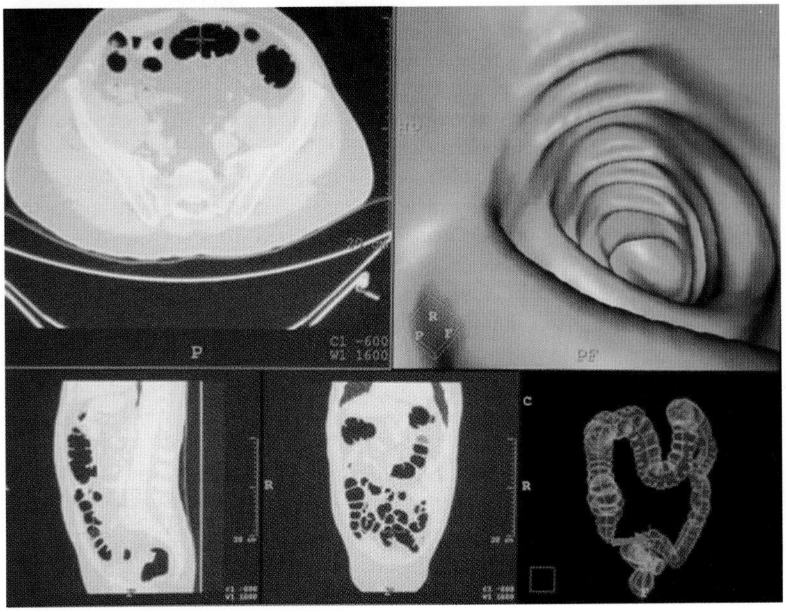

Fig. 4.3 cont'd

a

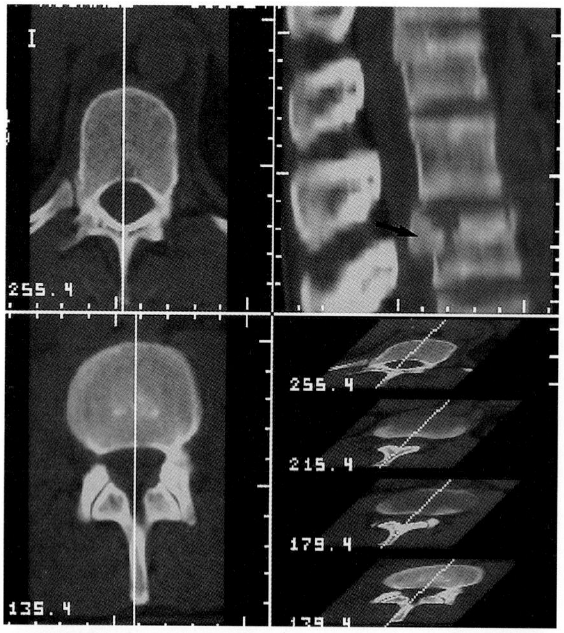

b

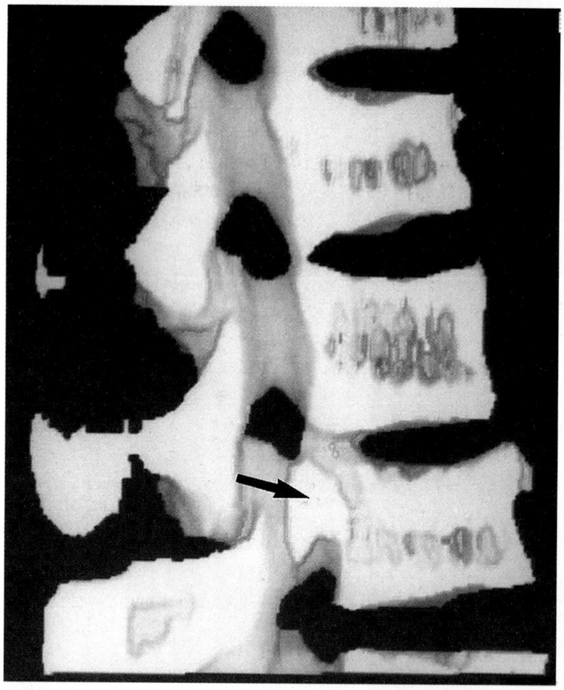

Fig. 4.4 Example of two- and three-dimensional reconstruction. (a) Sagittal reformatted image. (b) Three-dimensional reformatted image showing a large fragment of bone displaced posteriorly (arrow) into the canal.

- water-soluble
- ultimately excreted from the body
- associated with a low incidence of adverse effects.

To date, only iodine atoms packaged in various organic molecules have proved satisfactory.

There are three broad groups of intravascular contrast agents:

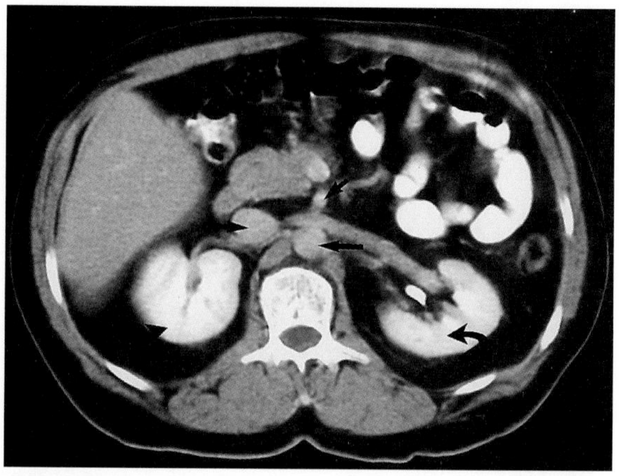

Fig. 4.5 Axial CT slice of the upper abdomen during the injection of intravenous contrast medium. Oral contrast medium opacifies the bowel. The blood vessels (arrowed) and kidneys (curved arrows) are also opacified, making them of high density (white).

- conventional
- ionic low osmolar
- non-ionic low osmolar.

These are described further in Table 4.5.

Reactions. In general, intravenous administration of contrast media is more liable to be associated with severe reactions than is intra-arterial injection. Severe life-threatening anaphylactic reactions to intravascular agents are idiosyncratic and occur in about 0.1% of intravenous administrations of conventional agents and 0.001% of low-osmolar non-ionic agents. The risk is greater in allergic individuals. It is becoming increasingly recognised that intravenous contrast can exacerbate renal failure. Other relative contraindications are given in Table 4.6. If a patient with one of these conditions is thought to require investigation, the matter should be discussed with the imaging department.

Intravenous injection is used for:

- contrast enhancement during CT scanning
- urography (IVU, see Ch. 33)
- venography (see Ch. 30).

Arterial injection is now almost always done by the Seldinger technique (Ch. 11). It is widely used for:

- direct imaging of the arterial tree (Ch. 29) and the heart (Ch. 17) to provide fine and precise details of vascular anatomy, both normal and abnormal, and to outline organs and abnormalities such as tumours
- interventional procedures – after a lesion has been identified, it may be possible to treat it by the intra-arterial route:
  - dilatation of coronary and peripheral arteries (angioplasty, Chs 17 and 29)
  - stenting of stenoses in peripheral vessels (Ch. 29)
  - embolisation of bleeding lesions in the GI tract (Ch. 18) and arteriovenous malformations.

There are no absolute contraindications to arteriography, but special precautions are needed in some patients.

Table 4.5 Types of intravascular contrast agents

Class	Nature	Examples	Problems
Conventional (up to 8 × concentration of plasma)	Salts of triiodinated benzoate anion	Sodium and meglumine iothalomate or metrisoate	Nausea and vomiting Endothelial and red cell damage Vasodilatation These conventional agents are now hardly ever used for intravascular studies
Ionic low osmolar	Mono- and dimmer compounds that can package the same amount of iodine at half the osmolarity	Sodium and meglumine ioxaglate	Much reduced osmolar effects Have an overall incidence of 0.05% of urticaria and mild hypotension (compared with 0.1% with conventional agents)
Non-ionic low osmolar	Replacement of carboxyl group by a non-ionising radical	Iopamidol Iohexol Iopromide	Bronchospasm, urticaria and mild hypotension – 0.02% compared with 1% with conventional agents Life-threatening reactions – 0.001% compared with 0.1% with conventional agents

Table 4.6 Relative contraindications to intravascular contrast media

Condition	Problem
Sickle cell disease	Sludging and thrombosis
Phaeochromocytoma	Paroxysmal hypertension
Myeloma	Renal tubular blockage
Asthma	Induction of bronchospasm
Renal failure	Exacerbation
History of idiosyncratic reaction	Further reaction

Other uses. Intravascular agents can also be used for investigations outside the vascular system, such as fistulography, hysterosalpingography and sialography.

Digital subtraction

The data that constitute an X-ray image may be either analogue or digital. Manipulation and comparison are much easier with the latter because arithmetic addition or subtraction within each small zone that has been assigned a numerical value based on digital code (a pixel) becomes possible. To achieve this, an original analogue image must first be converted into pixels, although a digitally acquired image is already in that form. Once the image is digital, a preliminary plain film can be subtracted from a subsequent contrast study of the same region so that the background is removed and the contrast is enhanced. The technique is widely used in vascular studies.

Intraluminal contrast agents for the bowel

Barium sulphate is relatively inert and is insoluble in water, characteristics that have made it the contrast medium of choice for bowel examination for more than 50 years. There are two types of study: single contrast (Fig. 4.6) and double contrast (Fig. 4.7). Both provide examples of the four different image types that can result – double-contrast (in which air is the other contrast medium), full column, compression and mucosal relief images – but the proportions differ. In single-contrast studies, full column, mucosal relief and compression views are utilised, with few double-contrast images; double-contrast studies consist mostly of double-contrast images with some full column and mucosal relief images.

The barium required for double-contrast studies is generally of much higher density than that for single-contrast films. In double contrast, a fine layer of radiographic density is required, whereas in single contrast the X-ray beam attempts to penetrate the barium column in order that protrusions of the wall into the lumen (filling defects) can be seen as dark (greater radio penetrance) areas within the barium image; conversely, ulcers and diverticula contain barium and appear as white (reduced radio penetrance) foci.

Double-contrast techniques have the potential to identify smaller abnormalities than single-contrast studies, but with the disadvantage of being more difficult to interpret (Fig. 4.8). The accessibility of the GI tract to endoscopic study has led to an inexorable increase in the use of endoscopy (see below). Endoscopy has the advantage that diagnostic biopsy is possible and therapeutic action, such as relief of oesophageal obstruction, can follow on direct observation. Comparisons between radiological and endoscopic techniques in the GI tract are given in Table 4.7. An important, but underused, advantage of barium studies over endoscopy is that they can also assess motility in addition to structure. A radiological study can also better demonstrate some subtle strictures (Fig. 4.9).

Other agents. Barium preparations are contraindicated where there is a risk of contamination of serous surfaces, in particular when an intraperitoneal perforation is suspected or impending. Barium in the peritoneal cavity causes a high mortality from peritonitis, and survival may be followed by extensive fibrosis. Barium sulphate is also regarded by many surgeons as not the best medium if an emergency or an early operation is contemplated, in that it remains for some time in the bowel and may become inspissated. The other contraindication to the administration of barium by mouth is when there is a risk of respiratory aspiration.

Water-soluble contrast media can be used when barium is inappropriate. They are the same as urographic contrast agents and, if spilled into the peritoneum, are absorbed and excreted by the kidneys. The commonest is a mixture of sodium and meglumine diatrizoate (Gastrografin), although it is hyperosmolar and, if aspirated, causes pulmonary oedema. When the risk of aspiration is present, the more expensive

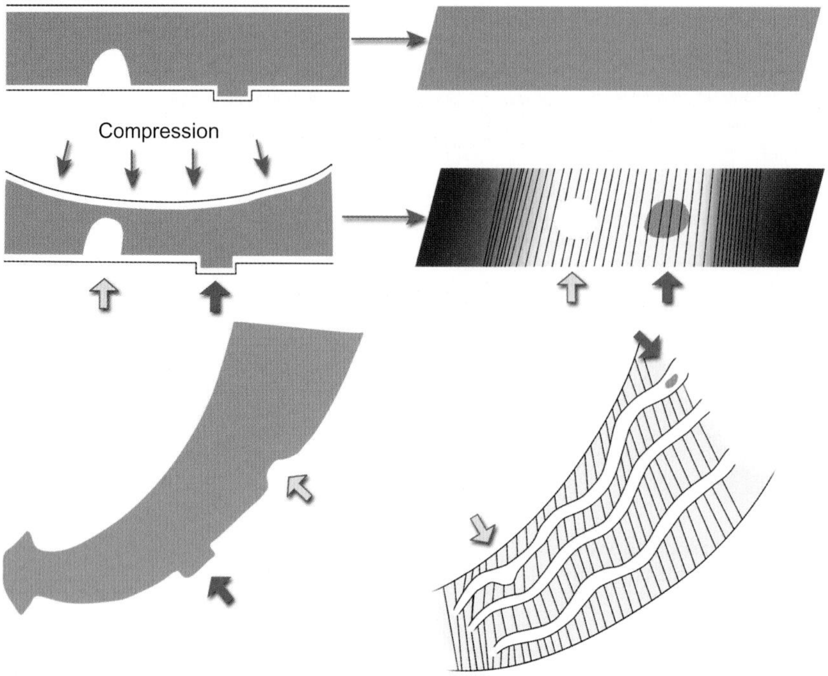

Fig. 4.6 Single-contrast barium images. The effect of compression (on the abdominal wall and therefore on the colon) can be seen in the upper images. A mucosal projection into the bowel lumen (e.g. a polyp) and a depression in the bowel wall (e.g. an ulcer or diverticulum) become visible and distinguishable. The lower images show the appearances of these lesions in tangential (mucosal relief) views.

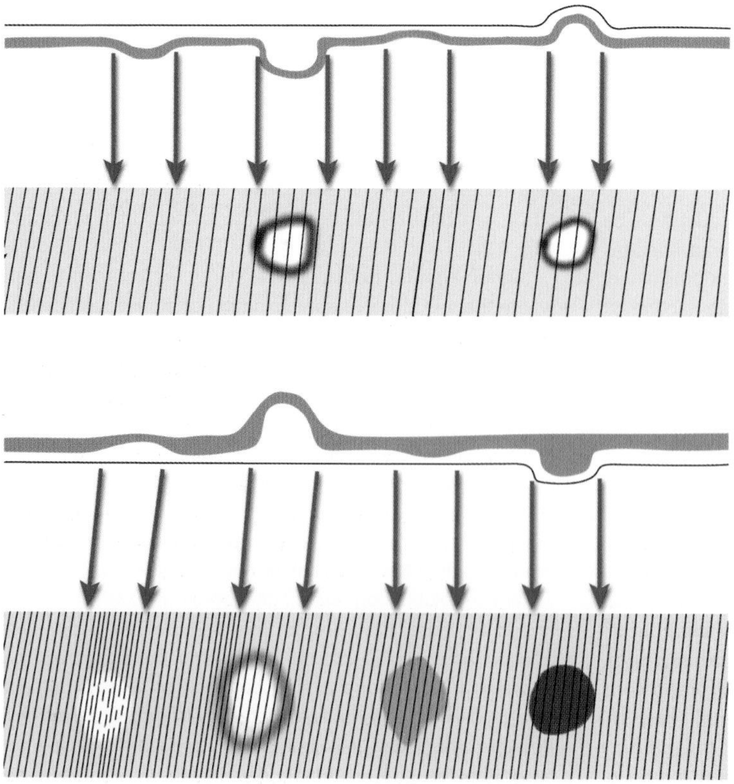

Fig. 4.7 Double-contrast barium images. The bowel lumen is filled with air and barium. The barium coats the mucosal surfaces and the air fills the rest of the lumen. The appearances of a projection on, or depression in, the mucosal surface vary with gravity – the same lesions on the upper and lower mucosal surface may produce different X-ray images.

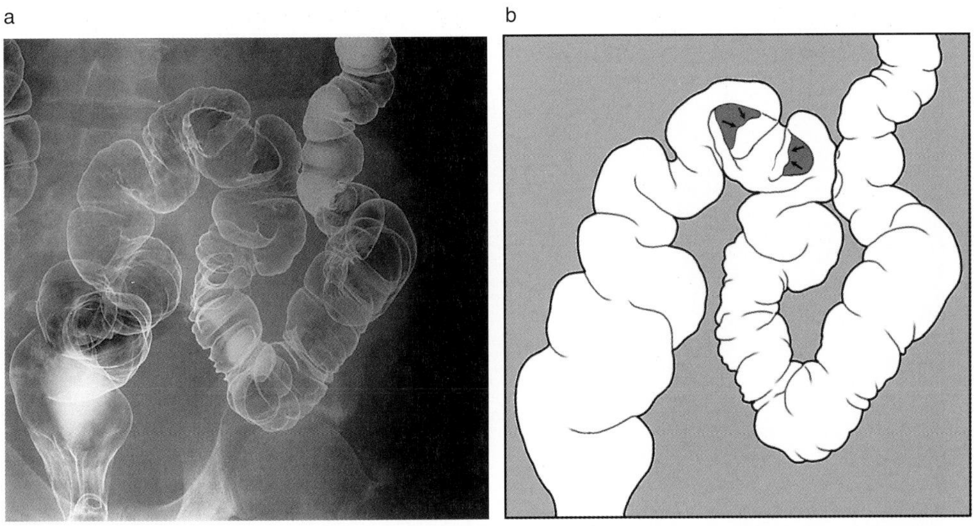

Fig. 4.8 This double-contrast study shows a carcinoma of the sigmoid colon with a saddle outline. It is recognised only by the presence of abnormal line or edge densities, emphasising that the double-contrast technique is the most sensitive but also the hardest to interpret.

Table 4.7 Comparison between barium contrast studies and endoscopy in the gastrointestinal tract

Factor	Barium contrast	Endoscopy
Safety	Higher	Lower
Overall diagnostic accuracy	Slightly lower	Slightly higher
Detection of superficial mucosal lesions	Lower	Higher
Detection and management of bleeding lesions	Lower	Higher
Biopsy	Not possible	Usually possible
Ionising radiation	Inevitable	Present only if X-ray examination is used as an adjunct
Hard copy	Automatic	Only if still photography or tape recording is used; video-endoscopies easily produce a permanent record
Subtle strictures	Better	May be missed
Overall topography and surgical mapping	Better	Poorer
Study of distal duodenum and small bowel	Prime method	Not easy as routine

but safer low-osmolarity agents are used. Only basic single-contrast studies can be performed with water-soluble agents, and their use is limited for the most part to the demonstration of perforation, fistula and obstruction.

Radiological interpretation

Precautions and preliminaries in interpretation

Many of these guidelines apply to all images, but some are specific to plain X-rays:

- Always look at the label that gives the patient's name and the date; it is very easy *for the wrong patient to be pulled up on a PACS screen.*
- Always check the marker that indicates side – right or left.
- Make an assessment of the adequacy of the image: does it include the entire part being examined; is it sufficiently penetrated; is it correctly positioned?
- Make a conscious effort to decide in what position the image was taken. Appearances may be altered dramatically by whether:
  - the patient was supine or erect
  - the part was weight-bearing or not
  - exposure was made in inspiration or expiration
  - the X-ray beam was horizontal or vertical – this is important because the demonstration of air–fluid or fat–fluid interfaces depends primarily on the orientation of the beam and not on the position of the patient (Figs 4.10 and 4.11).
- When fractures and dislocations are examined radiologically or when they are suspected, two images are needed, preferably taken at right angles to each other to allow a mental reconstruction of a three-dimensional assessment (Fig. 4.12). Some fractures are only visible on one of the two views.
- With a contrast-enhanced study, always remember that an opacity may have been present before the agent was administered, and review any plain images, which normally are taken initially (Fig. 4.13).

Principles

As already indicated, X-rays are interpreted by a biological or artificially created difference in contrast. This reflects the difference in penetration of the beam after its encounter with

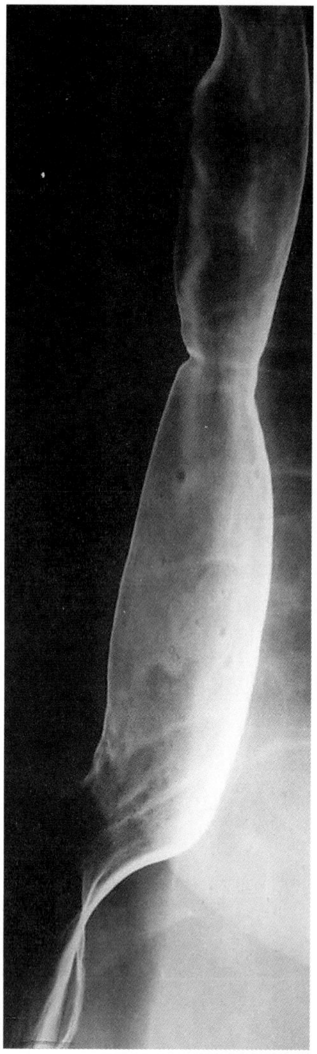

Fig. 4.9 Double contrast barium swallow. Stricture in the oesophagus in a patient who presented with difficulty in swallowing. Endoscopy had failed to reveal any narrowing.

tissues and therefore its ability to reach the detection device. There are biological contrasts – the difference in penetration of an air-filled organ such as the lung – which can be interpreted on plain films. However, from the point of view of differentiating many structures of comparable radiographic density (contrast resolution), plain films are not so adept. For practical purposes, four radiographic densities are distinguishable on plain films:

- gas – dark
- fat – relatively dark
- other soft tissue and body liquids – relatively light
- calcium/bone – light.

They can only be distinguished by contrasting one with another, e.g. an interface between gas and fat or liquid.

A basic radiographic maxim is the silhouette sign. Paraphrased, this states that if structures of similar radiographic density are contiguous with each other, then a radiographic boundary between them is not seen. At first sight, this seems obvious, yet it is difficult to explain in situations such as that illustrated in Figure 4.14.

The rule was initially formulated for the interpretation of chest X-rays, to explain, for instance, why a consolidated middle lobe (soft tissue density) can be inferred from loss of definition of the right heart border (also soft tissue density). However, it can also be used to explain signs such as the loss of the psoas border in acute pancreatitis because the fatty tissue adjacent to the psoas, which is normally responsible for delineation of the border of that muscle, becomes oedematous and necrotic with a density closer to soft tissue than to fat. Applying the silhouette sign, the two adjacent tissues are now of the same radiographic density and can no longer be distinguished. The application of this sign will also avoid radiographic misinterpretation such as believing you can diagnose a cyst within liver parenchyma without contour deformity or calcification.

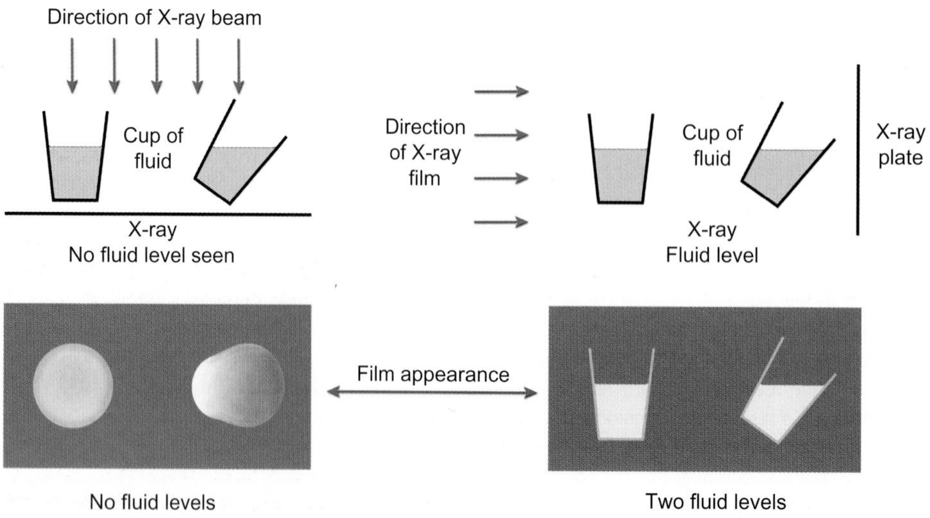

Fig. 4.10 For fluid levels to be shown on a film, it is the direction of the X-ray beam (which must be horizontal), rather than the position of the patient, that is important.

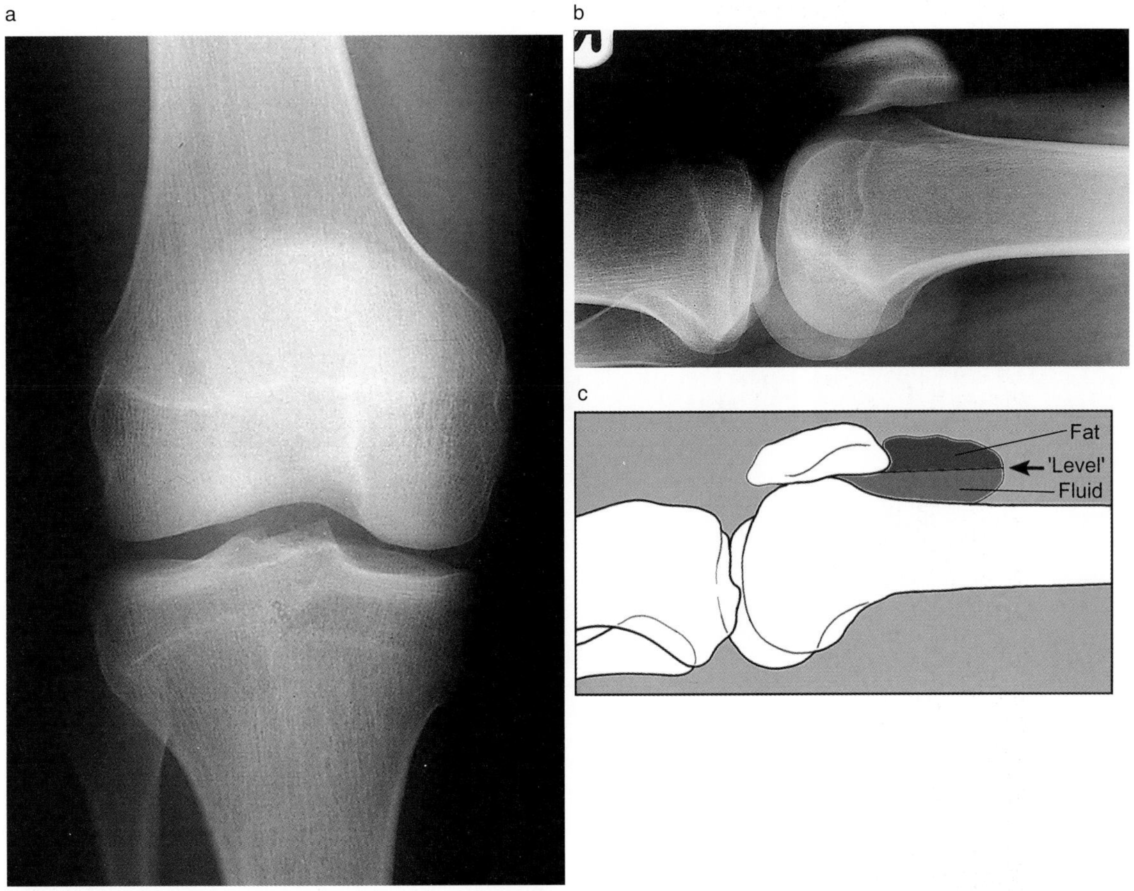

Fig. 4.11 (a) This AP view of a knee, taken after trauma, was considered normal. (b & c) A horizontal beam film was taken later, and a clear fat–fluid level was seen in the suprapatellar pouch of the joint. This indicated that there is a fracture, with blood and liquid bone marrow fat escaping into the joint space. A tibial plateau fracture was later confirmed.

ULTRASOUND

Physical basis

To create an ultrasound image, wave energy at a frequency above 20 kHz (the level of audibility to the human ear), but usually in excess of 3 MHz, is directed at tissues, liquids and gases from a transducer – often a small probe. Some reflection takes place that varies with the nature of the tissue and can be detected by a separate sensor at the ultrasound source. Because the velocity of sound in soft tissue is a constant, the time delay for an echo to return to the detector is an indication of the depth at which reflection takes place. After electronic processing, these echoes can be displayed on a screen.

The resolution of the image is directly related to the frequency of transmission – the higher the frequency, the better the resolution. However, penetration into tissues is inversely related to the frequency, which means that for reasonably deep penetration, as is needed in, say, the abdomen, a low frequency of 3–5 MHz has to be used with some consequential limits on resolution. However, for small parts such as the musculoskeletal system, thyroid, scrotum, eye and breast, it is possible to use higher frequencies (7–15 MHz) in that the probe can be placed very near to the area of interest. The development of *endoluminal* probes has also permitted higher-frequency scanning and hence better resolution of organs within the body: transvaginal for ovaries and uterus; transrectal for prostate and rectum; endoanal for the anal canal and sphincters; transoesophageal for heart and oesophageal wall; and transgastric/transduodenal for stomach wall, pancreas and biliary tree.

Tissue harmonic imaging (THI) has been introduced relatively recently. Defocusing and phase shifts of the reflected ultrasound beam caused by tissue inhomogeneities can compromise both the spatial and contrast resolution. Reflected echoes in an ultrasound examination are not only at the initial frequency (X MHz) of the inflected beam, but also contain multiples (harmonics) of that frequency ($2X$, $3X$, etc.). THI works by imaging the second harmonic reflection ($2X$). Although much weaker than the primary reflection, the image produced is much 'purer' with less interference.

Doppler effect

The movement of red blood cells towards or away from a transducer can be detected by the well-known frequency shift of returned echoes. The amount of shift is related to both the velocity and the angle of incidence of the ultrasound beam to the direction of flow. With duplex Doppler equipment, the imaging and Doppler analysing capability are

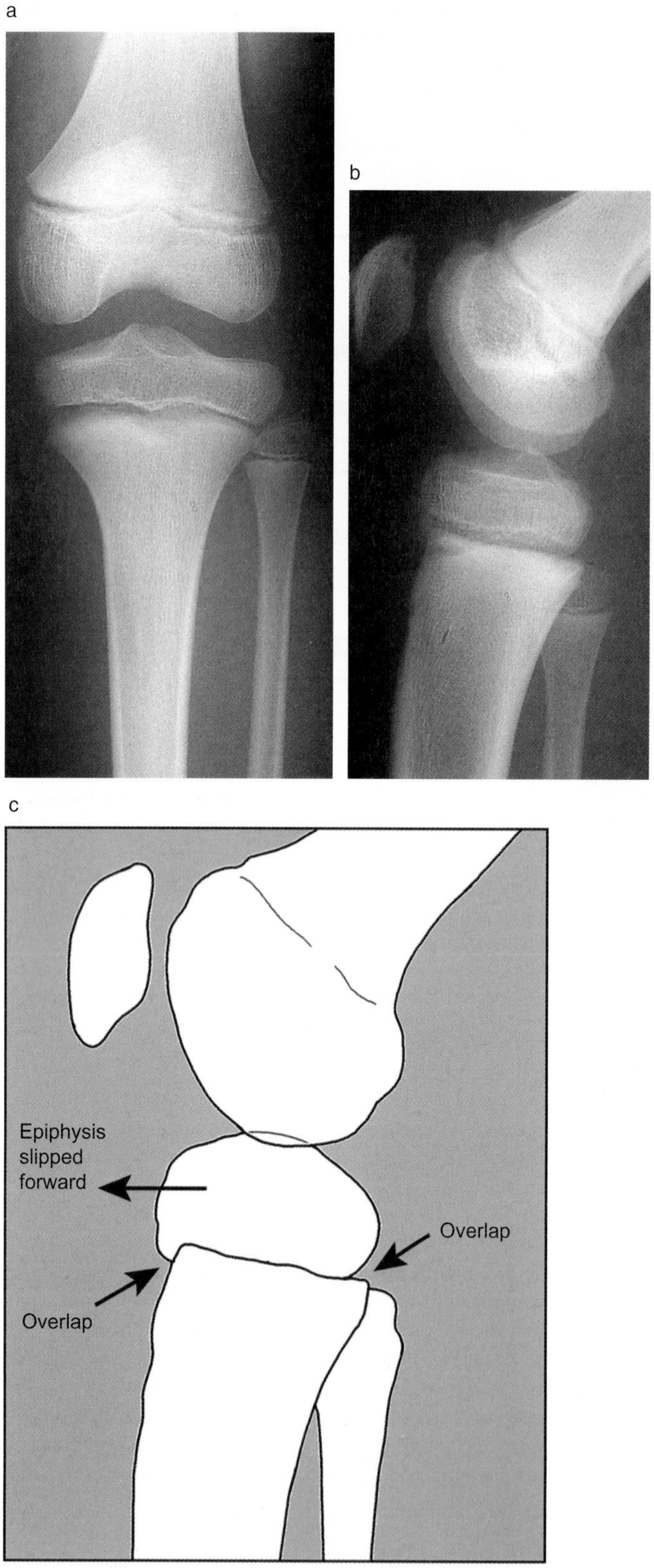

Fig. 4.12 X-rays give only a two-dimensional representation of a three-dimensional object. In many circumstances, particularly skeletal trauma, it is essential to obtain two views, ideally in orthogonal (right angle) planes. There is an injury to the epiphysis of the upper tibia. The AP view (a) appears to be normal, but the lateral projection (b & c) shows a forward slip of the epiphysis.

a

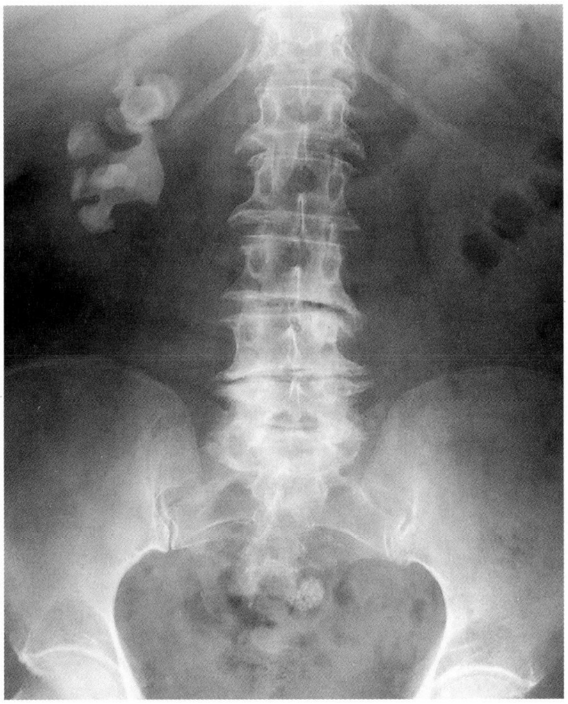

b

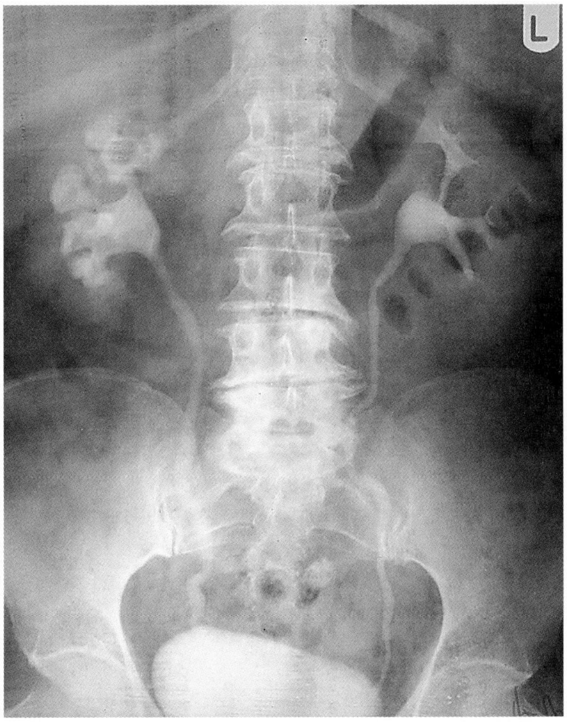

Fig. 4.13 It is important in many clinical circumstances to obtain a plain film (a) before contrast (b) is administered. In this patient undergoing an IVU, the large staghorn calculus is almost obscured by the medium that is being excreted by the kidney.

combined into one probe so that it is possible simultaneously to image a blood vessel and to measure the flow within it. The disadvantage is that it is only possible to assess flow in a small segment of a single vessel. Colour Doppler images are produced by detailed analysis of the frequency shifts over the whole area under study, and such images allow flow in all blood vessels within the field of view to be displayed. Blood flow is shown as varying shades of blue and red, depending upon the direction of flow with respect to the transducer and also the velocity (Fig. 4.15). Power Doppler is a more sensitive form of Doppler for detecting flow, but does not give any directional information. The signal depends on the quantity and acoustic impedance of the flowing blood. It does have the advantage of being almost independent of the angle between the beam and flow direction.

These methods have become of considerable importance in the investigation of the vascular system (see Chs 29 and 30).

Detection and display

The most usual method of display is brightness (B) mode in which the intensity of the spot on the screen is related to the amplitude of the echoes. By fast mechanical or electronic sweeping of the transmitted sound waves through a sector or rectangle, a real-time ultrasound image can be built up (Fig. 4.16). Its anatomical plane is determined by the angle at which the probe is placed to the skin surface. The thickness of the imaged slice depends on the width of the ultrasound beam, which in practice is a few millimetres. Motion (M) mode display is used to assess movement but without an accompanying real-time image. Echocardiography, for example, produces traces in which motion of the heart valves and other intracardiac structures is displayed as a varying position of the reflected echo from the moving structure (e.g. the cusp of heart valve) with respect to the baseline (Fig. 4.17).

With advances in the technical performance of probes and in processing of the signals, the quality of ultrasound images has improved substantially over the past 30 years. Three principles are important:

- The sound waves must be transmitted into the tissues by good contact between the transducer and the skin, which is achieved by using a contact jelly.
- Gas and areas of calcification (e.g. bone) do not transmit ultrasound waves; in consequence, the position and angle of the probe have to be constantly adjusted to avoid both (e.g. the bowel in abdominal examination) and to obtain the best image of a particular anatomical region and any disorder within it. Gas can also be displaced by compressing the gas-containing structure with the probe.
- The examination is taking place in real time, and therefore there is constant change in the image.

Endoluminal probes can also be used to overcome some of the obstacles to external ultrasound imaging.

The information obtained from an ultrasound examination and its interpretation are related to multiple real-time images.

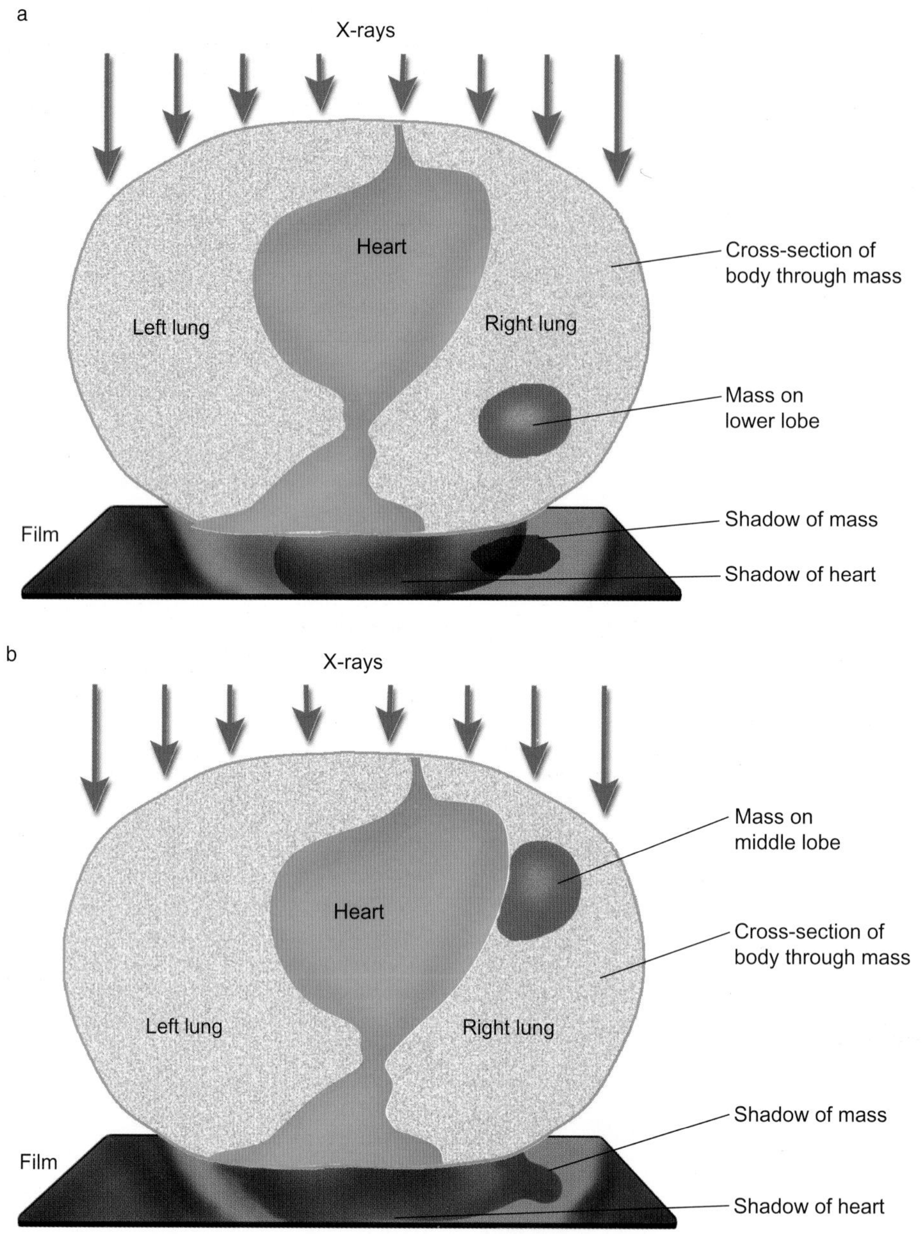

Fig. 4.14 The silhouette sign is not as obvious as it sounds. (a) The mass in the right lung is in the lower lobe and a border is seen between the heart and the mass on the film. (b) The same size mass is in the middle lobe abutting the heart and a border is not seen between the mass and the heart. In both instances, however, the X-ray beam has passed through the same mass of tissue.

Static or snap images are taken during the course of any real-time session, but the ultrasound operator eventually gives a report based on all the information that has been accumulated during the examination. Real-time ultrasound is thus very operator-dependent in both the acquisition and interpretation of data.

A variety of contrast agents have been introduced into ultrasonography over the last few years. They rely on tiny amounts of gas being encapsulated in a shell and injected intravenously. The gas is highly reflective and increases the ultrasonographic signal. Some microbubbles are designed to emit harmonic signals when imaged by THI. Others are designed to disrupt under the ultrasound beam and release the gas, which also increases the signal.

Dynamic scanning is possible with ultrasound. As ultrasound is performed in real time, it is possible to evaluate movement of joints, tendons and muscles (for example in shoulder impingement and snapping hip syndrome).

Recently **extended field of view (FOV)** image display has been introduced. This is achieved by producing a long image on the display screen as the ultrasound probe is moved slowly and smoothly along the whole length of a structure. It is particularly useful as a form of display for long structures such as the thigh muscles.

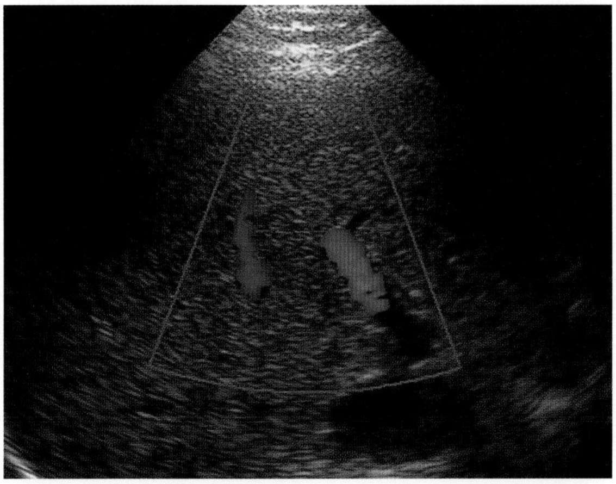

Fig. 4.15 Colour Doppler of the liver showing flow in the portal vein (red indicating flow towards the probe) and hepatic vein (blue indicating flow away from the probe).

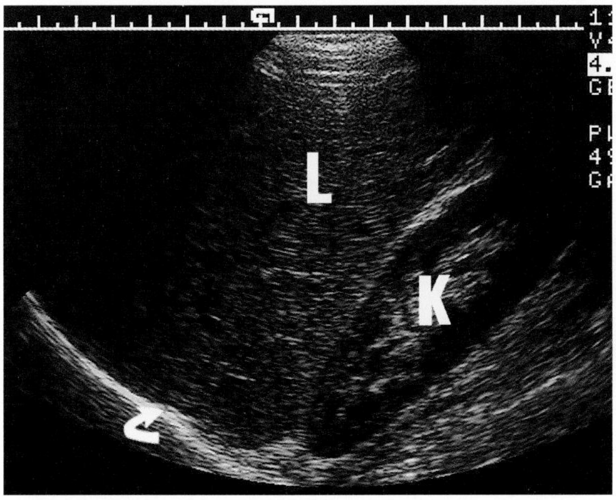

Fig. 4.16 Example of a real-time ultrasound image. A sagittal image of the right upper abdomen showing the right hemidiaphragm (curved arrow), liver (L) and right kidney (K).

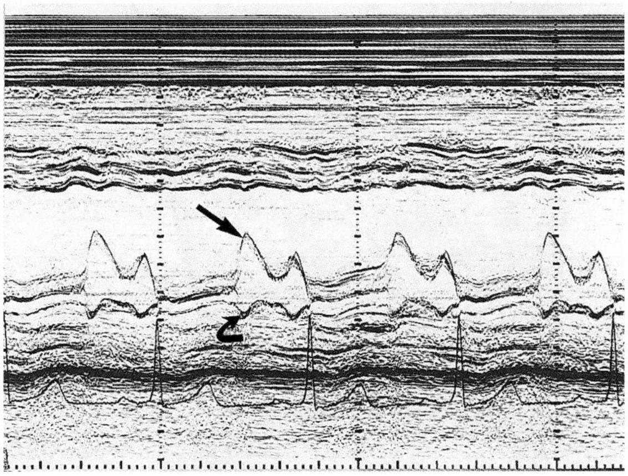

Fig. 4.17 Example of an M-mode image of the heart (echocardiogram) showing normal movement of the anterior (arrow) and posterior (curved arrow) cusps of the mitral valve. The ECG recording is shown at the bottom of the tracing.

3D (static three-dimensional images) and **4D** (moving 3D images) can now be produced with the computing power of modern ultrasound machines. Rapid acquisition of multiple scanning planes are combined to produce the 3D image. This is mainly used in antenatal scanning to assess fetal anatomic anomalies and in endoanal scanning to demonstrate the precise location and pattern of sphincter damage.

Elastography has recently been introduced into ultrasound imaging. This is based on the principle of physical elasticity or stiffness. A pressure wave exerted by the ultrasound probe is used to 'estimate' the induced strain distribution by detecting tissue motion. An image of the elasticity of tissue can be superimposed as a colour map on the 2D sonographic image. This was initially developed for detection and characterisation of breast lesions but is finding wider applications.

Safety

There is currently no evidence that ultrasound waves have any deleterious biological effects. However, an open mind must be kept because methods of detection of cell damage are still quite crude. Nevertheless, the perceived safety of ultrasound over X-rays, the lack of ionising radiation and the low cost make it the investigation of first choice in many circumstances, such as suspected biliary disease (Ch. 20), neonatal brain problems and gynaecology.

MAGNETIC RESONANCE IMAGING

The production of an image by MRI involves more complex physics than the production of radiological plain images, CT or ultrasound scans. Therefore only a brief description is given here, but further information can be obtained from texts listed in the 'Further reading' section.

Principles

MRI is based on the fact that nuclei spin and that those with uneven numbers of protons (particularly hydrogen, which is the most abundant nucleus in biological tissues) behave like small magnets with a north and a south pole. They align themselves along the main magnetic field to which they are exposed but can be sent 'off balance' by a radiofrequency pulse; they then subsequently resonate and realign. As this takes place, a radiofrequency pulse is emitted which can be detected by receiver coils. These can be exactly located in relation to the slice of tissue targeted. One great advantage of MRI is that any anatomical plane can be chosen for acquisition, and consequently the most diagnostically helpful orientation is employed for different clinical circumstances – sagittal and axial images of the spine; sagittal and coronal images of the pituitary; similar views for the knee; and oblique coronal and axial views for the shoulder (Fig. 4.18).

Detection and display

The signal produced from the targeted tissue depends on a number of variables, including the density of protons within the sample volume, and the way in which resonance stops

a

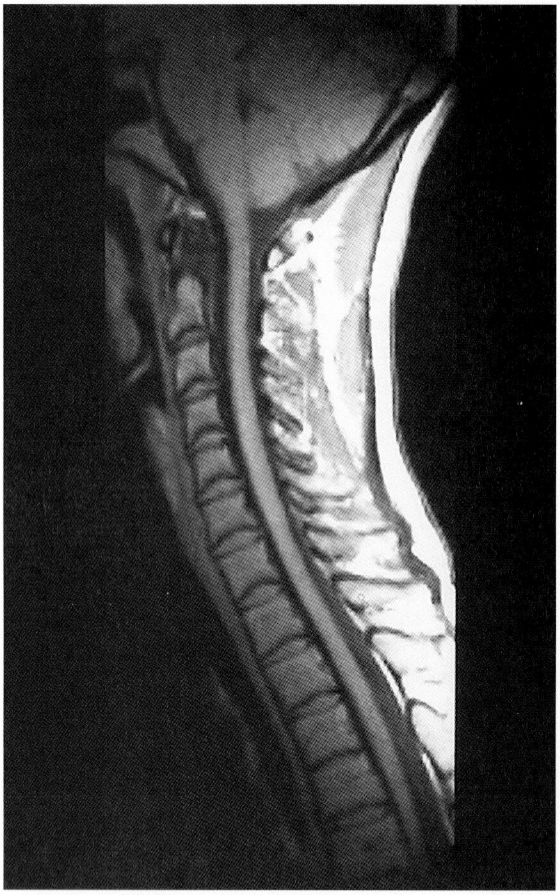

b

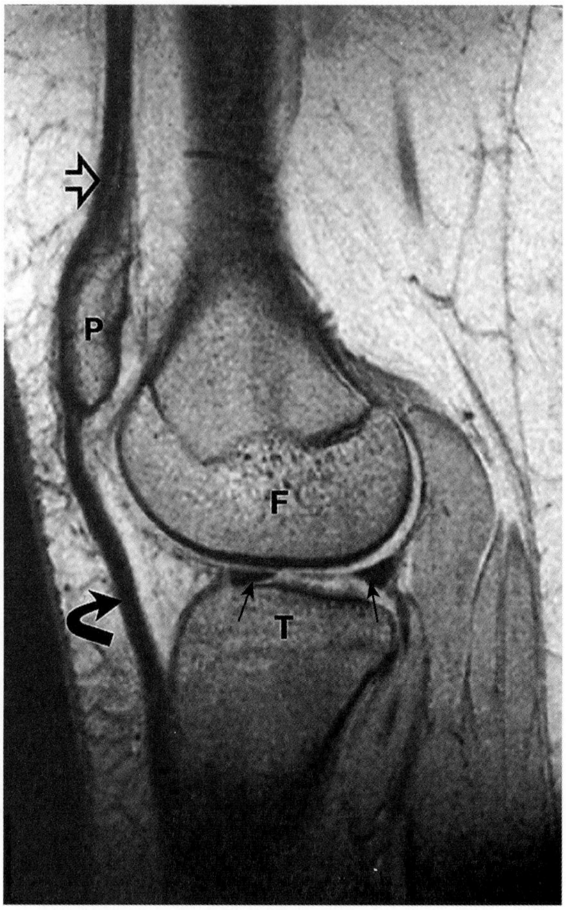

c

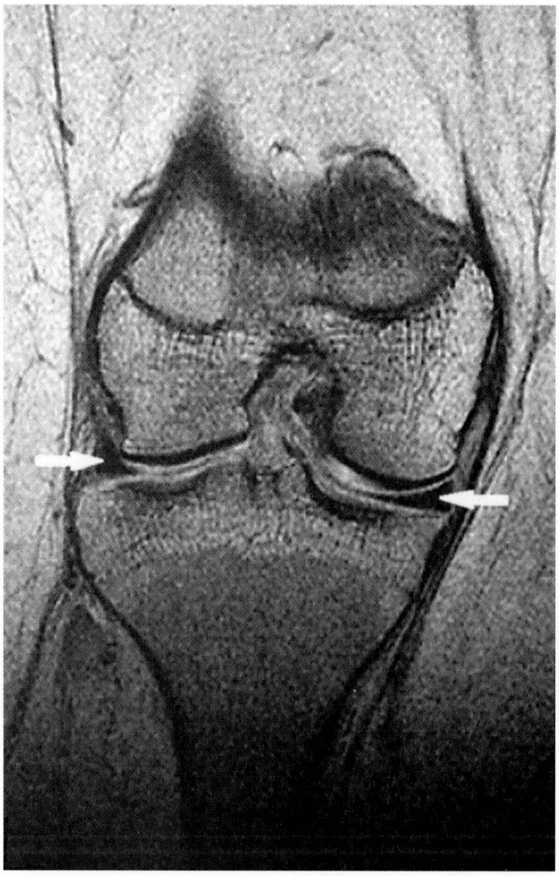

Fig. 4.18 Examples of different planes achievable with MRI. (a) A sagittal T1-weighted image of the cervical spine. (b) Sagittal image of a knee showing the black triangular-shaped anterior and posterior portions of the medial meniscus (arrows) lying between the medial femoral condyle (F) and the medial tibial plateau (T). The patella (P), patellar tendon (curved arrow) and quadriceps tendon (open arrow) are seen anteriorly. (c) Coronal image of a knee showing the menisci as black triangles (arrows).

when the radiofrequency pulse is switched off (relaxation). These determine two main phenomena which are used in clinical practice:

- T1 (longitudinal) relaxation time, which is the result of the resonating nuclei transferring energy to larger non-resonating macromolecules in the environment
- T2 (transverse) relaxation time, which is the interaction of energy transfer (dephasing) of the resonant nuclei with other adjacent nuclei.

Both of these occur simultaneously but, by varying the scanning criteria (so-called pulse sequences), it is possible to produce MR images with different tissue contrast – T1- and T2-weighted images. Furthermore, because different tissues have variable macromolecular contents, they can be differentiated on one imaging sequence or another; the intrinsic contrast resolution of MRI is thus very high. The way that a tissue behaves with different sequences also gives some idea of its water content. Another useful variant in MRI is to use sequences which cause fat saturation or fat suppression in which the signal from fat-containing tissues is suppressed, thus highlighting signals from adjacent non-fatty tissues. The general appearances of tissues on MRI are given in Table 4.8 and representative examples of T1 and T2 weighting are shown in Figure 4.19 (a) and (b).

An MRI system comprises:

- a main magnet of extremely high and uniform magnetic field (0.2–3 Tesla, which is 4000- to 60 000-fold greater than the Earth's magnetic field). Machines with even higher magnetic fields are now being developed
- gradient coils which can superimpose minor magnetic gradients on the main magnetic field in a defined manner along the x, y and z axes; these are turned

Table 4.8 Appearances of tissues and their contents on MRI

Tissue or content	T1-weighted image	T2-weighted image
Air	Black	Black
Liquid (CSF, urine, bile)	Dark grey to black	White
Bone cortex		
Fibrous tissue		
Tendon	Black	Black
Fat		
Fatty bone marrow	White	White
Cellular bone marrow	Dark grey	White
Neoplasms	Dark grey to grey	White
Haematomas	Variable (met-haemoglobin white)	Variable
Muscle	Grey	Grey
Brain		
–White matter	Light grey	Dark grey
–Grey matter	Dark grey	Light grey

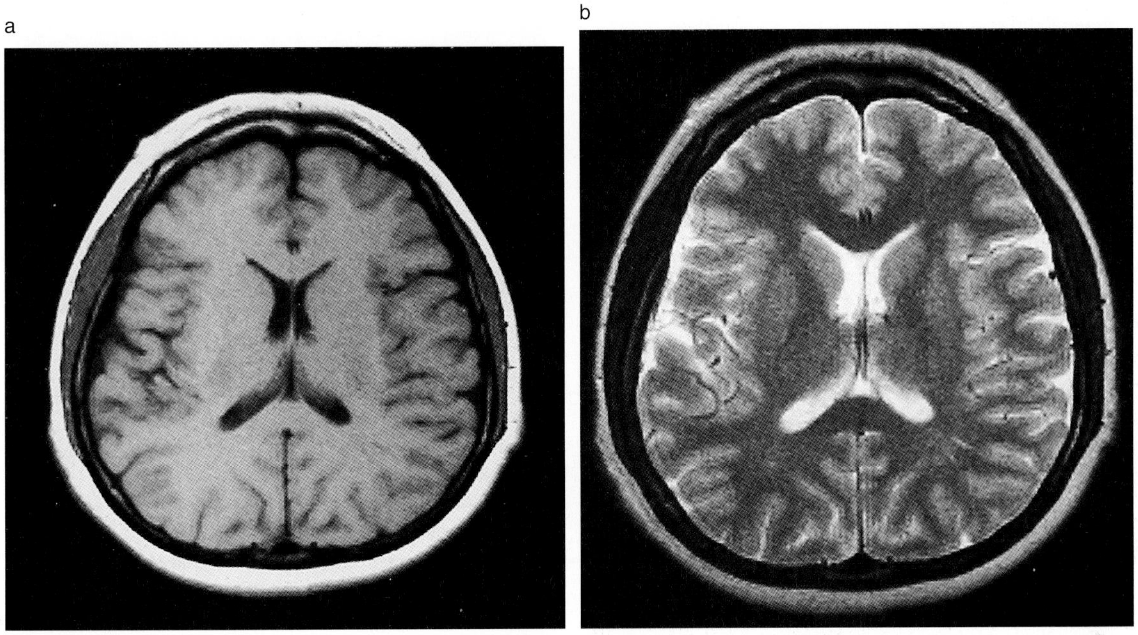

Fig. 4.19 (a) A T1-weighted axial image of the brain at the level of the lateral ventricles, showing CSF in the ventricles and cerebral sulci as low signal intensity (black). (b) On the corresponding T2-weighted image, the CSF has high signal intensity (white).

Table 4.9 Comparison of cross-sectional imaging techniques

	Computed tomography	Ultrasound	Magnetic resonance imaging
Uses ionising radiation	Yes	No	No
Speed	0.5–20 s	Real time, examinations typically lasting 5–15 min	15–60 min
Imaging plane	Axial but coronal in some circumstances	Variable at time of scan	Multiplanar
Portable	No	Yes	No
Capital cost (£1000)	200–600	20–150	500–2000
Operator dependency	Low	High	Low
Image degradation	Metal implants	Bone and gas and patient movement	Metal implants
Images			
–Bone	Yes – cortex	No	Yes – medulla
–Lungs	Yes	No	No
–Solid organs	Yes	Yes	Yes
–Gallbladder calculi	Only if radio-dense	Yes	Yes
Head and spine, including neonate	Yes	No – except neonatal and intraoperatively	Yes – best method
Liquid collections	Yes	Yes	Yes
Blood vessels	Yes but needs contrast medium	Yes with Doppler	Yes and does not always require contrast medium
Fetus with safety	No	Yes – ideal for routine scanning	No – research only at present time
Guided biopsy and drainage	Yes	Yes	Feasible and likely to increase
Contraindications	Same as for all X-rays	None known	Heart pacemakers; clips on intracranial aneurysms; metal in eye

on and off rapidly during imaging to produce spatial localisation

- radiofrequency transmitting and receiving coils which send, with great precision, radiofrequency pulses into slices of the patient and detect the resultant signal; these coils can be either large body coils or small surface coils for increased resolution of small areas of tissue
- computational facilities to process the raw data and provide storage, image display and manipulation
- methods for display of 'hard copy'.

Safety

MRI has no known deleterious biological effects (for contraindications, see Table 4.9).

Advantages and disadvantages

MRI has the advantage that it:

- is without ionising radiation
- can image in any plane
- provides very good images of soft tissues – better than CT.

MRI also provides images of blood vessels and is capable of producing angiograms without intravascular injections (Fig. 4.20), although the most detailed angiograms are performed with intravenous gadolinium-based contrast agents. The quality of MRI angiograms continues to improve with technological advance, and they are increasingly replacing conventional techniques. Gadolinium-based contrast agents in very dilute amounts can be injected into joints to improve visualisation of intra-articular structures (e.g. the labrum in shoulder and hip imaging); this is termed MR arthrography.

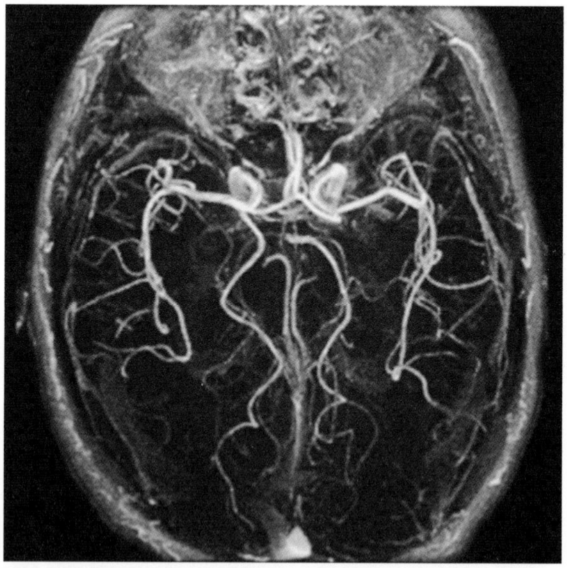

Fig. 4.20 MR angiogram of intracranial blood vessels.

Liver-specific contrast agents have been developed for MRI. Superparamagnetic iron oxide particles (SPIO) are taken up by the reticuloendothelial system Kupffer cells where they create a marked decrease in signal on T2-weighted images. Liver metastases and other tumours do not possess these cells and the contrast between normal liver and such masses is greatly enhanced with the use of SPIO. The other approach has been to develop agents that are taken up and excreted by hepatocytes. These include manganese compounds and some gadolinium chelates. These liver-specific agents have been developed to improve detection and characterisation of liver lesions. Many of the agents can be used in the dynamic phase (while the molecules are in the extracellular space) in much the same way as standard gadolinium chelates. The agents are then handled differently by the body. Those taken up by hepatocytes can demonstrate enhancement with functioning hepatocytes (normal liver, some well-differentiated hepatocellular carcinomas and focal nodular hyperplasia for example). If they are excreted in the bile in later phases, they can be used for positive cholangiography.

Diffusion-weighted imaging is now available on most modern MR equipment. This is particularly useful for assessing whether an infarct in the brain has occurred recently or is in fact old. MR spectroscopy is a technique in which the MR spectrum from a small targeted area of body tissue is acquired. The target is selected from an MR image so that the exact site can be identified. Research is ongoing to validate the usefulness of this technique in differentiating between normal and pathological processes (e.g. tumours).

Functional MRI (fMRI) is a technique looking for small changes in oxygenation of brain tissue to identify cortical activation. Research in this area is helping to both identify the function of different parts of the normal brain and also to identify areas of abnormally functioning brain.

The main disadvantage of MRI is that it is relatively slow and expensive compared with other techniques. Each sequence has until recently taken between 2 and 8 minutes to perform depending on:

- magnet strength
- pulse sequence
- image quality required.

With these times of scanning, movement of the patient, respiration and cardiac motion are all problems. Faster scanning is being developed and has already allowed some MR images to be obtained in seconds rather than minutes. As well as assessing blood vessels, MRI is being employed to assess the anatomy (chambers and wall) and function (including ejection fraction) of the heart. Respiratory and cardiac 'gating' can also improve these images.

Contrast agents can also be used to look for differing rates of uptake of contrast compared to normal tissue by repeating fast scan sequences over a period of up to 5–10 minutes. These so-called dynamic MR scans are being employed in many situations such breast imaging, prostate imaging and characterisation of liver lesions.

Interventional MRI techniques are also under development and, when combined with fast scanning, are beginning to allow the possibility of surgical procedures under real-time MRI control.

Comparison with other methods of cross-sectional imaging

The availability of CT, ultrasound and MRI for the creation of cross-sectional images makes the choice of method for individual circumstances quite difficult. Table 4.9 gives a comparison of the features of the three methods.

RADIOISOTOPE IMAGING

Principles

Radioisotope imaging studies provide information more about function than structure. Radioisotopes are isotopes which emit radioactivity, and most of the radioisotopes in medical usage emit gamma radiation, identical to X-rays, but a few emit particulate radiation in addition (alpha or beta radiation). Radioisotopes in common usage include ^{99m}Tc (technetium), ^{123}I and ^{131}I (iodine), ^{111}In (indium), ^{67}Ga (gallium) and ^{201}Th (thallium) although at the time or writing some isotopes (e.g. gallium) are difficult to obtain for manufacturing reasons. Radioisotopes may be administered to the patient as ions – e.g. pertechnetate (^{99m}Tc) scan for Meckel's diverticulum – but may also be incorporated onto more complex molecules (radiopharmaceuticals). These substances mimic a metabolic or biochemical pathway and localise in the target organs of interest, and their sites of distribution may be visualised using a special detector called a gamma camera. Although the radioisotopes produce radiation in all directions, spatial localisation is achieved by collimators permitting only radiation in one direction to interact with a large sodium iodide crystal (scintillation) detector in the camera. The radiation impact produces photons in the crystal, which are then amplified by photomultiplier tubes. Tomographic techniques can be used to improve spatial resolution, but in general such resolution is inferior to that of cross-sectional imaging techniques.

With *single-photon emission computed tomography* (SPECT), images are acquired in a similar manner to planar studies except that the camera head or heads rotate around the patient, collecting data over 180 or 360 degrees, and the data are analysed using similar computing techniques (back-projection) to those used in CT. SPECT studies take longer to acquire than conventional planar studies, but this disadvantage is often countered by administering a greater dose of the radiopharmaceutical. SPECT-CT is a further development of SPECT and an example of fusion imaging in which isotope activity can be directly localised to an area on the CT scan. It is proving useful in small joint disease and differentiation of benign from malignant vertebral collapse, the activity being confined to the vertebral endplates in the former.

Positron emission tomography (PET) is a newer and more expensive technique. Some radiographic substances emit positrons, which combine with an electron to convert their energy into two back-to-back photons. If these photons are detected in opposite detectors at the same time (coincidence), their position of origin in a line connecting the detectors can be assumed. Computer techniques are used to reconstruct a large number of these 'coincidences' into a cross-sectional image. Positron emitters are produced by cyclotrons and incorporated into biologically relevant and stable compounds, and physiological metabolism can be evaluated. PET is proving useful in imaging of physiological brain metabolism, tumour detection and functional cardiac imaging. More recently 'PET-CT' was introduced and this has largely replaced conventional PET scanning. In this technique a CT scan is produced at the same time as the PET image, and the site of PET activity is accurately anatomically localised. This has proven of particular benefit in oncological practice but recognising it has the potential for a high radiation dose study, particular attention to detail in technique is required. Currently most PET scanning is performed with ^{18}F-labelled 2-deoxy-2-fluoro-D-glucose, which is an analogue of glucose and is taken up by metabolically active tissue. In the future other substrates will be developed specific for different metabolic pathways.

Safety

The risks of radioisotope imaging are those of ionising radiation. The dose depends on the type of examination and the activity of isotope used, but in general many of the examinations have doses in the mid or high range compared with other radiological examinations. The incidence of allergic reactions to injected radioisotopes is exceedingly small.

Advantages and disadvantages

Although spatial resolution is relatively poor, radiopharmaceuticals can be tailored to be handled in different ways by various organs, and the amount of radioactivity passing through different systems can be quantified. Transport, distribution, metabolism and clearance can all be measured. The functional information supplied is often unique, and examples include:

- demonstrating osteoblastic activity for the detection of skeletal metastases and bone inflammation before radiographic changes
- distinguishing a dilated non-obstructed renal collecting system from an obstructed one
- localising foci of infection or segments of active inflammatory bowel disease with labelled leucocytes
- localising active gastrointestinal bleeding when angiography is negative
- detecting areas of reversible ischaemia or infarction in heart muscle
- identifying the first drainage node from tumours such as malignant melanoma or breast carcinoma in the sentinel node technique, which allows biopsy of that node to aid the decision as to whether surgical regional node clearance is necessary.

ENDOSCOPY

Endoscopy ranks as one of the most important technical advances in medicine of the last few decades. Not only has it added a new precision to gastrointestinal and pancreaticobiliary diagnosis, particularly when used in conjunction with cytology or biopsy but also it has been one of the earliest tools, along with interventional radiological techniques, in the advances of minimally invasive therapy.

Principles

There are two types of endoscope: rigid and flexible. Rigid instruments are usually more basic in design. Typical examples of rigid instruments are the proctoscope (for the anal canal; Ch. 26) and the sigmoidoscope (for the rectum up to the rectosigmoid junction; Ch. 26). Rigid bronchoscopes (Ch. 16) and oesophagoscopes (Chs 14 and 18) are now only infrequently used. The rigid cystoscope is still useful for diagnostic purposes, but most urological units rely on flexible cystoscopy for inspection of the bladder and reserve the rigid instrument for operative intervention (Ch. 33). Laparoscopy (inspection of the peritoneal cavity; Ch. 5) and arthroscopy (Ch. 33) are performed with a rigid instrument, partly because it is easier to work with a rigid instrument in a cavity which has been distended by gas (carbon dioxide) as is done in both instances.

The modern flexible endoscope is a complex but robust precision instrument varying in diameter from 7 mm (bronchoscope, arthroscope) to 15 mm (colonoscope). It has the following features:

- light source – in the handle with a fibreoptic bundle for the transmission of light to the area under investigation
- viewing system – originally a second bundle arranged coherently to transmit an image to a lens system; more recently, a silicon-based photosensor (charge-coupled device, CCD) made up of a grid of photosensitive elements. Photons impacting on this are converted into a digital video signal which can then be viewed on a screen; the endoscopist no longer needs to peer down an eyepiece. The video image can easily be stored for use in teaching and can be enhanced by electronic processing
- control and manipulative elements which are still mechanical and allow the tip to be deflected and instruments such as snares, stents, biopsy forceps, balloons and baskets to be passed along a working channel.

Flexible endoscopes are used in the following investigations:

- upper GI endoscopy (Ch. 18)
- retrograde biliary and pancreatic endoscopy (ERCP) (Chs 20 and 22)
- flexible sigmoidoscopy and colonoscopy (Ch. 25).
- nasal cavity and pharynx
- trachea and bronchi (bronchoscopy, Ch. 16).

Because endoscopy can be physically and emotionally unpleasant for the patient, many procedures are performed under sedation (which may vary from a small dose of a benzodiazepine to heavy sedation with a combination of a narcotic with a benzodiazepine) and, where necessary, local anaesthesia. Occasionally, full anaesthesia is used. The use of sedation means that patients need help to return home and need to take a day off work. Sedation itself does carry some risks; continuous monitoring of arterial oxygen saturation with pulse oximetry is now used routinely because, particularly in the elderly, there is a high incidence of hypoxia and cardiac dysrhythmias. Because of these concerns, there is increasing use of thinner and less traumatic endoscopes without sedation in upper GI endoscopy, and probably over half of simple diagnostic upper GI procedures are now performed this way.

Box 4.1 Potential complications of endoscopy

- Cardiac arrhythmias and respiratory arrest
- Cross-infection
- Bacteraemia
- Perforation of hollow viscus
- Aspiration of upper GI contents into the lung
- Bleeding from mucosal injury
- Rare events such as endoscopic impaction/knots, igniting intraluminal gas.

Complications

Diagnostic endoscopy is generally a safe procedure provided the endoscopist and his or her team are well trained. Potential complications are listed in Box 4.1.

Cross-infection

As with any procedure in which patients with potential pathogens are investigated, there is a risk of these being carried by instruments from one individual to another. Endoscopes are not the easiest of tools to clean, but there are satisfactory regimens and the hazard is currently low. Transmission of viral disease appears to be virtually non-existent.

Bacteraemia

Any instrumentation of a tract that normally contains organisms may cause transient bacteraemia, but the rate is low and the clinical manifestations are usually absent or minimal. The number of organisms in the blood is increased during procedures that require much tissue manipulation, such as dilatation of a stricture in a contaminated hollow tube. Particularly at risk and for whom antibiotic prophylaxis must be seriously considered are those with:

- prosthetic heart valves
- other prostheses, although the exact hazard is not fully established
- previous rheumatic fever with damage to heart valves
- immunosuppression.

There is a further theoretical risk of cross-infection because of a contaminated instrument, but careful cleaning eliminates this hazard.

Perforation of hollow viscera

This is most common following dilatation of strictures and during a difficult colonoscopy. The latter is particularly dangerous because symptoms of perforation are often delayed, so that a high morbidity and mortality may result.

Therapeutic endoscopy

There is now a wide range of therapeutic procedures that can be carried out under endoscopic (and sometimes additional fluoroscopic or ultrasound) control. These are considered throughout this text and include a variety of methods to control haemorrhage (Ch. 18), and dilatation (and stenting) of strictures in the GI tract and its tributaries (Chs 18, 20 and 22). Removal of foreign bodies is greatly facilitated (Chs 14 and 26), and percutaneous gastrostomy has made supplementary enteral feeding (Ch. 7) much more acceptable. Polypectomy for colonic lesions (Ch. 25) and injection therapy for oesophageal varices (Ch. 18) have changed management. The use of injection therapy and the heater probe applied endoscopically to bleeding peptic ulcers has reduced mortality.

In addition to these specialised endoscopic techniques, endoscopes (usually rigid) form the basis of minimal access surgery which is considered in Chapter 5.

Recent advances in gastrointestinal endoscopy

A number of developing techniques in endoscopy promise to improve its already excellent diagnostic performance: the wireless endoscopy or capsule, magnification endoscopy, chromoscopy, double-balloon enteroscopy and optical coherence tomography. In capsule endoscopy, a capsule the size of a pill is swallowed by the patient and transmits images to a receiver belt worn by the patient. The capsule can visualise the entire small bowel. The main disadvantages are the large amount of data produced and the inability to take specimens. There is a small risk of capsule impaction. The most established indication for capsule endoscopy is obscure GI bleeding. Magnification endoscopy has become possible following advances in CCD technology, and the use of this technique has helped in identification of abnormal mucosal patterns (for instance consistent with dysplasia) and is aided by chromoscopy, when various dyes are sprayed on the mucosa. Double-balloon enteroscopy is another technique for visualising the small bowel with an overtube placed and fixed in the small bowel by a balloon and the endoscope passed beyond this and then pulling back the small bowel in a concertina manner by a balloon attached to the tip. This procedure can visualise approximately 75 % of the proximal small bowel by an oral approach and the remainder by a retrograde approach from the colon. Optical coherence tomography is a new technique in which infrared light is passed down the endoscope onto tissue to provide an image akin to a histological sample. This may prove useful in identifying areas of dysplasia in high-risk patients or directing biopsies. Confocal microscopy is a newer technology which gives clearer and striking images even being able to 'see' *Helicobacter pylori* bacteria, but currently is expensive and impractical.

In endoscopic intervention a number of advances have also occurred. Upper GI endoscopic ultrasonography has been boosted by linear (or curved linear) probes with fine-needle aspiration capability. Nodal staging of tumours has been improved by this technique, and biopsy of retroperitoneal masses without transcoelomic seeding has been facilitated. Enteral stenting with self-expanding metal stents has proven useful in palliation of duodenal and colonic tumours. New endoscopic clips and loops have been developed to add to the armamentarium in dealing with gastrointestinal haemorrhage, and an endoscopic suture method has been developed to cure gastro-oesophageal reflux. Endoscopic mucosal resection (EMR) encompasses a number of techniques for removing superficial tumours from the gastrointestinal tract by either injecting the submusosa with saline to elevate the tumour or using a 'hood' into which the mucosa is sucked and then removed . Both techniques can be used together.

TISSUE SAMPLING

Cells for examination under the microscope may be obtained in four ways:

- body fluids, e.g. sputum (Ch. 16), urine (Ch. 33), effusions in the pleural and peritoneal spaces
- brushings or smears, e.g. cervical smear
- fine-needle aspiration (FNA)
- tissue biopsy, which can be either an open removal of a sample or of the whole identifiable lesion, or a core biopsy using a large-bore specially designed needle. This yields a core of tissue that can reveal not only the type of cells within a lesion but also their position in relation to other elements such as the basement membrane and vessels.

Brushing (or scraping) and fine-needle aspiration (FNA)

Brushing is suitable for the skin and endoscopically accessible parts of the GI tract. FNA is applicable to organs near the surface (such as the breast) but, under image control, can be applied to many deeper organs (see Box 4.2). Both techniques yield cells only from the organ being sampled and do not establish how these cells are related to tissue architecture.

Both may show cells that are obviously abnormal – with unusual nucleocytoplasmic ratios, increased mitotic activity and structural changes in the nuclei and nucleoli. Also, the presence of obviously malignant epithelial cells in an aspiration sample from a tissue which does not normally have epithelial elements (e.g. pleural cavity or lymph node) is as effective in confirming the presence of carcinoma as is a biopsy.

FNA has some disadvantages:

- Positive results are the only ones that can be evaluated with confidence; false negatives due to sampling errors are possible but can be reduced if the area of interest can be precisely targeted, e.g. under ultrasound control.
- In a solid organ, such as the breast, it is not possible to distinguish in-situ from invasive cancer.
- In the thyroid (Ch. 32) it is not possible to distinguish between follicular adenoma and carcinoma.

Biopsy

There are two forms:

- closed biopsy – this is an extension of FNA in which a wide-bore needle is used with the aim of removing a core of tissue which is suitable for histopathological examination (Fig. 4.21). Advances in imaging guidance

Box 4.2 Fine-needle aspiration

- A 22G needle is attached to a syringe inserted into the target issue (usually a lump), and aspiration is achieved by withdrawing the barrel of the syringe
- If the lesion is a cyst, liquid flows and the structure is emptied, if necessary by changing the syringe until no more can be aspirated
- If solid tissue is encountered, negative pressure allows a number of cells and tissue fluid to be aspirated into the needle, which can then be expelled onto microscopy slides and analysed cytologically

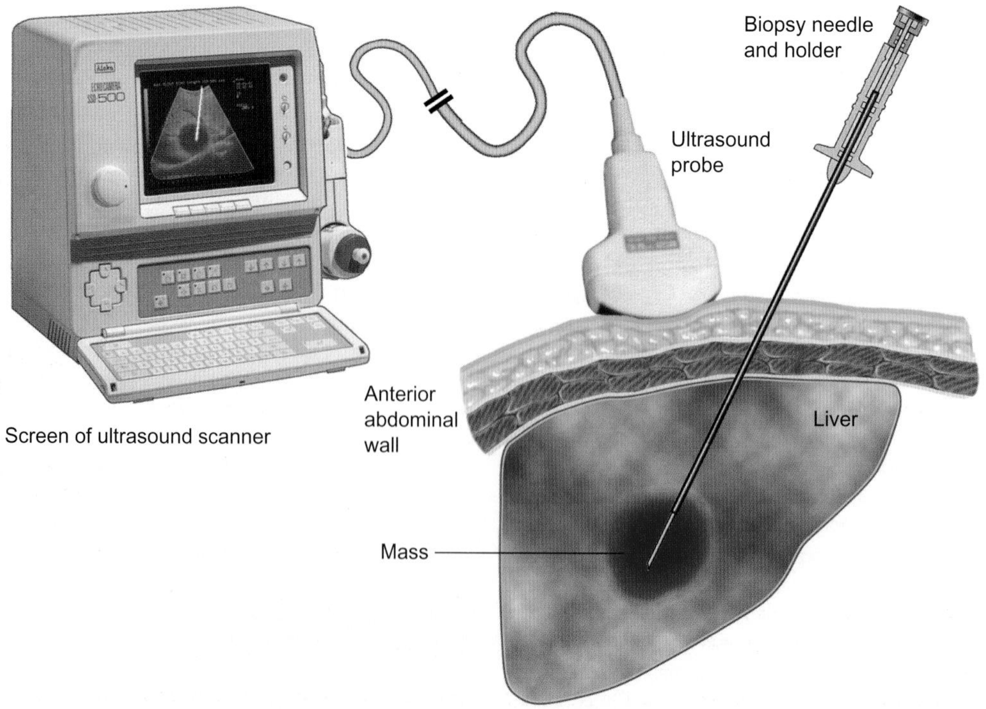

Fig. 4.21 Closed needle biopsy.

have made this technique more widely applicable to organs such as the prostate and the pancreas.

- open biopsy – a lesion is targeted and a formal incision is used to expose it and obtain a segment of tissue.

If the target of open biopsy is a lymph node, it is better to excise this intact rather than to cut into it, so as to avoid spillage of possible malignant cells which can cause a local recurrence. An intact node is also helpful to the pathologist because its architecture can be assessed (see Ch. 12).

In contrast to FNA, a biopsy may reveal that abnormal cells are transgressing natural boundaries such as the basement membrane of a mucosal surface or are invading blood vessels or lymphatics.

Biopsy may be contraindicated when it possibly transgresses the field of resection of a malignant growth.

Frozen section biopsy

Occasionally, histological diagnosis is required urgently while the patient is under an anaesthetic, because confirmation of malignancy may change the type of operation that the patient should undergo. In such circumstances, the usual tissue fixation techniques are too slow. Instead the biopsy is frozen in liquid nitrogen, which makes slicing and staining for microscopy possible within minutes.

Decisions based on frozen sections should be made only in broad categories such as malignant or benign; pathologists should not be asked to make fine distinctions on frozen sections.

FUNCTION TESTS

Measurement of the functional capacity of organ systems, with or without visualisation of anatomical structure, can provide a more accurate assessment of the risks of an operation. Assessment of cardiovascular, respiratory, renal and, in some circumstances, liver function are evaluations that can be useful.

Cardiovascular risk

Electrocardiogram and stress electrocardiogram

An electrocardiogram (ECG) should be obtained routinely for all elective surgery in those over 40 years of age. Younger patients require ECG if they are symptomatic or in a high-risk group for coronary artery disease. However, the sensitivity of an ECG in demonstrating asymptomatic coronary artery disease is not high. Major vascular operations (e.g. aortic aneurysm repair) often impose a specific physiological strain on the cardiovascular system; in consequence, the presence of asymptomatic coronary disease may be of significance. If present, correction prior to the vascular procedure should be undertaken.

In a stress ECG, clinical evaluation and serial readings are made while the patient walks on a treadmill at increasing speeds, and it may reveal subclinical myocardial ischaemia. This is indicated when the test induces chest pain (angina) or produces a fall in blood pressure (not usually seen on exercise), ischaemic changes in the ST segment of the ECG and/or ventricular ectopic beats.

Similar stress can be induced by administration of inotropic agents such as dobutamine.

Thallium-201 (or ^{99m}Tc-sestamibi) perfusion scintigraphy

This is a relatively non-invasive procedure which identifies areas of myocardial hypoperfusion, which may include infarcts. Other areas, apparently normal at rest, may not show increased uptake on exercise because they are supplied by narrowed coronary arteries that are unable to allow the increased flow that is physiologically demanded by exercise. Such abnormalities should be investigated by more detailed studies of left ventricular function (see labelled red cell ventriculography, below) and by coronary angiography; when a major procedure is under consideration, a preliminary angioplasty or coronary bypass operation may be necessary.

Technetium-labelled red cell ventriculography (MUGA)

If there are significant areas of abnormal isotope uptake on a perfusion scan, then ^{99m}Tc-labelled red cell ventriculography is indicated and provides information about left ventricular function, including ejection fraction and the presence of aortic regurgitation during diastole.

Echocardiography

This non-invasive investigation can also provide some assessment of the function of the left ventricle but it is not as accurate as radionuclide ventriculography.

Regional blood flow

See Chapter 29.

Lung function

Upper abdominal and thoracic operations produce the greatest impairment of respiratory function, but all procedures associated with general anaesthesia and pain cause some abnormality of respiratory function (Ch. 6). The risk of postoperative respiratory complications increases in:

- smokers
- obesity
- the elderly
- those with pre-existing respiratory disease – chronic bronchitis and emphysema, asthma and mucoviscoidosis.

In some circumstances, pre-existing respiratory dysfunction may require special measures or even contraindicate operation.

Function is assessed by the measurement of:

- arterial blood gas concentrations
- peak expiratory flow rate
- occasionally, the lung volumes.

Criteria for prediction of postoperative risk of respiratory complications include:

- forced vital capacity (FVC) less than 70% of that predicted
- forced expiratory volume in the first second (FEV_1) less than 70% of that predicted
- FEV_1/FVC less than 65% of that predicted
- arterial blood CO_2 tension (P_aCO_2) greater than 45 mmHg
- in upper abdominal procedures, a vital capacity of less than 1 l.

Cardiopulmonary exercise testing (CPX) is increasingly used to determine operative risk in patients undergoing high-risk procedures such as oesophagogastrectomy. Cardiopulmonary exercise testing is an objective method of evaluating both cardiac and pulmonary function. Cardiac function is evaluated in terms of aerobic capacity and respiratory function is evaluated by dynamic flow volume loops and VQ measurements actually performed during exercise. The patient is exercised preferably on a bicycle ergometer or failing that a treadmill. During exercise he breathes through a mouthpiece which is in fact a minaturised pressure differential pneumotachygraph. The inspired and expired gas is continuously sampled and both oxygen uptake and carbon dioxide elimination is computed. Not only is maximal aerobic capacity calculated but also the point during exercise where anaerobic metabolism is used to supplement aerobic metabolism as a source of energy. That point is very accurately measured via gas exchange data and is termed the anerobic threshold or AT. Cardiac failure may be very accurately assessed in quantified fashion by use of the AT. Anaerobic threshold (the point at which lactic acid levels rise in the bloodstream) appears to be a good guide to operative risk.

Gastric and intestinal function

See Chapters 18, 24 and 25.

Pancreatic function

See Chapter 22.

Endocrine function

See Chapter 32.

SCREENING FOR SURGICAL DISEASE

See Chapters 12, 18, 25 and 28.

Other surgical disorders such as abdominal aortic aneurysms by ultrasound

The general principles of screening outlined in Chapter 12 for malignant disease are applicable to all screening programmes.

FURTHER READING

Adam A, Dixon AK, Grainger RG, Allison DJ 2007 Grainger & Allison's diagnostic radiology: 2 volume set, 5th edn. Churchill Livingstone, Edinburgh

Banerjee AK 2006 Radiology made easy, 2nd edn. Cambridge University Press, Cambridge

Begg JD 2006 Abdominal X-rays made easy, 2nd edn. Churchill Livingstone, Edinburgh

Carne J, Carroll M, Delaney D, Brown I 2002 Chest X-ray made easy, 2nd edn. Churchill Livingstone, Edinburgh

Daffner RH 2007 Clinical radiology: the essentials, 3rd edn. Lippincott Williams & Wilkins, Philadelphia

Plaut S 1993 Radiation Protection in the X-ray Department, 1st edn. Butterworth-Heinemann, London

Raby N, Berman L, Delacey G 2005 Accident and emergency radiology: a survival guide, 2nd edn. WB Saunders, Edinburgh

5 The operation

For those entering the operating department for the first time, it can be a daunting experience (Ch. 2). It is an unfamiliar environment; there are specific regimented procedures that must be followed, a multitude of new terms, and unfamiliar techniques and equipment that have to be understood. In this chapter some of these matters will be demystified through discussion of the following: the working of the operating department, including its design and the way patients pass through it; the techniques used in operations in general; and technological innovations such as minimally invasive and robotically assisted surgery.

A list of commonly used suffixes in surgery is provided in Box 5.1.

DESIGN OF THE OPERATING DEPARTMENT

Principles

Although the physical features of operating departments often differ, they are all designed around some widely accepted principles, which are the outcome of the experience of surgeons, the impact of the biomedical sciences and accordance with clinical safety principles.

The individual principles upon which the design of each operating department is based are as follows:

- Scope of service – this depends on which surgical services are to be catered for
- Workload – this is largely the outcome of the scope of service, an estimate of which determines the number of operating rooms (known in the UK as theatres)
- Needs of special services – for example, the implantation of orthopaedic devices requires systems for ultraclean and smooth air flow, and the cardiac surgical team may need a perfusion room in which cardiopulmonary bypass equipment can be prepared
- Accessibility – there needs to be a speedy access to and from the intensive therapy unit, the accident and emergency department, the imaging department, local X-ray and the places where patients are accommodated both before and after an operation
- Safety – there must be protocols put in place to ensure safety for the patients and staff.

Supplies

Repeatedly used and disposable equipment (instruments, drapes and other special items) come either from an adjacent dedicated theatre sterile supply unit (TSSU) or the central sterile supply department (CSSD) which supplies the whole hospital; increasingly, these may be centralised for many hospitals.

Patient flow

In well-designed departments, patients enter at a central reception area. There they are handed over by the team responsible for preoperative care (Ch. 6) to the theatre staff (Box 5.2), and the following are checked ('sign in'):

- completed and correct identity bracelet and allergies
- consent form (Ch. 2) completed and the procedure the patient is having carried out and the site and side of surgery as applicable
- time of last food and drink
- impediments to safety, such as false teeth, make up, nail polish and jewellery, all removed.

From this point the patient may be transferred to a theatre trolley and then taken to the anaesthetic room. Before or after anaesthesia has been induced (Ch. 6), transfer is made to the operating table. Once the patient has been prepared for operation, he or she is transferred to the operating theatre (Fig. 5.1).

New guidelines have been introduced in the UK, for all clinical staff to undertake a 'time-out' (or 'surgical pause')

Box 5.1 Commonly used suffixes in surgery

-ectomy	Removal of a segment or all of an organ, e.g. appendicectomy; thyroidectomy
-otomy	Surgical incision into an organ or cavity, e.g. laparotomy (an incision into the abdominal cavity), enterotomy (an incision into the small intestine) Occasionally, cutting of a structure, e.g. vagotomy (division of the vagus nerve)
-ostomy	Surgically created connection between two organs, e.g. gastroenterostomy (a connection between the stomach and small bowel) Connection between an organ and the skin, e.g. colostomy (an opening between the colon and skin)
-oscopy	Visualisation of the inside of a duct, cavity or organ by means of an endoscope, e.g. gastroscopy, cystoscopy
-orrhaphy	A repair operation, e.g. herniorrhaphy (repair of a hernial defect)
-pexy	An operation to secure an organ or structure, e.g. rectopexy (reconstruction and fixation of the rectum to treat rectal prolapse)
-desis	An operation to fuse two structures together, e.g. arthrodesis (the fusion of a joint)
-plasty	An operation to alter structure or function, e.g. arthroplasty (remodelling a joint), pyloroplasty (dividing the pyloric sphincter), rhinoplasty (remodelling the nose)

Box 5.2 Theatre personnel

Theatre manager – usually a senior nurse in overall charge of normal day-to-day running of the department
ODP (operating department practitioner) – trained in all aspects of operating theatre technique, they typically assist the anaesthetist, especially during induction of anaesthesia and positioning of the patient
Scrub nurse – a nurse trained in theatre techniques who prepares the instruments and assists the surgeon during the operation
Runner – a nurse or healthcare assistant who prepares the theatre for each operation and fetches equipment required during the procedure
Porters – they transport patients to and from theatre and often assist in their transfer and positioning in the operating theatre

and go through a final checklist prior to the operation being carried out. This includes all staff introducing themselves, checking patient details, the site and side of surgery, mentioning any particular anticipated problems and whether antibiotics and thromboprophylaxis have been given (Fig 5.2).

Once the procedure is complete a further final check ('sign out') is made prior to exit to the recovery area, usually through a different path from that of entry. This one-way flow of traffic through the operating room prevents congestion, allows a continuous flow of patients and allows a second anaesthetist to deal with the next patient while the previous patient is leaving theatre. From the recovery room, the patient is transferred back to wherever it is thought appropriate:

- in-patient accommodation after major operations, which may be either to a routine bed or to an intensive or high-dependency care unit
- a holding area before returning home after day-case operations.

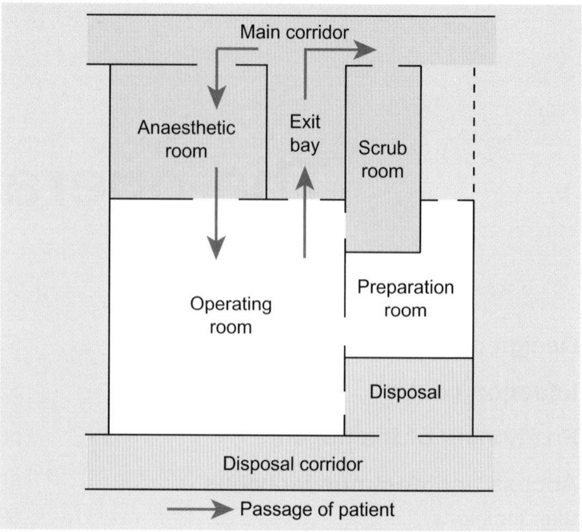

Fig. 5.1 Plan of an individual operating theatre with clean (blue), sterile (white) and disposal (pink) zones.

Operating department layout

An important aspect of theatre design is to keep bacterial contamination to a minimum – the concept of asepsis. Operating areas (Fig. 5.1) can therefore be divided into zones, as follows:

- transfer zone – includes the reception area where the patient arrives, the recovery and staff changing areas and the points of entry to the department from the rest of the hospital
- clean zone – a transition area between the transfer and sterile zones; it must also incorporate storage areas for theatre and pre-sterilised equipment
- sterile zone – the operating room and sterile preparation room where the equipment for individual operations is assembled
- disposal zone – the least clean area where the detritus, such as swabs and dirty instruments, is dealt with.

Although there is no strong bacteriological evidence that adhering to zones, or isolating each zone, reduces infection rates, it is a concept that should nevertheless be observed.

Structure

The operating complex is designed so that a high standard of cleanliness can be maintained. Junctures between walls, ceilings and floors are curved to prevent the collection of dust. All equipment should be movable so that the theatre can be cleared for cleaning and all surfaces should be smooth and easily washable.

Ventilation

The ventilation system of the operating department permits:

- control of temperature and humidity – typical figures are 20–22°C and 60% relative humidity; lower temperatures

Surgical Safety Checklist

World Health Organization | Patient Safety
A World Alliance for Safer Health Care

Before induction of anaesthesia → **Before skin incision** → **Before patient leaves operating room**

Before induction of anaesthesia

(with at least nurse and anaesthetist)

Has the patient confirmed his/her identity, site, procedure, and consent?
- ☐ Yes

Is the site marked?
- ☐ Yes
- ☐ Not applicable

Is the anaesthesia machine and medication check complete?
- ☐ Yes

Is the pulse oximeter on the patient and functioning?
- ☐ Yes

Does the patient have a:

Known allergy?
- ☐ No
- ☐ Yes

Difficult airway or aspiration risk?
- ☐ No
- ☐ Yes, and equipment/assistance available

Risk of >500ml blood loss (7ml/kg in children)?
- ☐ No
- ☐ Yes, and two IVs/central access and fluids planned

Before skin incision

(with nurse, anaesthetist and surgeon)

- ☐ **Confirm all team members have introduced themselves by name and role.**
- ☐ **Confirm the patient's name, procedure, and where the incision will be made.**

Has antibiotic prophylaxis been given within the last 60 minutes?
- ☐ Yes
- ☐ Not applicable

Anticipated Critical Events

To Surgeon:
- ☐ What are the critical or non-routine steps?
- ☐ How long will the case take?
- ☐ What is the anticipated blood loss?

To Anaesthetist:
- ☐ Are there any patient-specific concerns?

To Nursing Team:
- ☐ Has sterility (including indicator results) been confirmed?
- ☐ Are there equipment issues or any concerns?

Is essential imaging displayed?
- ☐ Yes
- ☐ Not applicable

Before patient leaves operating room

(with nurse, anaesthetist and surgeon)

Nurse Verbally Confirms:
- ☐ The name of the procedure
- ☐ Completion of instrument, sponge and needle counts
- ☐ Specimen labelling (read specimen labels aloud, including patient name)
- ☐ Whether there are any equipment problems to be addressed

To Surgeon, Anaesthetist and Nurse:
- ☐ What are the key concerns for recovery and management of this patient?

This checklist is not intended to be comprehensive. Additions and modifications to fit local practice are encouraged. Revised 1 / 2009 © WHO, 2009

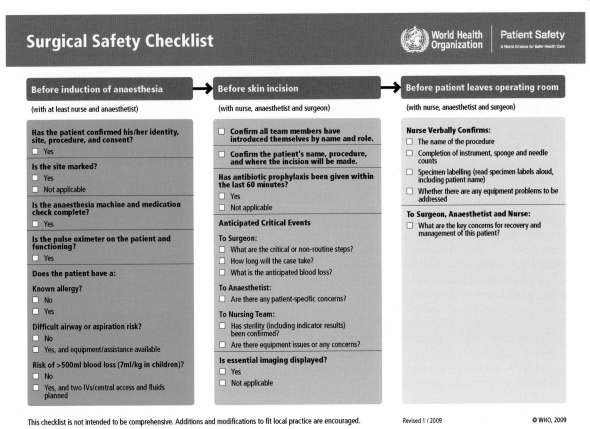

Fig. 5.2 The WHO Surgical Safety checklist (2009). Reproduced with the permission of the World Health Organization (www.who.int).

carry the risk of hypothermia for an anaesthetised patient in whom vasoconstriction is abolished, and higher ones make the work of the operating team uncomfortable (see also the special needs of neonates – Ch. 36)

- air filtration to remove microorganisms
- movement of air from clean to less clean areas within the department by creating overpressure in the most clean zones
- rapid and non-turbulent air change in the operating room; this dilutes the concentration of microorganisms inevitably released from patients and staff. In circumstances where infection of a wound is disastrous, e.g. orthopaedic prosthesis insertion (Ch. 9), special systems are used which direct a stream of clean air over the operating zone (laminar flow enclosures).

INFECTION CONTROL

Antisepsis places a barrier which destroys organisms between the wound and the external environment. In surgical operative practice the objective of asepsis is to have as few organisms as possible in the immediate vicinity of the operating field. This is achieved partly by ventilation control (as described above) but principally by ensuring that everything that comes into contact with the field is first rendered sterile by the complete destruction of all microorganisms, including bacterial spores. A number of methods of infection control are available (Box 5.3). There are three major factors of importance in the operating field:

- sterilisation of instruments and equipment
- skin preparation and draping of the patient
- preparation and clothing of the operating team.

Box 5.3 Infection control

Sterilisation – a process that involves the complete destruction of all microorganisms, including bacterial spores

Disinfection – reduces the number of viable microorganisms but does not necessarily inactivate viruses and bacterial spores

Cleaning – a process that physically removes contamination but does not necessarily destroy microorganisms.

Sterilisation

There are two types of sterilisation: heat and cold (Box 5.4). The process applies to instruments and equipment for use in a procedure where the skin is breached but not necessarily to gastrointestinal endoscopy (Ch. 18). Skin cannot be sterilised (see below).

Box 5.4 Methods of sterilisation

Heat sterilisation
- Autoclaving (steam under pressure)
- Dry heat
- Low-temperature steam/formaldehyde

Cold sterilisation
- Irradiation
- Ethylene oxide
- Glutaraldehyde

Heat sterilisation

Steam under pressure

Sterilisation is dependent on the temperature attained and the length of time for which this is maintained; the higher the temperature, the greater the lethal effect on microorganisms. An increase in ambient pressure raises the boiling point of water, so higher steam temperatures can be achieved at higher pressure. This process is carried out in an autoclave. The instruments or drapes to be sterilised are usually pre-packed in a container which is permeable to the steam but which will not subsequently let in organisms. Air is sucked out to create a vacuum and the instruments are then exposed to moist heat under pressure. Typical cycles are:

- 134°C and 30 lb/in^2 (20×10^3 N/m^2) for 3 min
- 121°C and 15 lb/in^2 (10×10^3 N/m^2) for 15 min.

Autoclaves are usually located in the CSSD, to supply the needs of the whole hospital, or in the TSSU, usually situated next to the operating department.

Dry heat

In this type of sterilisation a higher temperature for a longer period is required, e.g. 160°C for 2 hours. It is suitable for sterilising airtight containers and fine instruments that are susceptible to corrosion.

Low-temperature steam/formaldehyde

A combination of dry saturated steam and formaldehyde sterilises at a lower temperature (73°C) and is therefore suitable for heat-sensitive materials and equipment. It is important to remove all traces of formaldehyde at the end of the process.

Cold sterilisation

Irradiation

Gamma rays at high intensity are lethal to cells, including those of microorganisms. The method is not feasible in a hospital setting but is used by industry for the sterilisation of mass-produced disposable items such as syringes, catheters and sutures.

Ethylene oxide

This is a highly penetrative gas that, under controlled conditions, has good sterilising properties, killing most bacteria, spores and viruses. It is ideal for heat-sensitive, delicate items such as electrical equipment or endoscopes but is largely an industrial process for sterilising single-use plastic items.

Glutaraldehyde

Alkaline glutaraldehyde (Cidex) is a liquid chemical disinfectant used to clean lensed instruments such as flexible endoscopes or cystoscopes, which have many heat-sensitive components. It is, however, a highly toxic, irritant and allergenic substance, and its use should be carefully controlled by trained staff. Automated contained systems are now used to clean and sterilise flexible endoscopes.

Preparation of the patient's skin

Up to half of all wound infections are caused by bacteria resident on the skin. Their quantity can be reduced by having the patient shower on the morning of the operation with an antiseptic substance such as chlorhexidine. At the start of the operation a wide area of skin around the incision site is cleaned with a povidone-iodine or chlorhexidine solution. Either of these combined with ethyl alcohol gives better disinfection but organisms still persist in hair follicles and sweat glands. Pools of residual alcohol must be avoided because they can be ignited by a spark from an electrocoagulation instrument and cause a burn.

Shaving

Hairs get in the way during closure of the skin wound. Patients have traditionally been shaved for operations, but when a razor is used it can cause minor nicks and scratches, and increases the incidence of wound infections compared with the use of depilatory creams or clippers. If hair needs to be removed, then clippers or depilatory cream should be used.

Isolation of the operation field

The area to be operated on is isolated using heat-sterilised surgical drapes. These were traditionally cotton sheets, although cotton can quickly become wet and lose its protective ability. Newer impermeable materials and disposable drapes have been introduced, but they are more expensive. Self-adhesive plastic drapes are often used for irregular or extensive operation sites, but there is no evidence that they reduce wound contamination or infection rates. Newer drapes are also available that are made specifically for laparoscopic operating fields. These usually have the fields already cut out of the centre of the main drape. Drapes also serve to identify the aseptic operating zone in which the surgeon, assistants and scrub nurse work; any equipment, instruments or staff that come into contact with the drapes must also be sterile.

Preparation of the operating team

Scrubbing up

Scrubbing up is the term given to the hand and arm cleaning process undertaken at the start of an operation. It was formerly a ritualised process of alternate scrubbing and rinsing of the fingers, hands and arms with a brush for a defined period of time. This is now known not to be necessary and that brisk scrubbing of the skin with a brush can cause microtrauma to the epidermis and increase the bacterial count at the skin surface. An initial scrub of the fingernails at the start of an operating list is all that is required and should take about 3–5 minutes.

All jewellery should be removed. The fingers, hands and forearms are cleaned thoroughly using a medicated detergent such as chlorhexidine gluconate (Hibiscrub) or povidone-iodine (Betadine). Chlorhexidine is rapidly effective and has a prolonged action but is ineffective against bacterial spores. Povidone-iodine kills all organisms including spores but does not have a prolonged effect and has a higher incidence of allergic reactions. After washing, the hands are dried thoroughly with a sterile towel; this further decreases the bacterial count and makes donning of gowns and gloves much easier.

Gowns and gloves

Both of these are donned with a closed technique (i.e. the skin does not touch anything on the outside surface) so that the chance of contamination of a surface which is in contact with the patient's tissues is reduced.

Conventional sterile cotton gowns can soon become wet and pervious to bacteria. They also allow contamination of the surgical team by the patient's body fluids. One partial solution is to wear a disposable plastic apron beneath the gown. Newer materials such as Goretex™ or close-woven polyester have been developed to overcome the problem of permeability but have two drawbacks: they are expensive and their impermeability may cause discomfort. However, some form of impervious gown is essential when operating on high-risk patients (hepatitis B and C, HIV – see also below) to prevent transmission of the infective agent in the patient's body fluids to the surgical team.

Gloves were formerly lightly coated or the hands dusted with talc so as to make them easy to put on. However, talc is irritant, and a particularly difficult form of adhesive small bowel obstruction (Ch. 24) may follow contamination of the peritoneal cavity. Starch was then substituted, but it is now clear that there are individuals who are starch-sensitive who also form abdominal adhesions. Most surgeons therefore now use starch-free gloves. Double gloving is also often carried out by many surgeons, especially for the more high-risk cases. Eye glasses or shielded masks are also advisable.

Infected and other high-risk patients

Patients themselves can be a source of infection and pose particular problems when their tissues are exposed. The simplest instances are when infected patients, e.g. those having drainage of an abscess or those with infected open wounds, contaminate the operating room, which can lead to contamination of subsequent patients. It was previously common practice to put at the end of elective operating lists those regarded as being able to disseminate infection. However, if the theatre is adequately cleaned between each procedure, then this practice is not essential.

Specialties, such as orthopaedics or transplant surgery, which require ultraclean conditions should have dedicated theatres that are not used by others.

Dressings or bandages from infected patients and disposable equipment used in their operation should be carefully disposed of in plastic sacks. These should only be filled to three-quarters of their capacity (in case overfilling results in rupture) before being sealed and disposed of by incineration.

The usual measures to prevent cross-infection within the operating suite include:

- use of impervious gowns and drapes so that the operating table or surgical team do not come into contact with the patient's blood or body fluids
- a plastic apron under the operating gown if heavy contamination is anticipated
- latex operating gloves, although these provide little or no protection from injuries by sharp instruments such as knives or needles
- operating room discipline, e.g. passing needles or scalpels between the scrub nurse and surgeon in a transit dish to prevent injury from hand-to-hand passage
- careful disposal of all contaminated material at the end of the procedure into plastic sealable bags for incineration.

The term 'high risk' has now become applicable to patients positive for:

- HIV
- hepatitis B, or
- hepatitis C.

These agents are of most concern to the surgical team because of the risk of transmission through the patient's blood entering the body of a member of the team during an operation as a result of a surface injury such as a needle stick or a minor nick with a knife. The same applies to a lesser extent to other body fluids. Other transmissible agents may appear in the future.

At present, routine testing of patients for HIV or hepatitis B antibodies is not performed in the UK. The ethical and moral issues which relate to testing preoperative patients continue, but currently the only way to identify high-risk patients is by the patient's own admission of infection, a history of high-risk behaviour or the detection of significant physical signs, such as multiple injection marks from intravenous drug abuse.

The safest policy to adopt would be to consider all patients to be high risk, but this adds to costs and may slow down the work of the operating team. However, the majority of surgeons do take extra precautions when they are known or thought likely to be needed and modify their techniques to decrease the likelihood of injury by knives and needles.

Extra precautions when operating on high-risk patients include:

- *Double gloving.* Wearing two pairs of gloves reduces the likelihood of glove perforation; it is usual to wear the inner glove a half-size larger than the individual's normal size.
- *Eye protection*. Goggles or visors are essential to prevent splash contamination of the conjunctiva. They are most important when power tools are being used, because these can create a fine aerosol mixture of body fluids with a theoretical risk of viral transmission.

- *Surgeon.* The most experienced surgeon available should do the operation.
- *Staples.* Stapling devices (Ch. 8) should be employed for anastomoses and skin closure to reduce the risk of needle injuries.
- *Needles.* Hand-held needles should be avoided because the incidence of glove perforation is so high as to be unacceptable. Needles have been designed with blunted ends that will penetrate fascia but should not pierce gloves and are particularly useful during mass closure (Ch. 8) of laparotomy wounds, when the incidence of needle injury and glove perforation is greatest.

Prevention of cross-infection and the infection of healthcare workers by viral diseases depends on the efficacy of the barrier between patients and the surgical team; this consists of both the mechanical barrier (as outlined above, by the use of impervious materials) and that resulting from good surgical practice. At present there is no satisfactory prophylaxis against hepatitis C. Anti-retroviral drugs are usually prescribed after exposure to HIV. Hepatitis B can be protected against by immunisation, and this should be mandatory for all healthcare workers.

POSITIONING OF THE PATIENT

Once anaesthetised, patients lose the protective reflexes generally taken for granted in daily life. It is the responsibility of the operating room staff and, in particular, the surgeon and anaesthetist to make sure that no harm comes to the patient as a result. The surgeon is also responsible for positioning the patient so that good exposure may be achieved during the operation.

The operating table

In most rooms this is free-standing and may be moved out during cleaning. Some rooms have a fixed base built into the floor with removable top sections which can be changed according to the operation being done. The table must be heavy and stable enough to support the patient but also highly adjustable. The top of the table is divided into sections, each of which can be adjusted independently. The central section should be radiolucent, which is especially important in urological and general surgery when perioperative abdominal X-rays or the image intensifier are used. Operating tables have a soft sorbo-rubber padding on top so that pressure is widely distributed to avoid pressure points which could lead to skin breakdown. The common positions are listed in Table 5.1.

Precautions

Rigorous care must be taken to avoid:

- unintentional contact of the patient with metal – if monopolar diathermy (Ch. 8) is being used and the patient is in contact with metal, such as a part of the operating table or a support, the current will pass to earth through the exposed skin and metal, and a burn (usually full-thickness) at the point of contact will result
- possible points of pressure – padding should be placed around areas at risk of pressure such as the elbows or heels; in the supine position a rubber pad is placed under the ankle joints to relieve pressure on the skin of the heels and to avoid compression of the deep veins of the calf muscles.

Avoiding nerve and joint injuries are two other matters which depend on careful positioning.

Nerve injuries occur as a result of traction or pressure. It must be remembered that muscle paralysis may impose

Table 5.1 Common positions for operations

Position	Use
Supine	Suitable for many operations
Trendelenburg Supine, but the patient is tilted 30–40° head-down	Operations on pelvic organs; small intestine moves out of the way with gravity
Reverse Trendelenburg As Trendelenburg but the tilt is head-up	Operations on upper abdominal organs
Lithotomy Supine with hips and knees fully flexed and the feet in stirrups or straps	Access to the anal and perianal regions and the external genitalia, vagina and uterine cervix, urethra and bladder (endoscopic)
Lateral Position of extension on the right or left side with the uppermost arm raised above and in front of the head. The centre of the table may be angled (broken) to improve access	Operations on the kidney and in the chest
Lloyd-Davies As Trendelenburg but with the legs abducted and the hips and knees slightly flexed and the legs in rests	Combined procedures which involve the abdomen and perineum (usually on the distal large bowel)
Bowie or prone jack-knife Prone with flexion at the hips	Access to the perianal area

forces different from those in the unanaesthetised state. The nerves particularly at risk include:

- brachial plexus – abduction of the arm to greater than 90° can stretch the plexus
- ulnar nerve – from compression by a table support or other hard surface as the nerve passes behind the medial epicondyle at the elbow
- radial nerve – risk of compression where it winds around the shaft of the humerus
- common peroneal nerve – may be damaged by lithotomy supports where the nerve winds around the neck of the fibula.

Joint injuries are avoided by maintaining natural joint positions and not forcing the limbs to conform to what seems best for the surgical team; for example, hip joints can be damaged when putting a patient in the lithotomy position unless care is taken to lift both legs smoothly and together. Particular care should be taken in transferring patients with known back or joint problems or those at particular risk, such as patients with rheumatoid arthritis or those who have had a joint replaced. Long procedures where blood flow may be compromised to extremeties, such as when the patient is positioned with their legs up (or in the Lloyd-Davies position), have the potential for leading to compartment syndrome and so if there is an opportunity to put the legs down at an appropriate juncture in the procedure then this should be taken.

Temperature control

The unconscious patient has lost the ability to regulate body temperature because of vasomotor paralysis and also possibly inhibition of central mechanisms. Hypothermia will follow if the ambient temperature falls below 21°C for more than an hour or two. Measures to prevent this include:

- minimising the time the patient is left uncovered
- limiting the exposure of large areas of tissue to the atmosphere, particularly the contents of the abdomen or chest
- placing a heating mattress between the patient and the operating table, consisting of multiple long tubes which are electrically heated or filled with circulating warm water
- placing space blankets or warm-air-heated blankets over the patient and beneath the drapes, leaving only the area being operated on exposed
- humidification of inspired anaesthetic gases
- use of warming devices for the administration of blood or other fluids.

ACCESS AND COMMON INCISIONS

In order to do an operation well, the correct incision must be made. The most important aspect is that it allows adequate access to the operating field. Other important considerations are:

- sound healing
- minimum pain during the course of healing
- minimum complications
- satisfactory cosmetic result.

The ability to extend an incision to allow greater access is also necessary when unexpected problems or findings are encountered. In the abdomen, the classic example is when the appendix is exposed for appendicitis but a carcinoma of the caecum is found and a right hemicolectomy is needed. Some operations are approached through a standard incision (thyroidectomy, Ch. 32) while others may be done through a variety of approaches (see 'Abdominal incisions' below). For example, an open cholecystectomy (Ch. 20) may be performed via a right upper paramedian or midline incision, a transverse upper right incision or an oblique subcostal incision, depending on the patient's build and to a certain extent on the surgeon's preference.

SKIN INCISIONS

Although exposure is the most important principle in surgical access, cosmesis is also desirable because the skin incision is the patient's only visible reminder of the operation. The cleavage lines or lines of Langer show the 'grain' of the skin and represent the parallel sheets of collagen and elastic tissue fibres in the dermis. They run transversely or obliquely on the trunk and neck and circumferentially on the limbs (Fig. 5.3). Incisions made along the lines will heal with fine scars and minimal contraction, whereas those made across them retract maximally to leave ugly scars.

Joint crease lines are areas where the skin is more firmly attached to the underlying fascia and are more marked on the flexor aspects of the joint. As with skin cleavage lines, they should not be crossed perpendicularly because tethering of the skin may result in impaired joint function.

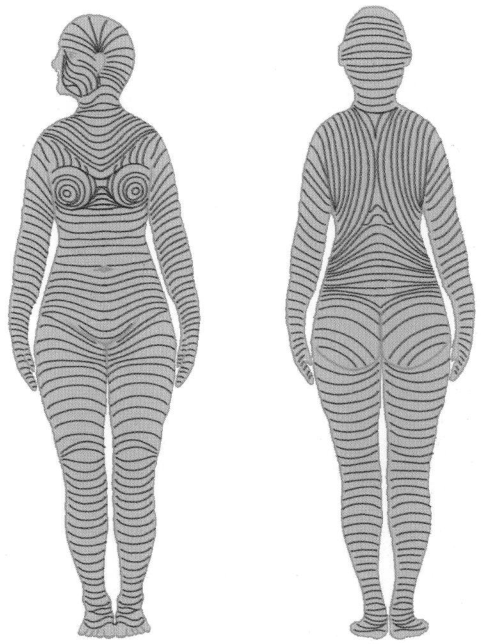

Fig. 5.3 Skin cleavage lines (Langer's).

ABDOMINAL INCISIONS

The trend to minimal access surgery (see below) means that many abdominal and thoracic operations are now performed through small incisions used for the placement of trocars. Through these trocars a video telescope and specially designed instruments are inserted. Trocars typically vary from 5 mm to 15 mm in diameter and are positioned for optimal access to the operative field. Skin crease incisions are usually used (Fig. 5.3).

When an open operation is necessary the abdominal incision chosen depends on the diagnosis or the organ involved and may be vertical, horizontal or oblique (Fig. 5.4).

Vertical incisions

Upper midline

This incision allows access to the stomach, duodenum, liver, gallbladder, pancreas and spleen. It divides the skin, subcutaneous fat, linea alba, preperitoneal fat and peritoneum; it is relatively bloodless and is also quick to make and close.

Lower midline

This allows access to the pelvic organs. As with the upper midline incision, it can be extended for greater exposure.

Full midline

This incision is used when greater exposure of the abdominal contents is required; e.g. for an abdominal aortic aneurysm.

Paramedian incision

A paramedian incision is made 2 cm either side of the midline depending on which organ or portion of the bowel is to be operated on. The skin and anterior rectus sheath are incised; the rectus muscle is retracted laterally and the posterior rectus sheath and peritoneum are then divided in the same line as the skin. It takes longer to open and close than a midline incision but is said to have a lower incidence of wound problems as the rectus abdominis muscle acts like a shutter to prevent hernia formation.

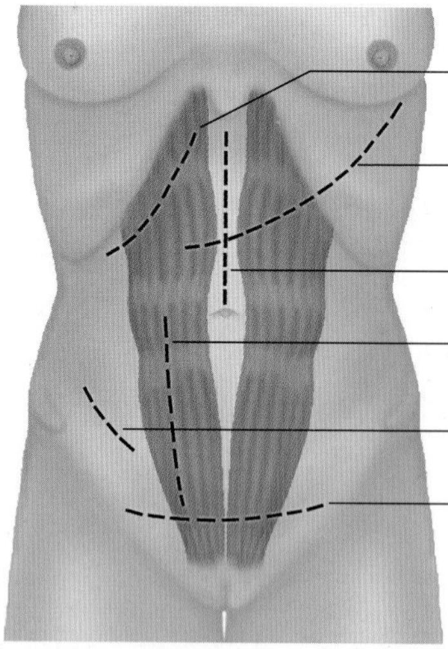

Fig. 5.4 Types of abdominal incision.

Horizontal incisions

Transverse abdominal incision

This type of incision heals well, with fine scars and less pain. It allows good access to the abdominal contents. It is either muscle-splitting or muscle-cutting, the former taking longer to open and close. Transverse abdominal incisions are often used in neonates or infants.

Pfannenstiel incision

This is a transverse incision 1 cm above the pubic symphysis. It is widely used by gynaecologists because it gives good access to the pelvic organs.

Oblique incisions

Right subcostal (Kocher's)

This type of incision begins below the xiphisternum and runs laterally 2 cm below and parallel to the costal margin, dividing all layers in the line of the incision. It gives access to the gallbladder.

Gridiron

This is the classical approach to the appendix, centred on McBurney's point, which is two-thirds of the way along a line from the umbilicus to the anterior superior iliac spine. The incision passes obliquely downwards from lateral to medial and splits the aponeurotic and muscle layers in the line of their fibres.

Closure of abdominal incisions

Midline incisions may be closed with a mass closure, which employs a strong, slowly absorbable (or non-absorbable) suture in a continuous over-and-over stitch, taking bites of all layers of the incision deep to the skin 1 cm from the wound edge and 1 cm apart. To reduce the incidence of wound dehiscence or postoperative hernia after mass closure, the ratio of suture material used should be four times the length of the wound (Jenkin's rule).

The closure of abdominal incisions is discussed in more detail in Chapter 8.

HAEMOSTASIS IN SURGERY

See Chapter 8.

DRAINS

Drains are inserted either to evacuate established collections of pus, blood or fluid or to drain potential collections that may follow operation because of continued oozing of blood or inflammatory exudate. They range from a simple gauze wick to low-pressure suction applied via tubing.

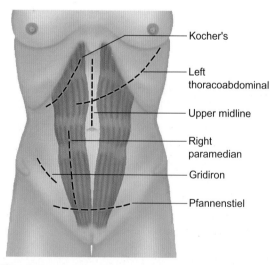

Abdominal incisions
Haemostasis in surgery
Drains
Minimal access surgery

The use of drains is contentious. Advocates maintain that:

- drainage of fluid collections removes a potential source of infection
- drains guard against further fluid collection
- drainage content may alert the surgeon to the presence of an anastomotic leak or to the possibility of secondary haemorrhage
- when removed, a track is left for any residual collection to discharge.

Opponents argue, supported by several recent meta-analyses from the Cochrane Foundation, that:

- the presence of a drain increases the chances of infection by acting as a route for bacterial entry
- damage can be caused by mechanical pressure and through the use of suction
- healing is delayed and, in certain circumstances, complications (such as leakage from an intestinal anastomosis) are more common
- in the peritoneal or pleural cavities, the majority of drains are sealed off within 6 hours and are therefore ineffective
- drains cause pain and may delay discharge from hospital
- there is little or no evidence of benefit for drains after many operations where they are still widely used.

There are many different types of drain, which may be either active or passive (Fig. 5.5). In active drainage, suction forces provided by vacuumed containers (disposable, e.g. Redivac™, or reusable) are used to draw out any collection. Passive drains function by differential pressures between the body and the exterior and are dependent on gravity or capillary action to drain fluid. Because these differential pressures are sometimes reversed, with intraperitoneal or intrapleural pressures lower than atmospheric pressure, fluid movements along the drain can be reversed, thereby increasing the risks of the introduction of bacteria from the outside.

Drains may also be open or closed. Open passive drains lead directly into drainage bags or external wound dressings (Ch. 26). They may be tubes or sheets – often corrugated – of rubber or plastic. Closed tube systems drain directly into a container with or without suction and avoid spillage and soiling of dressings and minimise the hazards if the drainage material is contaminated.

For many years tube drains were made from soft red rubber, but because this substance is irritant (bioreactive) it has largely been superseded by newer material such as polyvinylchloride, Silastic or polyurethane. All have the advantages that they are relatively inert and are transparent so the colour of the drainage fluid can be seen. However, a degree of reactivity can sometimes be advantageous because the fibrosis leaves a track when the drain is removed down which residual drainage can occur. T-tubes to drain the common bile duct after exploration (Ch. 19) are often still made of rubber for this reason.

Drains are discussed further in Chapter 7.

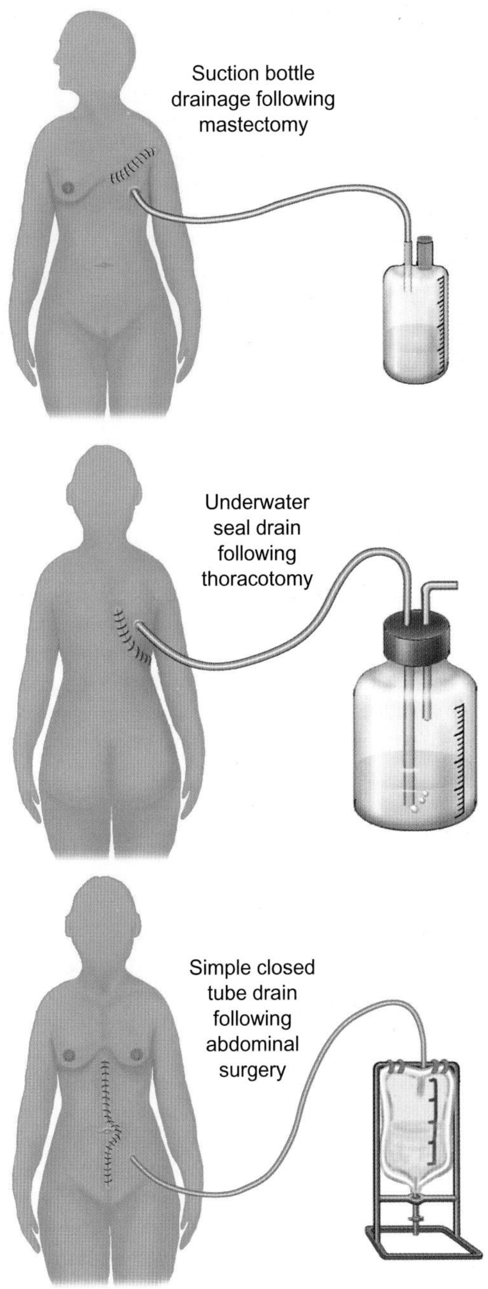

Fig. 5.5 Different types of drain.

MINIMAL ACCESS SURGERY

The term minimal access surgery partially overlaps with several others, including:

- endoscopic surgery
- minimally invasive surgery
- laparoscopic surgery.

Lay people refer to it as keyhole surgery. The student should realise that these words and phrases are often used interchangeably but that individual surgeons and surgical teams may have their own preferred definition. Operating room set-up has changed with the advent of laparoscopy

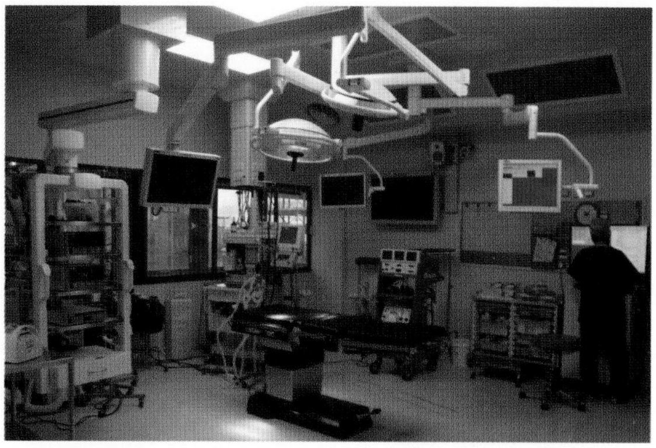

Fig. 5.6 A modern integrated minimal access theatre.

becoming more commonplace. Older stacks and screens are now being replaced with ready-built laparoscopic operating theatres with all the plumbing, wiring and connections being integrated and inbuilt with the design of the theatre itself (Fig. 5.6). This allows for a more ergonomic set-up and for less clutter in the operating theatre. New developments in technologies, especially for optics and for screen visualisation, have made the quality of the image more superior and continued progress will allow better picture and image capture during surgery itself.

TYPES OF PROCEDURE

Laparoscopy

Laparoscopy, i.e. minimal access to the abdomen for diagnosis and later for therapy, was invented in 1910 by a Russian gynaecologist (Isaac Ott). The peritoneal cavity is distended with a gas (usually carbon dioxide), and instruments, including a telescope, are introduced through trocars via small puncture wounds known as ports. Although some gynaecological procedures were performed laparoscopically, it took some decades for surgeons to adopt the technique for diagnosis and increasingly for therapy over the last 20 years.

Therapeutic application in areas other than gynaecology began in 1987 when a French surgeon (Philippe Mouret) performed the first laparoscopic cholecystectomy. Soon after, and with the advent of high-definition televideoscopy, a revolution began in abdominal and also in thoracic surgery (thoracoscopy) which is still in progress. The advantages of laparoscopic access for cholecystectomy (Ch. 20) are now well recognised. Its place in both diagnosis and management of the abdomen is discussed elsewhere in this book.

Diagnosis

Advances in the quality of view that can be achieved with the laparoscope now allow surgeons to perform an abdominal exploration that approximates very closely to that achieved through a large laparotomy incision. Applications include:

- assessment of liver disease
- unknown causes of ascites
- the acute abdomen, including acute appendicitis
- detailed diagnosis and staging of intra-abdominal malignancy
- diagnosis and staging of lymphoma
- preoperative assessment of both blunt and penetrating trauma.

Management

Laparoscopy is used commonly in the management of the following:

- cholecystectomy and appendicectomy
- oesophageal reflux (fundoplication)
- colon malignancy and other colorectal resections
- splenectomy
- retroperitoneal procedures, e.g. adrenalectomy and nephrectomy.

Also under development are flexible laparoscopes and ultrasound probes that can be introduced into, and manipulated within, the abdomen. These devices should add significantly to thorough evaluation not only of the peritoneal cavity but also of the retroperitoneum.

Thoracoscopy

See Chapter 16.

Urological minimal access surgery

See Chapter 33.

ADVANTAGES AND DISADVANTAGES OF MINIMAL ACCESS SURGERY

Advantages

- The large, painful wound of open access is avoided.
- The instruments used for dissection are small and fine, and so the tissue trauma of surgical dissection is further reduced.
- The operation is carried out inside the closed confines of the body cavity, which avoids cooling, drying, excessive handling and extensive retraction of internal organs.
- The overall disturbance to the patient, including pain and discomfort, is reduced.
- Recovery to full activity is accelerated.
- There is considerable reduction in all complications related to the wound; dehiscence and incisional hernia disappear (although an incision to create a port may result in a later port site hernia).
- There is reduced contact with the patient's blood and a consequent reduction in the risk of transmission of viral diseases (Ch. 9).
- There is a reduction in postoperative complications associated with recumbency and pain; e.g. chest problems (Ch. 16), deep vein thrombosis (Ch. 30).
- There is a possible reduction in postoperative peritoneal adhesions.

Disadvantages

These fall into categories of general and organisational and of physiological and pathological constraints.

General and organisational constraints

- *Time.* Procedures performed laparoscopically are generally slower, especially when setting-up time is included. This has important effects on scheduling and costs. Training and learning curves of surgeons and trainees are things to consider.
- *Skills.* Special technical expertise is necessary, and it is only recently that training centres have been set up.

Physiological and pathological constraints

- A large pneumoperitoneum may compress the diaphragm and lung bases and cause postoperative hypoxia.
- Previous adhesions may make a pneumoperitoneum impossible.
- There is a risk of gas embolism, although this is very small.
- Tactile feedback to the operating team is lost; this is important in some aspects of the evaluation of local disorder.
- Precise control of bleeding is undoubtedly more difficult to achieve through an endoscope because the bleeding point often retracts within surrounding tissues. Bleeding during minimally invasive surgery can considerably obscure the field of vision.
- Organ extraction may pose problems. In some instances use is made of natural pathways, such as the mediastinum for the oesophagus or through the rectum for the colon is possible. Other organs, such as the gallbladder or appendix, are small enough to be removed through a port site after they have been put into a bag to stop the consequences of rupture and possible contamination. Yet others (e.g. spleen) can be broken up (morcellised) in a bag prior to extraction from the peritoneal cavity.

CONVERSION FROM LAPAROSCOPY TO OPEN EXPOSURE

Minimal access surgery is only as safe as the skill and judgement of the surgeon. Conversion from a laparoscopic to open procedure does not constitute a failure. Part of the success of minimal access surgery rests on the ability of the surgeon to determine that the patient's interests are best served by converting a laparoscopic procedure to the same operation performed with open access.

FURTHER ADVANCES IN MINIMAL ACCESS SURGERY – ROBOTIC SURGERY

The technique of minimal access surgery/laparoscopy is hindered by having a two-dimensional view, reduced degrees of freedom of manipulation and little tactile feedback. Advances in optical technology, new lenses, cameras and computer software may provide the surgeon with three-dimensional views and thus an operative field with a sense of perspective. Such technology, coupled with a system which would allow seven degrees of freedom of movement within body cavities, would further enhance surgical technique.

This is now possible with robotic systems. General surgery, urology, cardiothoracic surgery and gynaecology have all been assessed and procedures shown to be safe and possible. The surgeon sits at a console and operates the minimally invasive instrumentation which has been adequately positioned for the procedure, thus creating a master–slave system. In theory this should allow more meticulous dissection, particularly with removal of human hand tremor, and better spatial awareness. Furthermore, with the development of motion scaling (where gross hand movements can be reduced and in which precision tasks on minute scales can be carried out), microsurgical technique and capability will continue to progress. Voice-activated systems also allow the operator to move the field of vision without further human aid. Obviously more skilled training is required for the operation of such systems. However this training can be integrated with 'virtual operations', thus allowing surgeons to train on artificial models prior to implementing their skills on patients. Such training also allows objective measurement of surgical skills and enables continuous assessment of developing techniques.

The use of virtual immobilisation (where the original motion of the target organ is eliminated by the optical systems and software combined) will facilitate surgery on moving organs such as the heart. This technique would allow further procedures on the beating heart and therefore reduce the need for cardiopulmonary bypass, which carries significant morbidity. Cardiac surgery in particular is a specialty where robot-assisted procedures benefit technique. Micro-anastomoses can be carried out, with the removal of hand tremor, on a moving target which can be made to appear motionless. The use of port site incisions instead of standard midline sternotomy would further reduce morbidity.

Minimal access and robot-assisted surgery has the potential to change many aspects of modern surgical treatment (Box 5.5). Continuing progress in optics and software developments will further aid the surgeon. Currently these machines are large, cumbersome and expensive, and few operators are trained in their use. However, the techniques are still being developed, and the potential for the future is immense.

Recently the laparoscopic approach has been modified to make it even less invasive – with the technique known as single port surgery or single incision laparoscopic surgery (SILS) or transumbilical laparoscopic surgery (TULA). This technique involves putting three (or more) laparoscopic trochars through the umbilicus for an un-triangulated view which allows virtually scarless surgery. This may be the stepping stone towards natural orifice surgery, also known as

Box 5.5 Areas where robotic surgery can take place

- GI surgery: e.g. laparoscopic cholecystectomy, laparoscopic fundoplication
- Cardiac surgery: e.g. CABG (Coronary Artery Bypass Grafting), valve replacements, septal defect repair
- Urology: laparoscopic radical prostatectomy, laparoscopic pyeloplasty, laparoscopic cystectomy
- Neurosurgery: possibilities but still in the early stages of trials

NOTES (Natural Orifice Translumenal Endoscopic Surgery). There have been a few reports in the literature of cases in humans of NOTES appendicectomies and cholecystectomies; however, this technique is still virtually in its infancy.

FURTHER READING

Argenziano M 2009 Robotic cardiothoracic surgery (current cardiac surgery), Humana Press, New York, USA

Berlinger NT 2006 Robotic surgery – squeezing into tight places. New England Journal of Medicine 354:2099–2101

Department of Health 2008 HIV post exposure prophylaxis: Guidance from the UK Chief Medical Officer's Expert Advisory Group on AIDS

Hemal AK, Menon M 2010 Robotics in urological surgery, Springer, London, UK

Purkayastha S, Athanasiou T, Casula R, Darzi A 2004 Robotic surgery: a review. Hospital Medicine 65(3):153–159

World Alliance for Patient Safety 2009 WHO Surgical Safety Checklist, World Health Organization

Zacharakis E, Purkayastha S, Teare J, Yang GZ, Darzi A 2008 Natural orifices translumenal endoscopic surgery (NOTES) – who should perform it? Surgery 144(1):1–2

6 Anaesthesia and pain control

The specialty of anaesthesia has expanded to take in many areas of hospital practice which now include not only the operating rooms (Ch. 5) but also the intensive care unit (Ch. 10), chronic pain clinics and the labour ward. However, this chapter concentrates on the management of patients who undergo surgical procedures.

The administration of a safe anaesthetic is the central purpose of the specialty, but equally important are careful preparation and appropriate postoperative care. This chapter includes information to help undergraduates not only during their anaesthetic attachments but also in their general understanding of the care of the surgical patient. Detailed descriptions of practical procedures are not given, in that these are best learned during a clinical attachment. Throughout, drugs are referred to which may be initially unfamiliar, and these are described in some detail (see 'Drugs used in anaesthesia' below).

HISTORY AND PRINCIPLES OF ANAESTHESIA

The introduction of anaesthetics in the 19th century was a major advance in the practice of surgery. Before it took place, the range and extent of procedures possible were limited. The first anaesthetic reported was given on the 16th October 1846 by W T G Morton of Boston in the USA. The patient was anaesthetised by inhaling ether. The practice spread rapidly, and in the UK the first anaesthetic was given later that same year to a patient undergoing dental extractions. Chloroform and nitrous oxide were soon added to the range of anaesthetics available, and simple techniques were initially used. Since then there has been a steady evolution of the specialty; some of the more notable landmarks are listed in Box 6.1.

What is anaesthesia?

It is difficult to give an all-encompassing definition for the term. The phrase 'reversible unconsciousness' has been popular but obviously does not include regional anaesthesia. A brief description of the purpose of anaesthesia is the best way to describe the scope of the subject.

Purpose

The purpose of anaesthesia is to allow patients to undergo surgical or investigative procedures in a safe and pain-free way. With general anaesthesia, the patient is unconscious and should not be aware of what is happening. This state, when associated with techniques to reduce the perception of painful stimuli, is now called balanced anaesthesia. The term recognises the fact that a number of different techniques and agents (drugs) can be used in combination to produce the desired state. Many procedures include the use of muscle relaxants, either to allow intubation of the trachea for protection from obstruction of the airway and to permit safe administration of inhaled gases or to aid surgical access (e.g. laparotomy). Paralysis is therefore often a feature of an anaesthetised patient but is not essential.

In the use of local or regional anaesthesia, it cannot be said that the patient is generally unaware; rather, there is a selective state of lack of recognition of what is being done in the area of the procedure. In this, as in all forms of anaesthesia, there is always a balance between ensuring a pain-free subject and the potentially undesirable effects of high concentrations of anaesthetic agents.

Box 6.1 Key events in the history of anaesthesia

1846 W T G Morton, a Boston dentist, demonstrated the use of ether
1853 John Snow, a London physician, gave chloroform analgesia to Queen Victoria at the birth of Prince Leopold
1884 Koller, Viennese ophthalmologist, demonstrated local anaesthetic properties of cocaine
1898 August Bier, first use of spinal anaesthesia
1917 Edmund Boyle, Guy's Hospital, described an early anaesthetic machine
1934 J S Lundy, US anaesthetist, popularised thiopental
1935 Introduction of the intravenous drip
1949 Introduction of muscle relaxants
1956 First clinical use of halothane, at the Manchester Royal Infirmary
1972 College of Anaesthetists formed

How do anaesthetics work?

Despite the highly scientific and technical growth of the specialty over the past 150 years, it is still not possible to give a definitive description of how general anaesthetics work, in the way that, for example, an endocrinologist can often describe the chemical pathways which account for the action of, say, insulin. However, there are a number of factors that allow some reasonable assumptions about the possible action of anaesthetic agents:

- The potency of anaesthetic agents is closely related to their lipid solubility – this points to the cell membrane as the likely site of action.
- Anaesthetic agents probably interfere with the propagation of nerve impulses through central nerves by an effect on the neuronal cell membrane at synaptic junctions.

Many of the assumptions made about the actions of general anaesthetics come from observing their effects on patients. The difficulty of defining exactly how anaesthetics work has made the measurement of the level of anaesthesia in individual patients difficult. There is much current research in this area.

The actions of local anaesthetics are more readily explicable, as will be described later in this chapter.

PREOPERATIVE PREPARATION

A crucial factor in the administration of safe anaesthesia is the correct preparation of the patient. The aim is always to have the optimum condition for an operation. For simple day-case procedures, preparation is relatively straightforward. However, in more complex circumstances, admission may be necessary several days in advance to organise investigations and optimise underlying medical conditions. The anaesthetist visits the patient during this period to make an assessment of likely problems; this is now usually known as pre-assessment.

PRE-ASSESSMENT

The elective patient is evaluated by a review of the history, physical examination and available investigations in the context of fitness for both anaesthesia and the operative procedure. If required, further investigations may then be ordered and specific therapy initiated to optimise the patient's condition before the procedure. This period also provides an opportunity to discuss the anaesthetic and to explore post-operative issues such as the need for analgesia, intravenous infusion and high-dependency care (Ch. 10). Most importantly, the preoperative visit gives patients an opportunity to voice any fears about the anaesthetic, and to receive informed reassurance from the person responsible (the anaesthetist) for their care during and often after the operation.

The assessment often begins with questions to assess the patient's understanding of the proposed procedure. Most individuals can understand the diagnosis and relate this to the site of the lesion; this is adequate for most minor and routine surgery. However, in unusual or major cases, the anaesthetist must always be in contact with the surgical team to discuss the intended procedure, how it might have to be extended and the requirement for blood products or more intensive postoperative care. It is not unusual for the simple closed reduction of a bone fracture, intended to finish in a few minutes, to progress to open fixation and nailing over several hours with considerable blood loss and the need for postoperative high-dependency care. Similarly, to know the site of the lesion and route of surgical access is important because operations on various sites – from lung and larynx to bladder and feet – require very different airway and anaesthetic management. For example, to maintain the airway in an anaesthetised patient by a mask over the face is not possible if the surgeon needs to work inside the mouth.

ASSESSMENT OF MEDICAL FITNESS

With the nature of the procedure clarified, the patient's present medical status may then be evaluated. Details of the past medical history should be recorded and existing disease documented with respect to duration, severity, medication, complications and hospital admissions.

Consideration may then be given to the requirement for further investigation and treatment. Within each of the physiological systems there are many conditions which influence anaesthetic management. Lack of cardiorespiratory reserve is a great concern because surgical procedures elicit a stress response with neuroendocrine changes which lead to alterations in metabolic function and, in major surgery, elevations in cardiac demands and oxygen requirements. Lack of cardiorespiratory reserve may mean that these demands cannot be met without decompensation in spite of the most effective balanced anaesthesia and most minor surgery. Therefore, for those with significant disease, the anaesthetist may require further investigations, specific treatment (even coronary artery bypass grafting before a major procedure on another system such as the gastrointestinal tract), more invasive perioperative monitoring and intensive or high-dependency postoperative care.

Assessment of the adequacy of cardiac and respiratory function is of overriding importance in that both are disturbed by anaesthesia and surgery and both may determine post-operative complications. Impairment is assessed clinically by evaluation of exercise tolerance to activities of daily living, such as walking, climbing stairs and carrying shopping. Known cardiovascular disease – congestive cardiac failure, angina, previous myocardial infarction (particularly within the last 6 months), arrhythmias, hypertension and valvular lesions (particularly aortic stenosis) – need not lead to cancellation, but it is helpful if the anaesthetist is given ample warning in advance so as to formulate an appropriate plan. Hypertension is defined as a systolic pressure greater than 140 mmHg and/or a diastolic pressure of greater than 90 mmHg. Hypertension so defined occurs in approximately 10% of the adult population and constitutes a serious perioperative risk to the patient of stroke or renal dysfunction. Hypertension is therefore a contraindication to elective surgery, and patients found to be hypertensive should be referred for a cardiological opinion.

Respiratory competence is assessed initially by clinical means – exercise tolerance and the occurrence of breathlessness under physical stress – and, for even minor surgery, it is essential that obstructive airways disease, asthma and infection should have been investigated and measures taken to reduce adverse factors. There is a higher incidence of perioperative and postoperative complications (e.g. hypoxic episodes, pneumonia) in patients with respiratory disease. The incidence increases significantly if the disorder is not controlled.

Pathological disturbances within other physiological systems may also be pertinent. A history of gastro-oesophageal reflux warns of patients who may have a hiatus hernia and who are therefore at much higher risk of aspiration. Such individuals can benefit from acid suppression prophylaxis (e.g. ranitidine) and from early tracheal intubation to protect the lower airway. A history of epilepsy may alter anaesthetic medication in that some anaesthetic drugs lower the seizure threshold. Evidence of peripheral nerve damage or neuropathy may dissuade the anaesthetist from employing regional techniques of nerve blockade. Patients with diabetes require varying degrees of management, dependent on the severity of the condition and the magnitude of the procedure; management ranges from simple monitoring of blood glucose by the BM stick procedure to precise metabolic control with frequent blood glucose determinations and intravenous infusions of dextrose, insulin and potassium which may begin some hours preoperatively.

Cerebrovascular disease is common. Stroke is responsible for death in 9% and 15% of the general population of adult men and women, respectively. A history of previous stroke, particularly in the presence of hypertension, means that particular attention should be paid to the state of the peripheral circulation, and the patient should undergo examination of the carotid pulse (palpation and auscultation) at the least before operation. If there have been recent transient disturbances of cerebral function, these patients should be referred for duplex Doppler examination with a view to possible carotid angiography.

Other system disease, such as renal failure, liver disease, haematological or musculoskeletal abnormalities, must also be defined because all may influence anaesthetic technique.

Existing medical treatment

An accurate medication and allergy history is vital. Diuretics may cause electrolyte imbalance that can lead to cardiac arrhythmias or dehydration, which on induction of anaesthesia may lead to hypotension. Beta-blockers may prevent cardiovascular compensation for hypotension caused by either bleeding or loss of sympathetic vasomotor control during both regional and general anaesthesia. Anti-arrhythmics (e.g. digoxin, amiodarone) may potentiate the bradycardic effects of anaesthetic drugs such as propofol, fentanyl or vecuronium (these agents are discussed later).

Bronchodilators and other sympathomimetics may increase the incidence and severity of tachyarrhythmias. If a course of systemic steroids has been taken within the last year, consideration needs to be given to steroid supplementation as prophylaxis against an adrenal crisis (Ch. 32). Those on monoamine oxidase inhibitors may experience severe cardiovascular and neurological disturbances if sympathomimetics (e.g. adrenaline) or opioid analgesics such as pethidine are used.

Those on the oral contraceptive pill may require measures to reduce the risks of developing deep vein thrombosis and pulmonary emboli (Ch. 16). In circumstances in which the patient is likely to be ambulatory soon after the operation (the majority of modern procedures), the risks of an unwanted pregnancy usually outweigh the chances of thrombotic complications, and patients are advised to continue on the contraceptive pill unless they are having major surgery for malignant disease.

Oral anticoagulants may need to be adjusted to a reduced dose, changed to intravenous heparin or stopped altogether. Drugs such as antihypertensive, anti-arrhythmic bronchodilator agents should be maintained at their usual schedule up to the induction of anaesthesia, and so may need to be included in the premedication.

Details of past anaesthetics should be sought from both the patient and the notes. A history of difficult intubation, allergy, malignant hyperthermia (a serious allergic reaction to certain anaesthetic agents) and postoperative nausea and vomiting are of great interest and influence the plan for subsequent anaesthesia. For those previously not exposed to an anaesthetic, a review of family experiences of anaesthesia complications may reveal congenital conditions of note, e.g. malignant hyperthermia, suxamethonium apnoea (see below) and sickle cell disease.

Questions should be directed towards cigarette and alcohol consumption – a social history which may yield very useful information about unrevealed problems, as well as indicators of the response to an anaesthetic. Premenopausal women should be asked if they could be pregnant, to avoid exposing the fetus to potentially teratogenic anaesthetic drugs.

A check that an appropriate period of fasting will have elapsed before induction of anaesthesia should be mandatory. A period of 6 hours following solid food and 4 hours following clear liquids is standard in most hospitals.

Box 6.2 Conditions which predispose to difficult endotracheal intubation

Congenital
- Pierre Robin syndrome
- Treacher Collins syndrome
- Achondroplasia
- Marfan's syndrome
- Noonan's syndrome
- Cystic hygroma

Anatomical
- Reduced mouth opening
- Reduced neck movement
- Small mandible
- Prominent teeth
- Obesity

Acquired
- Airway instability: trauma, rheumatoid arthritis
- Trismus, fibrosis: causing reduced movement of temporomandibular joint
- Reduced neck movement: arthritis, hard collar
- Swelling: tumour, abscess, haematoma
- Airway obstructed: bleeding, vomitus
- Scarring: burns, radiation

Airway examination

Examination of the airway is mandatory for the anaesthetist, particularly if the use of an endotracheal tube is contemplated – patients have died after induction of anaesthesia where there was, because of lack of previous knowledge, inability to ventilate the patient or site an endotracheal tube. Conditions that lead to difficulties with intubation are shown in Box 6.2.

The airway examination should include:

- mouth opening (two finger breadths or less is likely to lead to problems)
- jaw protrusion – can the lower incisors be placed in front of the upper?
- neck flexion and extension
- the presence of prominent or loose teeth
- a view of the posterior pharyngeal structures – this has been shown to be a valuable indicator of the ease of laryngoscopy.

Very occasionally, additional investigations of the airway are needed, such as lateral X-rays of the neck, flow-volume pulmonary function tests or awake fibreoptic examination. The known difficult intubation seldom causes severe problems, but the unexpected one may quickly become a medical emergency. Therefore patients who are known to be at risk of a difficult intubation should be referred to senior anaesthetists at pre-assessment.

Investigations

Further investigations may be required, the common indications for which are listed in Table 6.1. The list is not exhaustive, and many other examinations may be necessary. In addition, few of the indications are absolute and, if an investigation has recently been performed, then it is not of value to repeat it unless circumstances have changed.

Table 6.1 Indications for preoperative investigations

Investigation	Indication
Full blood count	History of bleeding, major surgery, cardiorespiratory disease, premenopausal women
Electrolytes	History of vomiting, diarrhoea, renal disease, cardiac disease, diabetes, diuretics, ACE inhibitors, anti-arrhythmics, steroids, hypoglycaemics
Glucose	History of diabetes, abscesses, steroids
Liver function tests	History of liver disease, alcoholism, bleeding, pyrexia of unknown origin
Clotting studies	History of liver disease, bleeding
Sickle cell test	Afro-Caribbeans if sickle cell status unknown
Electrocardiogram	History of hypertension, cardiorespiratory disease, age > 55 years
Chest X-ray	History of cardiorespiratory disease, heavy smoker, potential metastases, recent immigrants from area where TB is endemic
Pulmonary function tests	Respiratory disease, thoracic surgery
Arterial blood gases	Respiratory disease, thoracic surgery
Cervical spine X-ray	Rheumatoid arthritis, trauma

Box 6.3 Preoperative grading system of the American Society of Anesthesiologists

ASA I Healthy patient
ASA II Mild systemic disease, no functional disability
ASA III Moderate systemic disease, functional disability
ASA IV Severe systemic disease, constantly life-threatening
ASA V Moribund patient, unlikely to survive 24 hours with or without an operation

Preoperative grading

Following this assessment, the anaesthetist will be able to grade the patient. A commonly used system is that described by the American Society of Anesthesiologists (ASA), in which patients are allocated to one of five categories (Box 6.3); addition of an E denotes an emergency procedure, usually of higher risk. The scoring system allows easier communication between anaesthetists and is also a useful research tool. However, it gives only limited prognostic information about the chances of an individual surviving an operation. Significant factors, including the type of procedure, a history of difficult intubation and of obesity, are not included in the classification.

IMMEDIATE PREOPERATIVE PREPARATION

Although reflexes which protect the lungs are lost only under general anaesthesia, the requirements for preparation for general, local and regional anaesthesia are the same. An adequate history and examination must have been taken, fasting protocols adhered to, drugs and fluids for resuscitation and also a defibrillator must be readily available, and suction, oxygen and airway equipment must be to hand. Except for the simplest of procedures, it is sound to ensure that there is someone available other than the anaesthetist to monitor the patient, including pulse, blood pressure and oxygenation. The patient's identity should be confirmed and the procedure to be performed and completed consent form checked before anaesthesia is started in line with the WHO surgical checklist (see Ch. 5).

Premedication

Premedication is now prescribed only to individuals with a specific indication (Table 6.2).

THE PRACTICE OF GENERAL ANAESTHESIA

There are a number of ways to anaesthetise a patient, and the technique used depends on a number of factors, some of which have already been considered. The most important are:

- clinical condition and general health
- the type and extent of the procedure
- protection of the airway.

The last of these is integral to safe anaesthesia and should be an essential part of undergraduate practical training.

Table 6.2 Premedications

Indication	Class of drug used	Example
Sedation	Benzodiazepines	Temazepam, diazepam, lorazepam
	Opioids	Papaveretum, pethidine
	Butyrophenones	Droperidol
Acid aspiration prophylaxis	H_2 antagonists	Ranitidine, cimetidine
	Prokinetics	Metoclopramide
	Antacid	Sodium citrate
Reflex activity prophylaxis	Bronchodilators	Salbutamol
Bradycardia prophylaxis	Anticholinergics	Atropine
Anti-sialogues	Anticholinergics	Hyoscine, glycopyrronium, atropine
Anti-emetics	$5HT_3$ antagonists	Ondansetron
	Butyrophenones	Droperidol
	Antihistamines	Cyclizine
Analgesics	Opioids	Morphine, pethidine
	NSAIDs	Diclofenac
Amnestic	Benzodiazepines	Lorazepam
	Anticholinergics	Hyoscine

MANAGEMENT OF THE AIRWAY

After the induction of general anaesthesia, the patient's ability to maintain the airway is lost. There are many contributory factors, but the relaxation of the muscles of the tongue is central and can lead to physical obstruction of the airway which may be partial or complete. To avoid both, anaesthetists rely on careful positioning of the patient and special equipment.

Patient position

The patient is usually supine, with the head resting on one pillow and the shoulders flat on the theatre trolley or bed – the head is thus extended on the neck and the jaw is elevated (Fig. 6.1). This position lifts the base of the tongue away from the posterior wall of the pharynx and is sometimes called sniffing the morning air.

Equipment

Anaesthetic mask

All masks must fit snugly against the face to produce an airtight seal to ensure the precise delivery of gases. As with all apparatus it is important to select the right size: the average adult male requires a size 5 mask, adult females size 4 (Fig. 6.2).

Oral and nasal airways

These are the simplest aids to airway management. Oral airways (e.g. Guedel) come in different sizes and help to keep the tongue away from the posterior pharyngeal wall (Fig. 6.2). Nasal airways are useful if it is impossible or inappropriate to use an oral airway (Fig. 6.3).

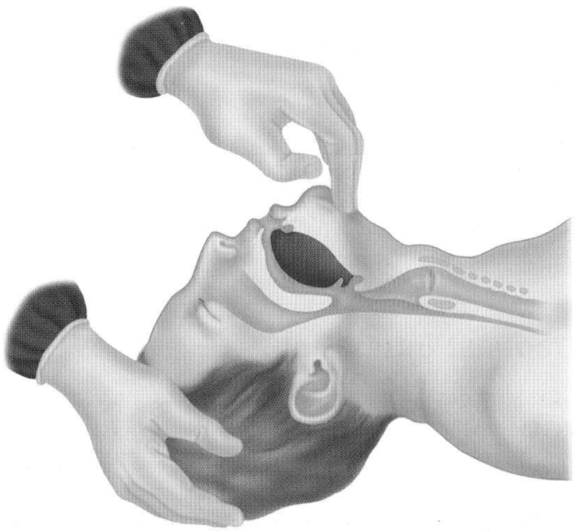

Fig. 6.1 Supporting the airway.

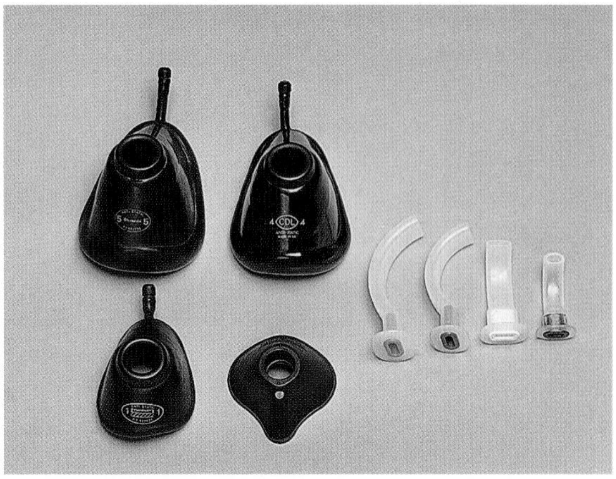

Fig. 6.2 Anaesthetic masks and oral airways.

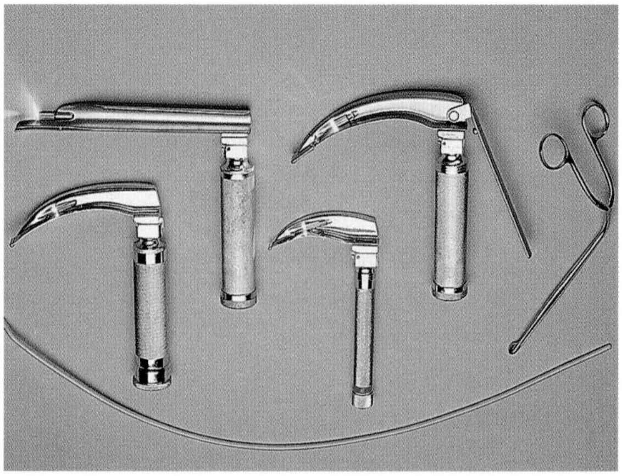

Fig. 6.4 Laryngoscopes and aids to intubation.

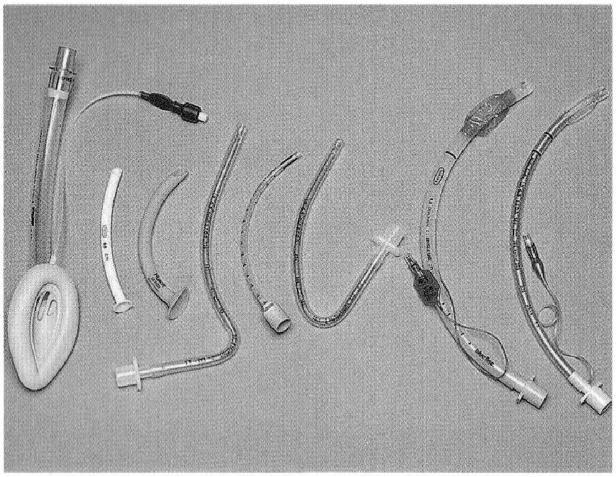

Fig. 6.3 Airways: laryngeal mask airway, nasopharyngeal airways, and different types of endotracheal tubes (with and without cuffs).

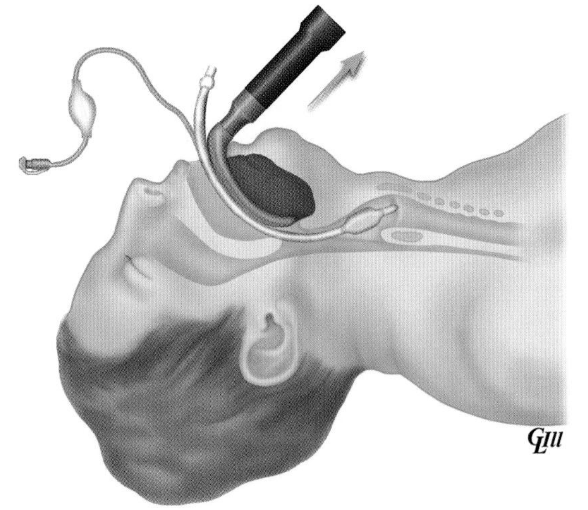

Fig. 6.5 Use of a laryngoscope to insert an endotracheal tube.

Laryngeal mask airway (LMA)

The LMA is a more complicated oral airway than the Guedel. Because of its design it can be directly attached to an anaesthetic circuit (Fig. 6.3). However, it is still an airway, and although it has an inflatable cuff, its position above the vocal cords does not provide protection against aspiration into the trachea.

Laryngoscopes

These are instruments used to facilitate tracheal intubation, and many types have been designed (Fig. 6.4) to suit many different situations (examples are paediatric and fibreoptic instruments for children and for difficult intubations).

Tracheal intubation

A specially designed tube is passed across the vocal cords into the trachea and guarantees a clear upper airway free from the risk of aspiration, particularly if, as is usually the case for adults, the tube has an inflatable cuff (Figs 6.3 and 6.5). Intubation is an essential skill for those involved in airway management, and students should gain hands-on experience during clinical attachments. This includes familiarity with equipment for intubation and the safeguards used to check that the tube is correctly placed in the trachea.

INDUCTION, MAINTENANCE AND RECOVERY FROM ANAESTHESIA

Induction

Induction usually takes place in an anaesthetic room adjacent to the operating room. Patients will have been checked to ensure they are properly prepared for surgery. The anaesthetist normally has an assistant who may be another specialist or a nurse. On arriving in the anaesthetic room, monitoring equipment is attached and, in most instances, an in-dwelling intravenous catheter is inserted at this stage. Usually an intravenous agent such as propofol is used to induce anaesthesia, although occasionally induction is by breathing anaesthetic gases (inhalational induction). While the patient is breathing 100% oxygen, the intravenous agent is injected slowly. Once the patient has lost consciousness,

Box 6.4 Indications for endotracheal intubation

- Provides clear airway
- Protects against aspiration
- Allows positive pressure ventilation
- Protects airway if operative site is near
- Patient in awkward position, e.g. prone
- Airway maintenance by mask difficult

Box 6.5 Indications for the use of muscle relaxants

- Facilitates intubation
- Facilitates ventilation
- Allows surgical access, e.g. laparotomy
- Allows control of CO_2 levels

the anaesthetist places an anaesthetic mask on the face and changes the gases to deliver an anaesthetic mixture which usually includes oxygen, nitrous oxide and a volatile agent such as isoflurane. During this period, the concentration of anaesthetic gases in the patient's tissues increases as the concentration of the intravenous agent decreases – induction gives way to maintenance. At this stage any additional ancillary procedures are done, such as intubation (the indications for which are listed in Box 6.4) or the insertion of additional intravascular lines for cardiovascular monitoring. During this time, attachment to an anaesthetic machine is usually necessary and, if paralysis has been induced (indications in Box 6.5), a ventilator is necessary.

Maintenance

The patient is either transferred into the operating room with the anaesthetic machine or reconnected to one in the room. The 'time out' section of the WHO checklist is now undertaken (see Ch. 5). The maintenance of anaesthesia requires constant vigilance (Fig. 6.6). It is essential to ensure that anaesthesia is deep enough (Box 6.6) to avoid the risk of awareness. The patient is monitored so that any complications of the surgery or anaesthesia not obvious clinically can be detected early and treated. During this period the anaesthetist tries to keep the patient's general condition in balance, which includes fluid management, replacement of blood loss, cardiorespiratory support and maintenance of body temperature. During the procedure other drugs are administered to supplement anaesthesia. In most instances an analgesic (e.g. morphine) and an anti-emetic (e.g. cyclizine) are given.

Recovery

As the operation comes to an end, the anaesthetist steadily reduces the concentration of anaesthetic gases and, once the last active painful stimulus is withdrawn, the anaesthetic agents are turned off and replaced with 100% oxygen. At this point it may also be necessary to give a drug to reverse residual muscle paralysis; this injection does not have any effect on the concentration of anaesthetic gases in the body and therefore does not influence wakening. Gradual awakening occurs as the concentration of gases is reduced by expiration. If possible the recovery position is adopted until full control of the airway has been achieved. As this occurs, adjuncts such as an endotracheal tube are removed and a simple oxygen mask applied. The 'sign out' section of the WHO checklist is performed at this stage (see Ch. 5). Transfer to a recovery area then takes place for further care.

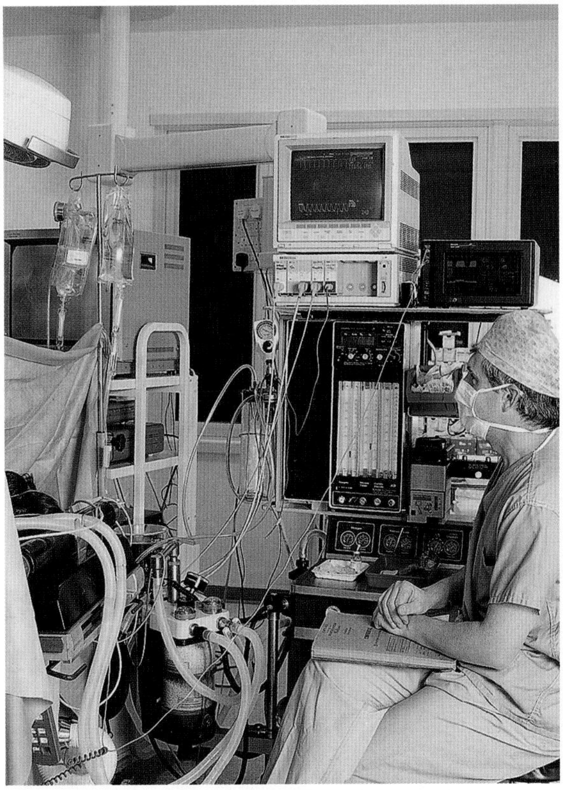

Fig. 6.6 Maintenance of anaesthesia. Note the extensive monitoring and vigilant anaesthetist.

Box 6.6 Signs indicating inadequate depth of anaesthesia

- Dilated pupils
- Tears
- Sweating
- Tachycardia and hypertension
- Patient movement
- Increased respiratory rate

COMPLICATIONS OF ANAESTHESIA

Emergency surgery and that undertaken at the extremes of age are more dangerous than that done as a routine on healthy subjects. Box 6.7 lists some of the complications. Here two potentially fatal matters are considered.

The difficult airway

In certain instances the airway may be difficult to maintain and therefore the delivery of adequate oxygen becomes a problem which can be life threatening. Prediction may be possible, and if a problem is anticipated, senior members of staff should be involved even though all anaesthetists are trained to cope with an airway problem – both one that is

Box 6.7 Complications of anaesthesia

- Hypoxia
- Hypercapnia
- Hypotension
- Arrhythmias
- Pulmonary embolism
- Allergic reactions
- Hypothermia
- Awareness
- Minor trauma, e.g. sore throat
- Headache
- Malignant hyperpyrexia
- Nausea and vomiting

Box 6.8 Advantages and disadvantages of regional anaesthesia

Advantages
- Avoids complications of GA
- Contributes to postoperative analgesia
- Less postoperative nausea and vomiting
- Patient satisfaction (e.g. caesarean section)
- Reduces incidence of DVT

Disadvantages
- Toxic effects of local anaesthetics
- Patient unhappy to be awake
- Inadequate anaesthesia
- Possible nerve damage
- Can be slow onset

expected and one that comes out of the blue. There are a number of techniques and instruments to help deal with these matters.

Aspiration of stomach contents

With the onset of anaesthesia, the reflexes that protect the airways – especially cough and gag – are lost. Therefore it is possible for stomach contents to reflux up the oesophagus and enter the lungs. The repercussions can be serious: either acute asphyxiation or aspiration 'pneumonia' (a progressive bronchopneumonic inflammation). Therefore elective patients are fasted to ensure that the stomach is empty. In an emergency where the stomach may be full, either because of a previous meal or because of the presenting condition (e.g. intestinal obstruction), an endotracheal tube is passed to avoid reflux and inhalation. However, there is a short period of time after the patient has become unconscious and before the endotracheal tube is sited when the lungs are still potentially at risk. A procedure known as cricoid pressure is used during this period. Pressure sufficient to occlude the upper oesophagus is exerted anteroposteriorly on the cricoid ring just below the larynx. Those in attendance on the induction of anaesthesia in such circumstances require training, and the technique is not without hazards.

LOCAL AND REGIONAL ANAESTHESIA

While most patients and many doctors will assume that anaesthesia automatically implies a state of unconsciousness, such loss of awareness is not always necessary or even desirable. Many procedures can be performed safely and comfortably under local or regional anaesthesia, under regional anaesthesia with sedation, or with a combination of regional and general anaesthesia. Regional anaesthesia is the term used to describe local anaesthetic blockade of a group of nerves or nerve roots (e.g. the brachial plexus) to produce anaesthesia of a specific area. There is often no clear-cut advantage of one technique over another: Box 6.8 lists some of the factors that influence the decision.

Box 6.9 Maximum safe doses of local anaesthetics

- Lidocaine (lignocaine) 4 mg/kg
- Bupivacaine 2 mg/kg
- Prilocaine 5 mg/kg

NB: 1% solution of drug = 10 mg/mL

How does a local anaesthetic work?

Local anaesthetics (LAs) block the generation and propagation of nerve impulses at several sites – the spinal cord, spinal nerve roots or peripheral nerves – by inhibiting sodium channels in nerve fibres, which are essential for the propagation of nerve impulses. In general, they are membrane stabilisers.

Local anaesthetic toxicity

As with any group of drugs, overdosage of local anaesthetics leads to toxic side effects. Box 6.9 lists the maximum allowable dose of some commonly used agents. Local anaesthetics are presented for use in percentage strengths, which can easily be converted into milligrams if it is remembered that *a 1% solution contains 10 mg of drug per millilitre.* Hence 10 mL of 2% lidocaine (lignocaine) contains 200 mg.

During a toxic episode, inhibitory cell membranes are first blocked, which leads to unopposed excitatory activity manifest as seizures. Other excitable cell membranes are also inhibited, most notably those of the conducting system of the heart, which results in arrhythmias such as ventricular tachycardia or fibrillation. Eventually coma and cardiovascular collapse ensue.

ROUTES OF ADMINISTRATION

Topical

EMLA (eutectic mixture of local anaesthetic) or Ametop cream may be used to provide skin analgesia before venepuncture, although the effect is best on the relatively soft skin of children. The conjunctivae, and the mucosa of the nose, throat and urethra can also be anaesthetised topically.

Subcutaneous infiltration

This is used, for example, before venepuncture and in the suturing of wounds. When local agents are infiltrated circumferentially around an extremity (the toe or finger), a ring block is produced which can have implications for the circulation.

Bier's block

Also known as intravenous regional anaesthesia, this has been classically used for reduction of Colles' fractures (Ch. 35) and is the exception to the rule that local anaesthetic should never be injected directly into the circulation. Systemic toxicity is prevented by the use only of prilocaine (the least toxic LA) and by separating the intravenous local anaesthetic in the limb from the general circulation by a tourniquet until the agent is bound in the tissues – about 20 minutes. Deaths have resulted as a consequence of tourniquet failure.

Nerve block

Individual nerves can be anaesthetised if local anaesthetic can be introduced close enough to the nerve; in theory, any nerve can be blocked, but in practice some nerves are difficult to reach even for those who are skilled and enthusiastic. In that most nerves pass close to arteries, these vessels can be used as markers to position the injection. A peripheral nerve stimulator can also be used if the nerve carries motor fibres: a small electrical current is produced which elicits muscle twitching if the needle to be used for the block is close to the nerve. Ultrasound is now being used to introduce local anaesthetic close enough to the nerve without damaging it or the surrounding structures. Blocks can be one-off single injections, or flexible catheters can be inserted to allow repeated injections ('top-ups') or continuous infusions. In this way, the block can be continued for as long as the catheter remains in situ.

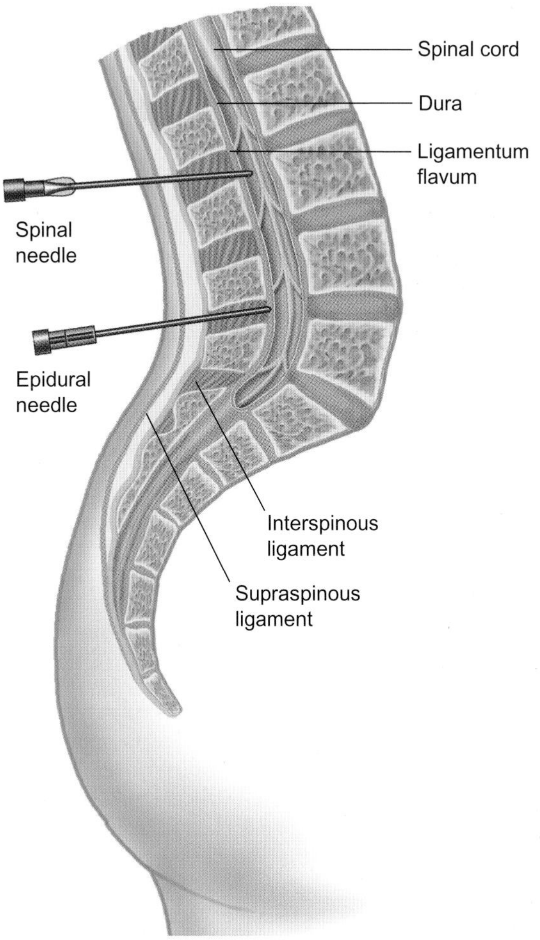

Fig. 6.7 The anatomy of spinal and epidural anaesthesia.

Epidural and spinal anaesthesia

In relation to nerve action, the introduction of local anaesthetic into the epidural or subarachnoid (spinal) spaces is similar to regional blockade, although the timescale and intensity differ. Both techniques involve the insertion of a needle into the midline between the spinous processes of adjacent vertebrae (Fig. 6.7). This form of anaesthesia is especially useful for surgery below the waist; blocks can be made as high as the mid-thoracic region, but associated abdominal and intercostal muscle weakness can interfere with the ability to breathe or cough.

The *epidural* space is the more superficial of the two and is classically identified by the loss of resistance to injection of air or saline. Because an epidural injection does not puncture the dura, and therefore is well clear of the spinal cord, it can be done at any level in the vertebral column. In addition, wider-bore needles can be used, which allow the passage of a catheter into the epidural space and either 'top-ups' or continuous infusions. The local anaesthetic introduced into the epidural space has to diffuse through the epidural fat towards the nerve roots as they emerge from the dura; as a result, the block can take up to 20 minutes to become effective and may miss some nerve roots, leaving unblocked segments. It is generally less dense than a spinal anaesthetic. Larger doses of anaesthetic agent are also needed than for a spinal because the anaesthetic is injected further from its eventual site of action.

With *spinal* anaesthesia, the dura is deliberately punctured to enter the subarachnoid space. The resulting persistent breach in the membrane can lead to leak of CSF and be a cause of debilitating 'spinal' headache. To minimise this complication, very fine needles are used. Spinal anaesthetics are usually 'single shot' and last up to 2 hours. The spinal cord ends at the level of the body of L1; at or above this level, the cord is tethered and is at risk of being skewered by a needle; below this, there is the freely floating cauda equina and a needle tends to push the nerves away. In consequence, spinal anaesthetics are administered below the level of L1. The anaesthetic introduced is close to the nerves, and very small volumes can produce satisfactory blocks with very rapid onset. The agent introduced into the subarachnoid space can be 'floated' in the CSF towards the desired level of block above the level of insertion by appropriate positioning of the patient.

Complications

Epidural and spinal anaesthesia carry the same hazards as all other nerve blocks, but local complications in the central nervous system can be catastrophic, as follows:

- Infection in the vertebral column can result in meningitis or cord compression secondary to abscess formation.
- Haematoma can also lead to cord compression.
- Epidural cannulae can shift over time or be misplaced from the beginning, so that inadvertent epidural venous cannulation can lead to rapid onset of local anaesthetic toxicity, and an unrecognised spinal tap can lead to an epidural dose being injected spinally, with dangerously high levels of block.
- Epidural and spinal anaesthetics block not only motor and sensory nerves but also vasomotor control; vasodilatation and a fall in the blood pressure may result.

Such anaesthetic blockade should never be performed without the same preparation and monitoring as for a general anaesthetic.

MONITORING AND CHARTING

All patients undergoing anaesthesia or sedative techniques should have their vital signs monitored. The range of monitoring information available to anaesthetists is vast, from fairly simple parameters such as temperature to complex data such as integrated electroencephalograms (EEGs). In this section we will concentrate on what are now accepted as standard monitoring requirements. We can usefully divide monitoring into devices that monitor the patient and those that monitor the anaesthetic machine and its function. However, in all cases the best monitor is the constant presence and vigilance of the anaesthetist (see Fig. 6.6). The anaesthetist should view the information he or she receives from the monitors in the context of the individual patient and the procedure the patient is undergoing.

MONITORING THE PATIENT

Clinical observations

The anaesthetist can obtain useful information by direct observation and examination. A warm, well-perfused, pink patient who is passing good volumes of urine is unlikely to be hypovolaemic. Likewise, observations of the pupils will guard against awareness (see Box 6.6). It is important for the anaesthetist to be aware of what is going on surgically. Measuring blood loss and predicting further losses will enable a more controlled replacement by transfusion if required.

Equipment

Standard monitoring is aimed at the cardiorespiratory systems (Box 6.10). The continuous recording of the ECG is mandatory and gives information on the heart rate and rhythm. Measurement of blood pressure is usually automated. The machines use the same principle as a manual blood pressure cuff used at the bedside. The automated mechanism and detecting devices allow the pressure to be measured at regular intervals (e.g. every 2 minutes). The pulse oximeter (Fig. 6.8) gives the anaesthetist a continuous measurement of oxygenation. The device measures the percentage of haemoglobin which is in oxygenated form, and isolates that measurement to arterial blood. These three devices give a lot of information about the patient's well-being. They are safe, easy to use and accurate. However, their interpretation requires some knowledge of physiology. For example, the oxygen saturation is related to the partial pressure (the important parameter) of oxygen in the blood by the relationship shown in the oxyhaemoglobin dissociation curve (Fig. 6.9). It can be seen from this diagram that, when the saturation falls below 90%, there is a rapid decline in the partial pressure of oxygen. Before use, these devices are programmed with what are considered normal limits for the patient. If the measurements fall outside these limits an alarm will sound.

Box 6.10 Standard monitoring

- ECG
- Non-invasive blood pressure
- Pulse oximetry
- End-tidal carbon dioxide levels
- Temperature
- Degree of muscle relaxation
- Inspired oxygen concentration

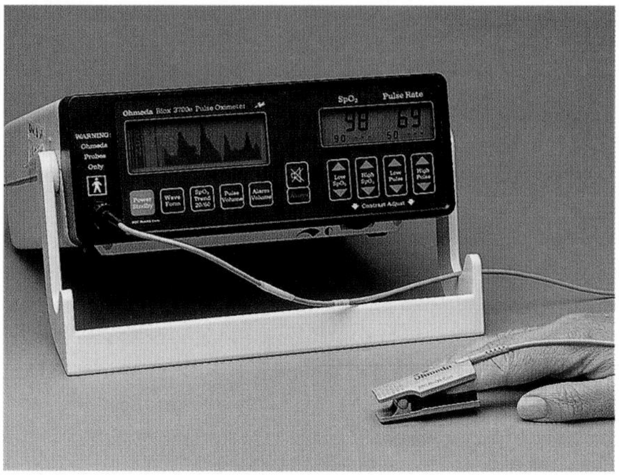

Fig. 6.8 A pulse oximeter.

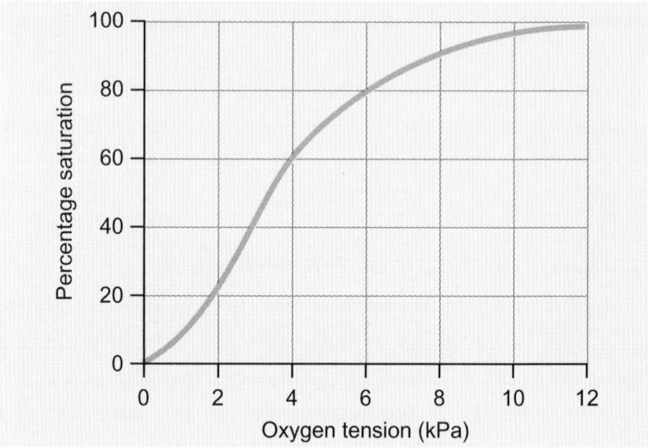

Fig. 6.9 Oxyhaemoglobin dissociation curve.

Standard monitoring also includes measurement of the concentrations of gases exhaled from the lungs (i.e. alveolar gas, which has a higher than ambient level of carbon dioxide). A capnograph enables measurement of the level of CO_2 in expired alveolar gases. In turn, this indicates if ventilation is adequate and also, importantly, whether controlled or spontaneous ventilation is happening at all.

In addition to the standard monitoring outlined above, anaesthetists have a number of other tools at their disposal. The degree of muscle paralysis can easily be assessed. In complex cases, the function of the cardiovascular system can be followed invasively with intra-arterial catheters, central venous lines and cardiac output devices. These also allow frequent blood sampling for measurement of haematological and biochemical variables.

However, one measurement which is not easy to make is the depth of anaesthesia. The bispectral index (BIS) monitor was introduced only in the last decade. It uses the effect of anaesthesia on the EEG to estimate the depth of anaesthesia and therefore decrease the risk of awareness under anaesthesia.

Throughout the procedure the anaesthetist charts the information received from the monitors; this allows observation of developing trends and also acts as a permanent record of events.

MONITORING THE ANAESTHETIC MACHINE

Once again the anaesthetist's vigilance is most important. The function of the machine will have been checked before the procedure is embarked upon, and regular observation throughout should detect problems. Within the machine there are devices to detect changes in pressure and flow throughout the system. Importantly, incorporated with the capnogram described above are devices which measure the concentration of gases that enter the patient. In particular, it is vital to know that a safe concentration of oxygen is delivered. The device also measures the concentrations of anaesthetic agents which leave the patient's lungs, so enabling approximate adjustment of the depth of anaesthesia.

The anaesthetic machine

The anaesthetic machine (Fig. 6.10) at first glance appears to be a baffling collection of cylinders, gauges, valves and monitors. However, it is really the modern descendant of the very simple systems used to deliver anaesthetics in the 19th century. At that time agents such as ether were dripped onto simple masks held over the patient's face, allowing the inhalation of the vapour produced. The modern machine is designed to deliver highly accurate concentrations of vapours and gases to maintain appropriate levels of anaesthesia while at the same time avoiding rebreathing of expired CO_2.

Flow meters

Anaesthetic gases are delivered to anaesthetic machines from pipelines connected to a central source or from cylinders at high pressures. The pressure is reduced by a series of valves, and the flow meters then accurately deliver the gases at atmospheric pressure at the flow rates required.

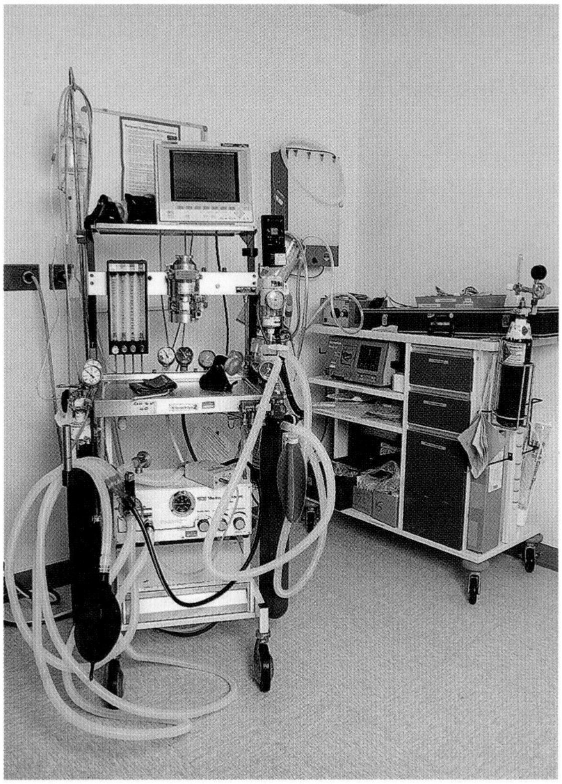

Fig. 6.10 Anaesthetic machine (left) and a difficult airway trolley (right).

Vaporisers

The liquid but volatile anaesthetic agents (e.g. isoflurane) are kept on the anaesthetic machine in vaporisers which allow delivery of accurate concentrations into breathing systems.

Breathing systems

The anaesthetic machine produces a mixture of gases and vapours. To deliver these to the patient without dilution by air, a breathing system is used. There are a number of systems available that have different characteristics and are designed for different circumstances (e.g. paediatric anaesthesia). The details of these systems are outside the scope of this chapter. Two of the most commonly used are the Magill and Bain circuits.

Ventilators

A ventilator is a device that takes over the work of breathing from the patient. Most use a phase of positive pressure to blow gases into the lungs. There are many different types with different characteristics. All ventilators are able to deliver a set volume of gases to the lungs at a set rate and usually have safeguards to prevent too high a pressure being delivered.

DRUGS USED IN ANAESTHESIA

INTRAVENOUS INDUCTION AGENTS

Ideally the agent used should have a rapid onset of effect, with rapid production of unconsciousness. It should have few side effects on the cardiovascular and respiratory systems and be quickly metabolised to aid speedy recovery.

Thiopental (thiopentone)

Introduced into clinical practice in 1932, this drug is a sulphur analogue of pentobarbitone (a barbiturate). It produces unconsciousness in less than one brain–arm circulation time (about 30 seconds). It is then redistributed to the fat and muscle compartments, so its effects wear off relatively quickly. Unfortunately it needs to be used very carefully because too large a dose can cause a severe fall in blood pressure, especially in those who have other factors which can contribute, e.g. hypovolaemia and impaired vasomotor tone. In common with all anaesthetic induction agents, it causes marked respiratory depression. Although painless on intravenous injection, extravasation into the tissues or accidental intra-arterial injection can cause pain and distal ischaemia.

Propofol

This simple molecule (2,6-di-isopropylphenol) has become extremely popular. It has a fast onset of action and is metabolised very rapidly by the liver and other organs. This means that the agent has very few hangover effects and results in a very bright, clear-headed recovery – it is ideal for day-care surgery. Its rapid metabolism also allows use as a continuous infusion, either for a short anaesthetic or as sedation on the intensive care unit. In common with thiopental (thiopentone) it can cause marked falls in blood pressure and markedly depresses respiration. Unfortunately it is sometimes painful on intravenous injection, and to prevent this, many anaesthetists add a small dose of local anaesthetic (lidocaine [lignocaine]) to the solution.

Ketamine

This phencyclidine derivative is somewhat different from the other agents. It can be used as a sedative or to induce anaesthesia. Interestingly, systolic blood pressure is usually raised by ketamine, and respiration is not depressed except by very large doses. It is also a good analgesic. Unfortunately it is associated with a high incidence of postoperative hallucinations. It may be used as the sole anaesthetic agent in those with shock and thus has a role in military surgery.

INHALATIONAL MAINTENANCE AGENTS

Once anaesthesia has been induced, it must be maintained, usually by inhalational agents. These are mainly ether derivatives (methyl-ethyl ethers) and hydrocarbons. They are mostly liquids at room temperature and are administered through special vaporisers on the anaesthetic machine, which are calibrated to allow specified concentrations of the vapour to be added to the oxygen and other gases in use for ventilation.

Sevoflurane, desflurane, isoflurane and enflurane

These modern ether derivatives are all useful agents because they have a rapid onset and offset of action. Sevoflurane is pleasant to inhale and is often used to induce anaesthesia by the inhalational route in children who are intolerant of needles. Desflurane is less pleasant but, because it has a very rapid offset of action, is quite frequently used in day-case surgery, where rapid recovery is desirable. Isoflurane is an older agent in common use which has a relatively quick offset of action and has low levels of cardiovascular side effects. Enflurane is similar to isoflurane.

Nitrous oxide

The gas is supplied in blue cylinders which can be connected to the anaesthetic machine. It is an analgesic gas (colloquially known as laughing gas). Special meters on the anaesthetic machine allow it to be mixed in known proportions with oxygen. Because of its analgesic properties it is widely used in childbirth.

NEUROMUSCULAR BLOCKING AGENTS

Muscle relaxant drugs are often used as part of a balanced anaesthetic to allow intubation of the trachea and controlled respiration by intermittent positive pressure ventilation. This is usually necessary for prolonged or major surgery, particularly in the abdomen or thorax. It is also necessary in some emergency situations.

Muscle relaxants may also be used to facilitate assisted ventilation for long periods of time in the intensive care unit.

There are two main types of agent:

- *Depolarising.* These first stimulate contraction by their action at the neuromuscular junction and then produce paralysis. The only clinically important depolarising muscle relaxant is suxamethonium chloride.
- *Non-depolarising.* By contrast, these do not cause any muscle activity before relaxation. These are competitive blockers (see below) at the acetylcholine receptors on the neuromuscular junction. Drugs such as atracurium, vecuronium and pancuronium are examples.

The effects of these drugs can be reversed by the administration of acetylcholinesterase inhibitors, such as neostigmine, which increase the concentration of acetylcholine in the neuromuscular junction by preventing its breakdown. The increased concentrations of acetylcholine then compete with neuromuscular blocking drugs (hence the term competitive blockers) for receptors at the neuromuscular junction, and muscle power returns.

Suxamethonium

Suxamethonium is a depolarising neuromuscular blocking agent which provides very rapid muscle relaxation (within 30 seconds). It is therefore very useful in emergency work where rapid control of the airway is essential to avoid aspiration of stomach contents. Its effects usually wear off in 2–3 minutes. It is metabolised by plasma cholinesterase (also known as pseudocholinesterase). It does have side effects as follows:

- postoperative muscle pain
- bradycardia
- release (e.g. in the severely burned) of potassium from muscle cells into the bloodstream, which may cause cardiac arrest
- suxamethonium apnoea – approximately 1 in 3000 of the population have an inherited defect in cholinesterase which causes the muscle-paralysing effects to be prolonged, and anaesthesia and respiratory support must be maintained until the effects wear off
- acute anaphylactic shock (rare)
- malignant hyperpyrexia – a rare condition in which temperature control fails and death may follow.

Vecuronium, atracurium, rocuronium and pancuronium

These are longer-acting, competitive muscle relaxants. They take longer than suxamethonium to relax the muscles (approximately 1–3 minutes) but their effects last longer (sometimes between half an hour and 1 hour). Vecuronium is a useful muscle relaxant with very few side effects. It is metabolised in the liver and excreted via the kidneys.

Atracurium is also commonly used but can, as a side effect, release histamine; however, it has the advantage that it is degraded spontaneously in the bloodstream by a process called Hoffman degradation, which is dependent on the temperature and the pH of the plasma and is independent of liver and renal function. It can therefore be used in patients with renal or hepatic failure. Rocuronium is chemically similar to Vecuronium but has a quicker onset time of approx. 60 seconds. It has therefore been used in place of suxamethonium.

Pancuronium is a much longer-acting muscle relaxant often used during prolonged procedures.

ANALGESICS

Opioid analgesics

Most balanced anaesthetic techniques use opioids for analgesia. Opioid analgesics mimic endogenous opioid compounds which act at opioid receptors. There are three types of receptor:

- OP1 or δ (delta)
- OP2 or κ (kappa)
- OP3 or μ (mu)

The μ-receptor agonists are most commonly used. Drugs such as morphine and diamorphine have medium-term effects which last 2–4 hours. Shorter-acting opioid derivatives, such as fentanyl and alfentanil, are used intraoperatively for shorter procedures. Opioids can be administered by a number of different routes (see the section on postoperative analgesia).

Morphine

Morphine has potent analgesic and euphoric effects. It also depresses respiration by decreasing the respiratory response to increased levels of carbon dioxide in the blood, and respiration may stop altogether. Among a host of other effects, morphine also causes nausea and vomiting and should be given with an anti-emetic. The effects of morphine and other μ-agonist opioids may be antagonised by naloxone (Narcan). Morphine is metabolised in the liver to active metabolites which are excreted via the kidneys.

Diamorphine

This drug is the di-acetyl ester of morphine and has very similar effects. It is more potent than morphine because of its greater lipid solubility and is therefore given in lower doses. It is said to have less emetic effects and to cause more euphoria than morphine.

Fentanyl

This is a synthetic opioid which is commonly used intraoperatively. It crosses the blood – brain barrier rapidly, and its effects wear off within a relatively short time (≈30 minutes). It is a potent respiratory depressant. In common with the other opioids it also causes nausea and vomiting.

Alfentanil

This short-acting opioid has an even faster onset of action than fentanyl. It is also a very potent respiratory depressant.

Remifentanil

This drug has the fastest onset and offset time of all the opioids. It is also the most potent respiratory depressant. These properties make it the ideal opioid to use as an infusion during long procedures.

Tramadol

This is an opioid analgaesic agent which has other non-opioid analgaesic properties. It has fewer problems with sedation and respiratory depression than morphine. It can be given orally or parenterally.

Simple analgesics

Although simple analgesics such as paracetamol and aspirin are of limited value on their own after major surgery, they are a useful adjunct to analgesic regimens and may reduce the dose of opioid drugs required.

Paracetamol

Formulations combining paracetamol and codeine are extremely useful in the management of day surgical operations and also if given on a regular basis for more extensive procedures (e.g. co-dydramol contains 500 mg of paracetamol and 10 mg of codeine).

NSAIDs

Non-steroidal anti-inflammatory drugs play an increasing role in the management of postoperative pain. They are effective analgesics and, as part of a balanced approach to pain control, reduce markedly the requirements for opioids. They can now be delivered by all routes (oral, rectal, intramuscular, intravenous and topical). Caution must be applied when using these drugs, as they have well-recognised, serious side effects in the vulnerable patient (e.g. gastric ulceration with bleeding [Ch. 22] and renal failure). The most popular drugs in current use are diclofenac sodium and parecoxib.

MISCELLANEOUS DRUGS

Many other drugs are used as part of a balanced technique.

Benzodiazepines

These drugs are used for premedication (e.g. temazepam) and for short-acting intravenous sedation during procedures carried out under regional anaesthesia (e.g. midazolam).

Anti-emetics

Different classes of anti-emetics are used to prevent and treat postoperative nausea and vomiting. Metoclopramide and domperidone act at dopamine receptors in the midbrain. Anticholinergic agents (e.g. hyoscine) affect the so-called vomiting centre, also in the midbrain. Antihistamines (e.g. cyclizine) are effective but can cause sedation. $5HT_3$ antagonists (e.g. ondansetron) are extremely effective, as are steroids (e.g. dexamethasone).

POSTOPERATIVE CARE

Recovery from anaesthesia

Immediate recovery occurs first in the operating room and then continues as the patient is transferred into the recovery unit, which should be a dedicated one, designed, staffed and equipped to deal with all aspects of recovery. Patients are managed in separate bays, each equipped with oxygen, suction and monitoring equipment and adequately staffed by specially trained personnel skilled in management of the unconscious patient, particularly in airway management. As recovery proceeds, vital signs are monitored and the management of fluid balance and oxygenation continues. A check is kept on the operative site to detect any immediate problems such as bleeding. Pain control is also assessed and treatment instituted in consultation with anaesthetic staff. Before a patient is considered fit to leave the recovery room and return to the ward, a number of criteria must be met (Box 6.11). Those who have undergone major procedures or who have complex medical problems may need transfer to a high-dependency unit (HDU) or an intensive care unit (ICU).

Special features of recovery from day surgery

In the UK there has been a considerable increase in day surgery in recent years (Ch. 5). In some hospitals, 60% of routine surgery is done in day-care units. It is crucial to the success of this type of service that recovery is sufficiently rapid to allow a safe return home. It is essential that suitable patients are chosen and that the procedures they are to undergo are relatively brief and unlikely to result in significant postoperative pain. The criteria used to discharge patients home after day surgery are similar to those used to discharge in-patients back to hospital wards. However, it is essential that patients and their carers are informed about what to expect when they are at home. In particular, they should be given clear instructions on the analgesia that has been prescribed. With careful patient selection and preoperative education, even fairly complex operations (e.g. laparoscopic hernia repair) can be carried out successfully without in-patient hospital admission.

Box 6.11 Criteria for discharge from the recovery unit

- Awake and cooperative
- Cardiovascularly stable
- Well oxygenated
- Pain controlled
- Surgical site uncomplicated
- Postoperative fluids and drugs charted

Complications during the recovery period

Hypoxia

There are a number of causes:

- respiratory depression caused by anaesthetic agents and analgesics
- unconsciousness with airway obstruction
- ventilation/perfusion mismatch – poorly controlled pain with inadequate expansion, particularly of the lung bases, and unresolved pulmonary collapse; most resolve in a relatively short time and can be treated easily with supplementary oxygen.

The requirement for oxygen after operation varies with the type of operation and the patient's pre-existing condition. However, all patients should receive postoperative oxygen even after minor surgery, and the decision to discontinue oxygen should be taken with care and in the light of objective evidence of adequate oxygenation.

Postoperative nausea and vomiting (PONV)

Both of these are common and distressing and are the result of a combination of many factors. Anaesthetic agents and analgesics are often implicated. It is recognised that certain procedures have a very high incidence of PONV (e.g. middle ear operations and gynaecological procedures). A past history of PONV is a common feature. Management is with the agents discussed above.

Postoperative pain

One widely used definition of pain is an unpleasant experience caused by a noxious substance, tissue damage or anticipated tissue damage: this produces a reaction consisting of withdrawal response, metabolic response, hormonal response and conscious aversion. To discuss treatment it is necessary to look briefly at how pain is produced. Tissue damage (e.g. surgical operation, trauma) causes the release of chemicals – so-called pain mediators (e.g. histamine, bradykinins) – at the site of injury. These stimulate nerve fibres which transmit the sensation of pain via the spinal cord to higher centres where the pain is experienced. Therefore it seems logical that there are several points along this pathway where it might be possible to interrupt and alter the pain message. Anti-inflammatory agents inhibit the release of pain mediators at the site of injury. Local anaesthetic agents can block peripheral and central nerves to prevent the impulses reaching the brain. Opioids (e.g. morphine) act centrally to alter the perception of pain.

Why should pain be treated?

The answer to this question may seem rather obvious. However, the effects of pain on the postoperative patient are diffuse. There is of course the unpleasant experience for the patient and the psychological upset this causes. However, poorly controlled pain can lead to a number of other unhelpful sequelae. Patients who have undergone abdominal or thoracic surgery find breathing and coughing difficult and painful. The consequent inadequate ventilation can lead to hypoxia in the immediate postoperative period and chest infections subsequently (Ch. 16). Chest infections can seriously complicate the recovery period. There is something of a vicious circle here because the prophylaxis and treatment of chest infection involve vigorous physiotherapy, which further exacerbates the problems of pain control. Postoperative pain can lead to hypertension and tachycardia which may stress a vulnerable myocardium. Poor pain control can lead to a slow recovery and delayed mobilisation with increased risk of other complications such as deep vein thrombosis (Ch. 29).

How should pain be treated?

A number of techniques and drugs are used. The drugs have been described earlier. Important underlying principles before prescription are as follows:

- Each patient should be treated as an individual and likely needs assessed preoperatively.
- The patient should be involved in and understand the decisions taken.
- Patient confidence in the plan for pain control is vital.
- An important part of pre-assessment is to evaluate which analgesics are safe and whether any technique (e.g. an epidural) is contraindicated.

There are two other important matters. First, postoperative pain is much easier to manage if the patient wakes up with pain already minimised; management should therefore begin during or even before surgery – so-called pre-emptive analgesia. Second, there are a number of different groups of drugs that are analgesic in action; good analgesia can best be achieved by a combination of these, which in turn enables smaller doses of each type to be used, so lessening the risks of side effects (balanced analgesia).

A fairly simple guide to postoperative pain management is given in Table 6.3. It is obvious that the major operations are those where the problems are most difficult.

Management of pain after major operations

A combination of drugs usually produces the best results. This may include the use of local anaesthetic agents either at the site of surgery or as part of a regional nerve block (e.g. epidural), plus NSAIDs and opioids. The administration of opioids has changed in recent years, and a closer examination of the place of morphine is a useful example.

For many years, morphine given intramuscularly at regular intervals was the mainstay of control. Although this method is not optimum, if morphine is given at regular intervals and at a correct dosage, good analgesia can be achieved. The method is also cheap and safe. However, on a busy surgical ward it can be difficult to make sure that administration is sufficiently frequent and adjusted to individual needs, and therefore other techniques were developed. Morphine by bolus intravenous injection is a good way of rapidly controlling acute postoperative pain, but its use further into the postoperative period is limited by safety factors and the intermittent nature of the analgesia achieved. Morphine by intravenous infusion allows a steady concentration to build up in the blood. Although this smoothes out some of the breakthrough pain experienced with intramuscular injections, it is difficult to select the correct infusion rate, and altering the infusion rate takes a significant time to achieve results. This has led to the widespread introduction of patient-controlled devices (patient-controlled analgesia, PCA).

Patient-controlled analgesia

The morphine is housed in the reservoir of a pump system and connected to an intravenous cannula; the patient controls the delivery of the drug by pressing a button which causes the device to deliver a predetermined dose (Fig. 6.11). There follows a period (lock-out time) when a further press is ineffective, which protects against over-administration. Use of such a device allows the patient to determine analgesic dose according to perceived pain. The device also gives the patient confidence that analgesia is readily available when necessary.

Opioids can also be administered as part of an epidural regimen, usually in combination with a local anaesthetic. However, it is important to note that more-involved pain management techniques such as this need more-intensive nursing and are probably unsuitable for most general surgical wards. The adverse effects of opioids are discussed above. Box 6.12 lists some suggested doses.

Table 6.3 Standard postoperative analgesia regimens (fit, adult, male, 70 kg)

Grade of surgery	Example	Postoperative analgesia
Minor	Lipoma removal	Paracetamol, 1 g, 6-hourly
Intermediate	Arthroscopy Hernia repair	Co-dydramol, 2 tablets, 6-hourly + diclofenac, 50 mg orally, 8-hourly
Major	Laparotomy Hip replacement	Morphine PCA, 1 mg bolus, 5 min lock-out + diclofenac, 50 mg orally, 8-hourly

PCA, patient-controlled analgesia.

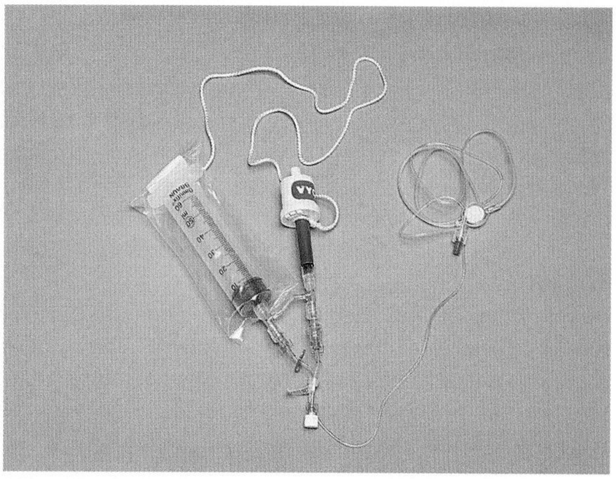

Fig. 6.11 A device for patient-controlled analgesia.

Management of chronic pain

There is a large group of patients who have continuous pain. The types, sites and causes of this pain are many and varied, and most specialties have some patients who experience chronic pain. Anaesthetists have now developed a major interest in this group. The practical skills and the knowledge of analgesics required for standard anaesthetic practice are readily transposed into the management of chronic pain. Most large hospitals now have a chronic pain clinic headed by an anaesthetist. However, it is important to note that the initial goal of management of any patient with chronic pain is to endeavour to achieve a diagnosis and then to treat the underlying cause. A chronic pain specialist uses the skills of a number of other practitioners to treat patients, e.g. psychologists, physiotherapists and acupuncturists.

In most cases, the management of chronic pain involves a multifaceted approach. In chronic back pain (a common condition), an epidural injection may be followed by a course of physiotherapy. At the same time, various analgesics may be prescribed and amitriptyline used for depression. Antidepressants, at the dosages used in chronic pain, seem to have several effects. They have a direct and indirect analgesic effect, the mode of action being unclear. They also help the patient to sleep, and the direct antidepressant effect is helpful.

Box 6.12 Standard opioid doses (fit, adult, male, 70 kg)

Morphine (i.m.)	10 mg, 2-hourly PRN
Morphine (PCA)	1 mg bolus, 5 min lock-out
Diamorphine (i.m.)	5 mg, 2-hourly
Pethidine (i.m.)	75 mg, 2-hourly

FURTHER READING

Aitkenhead AR, Smith G, Rowbotham DJ 2006 Textbook of anaesthesia, 5th edn. Churchill Livingstone, Edinburgh

Smith T, Pinnock C, Lin T, Jones R 2009 Fundamentals of anaesthesia, 3rd edn. Cambridge University Press, Cambridge

Allman K, McIndoe A, Wilson I 2009 Emergencies in anaesthesia, 2nd edn. OUP, Oxford

7 Perioperative management and postoperative complications

This chapter deals with the maintenance of patients before, during and after an operation and the complications which may ensue. For this purpose, an understanding of the physiological responses to injury (which are common to surgery, trauma and sepsis) is an essential foundation because the changes that occur influence management. The 20th century, particularly after 1930, has been noteworthy for the widespread application of new scientific knowledge and technology to improve perioperative care. Among the areas involved are anaesthesia (Ch. 6), ventilatory support (Chs 6 and 10), blood transfusion, renal dialysis, cardiopulmonary bypass (Ch. 17), antibiotics (Ch. 9) and parenteral nutrition (Ch. 10). Advances in all these and other areas have permitted major surgical procedures to become commonplace with minimal morbidity and mortality.

The growing therapeutic complexity of surgical care has led, as described in Chapter 1, to increased specialisation among doctors and the necessity for teamwork. However, the surgeon retains the primary responsibility for perioperative care.

Most complications that follow soon after operations are directly related to the operative procedure. Many can be avoided by good surgical technique. Careful perioperative care, however, can also decrease the incidence of complications and enhance the patient's chance of recovery.

PHYSIOLOGICAL BASIS FOR SURGICAL CARE

The biological response to injury can be thought of as a wake-up call to optimise performance and integrate the action of body systems (homeostasis) in the face of a potential threat to survival. Priorities are to ensure:

- oxygen delivery (Chs 6 and 10)
- tissue perfusion (Chs 6 and 10)
- acid–base equilibrium (Ch. 6)
- water and electrolyte conservation, balance and replacement
- availability of energy.

The injury response is phased and its effects include restrictions on the excretion of sodium and water, increased metabolic rate and protein catabolism. Mediators of the response include hormones (e.g. catecholamines, cortisol and glucagon), pro-inflammatory cytokines (e.g. tumour necrosis factor-alpha [TNF-α], interleukin-1 [IL-1] and interleukin-6 [IL-6]) and at the tissue level, arachidonic acid metabolites, oxygen free radicals, nitric oxide and the amino acid glutamine.

Water and electrolyte metabolism

In a 70 kg male, body composition is approximately:

- fat (15 kg)
- protein (12 kg)
- water (42 kg)
- glycogen and minerals (1 kg).

Total body water (TBW) is divided into two main compartments (Fig. 7.1):

- water around cells (extracellular fluid, ECF) – 19 L
- water in the cytoplasm (intracellular fluid, ICF) – 23 L.

The ECF (Fig. 7.2) is further subdivided into:

- interstitial – 15 L
- intravascular (plasma) – 3 L
- third space (transcellular – gastrointestinal and renal) – small (≈1 L) at any one moment but with a large rate of turnover: approximately 12 L/day for the GI tract and 170 L/day for glomerular filtration; an abnormal third space may develop if the normal transcapillary exchange is interfered with by, say, inflammation so that exudation exceeds reabsorption.

ECF contains sodium (Na) at 124 mmol/L and potassium (K) at 4 mmol/L. ICF has concentrations of Na and K opposite to that of ECF: Na at 10 mmol/L and K at 150 mmol/L maintained by the energy-dependent Na/K pump in the cell membrane. With the exception of 1 L of non-exchangeable water enfolded in the quaternary structure of protein molecules, all water molecules in the various compartments and most non-ionised small molecules (e.g. urea) are freely diffusible. The result is that osmolality (overall osmotic concentration in

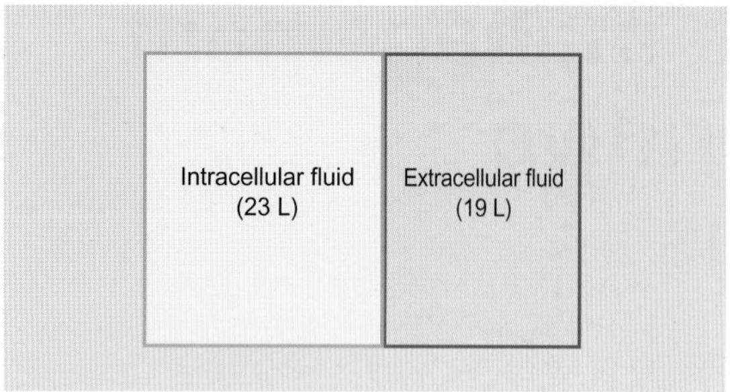

Fig. 7.1 Total body water.

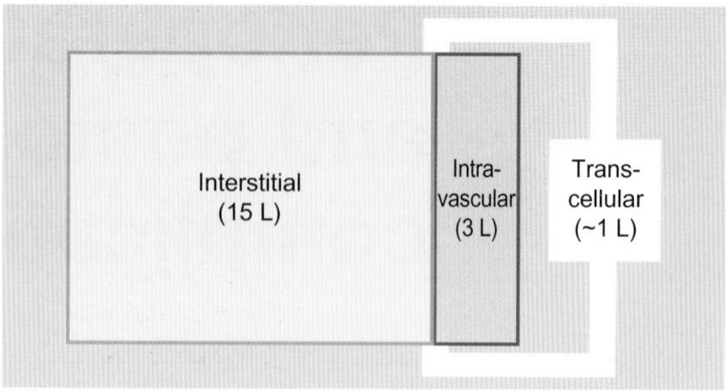

Fig. 7.2 Extracellular water.

Table 7.1 24-hour intake and output of water and electrolytes in health

Substance	Intake	Excretion and route
Water	2000–2500 mL (further 500 mL of water of oxidation which must be taken into consideration if renal excretion is limited)	Kidney (1500 mL) and insensible loss (respiratory and sweating, 1000 mL)
Sodium	100 mmol	Kidney (although sweat may also contain substantial quantities at up to 120 mmol/L)
Potassium	Up to 100 mmol	Kidney; restricted input is not followed by fall in excretion

mmol/kg) is maintained uniform throughout the body except at special sites such as the transcellular water in the kidney.

The 24-hour intake and output of water in health is shown in Table 7.1. Sodium intake varies widely with diet, but in the developed world is between 50 and 100 mmol/day. Excretion, mainly via the kidneys, is regulated by the distal renal tubule, which is the effector organ of the renin–angiotensin–mineralocorticoid endocrine axis. If input of Na falls, so does renal output and, in consequence, the volume of the ECF and tissue perfusion are maintained. If extrarenal losses – vomit, diarrhoea, increased sweating – occur, compensation is not possible (except by replacement by therapy) and the ECF shrinks. Requirements for K are of similar magnitude, approximately 40–80 mmol/day. Excretion is via the kidney and, in contrast to Na, persists even when intake is reduced.

During the perioperative period in major procedures, intravenous (i.v.) fluids are often required for a variable period until oral intake can be re-established. As part of the response to injury, the rate of secretion of cortisol, aldosterone and antidiuretic hormone (ADH) is increased, with the effects in the first 24–48 postoperative (or post-injury) hours of:

- reduction in renal excretion of Na and consequently of water, so that osmolality remains constant
- increase in renal excretion of K, some of which results from tissue damage and breakdown of cells
- decreased renal water excretion with a urine of low volume and high concentration, unresponsive to the normal effect of any increase in water intake.

After this time, and depending on the degree of surgical trauma and other factors such as sepsis, Na retention (and consequently water retention) may continue, with increased K excretion.

Management

Water and electrolyte therapy (indexed to a 70 kg adult male) are divided into: maintenance needs, restoration of pre-existing deficits and replacement of ongoing losses.

Provision of maintenance requirements

- Water – 100 mL/hour, adjusted upwards for fever and/or high ambient temperature
- Sodium – 75 mmol/day but can be further reduced over the first 2 days
- Potassium – 60 mmol/day.

Replacement of pre-existing deficits

Loss of extracellular fluid is combined loss of sodium and water (commonly called dehydration in clinical practice although that word literally means loss of water alone) and is replaced with fluids which have a sodium content close to that in the extracellular space, e.g. 0.9% saline or Hartmann's (Ringer's lactate) solution.

Loss from the stomach has special features. Although hydrogen ions are lost, renal compensation takes place, with reabsorption increased by the kidney and excretion of potassium and bicarbonate also raised. In consequence, hypochloraemic alkalosis and hypokalaemia may develop, and slightly more complicated therapy is required.

Pure water loss occurs only when either access to water is impossible (trapped patients after injury) or there is a high obstruction to the gastrointestinal tract (usually oesophageal). Replacement is enteral if the obstruction can be bypassed or by isotonic (6%) dextrose solution given intravenously.

Replacement of ongoing losses

The commonest such losses are:

- gastrointestinal – nasogastric aspirate or vomit, fistula and diarrhoea
- loss into an abnormal third space (see above), usually the result of inflammation, e.g. the retroperitoneal effusion that occurs in pancreatitis (Ch. 22).

Assessment is by careful recording of fluid balance, supplemented where possible by daily weighing. Measured upper GI losses are replaced with isotonic sodium-containing solutions – 0.9% saline or Ringer's lactate – supplemented by potassium.

In losses from gastrointestinal fistulae or diarrhoea, increased amounts of potassium are usually required in that the more distal in the intestine the source, the higher the potassium content.

Third space losses (which are not directly assessable) are replaced with Ringer's lactate solution; the volume administered is determined by observation of those clinical features which indicate a normal ECF volume (adequate filling of the veins and normal central venous pressure; satisfactory perfusion, including renal perfusion and normal urinary output).

Favourable or unfavourable responses to a fluid challenge may also be helpful.

Types of fluid

Fluids can be divided into crystalloids or colloids. Examples of crystalloids include 0.9% saline, dextrose saline, Ringer's lactate solution and Hartmann's solution. Colloids contain larger molecules, which are less readily filtered by the kidney and stay in the intravascular compartment, and there acting as a plasma expander by retaining extracellular fluid within the vasculature. Examples of natural colloids are blood and albumin; gelatin-based infusions are synthetic colloids. In general on the wards, crystalloids are used. Potassium can be added to the bags in the form of KCl.

Energy requirements

Assessment of energy requirements in surgical patients must be undertaken with the factors indicated in Box 7.1 in mind. Body energy stores contain approximately 2000 kcal of glucose as glycogen (stored by liver and muscle) and 125 000 kcal of free fatty acids (FFAs) and glycerol hydrolysable from fat (for a healthy weight adult).

Tissues (red blood cells, renal medulla, brain and healing wounds), which are largely obligate users of glucose, adapt gradually over some days of starvation to the use of ketones derived from FFAs. Once glycogen stores are exhausted (approximately 24–36 hours), a minimum of 500 kcal/day of glucose is generated by gluconeogenesis from amino acids (plasma protein, muscle and visceral sources). The term 'body protein reserves' is inaccurate; any but the most trivial loss of protein leads to impairment of function, e.g. muscle weakness and immune deficiency. The theoretical benefit of providing glucose in standard intravenous regimens, which reduces protein breakdown during starvation to a minimum, cannot be relied on in practice adequately to prevent or reverse gluconeogenesis from amino acids, because of the altered metabolic milieu of the injured surgical patient.

Box 7.1 Factors affecting energy requirements in the postoperative period

- Body weight (fat-free mass)
- Degree of surgical trauma
- Sepsis
- Nutritional status.

Energy expenditure

In health, total energy expenditure (TEE) is approximately 40 kcal/kg body weight per day. Resting energy expenditure (REE) is the baseline level of the body's metabolic machinery, i.e. basal metabolic rate (BMR) plus the thermic effect of ingested food (dietary-induced thermogenesis, DIT) – approximately 25 kcal/kg body weight per day. The difference between TEE and REE (15 kcal/kg body weight per day) is the net energy cost of exercise (activity energy expenditure, AEE).

Elevations of REE between 10% and 30%, often loosely referred to as hypermetabolism or hypercatabolism, are seen in the surgical patient and depend on the degree of surgical trauma and the presence of underlying sepsis. In surgery of low or intermediate severity, this increased REE is compensated for by a fall in AEE (the main cause is that ambulation is reduced perioperatively) and thus the energy requirement is unchanged at 40 kcal/kg body weight per day. In the more critically ill, considerable expansion of total body water (up to as much as 10 L) can be present; the energy requirement should then ideally be related to the metabolic body size, for which fat-free mass (FFM) is a good substitute, to give a figure of approximately 50 kcal/kg FFM per day. However, accurate methods of body composition analysis are not widely available, and body weight remains the usual index. Caution to avoid inadvertent overprescription of nutritional support is therefore required particularly in the obese and/or oedematous.

Management of energy provision

In most nutritional enteral or parenteral regimens, glucose and fat are usually delivered in roughly equal proportions, although for short-term supplementation (2 weeks), glucose as the sole energy source is acceptable. However, in major injury and sepsis, FFAs appear to be the preferred fuel source, and for this reason some fat should be provided. After 3–4 weeks, glucose-only regimens result in the clinical effects of essential FFA deficiency (a rash is the first sign), and subclinical effects are best avoided by the early provision of fat. Energy replacement may be enteral, provided that the gut is functioning, or parenteral, i.e. intravenous nutrition. Enteral nutrition has the advantage that the function of the cells of the gut is preserved, which may be of significance in the preservation of their metabolic role and also possibly in the prevention of mucosal atrophy and translocation of bacteria.

Respiratory function in relation to operation

The set of often-connected circumstances that threaten respiratory function in surgical patients includes:

- preoperative respiratory disease
- anaesthesia which may, because of a combination of positive-pressure ventilation (PPV) and the agents used, result in ventilation–perfusion (V/Q) mismatch and a fall in the arterial oxygen saturation (see also Ch. 6)
- correction of lowered arterial oxygen saturation by using an increased fraction of inspired oxygen. This reduces the biologically passive nitrogen skeleton of the inspired

gas mixture and leads to a patchy collapse of the bronchiolar–alveolar complex; further V/Q defects follow, and a vicious cycle is established
- hypoventilation and a reduced cough impulse after surgery, because of inadequate pain control, supine posture in bed, and the after-effects of anaesthesia and analgesia. Poor expansion of the lungs results, with the formation of mucus plugs to occlude bronchioles, leading to further collapse and atelectasis.

Pre-existing respiratory disorders are common because of cigarette smoking and the advanced age of many surgical patients. Restrictive and obstructive (reversible or otherwise) patterns are identifiable in patients with chronic emphysema, bronchitis and asthma. Otherwise healthy patients who have existing, or who are convalescent from, upper respiratory tract infections (URTIs) often have protracted periods of unusual bronchial hyperreactivity which puts them at increased risk of respiratory complications – these are avoidable if elective surgery is deferred. Preoperative treatment with incentive spirometry and chest physiotherapy appears to be of some value to improve overall pulmonary status in preparation for operation. Underlying pulmonary infections such as bronchitis or pneumonia should always be treated and operation delayed if possible because the ciliary paralysis that occurs with anaesthesia may cause severe postoperative pneumonia.

Routine preventative respiratory therapy is frequently used postoperatively to prevent pulmonary complications. Early mobilisation after operation is believed to improve the patient's overall respiratory status.

In high-risk patients, routine postoperative prophylactic chest physiotherapy has been shown to decrease the frequency of pulmonary infection significantly.

In seriously ill patients on respiratory support in the intensive care unit and who are on intravenous nutrition (IVN), high-energy infusions which utilise glucose as the sole energy source may lead to difficulty in disconnection from the ventilator; the cause is the high output of carbon dioxide when energy supply is from glucose (respiratory quotient 1) as compared with fat (respiratory quotient in the region of 0.75). The acidosis produced results in hyperventilation.

FEATURES OF PREOPERATIVE ASSESSMENT

Preoperative assessment is now often nurse delivered and led by the anaesthetists, it includes:

- screening (Ch. 4) to identify unexpected conditions or medications which may add to the risk and complexity of perioperative management
- evaluation of existing comorbid conditions and their potential impact on risk
- assessment of these comorbidities in planning the most appropriate operative procedure and care
- optimising pre-existing conditions to reduce the risk of operation
- initiation of standard perioperative regimens, e.g. preventative antibiotics (Ch. 9) and prophylaxis of deep vein thrombosis.

A routine history of the present complaint(s) and the illness for which surgery is planned must be recorded together with a past history of other conditions and enquiry in relation to other body systems. Additionally it is important to gain a social history and record a preoperative level of functioning in the elderly. During physical examination it is important both to confirm that the indications for surgery have not changed and to undertake a comprehensive examination particularly of the cardiovascular and respiratory systems. Finally, review the medications so that certain patients can be admitted early – e.g. insulin-dependent diabetics may need to be placed on an insulin sliding scale, and patients on warfarin will require that the warfarin be stopped and a heparin infusion started preoperatively

Investigations are considered in Chapter 4.

Assessment of risk

General and specific risk factors for operation are shown in Box 7.2 (see also Ch. 6).

Patient preparation for theatre

(See also Ch. 6.)

Psychological preparation

To undergo an operation is a major life event. In addition to the procedure itself, the underlying disease may be a cause

Box 7.2 Risk factors for operation

General factors
- Extremes of age
- Poor nutritional status
- Cardiovascular disease
- Diabetes mellitus
- Chronic respiratory disease
- Systemic infection
- Dehydration or other metabolic abnormalities
- Renal impairment
- Hepatic disease
- Obesity
- Malignant disease.

Specific factors
- Previous operation at the same site – increased operative difficulty and complication rate
- Local infection – wound or deep infection
- Bladder outflow obstruction – urinary retention
- Chronic airways disease – pneumonia
- Thrombotic tendency – deep vein thrombosis/pulmonary embolism
- Haemorrhagic disorder or anticoagulant therapy – wound haematoma or postoperative haemorrhage
- Previous radiotherapy – poor wound or anastomotic healing/dehiscence
- Steroid treatment or cytotoxic chemotherapy – infection, impaired wound healing
- Peptic ulcer disease or NSAID treatment – gastrointestinal haemorrhage

of considerable stress, especially in patients with malignancy, those needing to undergo life-threatening procedures such as coronary artery bypass (Ch. 17) and transplantation (Ch. 13), and those in whom the diagnosis is uncertain. These situations evoke a natural response of fear and anxiety with which even a well-adjusted individual with good support may find it difficult to cope. Surgeons, naturally enough, have a tendency to focus on the technical surgical problem but must also be able to recognise and respond appropriately to psychological distress. Excessive fear and anxiety are often the result of inadequate communication. The importance of clear and honest interchange of views and a willingness to spend time discussing the issues of greatest concern to the patient cannot be overemphasised. Sometimes specialised input will also be required, e.g. from support nurses or psychologists, and is best sought at an early stage. Such assistance is usually accepted if presented in a non-threatening way.

Somatisation – the exaggeration or invention of physical symptoms – is more common, and an operation should not be lightly recommended if symptoms are atypical. However, it is imperative to remember that people with psychological and mental disorders are not immune from physical illness and are entitled to the same consideration as others who present with similar clinical features.

Skin preparation

This is discussed in detail in Chapter 5.

Diet and bowel preparation

Common practice is that a patient who is to have a general anaesthetic is instructed not to have anything by mouth for 6 hours beforehand so as to minimise the risk of vomiting and aspiration, However, several studies have shown that a carbohydrate drink 2–4 hours preoperatively is safe and may have some benefit by modifying the stress response to surgery. Obviously these methods are not always either possible (emergencies) or effective (bowel obstruction, gastric stasis), and in such cases anaesthetists take specific measures to protect the airway, especially during induction (Ch. 6). For most operations, other specific dietary constraints are not necessary preoperatively. Elective operations on the large bowel are traditionally preceded by mechanical bowel preparation (see below) to reduce the risk of septic complications which may follow faecal contamination of the operative field. Recently, several randomised studies have called into question the need to do this for elective large bowel resection when systemic antibiotic prophylaxis is used, and a recent Cochrane Review concluded that there was no evidence to support this practice.

Mechanical bowel preparation

This combines a low-residue diet with either purgatives, isotonic lavage solution (e.g. polyethylene glycol) or osmotically active agents. The disadvantages of mechanical preparations include poor patient tolerance and fluid and electrolyte disturbances. Those who receive mechanical bowel preparation and who have cardiovascular or renal impairment are also given maintenance intravenous fluids with potassium supplementation overnight before operation to prevent dehydration and hypokalaemia. Many colorectal surgeons now limit bowel prepartion to a preoperative enema (e.g. phosphate) for left-sided resections only.

Informed consent

This is discussed in detail in Chapter 2.

THE POSTOPERATIVE PERIOD

Postoperative orders

Good communication between the team in the operating room and those responsible for postoperative care is essential. Verbal communication alone is not adequate, and a handwritten note of the procedure should be made immediately and leave the operating room with the patient accompanied by the anaesthetic chart and notes (Clinical Box 7.1). The procedures to be followed must be stated precisely, in uniform terms and with clear legibility. The team (including the anaesthetist) states the specifics of postoperative management to nurses and other members of the healthcare team via the postoperative orders. The preoperative work-up should already be available in the notes (whether these are held in hard copy or on a computer), and to these should be

Clinical Box 7.1 **Sample postoperative orders**

Date	Signatory	Notes
13/5/04	Hardy	*Operation:* Surgeon: Mr Laurel Assistant: Dr Hardy *Findings:* Tumour upper rectum No evidence of metastatic disease or other abnormalities Bowel preparation adequate *Procedure:* Anterior resection; stapled colorectal anastomosis; leak test OK, not defunctioned. Pre-sacral drain. Blood loss = 600 mL. Patient stable throughout *Postoperative orders:* i.v. fluids as charted NG tube free drainage Ice to suck Routine observations & hourly urine output measurement. Maintain output at greater than 30 mL/h Epidural analgesia – see anaesthetic chart for protocol Chest physiotherapy as ordered s.c. heparin to continue Early mobilisation in consultation with surgical team i.v. ranitidine as prescribed

NB No rectally administered medications and no NSAIDs.

14/5/04		Check FBC, urea & electrolytes, creatinine

added the operative procedure performed and postoperative orders.

Postoperative observations

Clinical signs

A variety of physical signs are important to recognise in the postoperative period (Table 7.2). Other physical signs may be present after specific operative procedures, e.g. changes in pulse characteristics after vascular procedures or neurological changes after neurosurgical procedures. The postoperative instructions must be sufficiently clear so that the nursing staff can notice and report the development of such specific features.

Monitoring

This is the term commonly used for routine observations undertaken on the assumption that deviations from normal values, particularly if they are progressive, indicate that something may be amiss. What is measured is guided by a thorough understanding of the preoperative status and medical history, the diagnosis that led to the operation, what procedure was done and the circumstances. The variables chosen (often called 'vital signs') are mostly in the cardiovascular and respiratory systems, and are often combined to form an 'early warning' scoring system (Table 7.3) such as the Modified Early Warning Score (MEWS).

If the patient is sent to the intensive care unit (ICU), this usually implies that there are grounds for believing that the postoperative course may be complicated and that additional monitoring is required. Table 7.4 shows the additional vital signs frequently monitored.

Laboratory investigations

A variety of laboratory tests may be routinely obtained postoperatively to assess the patient's course and detect changes that may require management to be altered (Table 7.5). However, these should not be a substitute for careful physical examination.

In interpreting laboratory findings after major surgical procedures, the following are important:

- A surgical procedure always tends to make diabetics more hyperglycaemic, although this does not necessarily mean that either insulin or an increase in the dose usually being administered is required.
- Haemodilution after haemorrhage takes up to 24 hours. A continued significant fall in haemoglobin after this time usually means that there is further bleeding (see 'Postoperative haemorrhage' below).
- The white blood cell count normally increases slightly for 2–3 days after operation; marked elevation during this period or persistent elevation beyond this time usually indicates an infective or inflammatory process.

Table 7.2 Specific signs that may be important in the early postoperative period

Sign	Possible meanings
Respiratory distress: tachypnoea, cyanosis	Hypoxia
CNS signs	
CNS depression	Oversedation
	Carbon dioxide retention
Agitation	Blood loss
	Hypoxia
	Pain
Disorientation	Inappropriate sedation
	Hypoxia
Severe inappropriate pain	Local complication at site of operation – bleeding, leakage of secretions, ischaemia
Wound	
Bleeding	Uncontrolled blood vessel
Soft-tissue haematoma	Clotting disorder
Irregular pulse	Unrecognised cardiac disorder
Skin pallor, empty veins, hypotension, tachycardia	Hypovolaemia

Table 7.3 Routine postoperative monitoring of clinical signs

Measurement	Possible significance
Temperature	Excessive heat loss during surgery
Low	Reduced metabolic rate possibly from poor peripheral perfusion
High	Core but not peripheral – peripheral vasoconstriction possibly from blood loss
	Core and peripheral – 1–2°C normal in first 24 hours but thereafter may mean sepsis
Pulse rate, blood pressure	Changes beyond minor variations imply possible circulatory instability
Central venous pressure	Usually a sensitive guide to venous return to the heart
Respiratory rate	
Increased	Possible carbon dioxide retention or hypoxia
Decreased	Oversedation
Pulse oximetry	Arterial oxygen saturation
Urine output (hourly)	Indirect measure of renal perfusion and therefore of organ blood flow
Fluid intake/output	Necessary to ensure that neither over- nor under-infusion takes place

Table 7.4 Additional vital signs often measured in the ICU

Sign	Possible significance
Direct measurement of arterial pressure (indwelling catheter usually in radial artery)	Earlier detection of changes in blood pressure
Continuous monitoring of CVP	Assessment of venous return
Pulmonary artery pressure (indwelling pulmonary catheter)	Detection of left heart strain (myocardial failure or artery over-infusion) Determination of cardiac output by dilution techniques
Pulmonary artery wedge pressure (Swan–Ganz catheter)	As for pulmonary artery pressure
Continuous ECG	Detection of arrhythmias

Table 7.5 Laboratory investigations in routine postoperative management

Investigation	Purpose	Frequency
Blood glucose concentration in diabetics	Control of insulin administration	4–6-hourly
Haemoglobin concentration	After blood loss in excess of 500 mL	Once after lapse of 24–36 hours and also after transfusion
White cell count	If there is suspicion of sepsis	Daily if initial value raised
Platelet count, clotting studies	Unexplained bleeding	Daily if abnormality identified
Serum sodium, potassium and urea concentrations	When parenteral fluids are required, e.g. after some gastrointestinal operations	Daily
Arterial Po_2, Pco_2 and pH	In borderline respiratory insufficiency	Daily or more frequently if respiratory failure is imminent or identified

- Mild thrombocytopenia normally accompanies major injury, massive transfusion and major operative procedures (e.g. cardiac bypass).
- In healthy individuals with normal renal function there is a slight fall in serum sodium concentration for the first 2–5 days after a major operation, which may be exaggerated or prolonged if there is over-infusion of water. In patients with chronic renal or hepatic disease or an illness that causes electrolyte derangement, concentration changes are difficult to predict and frequent measurements are indicated so that life-threatening hypo- and hyperkalaemia can be rapidly corrected.

Intravenous (parenteral) fluids

The major (normal) changes in water and electrolyte metabolism which influence management are:

- secretion of ADH in response to pain and other stimuli so that the normal response to water administration is suppressed and urine of high concentration and low volume is inevitable; the duration of such a response is usually 24–36 hours. However, careful assessment of any postoperative patient with a low urine output is necessary as this may be indicative of hypovolaemic or septic shock.
- reduction in renal sodium excretion, for 36–48 hours
- increase in potassium excretion, which may be greater if there is a considerable amount of tissue damage.

For two reasons, nearly all patients return from the operating room with an intravenous infusion in place:

- Replacement has been considered necessary because of losses (insensible water, blood) sustained during the procedure.
- A route is required for the administration of drugs such as antibiotics.

Box 7.3 Standard daily postoperative maintenance fluids

Nature	Amount (L)	Time period (h)
Glucose 5% + 20 mmol/L potassium	1	8
Sodium chloride 0.9% + 20 mmol KCl each bag	1	8
Glucose 5% + 20 mmol/L potassium	1	8
Totals:		
Water	3 L	
Sodium	140 mmol	
Potassium	60 mmol	

Continued parenteral fluid is normally required only until enteral absorption is restored, usually within a few hours. Circumstances in which a more prolonged period of intravenous fluid infusion may be required are:

- gastrointestinal procedures where recovery of absorption of fluid may be delayed
- unconsciousness.

In an adequately hydrated patient who has undergone a procedure with minimal blood loss and for whom the postoperative recovery period is expected to be short, maintenance fluids are sufficient (Box 7.3).

Pain and its relief (see also Ch. 6)

Surgical intervention almost always causes pain. Because it can have serious physiological and psychological consequences (Table 7.6), prevention is best, but if that cannot be

Table 7.6 Effects of postoperative pain

Effect	Outcome
Decreased respiratory excursion	Hypoventilation Pulmonary collapse/consolidation
Gastrointestinal atony	Ileus, nausea and vomiting
Bladder atony	Urinary retention
Catecholamine release	Vasoconstriction; increased blood viscosity, clotting activity and platelet aggregation; raised cardiac work

Table 7.7 Tubes and drains after surgical procedures

Purpose	Nature	Indications
Gastrointestinal decompression	Medium-bore nasogastric tube; gastrostomy	Controversial – see text: operations on the GI tract; need for enteral nutrition
Removal of blood and serous fluids	Open drainage by soft rubber or plastic wicks	Extensive dissections
	Closed drainage by tubes, preferably with suction	Large dead space
Drainage of pus found at operation	Wicks or (preferably) tubes	Persistent infected cavity
Channel for exit if leakage occurs	Usually small- to medium-bore tubes often with suction	Suture lines in the GI tract (often routinely used but little evidence to support this)

completely achieved, rapid and adequate relief is essential. The intensity of postoperative pain that is perceived by the patient is influenced by:

- cultural and family background, upbringing, personality, constitution, past experiences and motivation
- amount of information provided preoperatively – the more the better is a good guide
- psychological factors which are often situation-specific, such as emotional arousal and fear; a calm reassuring attitude from the team is of great value and is helped by close interpersonal relations with the patient
- preoperative and postoperative support provided by the whole team, which includes nurses and physiotherapists.

Management

Management has increasingly become a specialised province of either the anaesthetist or a pain management team (Ch. 6).

Prevention

A caring, sympathetic and informative approach by the team does much to reduce the patient's perception of pain, as does assurance that any pain felt will be relieved at once. Physical methods for preventing pain include:

- gentle surgical technique with minimal tissue damage
- adequate immobilisation of areas that have been operated on when this is possible – limbs in particular and after orthopaedic procedures
- blockade of nerve impulses, which may be achieved at a number of sites on the afferent pathway: e.g. local anaesthetic infiltration of the operative field, regional nerve blocks, epidural or spinal injections or infusions.

Therapy

Most agents are better given on a regular basis rather than withheld until relief is asked for, particularly in the early postoperative period.

Non-steroidal anti-inflammatory agents and drugs such as aspirin and paracetamol are often sufficient for mild postoperative pain provided the patient can swallow.

Narcotic (opioid) analgesics have long been the main agents used to counteract postoperative pain, and morphine sulphate remains the drug most widely used. Immediately after operation the drug is given by the parenteral route either intramuscularly or intravenously. It is now common for a continuous infusion to be used so that saturation of opioid receptors in the brain is achieved. Such an infusion may be supplemented by patient-controlled analgesia (PCA) in which the patient can trigger the administration of a small bolus of drug by a syringe driver, which is programmed so as to avoid excessive self-administration. This technique has obvious advantages in terms of satisfaction and in reducing the load on the nursing staff. More complicated regimens including epidurals are considered in Chapter 6.

Tubes and drains

The nature of tubes and drains placed at operation varies with the operation performed and the individual surgeon (Table 7.7). A more detailed consideration is given in Chapter 5.

Decompression of the gastrointestinal tract

The rationale is that, in abdominal procedures, a period of gastrointestinal paralysis follows:

- abdominal incisions and handling of abdominal organs
- retroperitoneal dissection.

As a result, gastrointestinal secretions accumulate in the stomach and proximal small bowel and may cause vomiting and aspiration into the respiratory tree.

However, in spite of a good deal of study, the exact circumstances when this occurs have not been accurately established and there is little clinical evidence to support the routine use of either nasogastric intubation or gastrostomy.

Nasogastric tubes in particular are uncomfortable for the patient and may contribute to respiratory complications by making coughing more difficult. Surgical teams now usually adopt a highly selective policy. Nasogastric decompression is appropriate in any patient in whom nausea, vomiting or gastric distension cannot be otherwise controlled.

Urethral drainage

A balloon urethral (Foley) catheter is commonly used after major procedures and serves two main purposes:

- It alleviates discomfort and prevents urinary retention.
- It allows measurement of hourly urine output using a urometer collection device; this can be used as an indicator of renal (and therefore of other vital organ) perfusion.

When hourly or frequent assessment of urine volume is no longer required and the patient is thought able to void spontaneously, the catheter is removed. Voiding is affected by postoperative pain, drugs (opiates, anticholinergics), regional anaesthesia (caudal, spinal, epidural blockade) and any pre-existing prostatism (Ch. 33). Males need to be comfortable enough to stand out of bed. Once the catheter is removed, documentation of adequate voiding is required. Even if voiding is successful, it is important not to allow the bladder to become overdistended, because this delays recovery of detrusor tone and may even necessitate the discharge of the patient with a catheter in situ and subsequent return for a retrial of voiding.

Parenteral and enteral feeding

This type of feeding is discussed in detail in Chapter 10.

POSTOPERATIVE COMPLICATIONS

All operations have a risk of complications. Complications can be divided into general or specific. General complications can occur after any operation, irrespective of its site, i.e. complications related to the general anaesthetic itself. Specific complications are the consequence of a particular surgical procedure.

This classification can be further subdivided into complications that occur immediately (in the operation or within the first 24 hours), early (within the first week) or late.

Good examples of immediate general complications are those that occur in the anaesthetic room, such as unexpected reactions to the anaesthetic agents or trauma to the mouth and teeth during intubation. Early general complications include chest infections, urinary retention, urinary tract infections, pulmonary emboli and deep vein thrombosis. An example of a late general complication includes pressure sores or problems in the healing process, such as keloid scars. Immediate specific complications are those that occur in the operation, such as damage to nearby structures. Early specific complications depend on the procedure and include abdominal or thoracic wound infections, anastomotic leaks or prosthetic infections. Late specific complications include incisional hernias or reoccurrence of the specific disease.

Trainees (interns) play an essential part in the recognition and management of impending or actual complications, as do nursing staff. In consequence, students, all of whom will become Foundation Programme trainees must understand what may happen in the immediate aftermath of a surgical procedure. Each of the important complications alluded to above will now be considered in more detail below.

Wound infection

Surgical wounds are categorised into four classes:

- clean
- clean–contaminated
- contaminated
- dirty.

A clean wound is achieved by aseptic technique (Ch. 5) and is not exposed to any additional contamination during the procedure (e.g. inguinal hernia repair, thyroidectomy). A clean–contaminated wound occurs when it is exposed during the procedure to known or potentially infected material (e.g. appendicectomy for uncomplicated appendicitis, elective bowel resection). A contaminated wound is exposed to more major contamination (e.g. after spillage of GI tract contents or operations on an infected urinary or respiratory tract). A dirty wound is one that is contaminated by established sepsis (e.g. laparotomy in peritonitis, thoracotomy in empyema).

In general, the rate of infection is lowest for clean and highest for dirty wounds; however, other patient factors (e.g. immunosuppression, shock) and surgical factors (e.g. duration of the operation, wound haematoma) also have an influence.

Surgical preventative measures

Wound management

Occasionally in contaminated wounds or if there is a delay in instituting management, the risk of wound sepsis is high and it is more effective initially to leave the wound open and then undertake delayed primary or secondary closure (Ch. 8).

Skin preparation

Any surgical wound, including abdominal wounds, can become infected with skin organisms such as *Staphylococcus aureus* (pus-forming) or *Streptococcus pyogenes* (wound cellulitis). Measures to reduce the risk are considered in Chapter 5.

Antibiotics

For clean and clean–contaminated wounds, antibiotic prophylaxis – by saturating the tissues with the agent before (in the case of an operation) or as soon as possible after the wound has been sustained (injury) – has been shown to reduce the incidence of wound infection by about two-thirds. The important issues to consider are:

- choice of agent
- route of administration

- timing
- duration of prophylaxis.

The choice of agent must reflect the likely spectrum of contaminating organisms. For operations that involve the upper GI tract, this is predominantly facultative aerobic Gram-negative bacilli such as *Escherichia coli*. Examples of antibiotics that provide prophylaxis against Gram-negative organisms include second- and third-generation cephalosporins, aminoglycosides and clavulinic acid/amoxicillin. In the lower GI tract, additional cover for anaerobes (mainly *Bacteroides*) is required. Selected second- and third-generation cephalosporins have some activity against anaerobes, but metronidazole is usually given in addition. Clavulinic acid/amoxicillin provides good prevention against anaerobes, but the aminoglycosides do not. Gram-negative bacilli often contaminate the obstructed urinary tract, and the spectrum of normal vaginal flora is similar to that found in the lower gut.

The route of administration depends on the drug and the patient. A non-functioning gut or a poorly absorbed drug contraindicates oral administration. Rectal administration is cheap and effective for some antibiotics (e.g. metronidazole). However, the intravenous route is most commonly used. Timing is important, as the aim is to achieve adequate tissue levels at the time of contamination. Rectal or orally administered antibiotics may be given with the premedication (about 1 hour preoperatively), whereas intravenous antibiotics are usually given on induction of anaesthesia.

In the past, prophylactic antibiotics were often continued for up to 72 hours postoperatively. However, more recent trials have shown that a single dose with a drug whose half-life is long enough to maintain effective levels for 6–8 hours is just as effective. In prolonged procedures a second dose should be administered after 6 hours.

Prosthesis infection

A wide variety of biomechanical devices are implanted surgically. These include:

- artificial heart valves (Ch. 17)
- vascular grafts (Ch. 29)
- joint replacements (Ch. 34)
- vascular access devices (e.g. for administration of drugs or renal dialysis)
- cardiac pacemakers.

Prosthesis infection can be life-threatening (e.g. an infected prosthetic heart valve) and is a disaster for the patient, which at least necessitates removal of the infected device. Therefore, whenever possible, prosthetic devices are inserted via surgical incisions made under ideal conditions (Ch. 5). Many surgeons, particularly for orthopaedic implantations (Ch. 34), routinely use antibiotics even though the procedure is clean. The most common contaminating organisms are derived from the skin or, more exceptionally, from the operating room environment. Infection subsequent to implantation may also occur from transient bacteraemia. Organisms that have become implanted in a prosthesis may remain silent for months or years before giving rise to symptoms.

Antibiotic prophylaxis

Antibiotic prophylaxis against prosthesis infection is combined with meticulous care to protect the operating field (Ch. 5). The agent should cover staphylococcal species, including *Staph. epidermidis*. The principles that govern timing, route and duration of therapy are similar to those for prophylaxis of wound infection.

A patient with a prosthesis already in place should be given antibiotics in any procedure that might cause transient bacteraemia (e.g. a dental extraction).

Taking all of these factors into account, there are a number of different antibiotic prophylactic regimens suitable for any given procedure. The final choice is usually dictated by local hospital policy, taking into account:

- known local antibiotic sensitivities
- need to reserve important therapeutic agents for use in therapy and to avoid the ever-present risk of the emergence of resistant strains
- the consequences of infection
- cost.

Most hospitals have an Infection Control Committee that monitors local trends and conditions and provides guidelines (Ch. 9).

Haemorrhage and circulatory complications

Correct diagnosis of circulatory failure (rapid low-volume pulse, hypotension) in the postoperative period is essential because management can be life saving and has to be instituted as a matter of considerable urgency. The possible aetiological factors that need to be considered are listed in Box 7.4.

Haemorrhage

Haemorrhage can be divided into primary (occurring during the operation), reactionary (at the end of an operation when cardiac output and blood pressure return to normal and a previous dry wound begins to bleed) and secondary haemorrhage that occurs several days after the operation.

Major postoperative bleeding can be recognised by:

- evidence of overt bleeding, including heavily bloodstained fluid from a drain if present
- cold and wet (clammy) peripheries together with other symptoms and signs of hypovolaemia including anxiety, tachycardia, hypotension, tachypnoea, and low-volume urine output
- distension after abdominal procedures.

Usually the diagnosis is self-evident, but occasionally it may not be apparent that major bleeding has occurred,

Box 7.4 Causes of postoperative circulatory collapse

- Haemorrhage
- Severe sepsis including septicaemia
- Myocardial infarction
- Pulmonary embolism
- Hypersensitivity reaction

Table 7.8 Quantifying hypovolaemic shock

	Blood loss (%)	Blood loss (mL) for 70 kg adult	Pulse	Pulse pressure	Blood pressure	Respiratory rate	Urine output	Mental state
Class I	<15	750	Normal	Normal	Normal	Normal	Normal	Mildly anxious
Class II	15–30	750–1500	↑	↓	Normal	↑	↓	Anxious ++
Class III	30–40	1500–2000	↑++	↓++	↓	↑ +	Almost nil	Confused
Class IV	> 40	>2000	↓+++	↓+++	↓+++	↑+++	Nil	Lethargic/ unconscious

particularly if the patient is obese or if the drain malfunctions because of obstruction by clot. In such circumstances the diagnosis may need to be confirmed by urgent, repeated haemoglobin estimation and by ultrasound examination.

Table 7.8 provides a classification of degree of hypovolaemic shock.

Management

The loss is stopped by control of the source of bleeding, correction of any coagulopathy, and the patient must be assessed for the need for a transfusion, guided in rate and quantity by the circulatory indices. Reoperation may be required to control a bleeding point.

SIRS and sepsis – see also Chapter 9

Septic shock is associated with:

- surgical procedures carried out in the presence of sepsis
- technical failure (anastomotic dehiscence) with intraperitoneal or intrathoracic leakage of gastrointestinal contents
- general spread from a focus, particularly if there is a reduced ability of the body to resist the multiplication of the organisms (impaired immunity, leucopenia)
- bloodstream contamination from a device, most commonly a central venous cannula.

A direct effect of circulating cytokines and other inflammatory mediators is to cause arteriolar dilatation so that, in contrast to other forms of circulatory failure, the peripheries may be warm. In addition there is loss of circulating blood volume as a result of capillary leak. If the infection is overwhelming, the blood pressure is profoundly reduced (<100 mmHg systolic) and the circulation resembles that of profound hypovolaemia.

Usually the clinical features are:

- high pyrexia
- hypotension
- tachycardia
- a warm periphery.

Investigation

Venous blood is sent for culture, but even if this proves negative, the diagnosis of severe sepsis may still be correct and treatment should be begun with a best-guess antibiotic combination. A search is made for a focus, e.g. a central venous catheter or an undrained abscess.

Management

Resuscitation is with intravenous fluids and intravenous antibiotics. Re-exploration may be indicated to deal with a septic focus or a technical failure.

Myocardial infarction and pulmonary embolism

This is not the appropriate place for a detailed description of these important central causes of shock. However, patients with established ischaemic heart disease are at significant risk of developing an acute myocardial infarction or dysrhythmia during the perioperative period because of the additional physiological stress. Ideally such patients should undergo detailed cardiological assessment before surgery.

Pulmonary embolism from a deep vein thrombosis is a common cause of postoperative death (see Ch. 29). Risk factors include immobilisation before and after operation, major or prolonged surgery, malignancy, obesity, old age, lower limb fractures especially fractured neck of femur, and prothrombotic disorders. Preventative measures include compression stockings, intermittent calf compression during surgery and the use of perioperative low molecular weight heparin injections.

Hypersensitivity reaction

This may develop as an immune response to a blood infusion or to drug administration, e.g. intravenous antibiotic. There is usually pyrexia, and the circulatory collapse may also be accompanied by respiratory distress and urticaria. Treatment includes discontinuing the drug/infusion, intravenous corticosteroids and circulatory support.

Deep vein thrombosis

This is discussed in detail in Chapter 30.

Complications associated with indwelling vascular catheters

Central venous catheters (single or multiluminal) and arterial catheters may be associated with bleeding, thrombus formation and infection. In one study, complications related to initial catheter placement occurred in 5.7%, sepsis in 6.5% and mechanical difficulties (commonly major venous thrombosis or nursing mishaps) in 9%. Careful technique and monitoring and the use of heparin-coated catheters can help keep the incidence low.

Complications of placement are haemorrhage and, for central venous catheters, pneumothorax (Ch. 11).

Management

Central venous thrombophlebitis and/or sepsis usually require immediate removal and parenteral antibiotic therapy; absolute indications are:

- continued fever without other cause
- repeated positive blood cultures despite antibiotic therapy.

An effective method of assessing catheter contamination in patients with central lines in place is routine catheter exchange and culture.

Respiratory complications

Pathophysiology

Pulmonary complications are common after general surgery and other operative procedures. In addition to any exacerbation of infection already present, the primary event is pulmonary collapse. In one study, dependent atelectasis (3–4% of lung volume) developed in 100% of patients 5–10 minutes after administration of anaesthesia; 1 hour later, collapse was present in 90%; and at 24 hours, it was still a feature in 50%. Up to 40% of the obese show evidence of basal pulmonary collapse on initial postoperative X-ray. Once an unrelieved segment of collapse is present, secondary infection is almost inevitable and pneumonia ensues. Factors that contribute to postoperative pulmonary collapse are shown in Box 7.5.

Those with pre-existing chronic lung disease and who smoke are particularly likely to progress to respiratory infection because they commonly harbour organisms in the lower respiratory tract, including *Pneumococcus* and *Haemophilus* species. If collapse persists, pneumonia in non-ventilated bronchoalveolar units is likely to follow.

Prophylaxis

The aim of prophylaxis is to prevent the development of postoperative respiratory infection:

- At-risk patients are identified preoperatively (Ch. 6) and, for elective procedures, every effort is made to improve respiratory function; physiotherapy, bronchodilators and specific antimicrobial therapy based on sputum cultures may all have a role.
- Antibiotic prophylaxis with an agent which covers most common pathogens in the gut, e.g. second- and third-generation cephalosporins, usually also provides adequate perioperative respiratory protection; established respiratory infection requires specific therapy (Ch. 9).
- Adequate pain relief is essential in the postoperative period (Ch. 6) and is combined with early mobilisation, chest physiotherapy and regular incentive spirometry.

Box 7.5 Factors which contribute to postoperative pulmonary complications

- Wound pain, particularly in the upper abdomen and chest
- Limitation of respiratory excursion
- Ciliary paralysis
- Drying of bronchial secretions
- Oversedation
- Obesity

Management

Chest physiotherapy and appropriate antibiotic treatment are used for established pulmonary collapse and infection. Oxygen supplementation and other forms of respiratory support may also be necessary (see Chs 6 and 10).

Urinary complications

Although a urinary catheter has advantages, its placement can lead to a number of complications, the most common of which is urinary tract infection.

The distal urethra is normally colonised with bacteria, and even a single catheterisation results in urinary tract infection in 1% of ambulatory patients. Bacterial colonisation of bladder urine develops within 3–4 days of catheterisation in 95% of those managed with indwelling catheters attached to open drainage systems. In general surgery patients, the overall infection rate after operation is 10%, and a quarter of these occur secondary to urinary tract infections; for example, 50% of orthopaedic infections and 75% of urological and medical infections are related to a urinary tract cause.

Escherichia coli is by far the most common pathogen, although other Enterobacteriaceae are also frequent. Staphylococci, streptococci and enterococci also cause urinary tract infection.

Management

The catheter should be removed as soon as it is no longer necessary. Appropriate antibiotic therapy and the maintenance of a high-volume urine output usually suffice unless urinary tract obstruction is present (see Ch. 33).

Gastrointestinal complications

Upper gastrointestinal bleeding

Before the routine administration of prophylactic acid supression therapy (H_2 receptor blocker) life-threatening upper gastrointestinal bleeding was a common problem in those with major stress, particularly head injury, burns or multiple trauma. With adequate prophylaxis, the incidence of massive upper GI bleeding is almost zero. Acid suppression therapy increases bacterial colonisation of the upper gastrointestinal tract and the risk of hospital acquired pneumonia.

Pseudomembranous enterocolitis

This complication may follow use of systemic antibiotics. The cause is colonisation of the large bowel with *Clostridium difficile* and the acute, sometimes fulminant, infection that follows.

The clinical features are diarrhoea usually 3–4 days after operation, which may be associated with abdominal distension, hypotension and shock. Blood and mucus, sometimes with a cast of the distal large bowel, may be passed per rectum. Diagnosis is confirmed by identification of *Clostridium difficile* exotoxin in the stool. Initial management is non-operative and with intravenous fluid replacement and oral metronidazole or vancomycin. The development of toxic dilatation may necessitate emergency colectomy.

Intraperitoneal abscess

The two common anatomical sites for this type of abscess are pelvic and subphrenic. Both are usually the consequence of leakage from the GI tract or from operations for intestinal perforation and peritonitis, e.g. perforated peptic ulcer (Ch. 18), perforated appendicitis (Ch. 25) and perforated diverticulitis (Ch. 25). The organisms involved are of enteric origin: *Bacteroides* (anaerobic) and usually *E. coli* (aerobic).

The clinical features common to either site are malaise and persistent or recrudescent fever from after the fourth postoperative day. The specific findings are given in Table 7.9.

Management

In the early stages, systemic antibiotics are given. However, evidence of obvious failure of the infection to resolve requires drainage either by percutaneous means or at open operation. Pelvic abscesses can usually be drained into the rectum.

Enterocutaneous fistula

This is characterised by a communication between the GI tract and the skin surface. The most common aetiological factors are listed in Box 7.6. The clinical features are usually systemic sepsis followed by the development of inflammation on the abdominal wall or in the abdominal wound. Initially, pus may be discharged, but this is rapidly followed by intestinal content, the quantity of which varies according to the level of the fistula.

Clinically, fistulae are usually classified as of either high or low output. The former occurs predominantly in the upper GI tract from stomach to terminal ileum, where output may be a litre or more a day and is further increased if distal obstruction is present. The latter is characteristic of large bowel fistulae or those which are not associated with complete division of the bowel or distal obstruction.

The local effects of fistulae are variable, but if the effluent contains digestive enzymes (stomach to terminal ileum), rapid digestion and secondary septic infection of the abdominal wall take place. The general effects are:

- water and electrolyte loss
- malnutrition from failure of absorption and the increased catabolism of the septic state.

Management

The management of fistulae is often complex, although many close spontaneously unless there is distal obstruction, mucocutaneous union or a persistent infective focus. Until closure takes place, nutritional and electrolyte support is necessary, as is protection of the skin from digestion. If any of the factors that prevent closure are present, operation is required once the fluid and electrolyte losses, malnutrition and sepsis have been corrected.

Box 7.6 Aetiological factors in enterocutaneous fistula

- Intestinal obstruction (distal to anastomosis)
- Chronic inflammatory disease (e.g. Crohn's, tuberculosis)
- Previous irradiation
- Intestinal ischaemia

Wound dehiscence

Wounds fail to heal and may then burst open because of:

- sepsis
- failure of adequate progression of healing
- distractive forces, especially in the abdomen
- poor surgical technique.

Table 7.9 Specific findings in intraperitoneal abscess

Features	Pelvic	Subphrenic	Elsewhere
Symptoms	Urgency of defection Mucous diarrhoea Sometimes blood in stool if abscess ruptures into rectum	RUQ pain (but often absent) Respiratory complications Hiccough	Vague Subacute intestinal obstruction
Findings	Abdominal – nothing or slight lower distension from coils of bowel above the abscess PR – tender (referred to anterior abdominal wall); boggy mass also felt PV in female	Upper abdominal tenderness Diminished diaphragmatic movement on affected side (usually right) Collapse/consolidation of lung, and pleural effusion	Nil or those of intestinal obstruction
Supplementary investigations	Straight X-ray for intestinal obstruction Ultrasound/CT scanning	Straight X-ray for lung signs and presence of gas under the diaphragm Ultrasound/CT scanning	Straight X-ray for intestinal obstruction Ultrasound/CT scanning Labelled leucocyte scan
Special points	Postoperative diarrhoea must be investigated	Pus somewhere, pus nowhere else = pus under the diaphragm	Re-exploration must be considered if there is poor recovery and features of sepsis after an abdominal procedure

There are three types of wound dehiscence:

- Superficial and revealed – occurs at about 2 weeks when the skin sutures are removed and the skin and subcutaneous layers separate; the cause is most often a wound haematoma or cellulitis.
- Deep and concealed – occurs at any time in the postoperative period and gradually, with separation of all layers of the abdominal wall with the exception of the skin. If not recognised while the patient is in hospital and given that the skin unites, an incisional hernia always develops at a later date.
- Complete and revealed – occurs on about the 10th day gradually or suddenly with the protrusion of a knuckle or loop of bowel or a portion of the omentum through a wound which is completely separated in the whole or part of its length (burst abdomen).

Burst abdomen was once a relatively common event in general surgery. The incidence is now very low as a result of mass closure of the abdominal wall using an appropriate suture material (slowly absorbed or non-absorbable, strong) and good technique (large, closely spaced bites of tissue – Jenkin's rule states that suture material four times the length of the wound should be used for closure). Rarely, abdominal disruption may be the consequence of a paroxysmal rise in intra-abdominal pressure (coughing) or the rapid accumulation of ascites (cirrhosis).

A complete dehiscence is usually heralded by serosanguineous or bloodstained discharge from the wound. In some instances, a concealed disruption may become obvious when superficial sutures are removed and bowel or omentum protrudes through the wound.

Management

This depends on the type of dehiscence (see Table 7.10).

Acute parotitis

Although now rare, this complication can occur in serious illness if mouth hygiene is deficient and dehydration develops. The gland swells rapidly with signs of local infection and early pus formation.

Initial management is by intravenous antibiotics. If there is no response, pus is likely and the gland may require drainage. Attention to mouth hygiene and a dental consultation are also required.

Pressure sores

Although pressure sores are not restricted to the postoperative period, age, obesity and immobility after operation do contribute to what should be regarded as a preventable condition. Other predisposing factors to the development of pressure sores include cachexia, increased sweating from pyrexia, which leads to increased risk of shear and friction. Decreased temperature in hypothermia can lead to decreased peripheral blood flow, both of which can promote the development of a bedsore. Sensory loss from stroke or epidural can leave the patient unaware of excessive pressure. Incontinence can lead to maturation breakdown due to moisture. Pre-existing disease, particularly diabetes, peripheral vascular disease, multiple sclerosis and spinal trauma can all be associated with the development of bedsores. Finally, medication, especially steroids and chemotherapy, can predispose.

Special considerations

Diabetes mellitus

The diabetic patient presents a number of management problems in the postoperative period. Precise control of blood glucose levels is necessary to avoid hypoglycaemia or hyperglycaemia with associated complications such as diabetic ketoacidosis and dehydration secondary to glycosuria.

Uncontrolled diabetes has a significant negative impact on wound healing. For patients whose disease is managed by diet alone, additional measures are usually unnecessary. In the postoperative period, careful monitoring, including finger-prick glucose measurements every 4–6 hours, is appropriate, with a sliding scale of regular insulin administered as needed. In those who are receiving oral hypoglycaemic agents, the medication is discontinued on the day before operation and insulin used as necessary to control hyperglycaemia. In those who normally require insulin, an intravenous dextrose infusion and one-half of the total daily dose of insulin as regular insulin is given on the morning of the operation.

Glucose is administered throughout the operation, as guided by repeated measurement of glucose levels. In those who require major procedures and extensive fluid administration, blood glucose is measured frequently during operation and insulin given intravenously as

Table 7.10 Management of abdominal wound dehiscence

Type	Management
Superficial and revealed	Lay skin and subcutaneous tissues open; treat infection. Once wound is granulating, either allow this to proceed to healing by secondary intention or carry out secondary suture
Deep and concealed	Usually only recognised late in convalescence; provided the skin remains intact, repair is deferred until recovery is complete unless there is a high risk of a strangulation through the incisional hernia
Complete and revealed	Urgent re-suture of all layers by mass closure

necessary. Postoperatively, glucose levels in some patients are well controlled by administration of insulin on a sliding scale based on finger-prick monitoring of blood glucose.

Steroid-dependent patients

These patients are at risk of an Addisonian crisis and of life-threatening hypotension and therefore often require extra steroid cover for major surgical stresses.

FURTHER READING

Hughes S, Mardell A 2009 Oxford handbook of perioperative practice (Oxford handbooks in nursing). Oxford University Press, Oxford

Leaper D, Whitaker I 2010 Post-operative complications (Oxford specialist handbooks), 2nd edn. Oxford University Press, Oxford

Woodhead K, Wicker P 2005 A textbook of perioperative care. Churchill Livingstone, London

8 Wound healing and management

Any breach in the surface of the body (which includes the gastrointestinal tract), or any tissue disruption deep to the skin produced by the application of energy, is a wound – open in the first instance, closed in the second (see also Ch. 35 for the application of the same classification to fractures of bones). Most often the energy is physical, but a burn (Ch. 10) is as much a wound as is an incision made with a knife. Both follow the same course towards the restoration of normality – the process of healing. The similarity of the response of the body to different modes of injury makes the task of understanding and managing this process that much easier.

PRIMARY WOUND HEALING

Healing is a natural and spontaneous phenomenon. Although the basic events have been observed for many years, the factors which initiate and control the process have become increasingly understood. The pattern of wound healing may be affected by cytokine, endocrine or pharmacological manipulation of the wound's environment.

Some wounds heal completely without surgical intervention. These include not only small lesions but also some larger tissue craters produced, for example, by drainage of an abscess or excision of a pilonidal sinus. Even if, as is often the case, such wounds are too heavily contaminated with bacteria for immediate surgical closure, they contract surprisingly quickly, providing local wound treatment is adequate.

Phases of healing

The overall healing process is illustrated in Figure 8.1. Healing can be divided into three phases:

- Inflammatory (preparative including haemostasis) – in this phase the early cellular reactions to injury take place. As the name implies, these responses prepare the site of injury for repair and are similar to the responses of tissues seen in acute inflammation from any cause.
- Reparative (proliferative) – the redevelopment of structural integrity. This does not usually mean the regeneration of functioning cells; rather it is by the laying down of collagen, and in epithelium by migration of living cells, to close a defect.
- Consolidative (remodelling) – once the tissue is knitted together by collagen, this substance undergoes changes which include reorientation and contraction to ultimately form a mature and relatively inactive scar.

These phases are not wholly separate but merge seamlessly one into the other. A complex series of cellular interactions are involved, controlled in part by growth factor and cytokines released within the wound itself (Table 8.1).

Inflammatory

Tissue and cell injuries lead to a cascade of events:

- bleeding followed by clotting and then clot lysis. Contact of blood with collagen triggers platelet aggregation and coagulation. A fibrin–fibronectin cross-linked plug forms, preventing further blood loss. The plug forms a matrix for later collagen deposition (see below) and cellular migration with clot lysis and replacement with granulation tissue. Thromboxanes and prostaglandins released by damaged cells cause a short-lived (5–15 minutes) vasoconstriction which also contributes to haemostasis.
- platelets release inflammatory cytokines, growth factors, extracellular matrix (ECM) proteins and other proinflammatory factors such as serotonin, bradykinin, prostaglandins, prostacyclins, thromboxane and histamine which result in vasodilatation, increased capillary permeability, intercellular oedema, cellular proliferation and migration of leucocytes into the damaged area.
- polymorphonuclear neutrophils (PNMs) migrate to the wound within an hour and are the predominant cell for the first 48 hours attracted by fibronectin, growth factors and pro-inflammatory cytokines. They phagocytose debris and bacteria and also kill bacteria by release of free radicals. Helper T-cells also migrate to the wound and release additional pro-inflammatory cytokines and activate macrophages.

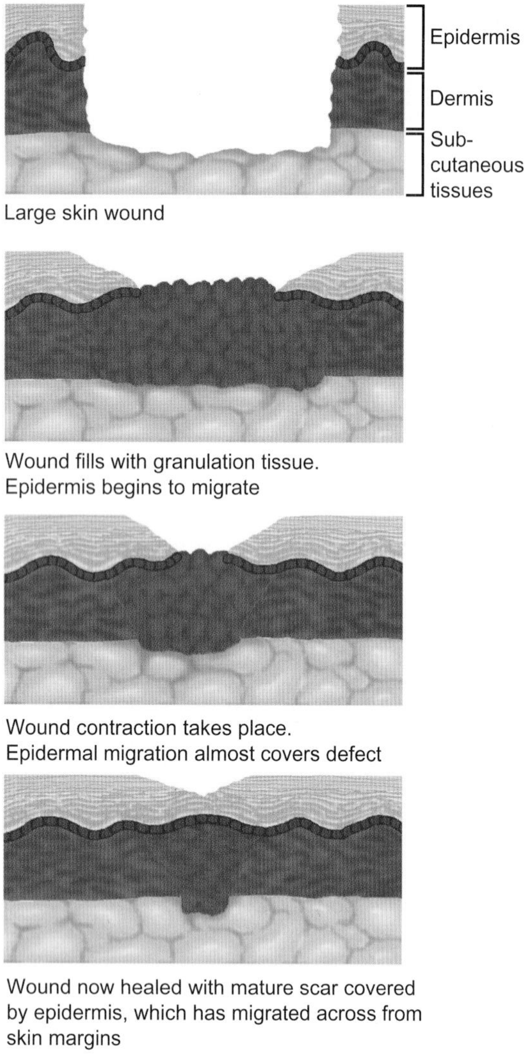

Epidermis
Dermis
Sub-
cutaneous
tissues
Large skin wound
Wound fills with granulation tissue.
Epidermis begins to migrate
Wound contraction takes place.
Epidermal migration almost covers defect
Wound now healed with mature scar covered
by epidermis, which has migrated across from
skin margins

Fig. 8.1 Phases of wound healing.

- macrophages replace and, indeed, digest apoptotic PMNs and become the dominant cell by 48–72 hours. They arrive largely as monocytes and rapidly mature into macrophages. They also phagocytose tissue debris and bacteria, and release proteolytic enzymes to break down damaged tissue. Macrophages release growth factors and cytokines that initiate the proliferative phase leading to angiogenesis, the formation of a new ECM, and epithelialisation.

The duration of the inflammatory stage is normally about 3 days. Any factor which interferes with the progress of this response may interrupt or delay healing.

Reparative (proliferative)

The following take place from about day 3 onwards:

- Capillary loops form in the damaged area by migration of endothelial cells to provide a new blood supply (angiogenesis). Endothelial cells are attracted by fibronectin, cytokines released by platelets and macrophages, and by tissue hypoxia and increased levels of lactic acid.
- The process of angiogenesis also requires clot lysis stimulated by plasminogen activators and breakdown of the early ECM by collagenases and metalloproteinases.
- Fibroblasts are also attracted to the wound at this stage (2–5 days) and they lay down strands of collagen. They migrate from surrounding tissue, attracted by growth factors (PDGF, TGB-β) and fibronectin, and initially adhere to the fibronectin in the ECM.
- Collagen, fibronectin, glycoproteins, glycosaminoglycans and hyaluronan are deposited to form a provisional ECM. Collagen is deposited at first in a provisional and apparently untidy manner but gradually becomes oriented along any lines of stress applied to the wound. It provides strength to the wound and a framework for cellular attachment and differentiation.
- The mass of new capillaries, fibroblasts, inflammatory cells and provisional ECM is known collectively as granulation tissue because of its visual appearance in an open wound. This granulation tissue then starts to contract, partly through the effects of specialised myofibroblasts.
- The combination of alignment of collagen fibrils, their cross-linkage and their subsequent contraction is vital to the restoration of tensile strength. Myofibroblasts (differentiated from fibroblasts under growth factor influence) also contribute to wound contracture. Contracture takes place at 5–15 days although it may last longer. The wound may reduce by 40–80% in size by this process. The myofibroblasts are attracted to fibronectin and migrate to the wound edges where they attach themselves to the cells and ECM within the wound. Contraction of these cells contributes to wound contracture. Collagen deposition from fibroblasts within the wound is occurring simultaneously. A distinction is drawn between this active process of *contraction* of the whole wound mass and the later shrinkage of mature collagen, which may lead to distortion of a healed area – known by the general term *contracture*.
- In addition, in an open surface wound, epithelial cells (largely basal keratinocytes) at the margins migrate across the surface of granulation tissue attracted by growth factors from fibroblasts, a lack of local cellular contact inhibition, and also by nitric oxide to cover the exposed area (epithelialisation). The keratinocytes detach themselves from their basement membrane and neighbouring cells by dissolving their desmosomes and releasing integrins from the cell's intermediate filaments. As the keratinocytes migrate, new cells are produced at the wound edges stimulated by growth factors so that tongues of epithelial cells cover the granulation tissue. The cells will migrate under any scab that has formed over the wound. The migrating keratinocytes also secrete growth factors and lay down proteins to form a new basement membrane. This process continues until the wound is completely re-epithelialised and the cells revert to normal epithelial form with attachments to neighbours and the new basement membrane.

As with the preparative phase, anything that interferes with or delays the steps described slows the whole process down.

Table 8.1 Some of the growth factors and cytokines involved in wound healing

Action	Factor/cytokine	Cell(s) of origin
PMN migration/activation	PDGF	Platelets, macrophages, T-cells, mast cells, endothelial cells, fibroblasts
	TGF-β	Platelets, macrophages, T-cells, keratinocytes, endothelial cells, fibroblasts
	IL-1	Macrophages, fibroblasts
	IL-8	Macrophages, endothelial and epidermal cells
Monocyte/macrophage migration/activation	PDGF	See above
	TGF-β	See above
Fibroblast migration/activation	PDGF	See above
	TGF-β	See above
	FGF-1 and FGF-2	Macrophages, T-cells, mast cells, endothelial cells, fibroblasts
	IL-1	See above
	IL-8	See above
Fibroblast proliferation	PDGF	See above
	FGF-1 and FGF-2	See above
	EGF	Macrophages, keratocytes
Angiogenesis/endothelial cell proliferation	VEGF	Mesenchymal cells
	HGF	Mesenchymal cells
	PDGF	See above
	TGF-β	See above
Keratinocyte migration	EGF	See above
	FGF-1 and FGF-2	See above
	KGF	Fibroblasts
	IL-1	See above
Keratinocyte proliferation	TGF-β	See above
	TGF-α	Macrophages, T-cells, keratinocytes
	EGF	See above
	KGF	See above
	HGF	See above
Metalloproteinase, fibronectin and hyaluronan production	PDGF	See above

PDGF: platelet-derived growth factor; TGF: transforming growth factor; IL: interleukin, FGF: fibroblast growth factor; EGF: epidermal growth factor; VEGF: vascular endothelial growth factor; HGF: hepatocyte growth factor; KGF: keratinocyte growth factor.

Consolidative

As collagen deposition is completed, the vascularity of the wound gradually decreases and any surface scar becomes paler as blood vessels are reduced by apoptosis. Although collagen turnover never ceases completely, the wound becomes relatively quiescent. The type III collagen deposited during the reparative stage is gradually degraded and replaced with type I collagen, which is stronger, more aligned with tension lines and cross-linked. The amount of collagen that is finally formed – the ultimate scar – is dependent upon the initial volume of granulation tissue. In an open wound with an epithelial gap, this may be large and scarring may be considerable. In some, the normal equilibrium between collagen synthesis and degradation is disturbed: instead of maturation with subsidence of cellular activity over a period of about 12 months, collagen may continue to be produced and results in a red, lumpy, hypertrophic appearance. If this extends into the surrounding tissues it is called a *keloid*.

Recovery of tensile strength

In some circumstances – such as the fascial layers of the abdominal wall after a surgical incision or at the site of tendon repair – the ultimate tensile strength (i.e. resistance to disruptive stresses) is important for tissue stability, for example the prevention of incisional hernia development or

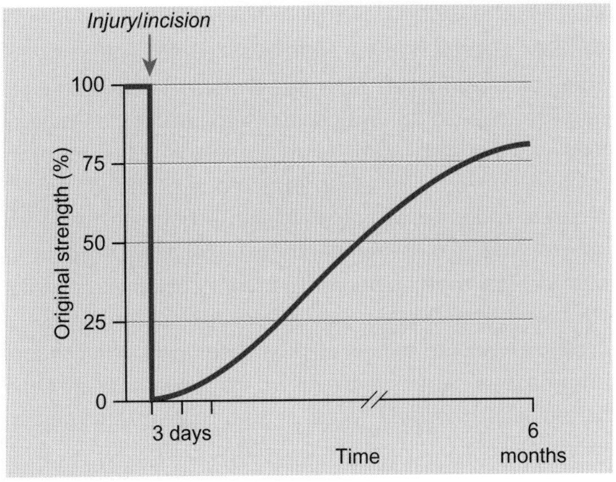

Fig. 8.2 Recovery of tensile strength in a fascial layer.

rupture of the repaired tendon. During the preparative phase in any wound, the opposed edges are merely adherent as a consequence of fibrin, and the intrinsic tensile strength is effectively zero. As collagen accumulates during the reparative phase, strength increases rapidly and reaches 50% of the original pre-injury tissues at 3 months, but it is many months before a plateau is reached at about 80% (Fig. 8.2). During this time, such wounds require extrinsic support – usually provided by sutures (see below). By contrast, in a wound in a viscus, e.g. the liver or intestine, where significant disruptive forces are not usually present, the scar rapidly exceeds the strength of the original tissue.

Clinical factors

The account given above is of the biology of wound healing. In surgical practice, wounds vary in four ways:

- causation
- contamination
- time interval between wounding and initial treatment
- biological factors in the individual.

Causation

The amount of damage within a wound is directly proportional to the force applied. An incised wound made by the deliberately applied scalpel of the surgeon causes very little surrounding damage; modern surgical technique is based on delicate incision and dissection to minimise tissue injury and so to permit smooth and rapid healing. At the other end of the scale are those wounds caused by large transfers of energy: shock waves are generated, tearing tissues or distracting them from their blood supply. Cells are destroyed and the tissue disrupted by bleeding. Such features are typical of wounds made by the weapons of war such as high-velocity missiles.

Contamination

Once the skin or other epithelial surface, for example the mucosa of the GI tract, is breached, a way is opened for the entry of bacteria. The circumstances in which the wound is sustained clearly influences the extent and type of bacterial contamination. Injuries sustained in the garden or in agriculture (including war wounds where the battle has taken place over cultivated land) are at high risk of contamination by the spores of *Clostridium* which can produce tetanus and gas gangrene (see Ch. 9). In hospital, surgical wounds may be inoculated not only with bacteria that originate from the patient's skin or other areas explored (e.g. the GI tract) – so-called endogenous contamination – but also by cross-infection from the environment – exogenous or nosocomial sources. The most important current problem is infection with methicillin-resistant *Staphylococcus aureus* (MRSA) – which can lead to failure of prostheses and other wound complications, although these are not usually fatal. Other contaminating bacteria found in the hospital environment include streptococci and *Bacteroides* (Ch. 9).

Time

Healing begins the moment a wound is sustained. However, in a contaminated wound, particularly if there is dead or damaged tissue, bacteria also multiply and increase in number. In most wounds, the first 4–6 hours is a period when bacteria are present but not in sufficient numbers to influence the healing cascade greatly; if they can be eliminated or their environment made unattractive during this time then healing proceeds normally. If this fails to occur, the balance from 6 to 18 hours tends progressively to tip in favour of the proliferating bacteria. By this time the bacteria are themselves influencing the inflammatory process, so that the wound must be regarded as infected.

Biological factors

Both local and systemic factors affect wound healing.

Local (Box 8.1)

- Bacterial infection as a consequence of contamination leads to further tissue damage and prolongs the inflammatory phase; abscess formation separates the wound edges and may be associated with dehiscence.
- If the local blood supply is inadequate there will be relative hypoxia which slows the rate of cell division; well-vascularised wounds on the face and neck heal quickly whereas those on the lower limb are slow and may be prone to breakdown. Ischaemia may also result from excessive tissue tension applied to achieve closure, from peripheral vascular disease (particularly in the lower limbs) and from an increase in tissue tension either secondary to infection or as a result of a compartment syndrome (see Chs 29 and 35).
- A foreign body within a wound can both separate healing tissues and, if it is contaminated, act as a focus for persistent infection and inflammation.
- Tissues infiltrated by malignant disease do not heal, e.g. a squamous carcinoma in a varicose ulcer or a pathological fracture of bone.

Systemic (Box 8.2)

- Malnutrition slows the healing process.
- Specific deficiencies, such as vitamin C (necessary for collagen synthesis and cross-linkage), zinc (an enzyme cofactor) and vitamin A, delay the healing course.
- Old age probably also slows down the reparative response to injury, although this is not a contraindication to necessary operation.
- Diabetes mellitus carries an increased risk of wound infection as well as being often associated with microvascular disease which reduces tissue perfusion and oxygenation.

Box 8.1 Local factors inhibiting wound healing

- Infection
- Ischaemia
- Foreign bodies
- Tumour

Box 8.2 Systemic factors inhibiting wound healing

- Malnutrition
- Old age
- Vitamin A and C deficiency
- Diabetes
- Jaundice
- Renal failure
- Steroid or cytotoxic treatment
- Radiotherapy
- Reduced tissue perfusion
- Haemorrhagic diatheses
- Immune deficiency states

- Jaundice is associated with delayed angiogenesis and reduced collagen synthesis.
- Renal failure suppresses cell division, neoepithelialisation and the formation of connective tissue.
- Treatment with corticosteroids or cytotoxic agents inhibits the inflammatory response and collagen synthesis.
- Radiotherapy interferes with cell division, but its effect is also to cause chronic damage to small blood vessels so that previously irradiated tissues are relatively ischaemic.
- Other general causes of reduced tissue perfusion and oxygenation are cardiac failure, chronic respiratory disease and severe anaemia.
- Haemorrhagic diatheses may lead to wound haematoma, delayed apposition of tissues and possible infection.
- Immune deficiency states (both acquired and inherited), particularly if severe, may increase the risk of infection and wound breakdown.

PATHWAYS OF WOUND MANAGEMENT

The objective of management is to ensure uninterrupted progress to healing with the minimum amount of scar formation. How this is achieved is dictated by the clinical factors described above. Wounds can be divided into four classes:

- *incised* – of recent origin and without significant contamination
- *lacerated* – of recent origin with tissue damage and/or contamination
- *late* – either incised or lacerated; strictly with a time interval of greater than 6 hours between injury and treatment but this may be extended up to 18 hours in some circumstances such as well-vascularised, lightly contaminated wounds in the face and scalp
- *infected* – wounds seen beyond 18–24 hours must be regarded as, and are often seen to be, infected, i.e. they are the site of an inflammatory response to the bacteria that are present.

Incised wounds

Typical examples of these are surgical incisions and accidental wounds from sharp agents such as knives and glass. After arrest of bleeding (haemostasis) they can be closed. This is known to surgeons as primary closure. However, all but the most superficial wounds must also be gently explored. There are two reasons for this:

- unsuspected foreign body – which may lead to later complications (e.g. infection)
- unsuspected deep penetration with damage to structures which requires either immediate or later treatment, e.g. nerves, blood vessels and viscera – an injury should be assumed to have damaged an underlying structure until this has been proven not to be the case.

Lacerated wounds

All dead and damaged tissue, visible contamination and foreign bodies must be removed by a combination of mechanical lavage and surgical excision using the knife or scissors to remove devitalised tissue and adherent foreign bodies – known as *debridement*. It may be difficult to be certain of viability, especially if the tissues are bruised and swollen as a result of injury; skin may be sheared off deep fascia in degloving injuries and so lose its blood supply; fat that initially appears normal may undergo late necrosis. Judgement may also be difficult if there has been much interstitial bleeding and swelling. In such circumstances the wound is best left open and reinspected at intervals before closure (delayed primary closure). However, if a thorough debridement can be achieved, the wound is now similar in biological nature to an incised one, and after exploration and arrest of bleeding it can be closed. This whole process is known as excision (debridement) and primary closure.

Late wounds

In the grey area of time between 6 and 18 hours, debridement and closure may be possible, particularly if antibiotic therapy is used (Ch. 9). However, it is now likely that the bacteria that are dividing cannot be wholly eliminated, so that the circumstances for their further proliferation should be made as unfavourable as possible. Bacteria welcome warmth, moisture and darkness – conditions that are found in a closed wound. If, after debridement and haemostasis, the wound is left open, the first two (and on occasion also the third – see Ch. 10) are less available. Provided infection does not become apparent within 3 days it is then biologically and practically reasonable to close the wound. Such management, known as debridement and delayed primary closure, is almost always used for war wounds and increasingly for complicated circumstances in peacetime. A wound managed in this way pursues the same path to healing as one closed primarily, because it enters the reparative phase at the same time as a primarily closed wound – therefore little is lost.

Infected wounds

Later than 18–24 hours, a wound is almost always infected. All that should be done is to open it widely, remove foreign bodies and detached tissue and treat the infection with systemic antibiotics. Because of the time involved, the wound now contains granulation tissue; the two granulating surfaces can then either be coapted or covered in some other way (e.g. skin grafting). This is known as secondary closure. In some circumstances, the amount of contraction of the wound during the management of infection makes formal closure unnecessary; perianal wounds such as those following incision of a perianal or ischiorectal abscess (Ch. 26) are good examples.

INFECTION PREVENTION AND MANAGEMENT

Bacteria can be assumed to be present in all accidental wounds and in those sustained at a surgical operation when an area that is colonised by bacteria is involved (e.g. the colon).

Good wound care is the first essential for the prevention of infection. In accidental injury, debridement and delayed primary closure are the two most important procedures. Incisions made by surgeons do not need debridement, but if there is contamination at operation (as may occur in an operation on the GI tract), delayed closure of the superficial layers is sometimes used. Many wounds can be assumed to be contaminated the moment they are sustained, e.g. when the abdomen is opened to deal with an intraperitoneal infection or when a limb is wounded in an accident. In the early part of the preparative phase of wound healing when bacterial proliferation is just beginning, it may be possible to eliminate these bacteria by establishing a high concentration of antibiotic in the tissues by parenteral administration. This prophylactic use of antibiotics over a short period of time is now common in many circumstances.

An established local bacterial infection, other than the special circumstances of *Clostridium* (Ch. 9), is dealt with as described above.

ARREST OF BLEEDING (HAEMOSTASIS)

A dry wound – i.e. one with minimal oozing – is an essential prerequisite for successful closure to achieve the best result with minimal formation of fibrous tissue. Failure to achieve adequate control of bleeding:

- keeps the wound edges apart and thus requires a larger gap to be bridged, which leads to a greater deposition of fibrous tissue
- may result in a haematoma – an accumulation of clot which is lysed and may require release before the wound edges can be opposed
- may lead to infection – a haematoma is an ideal place in which bacteria can multiply.

The three main traditional techniques used to stop bleeding have been extended by new products and technologies:

- compression
- ligation
- thermal coagulation
- clipping and stapling
- ultrasonic instruments
- haemostatic products

Compression

Packing a bleeding cavity with gauze swabs or applying pressure to a bleeding area are both particularly useful if there is widespread oozing. Five minutes of compression allows normal haemostasis to take place by contraction of the mouths of small vessels, platelet aggregation and coagulation. However, these processes must be normal for the effective arrest of bleeding.

Ligation

The mouth of the divided vessel which is bleeding is picked up with special forceps (haemostats, see Fig. 8.3) and tied off with a ligature; either absorbable or non-absorbable materials may be used. Absorbable sutures have a clear advantage in that, once the vessel has been occluded and has thrombosed behind the point of ligature, the suture material disappears so that foreign body reaction is minimal. However, the rate of disappearance may be too fast, particularly in the presence of sepsis and, in consequence, secondary haemorrhage may occur, particularly if there is infection which accelerates lysis of the suture material and interrupts the normal healing process. For this reason, large vessels are more often ligated with non-absorbable sutures, which are usually braided for easy handling.

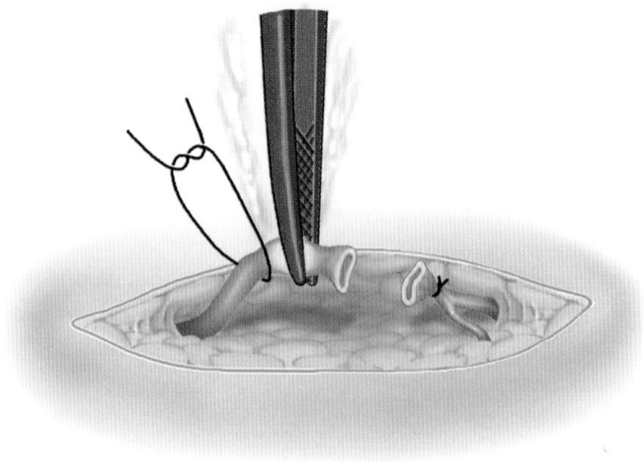

Fig. 8.3 Ligation of a bleeding vessel.

Thermal coagulation

Boiling oil and the hot iron have both been used since ancient times, although the amount of tissue damage they produced induced a famous surgeon of the 16th century (Ambrose Pare) to abandon them in favour of blander wound care which was equally successful. The modern, and much more refined, equivalent is high-frequency electric current – diathermy in Europe and cautery in North America. The pathway of current is either between two points of the instrument (bipolar, Fig. 8.4a); or from the point of application through the body of the patient to a large-area contact plate and thence to earth (unipolar, Fig. 8.4b).

Small blood vessels can be precisely dealt with using either technique, and the method is also used for cutting soft tissues with minimal bleeding when a continuous waveform is produced and an arc is generated between the electrode and the tissue. Vaporisation of the water in the cells occurs with disruption of tissue continuity (so-called 'cutting' diathermy).

Modern versions of diathermy use feedback-controlled systems to fuse blood vessels up to 7 mm in diameter with reduced collateral thermal tissue injury.

Clipping and stapling

Blood vessels and other small tubes (e.g. the cystic duct) may also be closed with metal or synthetic absorbable clips carried on a special forceps (Fig. 8.5). Larger vessels may be transected using vascular stapling instruments.

Ultrasonic instruments

High-frequency ultrasonic instruments produce cutting and coagulation of tissues at lower temperatures than those required by diathermy/cautery. They are widely used in both open and laparoscopic surgery.

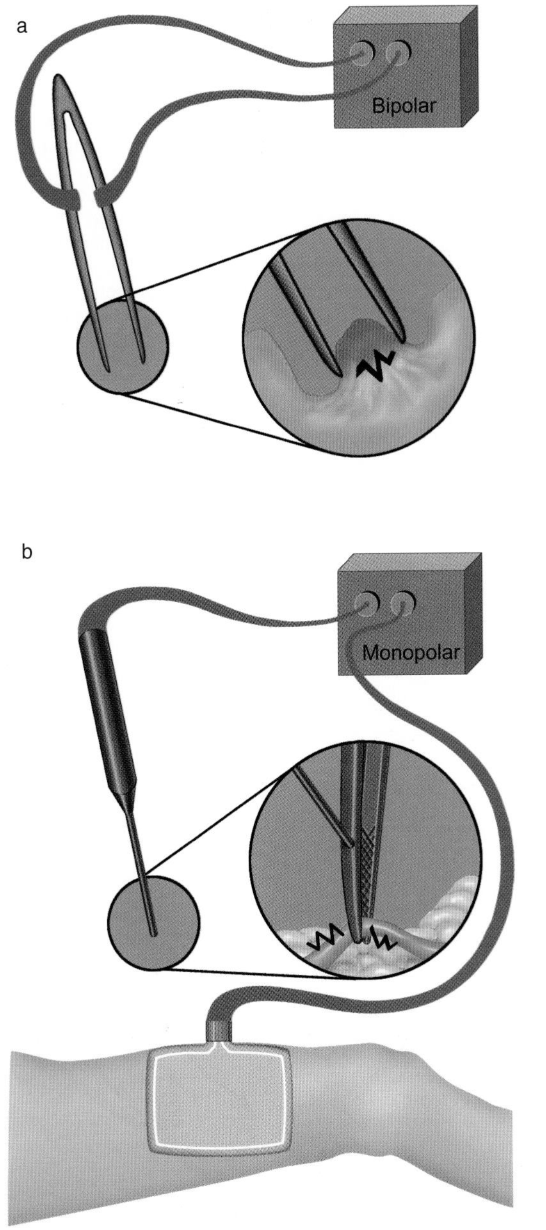

Fig. 8.4 (a) Bipolar diathermy. (b) Unipolar (monopolar) diathermy.

Topical haemostatic products

A number of topical haemostatic products are available in gel or membrane form for surgical applications to bleeding areas. These act in a number of different ways (Table 8.2).

WOUND CLOSURE

The methods of wound closure are as follows:

- suture with needle and the appropriate material
- techniques that mimic suturing, e.g. tapes, staples, glues
- plastic procedures – mainly to close defects that cannot be dealt with by the above two methods.

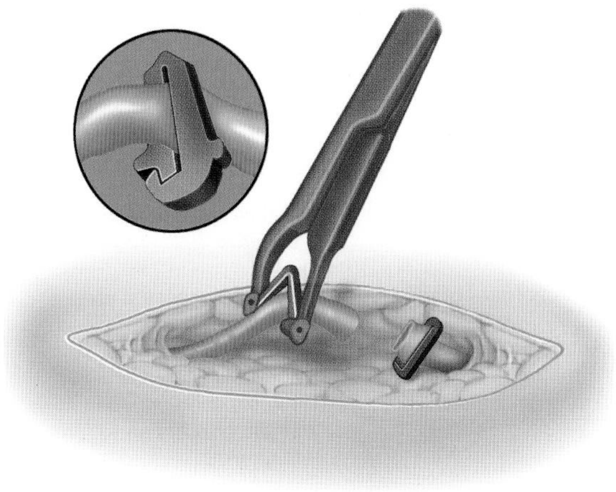

Fig. 8.5 Application of a clip to a bleeding vessel.

Needles and sutures

This classical method of bringing tissues together is based on the long-established techniques of the seamstress and tailor.

Needles

Straight needles are held in the hand and are very similar to those used in ordinary sewing. The two main differences are:

- The thread is swaged inside the hollow blunt end (Fig. 8.6b) instead of being passed through an eye.
- For closure of the skin and other tough collagen-containing tissues, the point has a triangular cutting edge behind it (Fig. 8.6b).

Curved needles in modern surgical practice are designed for use with a needle holder (Figs 8.6a and 8.7) and can either have a cutting edge or be round-bodied. Curved cutting needles may be large and are employed for closing wounds where they may have to penetrate tough fascial layers. Such needles are the commonest cause of needle-stick injuries to the hand of the surgeon or assistant. Many surgeons now use specially designed heavy blunt-tipped needles to avoid this risk. Round-bodied needles push the tissues aside and are often smaller and designed for precise work on viscera (such as the intestine), nerves and blood vessels. Microsurgical sutures, e.g. for vascular and ophthalmic surgery with an operating microscope, are of this type.

Sutures

Sutures are used both for the arrest of bleeding by ligation and for wound closure. They may be either natural or synthetic and absorbable or non-absorbable (Table 8.3).

Absorbable materials are broken down by proteolysis (catgut) or by hydrolysis (the newer synthetic absorbable polymers or monomers such as polyglycolic acid). Absorbables have the obvious theoretical advantage that they do not persist as a foreign body and therefore, if a wound becomes infected, bacteria cannot use the suture as a permanent hiding place. For many years, catgut (treated sheep intestinal submucosa – effectively, denatured collagen) was the only absorbable material. However, its rate of dissolution is such

Table 8.2 Locally acting haemostatic products

Agent	Mode of action	Uses	Risks
Bone wax	Tamponade	Bone surface	Infection, delayed bone union
Gelatin foams	Activates extrinsic coagulation system	Small vessel bleeding	Avoid closed spaces as pressure effects may cause nerve damage
Oxidised cellulose	Activates extrinsic coagulation system	Raw bleeding surfaces	Low pH may increase inflammation and interfere with thrombin-based agents
Microfibrillar collagen	Platelet adherence and activation	Bleeding surfaces	Not effective if thrombocytopenic
Thrombin (± gelatin matrix)	Converts fibrinogen to fibrin, activates coagulation	Raw bleeding areas	Allergic reaction especially to bovine products
Fibrin sealants	Thrombin and fibrinogen mixed at site of bleeding to form fibrin clots	Raw bleeding surfaces and tissue sealant, e.g. dura	
Polyethylene glycol hydrogels	Cross-linking polymers in wound	Sealing vascular anastomoses and adhesion prevention	Swells up to 4 times volume over 24 hours
Glutaraldehyde cross-linked albumin	Cross links albumin to cell proteins in wound to form protein scaffold for haemostasis	Seals vascular suture lines in arterial surgery	Allergy, constriction of nerves or other tissues
Fibrin dressings	Freeze-dried thrombin and fibrinogen on gauze dressing	Large raw surfaces	
Chitin/chitosan dressings	Vasoconstriction, mobilisation of red cells, platelets and clotting factors	Emergency control of wound bleeding	Allergy (shellfish product)
	Absorbs water and concentrates red cells, platelets and clotting factors	Emergency control of wound bleeding	Foreign body reaction to product

Adapted from: Achneck et al 2010 *A Comprehensive review of hemostatic agents: efficacy and recommendations for use*. Annals of Surgery 251: 217–228.

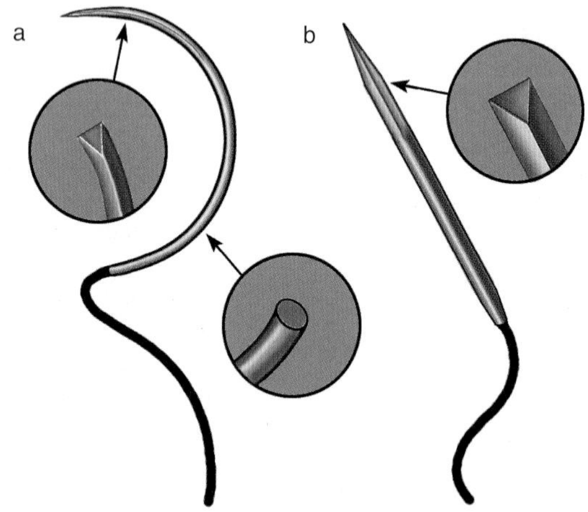

Fig. 8.6 The swaged attachment of the suture material to eyeless needles. (a) A curved needle with a different cutting profile at the tip compared with the main shaft. (b) A straight needle also with a cutting edge.

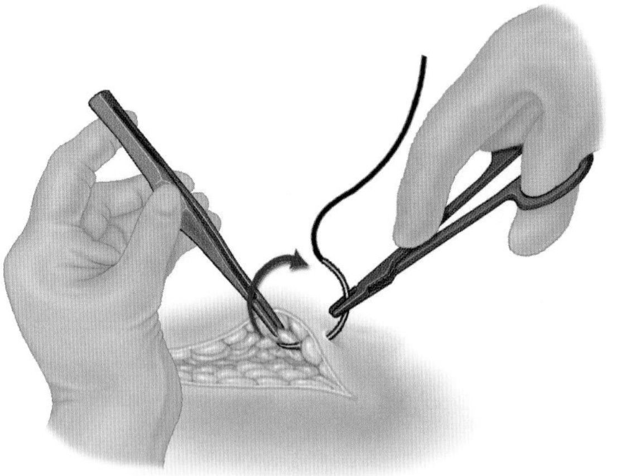

Fig. 8.7 Principle of the use of curved needles with a needle holder.

that it is unsuitable for wounds that are subject to any form of distraction, because it does not last long enough for intrinsic tensile strength to recover. Furthermore, in an infected wound catgut may disappear too quickly, which may result in secondary haemorrhage. Catgut is no longer used in the UK. The synthetic absorbables can have their rate of dissolution adjusted, and a range of products are available. These can be used effectively in different circumstances.

Non-absorbables are preferred by some surgeons because of the reassurance they provide about tensile strength until wound healing has progressed to an adequate stage. Non-absorbable materials are not subject to attack by proteolysis or hydrolysis and therefore retain their tensile strength for long periods – virtually permanently. However, they do promote a variable foreign body inflammatory reaction, which is greatest in natural materials such as linen or silk and least with synthetic materials such as polyamide (Nylon) and polypropylene (Prolene). Natural materials are available only in braided form which, although it makes them easy to handle, also provides a potential nidus in which bacteria can lurk. Infection which occurs in a wound with buried natural non-absorbables does not usually resolve until these are removed. The same is also sometimes true for synthetic non-absorbable materials; however, these are usually monofilaments, which means that they slide easily through the tissues and do not form such effective hiding places for bacteria.

Suture gauge

The original definition of suture diameter was based on 'gauge 1', which was, at the time, the finest available, with the numbers increasing for thicker threads. The development of finer sutures led to the introduction of gauge 0, 00 and so on down to 10/0, used in microsurgery. The modern metric gauge is 10 times the diameter of a suture material in millimetres: thus metric 3 corresponds to the old 000 or 3/0 and is 0.3 mm in diameter.

Other methods of closure

Although needle and suture closure has stood the test of time, surgeons are constantly looking for other methods either for novelty or to improve the quality of the end result.

Staples

Adaptations of the familiar office stapler have been developed which semi-automatically introduce a row or a circle of stainless steel staples. Titanium is generally used for internal staples as it produces less tissue reaction and is non-magnetic – and therefore MRI compatible. Stainless steel may be used for skin staples. They have found application in a number of sites (Table 8.4) including:

- skin – where they reduce the time taken for closure
- GI tract – where joining two cut ends of gut in anatomically difficult circumstances is easier and quicker, e.g. a low colorectal anastomosis
- lung – resections can be done using a stapler which delivers a staggered row of staples so that the line is airtight
- minimal access surgery – stapling techniques are widely used because suturing is technically difficult and time-consuming (see Ch. 5).

Tapes

These are applicable only to skin closure. They are useful in minor wounds and also where the cosmetic outcome is critical (e.g. the face) because the skin puncture marks of sutures are avoided. Once the wound has healed they can be peeled away rather than having to be removed.

Adhesives

Tissue glues, particularly enbucrilate preparations (Histoacryl), are sometimes used for the closure of minor skin wounds. They avoid suture marks and are particularly useful in children because injection of local anaesthetic can be avoided. Their mechanism is polymerisation on contact with tissue moisture to form a firm adhesive bond. A thin layer is used to avoid burns from the exothermic reaction. Their disadvantage is that incorrectly opposed tissues cannot be realigned.

Techniques of closure

The choice should be the simplest and safest; more complex and therefore more hazardous procedures are chosen only when the simpler methods do not meet reconstructive (and occasionally aesthetic) requirements.

Great attention to detail is required to ensure the most acceptable scar is achieved: haemostasis must be meticulous, tissue tension must be absent and suture material should be of narrow diameter unless high extrinsic strength is required.

Table 8.3 Suture materials

Natural	Synthetic
Absorbable	Absorbable
Catgut – plain or chromic (made from sheep intestine submucosa)	Polyglactin
	Polyglycolic acid
	Polydioxone
	Polyglyconate
Non-absorbable	Non-absorbable
Silk	Polypropylene
Linen	Polyamide
Stainless steel wire	Polyester

Table 8.4 Surgical staples

Use	Stapler design	Comments
Skin closure	One staple at a time with hand-held stapler	Often stainless steel
Transection of tissue/viscera including larger blood vessels	Linear automated stapling devices with or without a cutting mechanism between 4 or 6 rows of staples	Titanium Varying staple heights for different tissue thicknesses Open and laparoscopic/thoracoscopic instruments available
Gastrointestinal anastomosis	Linear or circular transection automated staplers	Titanium Various surgical techniques used Double or triple linear stapler firings required for closure Open and laparoscopic/thoracoscopic instruments available

Simple closure

The wound should first be converted to an ellipse whose long axis lies parallel to the skin creases – failure to do so may result in unsightly dog ears. The wound is closed so that the edges are precisely matched and slightly everted (Fig. 8.8). Fine-toothed forceps and skin hooks are used to minimise crushing damage by instruments to the skin edges. Tension is avoided by making sure that the tissues approximate easily; the support of buried subcutaneous sutures and the distribution of stress with adhesive tapes can both contribute to this. Given attention to these matters, the quality of the final scar is determined by the wound healing characteristics of the individual.

Closure of the abdominal wall

After a laparotomy (Ch. 5), the incision is under tension. A different closure technique is required to resist the tendency for the wound to pull apart. Heavy sutures are inserted through all layers deep to the skin and subcutaneous tissues ('mass closure') so that the disruptive forces are distributed over a large suture–tissue interface (Fig. 8.9). Continuous sutures are usually used and should be placed 1 cm apart and 1 cm deep into the tissues on each side of the wound. Using such a technique the length of the suture used should be approximately four times the length of the wound (Jenkins rule). Non-absorbable or slowly absorbable sutures can be used, usually of 0 or 1 gauge.

Deep tension sutures are passed through all layers of the abdominal wall including the skin. They have protective plastic tubes placed around the suture over the skin edges to prevent it cutting into the skin. They are primarily used for the resuturing of wounds that have broken down – dehisced – a relatively rare occurrence.

When it is not possible to safely close the abdominal wall because of distension or oedema of viscera, the abdomen may be temporarily left open (laparostomy) and packed with gauze dressings, or closed with a plastic sheet sewn to the wound edges. If possible such wounds are later closed by mass suture. Alternatively the wound may be left open and allowed to heal by secondary intention, a process that may be aided by vacuum wound dressing devices.

DRESSINGS

Surface wounds that are open or that have been closed are commonly covered. Apart from avoiding what may be a disturbing sight for the patient and others, the main purposes of dressings are:

- protection from further contamination
- absorption of discharge from a raw surface
- application of substances which may help eliminate infection and dead or damaged tissue and thus accelerate healing.

Protection and absorption

In a sutured wound, protection from further contamination after 48 hours is not usually required and hence many surgeons expose suture lines after this time; patients are often less enthusiastic, feeling (wrongly) that their wound is then at an unnecessary risk.

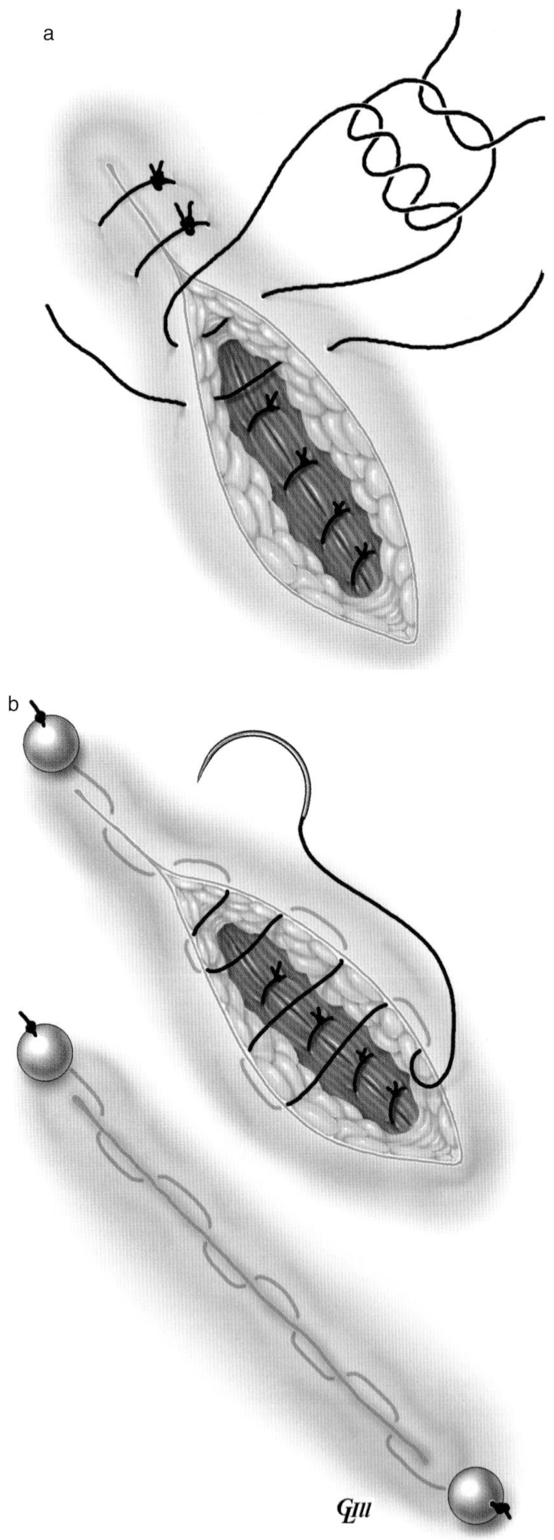

Fig. 8.8 The technique for closure of superficial wounds: (a) simple suture; (b) subcuticular suture.

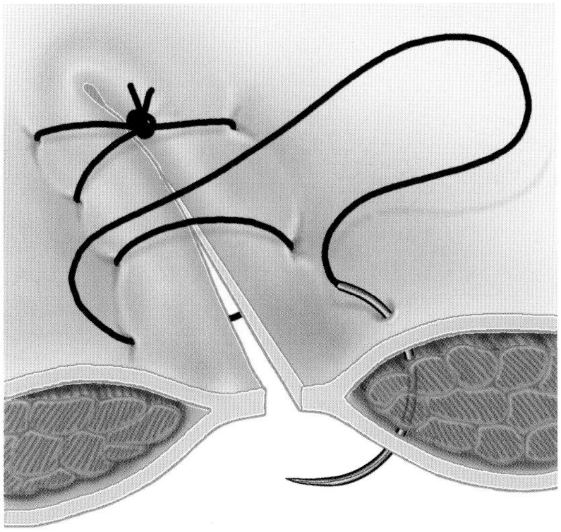

Fig. 8.9 Suturing of the abdominal wall with a continuous non-absorbable suture. Unlike most suturing, which aims to be fine and delicate, an abdominal wall suture line is subject to distraction and the bites are deliberately made large so that the forces are distributed over a large suture–tissue interface.

A wound which has not been closed for one or more of the reasons discussed above requires a barrier between it and the outside. Common ones are:

- plain cotton gauze with an outer layer of absorbent material – cotton wool is still the mostly widely used
- alginate mesh – an absorbent which is biocompatible and most suitable as a dressing for the donor site from which a split-skin graft has been taken
- gauze soaked in or impregnated with a bactericidal – an example is dressing of a burn with silver compounds
- a synthetic non-stick permeable membrane covered with an outer absorbent layer.

Plain gauze has the disadvantage that it adheres to the wound so that, if it is removed without anaesthesia, pain occurs in addition to surface injury. Both can be avoided if the dressing is moistened and removed only under general anaesthesia. Non-adherent dressings (e.g. gauze impregnated with petroleum jelly) are easily changed but they have little absorptive capacity and are unsuitable if discharge is profuse. In that circumstance, special polymer absorptive substances in bead form (Debrisan and Iodosorb) have a place when there is a cavity but are expensive. An alternative is an occlusive dressing which contains a water-absorbing compound (Sorbsan or Granuflex).

Therapeutic dressings

It has always been a goal of surgical management to find substances which hasten healing, but down the centuries this has been more often a search for the surgical equivalent of the philosopher's stone. Apart from the barrier function of certain materials in special circumstances (e.g. silver compounds in burns), dressings which contain ingredients thought to be active in removing dead tissue or promoting the formation of granulation tissue have not been shown to add anything to careful surgical and nursing care.

FURTHER READING

Granick MS, Gamelli RL (eds) 2007 Surgical wound healing and management. Informa Healthcare,

Bryant R, Nix D 2011 Acute and chronic wounds: current management concepts, 4th edn. Mosby, Edinburgh

Patterson-Brown S 2009 Core topics in general and emergency surgery: a companion to specialist surgical practice, 4th edn. Saunders, Edinburgh

9 Surgical infection

Every operation in surgery is an experiment in bacteriology

Berkely Moynihan, 1920

This chapter is in two parts. The first is an introduction to infection in general. The second is about specific infections that are common or important in surgical practice; it is not an exhaustive account, and the reader is referred to other sources for a more complete coverage of infectious diseases (see 'Further reading').

Surgical infections include both those which are established and present to surgeons and those that result from surgical interventions (often called iatrogenic).

INFECTION IN GENERAL

IMPORTANCE OF INFECTION

History

As recently as 100 years ago, surgeons had few methods for the elimination of contamination from potential causes of infections. There were no antibiotics to combat established infections and no supportive treatments that are now available for patients with severe sepsis (Ch. 10). Infected wounds were treated by radical operations, in the knowledge that amputation was often essential to save life.

Antisepsis and asepsis

Limb amputation during the Franco-Prussian war of 1870 resulted in death from infection in all 34 soldiers. Louis Pasteur hypothesised that organisms caused infection by being carried through the air. Joseph Lister (1827–1912) discovered that meticulous technique and a spray of carbolic acid into and around the wounds of compound leg fractures reduced the incidence of infection and could make amputation avoidable. This use of the technique of antisepsis (destruction of infective organisms by physicochemical means) was followed by the development of asepsis (the absence of infective organisms) in surgical procedures. Amongst others, William Halsted (1852–1922) promoted handwashing, the use of surgical gloves and the donning of clean clothes before an operation, as did Lord Moynihan (1865–1936). The discovery by Paul Ehrlich (1854–1915) of chemical agents which could kill organisms changed for ever the treatment of infection. In 1929, Sir Alexander Fleming (1881–1955) discovered that a mould (*Penicillium*) inhibited bacterial growth, published on its therapeutic effect in 1940 and won the Nobel Prize in 1945.

Improvements since have now led to almost absolute sterility in the operating theatre and the deployment of many powerful natural and synthetic antibiotics.

Incidence

The incidence of postoperative infection has fallen because of advances in sterilisation techniques, antibiotic prophylaxis and surgical awareness. The risk is related to the type of surgery performed and the physiological status of the patient. In general surgery, operations have been classified into four risk groups (Table 9.1).

Morbidity and mortality

Postoperative infections are responsible for high morbidity, significant mortality and a prolonged stay in hospital. Many deaths after operation are the result of uncontrolled or unrecognised sepsis. Prevention relies to a large extent on attention to detail in the perioperative care of the patient (Ch. 7).

Cost

An estimate of a 5% postoperative infection rate, with each incident resulting in an average increase of 7 days in hospital, leads to a cost of approximately £200 million a year in the UK. Thus any method of reducing postoperative infection rates has the potential of being cost-effective.

BIOLOGY OF INFECTION

Infection is defined as the proliferation of organisms in tissues and their invasion of various bodily pathways such as the blood. Colonisation of parts of the body – e.g. the gastrointestinal tract and upper respiratory passages – is normal and usually without harm; in some instances it is important for health. So-called commensal organisms may have a role in production of essential metabolites.

There is also frequent exposure of the body to contamination by other potentially invasive organisms, but infection remains comparatively rare. Its development depends on complex interactions between the organism, local factors and host defences (Fig. 9.1).

Organisms

Load

Experimental studies have shown that a certain concentration or quantity of organisms is required before infection results. For example, more than 100 000 *Staphylococcus aureus* organisms are needed in a wound for an abscess to develop. Any wound is inevitably contaminated from the surrounding environment. The basis of simple first aid in traumatic wounds is the application of agents that selectively kill the organisms (antiseptics), decrease the load and reduce the chance of the development of an infection.

Pathogenesis and virulence

Organisms capable of causing infection (pathogens) have varying virulence or power to proliferate and spread within the body. The factors responsible include:

- direct growth, which damages surrounding structures by pressure and/or ischaemic effects, e.g. abscess formation, hydatid disease of the liver
- production of bacterial toxins which cause a variety of effects – e.g. bacterial spread (streptokinase), cell damage (haemolysins), interference with metabolism (cholera toxin), stimulation of nerve impulses (tetanus toxin), activation of cytokine cascades (Gram-negative endotoxin)

Table 9.1 Classification of risk of wound infection

Type	Definition	Example	Infection risk (%)
Clean	No breach of GI tract	Hernia, varicose veins	2
Clean–contaminated	Prepared GI tract opened	Elective colectomy	6
Contaminated	Unprepared bowel opened	Emergency colectomy	15
Dirty	Pus at operation site; perforated bowel	Perforated appendicitis	40

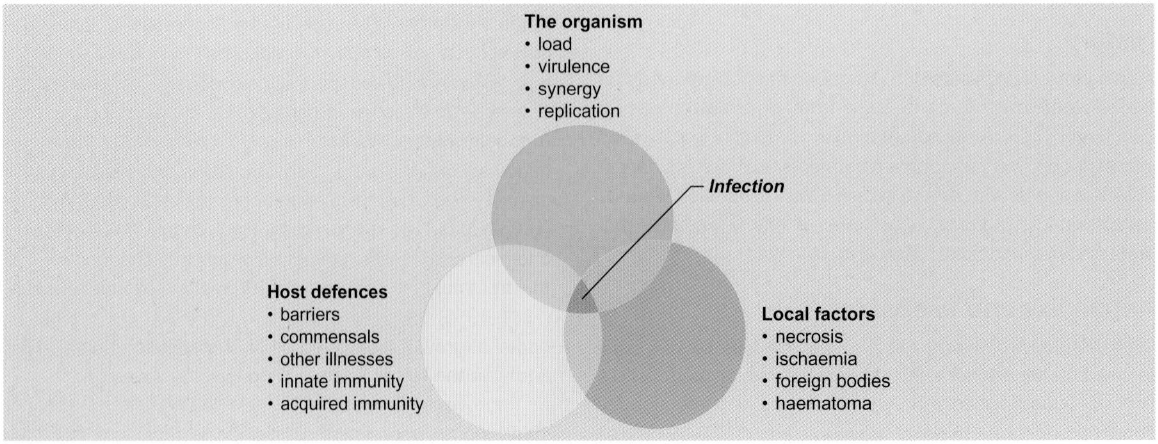

Fig. 9.1 Interaction between the factors that produce infection.

- synergy and interaction – e.g. combined promotion of infection by beta-haemolytic streptococci and anaerobic bacteria to produce rapidly spreading cutaneous gangrene (necrotising fasciitis) where hyaluronidase from the streptococci cleave the fascial planes and allow the infection to spread rapidly.
- replication – doubling rates of organisms can vary from less than 1 hour for most bacteria and viruses, to many days (tuberculosis) and even to years for some of the slow virus (prion) infections. Before antibiotics, a pneumococcal infection was a race between bacterial multiplication and host immune response. The patient died if the response did not keep up with bacterial replication.

Local host factors

The local environment has an impact on the chance of contamination resulting in an infection. Factors include:

- Tissue death – dead tissue can easily become infected, often with anaerobic organisms; in the absence of a blood supply, the host response is non-operative, and removal of necrotic tissue is essential in both the prevention and treatment of such infection.
- Reduction in oxygen supply (ischaemia) reduces the effectiveness of phagocytes and also aids the growth of anaerobic bacteria. Improvement in local tissue oxygen concentrations (e.g. the treatment of gas gangrene with hyperbaric oxygen and the management of infection in the lower limb by bypass grafting) can halt invasion.
- Diabetes mellitus is particularly associated with skin and soft-tissue infections – the mechanism is multifactorial: local hyperglycaemia, microvascular disease and peripheral neuropathy.
- Haematoma provides an ideal environment for bacterial growth – absence of blood supply and nutrition for the organisms. Prevention is by careful haemostasis during operations and appropriate use of drains.

Host defences

Mechanical, physical and chemical barriers

Invasion is discouraged wherever a natural interface occurs between the tissues and surrounding environment.

- Skin is a mechanical barrier against organisms and also secretes acidic sebum which can kill many pathogens.
- Cilia in the respiratory tract keep contaminated secretions in constant movement towards the exterior and so discourage local proliferation.
- The acidic pH in the stomach destroys many organisms so that the proximal small bowel is largely sterile.
- Peristaltic movement discourages local organism growth.
- A competent ileocaecal valve prevents reflux from the large to small bowel.
- Secretions such as tears and urine have a flushing action.
- Normal endogenous (commensal) flora on the skin and the GI tract provide a physical barrier by preventing the adherence of foreign organisms, and some also secrete mucus to produce a chemical barrier.

Concomitant illnesses

The general state of the patient can affect resistance to infection. The exact mechanisms are poorly understood but the disorders thought to influence the incidence and course of infection through effects on host defences are given in Box 9.1.

Natural immunity

Phagocytic cells: the macrophage and the neutrophil

Organisms that overcome the mechanical barriers of the skin or the respiratory and GI tracts are first attacked by these cells which ingest and then kill them using either oxygen-dependent methods (free radicals and superoxide molecules) or oxygen-independent mechanisms.

The complement system

A cascade of active proteins that attract phagocytic cells, increase vascular permeability and directly lyse pathogens (Table 9.2). Activation is either by the classical (antibody-mediated) or alternative (endotoxin-mediated) pathways. Defects in this system can lead to infection from normally non-pathogenic commensals.

Acquired immunity

There are two types of acquired immunity: antibody-mediated and cell-mediated.

Antibody-mediated

Not all organisms can be overcome by natural immunity. Those that evade the first lines of defence encounter lymphocytes. B-lymphocytes secrete antibodies which are classically divided into five classes: IgM, IgG, IgA, IgD and IgE. Stimulation of antibody production is most often T-cell-dependent but some polysaccharides can stimulate B-cells directly. Antibodies protect the host by simply binding to the foreign antigen or act with complement proteins to opsonise,

Box 9.1 Factors predisposing to infection

- Malnutrition
- Malignancy
- Jaundice
- Age
- Obesity
- Diabetes

Table 9.2 Complement proteins and their action

Active molecule	Action
C3a	Chemoattractant for neutrophils Liberates histamine
C3b	Enhances phagocytosis
C5a	Opsonisation
C8	Causes cells to leak
C9	Lyses antigens
C5–9	Chemoattractant for neutrophils

lyse and kill invading organisms. The classical pathway for complement activation involves the binding of C1-qrs, a calcium-dependent complex found in normal plasma, to IgG or IgM, which leads to the activation of C3 and consequent amplification of protein production; this in turn causes an increase in vascular permeability, attracts neutrophils and lyses foreign cells.

Cell-mediated

Two different processes are involved:

- CD8 T-lymphocytes kill cells which contain replicating invaders, usually viruses.
- CD4 T-lymphocytes help macrophages to kill phagocytosed organisms.

Cytokines

Cytokines are small peptides, released by white blood cells, which act like hormones for the immune system. They allow communication between the different cell populations and control the response to infection (Table 9.3).

Immune deficiency syndromes

Defects in the innate or adaptive immune systems illustrate the importance of both in protection from infection:

Innate

- Primary:
  - complement disorders
  - phagocytic cell deficiencies: chronic granulomatous disease, Chediak–Higashi syndrome.
- Secondary:
  - burns
  - trauma (including surgical procedures)
  - presence of foreign bodies
  - therapeutic corticosteroids.

Table 9.3 Cytokines and their actions in relation to infection

Factor	Source	Actions
IL-1	Macrophages	Pro-inflammatory
IL-4	T-cells	T- and B-cell proliferation Macrophage activation
IL-6	T-cells	B-cell differentiation
IL-9	T-cells	Mast cell growth
IL-10	T- and B-cells Macrophages	Cytokine inhibition
IFN-α	Multiple	Antiviral
IFN-γ	T- and NK cells	Antiviral Macrophage activation MHC induction
TNF-α	Monocytes	Cytotoxicity Cachexia, fever
TNF-β	T cells Macrophages	Inhibits T- and NK-cell activation
G-CSF	Macrophages	Granulocyte growth

G-CSF, granulocyte colony-stimulating factor; IFN, interferon; IL, interleukin; MHC, major histocompatibility complex; TNF, tumour necrosis factor.

Adaptive

- Primary:
  - B-cell deficiencies: Bruton-type agammaglobulinaemia
  - T-cell deficiencies: DiGeorge syndrome
  - combined: severe combined immune deficiency (SCID).
- Secondary:
  - humoral: immunosuppressive drugs
  - cell-mediated: HIV infection/AIDS
  - generalised: malnutrition, neoplasia.

Postsplenectomy

The spleen is part of the reticuloendothelial system and has three functions which oppose infection:

- specific immunity – T- and B-lymphocyte production
- phagocytosis of foreign antigens by macrophages
- opsonin production – two proteins (tuftsin and properidin).

Removal of the spleen leads to an increased risk of overwhelming infection by encapsulated organisms such as pneumococci (overwhelming postsplenectomy infection [OPSI]). If the spleen is to be removed electively, vaccination against pneumococci, meningococci and *Haemophilus influenzae B* should be done at least 2 weeks before operation. After operation, all patients need to be on lifetime prophylactic penicillin or amoxicillin (which is active against *H. influenzae*).

INFECTION CONTROL AND PREVENTION

Measures are required to protect the patient, other patients and healthcare personnel from infections which may be encountered during surgical management. Risks arise both from the environment and from the patient's own endogenous flora.

Disinfectants

Disinfectants are substances that can kill most pathogenic organisms but not bacterial spores or slow viruses. Their main use is for cleaning instruments (e.g. endoscopes) and surfaces which cannot be sterilised by other means. Examples in common use include:

- aldehydes, e.g. glutaraldehyde (Cidex)
- ethyl alcohol – 60–90%
- chlorine-releasing agents, e.g. sodium hypochlorite (bleach)
- clear phenolics, e.g. Clearsol.

Antiseptics

These are disinfectants that can be used on living tissue. Common examples include:

- aqueous or alcoholic 0.5% chlorhexidine
- aqueous or alcoholic 10% povidone-iodine.

Sterilisation

This process involves the complete destruction of all organisms, including spores and slow viruses (prions). A number of methods are available, and the choice depends on the resistance of the material to be sterilised and the quantity involved (for methods and details, see Ch. 5).

PROTECTION FOR THE PATIENT

The risk of infection of the surgical site (wound, anastomosis, peritoneal and other cavities) may be reduced in a number of ways.

Four factors associated with increased risk of infection are:

- operation of more than 2 hours' duration
- abdominal procedures
- contamination, either endogenous or exogenous
- more than three diagnoses for the patient.

When one or more of these is present, additional preventative measures should be considered. Prominent among these is the use of prophylactic antibiotics, although these are not a substitute for sound surgical aseptic techniques.

An assessment of the risk is made, based on the patient's medical state and the type of surgery to be done. Of the above four factors, if only one is positive, the risk of infection is less than 3%, and if all four are positive, there is a risk of 30%.

Theatre design and sterilisation of instruments and prostheses

This is discussed in detail in Chapter 5.

Aseptic surgical technique

Handwashing (Ch. 5) reduces the number but does not eliminate all organisms found on the hands. Gloves (also Ch. 5) are put on with minimal contact between their external surface and the hand. Likewise, surgical gowns are put on in such a way that the outside surface is never touched. Hair cover and masks are traditionally worn, although their role in preventing infection has been questioned.

Preparation of the skin and bowel

Skin

Antiseptics are used for the preparation of the skin before operation. Adherent plastic film placed onto the patient's exposed skin prior to incision may further reduce the chance of contamination from skin organisms.

Gastrointestinal tract

This is discussed in Chapters 18–27.

Antibiotic prophylaxis

Identification of patients at risk

Patients who are at high risk of infection, or in whom the risk may be low but infection would have serious consequences, should be given prophylactic antibiotics. There are operative and patient-related factors to consider:

- operative:
  - high risk of an infection – contaminated or dirty surgery (e.g. colectomy, trauma surgery)
  - placement of foreign materials, e.g. heart valve, arterial graft, joint replacement.
- patient:
  - immunosuppression
  - high-risk patients, e.g. previous foreign body implants, heart valve disease, peripheral vascular disease, obesity.

Choice of antibiotic

This is determined by the likely infecting organisms. Most units have agreed protocols tailored to suit the type of operations carried out and the local prevalence of particular organisms. The chosen antibiotic must be:

- effective for the likely organisms
- economical
- unlikely to promote resistance.

Cephalosporins are widely used for orthopaedic and general surgery, often in combination with metronidazole. Penicillins and aminoglycosides are also popular choices (Table 9.4).

Table 9.4 Examples of antibiotic prophylaxis

Operation	Infection site	Likely organisms	Prophylactic antibiotics
Colectomy	Wound	*E. coli* Anaerobes *Bacteroides*	Cefuroxime Metronidazole
Hip replacement	Prosthesis	*Staph. aureus*	Cefuroxime
Bladder instrumentation	Urinary tract	*E. coli* *Klebsiella*	Gentamicin
ERCP	Biliary tract	*E. coli*	Ciprofloxacin
Vascular graft	Graft	*Staph. aureus* *Staph. albus*	Cefuroxime

ERCP, endoscopic retrograde cholangiopancreatography.

Dose and timing

The highest tissue concentration of antibiotic is required at the moment of tissue contamination. For most procedures, parenteral administration at the time of induction of anaesthesia produces high local concentrations at the moment of incision and provides a satisfactory tissue level for the duration of the procedure. Two further doses at appropriate subsequent intervals completes 24 hours of prophylaxis, which is sufficient. Some argue that one dose is enough. Certain patients may require a longer course, such as those in intensive care units (Ch. 10), those with heart valve replacements or those with peripheral vascular disease undergoing arterial operations.

Route of administration

Intravenous

Adequate serum concentrations are guaranteed but the method is the most expensive.

Oral

The oral route is not widely accepted as effective except for prophylaxis in high-risk patients undergoing minor procedures, e.g. dental work on patients with prosthetic heart valves in whom an infection has serious consequences.

Rectal

Metronidazole suppositories are still used by some gastrointestinal surgeons and have the advantage of low cost. However, absorption kinetics are variable.

Topical

This route is used for specfic circumstances:

- gentamicin-impregnated cement for orthopaedic prostheses
- beads containing gentamicin which are implanted locally at sites of persistent sepsis
- tetracycline lavage of the contaminated peritoneal cavity.

Long-term prophylaxis

Certain groups of patients are at continuing risk of infection, and long-term prophylaxis may be appropriate to prevent recurrent (e.g. urinary) or overwhelming infections (see 'Post-splenectomy'). The hazard of the development of resistance can be overcome by rotation of those agents which are effective.

PROTECTION FOR OTHERS

Other patients

Continuous accurate monitoring of infections in the hospital environment as a whole can give important early warning of potential epidemic infections and so allow early measures to be taken such as temporary cessation of operations, isolation of patients and change in antibiotic regimens.

The routine and specially indicated measures used in the operating room are discussed in Chapter 5. On the ward those who are highly infectious to others are isolated in side bays. Clear instructions for staff and visitors about barrier nursing and the use of gloves, aprons and masks must be given.

The increase in hospital-acquired infection has led to a greater emphasis on hand hygiene and aseptic technique. A 'bare below the elbows' policy for all clinical staff has been widely adopted combined with handwashing or the use of antiseptic alcohol-based gels. Before and immediately after inspecting a wound (or indeed touching a patient or his/her belongings), all healthcare staff should clean their hands. If there is significant risk of infection, disposable gloves and aprons should be worn.

Patients who are admitted for elective joint surgery (Ch. 34) should not be placed next to someone with an infected wound; indeed, good practice would separate all elective clean surgery patients from those that are or might be infected. Many hospitals now screen all elective admissions for MRSA colonisation (see below), and test all emergency patients on admission.

In outpatient clinics, similar hygienic measures apply: paper covers to the examination couches; hand cleaning between patients; washing, disinfecting or sterilising examination instruments such as endoscopes; and, on microbiological if not economic grounds, the use of disposables.

Healthcare personnel

The spread of HIV drew attention to the protection of healthcare personnel, although hepatitis B has killed far more healthcare workers over the years. There have been few instances of HIV seroconversion following occupational injury. Almost all have been from hollow (syringe) needle injuries, often with deep penetration.

Surgical technique

This is discussed in Chapter 5.

Vaccination

All staff at risk (which implies all medical and paramedical personnel) should be vaccinated against hepatitis B, and it is desirable that they have had a recent serological test to show adequate antibody levels. While the vaccine for hepatitis B is very effective, other transmissible diseases such as hepatitis C and HIV do not yet have vaccines available.

Monitoring and reporting events

In order to monitor the incidence of occupationally acquired infection, injuries caused by sharps – knives and needles – must be reported and a serum sample obtained at the time, with another planned at 3 months. Post-exposure prophylaxis against HIV after injury from a high-risk patient is now routinely offered (see Ch. 5). Healthcare workers can contract many of the diseases associated with work in the same way as the general population; to prove a work-related cause, evidence of seroconversion following a reported injury is essential.

DIAGNOSIS AND MANAGEMENT OF INFECTION

Prompt identification of the source of infection and initiation of correct treatment are crucial to avoid the morbidity and mortality associated with delay. Blind treatment with broad-spectrum antibiotics before the causative organism is identified should, if possible, be avoided, although severe infections demand prompt antibiotic treatment on a best-guess basis while efforts are made to identify the cause.

Clinical features of infections in general

History

The timing of a postoperative infection gives clues as to its cause. Wound infections do not usually become clinically manifest in the first 48 hours, and chest infections are a more likely cause of sepsis in the early period after operation. A gastrointestinal anastomosis that leaks often presents with continuing low-grade fever after 4 or 5 days. Deep-seated prosthetic infection may not be apparent for weeks or months.

Direct questions for cough, dysuria or abdominal pain may focus further enquiry and investigation.

Established infections not clearly associated with surgical events should prompt the search for a history of recent travel, administration of antibiotics and determination of occupation. Evidence of immunosuppression or reasons for breakdown in the normal barriers to infection (e.g. intravenous drug abuse, diabetes) should be identified.

Physical findings

General

An assessment, with measurement of pulse, blood pressure and temperature, gives an indication of severity. Signs of systemic disturbance increase the urgency of treatment and may change the management plan. Resuscitation and consideration of transfer to an intensive care unit are necessary in severe instances, particularly if septic shock is present (see Ch. 10). In the elderly or those on corticosteroids, usual clinical features may be masked until circulatory failure develops.

Specific

Full examination is essential in a surgical patient with a pyrexia of unknown origin (PUO). Non-infective causes of PUO (deep vein thrombosis, haematoma, malignancy) should at this time be kept in mind. Likely causes of infection include:

- chest infection
- the surgical site (wounds, anastomoses) or areas adjacent to it (e.g. subphrenic spaces, pelvis)
- urinary tract infection, often secondary to catheterisation
- infection of intravenous lines.

Investigation of infection

Blood sampling

- *Full blood count.* A raised white blood cell count suggests the presence of infection and occasionally is the first sign of a deep abscess. Severe infections can suppress the bone marrow and cause leucopenia, anaemia and thrombocytopenia.
- *Blood culture.* It is important to take blood for both aerobic and anaerobic culture (and other samples as indicated such as CSF, urine, sputum) before antibiotics are started because interpretation of results afterwards may become difficult.
- *Serological examination* to detect antibodies can identify specific infections in their recovery phase but is sometimes useful for therapy (some viral infections, hydatid disease).

Microbiological analysis

All appropriate samples should be sent for microbiological analysis in an attempt to identify the causative organism(s), establish antibiotic sensitivities and guide therapy. Specimens may include:

- swabs from contaminated or infected wounds for microscopy, bacteriological culture and antibiotic sensitivity
- drainage fluid for microscopy, bacteriological culture and sensitivity
- urine for microscopy, bacteriological culture and sensitivity
- stool for microscopy, bacteriological culture and sensitivity and also for *Clostridium difficile* toxin testing
- tissue biopsies, particularly in chronic infections such as suspected tuberculosis when mycobacteriological studies (microscopy and culture) are requested in addition to routine bacteriological studies (see also amoebic disease of the bowel)

Methods of analysis include:

- Direct microscopy. Instant analysis can be performed but the information may be limited.
- Gram-staining of fluids can guide urgent treatment before a formal culture and sensitivity report is available.
- Culture and sensitivity currently takes 24–48 hours. Ideally the organism responsible for the infection should be grown and identified and the sensitivity of that organism to a range of antibiotics tested.

In severe infections, the time delay may not be acceptable, and treatment must be started according to likely sensitivities.

New microbiological techniques

- *Enzyme-linked immunosorbent assay (ELISA)* is used to detect antibodies to a particular organism and is the current technique to identify HIV and other viruses. A modified technique (ELISPOT) provides a useful rapid test for TB infection, although it may be positive in patients previously infected.
- *The polymerase chain reaction (PCR)* is increasingly used as a rapid test for a range of infections including TB, HIV and *Helicobacter pylori*.

Imaging

Localisation of the source of infection is often a challenge, and details of the techniques available are given in Chapter 4. Because of its ready availability and simplicity, ultrasound has become the first line of imaging in many circumstances, but other techniques such as CT scanning are often needed. Radionuclide imaging with labelled leucocytes has the particular advantage that it is a direct determinant of the presence of infection (or inflammation).

Management of infection

General measures

Basic treatment of infected wounds is summarised in Clinical Box 9.1. Other general measures include:

- resuscitation – see Chapter 10
- analgesia for pain
- anti-emetics
- paracetamol
- cooling fans for high fever.

Specific measures

Antibiotics

The decision as to which antibiotics to start and when to start them is not always easy. It may be beneficial to withhold antibiotics until the cause becomes apparent if the patient is not systemically unwell. Some fevers do not require antibiotics (e.g. postoperative pyrexia caused by DVT), and certain infections respond poorly to antibiotic therapy (e.g. an abscess). Antibiotics are described in more detail at the end of this chapter.

Drainage

A local collection of pus contains organisms that are inaccessible to systemic antibiotics. In addition, it acts as a toxic focus and may also exert pressure effects on surrounding structures. The collection should be removed, usually by external drainage. This can be achieved by:

- *Needle aspiration.* For abscesses that can be reached with a needle (sometimes under imaging control), aspiration and antibiotic therapy may be all that is required. The technique is particularly useful for areas where a scar is undesirable, such as on the face or breast. The disadvantage is that adequate drainage is often hard to achieve and the small puncture site is quick to close over, so allowing an abscess to reform.
- *Guided drainage.* Under image control with radiological or ultrasound techniques a tube drain can be inserted and left until the cavity has collapsed.
- *Surgical drainage.* This is the most certain method; not only can all loculi (subcavities with varying communication with the main one) be reached but also dead tissue (slough) can be removed. The cavity is then dressed regularly and left open to heal by secondary intention (see also 'Gas gangrene').

Clinical Box 9.1 Management of infected wounds

- Remove clips or stitches to open part of wound
- Surgically debride necrotic areas
- Take wound swab (although most wound infections do not need antibiotics)
- Mark area of cellulitis surrounding wound to assess efficacy of treatment
- Dress wound to keep it open, clean and comfortable
  - soaked gauze (saline, betadine or proflavin)
  - specialised dressings, e.g. Kaltostat, Aquacel, Iodosorb
  - avoid occlusive dressings which encourage anaerobic infection
- For complex or large wounds consider
  - stoma wound bag
  - vacuum dressing
  - sterile larvae (maggots)

SYSTEMIC EFFECTS AND SYNDROMES

Bacteraemia

The word 'bacteraemia' means simply bacteria in the blood. Blood is normally sterile but any minor trauma to a colonised area (even brushing teeth) can lead to transient contamination. This does not usually cause systemic colonisation, but in patients with a diseased heart valve or a valve prosthesis, bacterial endocarditis can result.

Septicaemia

In cases of septicaemia, bacteria are not just present in the blood but are using it as a culture medium and multiplying. The clinical manifestations are the response of the body to the event: fever, tachycardia, hypotension, oliguria, respiratory failure (ARDS) and multiple organ failure. Blood cultures are often positive, but the absence of a detectable organism does not preclude the diagnosis, because the clinical effects can be produced by the products of bacterial metabolism and their interaction with defence mechanisms such as cytokines (endotoxaemia – see below). Other causes of a negative blood culture include:

- low bacterial concentrations at the time of sampling – after the initial spike of fever
- prior administration of systemic antibiotics which prevent organisms in the blood sample from growing in culture.

Endotoxaemia

In some instances of severe sepsis, often with shock, organisms are not found, but circulating Gram-negative endotoxins can be demonstrated. Translocation of Gram-negative material from the gut and subsequent cytokine activation (notably tumour necrosis factor, TNF) have been proposed as the cause of this apparently sterile septic state.

Clinical features

Symptoms

Confusion and worsening general features of malaise during the course of a surgical illness are warning signs. There may be symptoms related to a focus from which the bloodstream has become involved.

Systemic effects and syndromes

Emergency Box 9.1

Emergency management of the septic patient

- Resuscitate if necessary with oxygen and i.v. fluids
- Identify likely cause – history, examination, case notes, temperature chart
- Take samples – blood cultures, swabs, urine
- Treat symptoms – lower fever with paracetamol or fans; analgesia for pain
- Treat infection – best-guess antibiotics i.v.
- Identify actual cause – arrange imaging: chest X-ray, ultrasound, CT scan
- Plan definitive treatment
  - Transfer to high-dependency area if in septic shock
  - Antibiotics according to microbiology sensitivities
  - Ultrasound- or CT-guided drainage
  - Surgical drainage

Physical findings

Fever, hypotension and oliguria are common findings. Focal sepsis may be evident, e.g. inflammation around the entry point of a central venous line. See also systemic inflammatory response syndrome (SIRS), below.

Investigation

Repeated blood culture is vital but may not always be positive, even if there is generalised sepsis. Raised white cell count is usual unless there is some systemic suppression of white cell production (immunocompromise by drugs, underlying illness, or overwhelming sepsis).

Management

Emergency management of the septic patient is summarised in Emergency Box 9.1. Best-guess antibiotic therapy should be started immediately after local and blood samples have been taken. Costly newer agents are often used (e.g. piperacillin or imipenem, because of their broad-spectrum efficacy). Restoration of the circulation is considered below. Any focus discovered should be eliminated as soon as possible, usually by drainage.

Systemic inflammatory response syndrome (SIRS)

Nomenclature

The systemic inflammatory response syndrome (SIRS) is the name given to a physiological state of septic collapse. It is often caused by an infection, but not always (Fig. 9.2). It therefore embraces the terms 'sepsis', 'septic shock' and 'toxic shock'.

Pathophysiology

The central mechanism appears to be activation of macrophages and release of TNF. Oxygen supply to the tissues is reduced, and the situation is aggravated by cell injury which leads to deficient uptake of oxygen. The result is general tissue hypoxia and a build-up of lactic acid. Cytokine activation also occurs; TNF can produce this clinical pattern experimentally. The clinical picture is characterised by fever, hypotension, respiratory failure, oliguria and multiple organ failure, with hepatic and bone marrow suppression occurring as late events.

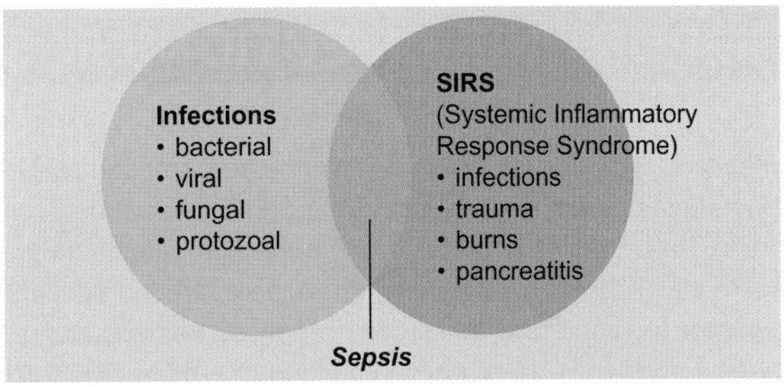

Fig. 9.2 Relationship between infection and systemic inflammatory response syndrome (SIRS).

Clinical manifestations

The clinical manifestations of SIRS are dealt with in detail in Chapter 10.

Generalised fungal infections

Causes are as follows:

- a severely compromised immune system, as in leukaemia, lymphoma or HIV infection
- extensive burns where immunocompromise may also be a factor
- prolonged administration of multiple antibiotics.

The commonest infection is with *Candida*.

Bacterial translocation

Some clinicians believe that ischaemic damage to the gut in the critically ill allows translocation of bacteria and toxins to maintain the appearances of sepsis; indeed, the GI tract has been called the undrained abscess of the abdomen. Once bacteria have crossed the bowel wall, they may translocate to the respiratory system, which becomes colonised with enteric organisms whose toxins can more easily escape into the systemic circulation.

Prevention

Selective decontamination

To reduce the endogenous bacterial load, selective decontamination of the digestive tract with topical, oral and intravenous antibiotics has been used. However, the technique has not lessened mortality, and in consequence it has not been widely adopted.

Immunomodulation

Artificial enhancement of immunity to endotoxins, and thus prevention of the systemic response, is an attractive idea that has yet to make a clinical impact. Immunoglobulins raised against the cell walls of Gram-negative organisms (antiendotoxin antibodies) have been protective in animal studies but have not improved mortality in humans.

IMPORTANT INFECTIONS IN SURGICAL PATIENTS

Infections which particularly concern the surgeon and surgical patients can arise as a result of surgical interventions or present as established infections that require surgical management. The infections considered here are particularly common or important to surgical practice. Bacteria, fungi, viruses and protozoa all cause infection that can present to the surgeon.

USE OF ANTIBIOTICS

Typical antibiotics and their uses are given in Tables 9.5 and 9.6. When to use antibiotics and which ones to choose is not always clear. Blind (rather than best-guess) treatment is often needed for sick patients, but may obscure the bacteriological diagnosis.

Table 9.5 Common antibiotics and their uses

Antibiotic	Common uses	Notes
Penicillin	All cocci: strepto-, staph-, pneumo-	85% of staphylococci are resistant because of beta-lactamase production Allergies are common: effects range from a simple rash to fatal anaphylaxis
Flucloxacillin	Active against staphylococci; should be included in treatment of cutaneous infections	
Meticillin	Similar antibiotic to flucloxacillin	Used to test bacterial sensitivity to flucloxacillin
Co-amoxiclav (Augmentin)	Broad spectrum: soft-tissue infections, pneumonia, UTI and for antibiotic prophylaxis	Combination of amoxicillin (amoxycillin) and clavulanic acid; latter acts to prevent action of beta-lactamases
Amoxicillin (amoxycillin, Amoxyl)	Active against both Gram-negative and positive organisms: urinary tract and respiratory infections	An amino group added to the basic penicillin molecule gives increased antimicrobial activity
Piperacillin (Tazocin)	Reserved for severe infections in combination with gentamicin (for Gram-negative, resistant organisms)	Later-generation penicillin that has activity against *Pseudomonas*
Cefuroxime	Broad spectrum: prophylaxis for bowel and biliary operations; treatment of GI conditions – cholecystitis, appendix mass, diverticulitis	Second-generation cephalosporin In common use in GI surgery often in combination with metronidazole; 10% of those allergic to penicillin are similarly affected by cephalosporins
Cefotaxime or ceftazidime	Second-line treatment for sepsis insensitive to cefuroxime	Third-generation cephalosporin Some improvement in activity against Gram-negative organisms but slightly poorer against staphylococci
Imipenem	Broad spectrum – reserved for use in ICU	A carbapenem–thienamycin beta-lactam best combined with cilastatin – an enzyme inhibitor of its metabolism by the kidney
Tetracycline	Pelvic inflammatory disease; other sexually transmitted diseases	Bacteriostatic rather than bactericidal; however, active against *Chlamydia*
Gentamicin	Severe sepsis (in combination with penicillin or metronidazole) Prophylaxis during urinary tract instrumentation	Aminoglycoside active against Gram-negative organisms and *Pseudomonas*; inactive against anaerobes and streptococci Potentially nephrotoxic, and serum levels must be regularly checked
Erythromycin	Soft-tissue and chest infections	Active against staphylococci and *H. influenzae* Useful in those allergic to penicillin
Clarithromycin	Similar to erythromycin	Used for *Helicobacter pylori* infections of the upper GI tract
Vancomycin	Gram-positive infections resistant to penicillins and cephalosporins (MRSA and pseudomembranous colitis)	Used orally to treat *C. difficile* infection
Teicoplanin	Similar uses to vancomycin	Requires administration by intramuscular or intravenous route
Trimethoprim	Urinary tract infections	
Co-trimoxazole	*Pneumocystis carinii* pneumonia	
Metronidazole	Anaerobic abdominal infections (including prophylaxis and usually in combination) Gas gangrene Amoebic infections Pseudomembranous colitis	Used orally to treat *C. difficile* infection
Ciprofloxacin	Gram-negative infections – *Salmonella, Shigella, Campylobacter*	4-Quinolone – the traveller's antibiotic

Table 9.6 Examples of typical antibiotic choices for particular clinical infections

Infection	First choice	Alternatives
Chest infection	Penicillin + erythromycin	Co-amoxiclav (Augmentin)
Wound infection (cellulitis)	Penicillin + flucloxacillin	Co-amoxiclav
Wound infection (abscess)	Drain collection	Flucloxacillin
Intra-abdominal infection (endogenous organisms likely)	Cefuroxime + metronidazole	Cefotaxime Gentamicin
Cholecystitis–cholangitis	Cefuroxime + metronidazole	Piperacillin (Tazocin)
Urinary tract infection	Trimethoprim	Gentamicin Co-amoxiclav
Pelvic inflammatory disease	Tetracyclines + cefuroxime + metronidazole	
Severe sepsis	Gentamicin + metronidazole + penicillin	Imipenem Ticarcillin
MRSA	Vancomycin	Teicoplanin
Pseudomembranous colitis *(C. difficile)*	Metronidazole	Vancomycin
Gas gangrene	Penicillin + metronidazole	Metronidazole

Box 9.2 Sources of hospital-acquired infections

- The operative site – the wound, any anastomosis, the cavity in which the operation was done (e.g. abdomen, pleura or within the central nervous system)
- In relation to a prosthesis – joint, cardiac, other vascular or more recently the mesh used to repair a hernia
- Respiratory or GI tract from translocation
- Urinary tract from procedures such as urinary catheterisation
- Infection from intravenous lines
- Cross-infection, particularly meticillin-resistant *Staphylococcus aureus* (MRSA) and *Clostridium difficile*

The selection of an antibiotic rests on:

- severity of the infection
- likely organisms and their sensitivities
- patient factors – allergies, pregnancy, renal function
- hospital policy.

More expensive antibiotics have a broader spectrum of activity but encourage bacterial resistance and are kept in reserve for severe infections or as second-line treatment.

Samples such as blood cultures must be taken if possible before treatment is begun. Other factors to take into account are:

- dose
- route of administration (i.v., oral, rectal)
- duration (up to 5 days' treatment is usually sufficient for common bacterial infections)
- potential side effects.

ACQUIRED INFECTIONS

Some infections arise as a consequence of an intervention or because of hospital admission. Common causes are listed in Box 9.2.

Clinical features

Most wound infections can be identified by simple inspection for erythema and by palpation, which should be done whenever there is postoperative pyrexia.

A deeper infection may present insidiously, again with pyrexia, a rise in the white blood count or organ dysfunction such as prolonged postoperative ileus. Some deep infections are hard to detect and require special imaging techniques (Ch. 4).

Management

Prevention

As described above, strict measures to reduce hospital-acquired infections must be observed. In particular the surgeon should:

- use meticulous technique to inflict minimal damage to tissues and to avoid a haematoma
- use prophylactic antibiotics – but not for prolonged duration in most cases
- avoidance of complications such as anastomotic breakdown
- maintain hand hygiene at all times
- comply with the 'bare below the elbows' policy
- ensure that peripheral and central intravenous cannulas are changed routinely (every 2 and 7 days, respectively)
- avoid prolonged antibiotic treatment whenever possible, and regularly review indication for treatment
- comply with hospital infection control policies
- screen elective cases for infection and MRSA colonisation prior to admission

Treatment

Antibiotics treat cellulitis surrounding a wound but cannot penetrate into an abscess. There is no substitute for drainage in presence of pus. For drainage, an infection of the wound can simply be laid open, the infection allowed to run its course and the wound left to heal by secondary intention (Ch. 8). More complex collections require drainage radiologically or surgically.

The common form of continued spread is peritonitis. If the infection has not localised, the only effective treatment is to re-explore and remove products of infection by lavage and control the cause of the infection. This is likely to be a leakage from an anastomotic suture line which requires repair or exteriorisation. The treatment of MRSA and *Clostridium difficile* infections are described below.

Infection of a prosthesis is a disaster. Although high-dose systemic antibiotics may work, the most effective treatment is to remove the prosthesis and not replace it until the infection has been controlled. Some prostheses cannot be removed without being immediately replaced (e.g. heart valves and peripheral vascular grafts with critical ischaemia beyond), and special measures may be necessary in these cases.

RESPIRATORY TRACT

Definition

Infection of the respiratory tract includes a range of conditions: bronchitis, pneumonia, lung abscess and empyema. An element of alveolar underexpansion (atelectasis) after operation is common (Ch. 6) and can cause mild pyrexia.

Organisms

The commonest organisms are *Pneumococcus* and *Haemophilus influenzae*. Gram-negative organisms can also be found in postoperative chest infections (see also 'Translocation').

Clinical features

Symptoms

- fever
- cough
- breathlessness
- confusion from hypoxia.

Physical findings

- cyanosis
- green sputum
- consolidation on chest examination.

Investigation

- chest X-ray
- culture of sputum or bronchial washings
- arterial blood gas tensions.

Management

Prophylaxis

- Do not undertake an elective surgical procedure in the presence of uncontrolled respiratory infection.
- In the postoperative period, provide adequate postoperative analgesia (epidural analgesia is particularly valuable for patients with painful abdominal or thoracic incisions – see Ch. 6), physiotherapy and early mobilisation.

Treatment

- Initial administration of oxygen with the aim of restoring normal blood gas tensions.
- Antibiotic administration; most hospitals have a policy on the treatment of chest infections – a combination of penicillin and erythromycin is a common first-line treatment which can be altered on the outcome of sputum culture.
- Drainage of focal collections such as purulent pleural effusion or an empyema.

URINARY TRACT (see also Ch. 33)

Definition

Bacterial contamination of the urine is common, and the clinical picture needs to be taken into account. Urinary tract infection (UTI) encompasses a range of clinical conditions which include cystitis, pyelonephritis and perinephric abscess.

Organisms

Escherichia coli is the most common organism. Other Gram-negative bacteria include *Klebsiella, Streptococcus faecalis, Pseudomonas* and *Proteus mirabilis*. Coagulase-negative staphylococci are an occasional cause.

Diagnosis

The urine of those with an indwelling catheter frequently contains organisms but not white cells. Unless the patient is systemically unwell, this does not require treatment. The urine will not become sterile until the catheter is removed.

Clinical features

Symptoms

Smelly urine, dysuria and, if a catheter is not in place, increased frequency and nocturia are all symptoms of a UTI.

Physical findings

In cystitis these are unusual. If proximal spread is taking place, tenderness in the renal angles may be found and is accompanied by fever. Established UTI can mimic an acute abdomen and be confused with appendicitis (Ch. 25).

Investigation

Midstream or catheter drainage specimens must be taken before any treatment is started, but the results of cultures do not have to be awaited before best-guess antibiotic therapy is begun.

Management

Common first-line antibiotics are trimethoprim, gentamicin, ciprofloxacin or co-amoxiclav until antibiotic sensitivities are known.

CLOSTRIDIUM DIFFICILE (PSEUDOMEMBRANOUS) COLITIS

This condition has appeared in the last two decades and its incidence has increased in patients who have a prolonged stay in hospital.

Aetiology and organisms

Disturbance of the normal colonic bacterial flora by antibiotics leads to colonisation with *Clostridium difficile*, an anaerobic spore-forming organism which produces an enterotoxin. Certain patients are at risk:

- prolonged admission (more than 4 weeks)
- elderly
- malignant disease
- broad-spectrum antibiotic treatment.

Respiratory tract
Urinary tract
Clostridium difficile (Pseudomembranous) colitis
Meticillin-resistant *Staphylococcus aureus* (MRSA)
Pyrexia of unknown origin (PUO)
Established infections in the surgical patient
Cellulitis

Clinical features

Symptoms

The patient develops profuse mucous diarrhoea after continued or repeated courses of antibiotics.

Physical findings

Fever and non-specific features of toxicity are common findings. The abdomen may be distended and slightly tender. Sigmoidoscopy reveals diffuse inflammation with contact bleeding and, in severe instances, the typical yellow membranous plaques.

Investigation

Culture of *C. difficile* is difficult (hence the name) and, although useful for research, it is not of practical value for diagnosis. A water-soluble contrast enema may give a characteristic picture of ulceration and mucosal plaques.

The diagnosis is made by the detection of the toxin in the stool. DNA typing may show a type 027 variant which has increased toxicity and mortality rate.

Management

Prompt recognition and treatment are necessary to avoid significant mortality and morbidity associated with toxic dilatation of the colon (see 'Ulcerative colitis', Ch. 25) and progressive systemic toxicity.

Stopping the antibiotics may be all that is needed in mild attacks. Oral metronidazole or vancomycin are the antibiotic treatments of choice. Colectomy may be needed for:

- failure to respond to medical treatment
- toxic dilatation
- perforation.

METICILLIN-RESISTANT *STAPHYLOCOCCUS AUREUS* (MRSA)

Meticillin (previously methicillin) is an antibiotic now only used to test bacterial sensitivity to flucloxacillin in the laboratory. Infection or colonisation with MRSA poses problems in management. Patients become colonised while in hospital, possibly by staff acting as carriers. The organism itself is no more virulent than its flucloxacillin-sensitive counterpart, but the increase in MRSA since 1990 has had considerable financial implications for the control and treatment of colonisation.

MRSA is particularly prevalent amongst elderly long-stay hospital or nursing home in-patients, and is now endemic in UK hospitals.

Clinical features

A patient may be colonised but have no signs of infection. Manifestations are those of low-grade staphylococcal infection, with wounds and prostheses being particularly affected.

Investigation

Swabs for culture from the wound, throat, nose, perineum, axilla and groin of the patient should be taken and may be used for pre-admission screening for colonisation. A rapid PCR-based test is also now available and may be particularly useful in testing emergency admissions.

Management

Most hospitals have a policy to deal with occurrences of MRSA, which consists of:

- isolation
- barrier nursing, including skin antiseptics
- topical mupirocin – an antibiotic agent related to vancomycin for local use only
- regular samples from the patient to ascertain if eradication has been achieved
- intravenous vancomycin or teicoplanin (an analogous agent) to treat serious infections.

Eradication of MRSA is possible by these methods, but lack of compliance with the treatment or ineffective barrier nursing methods leads to failure in over 50%. Colonisation of the throat is particularly difficult to eradicate. The problem is an important issue in orthopaedic, vascular and cardiothoracic surgical patients. Standard antibiotics used for prophylaxis do not deal with MRSA.

The incidence of MRSA-related deaths in the UK has been reduced by the prevention strategies described above, but there were still an estimated 1230 deaths in 2008.

PYREXIA OF UNKNOWN ORIGIN (PUO)

The cause of fever in the postoperative recovery period is not always apparent. Fever can be caused by exogenous factors such as Gram-negative endotoxin or by endogenous factors such as some cytokines (see Table 9.3). Nevertheless, a hidden infection is the cause in 50% of cases and should be looked for vigorously:

- intravenous lines
- abscess
- cholecystitis/pancreatitis in those convalescent from other disorders, particularly severe trauma
- pneumonia
- viral infections, e.g. cytomegalovirus.

Other less common causes of PUO include:

- unresected tumour
- factitious (Munchausen's syndrome)
- collagen diseases (systemic lupus erythematosus [SLE], rheumatoid arthritis).

ESTABLISHED INFECTIONS IN THE SURGICAL PATIENT

CELLULITIS

This presents as a diffuse reddening, usually of connective tissue, without pus formation (although cellulitis is present around an abscess). It can affect any part of the body but is commonly encountered as a primary event in the cutaneous or subcutaneous planes of the legs or face. Two special types, both uncommon, are worthy of mention:

- Erysipelas – intradermal infection with streptococci. The organism produces streptokinase and spreads rapidly.

The facial skin is often involved, and before penicillin the condition was potentially fatal.
- Ludwig's angina – submandibular cellulitis, secondary to dental infection.

Secondary cellulitis from intravenous lines or infected sutures is common.

Organisms

Causative organisms are streptococci, staphylococci and, occasionally, Gram-negative rods.

Clinical features

Symptoms

Pain and fever are common, often with tenderness in the regional lymph nodes.

Physical findings

These include a hot, tender, erythematous but non-fluctuant swelling with ill-defined margins and tender enlarged lymph nodes. There may be red lines leading proximally as a consequence of lymphangitis.

Investigation

It is rarely possible to obtain tissue or fluid specimen for culture.

Management

Treatment with appropriate antibiotics – penicillin for streptococci, flucloxacillin for staphylococci – should be started. Hospital admission for intravenous administration of antibiotics and pain control may be necessary.

ESTABLISHED ABSCESSES

Definition

An abscess is a collection of liquefied leucocytes, dead tissue (slough) and organisms.

Organisms

The commonest pathogen is *Staphylococcus aureus*. Depending on the site of the infection, other organisms are also common, such as gut bacteria (e.g. *E. coli* and enterococci in perianal and intra-abdominal collections). Tuberculous abscesses are a special case.

Clinical features

Symptoms

Abscesses close to the surface of the body cause pain from tension within the cavity. Deep-seated collections cause illness, fever and local pressure symptoms which depend on the site involved.

Clinical findings

A tense, painful, red, hot and occasionally fluctuant swelling in a patient with a fever is almost infallibly diagnostic. If there is any doubt as to whether pus is present (cellulitis can often mimic an abscess), needle aspiration of pus confirms the diagnosis and can sometimes be definitive treatment (e.g. breast abscess).

Investigation

Ultrasound and CT are useful to delineate deep-seated or multiloculated collections. A raised leucocyte count is usually present.

Management

Treatment is drainage, the technique used (aspiration, drain insertion under image control or surgery) being determined by the site and size of the abscess (see above). Antibiotics are relatively ineffective in an established abscess but can partially control the surrounding cellulitis.

GANGRENE

Definition

Gangrene is the presence of dead tissue, nearly always colonised by bacteria. Two types are described:

- non-infected or dry (often colonised by bacteria and usually caused by ischaemia of a limb)
- infected (organisms are proliferating) or wet.

Infected gangrene can be subdivided into clostridial and non-clostridial.

Clostridial gangrene (gas gangrene)

Organisms

Although other clostridia species can be involved, the predominant one is *Clostridium perfringens* (formerly called *Cl. welchii*) often in association with other anaerobes. The anaerobic Gram-positive clostridia are found in the GI tract of herbivores and omnivores and produce spores which survive in soil and faeces. In consequence, gas gangrene is likely to occur in contaminated wounds and was once common in wars fought over cultivated land. Modern surgical techniques and antibiotics have made it now almost unknown where proper facilities are available for the management of wounds.

The organisms multiply in dead muscle so that for the most part removal of this is an effective method of prophylaxis and also management.

Clinical features

Symptoms

In 50% of instances in civilian life, there is no history of trauma. The clostridia come from the GI tract of the patient affected. Severe pain and systemic illness lead rapidly to the features of septic shock and death if untreated.

Physical findings

Findings include a characteristic musty odour, blackening of the overlying skin and watery brown discharge from a wound or sinus. Digital palpation may suggest, from the sensation of crackling, the presence of gas (surgical emphysema) in the subcutaneous tissues. Prompt diagnosis is essential to avoid the high mortality associated with the condition.

Investigation

X-ray or ultrasound can demonstrate the presence of gas in the tissues. Gram-staining of wound discharge or tissue removed at operation shows the characteristic large Gram-positive rods, and these can be grown in anaerobic culture.

Management (see also Box 9.3)

Treatment is begun before the bacteriological diagnosis. Components of treatment include:

- resuscitation
- high-dose penicillin, usually with metronidazole
- urgent surgical debridement of all necrotic tissue back to bleeding and viable structures; urgent amputation may be needed
- oxygen therapy in hyperbaric chambers – this has been used to raise local oxygen tension and so kill the clostridia.

Non-clostridial gangrene

A number of different names have been used to describe this condition. The two main groups are:

- synergistic bacterial gangrene (Meleney's gangrene) – a mixed infection with a microaerophilic *Streptococcus* and *Staphylococcus aureus*, which spreads relatively slowly and affects chiefly the skin
- necrotising fasciitis (Fournier's gangrene) – infection by streptococci and anaerobes, which spreads quickly and causes necrosis of fat and fascia with overlying secondary necrosis of skin.

Organisms

Streptococci release toxins such as streptokinase and hyaluronidase which aid the spread of infection through the tissue planes.

Clinical features

Symptoms

In Meleney's gangrene, there is failure to control an episode of surface infection by conventional means. In Fournier's, there is very rapid development of severe toxaemia.

Physical findings

Black discoloration and breakdown of the skin without the crepitus of gas gangrene. Fournier's often affects the perineum (where it may have started as a small perianal collection).

Management

- Wide surgical debridement (Fig. 9.3)
- Penicillin and metronidazole.

Box 9.3 Prophylaxis of gangrene and tetanus

The text deals with the management of established gas gangrene and tetanus. However, real advances have come from the recognition that good practice can prevent nearly all infections. For gas gangrene and non-clostridial gangrene, early adequate excision of dead and damaged tissue, avoidance of primary suture of high-risk wounds and systemic prophylactic antibiotics have made the conditions vanishingly rare. For tetanus, immunisation programmes are in place – see Chapter 3.

There is no role for hyperbaric oxygen in either of these conditions.

TETANUS

Tetanus is a state of muscle spasm caused by an exotoxin (tetanospasmin) produced by the anaerobe *Clostridium tetani*. As with gas gangrene, wounds contaminated with soil or faeces are the main predetermining cause, and the disease is therefore more likely to be a complication of war wounds or agricultural work. Neonatal tetanus is caused by contamination of the umbilicus with organisms at division of the cord and is found only in developing countries where ritualistic dressing practices persist.

Organism

Clostridium tetani survives as a spore in soil and multiplies in the absence of oxygen.

Clinical features

The condition has an incubation period between an injury and the development of symptoms which varies from days to 3 months. A better prognosis is associated with a longer incubation period.

Symptoms

A sense of apprehension followed by jaw stiffness may be the first symptom, progressing to facial spasms (risus sardonicus) and back-arching convulsions with impaired ventilation. Autonomic dysfunction can present as arrhythmias and labile blood pressure.

Physical findings

Between episodes, findings may be normal. During an attack, muscle tone is increased and muscle spasm may be local or general. An obvious neglected injury may be present but may have healed. There is a high risk of cardiorespiratory arrest with brain damage or death.

Investigation

Drumstick spores can be found in wound tissue. However, treatment should be undertaken on the clinical diagnosis alone.

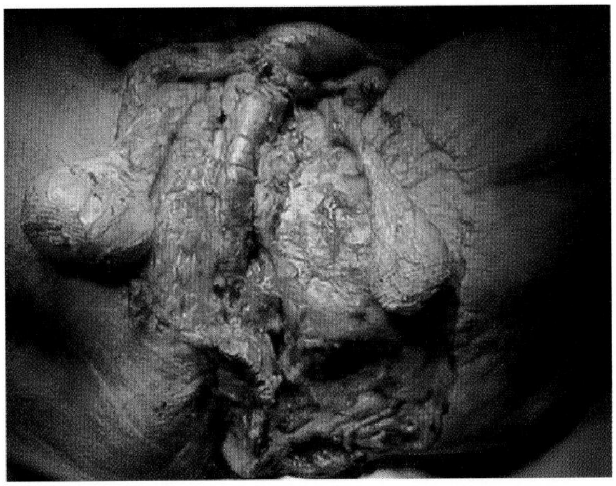

Fig. 9.3 Wide surgical debridement of scrotum and perineum needed to cure Fournier's gangrene.

Management (see also Box 9.3)

The disease only occurs after the migration of toxin along nerves to the CNS and its (irreversible) fixation to motor neurons. Nevertheless it is customary to give tetanus immunoglobulin (TIG) intramuscularly (150 μ/kg at multiple injection sites). Any neglected wound is treated and systemic penicillin and metronidazole administered to prevent bacterial multiplication. The spasms should be controlled by medical means: sedation with diazepam in mild cases, full respiratory paralysis and ventilatory support in severe cases.

CANDIDA INFECTION

Candida is an omnipresent fungus which can cause an opportunistic infection in patients who are ill for other reasons or who are taking antibiotics. A generalised fungal infection is life-threatening (overall mortality 30%).

Pathological features

The commonest sites are:

- oral and oesophageal – the elderly, the young, patients with steroid therapy, HIV infection or on chemotherapy
- perianal – a cause of pruritus
- vaginal – the contraceptive pill, in pregnancy and in diabetes
- endocardium – endocarditis in intravenous drug abusers
- generalised – immunosuppression (post-transplant, blood disorders such as leukaemia), multi-organ failure, long-term antibiotic treatment.

Clinical features

Symptoms

Symptoms are usually those of the accompanying disease or disorder.

Physical findings

Findings include clinical appearance of white plaques or white discharge. In generalised *Candida* infection, features of toxaemia and lack of response to conventional antibiotic treatment may be seen.

Investigation

- Microscopic evaluation of swabs or scrapings
- Blood culture.

Management

Local infection

Topical nystatin cream, mouthwash or pessaries suffice, although oral fluconazole is often used. A general review for any underlying disorder and consideration of changes in therapy should be undertaken.

Generalised infection

This is normally treated with intravenous agents, such as amphotericin, and correction of predisposing disease or treatments. Prophylactic systemic fluconazole (or other anti-fungal agent) is increasingly used in high-risk ICU patients.

TUBERCULOSIS

Organisms

Tuberculosis is mainly caused by *Mycobacterium tuberculosis*, a Gram-positive non-sporing bacillus.

Pathological features

The disease can affect the lung, skin, lymph nodes, bones, joints, genitourinary system, gut and the CNS. Two pathological types are recognised:

- Proliferative – affects solid organs (lungs, kidney)
- Exudative – affects serous cavities (pleural, peritoneal and pericardial cavities).

In both forms there is a slowly progressive inflammatory process which produces granulomas. In the proliferative form these tend to aggregate into an inflammatory mass. This leads to tissue breakdown, sterile caseation and a cold abscess which contains pus which may become secondarily infected if exposed on the surface of the body. In the exudative type, the granulomas cause inflammatory reaction on the affected surface with effusion into the involved cavity – peritoneal, pleural or subarachnoid. Haematogenous spread from a primary focus of either the proliferative or exudative type may set up metastatic foci or lead to generalised bloodstream invasion (miliary disease).

The disease is not on the decline as many would have hoped with the advent of chemotherapy in the years after the Second World War. Undernutrition, poor and overcrowded housing and the spread of HIV infections have kept the incidence high in both developing and developed communities, and this has been helped by undertreatment and the emergence of strains resistant to antibiotics.

About 90% of affected patients have lung involvement, but the common forms of surgical presentation are:

- cold abscesses in lymph nodes anywhere in the body but most frequently in the neck with a 'collar-stud' abscess
- scrotal sinuses from testicular disease
- acute or chronic tuberculous peritonitis (often regarded as miliary because it has arisen from haematogenous spread) when a diagnostic laparoscopy may be useful in confirming the diagnosis and providing tissue samples for culture and histology
- renal disease.

Clinical features

These are the consequence of the site of infection and are considered elsewhere.

Investigation

Histological examination of tissue obtained from an infected site may show classical granulomas and caseation. Staining by the Ziehl–Neelsen technique may identify acid-fast bacilli (AFB). The tuberculin skin reaction is positive with infection or with previous vaccination with TB antigens and is generally unhelpful in making a diagnosis in an individual.

Management

Prophylaxis

This is generally beyond the scope of this text, although, in the developed world, reduction in drug abuse and HIV infection are relevant.

Therapy

A current medical protocol is 6 months' therapy with a combination of:

- isoniazid
- rifampicin
- ethambutol.

Surgical management is outlined for individual organs and systems throughout this book.

HUMAN IMMUNODEFICIENCY VIRUS

Surgical presentation is the result of complications and is partially dependent upon the stage of infection. The risk of cross-infection to the healthcare team, although real, is very small provided certain precautions are taken (Ch. 5). Modern highly active anti-retroviral treatment (HAART) has greatly improved the prognosis for HIV-infected patients, but they remain at increased risk of developing various maligancies including lymphoma, anal and oesophagogastric cancer. Surgical involvement with these patients may take on a wide range of conditions, some of which are of increased prevalence including:

- anal diseases – warts, perianal abscess, carcinoma, and herpetic ulceration (Ch. 26)
- complications of injection of drugs – abscesses in relation to sites of injection, septic venous thrombosis and false arterial aneurysms
- lymph node biopsy for the diagnosis of associated disorders – e.g. tuberculosis, lymphoma

HYDATID DISEASE

The disease is endemic in the Mediterranean, South America, South Africa and Australasia. It is still seen occasionally in the UK wherever humans, dogs and sheep coexist or in immigrants from endemic areas. The dog is the definitive host of the parasitic worm *Echinococcus granulosus*, while sheep are the intermediate host. Close contact between an infected dog and humans allows humans to act as the intermediate host. Ingested ova hatch in the upper gut, enter the portal system and pass to the liver where they settle to form cysts.

Pathological features

Cysts in the liver and secondarily in other sites such as the peritoneum and the lung contain clear fluid; although many have become sterile over the years, they may contain active brood capsules which are the starting point for new scolices. The outer layer of the cyst is made up of compressed fibrous tissue. Cysts occasionally become secondarily infected by pyogenic organisms.

Clinical features

Symptoms

The patient may present with symptoms of a mass or of epigastric discomfort. Occasionally there is rupture into the peritoneum or biliary tree, the first of which causes an abdominal emergency and the second an attack of obstructive jaundice. Anaphylaxis may complicate either event.

Physical findings

Unless one of the above complications develops, physical findings are usually absent. The liver and/or an abdominal mass may be palpable.

Investigation

A plain abdominal X-ray occasionally shows calcification in the wall of a cyst, but ultrasound is more accurate in delineation. Eosinophilia is common but non-specific. Serological tests for the antibodies to hydatid are available but they have high false-positive and false-negative rates. Immunoelectrophoresis has a place in following medical treatment. CT gives detail on the site and size and is often used before a surgical procedure. The septae of the cysts can be clearly seen.

Management

Prophylaxis

Control of dogs – limiting the number of strays, repeated worming and denying access to offal – has succeeded in almost completely abolishing the condition in New Zealand.

Therapy

- Chemotherapy – albendazole is effective and may cause immunoelectrophoresis to return to normal, but it is a hepatotoxic compound that has to be used with caution.
- Conservative surgery – cystectomy, marsupialisation – using aspiration and hypertonic saline cyst injection to avoid spread.
- Radical surgery – partial hepatectomy.

FURTHER READING

Mazuski JE 2009 Surgical infections, an issue of surgical clinics. Saunders, Edinburgh

Taylor E, Williams J 2003 Infection in surgical practice. Hodder Arnold, London

Velmahos GC, Vassiliu P, Demetriades D et al 2002 Leave wound open if likely to be infected – it halves the risk of infection. American Surgeon 68(9):795–801

www.clean-safe-care.nhs.uk

NICE clinical guideline 74, Surgical Site Infection, October 2008

10 The seriously ill and injured patient

Some features of organisation for care of the surgical patient have been given in Chapter 2. There is an increasing awareness that as the hospital population changes with sicker patients and more co-morbidity the requirement for and expectation of specific critical care management have risen. Critically ill or injured patients presenting to hospital are referred to specialist units either initially or after rapid assessment in the Emergency Department (see Chs 2 and 3). Post-operative patients may also require critical care management after major surgery or if they have significant co-morbidity. There are also ward patients who deteriorate and are identified as requiring critical care. Among patients for whom critical care may be required are:

- general, vascular, trauma and other surgical problems with acute severe physiological disturbance
- burns – usually referred to a regional or supraregional unit which specialises in both the early (shock phase) care and later skin cover, plastic and reconstructive procedures (see Ch. 38)
- neurosurgical problems (especially head and spinal injury)
- transplantation – particularly in relation to liver and heart, where urgent action may be necessary to save life (Ch. 13)
- neonates and older children with critical illness or injury
- sepsis either on presentation or developing in hospital
- deteriorating co-morbidities in the ward.

CRITICAL CARE UNITS

A number of sites for the care of critically ill patients are available (Box 10.1).

BURNS UNITS

These units comprise facilities for the management of the whole range of burn injuries, from minor burns requiring little or no resuscitation or plastic surgery to those needing major resuscitation and extensive surgery. This specialist unit requires good critical care management associated with appropriate specialist burns treatment from plastic surgeons. As the results from well-run units are very good, there is no place for the management of occasional cases in non-specialist units.

HIGH-DEPENDENCY UNITS, INTENSIVE CARE UNITS AND THE FUTURE

With the increasing use of day-case surgery and outpatient management of patients who would previously have been admitted, it is inevitable that in-patients as a group will become an increasingly dependent and generally sicker population. As a result of this change, the level of nursing dependency will increase, as will the dependence on manpower-saving monitoring. Continuous monitoring on wards will become standard, and so part of the differentiation between the high-dependency unit (HDU) and the ward which currently exists will disappear. A gradation of illness

Box 10.1 Sites for the care of the critically ill

Intensive care/therapy unit (ICU/ITU)
An area where patients are treated for actual, impending or potential organ failure who require a high degree of organ support, including mechanical ventilation
Work style – 1 : 1 nursing; medical cover immediately available

High-dependency unit (HDU)
An area where patients at high risk are continuously and invasively monitored. Mechanical ventilation is not normally required
Work style – 1 : 2/3 nursing; medical cover immediately available

Ward
Intermittent clinical monitoring
Variable nurse:patient ratio

will still exist but the emphasis of applying appropriate care will relate to the availability of nursing and medical input rather than to the presence of monitoring. More complex interventions will remain in designated areas such as the intensive care unit (ICU) and HDU.

ICU and HDU admission criteria

This is a highly controversial area. Patients should receive a level of monitoring, nursing and medical care appropriate to the severity of their illness. However, the ability to sustain life in intensive care cannot be the only consideration; other important factors must be addressed:

- reversibility of the illness
- patients' and relatives' wishes
- quantity and quality of resources.

In light of the fact that 15–25% of patients admitted to general ICUs die – and in certain subgroups the mortality is much greater – it is important to pursue attainable and relevant goals. One approach is to apply intensive care medicine on the basis that the outcome realistically sought is to return patients to a state similar to that prior to their acute illness. This requires an assessment of the probability of achieving a successful outcome, not in isolation, but against the difficulties and discomfort likely to be imposed on the patient and the potential benefits to be accrued by the patient. Many individuals are unwilling to submit themselves or their family members to prolonged hospitalisation in the ICU, with its inherent discomfort, if the physician cannot state that there is a reasonable chance of survival. The physician must learn to predict when survival is possible and when death is inevitable. Despite attempts, invariably unsuccessfully, to approach this problem using scoring systems, it remains a difficult endeavour reliant on clinical experience.

The use of resources is a contentious issue. If a patient has advanced malignancy with limited life expectancy and a severe acute illness, it may mean that the acute illness can be treated but that it will take as long or longer than the life expectancy of the patient to return that person to a semblance of health. Age is not an issue but is part of the assessment of potential benefit. Each case needs to be sensibly appraised on its own merits. It is inevitable that intensive care will always be a limited resource and therefore it should be used efficiently and not abused.

Patient management

The nature of critical illness means that patients have complex, life-threatening conditions and the level of medical input should be appropriate to these problems. A multidisciplinary approach is required, but this has to be focused or it is counterproductive. The only way of achieving this is to have a team primarily involved in management who take consultancy advice from the various specialties involved. This implies that the primary team is trained and effective in the care of the critically ill patient, and in most countries intensive or critical care medicine is a recognised specialty.

Scoring systems

How sick is sick? Can we determine the likely outcome from the appearance of the patient on admission? Patients from a wide range of specialties develop critical illness and need intensive care. In such a heterogeneous group of patients it has always been difficult to compare clinical management and audit outcome, either between patients or between intensive care units. An essential prerequisite is a common language and measurement system by which one can gauge illness severity. A sickness severity score can also be used to predict outcome and to compare actual outcomes with predicted outcome.

Any scoring system has to allow for particular diagnoses which influence outcome, the physiological derangement at the time of admission, the health background of the patient prior to admission and, in more sophisticated systems, the way that the illness progresses once treatment has been initiated. Following recovery, the quality of survival may need to be measured.

The APACHE II (Acute Physiology and Chronic Health Evaluation II) scoring system is one of the most commonly used systems in intensive care (Table 10.1). The acute physiology score is derived from the worst values of 12 basic physiological indices in the first 24 hours, to which is added a chronic health evaluation. By evaluating outcome in large populations, the admission diagnosis can be given a prognostic value, which in combination with the APACHE II score can give an indication of the likelihood of death, the 'risk of death'. The predicted risk of death in a cohort of patients can then be compared with the actual death rate for that cohort and a standardised mortality ratio (SMR) can be derived. This provides a means of assessing the therapeutic efficacy of an individual ICU. The actual value of this score in the management or prognostication of an individual patient is very limited, but as a way of describing the general severity of illness it is in common use and therefore in this respect valuable.

Please note that the efficacy of a scoring system is heavily dependent on the individual who enters the data.

The number of scoring systems available is large and increasing. In trauma, TRISS, derived from the Revised Trauma Score (RTS) and the Injury Severity Score (ISS), can be used. The RTS is the score at the point of injury, scoring 1–4 for the Glasgow Coma Score, 1–4 for the systolic blood

Table 10.1 Acute Physiology and Chronic Health Evaluation II (APACHE II) scoring chart

	High abnormal range					Low abnormal range			
Physiological variable	+4	+3	+2	+1	0	+1	+2	+3	+4
Temperature, rectal (°C)	≥41	39–40.9		38.5–38.9	36–38.4	34–35.9	32–33.9	30–31.9	≤29.9°
Mean arterial pressure (mmHg)	≥160	130–159	110–129		70–109		50–69		≤49
Heart rate (ventricular response)	≥180	140–179	110–139		70–109		55–69	40–54	≤39
Respiratory rate (non-ventilated or ventilated)	≥50	35–49		25–34	12–24	10–11	6–9		≤5
Oxygenation: A–aDO$_2$* or P_aO_2 (mmHg)									
a. F_iO_2 ≥0.5 record A–aDO$_2$	≥500	350–499	200–349		<200				
b. F_iO_2 ≥0.5 record only P_aO_2					$P_aO_2 > 70$	P_aO_2 61–70		P_aO_2 55–60	$P_aO_2 < 55$
Arterial pH	≥7.7	7.6–7.69		7.5–7.59	7.33–7.49		7.25–7.32	7.15–7.24	<7.15
Serum sodium (mmol/L)	≥180	160–179	155–159	150–154	130–149		120–129	111–119	≤110
Serum potassium (mmol/L)	≥7	6–6.9		5.5–5.9	3.5–5.4	3–3.4	2.5–2.9		<2.5
Serum creatinine (mg/100 mL) (double point score for acute renal failure)	≥3.5	2–3.4	1.5–1.9		0.6–1.4		<0.6		
Haematocrit (%)	≥60		50–59.9	46–49.9	30–45.9		20–29.9		<20
White blood cell count (thousands/mm^3)	≥40		20–39.9	15–19.9	3–14.9		1–2.9		<1
Glasgow coma score (GCS): score = 15 minus actual GCS:									
A. Total acute physiology score (APS): sum of the individual variable points:									
Serum HCO$_3$ (venous, mmol/L) (Not preferred; use if no ABGs)	≥52	41–51.9		32–40.9	22–31.9		18–21.9	15–17.9	<15

B. Age points. Assign points to age as follows: ....

Age (years)	Points
≤44	0
45–54	2
55–64	3
65–74	5
≥75	6

C. Chronic health points

If the patient has a history of severe organ system insufficiency or is immunocompromised, assign points as follows:

a. for non-operative or emergency postoperative patients – 5 points
b. for elective postoperative patients – 2 points

Definitions

Organ insufficiency or immunocompromised state must have been evident prior to this hospital admission and must conform to the following criteria:

- Liver: biopsy-proven cirrhosis and documented portal hypertension; episodes of past upper GI bleeding attributed to portal hypertension; or prior episodes of hepatic failure encephalopathy/coma.
- Cardiovascular: New York Heart Association Class IV.
- Respiratory: chronic restrictive, obstructive or vascular disease resulting in severe exercise restriction, i.e. unable to climb stairs or perform household duties; or documented chronic hypoxia, hypercapnia, secondary polycythaemia, severe pulmonary hypertension (>40 mmHg) or respirator dependency.
- Renal: receiving chronic dialysis.
- Immunocompromised: the patient has received therapy that suppresses resistance to infection, e.g. immunosuppression, chemotherapy, radiation, long-term or recent high-dose steroids, or has a disease that is sufficiently advanced to suppress resistance to infection, e.g. leukaemia, lymphoma, AIDS.

APACHE II score

Sum of **A** + **B** + **C**

A, APS points: … … … … …
B, Age points: … … … … …
C, Chronic health points: … … … … …
Total APACHE II: … … … … …

*[A–aDO$_2$ is a calculated measure of the oxygen gradient across the alveolar membrane, i.e. how effectively oxygen is crossing the lung into the arterial blood.]

pressure and 1–4 for respiratory rate, giving a maximum score of 12 for a normal individual; a score of less than 4 indicates very severe injury. In the ISS, each injury sustained by a trauma patient is allocated a value from a large 'catalogue' of over 1000 injuries. The scores run from 1 to 6, where 1 is minimal and 6 is not compatible with life. The highest scores from all three body regions are taken, squared and added together, giving a maximum score of 75. A single score of 6 automatically leads to a maximal score of 75. The two scores are combined to produce TRISS, which can then be used to predict and audit outcome. Other scoring methods are being developed to measure the quality of life (QOL). This latter method is still in its infancy but may be useful in determining the efficacy of healthcare as assessed by the condition of the patient after critical illness.

Once in the ICU, the Therapeutic Intervention Scoring System (TISS) can be used to quantify the amount of intervention needed to treat or care for a patient. This system lists all the interventions, drugs, procedures and monitoring used for that patient and produces a score. This score can be costed and the amount of financial and other resources consumed by a particular patient derived. Many of these methods can be used as an audit system of the cost-effectiveness of healthcare. They are not, at present, used to determine suitability for ICU admission.

Probably of greater importance are the early warning score (EWS) used in the ward environment that indicate if a patient is physiologically deteriorating. It is usually far more effective to prevent problems than to have to treat them and so systems that indicate early intervention are proliferating. The MEWS is one such score, although there are many. It alerts the nurses to a deteriorating situation. Based on physiological measures, an example can be seen in Table 10.2. Each patient has a chart with a number of domains, each of which scores between 0 and 3. When the cumulative score of all domains reaches a set value (e.g. 5) it triggers medical assessment. Alternatively on some charts the aberrant scores are marked in red zones, with one or more red zones triggering a request for assessment. These systems have been introduced to try to reduce the number of patients deteriorating in ward situations without triggering intervention.

HISTORY AND EXAMINATION OF THE CRITICALLY ILL

As with every other area of medicine, the clinical history is extremely important but frequently overlooked while focusing on the specific episode (Box 10.2). The acute events leading to illness are important: Why did the patient present for surgery? Was it an elective or emergency procedure? If the patient presented with an acute abdomen, how long had the problem been there? In trauma, the mechanism of injury is very important: How fast was the car going? Did it stop gradually or did it hit a wall and stop immediately? In shooting incidents, other questions are relevant: What was the type of gun, the muzzle velocity and distance from weapon to the point of impact? How far did the patient fall? All these factors give indications as to the mechanism of injury, which may suggest the extent of damage and give clues as to patterns of injury likely to be encountered.

Postoperatively the nature, extent and duration of surgery are important. Was there contamination of the peritoneum? Was the surgery definitive? Was the bleeding stopped? Are there surgical packs in situ?

It is essential to have a clear idea of the mechanism and the full nature of the injury. The background of the patient is important; previous medical history, chronic illness and age may all impact on management and outcome.

In the examination of the critically ill patient it is important in the first instance to follow the ABC of resuscitation and assess the adequacy of respiratory and cardiovascular function. A quick glance will allow you to assess the patient's colour and identify obvious hypoxia and sweating, and whether the patient is pale, distressed, agitated or exhausted. The quick glance should tell you if the patient looks ill.

The airway and respiratory system must be evaluated for evidence of hypoxia, difficulty with breathing or abnormal patterns of breathing (Table 10.3). When the immediate problems have been corrected, examine the whole patient.

Box 10.2 Clinical history

Acute
- When – time to presentation at hospital
- Where – place of injury/illness
- How – mechanism
- Drugs/medications taken
- Episodes of hypoxia or hypotension
- Other events

Chronic
- Age
- Immunosuppression
- Malignancy
- Drug therapy – cytotoxics, steroids
- Normal health status and mobility

Table 10.2 Scores used in MEWS (Modified Early Warning Score)

Score	3	2	1	0	1	2	3
Resp rate (/min)	<8	9–14		9–14	15–20	21–29	>30
Pulse (/min)		<40	41–50	51–100	101–110	111–130	>130
Temp °C		<35		35–38.4	>38.5		
CNS				Alert	Voice	Pain	Unresponsive
Urine	Nil	<30	<60		>150		
Sys BP (mmHg)	<40	<70	71–80	101–199		>200	

A simple version of an early warning score (EWS). There are many variations of this system but the simple ones work best. Score each domain – add the scores and if it is greater than a set value, for example >5, then call for help.

Table 10.3 Signs of respiratory failure

Factor	Signs
Pattern of breathing	Rapid, shallow gasping
	Very slow, large-volume, sigh-like
Colour	Cyanosis, peripheral or central
Skin	Sweating, cool periphery
	Sweating, warm periphery (CO_2 retention)
Accessory muscles	Use of neck, shoulder and/or abdominal muscles to aid breathing
Saturation	Low
Arterial blood gases	$P_ao_2 < 7.5$ kPa, $P_aco_2 > 6.4$ kPa
	Respiratory acidosis, CO_2 retention
	Metabolic acidosis or mixed with hypoxaemia

The history alerts one to the potential problems, but the examination should allow the clinician to decide if the patient is sick, how sick and where the problem lies. The patient should be visually examined from head to toe: look at the skin, look for rashes and assess their colour. In the critically ill, the initial history and examination are part of the introduction to the patient, but management of that patient requires frequent re-evaluation of symptoms and signs throughout the course of the illness. From frequent reassessment the clinician is rapidly able to interpret trends, which facilitates greater sensitivity to any changes occurring in what is always a dynamic situation.

The cardiovascular system

A well-functioning cardiovascular system with an effective cardiac output (ECO) will result in a warm well-perfused normotensive patient with a normal pulse rate and signs of end-organ perfusion such as consciousness or urine output. The sympathetic system is very effective, especially in younger patients, at compensating for impaired cardiovascular function. Look for signs not only of decompensation, i.e. tachycardia, hypotension and poor peripheral perfusion, but also that the sympathetic system is working well. The normotensive, tachycardic, peripherally shut-down young patient is potentially misleading.

The important cardiovascular signs are:

- perfusion and capillary refill time (CRT); warm or cold; peripheral cyanosis
- pulse rate, volume, rhythm
- jugular venous pressure (JVP) – elevated or low
- blood pressure
- urine output.

Assessment of the pulse is always useful. The rate and nature of the pulse and their presence both centrally and peripherally can be used, in conjunction with the state of peripheral perfusion, to assess intravascular volume. Tachycardia, a low volume or thready pulse with cold hands and feet may indicate hypovolaemia. Hypotension, if present, is a late sign and always signifies cardiovascular derangement, i.e. hypovolaemia, pump failure or acute vasodilatation. However, a normal blood pressure can be misleading, especially in young patients, and may mask underlying hypovolaemia.

Table 10.4 Glasgow Coma Scale

Signs	Evaluation	Score
Eye opening	Spontaneous	4
	To speech	3
	To pain	2
	None	1
Best verbal response	Oriented	5
	Confused	4
	Inappropriate	3
	Incomprehensible	2
	None	1
Best motor response	Obeys commands	6
	Localises pain	5
	Withdrawal to pain	4
	Flexion to pain	3
	Extension to pain	2
	None	1

Look at the jugular venous pressure. If it is absent, it is a useful sign of potential hypovolaemia. If it is high with engorged veins, it provides information either on cardiac function and failure or on excessive fluid administration.

Feel the apex beat. In hyperdynamic septic patients with high cardiac output, there may be a bounding left ventricle which is easily palpable. Heart sounds may indicate rate and rhythm, and there may be a high-output systolic flow murmur. It may be possible to detect the murmur of tricuspid incompetence in a dilated heart. This would be associated with a large V wave on the JVP.

The central nervous system

Assessment of a patient's level of consciousness is an essential part of the initial examination. An unconscious patient is at risk for many reasons, but in particular there is a risk of aspiration and airway obstruction. Confusion, agitation or loss of consciousness may be indicators of poor cerebral perfusion or cerebral injury, both of which are important considerations in the injured patient. The critically ill patient with severe sepsis may present with a 'toxic' confusional state.

The conscious level can be evaluated using the Glasgow Coma Scale, and it is a reasonable way of appraising the critically ill (Table 10.4). Examine the peripheral nervous system. Motor and sensory function is particularly important after trauma.

Abdominal examination

In the unconscious patient, abdominal examination may be misleading and classical signs are not dependable. In the conscious patient, look at the shape and size of the abdomen and whether it is normal for that individual. Assess for guarding, rebound and localised pain. Are there any masses? Check the liver and spleen. Always examine the inguinal area. Look for lymph nodes and check for occult hernias. Bowel sounds are a difficult sign to interpret in the critically ill, but a change in the bowel sounds may be important, so a baseline assessment is essential. Examine the patient's back. It is often forgotten and there may be important signs, such as bruising or septic lesions.

The urological system

It is important to ascertain whether the patient is passing urine – if so what does it contain? The volume of urine is important. Following trauma, blood is an indicator of potential problems. Muddy urine may indicate the presence of myoglobin.

DIAGNOSIS

There are two aspects to diagnosis:

- identification of all the physiological disturbances which need urgent correction if life is to be sustained
- identification of the underlying problem that resulted in the patient becoming critically ill.

As with any medical diagnosis, history and examination should provide the general diagnosis. Defining the specific problem is important. The methods available are the same as those available to other specialties and should be used. However, some investigations, such as CT scanning, require the patient to be moved, which, in the critically ill, may be hazardous. Nevertheless, it may provide the information required to plan definitive treatment and so should not be ruled out. There is always a balance to be struck between the usefulness of the information that might be gained by an investigation and the cost, in terms of morbidity, of acquiring that information.

AETIOLOGY OF CRITICAL ILLNESS

Any patient from any specialty can become critically ill, although it is more likely in some specialties than in others. As the severity of illness increases, so do the levels of monitoring and intervention required. As a very general statement, the physiological derangement tends to follow common pathways, irrespective of the original specialty. Obviously there will be aspects of the original problem which will have an influence on the development and pattern of critical illness (Fig. 10.1).

SHOCK

Shock is a descriptive term based on the symptoms and signs which are secondary to one or more of a wide range of problems. Traditionally, each 'type' of shock was described by the symptoms and signs seen in that particular situation. It is more fruitful to look at the final common pathway and work back to the myriad causes. The final pathway is failure to adequately supply the peripheral tissues and cells with oxygen. At the cellular level it is the situation where cells are breaking down more ATP for energy than they are making because the oxygen supply is inadequate to maintain oxidative metabolism at an adequate rate.

When groups of cells become threatened with a reduction in oxygen supply, the body reacts vigorously to prevent this from happening. The manifestations of shock are partly those of the specific mechanism causing shock, partly the consequences of tissue hypoxia and partly those of the physiological protective mechanisms instituted to maintain oxygenation. These physiological mechanisms are the signs of sympathetic activity.

Shock should be considered in terms of:

- causes of shock
- consequences of shock
- physiological responses
- treatment.

Mechanisms

Anything that impairs the passage of oxygen delivery from the outside environment through to the oxidative metabolic system in the mitochondrion can result in shock. This can be

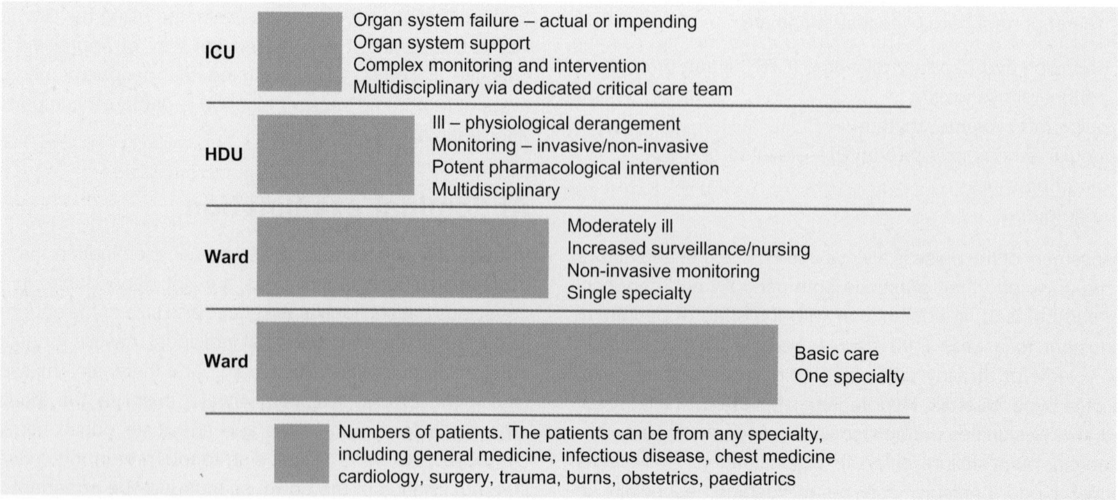

Fig. 10.1 Patient dependency within a hospital.

at any stage in the process, for example from breathing hypoxic air (e.g. at altitude) or through airway obstruction or ventilatory failure from causes such as muscle paralysis. Impairment of oxygen delivery sometimes occurs between the lungs and the tissues: there may be difficulty in the transfer of oxygen from the alveoli to the capillaries, as with pulmonary oedema, or failure to transfer the oxygen-carrying blood from the capillaries to the rest of the body (see Ch. 16). Exsanguination or hypovolaemia from any cause may reduce circulating volume (see Ch. 3). Cardiac 'pump' failure may reduce the blood and therefore effective oxygen supply to the tissues (see Ch. 17). At the tissue level, oedema in the interstitium may impede oxygen transfer from the capillaries to the cells; at the mitochondrial level, toxins such as cyanide may impede oxygen uptake by the cytochrome system. It is increasingly apparent that in sepsis mitochondrial dysfunction may have a prominent role. In short, any mechanism preventing a significant population of cells from receiving and using oxygen will result in a state of shock.

Consequences

The consequences of shock start at the cellular level. Cells need energy (from ATP) and use up their supplies very rapidly, producing hydrogen ions as a byproduct:

$$ATP = ADP + P + H^+$$

Hydrogen ions are taken up during oxidative metabolism at a rapid rate but only very slowly in anaerobic metabolism. If anaerobic metabolism increases, the rate of production of hydrogen ions from the cell using ATP far exceeds the ability of anaerobic metabolism either to use hydrogen ions or to produce ATP. There is a build-up of H^+ which coincides with a build-up of the base (lactate) from anaerobic metabolism. An acidosis develops intracellularly, and this moves out of the cell and is buffered. Eventually the buffering is used up and a systemic acidosis develops. This is known as lactic acidosis.

Other signs may reflect the primary cause. If the myocardium is deprived of oxygen, cardiac failure will ensue. Hypotension is the sign of losing intravascular volume or pump failure. If hypovolaemia occurs from blood loss, there will be signs of tissue hypoxia and poor perfusion associated with a fall in blood pressure. In sepsis, profound vasodilatation may result in a hot periphery, bounding pulses and hypotension ('distributive shock'). Usually these signs will be influenced heavily by the compensatory mechanisms that swing into action to protect the tissue oxygen supply.

Responses

The responses to cellular hypoxia are aimed at improving oxygen supply. The changes occurring from the mechanism of injury combined with the responses geared to increasing oxygen supply are the signs of shock. Air hunger and tachypnoea are attempts to increase gas exchange and oxygen availability. They also serve to excrete CO_2 and compensate for an advancing metabolic acidosis from cell hypoxia.

The cardiovascular system is stimulated to try to deliver more oxygen by delivering more blood to the tissues. This is achieved by increasing the heart rate and improving contractility, thereby increasing the cardiac output. All of this is mediated by the sympathetic system. Blood is diverted to perfuse vital organs. The periphery is non-vital and therefore becomes cold and 'shut-down'. The pulses tend to be rapid and of low volume in most situations, the exception being septic shock where vasodilatation is part of the underlying problem and the patient may have a large-volume, low-pressure pulse. With massive sympathetic compensation this may later become low in volume and low in pressure. Sweating is part of the sympathetic response, so the patient becomes cold and clammy. Renal perfusion is reduced and urine output ceases.

The patient in shock is very agitated. Failure to supply oxygen to the brain adds a picture of confusion and eventually loss of consciousness. This is superimposed on the agitation and irritation caused by the sympathetic system.

Treatment

Treatment is aimed at restoring oxygen delivery to the cell as rapidly as possible, and this is the primary intention. The cause of the shock should be determined and treated while ensuring the pathway between oxygen outside the body and the cell is unimpeded at all levels. The basic principles are to increase ambient oxygen, ensure a clear airway, facilitate adequate ventilation, guarantee an adequate circulating blood volume and improve cardiac performance – essentially the ABC of resuscitation: airway, breathing and circulation. Aim for an effective cardiac output (ECO) – warm well-perfused normotensive patient with normal pulse rate and signs of organ function such as urine output or consciousness.

Examples of shock

Three patients with shock of different aetiologies are described below to illustrate how the precipitating mechanisms may be different but the physiological pathways come together.

Myocardial infarction – cardiogenic shock

A 50-year-old man collapses at work complaining of severe chest pain and increasing shortness of breath. On arrival he is grey, cold and clammy with beads of perspiration on his forehead, and he is extremely anxious. He has peripheral cyanosis. His pulse is 120/min, regular but very weak and thready in nature. His JVP is markedly elevated. His blood pressure is low at 80/50 mmHg.

He has a myocardial infarct with reduced left ventricular function, and his heart is failing to pump adequately. Tissues are not getting enough oxygen. His sympathetic system is trying to compensate by increasing oxygen delivery. He is breathing faster to try to acquire more oxygen. His heart is failing and blood is backing up in his lungs and he is getting pulmonary oedema which worsens his oxygen transport further. His poor ventricular function is inadequate, and so he is developing a tachycardia to compensate. He is shutting down peripherally to divert blood to the central organs.

Management will involve treating both the shock and the condition: increasing oxygen, aiding breathing and improving cardiac output. Oxygen should be given, by mask, and a diuretic administered to try to reduce the fluid building up in his lungs. Thrombolytic therapy, percutaneous coronary intervention (PCI) or coronary bypass surgery should be considered urgently to reverse the infarct by establishing reperfusion of the occluded artery. A vasodilator may help, so that the heart is pumping against less resistance. An inotrope may be needed to boost left ventricular function if the BP is too low, but it has the negative effect of increasing the work on the heart, which may make the infarct worse.

Trauma – hypovolaemic shock

A 24-year-old man rides his motorbike into a bus. He sustains injuries to his pelvis, fractures his femur and tears his femoral artery. When the ambulance arrives he is lying in a pool of blood – conscious, in pain and very pale. He is sweating profusely. He is cool peripherally and feels clammy. He is breathing fast and he is agitated. His pulse is 150/min and his BP is 70/50 mmHg. JVP is not detectable, and his conjunctivae are white.

He is losing his circulating blood volume and cannot adequately deliver oxygen. He compensates by pushing it all round faster courtesy of his sympathetic system and a fit young heart. Agitation is a function of sympathetic outflow and to some degree hypoxia. He has diverted all his remaining blood to vital areas. Other areas will be getting hypoxic rapidly. His ability to compensate falls as his blood volume reduces.

The paramedics give him oxygen, and stop the bleeding. They insert large drips into him and pour in fluid to give him a circulating volume. You only need a few red cells to carry oxygen but they have to be carried by fluid. With adequate fluid he will get a circulating volume and will be able to deliver oxygen to the tissues. Extra blood will help.

Meningococcal septicaemia – septic shock

A 24-year-old girl on a working holiday in the UK and living in a crowded flat in Earls Court develops a flu-like illness. She has temperature and sore throat. Her flatmates go to work and she rings them there later to say she is feeling worse. When they get home she is lying on a sofa, very drowsy and confused. She feels hot all over. They notice a nasty purplish rash on her feet. The ambulance takes her to hospital, and she is unrousable on arrival. Her breathing is rapid and laboured, and she is hot and sweaty. She has photophobia and obvious neck stiffness. Her pulse is 150/min and her BP is 80/60 mmHg. Her neck veins are not visible.

She has septic shock. 'Toxins' are causing profound vasodilatation and they are probably affecting her cardiac contractility. At cell level, although oxygen is available, her cells either cannot get it or cannot use it as effectively as they require. Her white cells are activated and are using oxygen to produce oxygen radicals to combat infection. This all leads to increased oxygen requirements. Despite her heart working as fast as it can and a huge amount of blood being pushed around the circulation, her tissues are oxygen-deprived and need more. Her sympathetic system is struggling. It can push her heart but her toxaemia prevents her blood vessels from constricting to divert the blood to vital organs. With all the vasodilatation, her blood volume is inadequate to fill the space and her blood pressure falls.

Antibiotics will treat the meningococcus. Treatment is by support of her circulation and provision of oxygen to try to help her organs through a period of relative hypoxia. As inotropes will not work well at vasoconstriction, the only alternative is to try to fill the circulation with enough fluid to enable it to work in its dilated state and deliver oxygen. Inotropes may be necessary to push the toxic heart. The block of oxygen utilisation will improve as the septicaemia comes under control.

SIRS, sepsis and septicaemia

Following a wide range of insults, patients can develop a pattern of illness that has been defined as the systemic inflammatory response syndrome (SIRS) (see also Ch. 9). These patients demonstrate very similar problems to those with septicaemia, and for many years they were described as septic. However, while occasionally a causative organism was found, most of the time no organisms were found. This inflammatory response was probably sterile.

SIRS does not require an infective cause. The features of SIRS include having more than one of the following:

- body temperature > 38°C or < 36°C
- heart rate > 90 beat/min
- tachypnoea > 20 or a P_aCO_2 < 4.3 kPa
- white cell count of either >120 000 or <4000 with more than 10% of these being due to immature neutrophils.

Sepsis as a subset of SIRS can be defined in the same way but with the presence of infection.

'Septicaemia' is a term that has outgrown its usefulness. Bacteraemia is the presence of bacteria in the blood, and sepsis is the systemic inflammatory response to infection.

It has been suggested that SIRS is caused by an inflammatory cascade. A trigger factor – which can be a bacterial agent, another microbiological agent or an insult such as trauma, toxins, damaged cells or damaged tissue – can result in the activation of mediators from macrophages and other cells, including cytokines, prostaglandins and various peptides. These in turn lead to stimulation and release of other factors and mediators from other cells – a cascade.

The haemodynamic response in sepsis is vasodilatation, which is frequently described as a reduction in systemic vascular resistance associated with a fall in blood pressure, often with an increase in heart rate but not necessarily with any change in filling pressure. Changes in membrane permeability and a tendency to form oedema in various organs, especially the lungs, are examples of occasional features of the syndrome.

In practical terms, the vasodilatation and membrane permeability seen in sepsis mean that patients not only have a far bigger intravascular space than usual but also are losing fluid from that space into the interstitium. They have inadequate fluid in the intravascular compartment. The nature of sepsis means that the vasodilatation does not respond to their sympathetic system as it should, so they become hypotensive. These changes influence their haemodynamic management. With all the sympathetic activity, raised cardiac output and cardiac work, and increased white cell activity, the oxygen requirements of these patients rise. All of these features can exist with SIRS.

Having defined the term SIRS, it is important to appreciate that it is just a name and does not obviate the necessity of determining, if possible, the cause. The problem of acronyms in ICU is a serious one. It is easy to try to treat the acronym rather than the patient. Too often a diagnosis of, for example, ARDS (adult respiratory distress syndrome – see below) seems to imply that a set pattern of treatment is now appropriate and the underlying cause is no longer important. Nothing could be further from the truth. These acronyms should be an aid to description not an endpoint in diagnosis and management.

One of the reasons for defining these syndromes cautiously is that they often lead on to the development of other non-specific syndromes (which carry acronyms). SIRS is a systemic insult and potentially leads to problems throughout the body. Each and every organ system can be affected and damaged, each to a greater or lesser degree. As all organs are exposed to the generalised insult and some are overtly injured, this is grouped under the descriptive term of multiple organ system failure (MOSF). This is now called MODS (multiple organ dysfunction syndrome) because it implies that the alteration in function in each organ is not absolute at any particular point in time but describes some degree of malfunction or dysfunction which may be changing with time. Organ system dysfunction can be primary, as in an immediate response to a specific localised insult, e.g. contusion of the lung causing lung dysfunction. Alternatively, lung injury may occur as a consequence of repeated insults to all organs, including the lungs. In the first situation the injury is localised and, unless it triggers SIRS, will only affect the lung, while in the second situation all organs are affected to varying degrees and the acute lung injury is the manifestation of the generalised injury to that organ. Each organ will respond to a particular insult in an individual manner, with some organs being more susceptible than others. An example of this is hypotension and the kidney: a period of sustained hypotension will affect any perfused organ, but the kidney responds physiologically with a visible change in function. It may also be more sensitive. The effects of renal failure are easily seen, while liver or lung dysfunction may be less visible but still present.

The most important therapeutic intervention is treatment of the cause. This should be associated with appropriate organ support and then additional measures. As a non-specific insult results in a describable series of events, therapeutic strategies have been developed which aim to intervene in those patterns of events. If an initial insult liberates a cascade phenomenon, it gives us a rationale for treatment. The insult itself, whether infection, trauma, toxin or something else, should be contained and controlled and the impact of the insult minimised. For example, when treating hypovolaemia from haemorrhage, stopping the bleeding removes the insult, and prompt volume replacement minimises secondary effects. These simple measures may inhibit initiation of any cascade while sustained hypovolaemia may trigger the cascade.

If the cascade has started, there may be ways of impeding its development, i.e. mopping up the trigger factors. Endotoxins have been implicated, and there is considerable interest in the use of various antibodies for mopping up endotoxins, but to date the results are unconvincing.

An alternative approach is to block mediators within the cascade. Attempts have been made to use antibodies to block either the cytokines themselves, e.g. anti-TNF antibodies, or the cytokine receptors or to inhibit their production with the use of agents such as pentoxifylline. Prostaglandins have been implicated in the sepsis syndrome, and agents which inhibit them, such as ibuprofen, have been tried.

At capillary level, local production of nitric oxide is involved in capillary reactivity. This is often abnormal in sepsis. In the pulmonary vasculature, vasoconstriction can be reversed using exogenous nitric oxide, which may be helpful in oxygenating the patient. Paradoxically, there may be too much nitric oxide peripherally, and agents which block its production are being investigated.

Free-radical production is another area of current interest. White cell activation increases in SIRS. Oxygen radicals are produced and may account for some of the increased oxygen utilised in SIRS. Free-radical scavengers and antioxidants have been tried, but while there is a lot of evidence that free radicals are involved in some aspects of organ system damage, there is little or no data showing the efficacy of free-radical scavengers.

An important part of the management of the critically ill with or without SIRS is the prevention of recurrence of the primary problem and the prevention or reduction of secondary insults. These insults include nosocomial infection, haemodynamic instability and hypoxaemia. Management also involves minimising catabolism and trying to provide nutritional support.

MONITORING (see also Ch. 6)

It is important to consider what monitoring is for and what it is not for. Assessment and monitoring are in the first instance 'hands-on' phenomena. Equipment facilitates and supports clinical monitoring. From field to hospital, into the resuscitation room, to wards, operating theatre or ICU, the personnel looking after the patient are responsible for continual reassessment and monitoring of physiological parameters and should act on these assessments.

Monitoring systems provide several additional benefits (Box 10.3). However, they are always an adjunct and a help to the clinicians, not a replacement; they do not substitute

Box 10.3 Advantages of monitoring systems

- Confirm and support clinical monitoring; enhance accuracy and frequency
- Detect changes early
- Guide and follow clinical interventions
- Free up clinicians from repetitive, time-consuming tasks

for clinical acumen. This is in contrast to the alternative view that patient management requires total body monitoring and pan-scanning to provide maximum information and early warning of problems. This latter approach presumes that any kind of monitoring provides information and that all information is intrinsically beneficial. But remember: a small amount of relevant information is infinitely preferable to any amount of irrelevant information.

Monitoring is an adjunct to management, not vice versa, and a careful balance has to be struck when deciding which monitors to use, based on a cost–benefit analysis. One then has to decide what constitutes minimal requirements and build from that starting point. The question should be 'What do I need?' not 'What would I like?'. Monitoring should always assist and never hinder.

There are many monitoring facilities which can help considerably and, given the fundamental provisos discussed above, they can make management very much more effective.

MONITORING BY ORGAN SYSTEM

The central nervous system

Clinical appraisal is most important. Scoring is usually by the GCS, which gives a reasonable indication of level of consciousness irrespective of cause. Localising or lateralising signs may indicate the need for a CT scan providing the patient has been assessed and is stable in other respects. This is particularly pertinent in neurotrauma (see Ch. 3). CT scans provide anatomical information but do not indicate function. MRI scanning has a limited place in the critically ill but may be of assistance in the specific diagnosis of certain types of lesion. Intracranial pressure (ICP) monitoring may be useful in situations where there is intracranial damage and swelling or oedema is anticipated, e.g. following a closed head injury. Monitoring the ICP identifies and characterises the problem and may facilitate interventions designed to reduce the pressure. High pressure may impede the blood supply to the brain. If the ICP is known then the cerebral perfusion pressure (CPP) can be calculated (mean blood pressure minus ICP). Currently a CPP of greater than 60 mmHg is thought best to ensure adequate perfusion.

Electroencephalograph (EEG) monitoring may be helpful in determining if there is evidence of fitting or to assess the level of electrical activity. Cerebral function monitors, which allow continual assessment of electrical activity, are used in some situations to monitor the level of cerebral electrical activity.

Evoked-potential monitoring involves providing a stimulus and measuring the response to determine whether the central nervous connections are intact and the speed of response. These are specialised measurements and require careful expert interpretation.

A commonly used device is BIS™ or bispectral index monitoring that is popular in anaesthesia. It is meant to be able to indicate the awareness of the patient. As with all such devices it works well most of the time in most patients but is not yet foolproof.

The respiratory system

Clinical monitoring is of paramount importance. The pattern and rate of breathing, whether ancillary muscles have been recruited, the patient's colour and general condition all provide information as to the adequacy of respiratory function. Clinical awareness of 'tiredness', when a patient is struggling to breathe but seems too 'tired' to breathe effectively, is an important sign both off and on a ventilator. These clinical signs are of greater value than blood gases, which will usually help confirm a clinical impression.

Pulse oximetry (see Ch. 6) measures, by light absorption methods, the saturation of haemoglobin in arterial blood. It is non-invasive and easy and rapid to apply. It indicates oxygenation and pulse rate. Indirectly it indicates perfusion as a trace, which is an indication of blood flow. However, as most oximeters compensate for the signal and amplify low output, the trace is not a direct measurement. Therefore the presence of a trace indicates perfusion, but the compensatory mechanisms prevent extrapolation of the trace into qualitative values. There are several situations where the trace may be misleading. It is a late indicator of hypoxia, so desaturation means that hypoxia is present. Peripheral perfusion may influence accuracy. The presence of carboxyhaemoglobin in significant amounts will give an artificially high value at about 85% even if the oxyhaemoglobin is much lower. It is also unreliable in a very anaemic patient. The values from the oximeter must be checked by evaluating against clinical assessment. Genuine changes and artefacts are common, but it is still a very useful monitoring tool. In current practice it is extremely useful in ventilated patients and reduces dependence on blood gas analysis.

Airway pressure monitoring will show the peak pressures in the upper airway and give an indication of the pressures to which the lungs are exposed. High pressures (greater than 40 cmH_2O) are associated with barotrauma manifested as alveoli breakdown and pneumothoraces. This technique will also indicate and monitor residual pressure in the lungs when using positive end-expiratory pressure (PEEP) or continuous positive airways pressure (CPAP) modes of respiratory support. All patients on ventilators should have their airway pressures monitored routinely.

End-tidal carbon dioxide is easily measured on a breath-by-breath basis. The presence of CO_2 helps to confirm both tube placement and ventilation. It is also an indirect indicator of cardiac output, as the CO_2 delivered to the lungs falls with falling cardiac output.

The **chest X-ray** is also a monitor of the respiratory system, not just for acute events, e.g. pneumothorax or aspiration, but more importantly for following trends such as the development or resolution of pneumonia or oedema.

Arterial blood gases are a standard measurement in the critically ill patient. The partial pressures of oxygen and carbon dioxide are measured, as is the acid–base status. The carbon dioxide pressure indicates efficacy of ventilation. Oxygenation is indicated by the arterial oxygen partial pressure. The pH and the base deficit indicate the acid–base status and the likely cause of an acidosis, whether metabolic (low bicarbonate value) or respiratory (high CO_2 value). These measurements are invaluable in assessing a patient's condition. These measurements can also be used in combination with others, such as cardiac output, to measure oxygen delivery to the tissues.

The cardiovascular system

A simple **cardiograph** gives heart rate and rhythm, which is a valuable continuous clinical sign. The trace itself may give warning of ischaemia by monitoring the ST segment.

Manual blood pressure monitoring is labour-intensive, very intermittent and often unreliable. Automatic non-invasive systems are relatively cheap, easy to apply and an excellent example of how monitoring can be done more frequently and accurately and free up personnel at the same time. The monitors do not treat, but their presence gives clinicians more time. They are temperamental in the very unstable situation but useful once there is an element of control. They enable regular and reliable monitoring on an almost continual basis.

Invasive arterial monitoring is extremely helpful where there is instability. It is immediate and continuous. The trace can provide useful information as well as the absolute values. Fluctuations in amplitude with respiration show the reliance of cardiac output on venous return, which is accentuated in hypovolaemia.

Central venous pressure (CVP) monitoring can be helpful. A catheter placed in a central vein will give a pressure indicative of the pressure in the venous system returning blood to the heart, as does estimating the jugular venous pressure: low may indicate hypovolaemia whereas high may indicate overfilling. However, clinical judgement based on the signs of pulse rate (high), blood pressure (low) and peripheral perfusion (poor) tell you when a patient is 'empty', and confirmation with CVP is unnecessary. The value may be helpful with control of fluid administration. With rapid refilling it helps to prevent pushing the filling pressures too high, and this is its main use.

It is very important to remember that the CVP measures pressure not volume and does not indicate volume status of the patient. A young exsanguinated patient can compensate with vasoconstriction. A normal CVP can be achieved easily while that patient is tightly vasoconstricted, but if vasodilatation occurs, as with analgesia, the fluid deficit is rapidly and sometimes disastrously exposed. It is the assessment of CVP in association with other signs such as peripheral perfusion which gives some indication of intravascular volume status.

Monitoring of the left side of the heart gives an indication of left ventricular function, which may be significantly different from that indicated by the right side pressures in some circumstances. A pulmonary artery catheter can be introduced for this purpose, usually through a central vein, through the heart and into the pulmonary artery. If flow into the vessel containing the catheter is obstructed by inflating a balloon in that vessel, the pressure measured distal to the balloon reflects the pressure of the left atrium.

There is now a range of monitors, such as Lidco, Picco and Nico, that allow measurement of cardiac output without pulmonary artery catheterisation. The first two are based on dye dilution techniques to measure output whereas the third measures the carbon dioxide being excreted and uses that to derive the cardiac output. These are so-called 'non-invasive' methods.

Oxygen delivery and consumption can also be measured. Oxygen delivery is the volume of blood (cardiac output) multiplied by the amount of oxygen it contains (determined by knowing the haemoglobin, the saturation and the binding coefficient of haemoglobin). Cardiac output can be measured with a pulmonary artery catheter, the arterial blood gases will give the saturation, and the haemoglobin can be measured. The binding coefficient is a known constant. It is then easy to calculate the quantity of oxygen delivered by the heart per minute, i.e. the oxygen delivery. After passing around the body, the blood comes back to the lungs, depleted of oxygen. This can be measured by sampling a mixed venous sample from the pulmonary artery through the catheter. The difference between that delivered and that returned is the oxygen consumption.

A simpler and now popular means of deriving information is by using a central venous oxygen saturation measurement ($ScvO_2$) either continuously or by stat measurements. Arterial blood should be close to 100% saturated with oxygen. As oxygen is utilised by tissues the oxygen saturation of the blood decreases. If there is a reduced supply of oxygen to the tissues (i.e. poor perfusion) or if there is increased uptake of oxygen, then the oxygen saturation of the blood will be reduced. A value of 70% would reasonably be expected in the central venous circulation. Values lower than this may indicate inadequate perfusion and the need for further fluid resuscitation. $ScvO_2$ has to be used in the context of the clinical problems of the patient. The acid–base status or the lactate value may support the suggestion that the patient is inadequately resuscitated.

The gastrointestinal system

Gastrointestinal functional assessment starts with the physical examination of the abdomen. Conscious level is important, as in the unconscious, unresponsive or intubated patient, the flat, soft abdomen can be misleading. Passing a nasogastric tube can be informative in terms of stomach contents, the presence of gastric emptying with low-volume residue and also gastric pH. Some sources recommend using gastric tonometry, which measures intraluminal pH, to indicate gut perfusion. Intraluminal acidosis indicates poor mucosal perfusion, the implication being that increasing blood supply to that area may be of benefit.

The urological system

Renal function is easily monitored with a urinary catheter. The presence of albumin, glucose or blood in the urine can be ascertained. Urine volume is a useful indicator of general renal function. Tests such as short-term creatinine clearance measurements can give more accurate assessment of function, as can monitoring plasma urea and creatinine.

In impaired renal function the urea and creatinine both rise. In a dehydrated patient the urea may be reabsorbed while creatinine is not, leading to a greater rise in urea than in creatinine. Other causes of this are increased urea absorption from other sites, the most common example being gastrointestinal bleeding.

OTHER MONITORING

Temperature

Temperature is always measured in the critically ill. Core temperature is more useful than peripheral temperature. The differential between core and periphery is an indirect measure of general perfusion and can be a useful tool.

Pregnancy

Pregnant patients are rarely discussed, and yet they present a particularly difficult problem; there are two patients involved: mother and fetus. Both should be monitored as early as possible, as this may influence decisions regarding delivery. Monitoring can be clinical in the first instance, preferably with obstetric medical involvement, but use of continuous fetal heart monitoring assists during the various phases of resuscitation. It does not take priority over the ABC of resuscitation.

THERAPEUTICS

In the ICU every therapeutic intervention is performed to achieve benefit, but each and every intervention will have both positive and negative attributes. It is essential that each is evaluated in terms of potential benefits against potential harm prior to use. To do this, both positive and negative attributes need to be understood. The other fundamental principle is that it is better to prevent than to treat.

There are two parallel approaches necessary in the critically ill: resuscitation and diagnosis. It is essential to resuscitate the patient and correct life-threatening physiological disturbances. It is also vital to make a diagnosis so that the cause can be treated. All too often the diagnosis is ignored while the patient is salvaged, or alternatively the patient lost while the diagnosis is made. Both are essential in the management of the critically ill.

The goals of treatment are to:

- correct physiological disturbance and support normal physiology
- treat the underlying cause
- prevent secondary problems.

THE RESPIRATORY SYSTEM

Adequate oxygenation is a fundamental requirement. It is important to ensure that the patient is ventilating adequately and that the inspired oxygen is adequate to ensure oxygenation.

Ventilatory failure

Ventilatory failure is brought about by the inability of the chest wall to generate a negative pressure and therefore to ventilate adequately (Box 10.4). Management involves reversing the cause. An example of this is apnoea secondary to opiate overdose depressing ventilation. Naloxone reverses the opiate-induced respiratory depression, allowing the patient to breathe. Another example is apnoea due to airway obstruction; clearing the airway allows spontaneous ventilation.

Alternatively the patient may be ventilated. Mechanical ventilation is extremely effective for ventilatory failure, whether mechanical or neurological.

Box 10.4 Causes of ventilatory failure

- CNS failure and loss of respiratory drive – CVA, sedative drugs, head injury, spinal cord injury, infections (e.g. meningoencephalitis), sleep apnoea
- Peripheral nerves – phrenic nerve damage, neuromuscular blockade, myasthenia, Guillain–Barré syndrome
- Muscular problems – dystrophies, electrolyte disturbances (hypokalaemia, hypophosphataemia), disrupted diaphragm, disuse atrophy
- Chest wall – fractured ribs, thoracic surgery, kyphoscoliosis, obesity
- Airway – bronchospasm, obstruction, pulmonary fibrosis, air trapping

Box 10.5 Causes of respiratory failure

- Hypercapnic (ventilatory) failure
- Central nervous system (e.g. head injury, stroke)
- Peripheral nervous system (e.g. motor neurone disease)
- Chest wall/musculoskeletal (e.g. trauma or mesothelioma)
- Upper airways (e.g. tracheal stenosis)
- Lower airways (e.g. pneumonia)
- Hypoxaemic 'lung' failure
- Alveolar hypoventilation
- V/Q abnormality (e.g. pulmonary thromboembolism)
- Diffusion defects
- Right-to-left shunt

Respiratory failure (see Box 10.5)

This is lung failure or the inability to take oxygen up from the lung and to excrete carbon dioxide from the lung, because of problems within it. This occurs either because there is mismatch between ventilation (V) and perfusion (Q) or because there is an effective barrier between the gas space and the blood, which inhibits gas exchange. In the case of a mismatch there may be parts of the lung which are well ventilated but have no blood supply; a pulmonary embolus would do this. Alternatively there may be a good blood supply but no ventilation; severe pneumonia or atelectasis will cause this.

A barrier may be formed by fluid, pulmonary oedema or inflammatory or cellular infiltrates. There is a condition termed adult respiratory distress syndrome (ARDS), or more recently acute lung injury (also known as non-cardiogenic pulmonary oedema), which is essentially hypoxaemia in the presence of normal cardiac filling pressures; it is associated with diffuse alveolar infiltrates apparent on chest X-ray. In fact, the original definition was radiological. Any insult involving the lung (either local to the lung or general) may result in acute lung injury (see Box 10.6).

The main problems with ARDS lie in determining the underlying diagnosis in order to treat the problem and dealing with oxygenation. The pathophysiology is a combination of V/Q mismatch, some shunting and a barrier effect. Therapeutic measures include:

- methods to reverse the pathology by recruiting alveoli, thereby increasing the surface area of gas exchange
- methods to alter local perfusion by vasodilatation
- methods to improve the blood supply to ventilated alveoli, such as inhaled nitric oxide
- simpler methods such as increasing the inspired oxygen concentration.

Where gas exchange is poor, ventilatory failure is likely to become superimposed on respiratory failure and ventilation may help to alleviate the ventilatory component. Unfortunately it may aggravate part of the respiratory component, as the balance of V/Q abnormality is unpredictably altered by positive-pressure ventilation.

Lung failure is almost always a combination of different pathophysiological factors and is far more difficult to treat than ventilatory failure.

Box 10.6 Causes of acute lung injury (ARDS)

Local insult
- Smoke inhalation
- Airway burns
- Aspiration of gastric acid
- Near-drowning

Parenchymal insults
- Confusion
- Infection (bacterial and viral)

Systemic insults
- Septicaemia and SIRS
- Shock of any cause
- Pancreatitis
- Amniotic fluid embolus

Methods of ventilation

Spontaneous breathing is the physiological norm. The chest generates a negative pressure and entrains air. The negative pressure assists venous return to the heart. Ventilation and perfusion of areas within the lung are controlled by intrinsic mechanisms.

Mechanical ventilation is not physiological. It creates positive pressure in the chest, forcing air into areas that are most compliant (easily distendable). A number of modes of respiratory support and ventilation are used, as summarised in Table 10.5. However, it should be noted that there are negative aspects of positive-pressure ventilation:

- impairs venous return and depresses cardiac output
- induces endocrine changes, e.g. raised ADH
- worsens V/Q abnormality and gas exchange
- produces barotrauma
- creates a need for increased sedation or relaxants
- creates a potential for infection.

In very severe cases, it may be possible to manage oxygenation by putting the patient on extracorporeal membrane oxygenation (ECMO), but this is largely experimental at the present time. Current evidence shows that the efficacy of ECMO in adults is poor in comparison to adults; however, the ongoing CESAR trial suggests that there may be a subset of adult patients who would be likely to benefit from ECMO therapy.

THE CARDIOVASCULAR SYSTEM

Support of the cardiovascular system is a fundamental part of management of the critically ill patient. This is the system that delivers oxygen from the lungs to the tissues and ultimately to the cells. Failure of this system, either locally or globally, leads to tissue hypoxia. The areas which may be influenced are the heart and the vascular system.

The heart may fail for a number of reasons, including the failure to maintain adequate performance, either through impaired contractility or through an inefficient rate, whether

Table 10.5 Modes of respiratory support and ventilation features

Mode	Characteristics
Spontaneous	
Continuous positive airways pressure (CPAP)	Positive pressure overcomes resistance to inspiration, opens and keeps open alveoli which may otherwise collapse. Reduces work of breathing, recruits alveoli and improves oxygenation
Ventilation	
Continuous positive-pressure ventilation (CPPV)	Machine provides all ventilation
Intermittent mandatory ventilation (IMV)	Machine provides set number of breaths, and the patient breathes between
Synchronized intermittent mandatory ventilation (SIMV)	Patient can trigger machine breaths as well as breathe between mandatory breaths
Assisted spontaneous breathing (ASB)	Patient triggers machine which applies a preset pressure to assist the patient's breathing
Inverse ratio ventilation (IRV)	The inspiration:expiration (I:E) ratio is usually 1:2, but this reverses the ratio to 2:1. A longer inspiratory time allows longer for pressure to expand the lung and recruit alveoli. Helps oxygenation. Higher mean pressure in the airway
Positive end-expiratory pressure (PEEP)	Applied with most ventilation modes. Maintains positive pressure in the airway and helps prevent collapse of alveoli. Better oxygenation, worse venous return

high or low. Another mechanism of heart failure is where, despite performing well, the heart fails to meet the excessive requirements imposed upon it. The intravascular volume is a fundamental part of cardiac performance, and any cause of hypovolaemia will reduce cardiovascular performance.

Vascular changes influence the work that the heart has to perform. Vasoconstriction will tend to increase the work of the heart. Profound vasodilatation will reduce the work against resistance but may necessitate a larger cardiac output to sustain blood pressure.

The cardiovascular system obeys the rule V = IR, where V is pressure, I is flow or cardiac output and R is the resistance of the system. Each can be influenced by disease and each can be therapeutically manipulated. The key question is the volume status of the patient. This needs to be optimal. Assessment of volume is performed by evaluating perfusion (e.g. a warm periphery) and filling pressure (the JVP). This can be measured directly, as the CVP. The CVP does not indicate volume, only pressure, and an assessment of perfusion must be made.

If a patient is hypovolaemic, this should be corrected. The optimal filling pressure for the heart should be found. An easy test is to administer fluid to the patient until filling appears to be adequate. Then give small incremental boluses of fluid (200 mL in an adult) to see if the blood pressure improves. At the point where there is no improvement in blood pressure, the filling is probably optimal.

Cardiac performance can be improved by influencing contractility and, sometimes, rate. Various inotropes have effects on cardiac performance and on the vasculature (Table 10.6). The vasculature can be influenced by the vasoconstrictors listed in Table 10.6, but it is also possible to use a direct alpha-agonist such as phenylephrine or metaraminol as a potent vasoconstrictor. Vasodilators currently used include glyceryl trinitrate (GTN), sodium nitroprusside and prostacyclin.

Over the last few years there has been considerable emphasis on measuring oxygen delivery and attempting to increase delivery if thought inadequate. The difficulty is that, when grossly inadequate, it is obvious, but it has proved very difficult to define when a small enhancement of oxygen delivery might be of benefit. One of the problems is that there is a cost for increasing oxygen delivery by virtue of the other effects of the drugs used.

Methods of improving oxygen delivery

There are various methods of increasing the oxygen supply. At the lungs the inspired oxygen concentration can be increased. In the lungs, V/Q may be influenced by CPAP, ventilation pattern (see Table 10.5) or by agents such as nitric oxide. In the blood, oxygen carriage can be increased by changing haemoglobin concentration and guaranteeing intravascular volume. The delivery of oxygen can be enhanced by increasing cardiac output. This is achieved by volume loading or inotropes, or both. In the periphery, delivery may be influenced by venodilators such as GTN or prostacyclins.

An alternative approach to improving the ratio of supply to requirements is to reduce requirements by reducing consumption. The work of breathing is reduced by using a ventilator. Good temperature control, either by reducing hyperthermia or by generating hypothermia, will also cut the oxygen requirement.

THE KIDNEYS AND RENAL FAILURE

While the critically ill may develop renal failure for any of the reasons seen in the normal population, some causes are far more commonly seen. The mechanism is frequently prerenal due to effective hypovolaemia and hypoperfusion of the kidneys. Common causes include dehydration from poor fluid intake and inadequate replacement, and loss of fluid from any cause, e.g. diabetes mellitus or insipidus, bleeding, burns, diarrhoea and vomiting. Renal causes, including diseases such as glomerulonephritis, are relatively uncommon, although nephrotoxicity from drugs is frequently a component of renal failure in critically ill patients. Postrenal causes should always be excluded, usually by ultrasound.

As with many situations in the critically ill, there may be multiple causes. A kidney damaged by prerenal failure is more susceptible to nephrotoxicity, and potent and potentially dangerous drugs are more likely to be used in the critically ill. Due to alterations in drug kinetics, the use of these drugs is also far less predictable in this setting.

The principles of managing renal dysfunction are simple. Try to identify the cause of the problem, while ensuring that there is no prerenal element by maintaining a well-perfused patient with adequate blood pressure. An adequate blood pressure is one that is preferably close to the patient's normal value. This may require aggressive fluid management and sometimes inotropes. As perfusion is also important, it may be necessary to add a vasodilator to improve this.

There are also some other time-honoured methods of encouraging urine output. Diuretics should only be used if the patient is normovolaemic, as they can aggravate hypovolaemia. Osmotic diuretics are sometimes used – especially

Table 10.6 Cardiac inotropes – their effects on the heart and peripheral vasculature

Drug	Contractility	Rate	Vasoconstriction	Vasodilatation
Adrenaline (epinephrine), high dose	+++++	+++	++++	
Adrenaline (epinephrine), low dose	+++	++		++
Noradrenaline (norepinephrine)	+++	+	+++++	
Dopamine, high dose	+++	+++	++++	
Dopamine, low dose	+	+		+
Dobutamine	+++	++		+++
Dopexamine	+++	++		+++
Milrinone	++	++		++++

if there is jaundice, when patients are particularly susceptible to renal injury. Furosemide (frusemide) is also often used and acts by affecting the Na/K pump in the loop of Henle, encouraging a diuresis. It is currently thought that, at low dose, furosemide also reduces the oxygen requirement of the tubules and protects them from hypoxia. These methods are frequently advocated and regularly used, but remain of unproven benefit.

In the critically ill, renal failure is usually associated with generalised injury, and if the kidneys are failing there is usually damage to other organs, although it may be less easily detected. When renal failure is secondary to severe injury it carries a poor prognosis, and the mortality in the critically ill with renal failure is high: claimed to be 50–70% in most series and unchanged by recent advances. If the renal failure is genuinely an isolated phenomenon, associated with, for example, a nephrotoxic drug, it usually has a good prognosis.

Renal replacement

The principles of renal replacement are simple. The object is to remove toxic materials such as urea, creatinine and potassium from the blood. This can be done in two ways. The first of these is to remove or filter all the fluid containing the toxic waste and replace it with clean replacement fluid. This is filtration, and the removal of fluid parallels the glomerular filtration rate (GFR). A GFR of 20 mL/min needs $20 \times 60 = 1200$ mL/h or 28.8 L/day of replacement fluid.

The second method, dialysis, involves the use of the osmotic gradient. If the plasma with toxic waste is exposed to similar fluid with no toxins across a semi-permeable membrane, the toxins will pass down a concentration gradient into the clean solution. If a countercurrent is used, there is rapid transit of both urea and creatinine, and this is similar to the mechanism in the tubule. No replacement fluid needs to be given, and there is no contact between body fluid, plasma and the dialysis fluid except across the semi-permeable membrane. Creatinine clearances of 25–30 mL/min are easily achieved.

The blood flow through the filters can be driven either by blood pressure, using an arteriovenous shunt, or by venovenous pump. The latter is more dependable, independent of blood pressure and has minimal haemodynamic consequences. Standard dialysis with high flows can be used for much more rapid clearances but is more likely to result in haemodynamic instability.

THE CENTRAL NERVOUS SYSTEM

The central nervous system is very susceptible to injury and, in particular, to hypoxia. Once damage has occurred, reversal of damage is difficult or impossible. The main thrust of intensive care management of brain injury is to limit the damage that is taking place, prevent further damage and then attempt to reverse injury or at least provide an environment where recovery is more likely.

Fitting

There are two potential problems: hypoxia both from poor ventilation and from localised hypoxia around the area of the epileptiform activity in the brain, and injury from fitting itself. Treatment involves protection of the airway, ensuring adequate oxygenation and control of the fits. The latter is achieved with anticonvulsants, but, while they may control the fits, they may also depress ventilation.

Cerebral injury and cerebral oedema

The brain is in an enclosed space. Most kinds of injury result in localised oedema, and, if this is extensive, the brain will swell and then be constrained by the skull. Pressure in the brain will rise and blood flow will fall. Tissue hypoxia will result, accentuating the injury. The approach to treatment is to prevent a rise in intracranial pressure (ICP) but to try to ensure that the cerebral perfusion pressure (CPP, i.e. systolic blood pressure minus ICP) remains adequate to perfuse the brain.

Several mechanisms are likely to cause a rise in ICP (Boxes 10.7 and 10.8). Acute rises in blood pressure must be prevented. Hypercapnia also causes a rise in ICP. Excess fluid administration may increase oedema formation, as may a head-down posture. These should be avoided, but the CPP must be maintained, so hypotension must be avoided. Hypocapnia can result in cerebral vasoconstriction and reduced cerebral flow, so that should also be avoided.

Mechanisms for reducing intracranial pressure include diuretics such as mannitol. This will reduce pressure acutely and is useful in a crisis, as is hypocapnia, but sustained use of either will cause problems. In severe situations, using agents to reduce cerebral oxygen requirement to help protect the cells has been advocated, and drugs such as barbiturates have been used. The penalties associated with prolonged iatrogenic coma almost certainly outweigh the perceived benefit.

The key to cerebral treatment is cerebral protection.

THE GASTROINTESTINAL SYSTEM

Intestinal function consists of the absorption of nutrients, and the colon may also be involved in biosynthesis of short-chain fatty acids and branched-chain amino acids. The bowel is

Box 10.7 Factors affecting intracranial pressure (ICP)

Interventions which raise ICP
- ↑ Blood pressure
- ↑ Intravenous fluids
- ↑ $P_{a}CO_2$
- Head-down posture

Interventions which lower ICP
- ↓ Blood pressure
- ↓ $P_{a}CO_2$
- Head-up posture
- Barbiturates?

Box 10.8 Measures to prevent cerebral injury

- Prevent hypoxia and hypercapnia
- Maintain normocapnia or mild hypocapnia
- Maintain cerebral perfusion pressure
- Avoid acute changes in blood pressure

full of organisms; in the critically ill, it has been described as 'the sewer within'. The organisms are usually commensals with which the host lives comfortably under normal circumstances. Table 10.7 lists a number of factors which affect intestinal function in the critically ill.

The gut often becomes quiescent in the critically ill, and the milieu of the contents changes in terms of the substrates present. Antibiotics decimate gut flora and allow overgrowth of any organisms which are unimpaired by them. The flora changes completely to one which may be potentially hazardous to the host. An example of this is the high incidence of *Enterobacter faecalis* seen in ICUs since cephalosporins became routine for surgical prophylaxis, as this organism is resistant to cephalosporins.

Furthermore, in critically ill patients, gastric stress ulceration is a potentially lethal complication which is occasionally seen and, to prevent this, H_2 antagonists are used to reduce acid secretion. This increases intragastric pH and allows bacterial overgrowth of the upper GI tract, colonised from organisms which usually cannot thrive in the upper intestine. This may in turn, by spilling over into the respiratory tract, increase the incidence of nosocomial ('hospital-acquired') pneumonia. The stagnant gut also tends to undergo epithelial atrophy. The morphological and immunological barrier which exists in the gut wall may become impaired, and translocation of toxins and even bacteria may increase across the gut wall. These effects are accentuated by poor gut and liver perfusion in critically ill patients. Toxaemia and sepsis may then arise from the gut.

Various strategies are used to reduce these potential problems. H_2 antagonists are avoided by using mucosa-protecting agents such as sucralfate to prevent stress ulceration without altering pH. Early feeding prevents gut atrophy, reduces translocation and helps to sustain immunocompetence of the gut wall. Antibiotics should be avoided when possible to preserve commensal bacteria. Enteral feeding and the use of 'probiotic' cultures have been shown to enhance immune activity, delay gut colonisation by pathogenic organisms and improve outcome in antibiotic-associated diarrhoea and specific gastrointestinal infections such as *Helicobacter pylori*.

The issue of Selective Decontamination of the Digestive tract (SDD) describes a technique aimed at reducing the incidence of nosocomial infections (particularly ventilator-associated pneumonia) by the prevention of colonisation by, or the erradication of, pathogenic organisms from the upper gastrointestinal tract. These organisms may be carried 'silently' by healthy patients or may be opportunistic in the critically ill patient. The therapy involves the administration of a specific antibiotic regimen topically to the oropharynx, enterally and parenterally aimed at the culprit micro-organisms. It should be stressed that the widespread use of SDD is a contentious issue that should be seen as an adjunct to high standards of cross-infection control and prevention of infection rather than an alternative.

Early feeding

After major surgery the small bowel often starts peristalsis very rapidly – within a couple of days, as can be demonstrated with ultrasound. Unfortunately gastric emptying is frequently delayed, and so feeding via nasogastric tube may be futile. Some drugs, including dopamine, impair gastric emptying without influencing small bowel motility. Tubes may be placed in the jejunum from the nose via the stomach (nasojejunal) or a feeding jejunostomy catheter may be placed at operation. The benefits of early enteral feeding are better colonisation, less small bowel atrophy, better immunological function and less translocation.

Any approach to nutrition must take into account the pathophysiology of the patient at the time. There are three main categories of patient:

- the starved patient
- the hypercatabolic injured patient
- the starved hypercatabolic patient.

The starved patient has a specific response to starvation with a general slowing of metabolic rate, an adaptation to fat utilisation and an endocrine profile concomitant with this. Such patients are tuned to being able to survive by conservation of resources. Their energy expenditure is relatively stable and therefore predictable. These patients will adapt readily and rapidly to nutritional support and will utilise it efficiently. They will utilise both fats and glucose but are very well adapted to fat utilisation. In this regard, total parenteral nutrition (TPN) reverses starvation catabolism in skeletal muscle.

Table 10.7 Factors involved in the gut which can become a source of problems in the critically ill

	Effect	Consequences
H_2 antagonists	Reduced pH	Increased colonisation
Nil by mouth	Reduced gastric emptying Altered upper GI dynamics Reduced substrates in gut	Increased colonisation Cholestasis in gall bladder Changed flora Reduced biosynthesis
Antibiotics	Changed flora	Pathogenic organisms increased Reduced biosynthesis
Stasis	Overgrowth Villous atrophy Immunological incompetence	Translocation Toxaemia Infection
Poor perfusion in gut and liver	Barrier incompetence (morphological and immunological)	Toxaemia Translocation

The injured patient has an increased metabolic rate and a hormonal profile which enhances metabolic activity. While there is an adaptation of normal tissues towards fat utilisation, there is also an increased glucose requirement by the injured tissues. The endocrine profile is described as a stress response. The energy utilisation is extremely variable and unpredictable; indeed the energy utilisation calculated by indirect calorimetry can vary by 30% on consecutive days.

Under these conditions an overall change in metabolic status occurs. There is an increase in resting oxygen consumption, with a respiratory quotient (RQ) of 0.8–0.85, reflecting a mixed fuel source. Energy is derived from available glucose, proteins and some fats. There is an increase in all these substrates, but as fat utilisation increases, there is a relative decrease in the ratio of calories derived from glucose and from amino acids.

Nutritional support

There are two principles underlying nutritional support:

- everyone needs food
- the easiest, most normal route is best.

Nutrition is important not only because a small but significant proportion of patients are malnourished but also because the stress of major surgery or illness rapidly depletes nutritional resources. It is well known that operating on severely malnourished patients carries a high morbidity, and the fact that malnutrition is associated with poor outcome has led to the sensible assumption that nutritional support and correction are probably beneficial. Preoperative correction of malnutrition is probably relevant in less than 5% of patients admitted for major surgery, but it is important to note that it takes some time, probably about 10 days or longer, to make any impact on nutritional status.

In the critically ill, support of the catabolic patient during the acute phase of the illness may be crucial to survival. Malnutrition reduces the resistance to infection and slows down most healing processes. There is also an associated reduction in oxidation of pyruvate and an increase in release of alanine and lactate with oxidation of C_2 fragments from fat and amino acids. Carbohydrate metabolism is characterised by increased glycogenolysis, not suppressible with exogenous insulin or glucose, and an increase in glucose flow and utilisation by peripheral tissues, especially those that are injured. Insulin is increased but so is the glucagon:insulin ratio. The peripheral lactate byproduct is recycled through the liver. Fat metabolism is increased, with an increase in lipolysis and decreased lipogenesis. There is increased mobilisation of long- and medium-chain fatty acids, with a reduction in clearance of fatty acids. The increase in protein catabolism has already been mentioned, with the resultant massive mobilisation of amino acids. There is increased use of branched-chain amino acids, in particular glutamine, which is produced to transport available amino acids to sites of utilisation both as amino acids and as a calorie source to produce ATP via the Krebs cycle. Glutamine can be easily used as a primary substrate by many organs including the gut.

Nutritional assessment can be done at the bedside and should be part of the physical examination. Look for signs of weight loss. More sophisticated methods use arm muscle circumference, arm circumference and triceps skinfold thickness. This last measurement can indicate loss of muscle bulk but is better as a trend measurement than as an isolated reading, as it takes 3–4 weeks to show nutritional change. Measurements of serum albumin, total iron-binding capacity (TIBC), transferrin, thyroxine-binding pre-albumin and retinol-binding protein can all be used to assess nutritional status.

Administration

The route of nutrition is important. Enteral feeding is cheaper, safer and more efficient than parenteral feeding (Fig. 10.2). There should be a gradation from normal food at one end of the spectrum through to total parenteral nutrition (TPN) at the other. Efforts should be made to keep nutrition as simple as possible: simple is safe.

Enteral feeding

Enteral feeding keeps the gut functional, helps to maintain normal gut flora and may reduce the incidence of sepsis. The gut can assimilate and use nutrition from the gut lumen, and this may play a part in keeping the intestinal mucosa healthy. Current practice is to encourage early enteral feeding when tolerated. A number of different enteral feeds are available, and they may be delivered into the stomach or proximal jejunum.

Parenteral feeding

Intravenous supplementation should seek to provide the optimal combination of water, calories, protein, vitamins and trace metals for an adequate diet. This is in the context of the underlying problem and the ability of the patient to cope with not only the fluid load but also the nutritional load.

The two main components are calories and protein – the former as glucose or fat, and the latter as amino acids. In starvation, large calorie loads can be used, e.g. 55 kcal/kg per day with a kcal:N ratio (where N represents nitrogen, a measure of the protein content of feeds) of 200:1. In catabolic septic or injured patients, a calorie input of 30 kcal/kg per day and a kcal:N ratio of 100:1 (0.3 g/kg per day) are more appropriate.

Energy requirements are a controversial issue. After elective surgery, peak metabolism increases by 10–13% and returns rapidly to normal. After burns it may increase by 50%, largely determined by the temperature gradient between the patient and the ambient environment, as the calories are

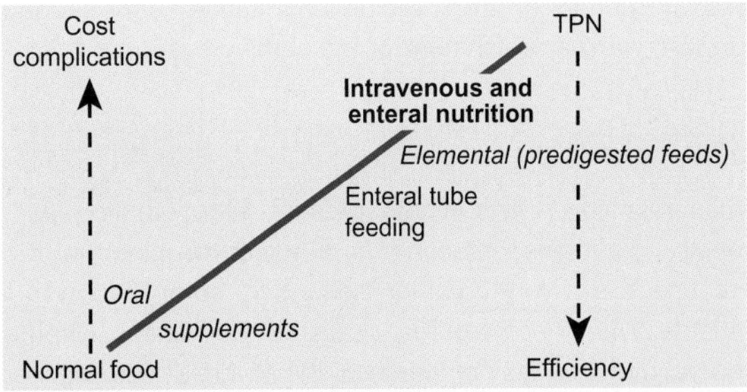

Fig. 10.2 Nutritional methods and their relationship to cost, complications and efficiency. TPN, total parenteral nutrition.

largely used to sustain body temperature. A calorie requirement of 34 kcal/kg per day is not unreasonable.

Glucose is a good calorie source, but after a maximum of about 5 mg/kg per minute, there is a tendency for glucose to become lipid through lipogenesis with a high output of CO_2 in the process. Glucose yields about 4 kcal/g. Lipid is easily administered and effectively used. Fat-soluble vitamins as well as essential phospholipids can be given with the lipid. The emulsion has chylomicron-size globules which are cleared from the circulation.

Protein is given in the form of amino acids at a rate of about 0.3 g N_2/kg per day. The range of available amino acids should include branched-chain amino acids, in particular glutamine.

Vitamins and trace elements should be supplemented in the critically ill. Folate deficiency is relatively common, as is thiamine deficiency. Selenium is also recognised as being commonly deficient and may play a significant role in prostaglandin pathways and in leucocyte function, via glutathione peroxidase. Zinc, iron, copper, manganese, cobalt, iodine, chromium and molybdenum are also important.

Complications of parenteral nutrition. The complications are all those of venous access, including pneumothorax, arterial puncture and, most importantly, infection. Parenteral nutrition is associated with sepsis, and line infection is a common problem with a significant morbidity. Disciplined asepsis when dealing with i.v. lines and rigorous surveillance are both essential. Other problems include cholestasis, which is also seen in the critically ill patient without parenteral nutrition.

COAGULATION

There are many causes of coagulopathy in critically ill patients. Postoperatively the commonest cause after a large haemorrhage and massive blood transfusion is exhaustion of clotting factors, often including platelets. This coagulopathy will respond to replacement therapy.

Abnormal coagulopathies include disseminated intravascular coagulopathy (DIC). In patients with major sepsis complicating the surgery, DIC may develop. Other causes include devitalised tissue or gross disruption of tissues. Brain contains cerebral thromboplastins, and massive disruption of cerebral tissue may result in release of thromboplastin and cause DIC; this is seen as deteriorating clotting studies with falling platelets and raised fibrin degradation products (FDPs). Clinically there may be bleeding from puncture sites, and blood samples taken fail to clot. Treatment is twofold: first, correction of the precipitating cause; and second, support, with replenishment of the clotting system.

INFECTION

While relatively few patients present with infection as a primary diagnosis, infection is a major problem in ICU because it is a very common secondary complication in ill patients. Whatever the primary cause of their illness, whether trauma, major surgery or infection, the severe stress imposed tends to threaten their immunocompetence. These patients undergo multiple procedures and have many breaches of their integument, such as wounds, intravenous lines and endotracheal tubes, all of which can serve as conduits for infection.

Because of the serious nature of infection in the ICU and the heavy use of powerful antibiotics, the unit tends to harbour pathogenic and often resistant organisms. The high intensity of nursing and medical attention predisposes to cross-infection. Handwashing is not only simple and sensible but is the only easily applied method of preventing cross-infection that has been shown to work.

General microbial surveillance is important so that the prevalent organisms in the ICU and in individual patients are known by both the microbiologist and the intensive care staff (Box 10.9). When a patient becomes infected it is better to be able to treat an identified organism than to be forced to use broad-spectrum therapy that may miss the relevant organism. It is also difficult to grow organisms from patients on antibiotics, and so avoiding antibiotics and using intensive surveillance constitute a logical approach to treatment.

The traditional approach in ICU of the widespread use of broad-spectrum antibiotics both prophylactically and to treat probable and possible infection may be partly responsible for the increasing emergence of super-resistant organisms. Cautious, controlled organism-specific use of antibiotics is more efficacious and less likely to lead to resistance.

ANALGESIA AND SEDATION

Patients in the ICU are frequently in pain, e.g. due to surgery or acute problems such as peritonitis, and they may suffer lesser discomfort from flatulence or constipation. Perceived oxygen lack or problems in the lung such as pulmonary oedema create anxiety and discomfort. Physical interventions such as intubation and positive-pressure ventilation are at best uncomfortable. There are three aspects of management that overlap, all of which need to be considered (Fig. 10.3):

- analgesia for pain
- anxiolytics for anxiety
- sedation for awareness.

The relative quantities of each are determined by the specific requirements of each patient at the particular point in his or her ICU management.

Sedation is a loosely used term to describe keeping a patient comfortable in ICU. In some circumstances it may be appropriate for this to mean unconsciousness, in others immobility, while at other times it may mean wide awake but not in discomfort and able to move, breathe and in particular

Box 10.9 Patient surveillance

- Clinical – clinical behaviour, temperature, white cell count, CRP
- Blood cultures – through central lines, peripheral sites
- Wound culture – wound sites
- Sputum – regular sputum culture
- Skin – skin swabs for MRSA
- Nares – nasal swabs
- Urine – midstream urine

CRP, C-reactive protein; MRSA, meticillin-resistant *Staphylococcus aureus*.

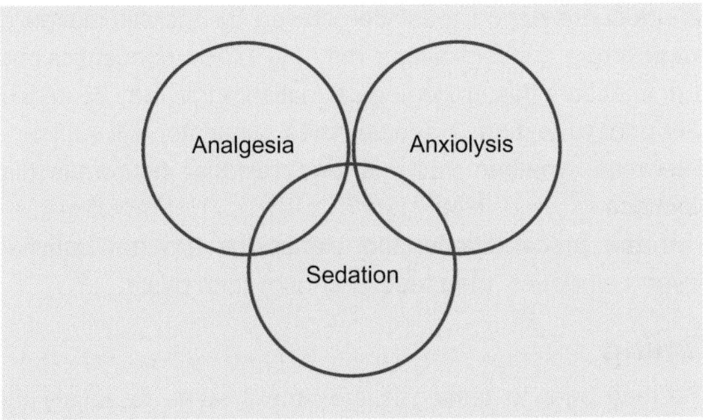

Fig. 10.3 Overlapping objectives in an intensive care unit.

to coordinate with the ventilator. There are several scoring systems available to attempt to quantify the level of sedation of a patient. While none is perfect, it is important to have some means of describing a level of sedation to aim for. There is considerable emphasis in regular 'sedation holds' where sedation is stopped to assess the patient so that over-sedation is now less common. This translates into shorter periods of mechanical ventilation and the inherent benefits therein.

Pharmacological considerations

The level of pharmacological control and the length of time for which it is required determine the choice of agent (see Table 10.8). Frequently a combination of agents works well because it enables smaller doses of individual drugs with differing pharmacodynamic profiles to be used.

Sedation

If rapid, reversible sedation is required then propofol is preferred. For longer periods the benzodiazepine midazolam may be more cost-effective, although it takes longer to wear off, especially in the presence of liver dysfunction.

It is recognised that sleep deprivation and disruption of the normal 'sleep/wake cycle' that is characteristic of intensive care admission (few completed cycles, frequent disturbances and awakenings for interventions and little in the way of 'deep' REM sleep) is detrimental to the patient's recovery and may be a factor in the development of acute delirium states and psychosis. Non-pharmacological techniques such as massage, relaxation therapy, reducing environmental disturbances and music therapy are often employed with variable success.

Analgesia

Opioids are powerful analgesics. They all work rapidly but cause respiratory depression. Diamorphine may have additional euphoric effects. For short-term requirements, alfentanil is effective and wears off rapidly. Most analgesic requirements are longer term in ICU, and, for this, diamorphine, morphine and pethidine are effective and cheap.

In renal failure, the metabolites of the opioids, especially pethidine, accumulate and cause neurological excitation. In some patients, ketamine, which is less cardiovascularly depressive, and in fact may increase the blood pressure, may be of benefit.

Table 10.8 Features of some sedative, analgesic and anxiolytic agents

Agents	Advantages	Disadvantages
Sedatives		
Propofol	Rapid onset Rapid offset	Expensive Haemodynamic disturbance
Midazolam	Rapid onset Accumulates Slow offset	Accumulates and can be a negative inotrope
Barbiturates	Rapid onset Long half-life Reduce metabolic rate	Accumulates Long time to wear off Haemodynamic effects
Analgesics		
Opioids		
Diamorphine	Good analgesia Long action	Accumulates
Fentanyl	Good analgesia Long action	Chest wall rigidity Accumulates
Pethidine	Good analgesia Long action	Accumulates, especially with renal dysfunction Neurological effects
Alfentanil	Good analgesic Short action	Expensive Accumulates if used by infusion
Non-opioids		
Ketamine	Good effect Long action	Hallucinations Agitation
Non-steroids	Anti-inflammatory Helpful adjunct No respiratory depression	Renal failure
Anxiolytics		
Benzodiazepines	Good effect Drowsiness	Tolerance develops rapidly
Haloperidol	Effective Long half-life	

Relaxants

There are occasions when immobility is important. In critically ill patients who are difficult to ventilate or when delicate practical procedures are being performed, it may be safer to paralyse the patient with muscle relaxants. For rapid control of the airway, the depolarising muscle relaxant suxamethonium is useful and produces a rapid onset of full paralysis. For longer-term relaxation, a non-depolarising agent such as atracurium or vecuronium can be used. As these agents are short-acting, a continuous infusion can be used. Atracurium is broken down by Hofmann degradation and is not dependent on renal or liver function for its metabolism, so it does not accumulate; however, it can release histamine, causing bronchospasm which may be a problem. Vecuronium is haemodynamically neutral, very unlikely to release histamine, but it is renal- and liver-dependent and can accumulate.

Pancuronium an old, relatively long-acting drug has sympathomimetic properties (increases heart rate), and this can be useful in cardiovascularly compromised patients.

BRAINSTEM DEATH

A patient is dead when declared to be so (using accepted criteria) by a doctor. Legally this is deemed to be the time of death. Classical criteria for the diagnosis of death have been: permanent cessation of breathing and of the heartbeat. With advances in medical technology, the function of organs other than the brain can be duplicated by machines. This has led to the ability to maintain vital organ function in a body with a non-functioning brain.

Therefore the nature of the criteria for diagnosing death have undergone reappraisal. The first step was the move from a classical 'cardiorespiratory' death to an understanding that a person is not dead until the brain has died. The second step was the acceptance that the permanent functional death of the brainstem constitutes brain death.

Cortical activation and consciousness depend primarily on the role of the brainstem nuclei and their global cerebral projections in the reticular activating system. All cortical sensory inputs and motor outputs traverse the brainstem. Hence the functioning brainstem is essential for meaningful function of the 'brain as a whole'. Any acute, massive, irreversible lesion of the brainstem prevents this function even if isolated parts may, for a short time, emit signals. Therefore a flat EEG is not a requirement for the diagnosis of brainstem death.

The testing of cranial nerve reflexes probes the brainstem slice by slice due to the compact arrangement of brainstem nuclei. No other area of the brain can be tested as thoroughly.

DIAGNOSIS OF BRAINSTEM DEATH

The diagnosis of brainstem death is not made in isolation but in the context of the clinical history and examination. It is a means of confirming clinical opinion.

Preconditions

These are as follows:

- apnoeic coma, i.e. unresponsive on a ventilator
- irreversible structural brain damage.

The primary diagnosis must be established in every case before proceeding to testing. This is usually not difficult, as 80% of cases where brainstem death is diagnosed in the UK have suffered a head injury or intracerebral haemorrhage. It is also important that no therapeutic manoeuvres have changed the patient's condition despite an adequate period having elapsed for observation.

Exclusions

Potential causes of profound but reversible changes in brainstem function must be excluded. These include:

- drugs – intoxication, sedation, poisoning
- neuromuscular blocking agents
- hypothermia
- acid–base disturbances
- electrolyte disturbances
- endocrine disorders.

An adequate period must be allowed for the elimination of drugs (brain concentrations may lag blood concentrations) and, to ensure this, toxicological investigation may be necessary prior to testing. A simple nerve stimulator will suffice to determine whether there is any residual neuromuscular blockade.

If the preconditions and exclusions are not satisfied beyond all doubt, then testing cannot take place.

Timing

The time prior to testing is the time it takes to satisfy the preconditions and exclusions, i.e. the time to establish an unequivocal diagnosis of structural brain damage and to become certain that the condition is irreversible.

The tests

Tests are carried out to prove that brainstem reflexes have been lost and to obtain precise confirmation of persistent apnoea. On examining the patient, observe for signs that the brainstem cannot be dead, e.g.

- seizure (generalised or focal)
- abnormal posturing (decorticate or decerebrate)
- the presence of doll's head eye movements.

All the above require live neurons in the brainstem.

The tests are carried out by two doctors, one of whom must be a consultant; the other may be a registrar (>5 years since full registration).

Tests of five brainstem reflexes

- No pupillary response to light. The pupil need not necessarily be dilated; mydriasis is not a feature of brain death.
- No corneal reflex. Use much firmer pressure than in a conscious individual.
- No vestibulo-ocular reflex. The auditory canal must be wax-free (verify with an auroscope). Use at least 20 mL of ice cold water in each ear. A normal response is for both eyes to deviate towards the irrigated side; for the brainstem to be dead there must be no movement of either eye. A basal skull fracture with CSF leak precludes the test, as do extensive facial injuries.
- No motor response within the cranial nerve distribution in response to adequate stimulation of any somatic area, e.g. grimacing in response to firm pressure on the fingernail.
- No gag or cough reflex. This is assessed by bronchial stimulation with a suction catheter passed down the endotracheal tube.

Testing for apnoea

Apnoea is confirmed by not observing any respiratory effort during a period of disconnection from the ventilator. Disconnection must be for long enough to ensure that the P_aCO_2 is high enough to drive any respiratory neurons still alive. It is therefore essential to avoid hyperventilation, and it is a prerequisite that the P_aCO_2 must be ≥ 5.3 kPa (40 mmHg) prior to testing.

Hypoxia during disconnection is avoided by preoxygenating the patient with 100% O_2 for 10 minutes, and on disconnection insufflating O_2 at 6 L/min via a catheter down the endotracheal tube. The P_aCO_2 will rise by at least 0.27 kPa (2 mmHg) per minute and reach 8 kPa (60 mmHg) after 10 minutes. The UK code recommends that during disconnection the P_aCO_2 should be >6.65 kPa (50 mmHg).

Patients dependent on hypoxic respiratory drive will not be able to undergo this test and will probably not be considered for a diagnosis of brainstem death.

Retesting

There is no legal requirement for a second set of tests. However, virtually all codes urge the tests to be carried out twice to rule out observer error. Retesting also ensures that the non-functioning brainstem is not just a single observation but has persisted over time. The interval between tests is left to the judgement of the doctors concerned but is usually 12–24 hours.

When applied correctly and performed precisely, the tests for brainstem function provide valid and unambiguous results.

ORGAN DONATION

If organ donation is envisaged, the 'beating heart cadaver' is reconnected to the ventilator, with organ removal then taking place at the convenience of the surgical team.

BURNS

Major burns should be dealt with in a specialised unit. Only the principles of management of a severe burn will be addressed.

Pathophysiology

Loss of integument and direct tissue injury lead to a generalised fluid leak into the burn area. This results in fluid loss and oedema formation. Secondary problems include myocardial depression, which usually recovers within 24 hours. There is also a degree of immunosuppression, with the major late problem of infection (Box 10.10).

Assessment

The area of burn should be determined. The method used is to assess the percentage of the total body surface area which has been damaged and the depth of the injury. This can be easily done from a chart (Fig. 10.4).

Management

The rules of ABC – airway, breathing and circulation – apply. The airway must be assessed and, if necessary, protected by intubation. Indications for endotracheal intubation include lung injury with hypoxia from inhalational burns; in the case of head and neck burns, oedema can develop rapidly, especially during resuscitation, and can occlude the airway.

Box 10.10 Problems associated with a large burn

- Fluid loss
- Myocardial depression
- Oedema formation – airway obstruction, compartment syndromes
- Airway burn – hypoxia
- Tissue damage – myoglobinuria
- Immunosuppression – infection

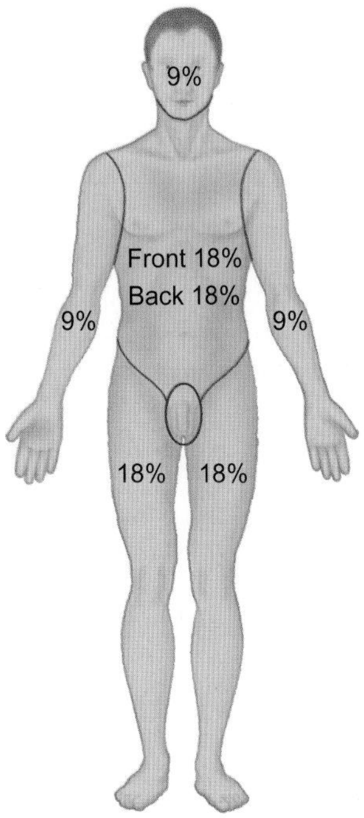

Fig. 10.4 Burn assessment. In an adult, the 'rule of nines' can be applied, in which the body surface is divided into sections of 9% or multiples of 9%.

There are massive fluid losses after burn injury, due to formation of oedema fluid and loss of the cutaneous barrier. Various formulae have been produced to guide fluid management in the resuscitation period, an example of which is the Parkland formula using Ringer's lactate solution:

$$\text{Volume (mL)}/24\text{ h} = 4 \times \text{weight (kg)} \times \text{percentage of total body surface area burnt (half in the first 8 hours)}$$

These formulae are rough guides, and resuscitation should be more accurately guided by clinical assessment using tissue perfusion, blood pressure and urine output. Fluid overload has replaced under-resuscitation as a major problem. It is also important to remember that burns patients may well have other injuries depending on the nature of the burn. History and full examination are very important.

The other important aspect of management is the control of pain and anxiety; as for any major injury the patient should be made as comfortable as possible. Pain may be very severe initially, but anxiety becomes a growing problem as the patient becomes aware of the predicament.

SEQUELAE OF INTENSIVE CARE TREATMENT

Traditional intensive care management has been focused on the endpoint of the patient being well enough to be discharged back to the ward environment. Increasingly, it is being recognised that from the patient's perspective, this is only the start of a long and multi-faceted recovery that involves not only physical rehabilitation but also psychological and social recovery.

The physical recovery will inevitably include some or all of the following aspects relating to reduced mobility as a result of muscle wasting and joint stiffness, chronic pain syndromes, possible tracheostomy issues (swallowing and speech), skin condition and wound healing and the worsening of premorbid conditions that may have been directly responsible for, or affected by, the intensive care treatment.

Common psychological consequences of prolonged intensive care management include anxiety, depression, post-traumatic stress disorders (PTSD) and chronic fatigue syndrome (CFS). Patients may become socially withdrawn, experience sleep disturbance, nightmares, poor structural memory, develop relationship difficulties and/or sexual dysfunction.

The management of these sequelae is often overlooked and requires a multi-disciplinary approach from a number of practitioners including physicians and surgeons, specialist nursing staff, pain specialists, psychologists, psychiatrists, physiotherapists, nutritionists, occupational therapists, speech and language therapy amongst others. The recovery from a prolonged period of critical care may take many months or even years despite the input of all these specialists.

ETHICAL CONSIDERATIONS IN THE CRITICALLY ILL

As with other fields of medicine the four key ethical principles of autonomy, beneficence, non-maleficence and justice apply. However, there are differences and considerations specific to the critically ill / intensive care patient that must be addressed including the withdrawal and withholding of treatments, the use of living wills.

Autonomy

Patients are often unable to make competent decisions for themselves as a result of either disease processes or the treatment that has been instituted (e.g. sedation, general anaesthesia). This has important legal implications regarding the consent process for interventions, procedures or surgery. Recent changes to the Mental Capacity Act include the provision of medical advocates for those without a legally appointed guardian / power of attorney whom are deemed unable to consent.

Beneficence

Treatments should only be carried out if the patient will benefit. It is this principle that is often cited in the withholding or withdrawal of futile treatments from critically ill patients. The Doctrine of Double Effect regards as morally 'right' the provision of a treatment that, although intended to provide a benefit, carries a recognisable risk to that patient. An example would be the end-of-life provision of opiates or sedation to a distressed patient with breathing difficulties with the intention of relieving suffering whilst recognising that the treatment may 'hasten' death.

Non-maleficence

The principle of 'cause no harm' underpins risk–benefit decisions regarding the treatment of critically ill patients on a daily basis.

Justice

Fair, equitable and appropriate treatment for all patients must take account of the market and available resources. Difficult clinical situations may be influenced by the utilisation not only of physical resources but also manpower issues. Does focusing one's attention and resources on patients who have a lesser chance of survival detract from the care of a larger population of patients who may benefit more?

The principles of medical ethics and particularly regarding end-of-life decisions are regularly encountered in an intensive care setting and therefore an understanding of the relevant issues is important.

CONCLUSION

The critically ill should be managed in an intensive care unit. It is an exciting environment where clinical signs abound. It is an area where acute medicine is managed by rapid pharmacological interventions to try to offset defined pathophysiological disturbances, and where sophisticated technology is regularly used to assist management.

FURTHER READING

Bernstein A, Soni N, eds 2008 Oh's intensive care manual, 6th edn. Butterworth-Heinemann, Oxford

Irwin RS, Rippe JM 2007 Irwin and Rippe's intensive care medicine, 6th edn. Lippincott Williams & Wilkins, Philadelphia

Singer M, Webb A 2009 Oxford handbook of critical care (Oxford Handbooks Series), 3rd edn. OUP, Oxford

11 Practical procedures

PRELIMINARIES

Informed consent

The general issue of consent is considered in Chapter 2. Consent is required for all invasive procedures and should be obtained in writing when the procedure carries any significant risk.

Explanation

Alternative methods of management should be discussed before the procedure in question is carried out.

Essential information that should be given to the patient includes:

- the nature of the procedure
- what is going to be removed, cut, changed or inserted
- non-specific possible complications – haematoma, infection
- specific possible complications – nerve, arterial and venous injury; cosmetic effect
- explanation of type of anaesthesia (general, local, regional) and risks involved.

Additional beneficial information includes:

- the position of the scar
- what cannulas, drains and catheters will be in place after the procedure
- postoperative pain control
- when food and drink may be resumed
- what may happen during the hours or days after the procedure and for how long a period such events may last
- how long before work can be resumed.

Documentation

All procedures should be recorded in the notes, with comments pertinent to the individual manoeuvre, e.g. the volume of residual urine found on urethral catheterisation or, after a biopsy, the dispatch of a specimen to the pathological laboratory.

Asepsis

There are varying degrees of aseptic technique (see also Ch. 5) according to the procedure and the possible subsequent effects of sepsis.

Gloves

Gloves and an impermeable disposable apron should be worn for every procedure that involves contact with a patient's secretions or blood. Non-sterile (but clean) gloves are indicated when there is a risk of contamination from patient to medical attendant (e.g. HIV, hepatitis B). Sterile gloves are part of the normal procedure to prevent access of organisms to the patient. The possibility of transmission of infection by the hands should always be maintained at a low level by keeping them clean, with short nails, everyday maintenance of hand hygiene, and washing with soap or using alcohol-based gels every time a clinician is in contact with a patient. The arms should be covered by a sterile gown or exposed and clean from above the elbows.

Superficial procedures

An example of such a procedure is superficial venous cannulation. An alcohol–chlorhexidine solution is used to clean the skin area. However, the operator requires protection against the possibility of infection from the patient. The wearing of gloves – either clean or sterile according to the circumstances – is recommended for every procedure.

Deeper and more complicated procedures

If the procedure is likely to leave a cannula, a drain or other device (e.g. pacemaker, central line) in situ, then sterile gloves, towels and handwashing and full skin preparation must be used.

Immunocompromised patients

In certain circumstances (e.g. AIDS, bone marrow transplantation, chemotherapy), immunocompromise may be present, and in such patients strict aseptic techniques should be used even for minor superficial procedures.

Handwashing and skin preparation

These are discussed in detail in Chapter 5.

Anaesthesia

Nearly all small procedures can be undertaken with local anaesthesia (LA). If general or regional anaesthesia (Ch. 6) is a possible alternative, two factors will determine which is chosen: the relative risks (regional anaesthesia usually has a marginally higher risk) and patient preference.

General features relating to the pain of administration of LA are summarised below:

- The initial needle prick is painful but, especially in children, can be lessened by the use of local anaesthetic creams or sprays.
- Rapid injection causes pain from increased pressure in the tissues; the slower the injection, the less pain there will be. Injection into dense tissue (such as the fibrous tissue of the sole of the foot) should always be slow.
- The smaller the needle (preferably 25 G or 27 G), the less pain the patient will feel upon insertion and also the slower will be the rate of injection; fine needles are often short but long ones are also available.
- The elderly often experience less pain on the injection of local anaesthetic, probably because of the laxity of their tissue.

Choice of local anaesthesia

Ethyl chloride spray can be used to numb the skin before a limited lance for a small abscess or for initial injections of LA. Local-anaesthetic creams, e.g. EMLA cream (a mixture of the un-ionised base forms of lidocaine and prilocaine) or Ametop cream (tetracaine 4%), are useful for paediatric venepuncture and for adults who have a phobia about needles, although it should be noted that they take up to an hour to become effective.

Commonly used local anaesthetics – with their maximum safe dose – are:

- lidocaine – 3 mg/kg
- bupivacaine – 2 mg/kg (it is 2–4 times more potent than lidocaine) (see Table 11.1)
- prilocaine – 5 mg/kg
- cocaine – used in ENT surgery for its local vasoconstrictor action.

Table 11.1 Concentration of bupivacaine for local and regional anaesthesia

Procedure	Concentration
Skin infiltration	0.5%
Minor nerve block	1%
Brachial plexus block	1–1.5%
Sciatic/femoral block	1–1.5%
Epidural	1.5–2%
Spinal	2–5%

Box 11.1 Contraindications to use of adrenaline (epinephrine) with local anaesthetic

- When the injection is close to end arteries
- Ring block of the digits (fingers and toes) and of the penis
- Intravenous regional anaesthesia (so-called Bier's block) which reduces venous drainage by the use of a tourniquet and so generates a high concentration of local anaesthetic; there is an unacceptable risk of ischaemia and of the escape of large concentrations of agent into the general circulation

Addition of adrenaline

Adrenaline (epinephrine) – a potent vasoconstrictor – added to a local anaesthetic slows the rate of absorption into the systemic circulation, reduces systemic toxicity and therefore prolongs the duration of action and may result in a more profound block. For this reason, the doses of both lidocaine and prilocaine quoted above can be increased if 1 in 200 000 adrenaline is added to the solution (e.g. lidocaine 5 mg/kg and prilocaine 8 mg/kg). The dose of bupivacaine should not be increased when adrenaline is used (see also Ch. 6).

If the patient has cardiac disease or is elderly, adrenaline needs to be used with caution as the patient may develop a tachyarrhythmia.

There are, however, absolute contraindications to the use of adrenaline with local anaesthetic agents, as listed in Box 11.1.

Principles of suturing

This is discussed in detail in Chapter 5.

Equipment

The best way to be certain that everything is available for any minor procedure is to run through the steps in your head beforehand, checking the equipment against that required for each step (see also the various procedures described throughout this chapter).

VENOUS ACCESS

Choosing the site

The ideal area for injection and short-term cannulation is the forearm. However, if the patient is obese, there can be difficulties with this. Sites that are not suitable include:

- The dominant arm is avoided if possible.
- The arm which carries an arteriovenous (AV) fistula for renal dialysis is never used.
- Poor venous or lymphatic drainage in a limb (e.g. after an axillary lymph node clearance) carries a higher incidence of infected lymphangitis, and such limbs must not be used.
- Avoid foot veins whenever possible because they thrombose easily and are prone to infection.
- A skin fold which crosses a joint should be avoided, although the antecubital fossa can be used for diagnostic venepuncture.

Choice of vein (Fig. 11.1)

Look where veins commonly occur; there is often a large vein running along the radial aspect of the forearm. Veins can sometimes only be felt rather than seen, even after the application of a tourniquet. **NB: The aim of the tourniquet used for venepuncture is that there is arterial inflow into the vein but no venous outflow.** Should there be uncertainty as to whether the structure is a vein, the tourniquet should be released. If the structure becomes impalpable, it is almost certainly a patent vein – arteries or thrombosed veins do not change shape or size when a tourniquet is removed.

To insert a cannula, the vein should be immobilised by stretching the skin, which includes positioning the adjacent joints. If the veins are difficult to cannulate because of mobility, then placing the cannula at a point of junction of two veins can help. If there is substantial subcutaneous fat, then often the dorsum of the hand may be the only suitable place; this area is not particularly convenient for the patient and can be painful during insertion. The antecubital fossa is also not particularly convenient for the patient, but for emergencies it is ideal as there are large, reasonably accessible veins which can take large cannulae.

There are methods which can be used to help locate a vein; these are listed in Clinical Box 11.1.

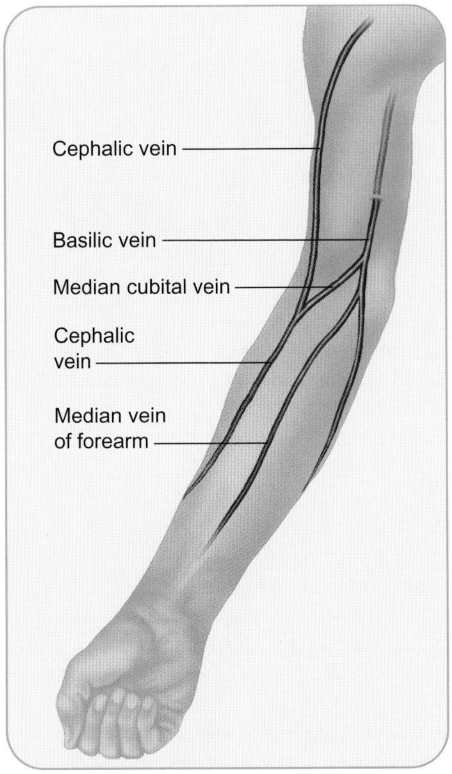

Fig. 11.1 Common sites in the arm for venous access.

Choosing a needle or cannula

The types of intravenous cannulae available in the UK (and in many other places in the world) are shown in Table 11.2.

VENEPUNCTURE

Equipment

Equipment required is:

- clean gloves
- tourniquet – either a short length of latex rubber tube or, preferably, a sphygmomanometer
- appropriate needle or cannula (see Table 11.2) but there may be need for a back-up if difficulties are encountered
- strapping to hold a cannula in place – adhesive tape
- 5 mL syringe
- 0.9% saline flush
- occasionally, cotton wool and adhesive tape to secure the site of unsuccessful cannulation
- bandage and tape for the same reason.

Clinical Box 11.1 Aids to location of a vein

- Use a sphygmomanometer and inflate it to below diastolic pressure to allow arterial inflow but not venous escape of blood
- Hang the patient's arm over the edge of the bed or couch and tap (not slap) the back of the hand to cause venodilatation
- Immerse the forearm in a bowl of warm water for 2 minutes and place the tourniquet before removing the hand from the bowl

Additional hint
In paediatrics or for anxious adults, EMLA cream can be helpful; apply over selected veins and cover with an occlusive dressing; wipe off after 45–60 minutes. After EMLA cream has been applied, veins do not distend as easily

Table 11.2 Types of intravenous cannula

Size	Colour	Use
22 G	Blue	Children, small fragile veins
20 G	Pink	Low-flow intravenous infusions such as analgesia, sedation
18 G	Green	Intravenous fluids and drugs
16 G	Yellow	Blood transfusions
14 G	Grey	Rapid fluid administration – shock, major trauma and GI bleeding
12 G	Brown	Rapid fluid administration – shock, major trauma and GI bleeding

Procedure

- Choose the preferred site.
- Place the tourniquet above the site of insertion.
- Swab the intended insertion area with antiseptic solution (allow alcohol to dry).
- Advance the needle or cannula-and-needle combination into the vein until a flashback of blood into the base of the cannula is seen.
- Advance the plastic cannula into the vein over the needle ensuring that the needle remains in the same position and is not pushed further into or through the vein (Fig. 11.2).
- Remove the tourniquet.
- When venepuncture alone has been done, elevate the arm above the right atrium, remove the needle and apply a small stabilising dressing.
- For a cannulation, occlude the end or connect the infusion immediately.

Complications

Thrombophlebitis

Inflammation at a peripheral site of cannulation (which may be caused by chemical irritation or infection) is manifest by pain, tenderness and a red line which spreads proximally. The cannula must be removed immediately. To prevent this complication it is best to change the site of a peripheral infusion at intervals no longer than 24 hours. There is some evidence that small amounts of heparin added to the infusion can also help to prevent this complication.

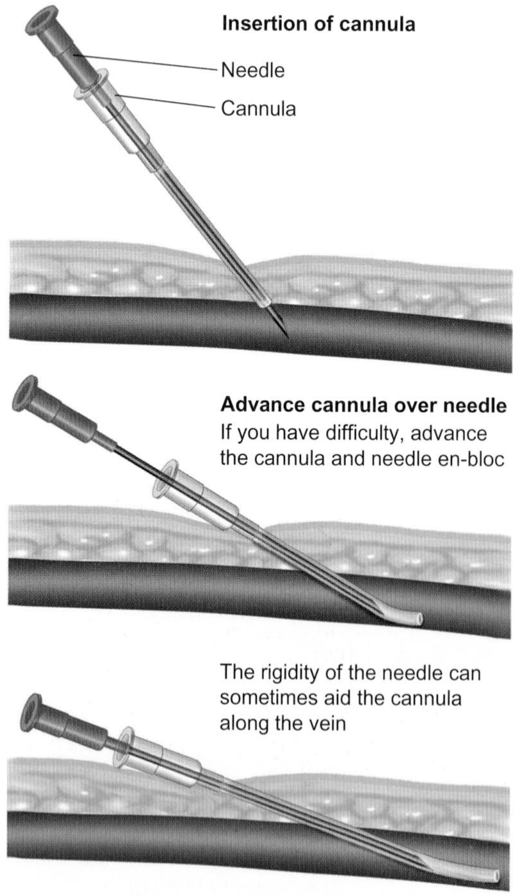
Insertion of cannula
Needle
Cannula
Advance cannula over needle
If you have difficulty, advance the cannula and needle en-bloc
The rigidity of the needle can sometimes aid the cannula along the vein

Fig. 11.2 Technique for venous cannulation.

Blockage

Sometimes patency can be restored with a flush of normal or heparinised saline (2–5 mL). The smaller the diameter of the syringe, the higher the pressure that can be attained (use a 5 mL rather than a 10 mL syringe).

VENOUS CUT-DOWN

Venous cut-down is the open exposure and cannulation of a subcutaneous vein. It is used when venous access cannot be obtained by percutaneous puncture (see above) and is an alternative to central venous catheterisation (see below) in some patients.

The most commonly used sites for this procedure are (Fig. 11.3):

- basilic vein – approximately 2.5 cm lateral to the medial epicondyle of the humerus at the flexion crease of the elbow
- saphenous vein – either at the saphenofemoral junction (2.5 cm lateral and inferior to the pubic tubercle) or 2 cm anterior and superior to the medial malleolus at the ankle.
- other sites include the cephalic vein at the wrist and the external jugular (Fig. 11.3).

Equipment

Equipment required is:

- sterile towels
- orange needle (25 G)
- scalpel (10 blade)
- fine scissors
- artery forceps
- two ties (4/0 vicryl)
- cannula 12 G or 14 G
- skin sutures (Prolene or silk 3/0)
- dressing.

Procedure (Fig. 11.4)

- Prepare the skin with antiseptic solution.
- Drape the area.
- Infiltrate the skin over the vein with 0.5% lidocaine, but take care not to inject local anaesthetic into the vein.
- Make a transverse full-thickness skin incision (2.5 cm) through the infiltrated area.
- By blunt dissection with the tip of an artery forceps, identify the vein and release it from any fat and fibrous tissue.
- Free the vein for at least 2 cm.
- Ligate the mobilised vein at its most distal exposed part and leave the tie attached for traction.
- Place a tie around the vein proximally but do not tighten this.
- Make a small transverse incision with scissors into the vein sufficient to accept the cannula, and dilate this opening with the tip of an artery forceps.

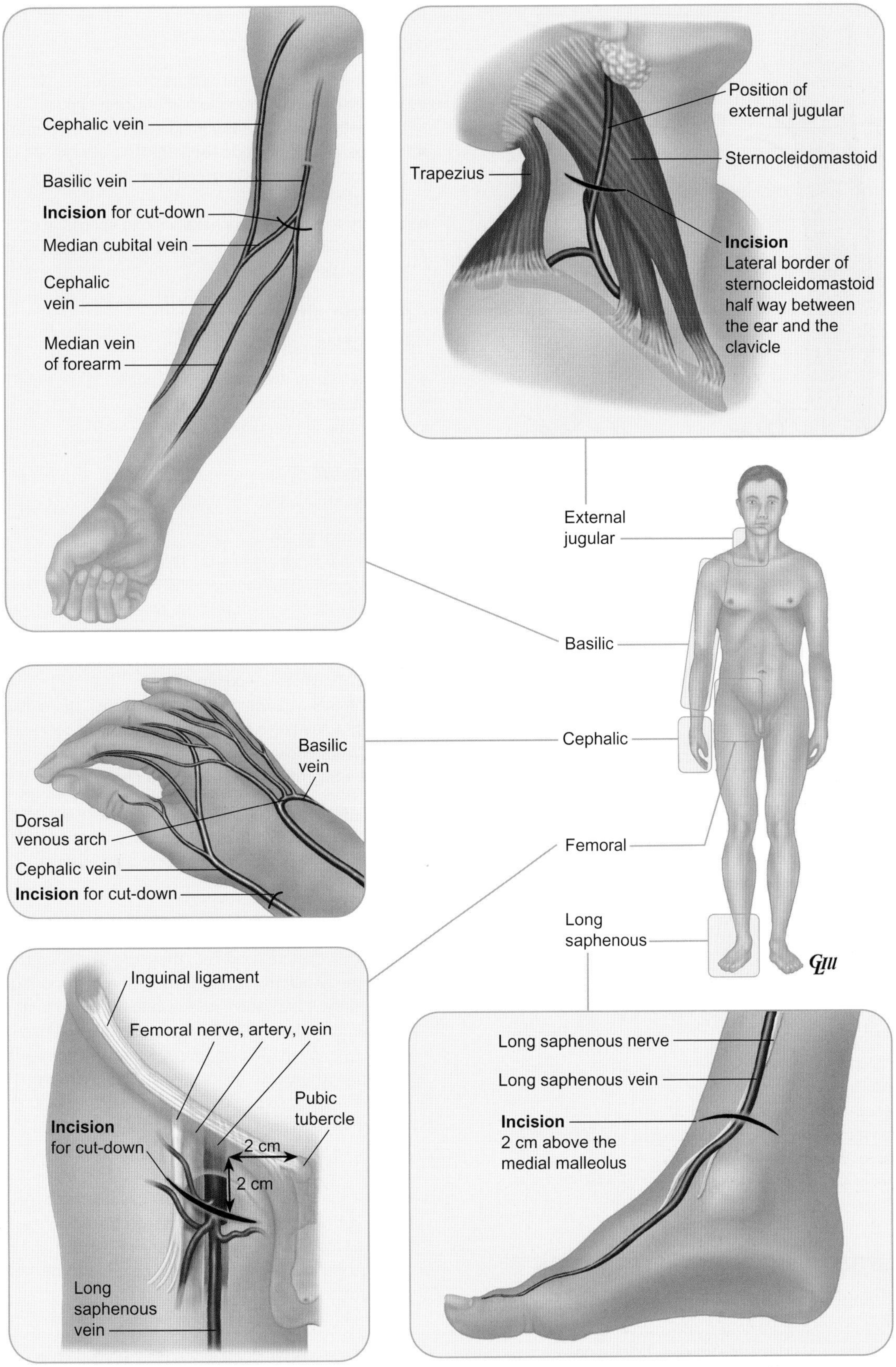

Cephalic vein
Basilic vein
Incision for cut-down
Median cubital vein
Cephalic vein
Median vein of forearm
Trapezius
Position of external jugular
Sternocleidomastoid
Incision
Lateral border of sternocleidomastoid half way between the ear and the clavicle
External jugular
Basilic
Cephalic
Femoral
Long saphenous
Basilic vein
Dorsal venous arch
Cephalic vein
Incision for cut-down
Inguinal ligament
Femoral nerve, artery, vein
Pubic tubercle
Incision for cut-down
2 cm
2 cm
Long saphenous vein
Long saphenous nerve
Long saphenous vein
Incision
2 cm above the medial malleolus

Fig. 11.3 Sites used for venous access.

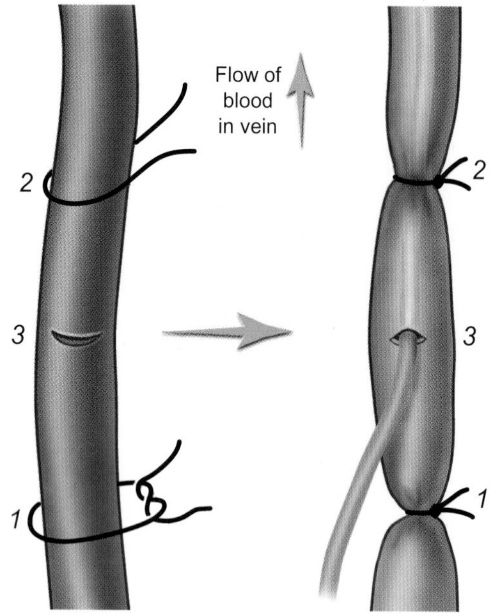

Fig. 11.4 Technique for venous cut-down.

- Introduce a large plastic grey (14 G) or brown (12 G) cannula which has, if necessary, been separated from its needle.
- Tighten the proximal tie around the vein and the cannula firmly but be careful not to constrict the lumen of the cannula.
- Attach the intravenous apparatus and check that flow takes place.
- Close the wound with interrupted sutures and apply further antiseptic solution and a securing dressing.

Complications

Complications include:

- perforation of the posterior wall of the vein
- haematoma
- phlebitis
- cellulitis
- venous thrombosis
- transection of a neighbouring nerve (e.g. saphenous nerve at the medial malleolus)
- mistake of an artery for a vein and arterial transection.

CENTRAL VENOUS CATHETERISATION

The objective of central venous catheterisation is to insert a hollow line into the proximal (usually superior) vena cava. The Seldinger technique is often used, in which a needle is placed in the vessel and an internal guide wire inserted into the vein first. The needle is then removed, the track into the vessel dilated and the cannula threaded along the wire into the lumen.

Indications

Indications include:

- measurement of central venous pressure
- infusion of certain drugs, e.g. inotropes, high concentrations of potassium (greater than 40 mmol/L)
- total parenteral nutrition (Ch. 10)
- insertion of a Swan–Ganz catheter (see below) or cardiac pacing wires
- inability to achieve peripheral venous access, e.g. intravenous drug use with extensive previous venous thrombosis.

Common sites

Common sites include:

- internal jugular and subclavian (usually on the right)
- femoral in the groin
- median basilic vein at the elbow.

Equipment

Equipment required is:

- fine scalpel blade
- orange (25 G) and green (21 G) needles
- two syringes (preferably of differing sizes, 5 and 10 mL) – one for local anaesthesia the other for heparinised saline
- heparinised saline flush (10 mL)
- central line infusion equipment
- suture material (2/0 or 3/0 silk or Prolene), preferably on a straight needle so that a needle holder is not required
- transparent occlusive dressing
- one-litre bag of 0.9% saline and a giving set.

Prepackaged central line sets often contain not only the infusion apparatus but also many of the items mentioned above; check before looking for the rest of the materials.

Procedure

Many patients who require a central line are seriously ill and cannot easily tolerate lying flat. Therefore all the equipment must be ready before placing them in the best position for the procedure. If the patient is known to be short of intravascular volume, 500 mL of colloid or crystalline solution given through a peripheral infusion just before the procedure is often helpful to increase the diameter of the vein to be used.

The patient should be positioned in a supine position with no pillows, or with no more than one pillow. The bed should preferably be in a 15° head-down tilt at the moment of puncture of the vein. The patient's arms should be placed at the side of the trunk. For subclavian vein cannulation, an assistant holding the arm on the side of the proposed cannulation, with downward traction, opens the space between the clavicle and the first rib; again, this should be done at the moment of puncture.

The procedure for cannulation is now as follows:

- Central venous puncture is normally preceded by ultrasound scanning to locate the internal jugular or subclavian vein and to guide venous puncture.
- Use an orange needle (Table 11.2) to insert local anaesthetic over the proposed point of entry into the

skin and infiltrate the proposed route towards the vein with a larger (green) needle.

- While allowing the anaesthetic to take effect, prepare the central line: all ports of entry on the apparatus are flushed through with heparinised saline and tested for patency; all are then closed either with a bung or a tap that is switched off, except for the distal one (usually labelled and in the centre of the cannula), which is left open.
- The guide wire should be prepared by checking that the end is hidden in the introducer and that it can be easily advanced (practise beforehand). Often the introducer has to be released from the sheath in which the wire is coiled.
- Flush the needle and syringe to be used to identify and cannulate the vein with heparinised saline to ensure fluid runs freely.
- Make a small (5 mm) incision through the skin at the proposed entry site.
- Insert the needle and, once deep to the skin, aspirate with the syringe and advance it under ultrasound guidance until venous blood is easily aspirated.
- Detach the syringe and ensure that blood flows freely out of the needle.
- Insert the wire and its introducer (if present – depends on the type of apparatus) into the end of the needle while grasping it to ensure that it does not move as the wire and introducer are advanced. The wire should be easily introduced without force (which should never be applied); sometimes rotation can help in that many of the wires have curled ends (if the wire does not have a pigtail end then the soft end of the wire should be introduced – the rigid end can perforate the vein).
- Once the wire is inserted to approximately 50% of its length, the needle is removed.
- The track is dilated by the introduction of the dilator over the wire, pushing it in until it is well inside the vein.
- Remove the dilator; this is usually associated with an increase in bleeding from the entry site – a good sign as it implies that the track is well dilated.
- The central line is introduced over the wire while this is held steady; often the wire must be pulled back slightly to allow it to come out of the end of the distal port. Again, the wire must be grasped before the cannula is further advanced; otherwise it can be lost into the right side of the heart.
- Push the central venous line in; the tip should ideally lie in the superior vena cava, judged according to the size and shape of the patient.
- Aspirate the line with a syringe to ensure that its position is truly in the vein as indicated by free flow of blood. If there is uncertainty, an infusion of 0.9% saline can be connected and checked to see if flow is free.
- Suture the line in place, if necessary after infiltrating further local anaesthetic.

Use of the subclavian vein

There are numerous techniques for cannulation of this vessel, which differ in detail, but all insertions start in the area 1 cm below the clavicle between its medial and lateral thirds (points a to b in Fig. 11.5) and the aim is to cannulate the vein as it passes over the first rib. Two differing approaches are described: the lateral and the medial.

Lateral

This is carried out at the point at which the lateral third and medial two-thirds of the clavicle intersect. The needle should

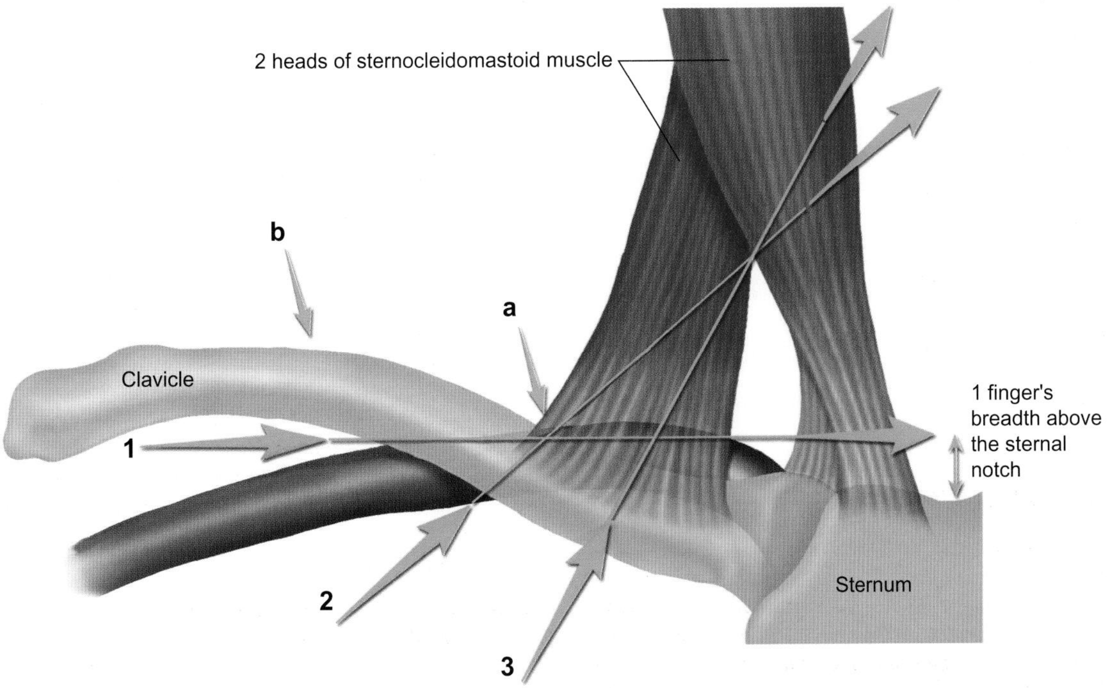

Fig. 11.5 The approach used for lateral (1) and medial (2 or 3) cannulation of the subclavian vein.

be aimed at a point 2 cm above the suprasternal notch and towards the opposite shoulder; it then runs in a straight line from the insertion point, passes just inferior to the clavicle and flat to the skin; if the needle is felt to bend away from this path, the usual reason is that the tip is below the first rib and towards the apex of the pleura; in this case the advice is to withdraw and start again, using a slightly higher angle.

Medial

This is carried out at the point of intersection of the medial third and lateral two-thirds. The needle goes in initially at right angles to the clavicle, just inferior to it and towards the division of the two heads of the sternocleidomastoid muscle (Fig. 11.5). Once the vein is punctured the cannula is advanced into the vein at the angle used for the 'lateral' technique. The medial method may have a reduced risk of pneumothorax.

Use of the right internal jugular vein

(Fig. 11.6)

Procedure

- Feel for the pulse of the carotid artery on the right side with the right hand (right-handed operators) or left hand (left-handed operators).
- Infiltrate a small area lateral to the carotid pulse at the level of the thyroid cartilage with local anaesthetic. If you attempt a lower insertion there is an increased risk of pneumothorax. Localise the vein with ultrasound scanning.
- Guard the carotid artery with the left hand and insert the needle at a 45° angle to the neck and pointing towards the nipple in the male or the anterior superior iliac spine in both males and females. Advance the needle slowly, preferably under ultrasound guidance, while applying negative pressure with a syringe. If there is no flashback of venous blood, release the finger from the carotid pulse and withdraw the needle slowly. This is sometimes successful because the compression had flattened the vein. Should the carotid artery be punctured, withdraw the needle immediately and apply digital pressure for at least 5 minutes.

Post-cannulation checks

After all central cannulations, the radial pulse should be checked. If there are frequent ectopic beats then it is likely that the line is in the right ventricle. A chest X-ray should be performed to verify the position of the tip of the line, which should be in the superior vena cava, and also to check for any complications (especially pneumothorax and haemothorax). If the line is not correctly placed, then adjustment is most easily performed under radiological control. Other means of ensuring that the line is within the vein are:

- Check easy aspiration of venous blood from all ports.
- Place the connected 0.9% saline bag and tubing beneath the patient with the tap open; blood should track back easily even if the patient has a low central pressure.
- If the blood travels up the line while above the place of insertion, it is likely you are within the artery.
- If you are uncertain, then a pressure-transducing device can be attached to the line.
- Sometimes the distal opening rests on a valve and therefore blood cannot be aspirated. If the line is pulled backwards a few centimetres, blood should then be easily aspirated.

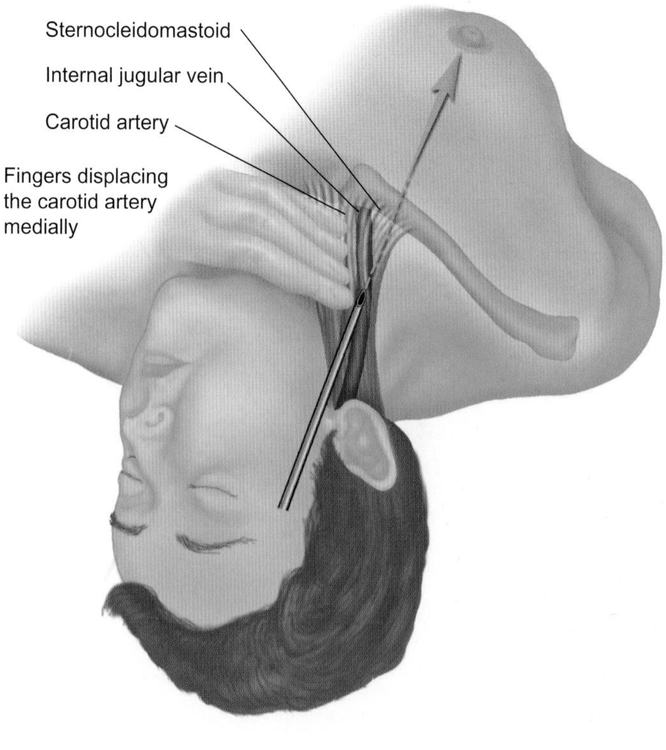

Fig. 11.6 The approach used for cannulation of the internal jugular vein.

Subcutaneous tunnelling

Temporary lines inserted as described above are, as time goes by, increasingly difficult to protect from the entry of bacteria. Sepsis is likely after 5–10 days, although careful care and strict asepsis decrease the incidence. However, some intensive care units judge it wise to change all central lines every 5 days. If the line is needed for long-term therapy (e.g. chemotherapy or TPN), then a subcutaneously tunnelled line should be used (Fig. 11.7). An alternative for intermittent therapy is to place a port with venous access subcutaneously (Portacath).

The number of lumens available per line ranges from one to four. When placing a subcutaneous tunnelled line, two different methods can be used: one is the Seldinger technique; the other is to cut directly down onto a vein (either the cephalic vein for a subclavian approach or the internal jugular vein), then insert the cannula and create a separate exit point which lies on the anterior chest wall away from the shoulder joint.

Complications of central line insertion

Complications include:

- haematoma
- cellulitis
- line infection (bacteraemia, septic shock)
- thrombosis
- phlebitis
- nerve damage including transection
- arterial puncture – more common in the internal jugular approach
- pneumothorax – more common in thin patients and if the subclavian approach is used
- haemothorax
- chylothorax
- arteriovenous fistula
- peripheral neuropathy
- lost wires or catheter in the venous system
- improperly placed catheters.

Swan–Ganz catheter

Uses

The Swan–Ganz catheter is a pulmonary artery flotation catheter which can be used to measure directly a number of cardiovascular parameters. Its use has diminished as less invasive methods of measuring cardiac output are now available – for example, transoesophageal Doppler probes – and its value has been disputed. The parameters that can be measured with a Swan-Ganz catheter include (normal range of values is shown in parentheses):

- pulmonary artery wedge pressure (12–20 mmHg)
- blood pressure
- central venous pressure (5–10 mmHg)
- cardiac output (4–8 L/min)

and to derive the following parameters:

- mean arterial pressure (70–90 mmHg)
- cardiac index (2.5–4.2 L/min/m^2)
- systemic vascular resistance (900–1600 dyne-s/cm^5)
- pulmonary vascular resistance (20–120 dyne-s/cm^5).

Measurement of cardiac output

Cardiac output is stroke volume × heart rate. It is measured using the thermodilution method. The change in temperature of 10 mL of 5% glucose between two given points on the catheter (CVP lumen and the tip of the catheter) is measured and cardiac output subsequently calculated.

Insertion

Insertion is as for a central venous catheter in the neck. The catheter is passed through the subclavian vein, right atrium, right ventricle and wedged in the pulmonary artery (Fig. 11.8), and then unwedged to lie in the pulmonary artery while other parameters are measured.

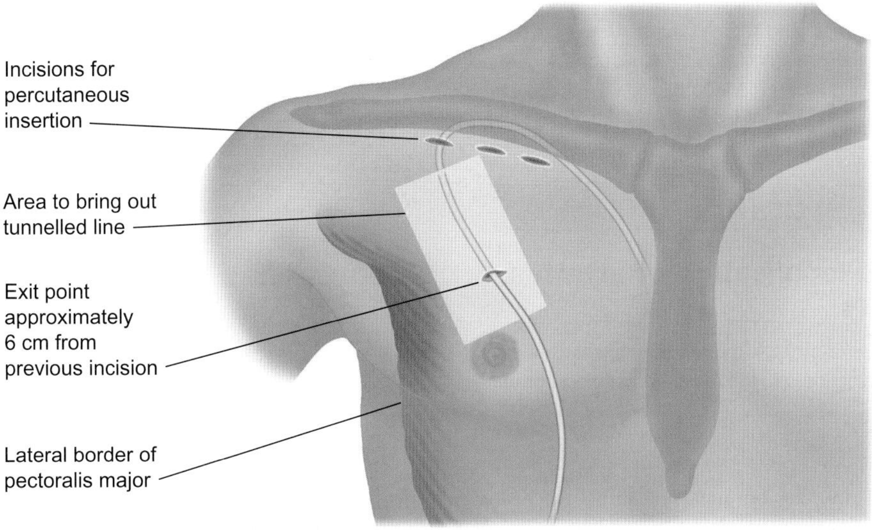

Fig. 11.7 Subcutaneous tunnelling of an intravenous catheter.

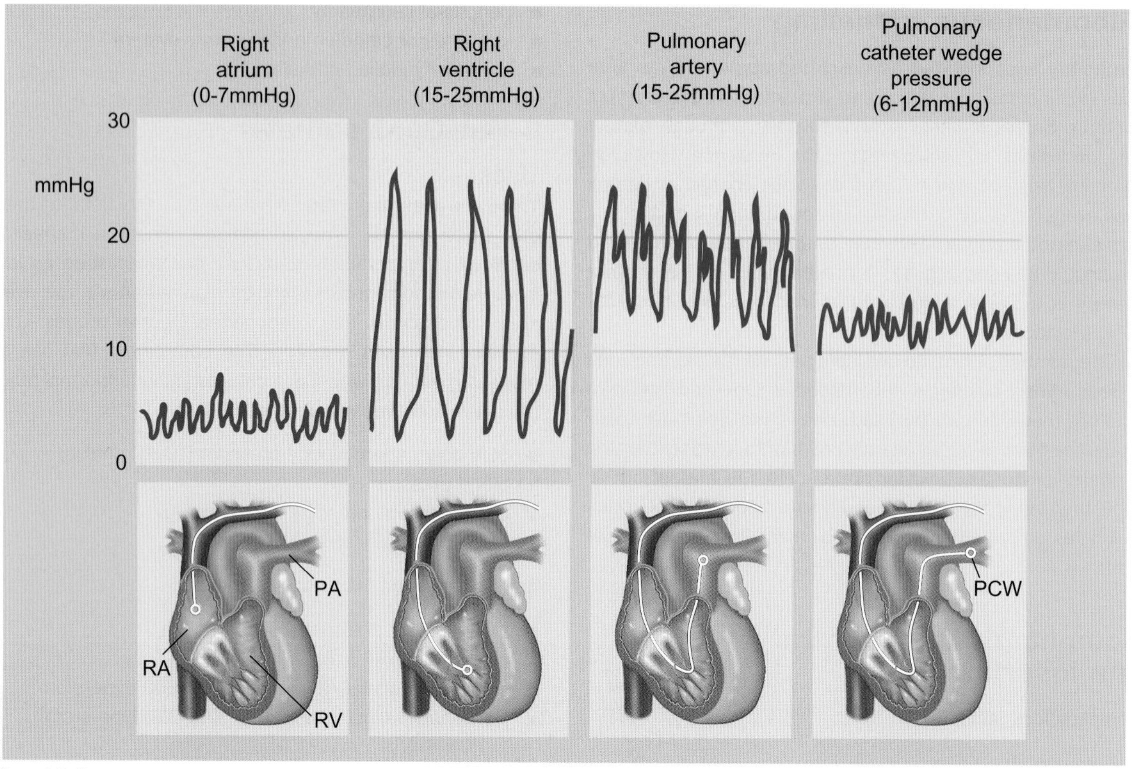

Fig. 11.8 Characteristic intracardiac pressure waveforms of a Swan–Ganz catheter during passage through the heart.

Pulse-induced contour cardiac output (PiCCO) measurement

PiCCO is a technique used in the ICU to measure cardiac output and the other parameters mentioned in the previous subsection.

Principles

Measurement requires the insertion of both a central venous catheter and an arterial catheter (see the next section). A large artery is needed, usually femoral or brachial.

The arterial catheter outputs an arterial waveform, the pressures of which are known. One thermodilution assessment is first performed and then, using volumetric assessments of the arterial waveform, the transpulmonary cardiac output can be continuously monitored.

ARTERIAL BLOOD SAMPLING

Choice and localisation of arteries for puncture

Vessels of choice, in order of preference unless there is a specific contraindication, are the radial, femoral and brachial arteries.

Radial artery

This artery (Fig. 11.9) can be found medial to the styloid process of the radius at the wrist. Before it is used for a sample, the ulnar collateral supply should be checked

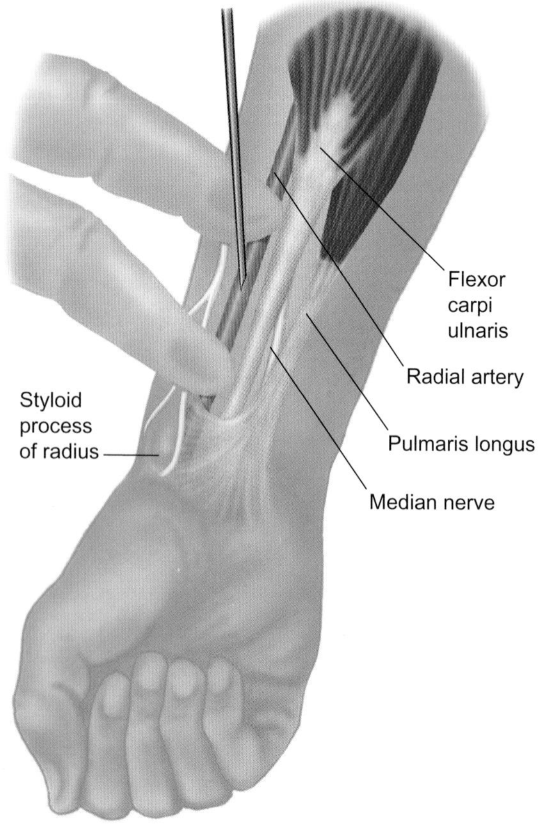

Fig. 11.9 The position of the radial artery at the wrist.

(especially if there is a history of previous wrist trauma); this is done by asking the patient to repeatedly make a tight fist while occlusive pressure is applied over the radial artery and ulnar artery. The ulnar artery occlusion is then released. The hand is then relaxed and, if it remains white for 10 seconds or more, collateral refill is inadequate and the other hand should be used (provided the same test is also negative).

Isolation is best achieved between the operator's index and middle fingers of the non-dominant hand, both fingers feeling the pulse over the tips of their palmar surfaces.

Femoral artery

The artery is at the midinguinal point (a point on the inguinal ligament halfway between the pubic tubercle and the anterior superior iliac spine). It is best isolated with the index and middle fingers of the non-dominant hand on either side of the artery just below the inguinal ligament, to prevent puncture of either the femoral vein (medially) or the femoral nerve (laterally) (Fig. 11.10).

Brachial artery

The brachial artery (Fig. 11.11) is only used if all other punctures are impossible or have failed. There is a risk of injury which could lead to peripheral ischaemia or of damage to the median nerve which lies on the medial side.

Equipment

Equipment required is:

- syringe, 2 mL – a special syringe is often available
- 22 G needle (blue) or smaller
- heparin 1000 U/mL (1 mL) – standard in many hospitals
- alcohol swab
- sterile cotton wool balls/gauze swabs
- syringe cap
- plastic bag full of ice.

Procedure

- Draw up 0.5 mL of heparin into the 2 mL syringe, withdrawing the plunger fully to coat the syringe walls – or use a special pre-heparinised syringe.
- The heparin in both the pre-prepared and self-heparinised syringes must be expelled completely to

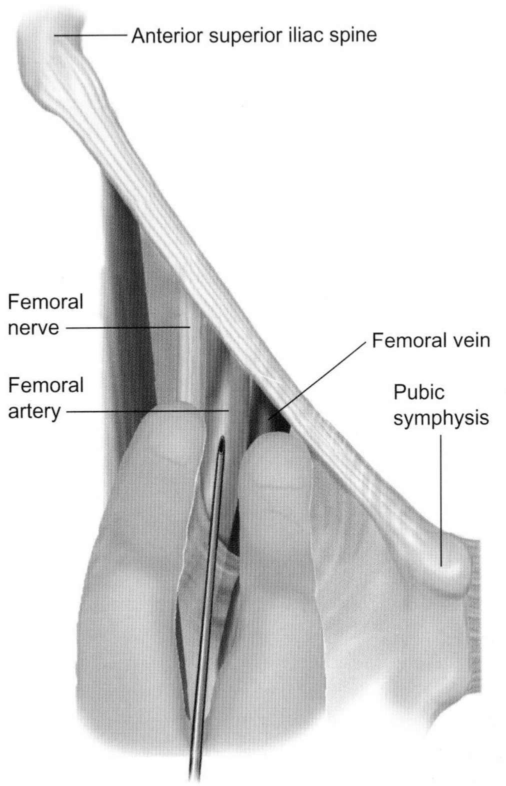

Fig. 11.10 The position of the femoral artery in the groin.

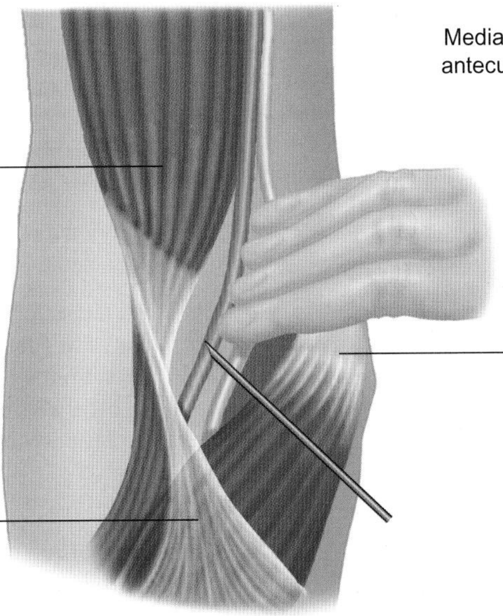

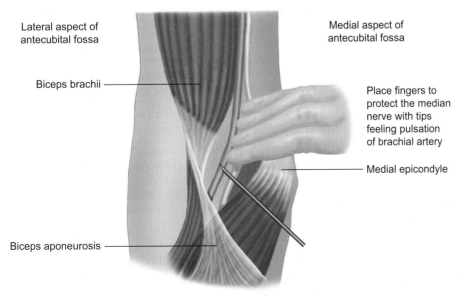

Fig. 11.11 The site for puncture of the brachial artery.

leave the plunger just moistened; large amounts of heparin in the syringe affect the pH of a sample taken for the determination of blood gas tension.

- Hold the syringe at a 60–90° angle to the skin and slowly advance the needle, maintaining a very slight negative pressure. When a flush of blood occurs, release the negative pressure; if the syringe then fills spontaneously, the artery has been entered.
- Once 2 mL of blood have been obtained, remove the syringe and needle and immediately apply pressure for at least 3 minutes.
- Tap bubbles to the needle end and expel all air that may have accumulated. Then, either take the sample immediately to the arterial blood gas analyser or place it on ice to slow down cellular use of oxygen in the sample (maximum 1 hour for reliable readings).
- If puncture fails, this may be because the artery has been transfixed; slow withdrawal of the needle sometimes yields free flow of arterial blood. If success does not follow, the arterial pulse is repalpated and a fresh attempt is made, preferably without coming out of the skin.

Understanding arterial blood gas results

Preliminaries

The percentage concentration of oxygen in the inspired air (e.g. 21% if the patient is inhaling air only) should be noted. It may take up to 20 minutes for the arterial blood gases to equilibrate after an adjustment to the oxygen supply. There may sometimes be difficulty in distinguishing between an arterial and venous sample: if the oxygen saturation (derived from the P_aO_2) is less than 50%, the blood is probably venous; 80% or above is certainly arterial. All indices should be considered together, i.e. P_aO_2, P_aCO_2, pH, base excess and H_2CO_3 (normal values are given in Table 11.3).

P_aO_2

Low values

The patient's usual level should be known – those with chronic respiratory disease can have a P_aO_2 as low as 7.5 kPa. A common cause of a truly low P_aO_2 in a surgical patient is a right-to-left shunt of blood through collapsed or consolidated lung tissue, in which instance the highly diffusable CO_2 is also low because of hypoxia-induced tachypnoea and hyperventilation. However, if the associated P_aCO_2 is high, there is chronic respiratory disease and/or acute respiratory failure (inability to ventilate). Those with known chronic respiratory disease who need oxygen to correct hypoxia must be given it carefully, starting with 24% O_2 and measuring the blood gases after 30 minutes to ensure that respiratory drive is maintained and that the P_aCO_2 does not rise. It should be noted that those with chronic respiratory disease can tolerate a much higher P_aCO_2 than normal.

The oxyhaemoglobin dissociation curve (see Fig. 6.9) means that small changes in P_aO_2 may have a large effect on oxygen saturation.

Table 11.3 Normal arterial blood gases

Measurement	Units	Level
pH	$-\log_{10}$ concentration hydrogen ion	7.35–7.45
P_aCO_2	kPa	4.3–6.0
	mm Hg	32–45
P_aO_2	kPa	10.5–14
	mm Hg	79–105
H_2CO_3	mmol/L	22–26
O_2 saturation	Percentage	95–100
Base excess	mmol/L	±2

High values

Hyperventilation without added oxygen cannot significantly increase the P_aO_2. The much more likely cause is that there is too high a concentration in the inspired air, and this should be adjusted provided the P_aCO_2 is normal.

P_aCO_2

Low values

The patient is usually hyperventilating. The causes are:

- hypoxia
- anxiety – there is an accompanying respiratory alkalosis
- compensation for a lowered pH – metabolic acidosis.

Hyperventilation from anxiety leads to a respiratory alkalosis (increased pH). If there is obvious hyperventilation, then a paper bag over the patient's mouth and a suggestion that respiratory rate is reduced is usually effective, as may be an instruction to hold the breath.

If the clinical state is a compensation for a metabolic acidosis, then the pH will be either normal or low and there will be a negative base excess.

High values

There is retention of CO_2 because of hypoventilation from one of the following:

- chronic respiratory failure (often with an associated low P_aO_2 and normal pH – chronically compensated)
- respiratory suppression from drugs (often opioids)
- exhaustion of the respiratory muscles (associated with a low P_aO_2 and inappropriately reduced respiratory rate) – the chief cause of acute respiratory failure in surgical patients
- brainstem malfunction, often with varied rates of ventilation; conscious level is decreased.

Respiratory support, such as ventilation, needs to be considered in acute respiratory failure:

- if the respiratory rate is either very high (greater than 25) or very low (less than 8) on maximum supplementary oxygen from a mask and the patient is not maintaining P_aO_2 of 10 kPa.
- in a previously normal patient if the P_aCO_2 is greater than 8 kPa.

pH and base excess

If the pH is less than 7.35, there is acidosis; if greater than 7.45, there is an alkalosis. It is necessary to decide if either is metabolic or respiratory in origin and whether compensation is present. Compensation suggests a more chronic disease process (days or weeks), whereas an uncompensated disorder suggests an acute disease process. Compensation usually occurs by a change in the respiratory rate (e.g. in a metabolic acidosis, hyperpnoea causes increased excretion of CO_2) or by renal regulation of the amount of HCO_3 that is excreted.

INSERTION OF A NASOGASTRIC TUBE

Indications

Indications include:

- vomiting from small-bowel obstruction or pyloric stenosis
- acute gastric dilatation
- the prevention of gastro-oesophageal reflux which could cause aspiration in patients with impaired gastric emptying
- enteric feeding (a nasojejunal tube may also be used)
- possible protection of an anastomosis distal to the pharynx – usually in the oesophagus (nasogastric tube usually positioned at operation).

Equipment

Equipment required is:

- non-sterile gloves
- nasogastric tube size 10 (small) to 16 (large)
- catheter drainage bag
- lubricant
- glass of water.

Procedure

- Inform the patient what is planned and how cooperation can help. Verbal consent is obtained.
- Sit the patient upright with the chin on the chest; if this is not possible then the alternative is on the side with the head propped up.
- Lubricate the tube and insert into one nostril directly backward towards the occiput – a patient may be aware which side is more likely to be successful. Gently advance the tube.
- If you are unable to advance, try the other nostril or reposition the patient.
- When the patient feels the tip in the pharynx, ask for a swallow and, as the tube moves, its advance is continued. Swallowing may be helped if a sip of water is given but there must not be any chance of aspiration, because of an inactive gag reflex.
- Should the patient cough or becomes cyanotic, it is probably because the tube is astride the larynx or trachea. Withdraw quickly, into the hypopharynx, let the patient settle and try again (unfortunately the tube is often then pulled out completely because of a feeling of impending suffocation).
- After apparently successful insertion, check that the tube is not simply curled up in the back of the mouth. To do this, attach a 20 mL syringe to the proximal end and, with a stethoscope bell just below the left costal margin, quickly inject air; a loud borborygmus confirms that the tube is in the stomach.
- If fluid can be aspirated from the nasogastric tube, it can be tested with pH indicator paper (not litmus paper). It should be acidic (pH <5.5).
- Secure the tube to the nose with strong adhesive tape.
- If there is any doubt the position of the tube should be checked by X-ray.

Extra hints

- A cold tube (one that has been in a refrigerator for at least 30 minutes) is stiffer and more easy to direct down the oesophagus.
- A change in the position of the patient – as indicated above – can sometimes secure success.
- If the patient has a poor gag reflex then sometimes a laryngoscope and a Magill's forceps can be used to direct the tube into the oesophagus.

Fine-bore tubes for enteric feeding may be easier to insert because they are of smaller diameter and are equipped with guide wire. However, their rigidity may, if they are forced down against resistance, lead to an abrasion or, rarely, perforation of the oesophagus. Furthermore, in an unconscious patient, it is easy to insert them into the trachea and bronchi. The final position of the tube should always be confirmed by a chest X-ray.

URINARY CATHETERISATION

Material

Urinary catheters are usually made of either latex or silicone rubber. Silicone is less irritant and should be used if the catheter is to be left indwelling for some days or weeks.

Special catheters

A Foley catheter is self-retaining because of an inflatable balloon (Fig. 11.12) and is usually but not invariably made of latex.

Three-way catheters are used for irrigation of the bladder, e.g. after prostatectomy.

Size

- 8–10 F: children and adults with tight urethral stricture
- 12–14 F: normal urethra or in the presence of mild prostatic hypertrophy
- 16–18 F: moderate prostatic hypertrophy
- 20–24 F: after prostatectomy for free drainage and in other circumstances where bladder irrigation is required with the use of a three-way catheter.

The smallest size feasible should always be used.

MALE CATHETERISATION (FIG. 11.13)

Indications

Indications include:

- urinary retention
- to assess hourly urinary output
- incontinence.

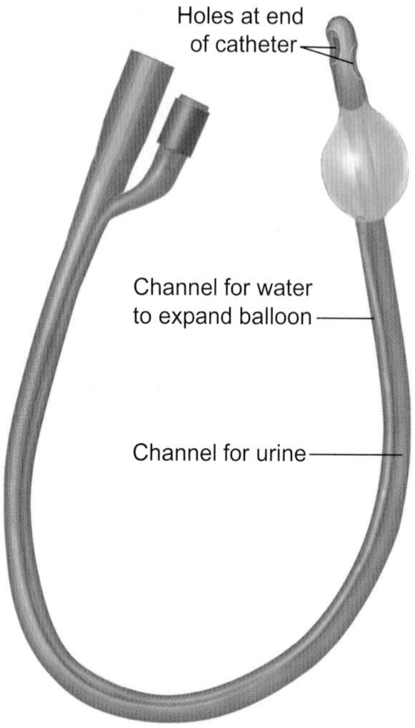

Fig. 11.12 A Foley urinary catheter.

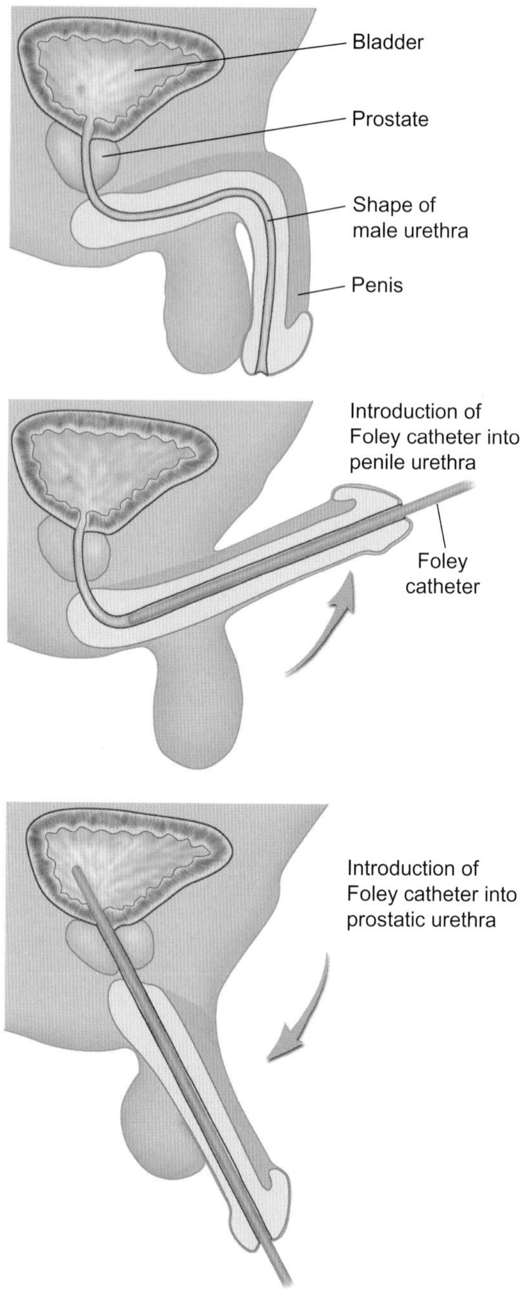

Fig. 11.13 Technique for male catheterisation.

Equipment

Equipment required is:

- urinary catheter
- sterile gloves
- lidocaine gel 0.5%
- bland antiseptic solution (e.g. cetyl trimethyl ammonium bromide) or sterile 0.9% saline
- pre-prepared catheterisation pack – kidney dish, gauze swabs, sterile towels
- 10 mL syringe and 10 mL of sterile water
- urine drainage bag.

Procedure

- Wash hands and don sterile gloves.
- Open out everything that is needed onto a sterile towel, usually on a trolley.
- Lay the patient flat – the more supine the position, the easier is the catheterisation.
- Drape the sterile towels or paper sheets to leave the penis exposed (a self-made hole in the centre of the paper sheet is often an easy way to expose just the penis).
- If right-handed, hold the penis with a sterile gauze swab with the left hand to prevent the penis from slipping; then retract the foreskin and clean the urethral opening with a swab.
- Gently squeeze the contents of a tube of lidocaine jelly into the urethra; in anyone of age less than 50, the sensitivity of the urethra often requires the content of two tubes.
- Open the plastic sheath which contains the catheter at the tip with the right hand and place a kidney bowl just below the urethral orifice of the penis.
- Hold the penis in the left hand and gently insert the catheter into the urethra using the right hand while withdrawing the plastic covering; ideally the catheter remains untouched, but this almost always proves impossible and the catheter has to be advanced without its plastic covering using the clean right hand. During insertion the external end of the catheter remains in the kidney bowl because, when the bladder is entered, urine usually spills out.

- If resistance is felt along the penile urethra or before the prostatic urethra has been traversed, pulling the penis gently upwards can help.
- Most often, resistance is found within the prostatic urethra, and pulling the penis downwards at this point can assist. Sometimes the cause is failure of relaxation of the external sphincter and, if the tip of the catheter is held at this point of resistance for 10 seconds, this is often enough to allow the sphincter to relax spontaneously.
- Force must not be used, because a false passage through the wall of the urethra can be made.
- A Foley catheter should be inserted fully to ensure that the balloon is within the bladder before inflation.
- Check the capacity of the balloon – it is usually 5–10 mL but for most three-way catheters is 30 mL. Usually only 5–10 mL capacity is needed; if the patient has just had a prostatectomy, then 20–30 mL are required so that the catheter can sit at the bladder neck and not move into the resected prostatic cavity.
- Either squeeze the already dilated water-filled area at the distal end of the catheter (after removing the clip) or insert the 5–10 mL of sterile water gently into the injection port for the balloon. If this generates pain or discomfort, stop at once, withdraw any water and advance the catheter further into the bladder.
- Once the balloon is inflated, the catheter is withdrawn until resistance is felt as the balloon lodges against the bladder neck.
- Replace the foreskin over the glans to avoid the possibility of a paraphimosis.
- Attach the catheter to the drainage apparatus.
- Send a urine sample for microscopy and culture.

If the catheter is to be in place for a considerable time – several days or more – the smallest diameter and the minimal amount of water in the balloon (5 mL) both help to decrease the likelihood of bladder spasm.

Extra hints

- If the catheter is in the bladder but urine does not flow, blockage by the lubrication jelly is a possibility. Aspiration with a 50 mL catheter syringe and/or injection of sterile water or 0.9% saline usually unblocks the catheter.
- If a stricture is encountered in either the penile or prostatic urethra, a narrower catheter (10–12 F) should be used.
- In a patient beyond 55 years with a history suggestive of benign prostatic hypertrophy, a larger-diameter catheter is paradoxically more likely to succeed.
- If the catheterisation fails, no more than two attempts should be made before more experienced help is sought. For the second, try to use a different-sized catheter (depending on the probable cause of difficulty) and extra lidocaine gel. Further failure should lead to consideration of suprapubic drainage (see below).
- If the patient bleeds from the urethra, abandon the procedure and summon help to decide how to proceed, which may mean the use of suprapubic catheterisation.
- If phimosis makes the external meatus difficult to find, gently dilate the narrow opening in the foreskin with the nozzle of the tube which contains the lidocaine jelly.

Removal of a urethral catheter

This is usually done by nursing staff. Failure to decompress the balloon calls for special manoeuvres.

Faulty valve

Sometimes the valve end can be cut off. If this fails, a needle inserted into the valve channel and aspirated may release obstruction.

Persistent impaction

Ultrasound identifies the balloon in the bladder, which can then be punctured with a fine spinal needle passed percutaneously under image control.

Catheterisation in relation to prostatic hypertrophy and prostatectomy

Size of catheter

As mentioned above, the prostatic urethra may, in the presence of prostatic hypertrophy, be more easily negotiated with a larger rather than a smaller catheter.

Bleeding

Initial rapid decompression of a dilated bladder may lead to rupture of distended veins at the bladder neck. A three-way irrigation system may be necessary until the condition settles, which it usually does.

Chronic retention

The presence of chronic retention with a considerably distended bladder before prostatectomy makes the necessity of prolonged drainage extremely likely; a 12–14 F silicone catheter which can be left in place for 6–8 weeks allows the bladder to recover tone. Long-standing obstruction at the bladder neck without acute retention leads to back pressure on the kidney and a presentation with features of chronic renal failure and creatinine levels in excess of 1000 μmol/L, although the electrolyte levels are remarkably normal when there is only an obstructive cause. Catheterisation in such circumstances means that there is the likelihood of the development of a polyuric phase because damage to the kidneys' distal tubules results in an inability to concentrate urine. Some 200–400 mL of urine an hour can be passed, and dehydration develops quite rapidly. The most practical way to adjust fluid balance to compensate for the polyuria is to give the amount of fluid passed out in 1 hour back intravenously over the next hour. Such polyuria may be accompanied by hyponatraemia and hypokalaemia, and replacement must be adjusted accordingly. The polyuric phase usually lasts for about 12–24 hours; continuation beyond this may mean over-replacement, with a vicious circle of water and electrolyte-induced diuresis. The hour-on-hour replacement of urinary losses is discontinued and the situation reassessed.

Post-prostatectomy failure of micturition

Withdrawal of the initial drainage catheter after transurethral prostatectomy may not be followed by micturition. In such circumstances, first check the fluid balance chart – the bladder may not be sufficiently full to initiate micturition. Also, pain and the feeling of inability to micturate are not always caused by an overfull bladder; severe pain is often the consequence of detrusor muscle spasm within the bladder and is best treated not by catheterisation but with a smooth muscle relaxant such as oxybutynin. If the patient has been bleeding significantly and the bladder is truly distended, this may be the result of clot retention. Catheterisation with a large-bore, three-way catheter and irrigation with 0.9% saline are necessary.

At transurethral prostatectomy it is relatively easy to dissect under the bladder neck and therefore possible to make a false passage on re-catheterisation. If the catheter easily advances its full length then this is unlikely; a check can be done by the insertion of 50 mL of water, which should readily be re-aspirated.

FEMALE CATHETERISATION

Anatomy

The female has a more easily traversed urinary tract than has the male. Only the muscles of the pelvic floor control access, and once the external meatus has been identified the short urethra is straight (Fig. 11.14).

Equipment

The equipment is the same as for male catheterisation except that there are some female catheters that are shorter than those used in males. Female catheterisation is often performed by the nursing staff, and doctors are asked to assist only when nursing staff have been unsuccessful.

Procedure

- Collect all equipment and set up the trolley
- Position the patient as for a vaginal examination – flat on the back with the heels together and the knees apart (hips in abduction and external rotation)
- Put on sterile gloves
- Part the labia minora and majora with the non-dominant hand and, using the dominant hand, clean the area with a cotton wool ball soaked in sterile 0.9% saline or a bland antiseptic solution
- Locate the urethral opening (Fig. 11.14) behind and below the clitoris and introduce a well-lubricated catheter tip; a small amount of lidocaine jelly applied around the opening can aid entry
- Successful catheterisation is followed by the procedures listed above for male catheterisation.

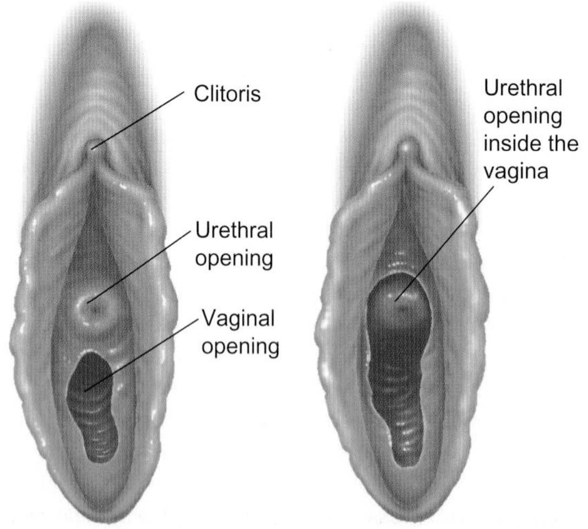

Fig. 11.14 Technique for female catheterisation.

Difficulty

If catheterisation has not been achieved this is usually because the urethral opening has not been identified and the vagina has been catheterised instead. The labia minora must be opened generously and usually the urethral opening can be seen pouting on the anterior aspect of the vaginal wall. A focused light and lying the patient on the side can both help, as can, occasionally, a vaginal speculum.

SUPRAPUBIC BLADDER DRAINAGE

Indication

Suprapubic bladder drainage is required when urethral catheterisation has failed and the patient has a full bladder.

Equipment

Equipment required is:

- sterile towels
- catheterisation pack – gauze, cotton wool balls
- skin preparation
- suprapubic catheter
- needles – orange, green and white
- 1% lidocaine 10–20 mL
- 10 and 20 mL syringes
- blade or knife
- suture to tie the catheter to the abdominal wall – 3/0 or stronger
- catheter bag.

Procedure

- Place the patient supine and make sure that the bladder is distended by percussion from the umbilicus downwards in the midline or by ultrasound scanning.
- Open the pack and all the equipment; if a Foley catheter is to be used, check the balloon. Use another type only if familiar with its mechanism of insertion.
- Clean the area in the midline between the umbilicus and symphysis pubis.
- Arrange the sterile towels around this area.
- Infiltrate the skin in the midline 2 cm above the pubic symphysis using the local anaesthetic and an orange needle and continue this through the layers of abdominal wall (the subcutaneous tissue and linea alba only) with the larger (green) needle.
- At the completion of infiltration, the needle is passed into the distended bladder and urine is aspirated; occasionally the longest (white) needle is required to achieve this (urine must be aspirated before suprapubic catheterisation is attempted).

- Make a stab incision in the skin large enough to take the chosen catheter.
- Insert the suprapubic trochar directly posteriorly in the same direction as that used for the final aspiration of urine.
- Once urine is obtained, advance the catheter over the trochar.
- Remove the trochar and advance the catheter further to the indicated marker; ensure that easy aspiration of urine occurs and that the patient is free from pain.
- Clean and dry the entry point and then secure the catheter – preferably at more than one point.

If the catheter falls out before 2 weeks have elapsed and the patient needs re-catheterisation, this must be done within 8 hours, otherwise the track will have closed. After 2 weeks, the track will have become lined with epithelium and therefore a new catheter (often a simple silicone-covered urethral catheter) can be easily inserted.

CHEST PROCEDURES

PLEURAL DRAINAGE (AIR AND/OR FLUID)

For all chest drainage procedures:

- First check the clinical signs and the X-rays.
- Ensure that the upper level of the pleural effusion is clearly established by percussion and mark this on the chest wall.
- Position the patient comfortably in a sitting position leaning slightly forward either in bed or on a chair. Ideally a table should be placed in front with a pillow or blanket to rest on, elevated to the level of the axilla (Fig. 11.15).
- Usually a site for aspiration/drainage is identified by ultrasound scanning.

Diagnostic aspiration

Indications

Indications include:

- infection
- malignancy.

Equipment

Equipment required is:

- dressing pack
- sterile gloves
- 20 mL syringe
- orange (25 G) and green (21 G) needles
- 1% lidocaine, 10 mL
- three sterile specimen bottles.

Procedure

- Confirm the signs and X-ray findings.
- Select the insertion site by ultrasound scanning or percussing out an effusion and mark the point of

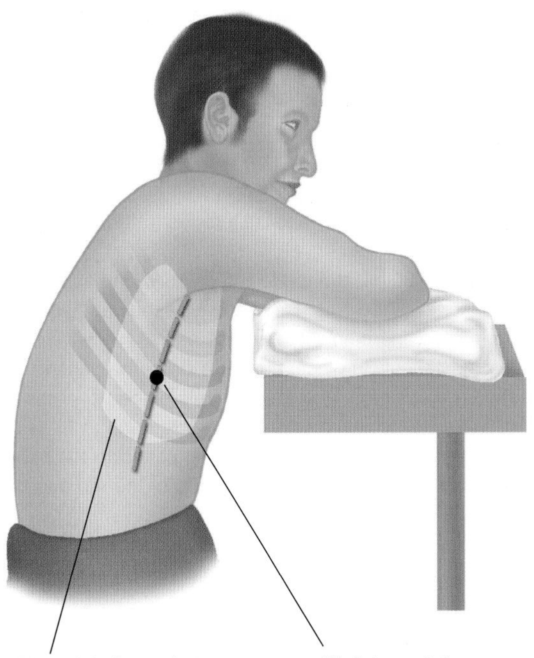

Fig. 11.15 The position of a patient during pleural drainage/chest drain.

dullness – ideally done between the midaxillary and posterior axillary lines and at a point three finger breadths below the tip of the scapula.
- Infiltrate the skin over the chosen point with local anaesthetic using an orange needle and then infiltrate deeper with a green needle; the needle should pass just superior to the rib to avoid the neurovascular bundle. Always withdraw before inserting local anaesthetic. On average, fluid should be aspirated at the full depth of a green needle, but a longer needle may be required for larger or more obese individuals.
- Attach the 20 mL syringe to the appropriately sized needle and insert it through the area that has already been anaesthetised while aspirating as the needle is advanced. When flashback of fluid occurs, gently aspirate 20 mL to send for laboratory analysis: culture and sensitivity, auramine stain and TB culture; protein, glucose and amylase; and cytology. When aspirating for cytological examination, the more fluid there is, the better (>40 mL).

Therapeutic aspiration

Indications

Indications include:

- relief of shortness of breath from a pleural effusion
- removal of a small pneumothorax.

Equipment

Equipment is as for diagnostic aspiration, plus the following additional items:

- large-bore i.v. cannula (brown or grey)
- a three-way tap
- 50 mL syringe
- i.v. giving set and an empty sterile bowel or saline bag.

Procedure

Fluid

- Larger cannulae need a small incision in the skin before their insertion.
- Attach the 50 mL syringe to the cannula and aspirate on insertion. After flashback, advance the cannula over the needle and then withdraw the needle, to leave the flexible cannula in place; as this is done the patient should breathe out and the thumb is placed over the cannula hub to prevent air being sucked in.
- A closed three-way tap is quickly attached to the hub.
- Attach the 50 mL syringe to one hub of the tap and the empty saline bag to the other.
- Aspirate 50 mL at a time, switching the three-way tap settings to allow the syringe to empty into the saline bag.
- Withdraw the cannula while the patient breathes out.
- Apply an occlusive dressing to the site of puncture.

Air

- The position of insertion of the cannula should be either in the second intercostal space in the midclavicular line (Ch. 16) or in the midaxillary line in the fifth intercostal space.
- Infiltrate as already indicated just superior to the rib and ensure aspiration of air.
- Make a small incision in the skin and insert the needle/cannula through the infiltrated area. On aspiration of air through the needle, advance the cannula quickly while the patient breathes out.
- Remove the needle immediately and, with the thumb, occlude the hub until a closed three-way tap is attached.
- Air is aspirated 50 mL at a time and expelled through the spare exit on the tap. Care must be exercised to avoid the open tap coming into direct communication with the chest cavity.
- Once there is resistance to further aspiration, withdraw the cannula slightly to see if there is still residual air. It is important never to force aspiration because to do so may suck lung tissue against the end of the cannula.
- Withdraw the cannula and apply an occlusive dressing.

For a therapeutic aspiration it is advisable to halt the procedure after 1000 mL of air or fluid has been withdrawn to avoid rapid shift of the mediastinum. If cardiorespiratory signs are absent, removal of air or fluid is resumed after an hour. Failure of a chest aspiration is usually the result of a localised effusion or empyema. Ultrasound scanning and guided aspiration should be used.

RELIEF OF TENSION PNEUMOTHORAX

The causes and mechanisms are discussed in Chapters 3 and 16. The diagnosis is clinical rather than radiological (Fig. 11.16), and urgent decompression is required.

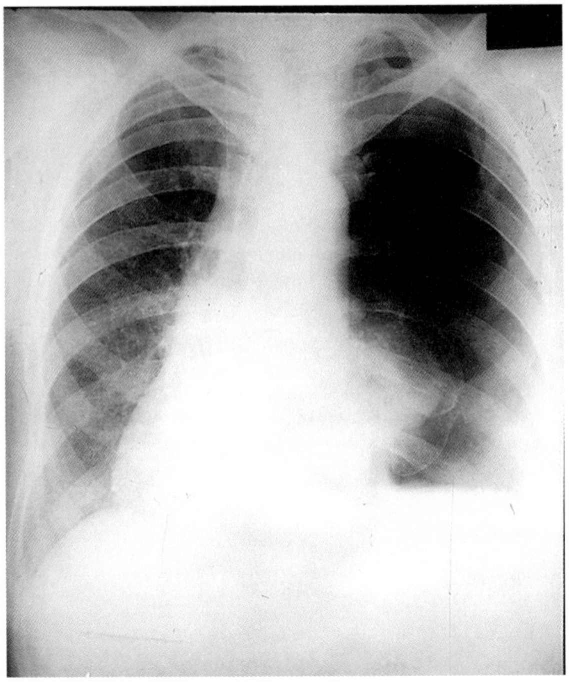

Fig. 11.16 Left-sided tension pneumothorax with mediastinal shift and complete collapse of left lung.

Equipment

Equipment required is:

- large-bore needle or needle/cannula
- 20 mL syringe.

Procedure

- Assess the patient's chest and respiratory function.
- Administer oxygen at 12 L/min by mask.
- Identify the second intercostal space in the midclavicular line on the side of the pneumothorax.
- If the patient is conscious and time permits, introduce local anaesthetic with an orange needle.
- Insert the needle with the 20 mL syringe attached – a small incision in the skin makes the insertion of a needle or cannula easier.
- Aspiration of air confirms the diagnosis: the syringe is removed and, in tension pneumothorax, a hissing sound is usually heard as the air is rapidly expelled; a hand held 5 cm from the needle or cannula can detect this rush of air.

The urgent procedure described converts a tension pneumothorax into an ordinary one. If air starts to enter the thorax, a three-way tap should be placed on the needle or cannula hub and sealed, which then enables further release of air before a chest drain is inserted – this is always done.

INSERTION OF A CHEST DRAIN

Indications

Indications include:

- large pneumothorax and after urgent release of a tension pneumothorax

- spreading surgical emphysema – sometimes an X-ray shows no sign of a pneumothorax, but a chest drain should be inserted on the assumption that there is a continuing leak of air into the pleural space
- large haemothorax with a possible continued source of bleeding
- large pleural effusion
- empyema.

Equipment

Equipment required is:

- chest drain between 22 F and 32 F but *without* an integral trocar
- 0.5% lidocaine, 20 mL
- underwater seal apparatus including bottle
- sterile water
- surgical blade
- small and large artery forceps
- heavy suture, e.g. silk 0
- adhesive tape – a waterproof variety is best.

Position

The position for insertion is the fifth intercostal space in the midaxillary line on the affected side – usually approximately at the level of the nipple in a male. This site is suitable for drainage of both a pneumothorax and a haemothorax and should always be used in trauma. Drainage of a pleural effusion or an empyema may need to be slightly lower, but the site should be carefully checked against the available imaging, with particular attention to the possibility of the dome of the diaphragm being raised. The distance between adjacent ribs determines the size of the intercostal drain tube; the largest drain possible is advisable, particularly in trauma.

Procedure

- Position the patient as for pleural aspiration.
- Make a final check of the clinical signs and the chest X-ray.
- Mark the proposed site of insertion.
- Prepare an area over two to three ribs in the midaxillary line and drape it.
- Anaesthetise the skin and the tissues down to the upper border of the chosen rib – not all the allocated lidocaine is used, because more is often needed later.
- Make a 2–3 cm transverse incision over the proposed site of insertion.
- Use the artery forceps to dissect bluntly through the subcutaneous tissues, going down onto the superior margin of the rib and dissecting through the intercostal muscles and then the parietal pleura (Fig. 11.17a) – this is where more local anaesthetic may be required.
- When the parietal pleura is punctured with the tip of the artery forceps, there is usually the escape of fluid and/or air. Sweep the gloved index finger down the line of blunt dissection to free any adhesions within the pleural space so that injury to the lung is avoided.
- Grasp the drainage tube at its tip with artery forceps and guide it down the track with the index finger. Once the drain is within the pleural cavity, remove the forceps and advance the drain gently.
- Attach the outer end of the drain to an underwater seal drainage apparatus.

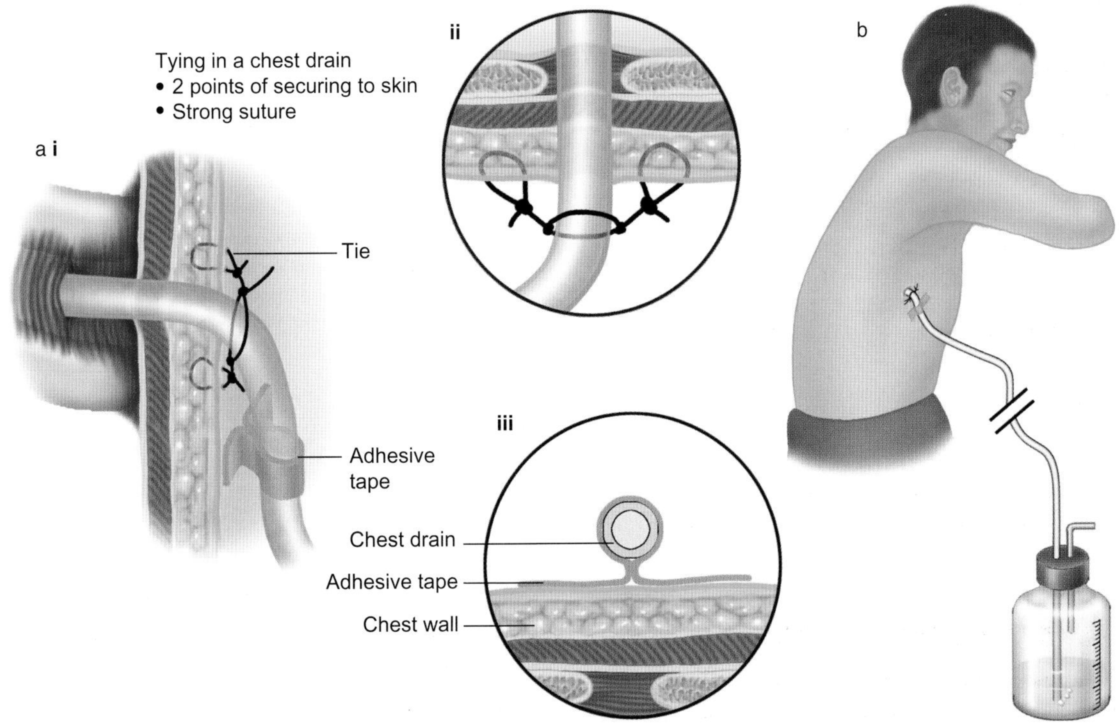

Fig. 11.17 (a) Technique for securing of a chest drain. (b) Chest drain in position with underwater drainage.

- Close the incision with interrupted sutures and a tight tie around the drain itself – there should not be leakage around the tube or through the incision.
- Insert a purse string suture around the drain or two interrupted sutures across the tube site, leaving the ends untied for final air-tight closure when the drain is removed.
- Check that the drain is working – fluid or air according to circumstances – or that the water is rising into the tube above the level in the bottle (swinging) with respiration; failure to swing may mean that the tube is misplaced.
- Secure the connection between the drain and the underwater seal with strong adhesive tape and, after wiping dry around the insertion site and applying a sterile dressing, tape the drain to the chest wall (Fig. 11.17b).
- Check the position of the drain by chest X-ray.

Complications

Complications include:

- damage to an intercostal artery or vein which causes either continued bleeding at the site of insertion or a haemothorax
- damage to an intercostal nerve which may cause later intercostal neuritis/neuralgia
- pleural empyema
- laceration or puncture of intrathoracic and/or abdominal organs – prevented by using blunt dissection
- local cellulitis
- local haematoma
- mediastinal emphysema
- subcutaneous emphysema.

Further hints

- Strong and long dissecting artery forceps are extremely useful.
- Do not use any trocar supplied with a drain – it is a common cause of injury to deep structures.
- The more subcutaneous fat that is present, the bigger the incision that is required; a good guide is that the incision needs to be as long as the subcutaneous fat is deep.

If the first drain does not resolve the pneumothorax or there is a large and continuing leak, further drains may well be required. The same applies if surgical emphysema continues to spread after the insertion of a chest drain.

If after pleural drainage for acute haemothorax more than 200 mL of blood (as distinct from bloodstained pleural effusion) drains every hour, thoracotomy may be indicated for control of bleeding.

Removal of chest drain

The chest drain does not have a continued role if it fails to swing with breathing or is not draining any fluid; these are the chief indications for its removal. Before this is done the patient should be asked to cough and, if the drain does not bubble, then any leak from a hole in the lung has almost certainly been sealed; however, for certainty, the test should be repeated after 12 hours. A check X-ray before removal can be useful to confirm that the lung is completely re-expanded and that any pleural effusion has been fully drained.

Large pleural effusions should be drained over several days. The maximum should be 1 L per hour and not more than 4 L per day, otherwise there is a risk of reflex pulmonary oedema.

Equipment

Equipment required is:

- sterile gloves
- suture cutters
- local anaesthetic and, if occluding sutures have not been pre-inserted, a closure suture
- occlusive dressing.

Procedure

Ideally this should be done with two people: one to tie the suture and the other to remove the drain. Local anaesthetic and a standby suture should be available.

- Undo the adhesive dressing and check whether there is a purse string suture in situ; if there is, release the suture and place a half knot.
- Release the suture holding the drain.
- Ask the patient to take two large inhalations and then momentarily to hold the breath in expiration (Valsalva manoeuvre to raise intrathoracic pressure); now pull the drain out quickly.
- Tie the purse string immediately and cover the site with a sterile dressing and occlusive tape.
- If there is any concern after the removal of the chest drain, a chest X-ray is indicated.
- If the occluding suture is ineffective, then gauze should be available to place over the hole and prevent a sucking chest wound.

PERICARDIAL PARACENTESIS

Indications

This procedure is used to relieve cardiac tamponade (Ch. 17), which most commonly occurs after penetrating injuries to the chest, although a blunt injury – such as a steering wheel – can also be responsible. The removal of a small amount of blood or fluid can make a dramatic difference to the cardiac output and the patient's condition. Also, rarely in surgical practice, a chronic effusion may require aspiration. The pericardial sac is a fixed fibrous structure which, distended by only a small amount of blood, restricts cardiac filling. The removal of 15–20 mL of effusion – blood or other fluid – may save the patient's life.

Equipment

Equipment required is:

- long plastic-sheathed needle 16–18 gauge – a single-lumen central line cannula is ideal; if this is unavailable then a needle is sufficient, but, if repeated aspiration is required, the procedure has to be repeated rather than re-aspirating from a cannula that remains in situ

- three-way tap
- 20 mL syringe
- small scalpel blade (if a cannula/needle is to be used).

Procedure (Fig. 11.18)

- Continuous recording of blood pressure, pulse rate, central venous pressure and ECG throughout the procedure is ideal, but in the urgent circumstances usually encountered this can be omitted.
- If time allows, prepare the xiphoid and subxiphoid areas.
- Attach the syringe to the three-way tap and needle/cannula.
- Feel for the apex beat to ensure that there has been no marked mediastinal shift; this may be difficult or impossible when there is cardiac tamponade.
- Anaesthetise the area and incise the skin over a point 1–2 cm inferior to the left of the xiphochondral junction at a 45° angle to the skin.
- Advance a long needle and cannula towards the head, aiming towards the tip of the scapula or shoulder. Aspirate as the needle is advanced and watch the ECG continuously in case needling the myocardium causes any irregularities, including an injury pattern, e.g. extreme ST changes or a widened and enlarged QRS complex. Premature ventricular contractions may also occur, secondary to irritation of the myocardium.
- When the needle enters the blood-filled pericardial sac, withdraw as much non-clotted blood as is possible, although it must be remembered that the epicardium will approach the inner aspect of the pericardial sac, and ECG changes may then occur.

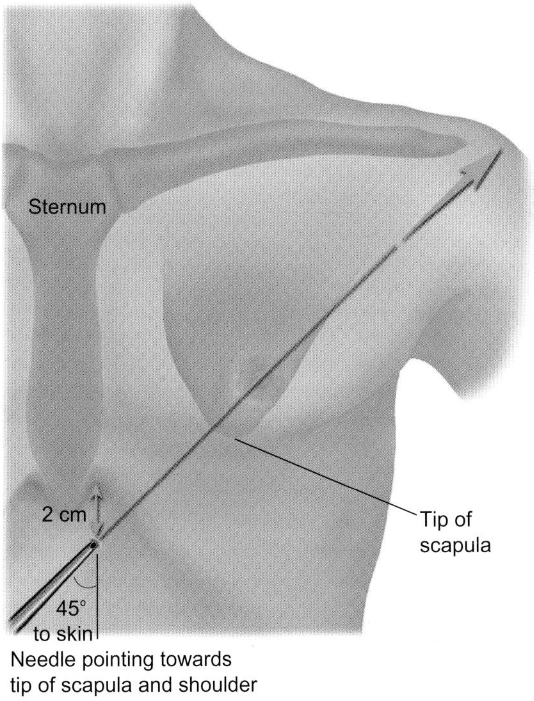

Fig. 11.18 Technique for pericardial aspiration.

- After aspiration is complete, slide the cannula over the needle and reattach the three-way tap, closing it off. Secure a catheter in place with adhesive tape.
- If the symptoms of cardiac tamponade persist, re-aspiration or a thoracotomy may be needed.

Complications

Possible complications are:

- aspiration of ventricular blood
- laceration of coronary artery or vein
- pericarditis
- cardiac arrhythmias – ventricular fibrillation, tachycardia
- puncture of aorta, inferior vena cava, oesophagus.

PERITONEAL LAVAGE

Indications

Peritoneal lavage may be useful in a patient with multiple injuries if:

- abdominal examination is equivocal because other injuries (fractures of ribs, pelvis and lumbar spine) may be obscuring physical findings
- abdominal examination is unreliable because of severe head injury, endotracheal intubation, intoxicants or paraplegia
- there is unexplained hypotension and/or blood loss.

However, urgent CT scanning is now often available and has reduced the need for peritoneal lavage.

Equipment

Equipment required is:

- peritoneal dialysis or peritoneal lavage catheter
- 1 L of 0.9% saline
- intravenous giving set
- scalpel
- local anaesthetic – 1% lidocaine with adrenaline 10 mL
- skin cleaner
- dressing pack and sterile towels
- instruments – tissue forceps, Allis clamps, arterial forceps.

Procedure (Fig. 11.19)

- Decompress the bladder by the passage of a urinary catheter.
- Prepare the area around the umbilicus (15 × 15 cm).
- Infiltrate local anaesthetic just inferior to the umbilicus and along the midline for approximately 2–5 cm, depending on the amount of subcutaneous tissue. Continue dissection through the linea alba to grasp its edges with the Allis forceps so as to provide countertraction.
- Expose the peritoneum and pick it up with arterial forceps.
- Insert the peritoneal dialysis catheter into the peritoneal cavity, advancing it towards the pelvis.
- Connect the catheter to a syringe and aspirate.

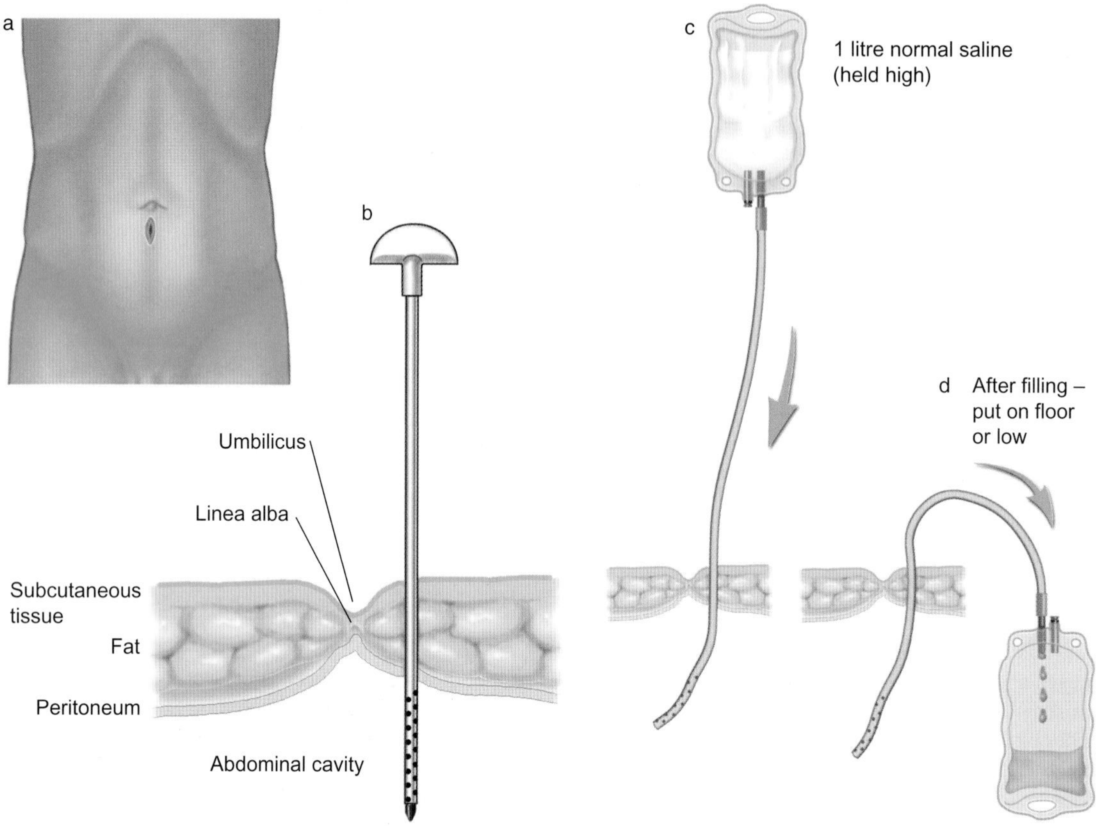

Fig. 11.19 Technique for peritoneal lavage.

- If gross blood is not aspirated, use the i.v. apparatus to instil 500–1000 mL of warmed saline.
- Given the patient is haemodynamically stable, allow the fluid to remain in the abdomen for 5–10 minutes before siphoning it off by putting the empty 0.9% saline container on the floor and allowing the peritoneal fluid to drain from the abdomen (which can take up to 20–30 minutes). A suture secures the catheter if some time elapses before the fluid is removed and it is necessary to make sure the container is vented to allow free flow.
- After return of the fluid, remove the peritoneal catheter and repair the fascia with interrupted sutures (e.g. Prolene 0 on a J needle) and the skin (e.g. Ethilon 3/0).

Indications for laparotomy after peritoneal lavage

Indications include:

- aspiration of more than 5 mL of obvious blood
- aspiration of enteric contents
- laboratory analysis of the peritoneal lavage fluid: >10 000 red blood cells/mm^3; >500 white blood cells/mm^3, bacteria and vegetable matter (usually associated with a raised WBC count).

False-negative results are obtained in 2% of peritoneal lavages, usually the consequence of isolated injury to retroperitoneal organs such as the pancreas, duodenum, diaphragm, small bowel and bladder.

AIRWAY MANAGEMENT

Any patient who is semi-conscious or unconscious must have an adequate assessment of the airway:

- Look for agitation, cyanosis, difficulty in respiratory effort and choking motions.
- Listen for snoring, gurgling, stridor and gargling sounds.
- Feel with the back of the hand for the exit of air with respiratory effort or see fogging of the oxygen mask on expiration.

Simple management

Blood secretions should be removed from the nose and mouth with a rigid suction device. A cribriform plate fracture must be considered, and gentleness is essential.

Chin lift

First complete clearance of the mouth, if indicated, by sweeping a finger between the tongue and the upper palate; be wary of the tendency of a semi-conscious patient to bite. Chin lift (Fig. 11.20) is a simple procedure which can be done on any patient without interfering with the cervical spine: the fingers of one hand are placed under the mandible in the midline, and are then lifted gently upwards to bring the chin forwards.

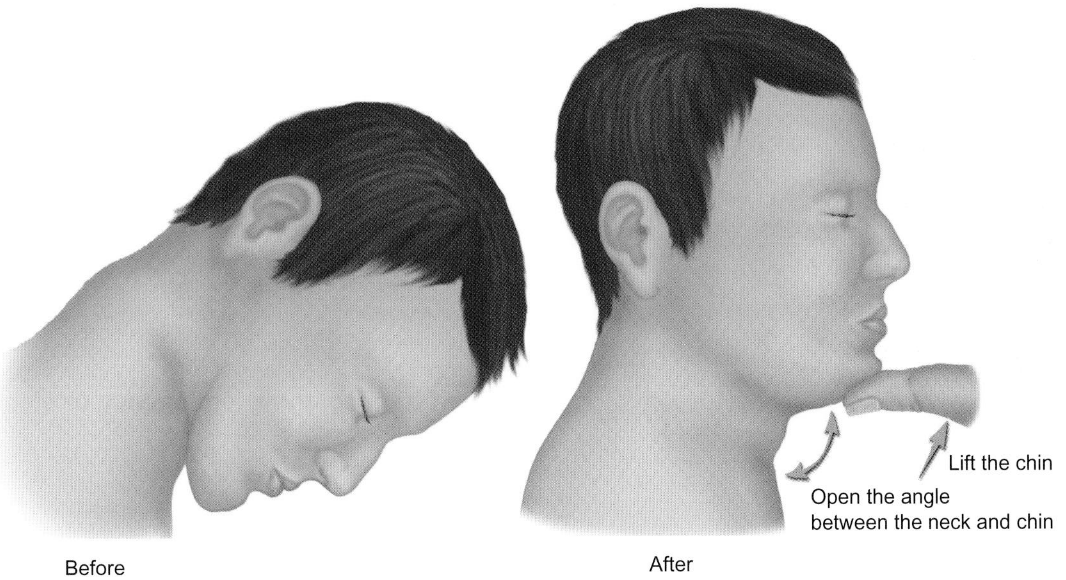

Fig. 11.20 Chin lift.

Jaw thrust

The angles of the lower jaw are grasped and the mandible displaced forwards. This is the method used with a mouth-to-face mask with a good seal.

Oropharyngeal airway (see Ch. 6)

A semi-conscious or agitated patient may cause difficulty, but an unconscious one usually accepts an oral airway. This should be inserted upside down with the concavity directed upwards until the soft palate is encountered. Rotation through 180° is then done, which places the concavity downwards and around the back of the tongue.

Nasopharyngeal airway (see Ch. 6)

This is useful when a patient has an upper airway obstruction but is unable to tolerate an oropharyngeal airway. The nasal airway is inserted into one nostril. It needs first to be lubricated and then inserted into the less obstructed nostril (often it is easier to insert through one or other nostril). If difficulty is encountered with one nostril, the other is used. The turbinates are often felt to fracture as the catheter is inserted, but little force is needed for this to occur and fracture is usual. If there is a suspicion of a base of skull fracture, a nasopharyngeal tube should not be used.

SURGICAL AIRWAY

Indications

An inability to intubate the trachea is the only indication for creating a surgical airway, and this can occur for various reasons:

- oedema of the epiglottis
- fracture of the larynx
- severe oropharyngeal haemorrhage
- when an endotracheal tube cannot be placed through the cords.

Cricothyroidotomy

Anatomy (Fig. 11.21)

The cricoid cartilage is the only circumferential support to the upper trachea in children and therefore surgical cricothyroidotomy is not recommended in children under 12 years. A 14 gauge needle/cannula can be used instead and is inserted through the cricothyroid membrane with intermittent oxygen jet insufflation. This method can lead to carbon dioxide retention and therefore should not be used for more than 40 minutes.

Equipment

Equipment required is:

- cricothyroidotomy set – often easily available in most resuscitation areas
- surgical blade
- curved arterial forceps and tracheal dilators
- small endotracheal tube of internal diameter 5–7 mm; if not available, then use any type of tube – metal, rubber or plastic.

Procedure

- Feel for the laryngeal prominence of the thyroid cartilage (Adam's apple) – more prominent in men than women. If it is difficult to be certain, then identify the hyoid bone and work the finger downwards; if it is still impossible to identify anything above what is thought to be the thyroid cartilage, it is possible that what was thought to be the thyroid cartilage is in fact the hyoid. As the finger descends in the midline, there is a palpable gap between the thyroid cartilage and the cricoid. It is through this window that emergency cricothyroidotomy is carried out. (Beneath the cricoid ring it is sometimes possible to feel the rings of the trachea but this depends on how much subcutaneous tissue is present.) (See Fig. 11.21.)

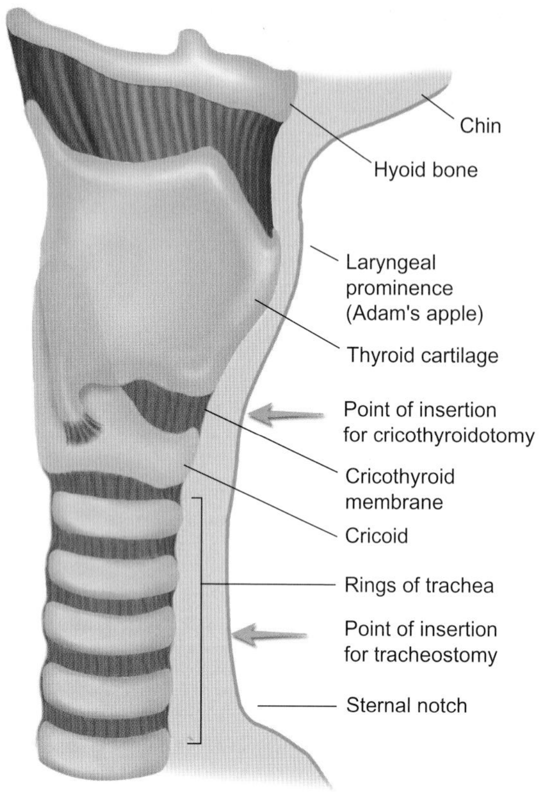

Fig. 11.21 Cricothyroidotomy and tracheostomy incision points.

- If time permits and the patient is conscious, insert local anaesthetic into the skin and subcutaneous tissues.
- Make a small transverse incision through the skin and extend this through the cricothyroid membrane; a hissing sound is audible once the trachea is penetrated. Alternatively, a Seldinger technique can be used.
- Use tracheal dilators and/or arterial forceps to expand the hole by separating the cricothyroid fibres (cricothyroidotomy set has appropriate instruments).
- Insert a small endotracheal tube (5–7 mm internal diameter) or any other appropriate tube that is available (normal tube sizes for adults are 8–8.5 mm for women and 9–10 mm for men).

Tracheostomy

This may be:

- emergency or elective
- percutaneous or open.

Indications

Indications include:

- airway obstruction
- head and neck surgery
- laryngeal trauma
- failed endotracheal intubation
- prolonged tracheal intubation
- prevention of pulmonary aspiration.

Emergency tracheostomy

This is rare because cricothyroidotomy is the preferred emergency procedure. If the larynx has been completely disrupted by injury and the cricothyroid membrane is not intact, then an emergency tracheostomy is indicated. The tracheostomy procedure is the same as for an elective procedure except where indicated.

Elective tracheostomy

It is preferable to relieve acute airways obstruction by endotracheal intubation or cricothyroidotomy and then to do an elective tracheostomy.

Open tracheostomy (emergency or elective)

Equipment

Equipment required is:

- tracheostomy set – usually obtained or used in the operating room (an operating room scrub nurse usually comes with the set)
- tracheal tubes of internal diameter 8–8.5 mm for women and 9–10 mm for men. If the neck is very large in diameter and the tracheal rings almost retrosternal, then a long tracheal tube should be considered.

Procedure (Fig. 11.22)

The procedure can be done under general or local anaesthetic (preferably the latter) and should be performed by an experienced surgeon:

- Ensure the patient's neck is extended as far as possible (in trauma the possibility of injury to the cervical spine must be remembered and ideally an assistant should keep the head and neck central).
- Oxygen should always be given to the patient even if you think the airway is completely obstructed, because sometimes this gives the patient a few extra minutes without severe hypoxia.
- Make a transverse incision halfway between the cricoid and the suprasternal notch and between the medial borders of sternomastoid muscles. In an emergency, if the anatomy is unclear, a vertical incision can be made from the laryngeal prominence of the thyroid cartilage to the suprasternal notch.
- Separate the strap muscles vertically in the midline through the investing fascia.
- Identify the thyroid isthmus, although it rarely needs to be divided in the adult and can usually be retracted upwards; in the child it is more likely to require division.
- Find the second, third and fourth tracheal rings.
- Incise the trachea vertically through the second, third and fourth rings; dilate the opening with either tracheal dilators or arterial forceps and insert an endotracheal tube (ideally 7–8 mm internal diameter) and attach the oxygen supply immediately.

In an emergency

- After the insertion of the tracheostomy tube, bleeding is controlled with artery forceps and ties; often the anterior jugular vein bleeds as well as the divided thyroid isthmus.
- Use a fine-bore suction tube to suck out the trachea.

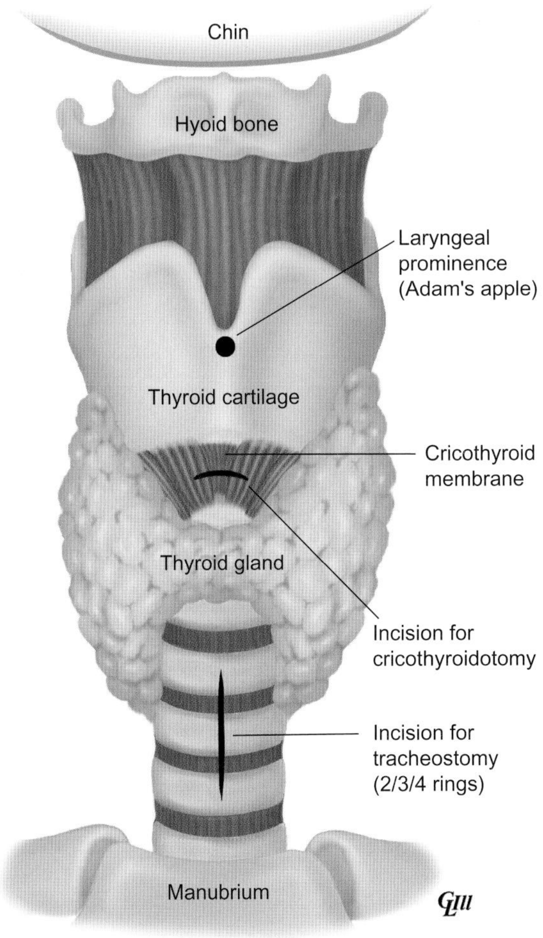

Fig. 11.22 Tracheostomy technique.

Elective and semi-elective open tracheostomy

- Before the incision into the trachea is made, check the tracheostomy tube: inflate the cuff and make sure there are no leaks; deflate the cuff and then gently lubricate the cuff and tube with lubricating jelly. Check that the connector is compatible with the anaesthetic tube and oxygen supply.
- Insert the tube at the same time as the endotracheal tube is withdrawn; make an immediate connection to the oxygen supply.
- Do not allow anyone to remove the endotracheal tube completely until you are certain your tracheostomy tube is in the correct position.
- In a child no part of the trachea should be excised, as there is a high risk of subsequent stenosis. Therefore a vertical incision is made over the second, third and fourth tracheal rings and a heavy suture is inserted through each side of the tracheal incision; this aids dilatation with the tracheal dilators and allows the tube to be inserted. The ends of the sutures should be left long so that they protrude through the incision to facilitate re-intubation should the tracheostomy be accidentally removed.

The same method can be used with advantage in adults. Some surgeons excise a circular piece of trachea anteriorly and others use a distally based flap. Subsequent stenosis is less likely in the adult, whichever method is adopted.

Percutaneous tracheostomy

Techniques

Techniques include:

- serial dilatation
- single tapered dilator
- guidewire dilatation
- forceps or screw.

Indication

Percutaneous tracheostomy is indicated for prolonged endotracheal intubation to facilitate weaning and nursing care.

Equipment

Equipment required is:

- bronchoscope
- 100% O_2
- sedation
- analgesia
- neuromuscular blockade.

Procedure

- Same position as for open tracheostomy.
- Infiltrate with lidocaine with adrenaline (epinephrine) over the incision site (1st and 2nd tracheal rings).
- Dissect down to trachea.
- Puncture trachea and insert guide wire or introducer.
- Check position of introducer/guide wire bronchoscopically.
- Dilate tract and introduce tracheostomy tube.

Complications of tracheostomy

Potential complications include:

- loss of airway
- malposition or displacement of tube
- haemorrhage
- bacteraemia
- surgical emphysema
- pneumothorax
- occlusion of tube
- oesophageal injury
- tracheal injury.

12 Principles of surgical oncology

The management of patients with cancer usually involves more than one specialist. Management decisions are made within a multidisciplinary team meeting (MDM or MDT) including surgeons, medical and clinical oncologists, radiologists, pathologists and specialists in palliative care. Increasingly, nurse specialists are also intimately involved in coordinating this multidisciplinary activity. Oncology therefore cuts across the traditional specialties, and the development of multidisciplinary teams provides a more efficient and complete service for patients. The surgeon may be called upon to assist with diagnosis, assessment of tumour staging and removal of tumour bulk and to perform surgical procedures to deal with mechanical complications. The diverse nature of surgical intervention demands considerable familiarity with the pathological basis of malignancy and the therapeutic options available.

A further aspect of oncological practice is the detection of malignancy before it has caused symptoms, or the identification of which patients or groups of patients are at high risk of developing malignant diseases. Both these roles are examples of screening, which is considered at the end of this chapter.

As in many other areas of medicine, the definition of terms can cause confusion. Malignancy means that a cell type has escaped normal control and is proliferating unchecked; the tissue of origin is not specified. Cancer used to mean a malignant tumour which had its origin in epithelial tissues, e.g. a squamous carcinoma of the skin or a transitional cell carcinoma of the bladder. However, this distinction has largely been lost and the terms 'cancer' and 'malignancy' are now used interchangeably.

GENERAL FEATURES OF MALIGNANT DISEASE

Incidence

Figures from the NHS in the UK show that malignant disease accounts for just over a quarter of all deaths (27%) in 2007, being second only to cardiovascular disease (approximately one-half). Table 12.1 shows the incidence of different types of malignancy in the UK in 2005.

Lung cancer still causes the greatest number of deaths for both men and women. Breast cancer is the second commonest cause of cancer death in women. Cancer of the gastrointestinal tract is the next most common cause. Total cancer deaths continue to increase, but the incidence of deaths from certain tumours, such as stomach cancer, is declining.

Aetiology

Malignancy is of diverse and multifactorial cause. No single chemical or biological factor has been definitively shown to cause human cancer. However, combinations of individual factors, such as genetic susceptibility, chemicals, occupation, lifestyle and viruses, may together induce malignant change in exposed or susceptible tissues. The assessment of a patient with suspected malignancy should include a family history and an enquiry of possible exposure to aetiological factors (Table 12.2). Their continued identification will inevitably lead to further preventative measures, comparable to the efforts being made to reduce the use of tobacco.

Epidemiology

Study of the population dynamics and distribution of malignancy helps in the appropriate planning of healthcare services and resources. In addition, detailed statistics can highlight trends in incidence that point to aetiological factors and geographical variations in the occurrence of tumours. The identification of causal occupational factors (e.g. exposure to industrial carcinogenic chemicals) has been largely the result of epidemiological study. In addition, epidemiological studies can identify groups with a high risk or a poor prognosis. These can then be subject to screening or rigorous follow-up after treatment.

Table 12.1 Incidence, per 100 000 population, of cancer in UK in 2005

	Men	Women
All cancers	523	430
Oesophagus	14	6
Stomach	14	6
Pancreas	10	8
Colon/rectum	56	36
Lung/bronchus	61	37
Breast	1	123
Kidney	13	7
Prostate	95	–
Non-Hodgkin's lymphoma	16	12

Table 12.2 Aetiological factors associated with malignant disease

Factor	Tumour
Genetic:	
Retinoblastoma (*Rb*) gene	Childhood retinoblastoma
Wilms' tumour gene	Nephroblastoma
p53 oncogene	Prevents malignant transformation unless mutated
FAP gene	Colonic carcinoma in patients with familial adenomatous polyposis (FAP)
Polyp–cancer sequence (multiple sequential genetic mutations)	Colorectal cancer
Environmental:	
Ultraviolet light	Basal cell carcinoma, malignant melanoma
Chemicals:	
Benzene	Leukaemia
β-Naphthylamine	Bladder carcinoma
Vinyl chloride	Hepatic angiosarcoma
Asbestos	Mesothelioma
Tar, crude oil	Squamous carcinoma
Tobacco smoke	Lung carcinoma
Ionising radiation	Skin tumours, leukaemias
Diet:	
Aflatoxins	Oesophageal carcinoma
Smoked foods	Gastric carcinoma
Alcohol	Oropharyngeal and oesophageal cancer
Drugs:	
Alkylating agents (in patients treated for other malignant disease)	Leukaemias
Viral:	
Hepatitis B and C virus	Hepatocellular carcinoma
Epstein–Barr virus	Burkitt's lymphoma, nasopharyngeal carcinoma
Human papilloma virus	Cervical carcinoma, anal cancer
Human immunodeficiency virus	Kaposi's sarcoma, B-cell lymphoma

BIOLOGY OF MALIGNANCY

Carcinogenesis and growth

Controlled cellular proliferation occurs during embryogenesis, hypertrophy, healing, regeneration, repair and during the metabolic response to trauma and sepsis. In many instances, cellular replication occurs because growth factors bind to specific receptors on the cell surface and induce intracellular signals which activate the nucleus and cause cell division. Within the nucleus, nucleoproteins ensure accurate DNA replication, DNA repair and DNA transcription to messenger RNA. However, these biochemical processes are susceptible to damage and malfunction by mutations, deletions or amplifications of the genes which code for many of the normal regulatory factors or their receptors. Mutations can occur either spontaneously or as a result of the interaction of aetiological factors with the DNA of the host. Malignancy is the consequence of escape from the normal controlling factors for cellular replication. At some point in the multi-step process of carcinogenesis, the transforming cell undergoes a number of genetic changes which result either in the unchecked expression of proto-oncogenes or in abrogation of the function of tumour suppressor genes. These are constituents of the human genome which are associated with normal cellular proliferation and differentiation. They become implicated in carcinogenesis when their encoded proteins are overproduced, mutated or otherwise modified so that their function is abnormally expressed, rather than regulated. This unregulated expression of normal genes may be responsible for the capacity of certain tumours to secrete proteins known as tumour markers into the circulation, e.g. carcinoembryonic antigen (CEA) for colorectal cancer and alpha-fetoprotein (AFP) for hepatocellular carcinoma.

Unlike normal tissues where, in general, a cell divides only in order to replace one which has been lost, tumour cells fail to respond to the signals which regulate normal replication. The belief that all tumours contain cells proliferating more rapidly than those in normal tissues is false. Most tumours enlarge because either the proportion of cells in the proliferative phase of the cell cycle (growth fraction) is greater than normal, or there is decreased cell loss from apoptosis (physiological cell death). It has been estimated that up to 50% of tumour cells are lost as a consequence of hypoxia, exfoliation, metastasis and destruction by host defences. Despite these losses, tumour cells adapt to the physiological selection pressures of their surroundings to achieve continuous advantage over the host. A further development of this adaptive nature is progression by which tumours become more aggressive with time and contain fewer cells which resemble their parent tissue, so producing cells with metastatic potential.

A fundamental concept is that change to malignant behaviour on the part of cells does not result in a single disease process. Tumours from the same tissue of origin may behave quite differently with respect to growth, invasion and metastases. This is frequently demonstrated by colonic tumours appearing as either bulky, locally invasive primary tumours without metastases or as small asymptomatic primary tumours with dissemination to other parts of the body. Carcinogenesis proceeds through multiple stages involving the interaction of different aetiological and host factors, each of which influences the tumour's final biological behaviour and clinical manifestations.

Influence of biology on clinical course

In general, a tumour is of sufficient size to be clinically palpable when it contains 10^9 or more cells; however, at clinical presentation most tumours have many more cells than this. Even the smallest radiologically detectable breast carcinoma contains 10^7–10^8 cells. Patients usually die when the total has reached 10^{12}. This natural history is shown diagrammatically in Figure 12.1.

Invasion and metastasis

Carcinoma in situ is a collection of malignant cells confined by their normal basement membrane. This is the earliest stage at which a tumour may be histologically identified and implies that the tissue has changed under carcinogenic influences. The cells are both functionally and structurally altered – a state of dysplasia. This process may be multifocal, which implies that the remaining apparently normal cells are at increased risk of malignant transformation (e.g. the normal mucosa surrounding a colonic carcinoma). The advance of malignant disease is by:

- local tissue invasion through and beyond the basement membrane
- distant spread of cells (metastasis) to form autonomous tumour deposits.

Invasion occurs when tumour cells start to secrete enzymes capable of digesting intercellular matrix. Many of these enzymes are now being characterised and their physiological or pharmacological inhibitors identified. Prominent among these enzymes are the matrix metalloproteinases. Through continued growth, suitably equipped cells can encroach upon and destroy adjacent organs (e.g. duodenal and bile duct obstruction from a pancreatic carcinoma). Tissue resistance to invasion is variable: arteries and tendons are rarely destroyed, but lymphatics and veins are commonly breached.

Tumour cells have metastatic capacity when they are able to:

- invade adjacent tissues (especially veins and lymphatics)
- survive in unfamiliar tissue environments – bloodstream, peritoneal cavity
- sustain their own proliferation to form a focus of tumour cells.

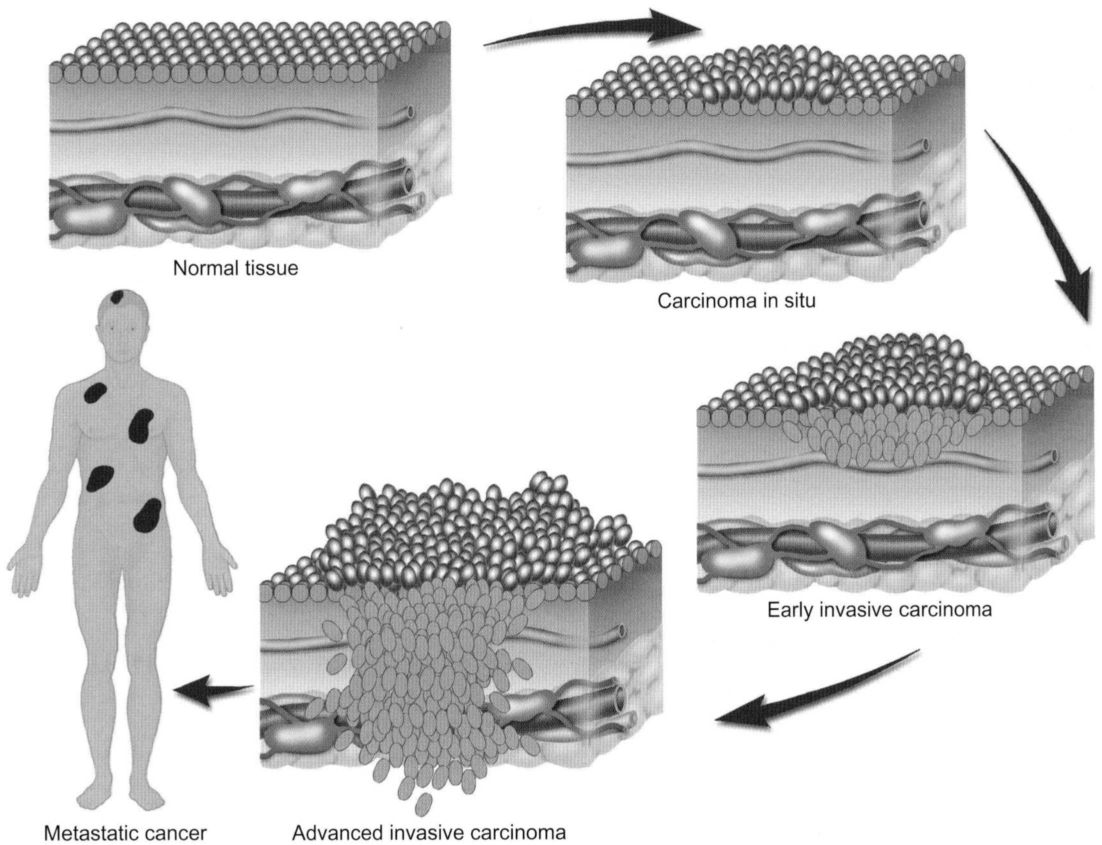

Fig. 12.1 The natural history of the development of malignant disease.

Although only about 1 in 10^6 tumour cells may have metastatic potential, many thousands of cells are shed from a tumour each day. Palpation or surgical manipulation of a tumour is known to increase shedding.

Tumour metastases may themselves undergo further malignant progression and bear little pathological resemblance to the primary tumour.

Routes of metastasis

Metastasis occurs by three routes (Fig. 12.2). Invasion of the lymphatics or veins allows the transport of viable invasive tumour cells to distant sites. The pattern of spread can be predicted for most tumours (e.g. breast and large bowel) and may be used to plan surgical removal of the primary tumour and possible sites of distant spread. Lymphatics usually accompany the arterial supply to an organ and so, in many instances, surgical removal of an organ which contains a tumour involves dissection of the arterial supply and removal of these vessels and their associated lymphatic tissue (e.g. radical gastrectomy, colectomy). Similarly, the venous drainage of an organ is an important determinant of venous metastatic spread. Because surgical manipulation of any malignant tumour causes shedding of tumour cells into lymphatics and veins, some surgical procedures have been designed to reduce this by initially dividing the blood supply, especially the veins (e.g. ligation of the inferior mesenteric vessels before mobilising a left-sided colonic tumour using a 'no-touch' technique – Fig. 12.3).

Distribution of metastases

The organ distribution of metastases varies with the type of tumour and is related to complex interactions between the migrating tumour cell and the capillary endothelium of the organ. Metastatic deposits may become sites from which tumour cells gain access to further vessels – metastases from metastases. In this way, tumours spread from the primary to predictable local metastatic sites, and then on to other less predictable places.

Some tumours have a predilection for particular metastatic sites. Gastrointestinal malignancy tends initially to metastasise to the liver via the portal venous circulation; renal and breast carcinoma to the lungs. Bony metastases are relatively common in all terminal disease but there are five tumours that commonly metastasise to bone:

- breast
- prostate
- lung
- kidney
- thyroid.

Occult micrometastases

Microscopic tumour deposits, present at the time of original diagnosis and treatment but which escape detection, may emerge as metastases or recurrent disease some time later. They are of considerable importance in surgical oncology. Although they are often called recurrence, they are in fact the continued growth of residual tumour. Modern oncological management aims to include adequate treatment to deal with

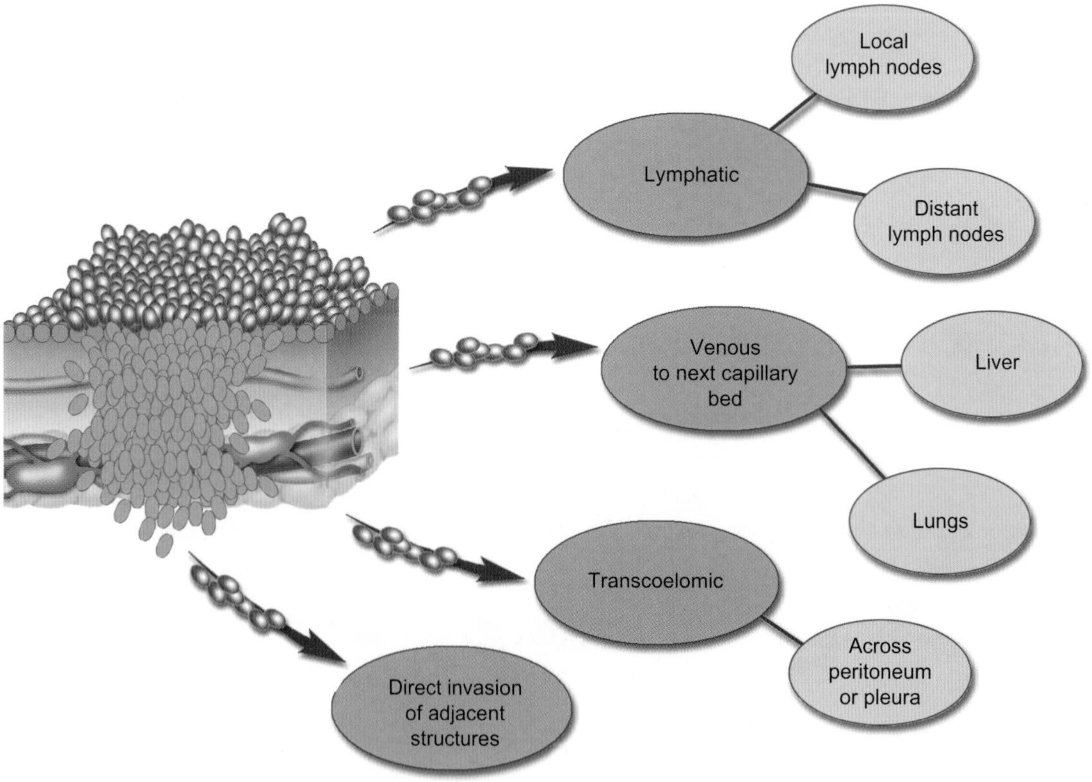

Fig. 12.2 Routes of tumour spread.

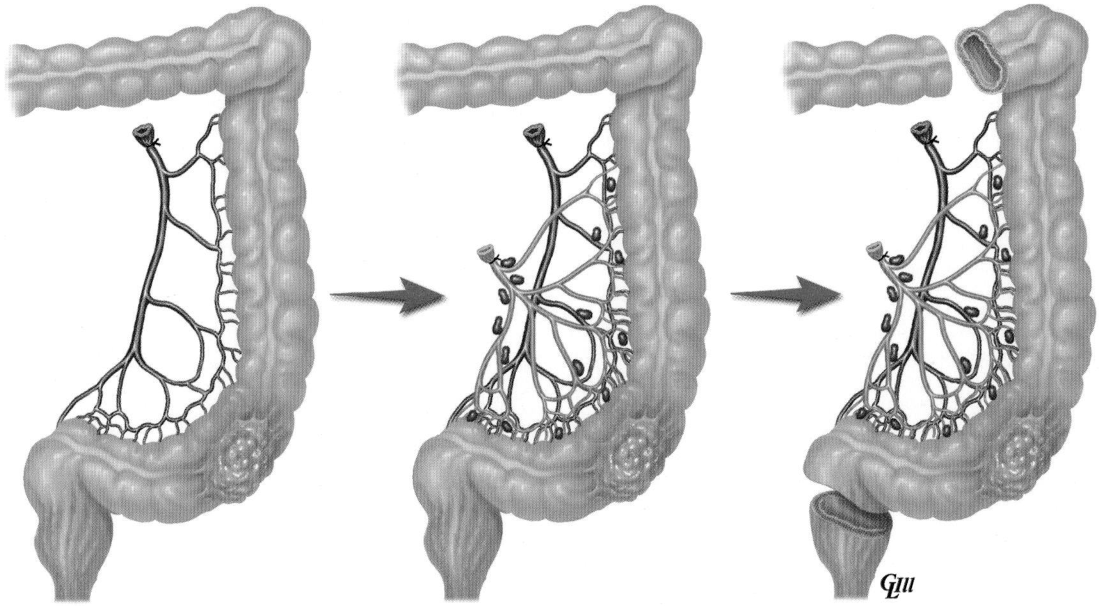

Fig. 12.3 Isolation of the tumour before surgical resection – the 'no-touch' technique.

such micrometastases. This involves systemic therapy additional to local surgical measures – adjuvant therapy, if given after the operation, or neoadjuvant therapy if given prior to surgical extirpation.

CLINICAL FEATURES OF MALIGNANT DISEASE

Most of these will be found in the individual chapters of this book devoted to regions or systems. The important clinical features of 'malignancy in general' are given in Box 12.1.

MANAGEMENT OF MALIGNANT DISEASE

Decisions about management must be made only after a full explanation of the condition and treatment options have been given to the patient and often also to his/her relatives. The advantages and risks of each treatment option, including where appropriate symptomatic treatment only, should be discussed before a treatment plan can be agreed.

PATIENT EVALUATION

The following components are involved:

History

- Duration and progression of symptoms – often symptoms last for months (rarely years) and are progressive
- Presence of non-specific symptoms such as fatigue, loss of appetite and weight
- Exposure to risk factors
- Family history of cancer.

Examination

- Identification of primary site (as suggested by the history)
- Evidence of local invasion (mobility or fixation, damage to local structures)
- Use of special techniques for individual circumstances – e.g. rectal examination, sigmoidoscopy
- Evidence of distant spread – palpable lymph nodes, enlargement or malfunction of organs (e.g. liver enlargement and jaundice), accumulation of effusions.

Investigation

Simple

- Full blood count – may reveal blood loss, marrow failure or infiltration
- Serum concentrations of urea and electrolytes – evidence of renal tract obstruction or dehydration
- Liver function tests – the presence of hepatic metastases or biliary tract obstruction
- Examination of urine for cytology and/or for the presence of tumour markers
- Plain X-ray, especially of the chest, for primary tumour or metastases
- Measurement of serum tumour markers, e.g. CEA, CA 125.

More complex

These investigations are determined by the suspected clinical diagnosis and include:

- contrast examination of the GI tract
- ultrasound scan, usually of solid organs

Box 12.1 Clinical features suggestive of malignant disease

Palpable swelling
This is most often painless. It is usually irregular and firm (unless bony in origin). It may be invading local structures and therefore fixed.

Anaemia
Loss of blood occurs readily from disorganised capillaries and other vessels in the tumour. Continued bleeding from a surface lesion should be viewed with suspicion. Internal bleeding (e.g. into the gut) is most often chronic and concealed; the result is iron deficiency anaemia of unknown origin.

Consequences of local invasion
Hollow tube obstruction is a sinister development in the natural history of a tumour. Examples of manifestations are dysphagia (oesophageal), abdominal colic (small and large bowel), jaundice (bile duct), hydronephrosis (renal tract) and bilateral leg oedema (inferior vena cava). Perforation of a hollow tube can follow invasion, with development of an acute emergency (e.g. perforation of a gastric carcinoma). Local invasion may also lead to destruction of tissue (e.g. nerves and bone) with pain.

Metastatic spread
This is common. Presentation is with a history of progressive general tiredness, weight loss and anorexia. Examination may reveal the signs of metastatic deposits: irregular hepatomegaly, lymphadenopathy, ascites, pleural effusion, pathological fracture, focal headache and epileptic fits (cerebral deposits).

Biochemical effects
This relates to the production of substances associated with clinical effects:

- *parathyroid hormone analogue* (PTH-rp) causes malignancy-related hypercalcaemia; it is not uncommon in breast and neoplasms but may be seen in any tumour causing significant bone destruction
- *antidiuretic hormone* in bronchogenic carcinoma
- *adrenocorticotrophic hormone* in pituitary tumours, leading to increased corticosteroid output
- *5-hydroxytryptamine* in carcinoid tumours
- *adrenaline* in phaeochromocytoma.

Asymptomatic detection
During routine assessment of other conditions (e.g. preoperative check before herniorrhaphy), never overlook the possibility of malignant disease.
Do not forget: *if you do not look you cannot find.*

- computed tomography
- magnetic resonance imaging
- positron emission tomography – PET scanning, usually with fluorodeoxy-glucose (FDG).

Invasive

These are usually directed both towards reaching a definitive diagnosis and assessing the extent of the problem:

- endoscopy, including the upper and lower GI tracts, the biliary tree and the air passages, all of which can include biopsy
- laparoscopy and thoracoscopy, also with biopsy.

Aspiration cytology and tissue biopsy (see also Ch. 4)

These are techniques that allow a pathological diagnosis to be reached – an essential preliminary to treatment. Aspiration cytology gives an assessment only of the shape and other features of individual cells. Histological examination of a tissue sample shows the pathological architecture (the relationship between cells and their surroundings).

Aspiration is done by passing a fine needle into the lesion and applying suction with a syringe. Small fragments are drawn back into the barrel and can be extracted and stained for examination under the microscope.

Needle biopsy uses a needle of larger calibre often equipped with a cutting device. A tissue core is extracted, processed and sectioned, so providing an histological section.

Open biopsy exposes the lesion and either removes part (incisional) or all (excisional) of it for histopathological examination. Biopsies of this nature can be processed immediately (frozen section) or by standard paraffin-embedded sections.

Guidance

All the above methods may be undertaken under some form of guidance. X-ray, ultrasonography or CT scanning may have been done previously and the site marked; more commonly the needle biopsy or incision may be performed under real-time image control, most commonly by ultrasound.

Tumour staging and prognosis

Staging

Staging is the attempt to classify tumours into categories (stages) of their natural history by using agreed criteria which are known to be relevant to prognosis. To categorise a patient into the appropriate stage is an essential part of the decision-making process for correct treatment. Many systems have been devised for tumours of different organs or anatomical regions. Most were originally based solely upon clinical findings or sometimes upon additional findings, such as the histopathological features for an individual tumour group, e.g. the clinical staging for breast carcinoma (Ch. 27) and the Dukes classification for colorectal cancer (Ch. 24). However, the more recent and widely adopted TNM (tumour, nodes, metastases) system (Box 12.2) allows a single generic method to be applied to almost all tumours, which has the advantage of allowing for different biological behaviour because each value of T, N and M is scored independently.

Histological grade (Table 12.3)

The histological grade, obtained either from a tumour biopsy or from the excised specimen, can be used in conjunction with the TNM stage to give a more accurate assessment of prognosis for an individual patient. This information allows more precise evaluation of the efficacy of different treatments on tumours of comparable stage. For example, a radical mastectomy (Ch. 28) for a histological grade 1 breast carcinoma of stage T1–N0–M0 may lead to cure, but the prognosis for long-term survival is more guarded in a tumour of similar stage but which is grade 3.

Prognostic markers

Both molecular and genetic markers which give prognostic information have been identified for some tumours. In breast

Box 12.2 The TNM staging system

Tumour
- T0: primary unknown (Tis: tumour in situ)
- T1: tumour < 2 cm metastases present
- T2: tumour > 2 cm
- T3: tumour > 5 cm (or reaching serosa in GI tract)
- T4: tumour infiltrating local tissues, e.g. skin, vessels, nerves

Nodes
- N0: not involved
- N1: local nodes involved
- N2: distant nodes involved

Metastases
- M0: no metastases
- M1: metastases present
- Mx: status unknown

Postoperative
R0: no residual tumour
R1: microscopic residual disease
R2: macroscopic residual disease

Table 12.3 Histological classification

Differentiation	Features
Grade 1 – well differentiated	Forms recognisable structures of parent tissue
Grade 2 – moderately differentiated	Some degree of organisation
Grade 3 – poorly differentiated	Architecture totally disorganised; cells not recognisable from parent tissue

cancers, the presence of nuclear receptor for oestrogen indicates a good prognosis, whilst those tumours which express an excess of receptors for epidermal growth factor or the oncogene c-erbB2 have a worse prognosis. Many new 'markers' of prognosis are described each year.

OPERATIVE SURGERY FOR MALIGNANT DISEASE

Histological confirmation

Before definitive elective treatment of a tumour there must (usually) be unequivocal histological confirmation of malignancy and an accurate assessment of the stage. However, some patients present with a surgical emergency (e.g. an obstructing carcinoma of the colon) which requires surgical intervention without either of the above items of information. In these cases a decision about the extent of surgical treatment is made on the operative findings, supplemented if possible by urgent pathological examination of tissue during the course of the procedure (frozen section).

Aim

The aim of surgical management is either curative or palliative. Those with obvious widespread tumours should not be treated by a surgical effort to achieve cure; a lesser procedure may be performed (e.g. bypass of a gastrointestinal tumour) to relieve distressing symptoms such as pain or gastrointestinal obstruction. Referral for non-surgical treatment or for palliative care is then appropriate.

Surgical attempt at cure involves the total excision of all tumour-bearing tissues together with the associated lymphatic and venous drainage (e.g. radical gastrectomy). Invasion of adjacent vital structures (e.g. invasion of the trachea by an oesophageal cancer) may determine the feasibility of removing a tumour (its *operability*, which is not the same as *curability*). By contrast, involvement of non-essential structures does not prevent resection of a tumour with the invaded structures (e.g. a colonic tumour that has invaded the small bowel). How far to place the resection away from the visible growth (*resection margin*) is decided by knowledge of the behaviour of the tumour and its propensity to local invasion. Both are described in the appropriate sections of this book. For most neoplasms treated by surgery the technical aim is to remove the tumour, the organ in which it is contained and the regional lymph node drainage (lymphatics and nodes) all in one piece: *en-bloc*.

Reconstruction after curative surgery is an important aspect of surgical technique. Most patients naturally wish to regain as near normal a lifestyle and self-perception as possible. An ileostomy (Ch. 24) requires more departures from usual habits than does a successful ileo-anal pouch (Ch. 26). Reconstruction after mastectomy (Ch. 28) restores body image and self-confidence. A careful, informed and sympathetic discussion with the patient is needed to reach a joint conclusion about the course of action.

ADJUVANT THERAPY

One of the most challenging areas in surgical oncology is the treatment of patients with apparently early disease. Clinical experience over the last 50 years has clearly shown that curative surgery alone for tumours that seem to be localised leads to cure in only a proportion of patients. This indicates either that some patients may have undetected micrometastases at the time of presentation or that surgical intervention triggers the release and seeding of tumour cells to distant sites where their growth becomes clinically evident some time after the initial surgery. Adjuvant therapy is additional anti-neoplastic treatment which is used for some patients with tumours that are thought to have been completely removed by surgical excision. Adjuvant chemotherapy, local radiotherapy or hormone therapy, or sometimes various combinations of these, aim to destroy occult micrometastases. Success in this effort must always be balanced against the fact that adjuvant treatment will be given to a varying proportion of patients who do not have micrometastases and who therefore do not need it.

Accordingly, adjuvant treatments must:

- be relatively non-toxic
- have been demonstrated to have efficacy against the same tumour, usually in patients with advanced disease
- have been proven to improve survival in randomised trials unless being given within such a trial.

Timing of adjuvant therapy

Adjuvant therapy was traditionally used only after curative surgery. More recently, treatment has been used before

Table 12.4 Adjuvant and neo-adjuvant therapy

Tumour	Adjuvant protocol	Timing
Breast	Epirubicin, cyclophosphamide and 5-fluorouracil	Postoperative
Oesophagus	Cisplatin and 5-fluorouracil, *or* epirubicin, cisplatin and 5-fluorouracil	Pre-operative
Colorectal	5-fluorouracil and oxaliplatin with folinic acid FOLFOX	Postoperative
Rectum	Chemoradiotherapy	Pre-operative

operation – neo-adjuvant therapy. Some examples of the protocols currently in use are shown in Table 12.4. A useful shrinkage of some tumours – oesophageal, rectal and breast – can be achieved by preoperative radiotherapy, and some of the many protocols for the treatment of breast cancer include postoperative radiotherapy.

NON-OPERATIVE THERAPY

Radiotherapy

Knowledge of the radiotherapeutic options for a particular tumour is essential for the practising surgeon. Unfortunately, a large number of tumours are relatively radio-resistant. Examples are clear cell carcinoma of the adult kidney, adenocarcinoma of the stomach and malignant melanoma.

Principles

The unit of absorbed radiation energy is the gray (Gy), 1 Gy being equivalent to 1 joule per kilogram (J/kg). Radiation acts by inducing chemical changes within the nucleus of the cell that cause damage to DNA. Irradiation depopulates a tumour of its malignant cells mainly via direct effects during mitosis, and thus its efficacy is determined by:

- the number of viable cells present
- intrinsic radiosensitivity of the cells
- mitotic rate.

Because irradiation damage takes place during mitosis, it follows that normal tissues, which have a high cellular turnover (such as the bone marrow and enterocytes), will also show evidence of damage within hours of irradiation. For the same reason, it may be weeks or months before the maximum effect of radiotherapy is apparent in a more slowly proliferating tumour such as basal cell carcinoma of the skin.

Dose and fractionation

The total dose of radiotherapy for a tumour is calculated for each individual site and size. Modern therapy is now given in fractions of the total dose, because this minimises the unpleasant side effects of treatment, i.e.:

- local soreness
- skin changes
- lethargy
- nausea and vomiting.

The spectrum of electromagnetic radiation can be adjusted to increase penetration into deep tissues. Newer 'supervoltage' apparatus is based on this principle. This can be used to focus treatment at a tumour site from different directions, thus enhancing the destruction of tumour cells without damaging surrounding structures. The level of expertise with this fractionated radiotherapy is now such that not only is it used as palliative therapy for certain unresectable or metastatic lesions but also it is employed as an adjuvant to surgery (e.g. following wide local excision of T1–T2 breast carcinomas or before excision of a rectal carcinoma).

Other methods of application

In addition to external beam irradiation mentioned above, radiotherapy can be applied in other ways.

Radioactive implants

These may be inserted into tumours to achieve maximum dose (brachytherapy):

- endoluminal radiation for oesophageal and rectal tumours
- iridium wires for cervical carcinoma
- yttrium implants for pituitary tumours.

Systemic administration of radioactive substances

This can be used if the tumour is known selectively to take up known chemicals. Radioactive iodine can be taken up by cells of thyroid tumours, which incorporate it as they synthesise thyroxine.

Chemotherapy

Cytotoxic drugs interfere with cell division in normal and malignant cells. Therefore the success of their use depends on:

- intrinsic resistance of the tumour cell to the agent
- the toxic effect on normal tissues, which limits the dose.

The gap between the two may be very narrow.

Types of chemotherapeutic agents

There are four main groups as well as additional miscellaneous agents. Many of these agents are used in varying combinations which have been developed empirically to maximise therapeutic efficacy without excessively increasing toxicity. However, their effects on normal proliferating cells result in bone marrow and intestinal toxicity.

Alkylating agents

Examples of these are the nitrosoureas and epoxide compounds – cyclophosphamide, melphalan, chlorambucil – which combine with intracellular molecules such as nucleic acids, proteins (especially enzymes) and cell membranes. Damage to the enzymes which link DNA strands, critically disrupts mitosis.

Antimetabolites

Antimetabolites – methotrexate, 5-fluorouracil, cytosine arabinoside and 6-mercaptopurine – disrupt the sequence of

DNA by being incorporated instead of the normal nucleotide or by irreversibly binding to the constituting enzyme in order to render it ineffective.

Vinca alkaloids

These bind to intracellular tubulin and inhibit microtubule formation. The latter is the spindle during mitosis, and in consequence this is arrested at metaphase.

Antimitotic antibiotics

These include doxorubicin, epirubicin, actinomycin D, mitomycin C and bleomycin. The first two intercalate between opposing DNA strands and disturb DNA function. Actinomycin D and mitomycin C are inhibitors of DNA and RNA synthesis, respectively, and also generate free oxygen radicals which are toxic.

Miscellaneous agents

There is a further group of agents whose mechanisms of action are varied or unknown. Cis-platinum and its less toxic derivative carboplatin react with the guanine in DNA and form cross-linkages along the DNA chain as well as between DNA strands. Other agents, such as etoposide, are tubular poisons derived from podophyllotoxin.

Biological response modification

Endocrine manipulation has been used for many years to control tumours which arise from cells that are dependent on hormones for their normal growth and division. The effect is obtained in a number of ways:

- removing the endocrine organ or organs that produce the hormone – orchidectomy for prostate cancer
- inhibiting hormone production with antagonists to releasing hormones – genetically engineered luteinising hormone release hormone (LHRH) for prostate cancer
- blocking the stimulatory action of the hormone by using the endocrine antagonist – oestrogens in large doses for prostatic cancer to exhaust testosterone production from the testis
- blocking the receptor site for the hormone on the malignant cell – tamoxifen prevents oestrogen binding in breast cancer.

The discovery of receptor sites for autocrine hormones on many different tumour cells will undoubtedly lead to the construction of synthetic analogues which block receptor binding and activation.

Biological therapies may also use the body's immune system to fight the cancer. Agents used include interferon, interleukins and colony-stimulating factors.

Monoclonal antibodies directed against cell growth factors have been introduced: e.g. trastuzumab for patients with HER-2 positive breast cancers, and cetuximab and bevacizumab for advanced colorectal cancer. Other monoclonal antibodies attach to the surface of tumour cells and stimulate the patient's immune system to destroy these cells: e.g. rituximab for non-Hodgkin's lymphoma. Monoclonal antibodies can also be used to deliver drugs or radiation directly to cancer cells and a number of clinical trials are underway.

ASSESSMENT OF RESPONSE TO TREATMENT

Clinicians must assess their therapeutic performance in two ways:

- review treatment outcome in their own patients – clinical audit
- study the publications that compare current treatment with new experimental protocols.

Such periodic appraisal allows advances to be incorporated into practice and outmoded treatments to be discarded.

Methods of assessment

Five-year survival

This has been the traditional method of outcome assessment. The figure is helpful in studying groups of patients who may receive different forms of treatment, but it gives little information that is relevant to the individual patient.

Median survival time (or median time to recurrence)

This information is more useful to clinician and patient than 5-year survival and is the preferred method. For example, the 5-year survival rate for pancreatic carcinoma treated by resectional surgery is approximately 25%, but the median survival is approximately 18 months.

Serial imaging of progression

The response of inoperable or metastatic tumour to non-surgical treatment can be gauged by serial imaging (ultrasound, CT or MRI) of the tumour. In such circumstances, duration of response is of equal importance to magnitude and is measured as the median duration of response in the patients treated. Accepted grades of response are given in Table 12.5.

Patient well-being

How a patient 'feels' is a subjective marker of response to reduction in the bulk of a tumour and of the side effects of the treatment that is being used. A number of scales have been formulated to assess this aspect of treatment (see Box 12.3).

Table 12.5 Grading of tumour response to non-surgical therapy for solid tumours (RECIST) criteria

Grade	Assessment
Complete response (CR)	Disappearance of all known lesions, confirmed at 4 weeks
Partial response (PR)	Decrease in tumour size by more than 30%, confirmed at 4 weeks
Stable disease (SD)	Less than 30% decrease or 20% increase in tumour size
Progressive disease (PD)	Greater than 20% increase in tumour size or of a deposit, or new lesions

Box 12.3 Scales for measurement of patient well-being

Karnovsky Performance Status scale
This scale provides a score, e.g.:
100 – Well, no complaints
50 – Requires considerable assistance and medical care
10 – Moribund

European Cooperative Oncology Group scale
ECOG 0 – asymptomatic
ECOG 1 – minor limitation
ECOG 2 – moderate limitation
ECOG 3 – severe limitation
ECOG 4 – moribund

Quality of life score
This is obtained from a multiple-field questionnaire

TERMINAL CARE

Terminal care should be seen as an integral part of oncological management and of equal importance to any of the other therapeutic disciplines. Accurate assessment of the disease will enable a prediction of the likely sequence of terminal events. Some of these (e.g. nausea) can be anticipated and prophylaxis undertaken.

Informing the patient

When treatment for cure fails or when treatment for palliation begins, a full and frank discussion about the prognosis and the plan of management is essential. The patient has an absolute right to this information, which can never be justifiably withheld, even if disclosure is against the wishes of relatives. Once the patient is fully aware of the situation, referral to a team which can provide palliative care should be sought. Although not necessarily about to die at this stage, many patients are apprehensive for their future and appreciate an introduction to those who may treat them in a later phase.

Fear of death and dying

For most patients with malignant disease, their abiding fear is of a painful, lingering death. Terminal care exists to alleviate both the psychological torment of impending death by counselling of patient and family and the physical problems posed by progressive malignant disease. Foremost in the aims of terminal care is keeping the patient in the familiar surroundings of home. Adequate facilities and the provision of satisfactory analgesia and nursing management must be available. There are a number of charity-based cancer nursing agencies in the UK for this purpose; they are staffed by nurses specially trained in the management of malignant disease and in dealing with its psychological impact on the patient and relatives.

SCREENING FOR MALIGNANT DISEASE

Tumours might either be foreseen in those who are known to be at high risk or detected early by examining in some way or other those in the population who might be susceptible. Such activities are called screening.

Table 12.6 Screening programmes

Method	Tumour
Mammography (high risk, 50–65 years)	Breast
Faecal occult blood (FOB) testing	Colorectal
Colonoscopy (genetic high-risk groups)	Colorectal
Oesophagogastroscopy (dysplasia – high-risk groups)	Oesophagus, stomach
Serum prostate-specific antigen	Prostate

Population screening. The knowledge that a large proportion of patients present with advanced disease has prompted the idea of screening the entire population. However, population screening often yields relatively few unsuspected tumours at a pathological stage which would make cure more likely. The cost of these huge projects is high.

Targeted screening of high-risk groups significantly increases the number of patients detected in relation to the cost of the procedure. The cost/benefit ratio is consequently improved.

Desirable criteria for a screening programme

For a screening programme to be effective, the following points are essential:

- The disease should be common or have defined high-risk groups.
- The natural history of the disease should be known, in order to define lesions which are truly localised and identify opportunities for curative treatment.
- Sensitive and specific methods of early detection must be available.
- Detection methods should be cheap, easy to use, and have a high patient compliance.
- Effective treatment for early disease should be available.
- The screening procedure must not involve significant hazard to the population tested.

Table 12.6 lists a number of tumours for which screening programmes are undergoing evaluation. However, few meet all of the above criteria.

Screening for recurrence of tumour

What is often called 'recurrence' of a tumour is in fact the progression of 'residual disease'. In some cases, the latter may be amenable to further surgical treatment (e.g. excision of a metastasis in the liver after primary resection of a colorectal carcinoma).

Simple methods

In those treated with the intention of cure, clinical assessment to detect residual tumour is often undertaken on a regular basis by follow-up and periodic examination. Features indicating the presence of disease, such as return of symptoms, enlargement of the liver or the development of

Table 12.7 Tumour markers in serum

Marker	Tumour
Prostate-specific antigen (PSA)	Prostate
Carcinoembryonic antigen (CEA)	Colorectal
Alpha-fetoprotein (AFP)	Hepatocellular
Beta-human chorionic gonadotrophin (β-hCG)	Testicular, gestational
CA 19-9	Colorectal, pancreatic
CA 125	Ovarian

palpable lymph nodes are sought. When such features are found, further investigation for evidence of tumour should follow. However, by this time the disease is often re-established and incurable. Earlier diagnosis of residual or recurrent disease may allow for more effective treatment. The techniques used in population screening are appropriate, because patients who have been treated for malignant disease are, by definition, a subpopulation with a high risk of recurrence, e.g. metachronous cancer of the colon or breast.

Tumour markers

These molecules (Table 12.7) are products of tumours which may be detected in body fluids or sometimes in urine in abnormally high levels. Their use in diagnostic screening is limited by the incidence of false positives in patients with benign disease.

Other methods of detection of residual disease

Monoclonal antibodies against tumour antigens can be radiolabelled. The antibodies seek out the tumour cells and can then be detected by gamma camera scanning for sites of increased uptake (e.g. colorectal tumour deposits in the liver).

FURTHER READING

Chaudry MA, Winslet MC 2009 Surgical oncology (Oxford Specialist Handbooks in Surgery). OUP, Oxford

Silberman H, Silberman AW 2009 Principles and practice of surgical oncology. Lippincott, Williams & Wilkins, Philadelphia

Poston GJ, Beauchamp RD, Ruers TJM 2007 Textbook of surgical oncology. Informa Healthcare, London

13 Organ transplantation

Over the past 30 years, organ transplantation has become a rapidly expanding and important surgical specialty. More than any other branch of surgery, organ transplantation requires the close cooperation of several disciplines – surgeons, anaesthetists, immunologists and physicians – to achieve a successful outcome. A synopsis of its historical landmarks is provided in Box 13.1.

Essential definitions

Autograft. Free (i.e. after disconnection of the blood supply) transplantation of tissue from one part of the body to another in the same individual.

Isograft. The transfer of tissue between genetically identical individuals – in humans this is between identical twins (rejection is not a feature of auto- or isografts).

Allograft. An organ or structure transplanted from an individual of the same species. Allografts are at the moment the main class of transplant in humans.

Xenograft. The transfer of organs between dissimilar species. Presently limited to tissues that have been chemically processed to make them non-antigenic, e.g. porcine heart valves. However, this is potentially the most exciting technique because, should it prove successful, the present acute shortage of organs for transplantation would be overcome. Great progress is being made in understanding the nature of the difficulties that form a barrier to xenografting.

Orthotopic graft. The donor organ is transplanted to the same site as the recipient's diseased one. The removal of the latter is first required, e.g. liver transplantation.

Heterotopic graft. The donor organ is inserted at a site different from its normal anatomical position, e.g. kidney transplantation to the iliac fossa.

Artificial (hybrid) organ implantation. The transplantation of bio-artificial organs, which are a combination of biomaterials and living cells, e.g. a hybrid artificial pancreas. At present this technique is experimental. Success would, as with xenografting, open a new chapter in transplantation.

Organ donation

Cadaver graft. An organ or tissue retrieved from an individual who has been pronounced dead according to criteria which differ from one culture to another (see below). There are currently three systems of cadaveric organ donation in use: 'required request', 'opting out' and 'opting in'. These are summarised in Box 13.2; however, no matter which system is adopted, the wishes of the family of the donor are the most important factor.

Living donors. There are two classes:

- *related donors* – parents or siblings who may have some genetic advantages and a sense of family or social obligation
- *unrelated donors* – In UK most of these are spousal or transplants from partners or friends. A small number are kidneys from individuals with a high philanthropic sense. In contrast to UK practice, internationally many kidneys come from donors who wish to make money. Although selling a kidney is outlawed in the West there is a thriving trade in other parts of the world and the moral issues are complex.

With the continued rise in the number of patients on waiting lists in the presence of a static or falling number of available organs, a number of patients from the UK are travelling abroad, mainly to countries in Asia, for their transplants. Most UK transplant centres will now support travel by potential related donors to the UK, where the pre-donation investigations are carried out prior to transplantation if the donor is suitable.

Box 13.1 Some landmarks in transplantation

Date	Event
c. AD 300	*Cosmos and Damian:* believed to have attempted a leg transplant
1778	*John Hunter:* coined the term transplant
1863	*Bert:* observed ingrowth of vessels into skin grafts and defined autograft, allograft and xenograft
1905	*Guthrie and Carrel:* developed vascular anastomotic techniques
1933	*Voronoy:* first human renal transplant – failed because of ABO incompatibility
1945	*Hume:* first short-lived functioning renal allograft
1950	*Lawler:* first long-term survivor from renal grafting
1963	*Starzl:* first human liver allograft
1966	*Lillehei:* first human pancreas transplant – technical success
1967	*Lillehei:* first human bowel transplant – failed
1967	*Starzl:* first long-term survivor from liver transplantation
1967	*Barnard:* first successful heart transplant
1981	*Shumway:* first successful heart-lung transplant
1988	*Grant:* first long-term survivor of small-bowel transplantation

Box 13.2 Systems currently in use for organ donation

- *Required request:* doctors looking after the potential donor have to ask, or refer the patient to, a retrieval coordinator who will enquire about donation.
- *Opting out or presumed consent:* all donors are presumed to have consented unless the family on approach refuse consent or the patient has previously registered his or her wish not to consent. This system produces the highest number of donors.
- *Opting in or required consent:* this is the system in use in the UK. Medical or nursing staff approach the family to ask about organ donation. Approximately one-third of the families refuse donation. To reduce this proportion, currently people are encouraged to register their desire for donation in the event of death on the NHS organ register. The register can be accessed prior to talking to the family.

BASIC IMMUNOLOGY OF ORGAN TRANSPLANTATION

Successful organ transplantation (with the exception of the cornea) requires the manipulation of the immunological defences of the recipient so as to overcome rejection. Because auto- and isografts do not elicit an immune response, it must be the genetic differences between the donor and the recipient that are of major importance in this process. These differences are expressed as *tissue or histocompatibility antigens*. The latter stimulate and lead the activation and proliferation of the immune cells and also identify cells which are the targets of the effector mechanisms induced by the immune reaction. The key cells involved in the rejection process are lymphocytes and antigen-presenting cells.

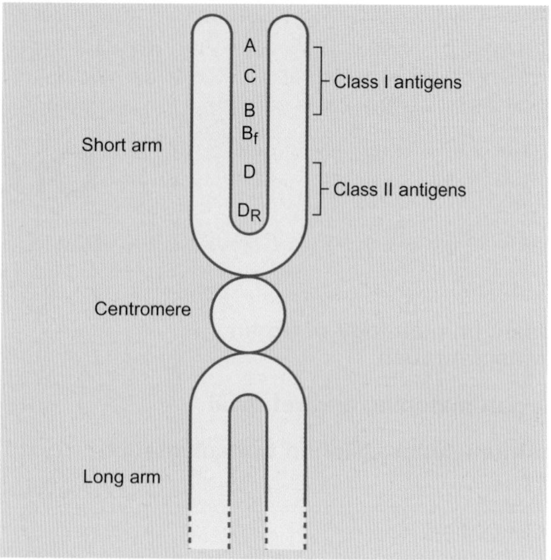

Fig. 13.1 Position of the major histocompatibility locus on the short arm of chromosome 6.

Major histocompatibility complex (MHC)

A large group of genes is present on the short arm of human chromosome 6 (Fig. 13.1), including those that encode the class I and class II MHC molecules which are involved in the presentation of antigens to T-cells. Class I molecules are integral membrane proteins found in all nucleated cells and platelets – the classical transplantation antigens. Class II molecules are expressed on B-cells, macrophages, monocytes, antigen-presenting cells (APCs) and some T-cells.

Human leucocyte antigen (HLA) loci

There are four of these on the short arm of chromosome 6:

- HLA-A – over 20 alleles have been identified
- HLA-B – over 30 alleles have so far been characterised
- HLA-C (between A and B) – seems not to have a role in mounting the immune response
- HLA-DR – appears to be clinically most important in that, if donor and recipient match for it, graft survival is improved.

Cells involved in the immune response to a transplant

Lymphocytes

These are the key cells controlling the immune response. They specifically recognise foreign (non-self) material as different from the tissues of the body. Lymphocytes are of two main types: B-cells and T-cells.

B-cells develop in the fetal liver and subsequently in bone marrow. Mature B-cells carry surface immunoglobulins which constitute their antigen receptor. The response to an antigenic stimulus is cell division and differentiation into plasma cells under the control of cytokines released by T-cells.

T-cells develop in the thymus, which is seeded during embryonic development with lymphocytic stem cells from the bone marrow. T-cells then develop their antigen receptors and differentiate into two major peripheral subsets: one expresses the CD4 marker, and the other the CD8. T-cells have a number of functions, including:

- helping B-cells to make antibody ($CD4^+$)
- recognising and destroying cells infected with viruses ($CD8^+$)
- activating phagocytes to destroy ingested pathogens ($CD4^+$)
- controlling the level and quality of the immune response ($CD8^+$).

Antigen-presenting cells

These are a group defined functionally by their ability to take up antigens and present them to lymphocytes in a form the latter can recognise. Some antigens are taken up by APCs in the periphery and transported to secondary lymphoid tissues. Others are intercepted as they arrive by APCs normally resident in lymph nodes and other lymphoid aggregates. B-cells recognise antigen in its native form, but T-cells recognise antigenic peptides that have been associated with self MHC molecules. In consequence, to present an antigen to a T-cell, an APC must internalise it, process it into fragments and re-express these at the cell surface in association with class II MHC molecules. In addition, many APCs provide additional stimulatory signals to lymphocytes either by direct cellular interactions or via cytokines (Fig. 13.2).

Rejection

Rejection is a destructive reaction initiated by the host to foreign HLA and other non-shared antigens. The process involves:

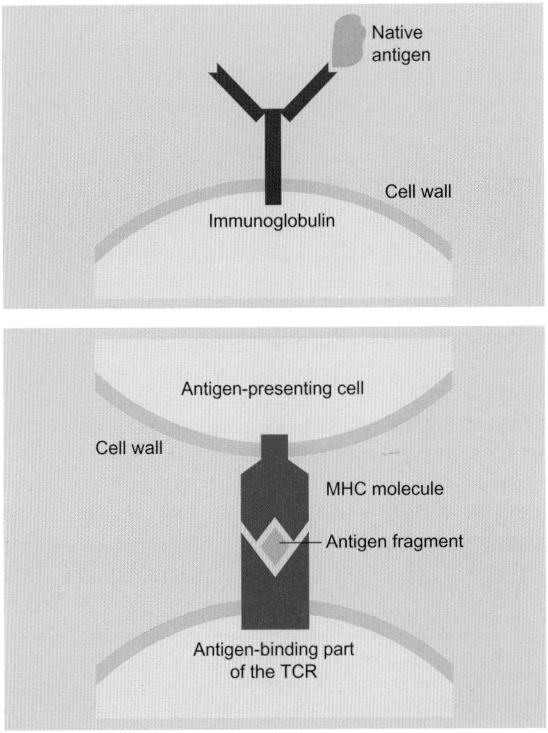

Fig. 13.2 Antigen handling by B- and T-cells. TCR, T-cell receptor.

- antigen recognition (afferent arc)
- activation of selected clones of T-cells and the effector mechanisms (efferent arc).

Afferent arc

Two routes lead to activation:

- foreign antigen or donor antigen-presenting cells (e.g. dendritic cells) which are directly recognised by the recipient's T-cells
- intracellular processing of foreign antigens by host antigen-presenting cells and subsequent presentation of peptides to T-cells.

Class II HLA antigens activate T helper ($CD4^+$) cells, and class I HLA antigens activate cytotoxic ($CD8^+$) T-cells.

Efferent arc

There is proliferation and differentiation of the selected T-cell population. $CD4^+$ cells (T helper – Th cells) produce interleukin-X (IL-10) which induces macrophages to produce IL-1, which in turn stimulates Th cells to produce IL-2 and other cytokines (e.g. IL-4, IL-5, IL-6). The latter cause B-cells to differentiate into plasma cells and to secrete antibody. Cytokines also stimulate $CD8^+$ cells to become cytotoxic. The coating of target cells by antibody allows K cells (large granular lymphocytes), macrophages or granulocytes to recognise and destroy them through a variety of mechanisms (release of enzymes, reactive oxygen mediators and perforins).

Clinical patterns of rejection

There are three patterns of rejection:

- *hyperacute and acute accelerated rejection* – this is the result of preformed IgG antibody and occurs within hours of exposure
- *acute cellular rejection* – this is infiltration by activated T-cells with recruitment of acute inflammatory cells; generally seen at 7–14 days post-transplant.
- *chronic rejection* – this is a major cause of graft attrition and is probably antibody-mediated. There is intimal hyperplasia and endarteritis obliterans. In liver transplants it is associated with loss of bile duct radicles.

Chronic rejection is difficult to treat, but strategies that involve the newer anti-B-cell drugs (e.g. mycophenolate mofetil) or rapamycin, which is not nephrotoxic, may have a role in the future.

ORGAN MATCHING AND RETRIEVAL

Organ matching

ABO compatibility

The biological rules are the same as those which govern blood transfusion. Because ABO red cell antigens are expressed on most tissue cells, ABO-incompatible allografts undergo hyperacute rejection. However, the rhesus factor is expressed only on red blood cells and therefore a match for it is not required for successful transplantation.

HLA-A, HLA-B and HLA-DR matching

Tissue typing (identification of the A, B and DR antigens) is carried out on the donor and the recipient by the separation of lymphocytes out of heparinised whole blood and their exposure to antibodies of known HLA-A, HLA-B and HLA-DR specificity. The technique is particularly relevant in the investigation of a family where a living donor may be available, and it also enables HLA-identical siblings to be identified. The influence of matching by tissue type on the successful outcome of organ transplantation is best established in renal transplantation, and its role in cardiac, liver and pancreatic transplantation is not yet clear.

Direct cross-matching

After a suitably matched recipient has been selected, a direct cross-match is set up because any recipient may have preformed circulating antibodies capable of reacting against donor cells. These antibodies may be the result of previous blood transfusion, pregnancy, viral infections or transplants. A direct cross-match incubates donor lymphocytes with the serum of the recipient in the presence of complement, to exclude cytotoxicity from circulating antibodies.

Exchange transplantation and desensitization programmes

In the United Kingdom at least 500 living kidney transplants are cancelled each year because of preformed cytotoxic antibodies. In approximately half, the cause is blood group incompatibility with the remainder presenting unacceptable anti HLA antibodies. At present there are two methods that allow these individuals to receive a transplant. One is exchange transplantation where donor A gives a kidney to recipient B and donor B donates a kidney to recipient A, thus overcoming the positive cytotoxic test. Individuals willing to exchange transplants are put onto a national register to increase the chances of finding a compatible combination. The 2nd option is a desensitization programme where over a number of session using filters or antigen columns, anti HLA antibodies are removed until their level is low enough to allow an initially incompatible transplant to proceed. There is, however, a significant risk of early rejection in these patients.

Organ retrieval

Most organs for cadaveric transplantation come from those who have suffered irreversible structural brain damage after road traffic accidents or cerebrovascular catastrophes and have been diagnosed brain dead by agreed criteria (see Ch. 10). In most countries that accept this practice, organs are then retrieved while the heart continues to beat and the donor receives ventilatory and other support. Such conditions are absolute requirements for transplantations of heart, heart-lung, and small bowel. Although organs can be retrieved from brainstem-dead individuals in whom coroners have determined the need for a postmortem, in practice many coroners refuse permission. The majority of transplant centres are developing links with pathology departments so that organ retrieval can take place in the presence of a pathologist in a way acceptable to the coroner. As the number of brainstem-dead donors continues to fall, many centres will now accept kidneys, livers, lungs and pancreas organs retrieved from controlled non-heart-beating donors. At present the only organs transplanted from non-controlled non-heart-beating donors (for example, individuals brought to the emergency department in asystole) are renal allografts (see Box 13.3).

Box 13.3 Sources of organs for transplantation

- Cadaveric heart beating and brainstem dead
- Cadaveric controlled non-heart-beating (non-brainstem dead)
- Cadaveric non-controlled non-heart-beating
- Living related and unrelated donors

Contraindications to organ donation are:

- history of disease or trauma involving the organs being considered
- long-standing history of diabetes mellitus, hypertension, cardiovascular or peripheral vascular disease (donors with the last three conditions are now accepted for donation but the organs are carefully assessed after retrieval to ensure they are of a satisfactory quality)
- prolonged periods of ischaemia because of profound hypotension or asystole (increasingly only a relative contraindication)
- malignancy – other than a primary brain tumour
- untreated systemic bacterial, fungal or viral infections – however, donors who have had bacterial infections adequately treated may still be suitable.

Chronological age in donors is usually less important than biological age. The age limit for each organ is given in Table 13.1.

Organ function in donors

Function of the organ which is to be transplanted must be established. A satisfactory past medical history and physical examination are essential. A well-perfused organ – as indicated by adequate blood pressure and normal arterial blood gas tensions – is also highly desirable.

Heart

Requirements are: normal blood pressure, ECG, chest X-ray and arterial blood gas tensions.

Lung and heart–lung

Requirements are:

- negative Gram stain on sputum
- absence of pathogens on sputum culture.

Liver

Requirements are:

- adequate liver perfusion – arterial blood pressure, blood and arterial gas tensions

Table 13.1 Age range for donors

Organ	Range (years)
Kidney	3–75
Liver	Neonate to 70
Heart and/or lung	Neonate to 50
Pancreas	Neonate to 50

- normal values for serum bilirubin, transaminase and alkaline phosphatase concentrations and a normal prothrombin time.

Kidney

Requirements are:

- normal urine output and urinalysis – however, oliguria may be pre-renal because of dehydration
- normal serum creatinine and urea concentrations.

Pancreas

Requirements are: normal serum concentrations of amylase and glucose – hyperglycaemia often develops in acute brainstem injury because of steroid administration and intravenous infusion of crystalloid containing glucose; elevated serum glucose alone is not necessarily a contraindication.

Retrieval after cardiac arrest

The continued shortage of organ donors has provided an impetus to re-examine retrieval from donors who do not have a beating heart. This may be in the controlled situation of an operating theatre where patients are moved from intensive care prior to cessation of ventilatory support or in a non-controlled situation where patients are seen in the emergency department after a cardiac arrest. Provided rapid organ perfusion with cold preservation solution can be achieved immediately after cardiac arrest, the lungs, liver, pancreas and kidneys may be usable.

Live related donation

Live related donor organs can be used for kidney, liver, pancreas, lung and small-bowel transplantation. Clearly the requirement for any organ other than the kidney must justify the operative risk of the partial resection of the relevant organ that is required. The increasing number of non-cadaveric transplants in the UK is illustrated in Figure 13.4. In Scandinavia and the USA up to half of transplants are from living donors.

Donor operation

Retrieval is becoming increasingly complex because many donors are now considered, and consent is obtained for multi-organ donation. Frequently there is a harvest from one individual of: corneas, heart, lungs, liver, pancreas, kidneys, bone and skin. With the recent success of small-bowel transplantation, the retrieval of the small bowel and the right colon may also be included. A number of transplant teams are involved, and it is essential that they fully agree the order of retrieval to be used before the start of the operation.

Retrieval procedure

Currently, the local kidney/liver team starts the procedure and is followed by the heart/lung team. The procedure for the abdominal organs is illustrated in outline in Figure 13.3. Organs are cold-perfused before removal, examined after removal to ensure they are anatomically satisfactory and then cold-preserved within double plastic bags and stored on a bed of crushed ice for transfer to the chosen transplant centre.

IMMUNOSUPPRESSION IN TRANSPLANTATION

There is a difficult balance to achieve between the prevention or reversal of rejection and the morbidity that can result from loss of host defences against infection – and also, in the long term, the development of malignant disease.

Immunosuppressive agents

Azathioprine. Metabolised in the liver to 6-mercaptopurine, this substance is a purine antagonist and reduces the synthesis of DNA and RNA in dividing cells.

Ciclosporin and tacrolimus. These act within the cell to prevent transcription of the gene for interleukin 2 (IL-2), a cytokine involved in the efferent arc of rejection.

Corticosteroids. These agents produce potent but non-specific immunosuppression and also have an anti-inflammatory action. They work by decreasing macrophage motility and phagocytic activity and also block both IL-2 release from macrophages and its generation by Th cells.

ATG. Thymoglobulin is a rabbit anti-human thymocyte immunoglobulin. It is polyclonal in nature and depletes lymphocytes in the circulation and lymphoid organs and also masks T-cell antigens non-specifically.

Monoclonal anti-CD25 antibody. Basiliximab and daclizumab are humanized monoclonal antibodies that target the IL-2 receptor. They have largely replaced ATG.

Monoclonal anti-T-cell antibody (OKT3). This is a murine antibody to the T3 antigen of human T-cells. It produces destruction of CD3-positive T-cells which are associated with graft rejection. There are other similar monoclonal antibodies, but OKT3 is the one most widely used.

Mycophenolate mofetil (MMF) inhibits proliferation of T- and B-lymphocytes and may prove more potent than azathioprine. It may also have a role in the prevention of chronic rejection because B-lymphocytes are thought to be important in this process which now accounts for the majority of renal transplants lost in the long term.

Anti-IL-2 receptor antibody. This is a monoclonal antibody to the IL-2 receptor on human lymphocytes. By binding the

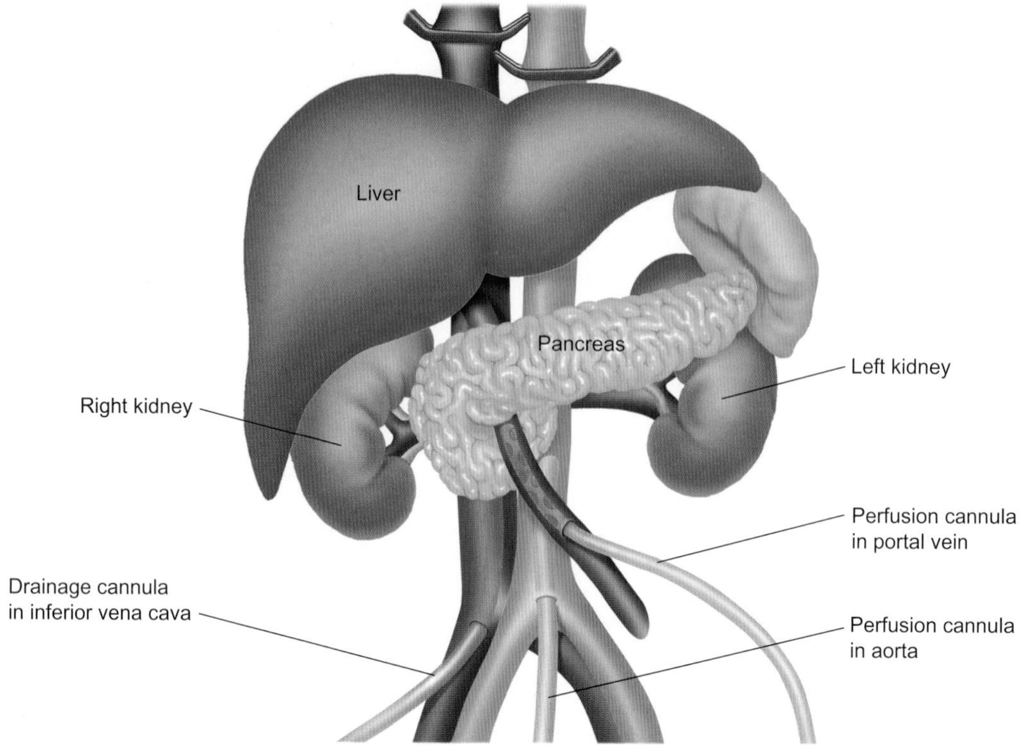

Fig. 13.3 Retrieval procedure for the abdominal organs.

IL-2 receptor it blocks the pathway of activation mediated through the release of IL-2.

Monoclonal anti-CD20 antibody. Rituximab is a monoclonal antibody directed against the CD20 antigen on B-cells. It may have a role in treatment of some forms of antibody-mediated rejection.

Sirolimus. This macrolide antibiotic binds the FK-binding protein, but its mechanism of action is via the 'target of Rapamune', or TOR. It inhibits G1- to S-phase cell division and, therefore, cell proliferation, and is used for maintenance immunosuppression and the treatment of chronic rejection.

Rapamycin. This drug reduces T-cell activation at a later stage in the cell cycle than ciclosporin or tacrolimus although still affecting the IL-2 signal transduction pathway. One of its main advantages is that it is not nephrotoxic (see Table 13.2).

Alemtuzumab is a recombinant DNA derived humanized monoclonal antibody that is directed against CD52, a protein which is present on the surface of mature lymphocytes. This drug is gaining popularity for use in desensitisation programmes or in regimens intending to induce immune tolerance to the transplanted organ.

Clinical regimens

These vary greatly from centre to centre but can be approximately categorised as follows.

Table 13.2 Immunosuppressive agents

Agent	Principal mode of action
Corticosteroids	Block IL-2 release
Ciclosporin/tacrolimus	Block IL-2 gene transcription
Rapamycin	Blocks T-cell proliferation in response to IL-2
Azathioprine	Reduces synthesis of RNA and DNA
Mycophenolate mofetil	Inhibits proliferation of T- and B-lymphocytes
IL-2 receptor antagonist	Blocks IL-2 receptors on T-cells
Antilymphocytes	The monoclonal OKT3 blocks the CD3 component of the T-cell receptor The polyclonal ATG depletes lymphocytes in circulation

Triple therapy

This is the most common standard induction and maintenance therapy, particularly in renal transplantation, and consists of:

- azathioprine – 2 mg/kg body weight, reduced to 1 mg/kg at the end of the first week
- ciclosporin – 8 mg/kg body weight adjusted according to the trough (pre-dose level) of free drug in serum
- prednisolone – 0.3 mg/kg body weight.

The mainstay is ciclosporin. Measuring its trough level is important because an excess can be nephrotoxic, although there is recent evidence that measurement of the peak level of ciclosporin (the C2 level) may provide a more accurate measure of the exposure to the drug. Further reductions in dose follow satisfactory progress over 3 months.

Another triple therapy regimen, based on tacrolimus (0.2 mg/kg) instead of ciclosporin and adjusted according to the trough level, is now being used in a number of centres and may be more effective in reducing acute rejection rates than ciclosporin.

Many American centres now also use MMF in place of azathioprine in triple therapy at a dose of 2 g/day.

Polyclonal and monoclonal agents against T cells

Basiliximab, alemtuzumab, OKT3 and ATG are agents used in some protocols for induction immunosuppression; however, OKT3 and ATG are very useful agents in treatment of steroid-resistant rejection.

Experimental regimens

There are a number of strategies for inducing tolerance to the transplanted organ – the aim being stopping most of the immunosuppression long term. An example is combined bone marrow and solid organ transplants together with the use of alemtuzumab, OKT3 or ATG as induction therapy.

Complications of immunosuppression

The most serious complication is an increased susceptibility to infections (see Box 13.4). Long-term immunosuppression also increases the risk of developing malignant disease, particularly squamous cell carcinoma of the skin and some forms of lymphoma. Other complications are the outcome of the specific side effects of individual components of the suppressive regimen (see Box 13.5).

Box 13.4 Infective complications of immunosuppression

Bacterial
- *Mycobacterium tuberculosis*
- *Listeria monocytogenes*

Fungal
- *Candida albicans*
- *Aspergillus* – various species

Protozoal
- *Pneumocystis jiroveci*
- *Cryptosporidium*

Viral
- Cytomegalovirus
- Epstein–Barr
- Measles
- Herpes simplex and zoster

GENERAL COMPLICATIONS OF TRANSPLANTATION

Apart from graft rejection and problems with drug toxicity, organ transplants of most kinds share a variety of complications which are summarised in Table 13.3. Technical problems are directly related to the quality of surgery and show a steady decline with increasing experience.

Monitoring the progress of a transplanted organ

The monitoring methods available are as follows.

Transplant function

- Kidney – serum urea, electrolyte and creatinine concentrations

Box 13.5 Complications of agents used in immunosuppression

Corticosteroids
- Reduced growth in children
- Impaired wound healing
- Bone – osteoporosis and avascular necrosis
- Diabetes mellitus
- Peptic ulceration
- Acute pancreatitis
- Hypertension
- Psychosis

Azathioprine
- Myelosuppression
- Liver – toxicity and cholestatic jaundice
- Acute pancreatitis

Ciclosporin
- Nephrotoxicity
- Hepatotoxicity
- Neurotoxicity
- Gingival hypertrophy
- Hypertrichosis

Table 13.3 Complications of transplantation

Category	Nature	Possible effects
General surgical	Wound – infection, dehiscence, incisional hernia	Occasionally life-threatening Further surgery required
Systemic infection	From i.v. lines, especially in liver transplantation Consequent on immunosuppression	Septicaemia
Vascular suture lines	Thrombosis Stenosis	Loss of graft In kidney – hypertension
Visceral suture lines	Leakage Stenosis	Fistula Interference with graft function (hydronephrosis, obstructive jaundice)

- Liver – urea and electrolyte concentrations, liver function tests and measures of clotting activity
- Pancreas – measurement of amylase and pH in urine (if the transplanted pancreas is implanted into the bladder).

Evidence of dysfunction (from the above)

- Kidney – Doppler ultrasound examination to exclude collections around it, obstruction of the ureter and arterial or venous thrombosis. In the absence of such findings, carry out percutaneous biopsy under ultrasound guidance.
- Liver – ultrasound to eliminate technical problems such as bile duct obstruction or vascular thrombosis; biliary contrast studies; biopsy if an immunological problem is suspected.
- Pancreas – the blood glucose level is not of value. Most transplants in the UK are combined kidney and pancreas, and the progress of the kidney can be used to monitor the pancreas.
- Small bowel – see below.

TRANSPLANTATION OF INDIVIDUAL ORGANS

End-stage failure means that the organ is no longer able to sustain life.

Kidney

With increasing success, the number of allografts transplanted increased every year, but the numbers have now reached a plateau because of the limited availability of donors. However, more and more patients are being admitted to dialysis programmes and are subsequently added to an ever-increasing list of patients waiting for a suitable allograft (Fig. 13.4).

Indications

Indication for kidney transplantation is renal failure from the following causes:

- chronic glomerulonephritis (55%)
- reflux nephropathy (25%)
- polycystic disease (8%)
- diabetic nephropathy (2%)
- malignant hypertension (1%)
- other causes, e.g. analgesic nephropathy (9%).

Operation

The transplant is heterotopic, with the kidney placed usually in the right iliac fossa and attached to the iliac artery and vein. The ureter is joined to the bladder to make a new ureterovesical junction (Fig. 13.5). The recipient's own kidneys are left in situ unless they are a source of recurrent urinary infection which may place the transplanted kidney at risk.

Results

There is intercentre variability in graft survival, but current cadaveric graft survival rates are 80–95% at 1 year, 60–70% at 5 years and 49–56% at 10 years (Fig. 13.6).

Liver

The procedure for liver transplantation is more recent than for kidney transplantation: However, it is now an established treatment of end-stage parenchymal liver disease, including congenital metabolic disorders. Survival figures have improved because of better patient selection and clinical support, organ preservation and immunosuppressive agents. In major transplant centres, a 70–90% 1-year survival is obtained and, in those transplanted for benign disease, survivors of the first year are likely to be alive at 5 years. The

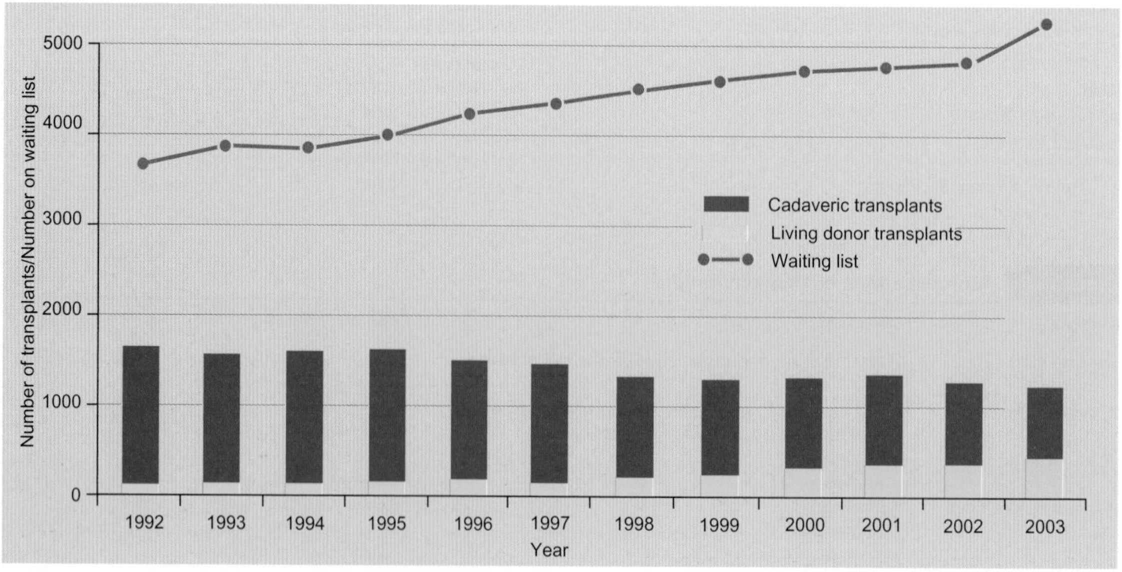

Fig. 13.4 Numbers of kidney-only transplants and active waiting list in the UK at year end, 1992–2002.

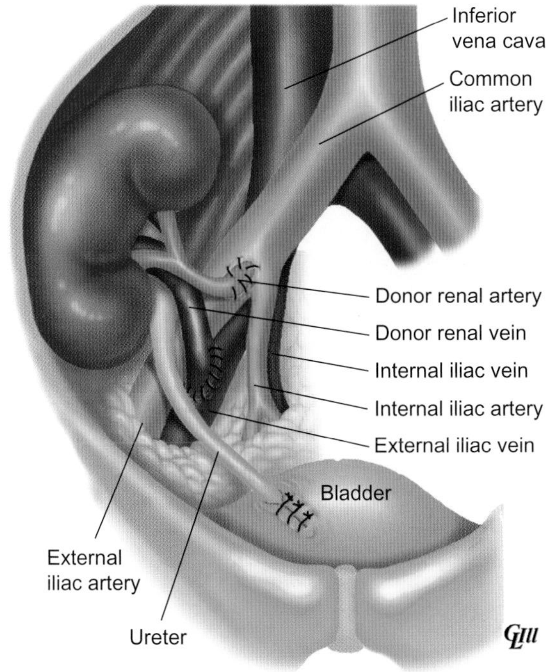

Fig. 13.5 Completed renal transplant in right iliac fossa.

results of liver transplantation in the management of primary liver tumours are universally poor, and its role in this situation remains controversial.

Unlike kidney transplants, the number of organs available has been better matched to the number of recipients. However, widening indications for the transplantation of the liver and the increasing awareness by clinicians of liver transplantation as a therapeutic option will undoubtedly result in a waiting list in the near future.

Indications

Transplantation is indicated in the presence of liver failure from any of the conditions shown in Table 13.4. Although these are all disorders which make the patient a candidate, many of them are rare and thus form only a small part of the liver transplant population.

Operation

The operation is a major procedure because the diseased liver may be difficult to remove and there are a number of vascular anastomoses to be made during which venous return to the heart must be maintained by bypass (Fig. 13.7).

Primary failure of function may occur in up to 10% of allografts. The morbidity and mortality of this complication is high. Survival following re-transplantation for primary non-function is only half that seen when the first graft functions successfully.

Results

The results of liver transplantation are rapidly improving. Currently the majority of centres report 1-year graft survival in excess of 70%. It is of note that over 85% of patients surviving more than 6 months after liver transplantation return to active life either at school or at work.

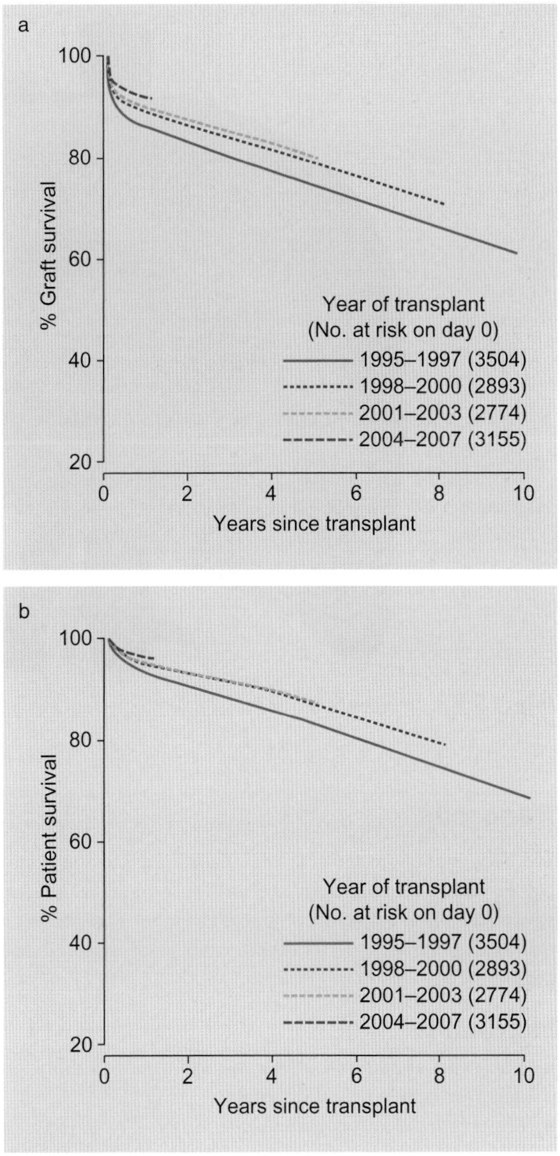

Fig. 13.6 Survival for patients and transplants after kidney transplantation.

Table 13.4 Indications for liver transplantation

Disease process	Suitable subgroups
Cirrhosis	Primary biliary Alcoholic liver disease Cryptogenic Secondary biliary
Hepatitis B and C virus infection	Chronic
Cholangitis	Sclerosing
Congenital anatomical disorders	Biliary atresia Budd–Chiari syndrome
Inborn errors of metabolism	Alpha-1-antitrypsin deficiency Galactosaemia Wilson's disease
Primary liver tumours	Hepatocellular carcinoma
Rare secondary tumours, e.g. neuroendocrine	A relative indication depending on the size of the tumour and absence of extrahepatic involvement

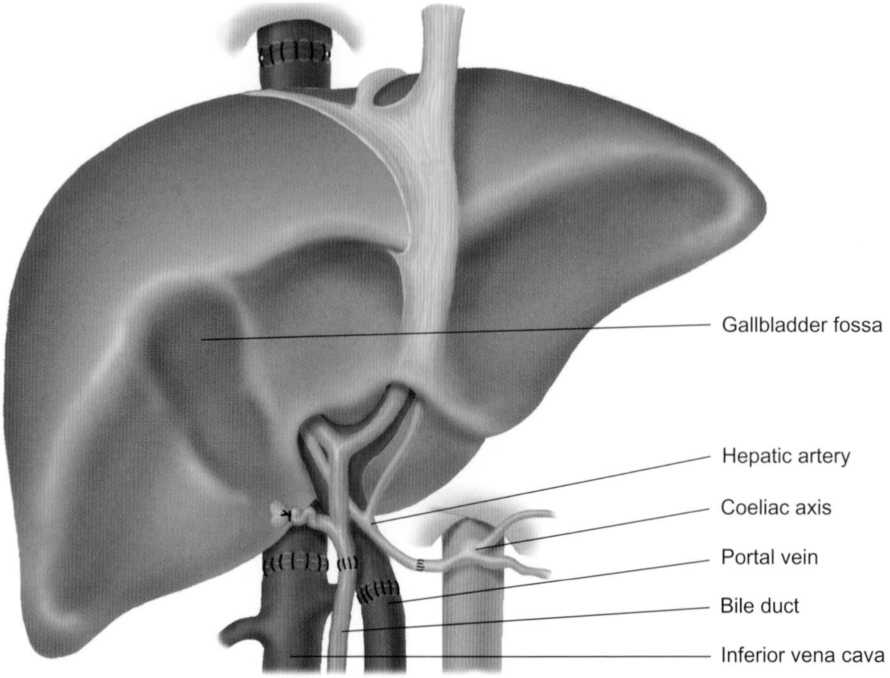

Fig. 13.7 Completed liver transplant. Note the numerous suture lines. The gallbladder is removed.

Pancreas

The large number of patients with diabetes has made transplantation of the pancreas a worthwhile goal. However, severe diabetes is often accompanied by renal disease which makes concurrent renal transplantation necessary if the patient is to be restored to health.

Indications

- Insulin-dependent diabetes with renal failure – combined pancreas and kidney transplant
- Pre-uraemic diabetic with severe complications, e.g. neuropathy, retinopathy and poor control of the disease – a pancreas-only transplant is needed.

Operation

The technique depends on whether a whole organ or a segmental graft is to be used. The latter is removed on a pedicle of splenic artery and vein and is revascularised using the external iliac artery and vein, with the pancreatic duct either occluded or drained into the urinary bladder. The whole organ is removed with the segment of duodenum which drains the pancreatic duct. Revascularisation is by a similar method to the segmental graft, with the duodenal loop drained into the bladder (Fig. 13.8). The latter technique has the least complications and the highest success rate. However, as experience with pancreas transplantation has increased, many centres are changing to an enteric drainage (anastomosis of donor pancreas or duodenum to the GI tract) but complication rates are high.

Results

With increasing experience, 1- and 5-year graft survivals of 70% and 40%, respectively, are being reported. However, transplantation of the whole pancreas is likely in the future to be replaced by transplantation of islet cells only.

Small bowel

Small-bowel transplantation presents particular difficulties because:

- the transplant contains a large volume of lymphoid tissue (see graft–versus–host reaction below)
- MHC class II antigens are constitutively expressed by the bowel epithelium
- the transplanted organ is colonised with microorganisms.

As a consequence of the last of these, there is breakdown of the intestinal barrier and the release of bacteria into the circulation (translocation), with consequent infection as well as an increased presentation of immune signals to the recipient.

Indications

The indications in adults and children are given in Box 13.6. A combined liver and bowel replacement may be necessary if there is coexistent irreversible structural damage to the liver, such as may occur with prolonged parenteral nutrition.

Operation

Proximal anastomosis of the graft is to the recipient's jejunum; distally the new gut is brought out as an end-ileostomy (Fig. 13.9).

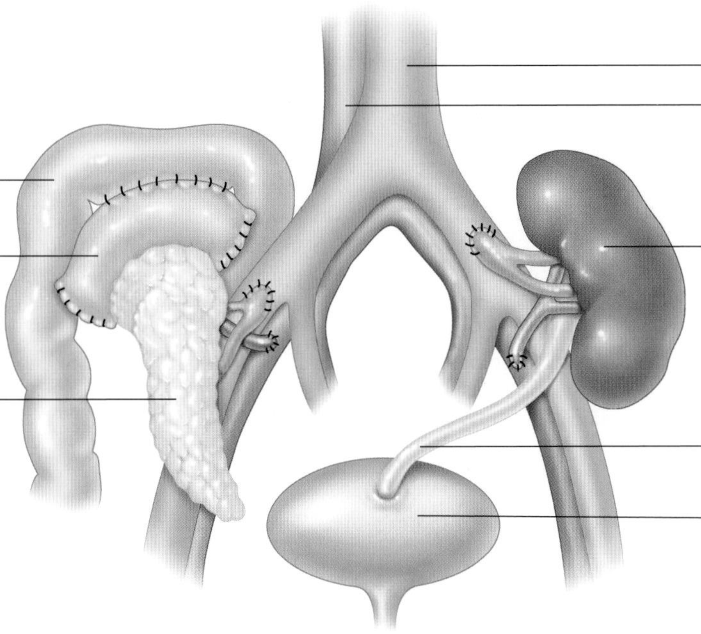

Fig. 13.8 Whole-organ pancreas transplant.

Box 13.6 Indications for small-bowel transplant

Adults
- Vascular
  - Superior mesenteric artery or vein thrombosis
  - Volvulus with irreversible damage to the gut
  - Desmoid tumour in the mesentery
- Crohn's disease with loss of function but without active sepsis

Children
- Intestinal atresia with loss of most of the small bowel
- Pseudo-obstruction – neurogenic failure of intestinal function
- Microvillus inclusion disease
- Gastroschisis with loss of small bowel
- Necrotising enterocolitis – extensive resection

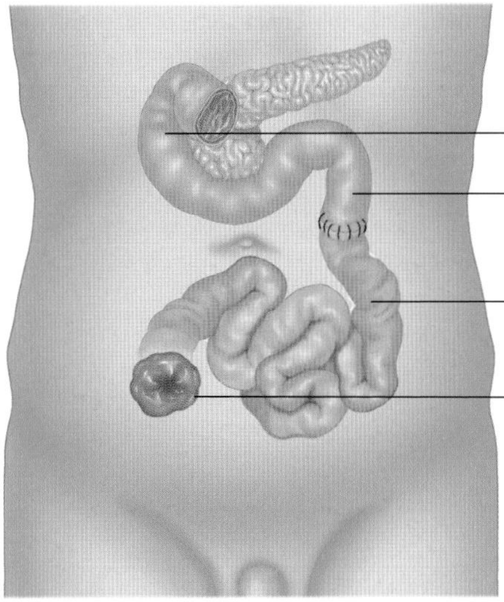

Fig. 13.9 Small-bowel transplant.

Results

The most encouraging results have been reported in Canada where the last five small-bowel transplants have all been successful with the use of the immunosuppressive drug tacrolimus. In the USA, survivals are now at 65% at 1 year and 43% at 2 years.

Heart, lung and heart–lung

This is discussed in Chapters 16 and 17.

Cornea

The cornea was the first solid tissue successfully allografted in humans. In recent years, a high success rate has made corneal transplantation the most commonly performed transplant.

Indications

- Opaque cornea from any cause
- Thin or distorted cornea
- Corneal loss – necrotising ulceration or trauma.

Operation

A button of the recipient's cornea is removed and replaced with a corresponding graft from the donor using very fine nylon sutures. Because the cornea is avascular, rejection is not a common problem unless the recipient's cornea has undergone neovascularisation before the transplant takes place.

Results

Worldwide, the survival of the graft is 95%, and it may be expected to last for life. Close HLA matching correlates with an improved long-term result.

TRANSPLANTATION IN CHILDREN

In older children with a weight in excess of 20 kg, most transplant procedures are the same as for adults, although specially skilled personnel such as paediatric anaesthetists are required to deal with the haemodynamic problems that may arise during clamping of major vessels. Such problems are greater the younger and the smaller the child.

Kidney

The results of transplanting paediatric kidneys into paediatric recipients are worse than if an adult kidney is used. Accordingly, most centres now transplant the best-matched organ, provided its size is not too discrepant; access may be modified to make the procedure feasible.

Other organs

For liver, heart and lung, the constraints of size are more relevant, and age matching is done. However, the increasing success of using a reduced-size liver graft has overcome the problem of supply in that area.

THE FUTURE

Despite the great success of current multi-organ transplant programmes, further developments are required to improve the long-term outlook of recipients. It is difficult to imagine that there will be many more technical improvements in transplant surgery. Advances in immunology, formulation of new less-toxic immunosuppressive drugs, xenografting and the development of cellular or biomechanical approaches to organ replacement therapy are clearly the most important areas for the future.

FURTHER READING

Abbas AK, Lichtman AH, Pillai S 2009 Cellular and molecular immunology, 6th edn. Saunders, Philadelphia

Forsythe JLR 2009 Transplantation: a companion to specialist surgical practice. Saunders, Philadelphia

Hakim N, Danovitch G, Dausset J 2010 Transplantation Surgery – Springer Specialist Surgery Series, Springer, New York

Hornick P (ed) 2006 Transplantation immunology: methods and protocols (Methods in Molecular Biology). Humana Press, Totowa

Morris PJ, Knechtle SJ 2008 Kidney transplantation: principles and practice, 6th edn. Saunders, Philadelphia

SECTION 2
REGIONAL SURGERY

14 The neck and upper aerodigestive tract

SWELLINGS IN THE NECK

The most common cause of a neck swelling is lymph node enlargement. The majority of such swellings are secondary to infection, the minority are the consequence of malignant disease. Making the correct diagnosis depends initially on a careful, thorough clinical assessment.

Clinical features

History

Important features are:

- the duration of the swelling
- progression in size
- associated pain
- other symptoms in the upper aerodigestive tract – hoarseness, dysphagia, localised sore throat, deafness
- systemic symptoms – weight loss, night sweats
- exposure to alcohol and/or tobacco – squamous carcinoma with a cervical lymph node metastasis is rare below the age of 40 in those who have not been exposed to either of these agents.

Physical findings

Examination of an individual lump should produce the following information:

- site and size
- relationship to other anatomical structures such as the great vessels
- fixation to other structures
- special features such as pulsatility, the presence of a bruit or thrill, tenderness or fluctuation.

A thorough orodental examination must be carried out. The oral cavity and oropharynx can easily be examined using a tongue depressor and bright light. The nasopharynx and laryngopharynx used to require indirect examination with a mirror, but the advent of the fibreoptic nasoendoscope has made these sites much easier to view directly. However, even with this instrument a very small submucosal primary tumour may be overlooked. If a lymphoma is suspected then the axillae, groins and abdomen should also be examined.

Clinical diagnosis

After the completion of the local examination, a first attempt can often be made at a clinical diagnosis.

Site

The site often indicates a possible origin (Fig. 14.1):

- Parotid swellings occur immediately in front of the tragus, over the angle of the mandible or just below the lobe of the ear. An associated facial palsy suggests a malignant tumour of the gland.
- Submandibular gland swellings are sometimes indistinguishable from regional lymphadenopathy. In either case, fixation to the mandible may make it impossible to get above the mass. A submandibular swelling is more likely to be palpable bimanually (via the mouth).
- Midline submental swellings are nearly always benign and, if cystic, are commonly a thyroglossal cyst, a midline dermoid cyst or a pyramidal lobe of the thyroid, if lower in the neck.
- High anterior triangle swellings can be metastatic in origin, with the likely primary site in the oral cavity or oropharynx. Alternatives are a branchial cyst or carotid body tumour.
- Low anterior triangle swellings are either related to the thyroid gland or are metastatic nodal deposits from a primary tumour in the larynx or hypopharynx. Such lymph node masses do not move on swallowing unless they are fixed to the thyroid gland or the larynx.

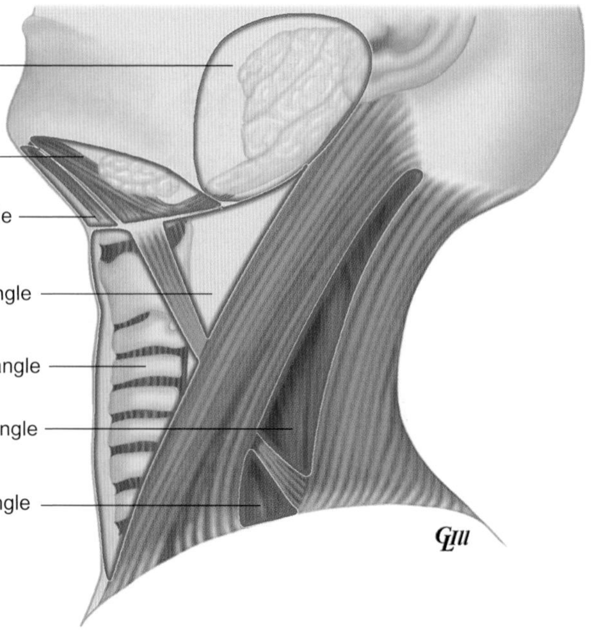

Fig. 14.1 Sites of swelling in the neck.

- Supraclavicular swellings are more common on the left side of the neck and are often caused by disease below the level of the clavicle, e.g. carcinoma of the lung or stomach.
- Posterior triangle swellings are rarely the result of metastatic carcinoma unless there are also palpable lymph nodes in the anterior triangle on the same side. More common causes are tuberculosis, toxoplasmosis and lymphoma. The last may occur in an otherwise fit and asymptomatic young adult.

Multiple cervical masses

These are almost always nodal and, if accompanied by an acute systemic illness, may be caused by viral infections such as infectious mononucleosis. A more chronic presentation can be produced by tuberculosis.

Time course

The time course of the swelling may be helpful in suggesting the diagnosis. Enlargement of a cervical lymph node(s) which has taken place over a few days, and which is tender, is almost always inflammatory. Lymphomas occasionally present in this way, but more commonly develop over a period of several weeks and are usually painless. Metastatic nodes have a similar pattern; although they may be tender on palpation, they rarely cause spontaneous pain unless there is invasion of the cervical or brachial plexus.

Investigation

Fine-needle aspiration

Fine-needle aspiration (FNA; Ch. 4 and Fig. 14.2) to obtain cell or tissue samples is the first invasive investigation to confirm a diagnosis and is best done immediately after clinical examination has been completed unless there are clinical reasons to think that it is potentially dangerous, e.g. evidence of considerable vascularity such as a bruit or thrill. A fluctuant swelling may yield pus, which is sent for culture, or either clear or opalescent liquid which suggests a branchial or other cyst. In both instances, a sample should be sent for cytological examination. A solid lump produces an aspirate which is examined cytologically and is likely to give an indication of the pathological cause. However, confirmation must nearly always be sought by other means such as endoscopy with biopsy for histology and imaging (see below) before treatment is undertaken. Cytology is not infallible.

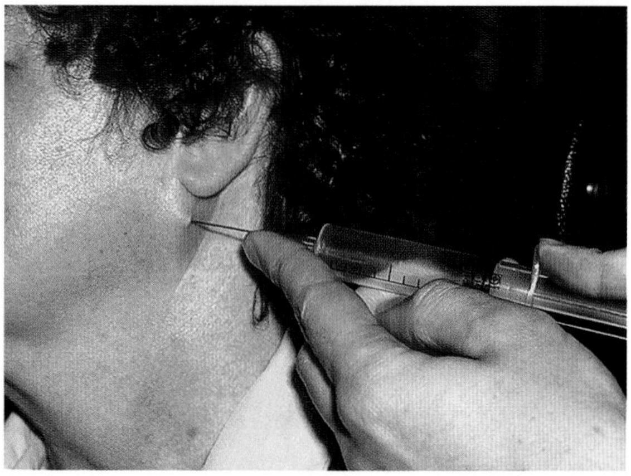

Fig. 14.2 Fine-needle aspiration of a parotid lump.

MRI scanning

This is valuable when the likely diagnosis is of metastatic nodal disease. The scan should extend from the base of the skull to the clavicles. Information is obtained about the relationship of the mass to other structures, and other impalpable swellings may be found. Indeed the scan may demonstrate the site of a primary tumour. CT and ultrasound scanning are also useful in certain clinical situations. Ultrasound-guided FNA is useful for small or deeper lesions in the neck.

Other investigations

These are based on the probable clinical diagnosis, particularly if the swelling(s) is thought to be of lymph node origin. The usual procedures are indicated in Table 14.1.

Further diagnostic strategy

The above investigations usually provide enough information to decide whether the patient requires formal endoscopy of the upper aerodigestive tract. The diagnostic pathways are decided from the outcome of the result of FNA and endoscopy, as follows.

Cytology suggests squamous carcinoma

Regardless of whether or not the primary is apparent, a formal upper aerodigestive tract endoscopy is undertaken, and must include examination of (Fig. 14.3):

- nasopharynx
- oral cavity/oropharynx (with inspection of ipsilateral tonsil)
- hypopharynx
- larynx and trachea
- bronchi
- cervical oesophagus.

Table 14.1 Supplementary investigations to be considered for a lump in the neck

Possible cause	Investigation
Acute infection	Full blood count (FBC)
Tuberculosis	Chest X-ray, Mantoux test
Infectious mononucleosis	Monospot, FBC
Lymphoma	FBC, bone marrow
Malignancy in lung	Chest X-ray, CT scanning

A biopsy is taken from any suspicious lesion. Such an endoscopy will uncover a primary tumour in approximately one third of cases. In approximately 2%, a second primary is found elsewhere. If the nodal mass contains squamous carcinoma but endoscopy and scanning fail to identify a primary tumour, then treatment of the neck should be by radiotherapy (for nodal disease < 2 cm in diameter) or neck dissection (where nodes > 2 cm in diameter).

PET-CT scanning should be undertaken as part of the diagnostic assessment of metastatic cervical lymphadenopathy, when no primary is clinically apparent. Ideally, the scan should be undertaken before mucosal biopsies are undertaken.

Cytology suggests lymphoma

Incision or excision biopsy of an enlarged node is almost always necessary to obtain sufficient tissue to identify with confidence the histological type of lymphoma (see also below). Excisional surgery is diagnostic, not therapeutic.

Cytology is unhelpful

A normal endoscopy and lack of information from FNA together indicate the need for surgical excision/incision biopsy as a last resort. The reason for trying to avoid this is that local surgery for diagnosis of a lump which is malignant may lead to seeding of tumour cells at the biopsy site. Whenever feasible, excision biopsy should be performed to reduce this hazard. Furthermore, it is best to obtain a frozen section at once and, if metastatic squamous carcinoma is confirmed, to go straight on to a radical neck dissection. If fixity of the node(s) makes this unfeasible, the wound is closed and alternative treatment, usually by radiotherapy, is undertaken.

Incision, as opposed to excision, biopsy of a benign lesion should be avoided whenever possible, as it makes subsequent surgery that considerably more difficult.

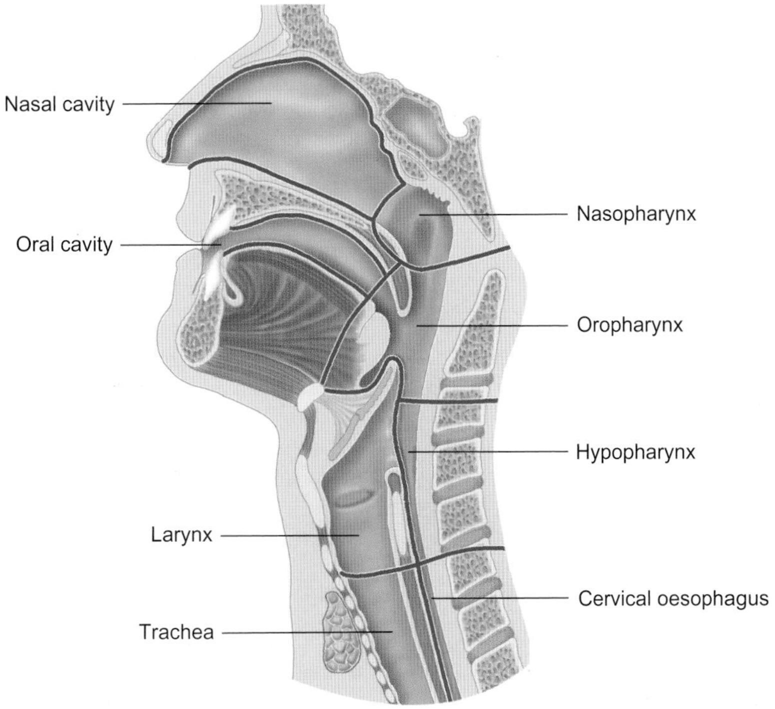

Fig. 14.3 Regions of the upper aerodigestive tract.

A primary tumour is found at endoscopy

If a primary tumour is found at endoscopy, the type of treatment recommended will depend on the site and size of both the primary and the cervical node metastases. A radical neck dissection should not be undertaken if the primary is known to be below the clavicle.

BENIGN CYSTIC SWELLINGS

Thyroglossal cyst

Aetiology

The embryonic mesoderm which ultimately develops into the thyroid gland descends from the foramen caecum of the tongue to the normal pretracheal site of the gland. The tract usually disappears, but islands of thyroid tissue may be deposited at any point along its course and develop into a cyst.

Clinical features

Presentation is commonly during the second or third decades of life. The mass is usually midline, between the thyroid notch and hyoid bone, and moves upwards on protrusion of the tongue (Fig. 14.4).

Management

The cyst is removed surgically. To avoid recurrence, which may be associated with sinus formation, the central portion of the hyoid bone is included in the excision because the tract can run either deep or superficial to the bone (Sistrunk's operation).

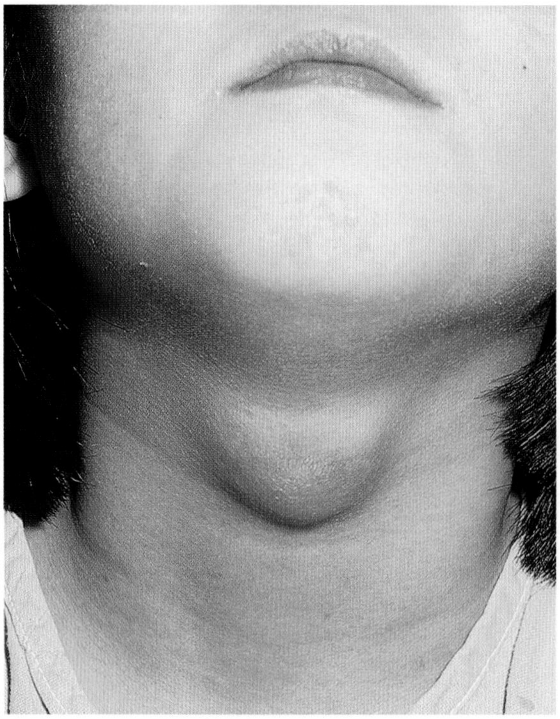

Fig. 14.4 Infected thyroglossal cyst.

Branchial cyst

Aetiology

The cause is uncertain. It is considered by some to be a remnant of the branchial complex which contributes so much to the development of the neck structures.

Clinical features

Presentation is typically between the ages of 15 and 35 years with a cyst in the upper part of the anterior triangle with its posterior portion deep to the sternomastoid muscle. It is smooth, mobile and, unless infected, not tender. Occasionally the cyst communicates with the skin via a sinus. The diagnosis can be confirmed by FNA, which characteristically produces pale creamy fluid, and ultrasound scanning. Further imaging is rarely necessary. Treatment is by excision together with any sinus tract that may run from it.

VASCULAR TUMOURS

Chemodectoma – carotid body tumour

Aetiology

There is sometimes a family history and these tumours are more common in those who live at high altitudes. Not much else about the cause of this rare tumour is known, except that it is derived from paraganglionic cells.

Clinical features

The patient usually presents in adult life with a history of a lump which is ovoid, non-tender, pulsatile and which is in the upper anterior triangle of the neck. Characteristically, it is mobile in the horizontal but not the vertical plane. However, it may be difficult to distinguish a carotid body tumour from a branchial cyst without appropriate investigation. Auscultation may reveal a bruit. A CT scan demonstrates the lesion but confirmation is best made by carotid angiography, which shows a highly vascular mass. Treatment is by surgical excision, which is usually preceded by embolisation of the tumour.

TUMOURS OF THE UPPER AERODIGESTIVE TRACT

Malignant tumours are more common than benign ones and almost all are primary as opposed to secondary. Squamous carcinomas are the most common (more than 90%), followed by lymphomas, salivary gland tumours, melanomas and sarcomas.

SQUAMOUS CARCINOMA

Aetiology

The most important predisposing factors are:

- smoking
- high alcohol intake, especially of wines and spirits
- presence of pre-malignant conditions.

Other factors include:

- chronic irritation from a jagged tooth
- chewing betel nut (common in the Indian subcontinent)
- oral syphilis (very rare).

Pre-malignant conditions

Leucoplakia

This is a descriptive term for a white patch or patches on the mucosa, usually of the oral cavity and larynx. It usually results from chronic irritation, although in 10% it is of unknown cause. The histological picture is often one of dysplasia, but the condition may be associated with frank malignancy.

Management should be conservative, once malignancy has been excluded by biopsy. Close follow-up of the patient is essential, and further biopsies may be necessary. Causative factors should be removed if possible.

Erythroplakia

These are fiery red patches of mucosa that bleed easily. They imply severe dysplasia and are often associated with the presence of an in-situ carcinoma.

Sideropenic dysphagia

Erythroplakia may be associated with this syndrome in postmenopausal women; it involves dysphagia, iron deficiency anaemia and a web in the postcricoid hypopharynx. A barium swallow demonstrates the web, which may be associated with a locally dysplastic mucosa. Endoscopy and biopsy are therefore necessary, the passage of the endoscope often temporarily relieving symptoms. The condition is not, however, reversible with correction of the anaemia. Subsequent development of a postcricoid carcinoma is a distinct possibility, and the patient should be kept under observation.

Clinical features

These are site-specific (see Fig. 14.3).

Symptoms

Nasal or sinus tumours can cause local problems, such as unilateral nasal obstruction and epistaxis, or can invade adjacent structures and give rise to clinical features that are misleading, such as diplopia, middle ear effusion or loosening of teeth. Oral cavity and oropharyngeal tumours commonly present with symptoms of local pain, referred otalgia or difficulty eating but, as with tumours of the hypopharynx, the primary may be asymptomatic and it is the presence of metastases which draws attention to the lesion.

Tumours of the larynx characteristically result in hoarseness, and compromise of the airway only occurs in very advanced cases. Referred otalgia, mediated by the vagus nerve, may also be a presenting symptom. Laryngeal, hypopharyngeal and cervical oesophageal neoplasms may also cause dysphagia, initially to solid food. This is in contrast to dysphagia of neurological origin e.g. (motor neurone disease or after a cardiovascular accident), when swallowing is initially more difficult with liquids.

Clinical examination

The sequence of examination is outlined above. The primary may be readily apparent on inspection, usually as an ulcer with a raised edge. Examination is not complete without careful palpation of the neck.

Investigation

The choice of investigations depends on the known or likely site of the tumour. The principles have already been outlined.

The presence of an unexplained hoarse voice for longer than 6 weeks and inability to assess the larynx fully as an outpatient is an indication for direct laryngoscopy under general anaesthesia. A similar principle is observed for persistent dysphagia and the need for oesophagoscopy; a diagnosis of functional dysphagia (globus pharyngis or globus hystericus) should never be made until both a barium swallow and an oesophagoscopy have been shown to be normal, thus excluding both strictures, mucosal disease and motility disorders.

Management

A multidisciplinary approach (MDM or MDT) is required. Surgery and radiotherapy are the two principal treatments, used either alone or in planned combination. The role of chemotherapy remains unclear. Eradication of the tumour is the first priority, but preservation of function (particularly of speech and swallowing) and of appearance are also important factors.

Approximately 20% of patients with head and neck cancer present with such advanced disease that it is wisest and kindest to do nothing more than provide supportive care and analgesia. Whilst this may initially be at home, hospice care usually becomes necessary later because of swallowing and respiratory problems, and intractable pain. A gastrostomy or tracheostomy may be useful in referring severe digestive or respiratory tract obstruction.

Small tumours

For small or early cancers radiotherapy and surgery are equally effective and, in view of the wish to preserve function, radiotherapy is often the treatment of choice. Once a full course (60–65 Gy) of radiotherapy has been given, the irradiated volume cannot be retreated, and recurrent or new tumours, however small, which occur within the irradiated field have to be treated by surgery.

Using a microscopy and CO_2 laser, certain small volume carcinomas of the larynx can be excised endoscopically, with preservation of the voice.

Large tumours

The bigger the tumour, the less likely it is to be cured by radiotherapy, and this is particularly so if there is invasion of bone or cartilage. Primary surgery is better in such cases. The decision as to whether or not to add planned postoperative radiotherapy may be made before surgery or may depend on histological factors revealed by study of the operative specimen. Very close or positive margins of excision of the primary, extracapsular rupture of a lymph node or involvement of multiple levels of the neck would merit planned postoperative radiotherapy.

Given the propensity for these tumours to metastasise to the cervical nodes, these may need to be treated at the same time as the primary tumour. Small nodes can be treated by radiotherapy or surgery, and the appropriate choice may well depend on the treatment modality chosen for the primary site. Large nodes should be treated by a neck dissection. Some primary sites (e.g. tongue, bone and tonsil) carry such a high risk (50%) of microscopic nodal disease that prophylactic treatment of the ipsilateral neck should be undertaken even when there is no clinical evidence of metastasis. The modality used will usually be the same as that employed for the primary site.

Prognosis

Survival rates depend on the site and size of the primary tumour, and the presence or absence of metastatic nodal disease. A patient with a tumour of the larynx is likely to fare much better than one with a tumour of the same size in the hypopharynx. This is partly the result of more ready spread of the latter to the regional lymph nodes. Once lymph node metastases have developed, the prognosis for any tumour, no matter how small the primary, worsens considerably. Failure to control the disease is almost always because recurrence takes place loco-regionally; distant metastases are unusual unless there is already advanced disease above the clavicles. Such loco-regional recurrence is most likely to occur within 2 years of the initial treatment. Overall, the 5-year survival rate for all head and neck malignancies is approximately 40%.

Surgical management

Reconstruction

The defect after surgery for a large aerodigestive tract tumour is often of considerable size, and it may be difficult to achieve a satisfactory cosmetic and functional result by direct closure. Recent advances in plastic surgical techniques have provided a variety of options, which include:

- *Simple free grafts of split or full-thickness skin.* These are only appropriate for small defects, as they rely on the tissue bed for their revascularisation.
- *Pedicled skin flaps.* These may be random, where there is no specific nutrient artery, or axial, where the flap has a named blood supply (e.g. the pectoralis major myocutaneous flap supplied by the thoraco-acromial artery). Axial flaps are much more reliable and are not limited by the width/length ratio of the flap.
- *Free skin flaps and jejunal segmental transplant.* A piece of forearm or lateral thigh skin or a segment of jejunum can be dissected with its own arterial supply and venous drainage which can then be anastomosed to appropriate vessels in the neck, so restoring the graft tissue's circulation. The radial forearm flap has the great advantage that it can be raised in continuity with a piece of radial bone, which will restore continuity following resection of a segment of mandible for an oral cavity carcinoma. A transplanted length of jejunum can be used as an oesophageal replacement.
- *Transposed viscus.* Following a laryngopharyngo-oesophagectomy for a postcricoid carcinoma, the stomach can be mobilised and brought up through the mediastinum for anastomosis to the pharynx in the neck (stomach pull-up procedure). Another less reliable option is to bring up a vascularised segment of transverse colon.

Restoration of speech

One of the greatest handicaps which can result from the surgical treatment of head and neck tumours is the loss of voice which follows total laryngectomy. Until relatively recently, adequate speech after laryngectomy was often not achievable, the patient being doomed to a life of silence and a pen and paper. However, the last decade has seen the advent of surgical speech restoration.

A tracheo-oesophageal fistula is created surgically through the posterior wall of the trachea, approximately 5 mm below the mucocutaneous junction (Fig. 14.5). A one-way valve can then be introduced into the tract, where it can be left for several months before replacement. By occluding the tracheostomy with a finger during expiration, the patient can divert air up through the valve into the pharynx. The air is set in vibration by the valve and speech can be produced.

LYMPHOMA

Pathological features

The majority of lymphomas in the head and neck region are non-Hodgkin's in type. They can be nodal or extranodal, and those found in Waldeyer's ring (the lymphoid tissue ring located in the pharynx and to the back of the oral cavity which includes the tonsils) characteristically form a protruding mass, unlike squamous carcinomas.

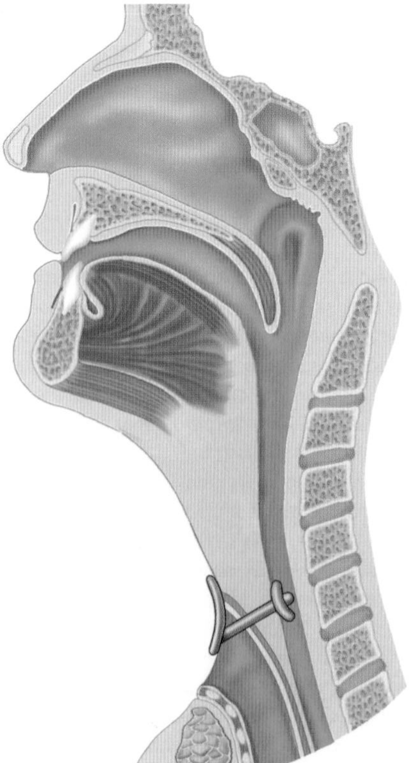

Fig. 14.5 Restoration of speech after tracheostomy.

Lymphoma
Diseases of the salivary glands
Non-neoplastic salivary gland disease

Clinical features

The patient presents with a local lesion or enlarged lymph node(s).

Diagnosis

Biopsy is the only method of making an exact diagnosis.

Investigation

The studies to be done are the same as for lymphomas at other sites (Ch. 30). Surgery plays only a diagnostic role in management.

DISEASES OF THE SALIVARY GLANDS

There are three paired salivary glands: the parotid, the submandibular and the sublingual glands. Scattered throughout the mucosa of the oral cavity and pharynx are millions of other tiny minor salivary glands. Although tumours may arise in the latter, they are rarely a site of inflammatory disease.

NON-NEOPLASTIC SALIVARY GLAND DISEASE

Bacterial infection

Infections in the parotid or submandibular salivary gland are relatively uncommon. Bacterial parotitis tends to occur in elderly debilitated patients, probably as the result of poor oral hygiene and dehydration. Bacterial infection of the submandibular gland is more common and can occur in an otherwise well patient. Infection is frequently due to a stone lodged in the gland's duct.

Clinical features

Parotitis

The gland swells, becomes acutely tender and the overlying skin may be erythematous. A plain X-ray may demonstrate a stone in the duct, but a contrast examination should not be done while there is acute inflammation.

Submandibular sialadenitis

The appearances are the same as for parotitis. A stone may be palpable on bimanual examination. Alternatively, a stone may be identified on an intraoral dental X-ray (Fig. 14.6).

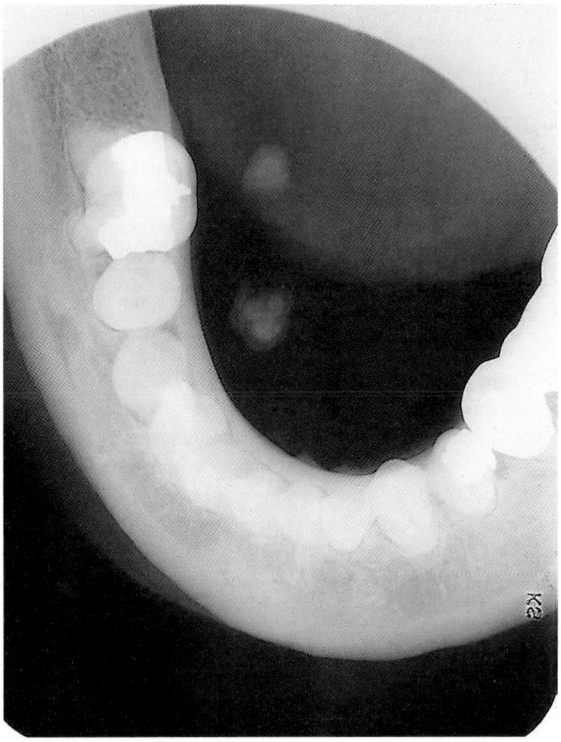

Fig. 14.6 Oblique X-ray of the floor of the mouth showing two stones in the submandibular salivary duct.

Management

Parotitis

Parotitis requires energetic care of the mouth, rehydration and antibiotics. If fluctuation develops, incision and drainage of the abscess is necessary, ensuring that the facial nerve is not damaged.

Submandibular sialadenitis

This is treated in the same way as parotitis, but if a stone is obvious, then intraoral incision of the duct and removal of the stone under local anaesthesia may be all that is required. However, a submandibular duct stone can be very mobile and difficult to remove, particularly if it is lodged far back in the duct, where damage to the adjacent lingual nerve may occur. In such circumstances, it is better to allow the infection to resolve with antibiotic treatment and then remove the entire gland.

Viral parotitis

This is a common disorder usually caused by the mumps virus. Other agents include the cytomegalovirus and Coxsackie virus. Although the gland may swell considerably, there is not as much pain or systemic upset as in bacterial infection.

Sialectasis

This is primarily a disease of the parotid gland and may be a forerunner to stone formation. Epithelial debris mixes with the saliva to produce sediment in the ducts, which in turn leads to stasis and poor emptying of the ducts when secretion is stimulated.

Clinical features and investigation

Painful swelling of the gland occurs at mealtimes and can last several hours. Sialography characteristically demonstrates a snowstorm appearance of the duct system, caused by patchy cystic dilatations of the ducts interspersed with areas of stricture formation.

Management

Salivary flow is increased by the use of sialogogues, such as lemon juice. Parotidectomy should be avoided if at all possible because of the risk of damage to the facial nerve.

Connective tissue disease

Keratoconjunctivitis sicca and rheumatoid arthritis (Sjögren's disease)

Salivary gland swelling occurs in about one-third of affected patients. Because the disease is associated with an abnormality in lymphocyte function, the patient is at risk of developing a lymphoma.

Benign lymphoepithelial infiltration

This causes general enlargement of the submandibular and parotid glands without any of the other features of Sjögren's disease. A sublabial mucosal biopsy demonstrates a dense lymphocytic infiltrate of the minor salivary glands. Again, there is an increased risk of lymphoma, and any further increase in size of any of the salivary glands should be viewed with suspicion and FNA carried out.

Drug-induced salivary gland swelling

Certain antihypertensives, monoamine oxidase inhibitors and iodide-containing drugs can cause enlargement of the parotid, as may the contraceptive pill.

SALIVARY GLAND NEOPLASMS

Most salivary gland tumours are benign. However, the smaller the gland, the higher is the chance of a tumour being malignant. Although 70% of parotid tumours are benign, 70% of minor salivary gland tumours are malignant.

Pleomorphic adenoma

This is the most common benign tumour, so-called because histologically it can mimic a variety of tissues. If left untreated for many years, it can undergo malignant change, which is usually signalled by a sudden increase in the rate of enlargement.

Clinical features

The history is of a painless mass, usually in the parotid, which may enlarge very slowly over a period of several years. The lump is discrete and mobile. If it occurs in the parotid it rarely results in a facial palsy (unlike a malignant tumour).

Management

Surgical excision is the standard treatment. The tumour has a capsule, and rupture of this can lead to tumour seeding and recurrence. As most parotid adenomas are in the bulkier superficial lobe of the gland, a superficial parotidectomy with preservation of the facial nerve can be undertaken. A submandibular adenoma is best managed by removal of the whole gland.

Cystadenoma lymphomatosum (Warthin's tumour or adenolymphoma)

This is another common benign tumour found only in the parotid gland. It is bilateral in 10%, does not undergo malignant change and bears no connection with lymphomas.

Malignant neoplasms

Malignant salivary gland tumours are rare and histologically diverse. *Muco-epidermoid carcinomas* can be high grade (and mimic squamous carcinoma in clinical behaviour) or low grade (when they behave in a relatively benign way). *Squamous carcinoma* is an aggressive tumour, which, in the parotid gland, often produces a facial nerve palsy. It is important to differentiate this disease from metastatic squamous carcinoma in an intraparotid lymph node. *Adenocarcinomas* and *adenoid cystic carcinomas* can also develop in the salivary glands. The latter has a tendency to infiltrate along nerves for considerable distances.

Management

Surgical removal is the main treatment. If a malignant parotid tumour is found to directly involve the facial nerve, then that structure must be sacrificed and continuity of the nerve re-established using a segment of greater auricular or sural nerve as a graft. Unfortunately, both fine needle aspiration biopsy and frozen section biopsy are notoriously unreliable at providing an accurate morphological diagnosis of a salivary gland malignancy.

Lymphomas

These tumours may develop in any of the larger salivary glands. Once the diagnosis has been made by either FNA or biopsy, treatment is by conventional methods (see Ch. 30).

NECK SPACE INFECTIONS

Peritonsillar abscess (quinsy)

Anatomy and pathological features

The faucial tonsil lies medial to the pharyngeal constrictor muscle and has a pseudocapsule of fibrous tissue around its deep surface. A peritonsillar abscess develops when this potential space becomes infected by direct spread from acute tonsillitis. The problem is usually unilateral, and in the early stages there is a local cellulitis rather than overt abscess formation.

Clinical features

History

There is a background of acute tonsillitis that suddenly progresses with increasing unilateral pain and dysphagia. The patient may be unable to swallow saliva and usually has marked trismus because of reflex spasm in the adjacent pterygoid muscles.

Physical findings

A fluctuating pyrexia is invariable. The tonsil is displaced downwards and medially. There may be obvious cervical lymphadenopathy or just a vague fullness on that side of the neck.

Management

In the early stages, intravenous antibiotics (penicillin and metronidazole) are given. However, if there is any suspicion of a local collection of pus, then the inflammatory mass should be drained. This is best performed with a 14 G needle and 10 mL syringe or a fine blade on a long-handled scalpel, having first sprayed the palate with lidocaine. The site of the puncture is shown in Figure 14.7.

Parapharyngeal abscess

Anatomy and pathological considerations

The parapharyngeal space is a potential one that is triangular in cross-section (Fig. 14.8). It lies lateral to the pharyngeal constrictors, anterior to the prevertebral fascia and deep to the deep cervical fascia. Its chief contents are the carotid tree, the internal jugular vein and the last four cranial nerves. Infection of this space is usually the consequence of dental sepsis or uncontrolled tonsillitis. Two dangerous complications may result:

- spread of the infection inferiorly into the mediastinum
- mucosal oedema in the adjacent larynx and pharynx with airways obstruction.

Clinical features

There is fever with diffuse swelling of the affected side of the neck and loss of the normal gutter anterior to the sternomastoid muscle.

Management

Prompt treatment is essential because of the risk of complications. Intravenous antibiotics should be administered and a CT scan obtained to ascertain whether or not there is a collection of pus. When present, pus is drained through an incision running down the anterior border of the sternomastoid muscle.

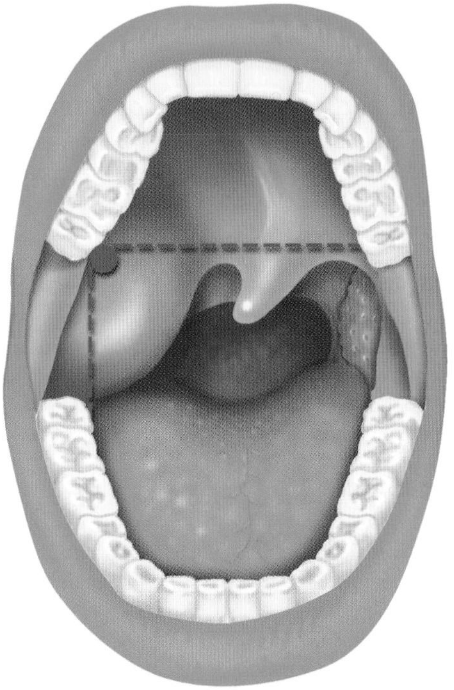

Fig. 14.7 The site of a right-sided peritonsillar abscess, with the point of incision.

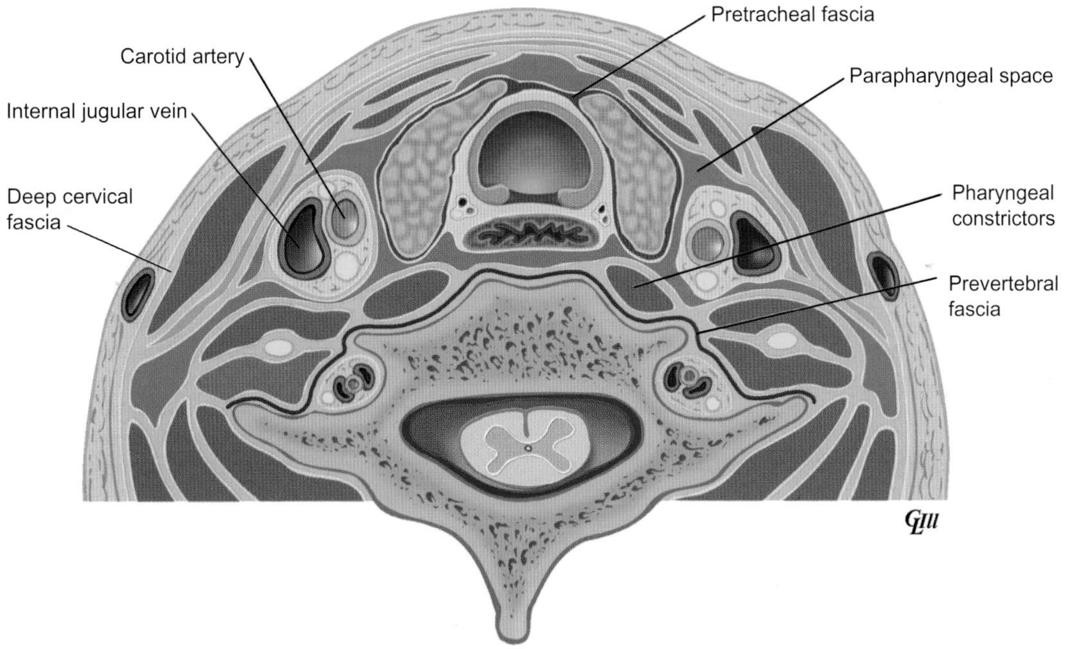

Fig. 14.8 The parapharyngeal space.

Emergency Box 14.1

Acute airways obstruction

Any neck space infection is a potential cause of acute airways obstruction. Failure to improve after 24 hours of intravenous antibiotics may necessitate surgical drainage and/or a tracheostomy.

Ludwig's angina (Emergency Box 14.1)

Anatomy and pathological considerations

Soft-tissue infection of the floor of the mouth on both sides of the mylohyoid muscle usually results from gross dental sepsis. A combination of bacteria, which may be anaerobic, is often involved.

Clinical features

A brawny swelling of the submandibular and submental triangles is present. On intraoral inspection, there is gross oedema of the mucosa of the floor of the mouth, with upward and posterior displacement of the tongue. The latter is potentially fatal, in that the tongue may obstruct the airway.

Management

Treatment is initially with antibiotics, which should be chosen to include cover for anaerobic infection. Any collection of pus should be drained, if necessary using through-and-through incisions running from the floor of the mouth medial to the mandible and out into the neck. It may be necessary to maintain the airway by nasopharyngeal or nasotracheal intubation. If this is unsatisfactory, a tracheostomy is required.

Tonsillar swelling from infectious mononucleosis

Alarming swelling of both tonsils may occur and, in extreme cases, compromise the pharyngeal airway. However, peritonsillar abscess does not occur unless a bacterial tonsillitis supervenes. Impending airways obstruction can often be prevented by using steroids.

VOCAL CORD PARALYSIS AND UPPER AIRWAYS OBSTRUCTION

Paralysis of a vocal cord is usually the consequence of damage to the ipsilateral recurrent laryngeal nerve, which is a branch of the vagus nerve.

Anatomy and physiological features

The left nerve runs a significantly longer course than the right, down into the superior mediastinum and around the arch of the aorta. Therefore it is three times more likely to be affected. When the recurrent laryngeal nerve is damaged or divided, the cord assumes a paramedian position. This may be asymptomatic or result in hoarseness; however, if both recurrent nerves are affected then acute airways obstruction is almost inevitable. Damage to or division of the main vagus nerve at the base of the skull is more likely to cause the ipsilateral cord to assume a more lateralised position. Although this does not threaten the airway, it results in a very poor breathy voice and serious problems with aspiration of saliva and food.

Aetiology

Common causes of distal disruption of the recurrent laryngeal nerve are:

- thyroid surgery (Ch. 32)
- cardiac (aortic arch) surgery
- carcinoma of the bronchus
- carcinoma of the thyroid
- carcinoma of the oesophagus.

There is, in addition, a large idiopathic group in which the cause is never found and where spontaneous recovery is relatively common.

Diagnosis

The development of a recurrent laryngeal nerve palsy should lead to a detailed search for the cause, which may require a variety of special investigations to find or exclude an intrathoracic cause.

Management

The frequency with which an idiopathic palsy occurs and its likely spontaneous recovery mean that elective surgery for hoarseness, airways obstruction or aspiration should only be undertaken in those patients who have an identifiable, non-reversible cause or who have had symptoms for at least 9 months and are therefore very unlikely to recover. Patients with a unilateral palsy very rarely require a tracheostomy.

Surgical treatment

There are two categories:

- medialisation of the vocal cord
- lateralisation of the vocal cord.

Medialisation is used when one cord is paralysed and the other unable to provide complete closure of the glottis. The affected cord is moved medially to improve the voice and reduce aspiration. Either a paste is injected endoscopically at two or three sites immediately lateral to the cord, or a piece of thyroid cartilage is wedged between it and the thyroid ala (thyroplasty).

Lateralisation is used in an attempt to improve the airway in bilateral palsy when the cords lie in the paramedian position. A type of laser cordectomy can be undertaken, although this treatment is inevitably a compromise; as the gap between the cords is increased, the airway improves, but the voice deteriorates and aspiration becomes an increasing problem.

In bilateral paralysis, a permanent tracheostomy is usually the best management. A cuffed tube will be necessary if aspiration is a serious problem.

Obstructive sleep apnoea

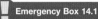

Obstructive sleep apnoea (OSA) is an increasingly recognised condition where blockage occurs in the upper airways during sleep. This results in repeated episodes of apnoea and is particularly common in the morbidly obese. Other risk factors include male sex and age over 40 years. Diagnosis is suspected on history and confirmed by sleep studies. OSA may lead to daytime sleepiness, hypertension, cardiovascular disease, memory problems, weight gain and headaches. Treatment is usually non-surgical with the use of a dentally fitted mandibular advancement devices (MDA) or continuous positive airways pressure (CPAP) masks which help to prevent airways obstruction at night. Weight loss should be achieved in the obese patient if possible. Morbidly obese patients may benefit from bariatric surgery (see Ch. 19). In children tonsillectomy and adenoidectomy may cure the condition. In some adults surgery to reconstruct the soft tissues of the upper airway, and occasionally the bony structures may be recommended. Options include uvulopalatopharyngoplasty (UPPP – which involves removal of the tonsils, adenoids, and part of the soft palate and uvula), laser assisted uvulopalatoplasty, and radiofrequency ablation (RFA) treatment to the soft palate and tongue.

COMMON SURGICAL PROCEDURES ON THE NECK

Tonsillectomy

The indications for tonsillectomy are given in Box 14.1. Although the frequency of this operation has reduced, it is still a commonly performed operation, which is not without complications. Haemorrhage is the most important and may be primary (within 24 hours of surgery) or secondary (days 5–10), when it is usually the result of infection at the site of excision. A bleeding diathesis, such as von Willebrand's disease, may present with bleeding during or after tonsillectomy.

Tracheostomy

There are two types of tracheostomy (Fig. 14.9):

- After a laryngectomy, the divided trachea is brought out and sutured to the skin.
- More frequently an opening is made, into the front wall of the trachea, the larynx remaining in situ. It may be a temporary or permanent, elective or emergency procedure.

Whenever possible, a tracheostomy should be performed with an endotracheal tube in situ. This way, the airway

Box 14.1 Indications for tonsillectomy

- Recurrent tonsillitis with more than four attacks per year
- Obstructive sleep apnoea with tonsillar hypertrophy in children
- Peritonsillar abscess with a past history of recurrent tonsillitis
- Unilaterally enlarged tonsil with lymphoma a possibility
- Malignant ipsilateral lymphadenopathy due to squamous carcinoma, with no known primary

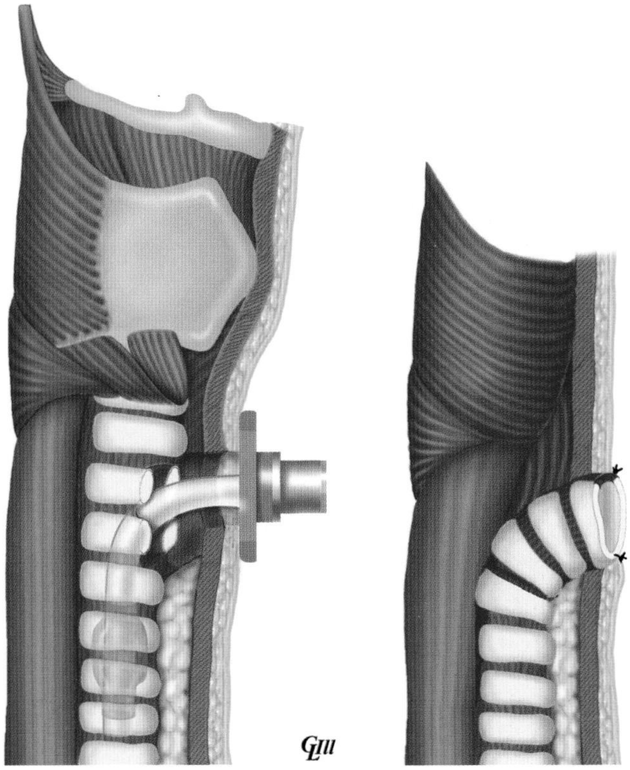

Fig. 14.9 The two types of tracheostomy.

Box 14.2 Indications for tracheostomy

Supralaryngeal obstruction
- Ludwig's angina
- Severe facial fractures
- Glandular fever
- Laryngeal obstruction
- Epiglottitis
- Laryngeal tumour
- Bilateral vocal cord palsy

Recurrent aspiration
- Coma
- Myasthenia gravis
- Bulbar or pseudobulbar palsy

Respiratory support
- Injury to the chest wall
- Seriously ill or injured patients (ARDS)
- Prolonged endotracheal intubation

remains secure throughout the procedure. In adults, a window should be excised from the anterior tracheal wall: a trap door flap is dangerous as it can become inverted and obstruct the tracheal lumen. In children, a vertical slit controlled by stay sutures should be employed.

The indications for tracheostomy are given in Box 14.2.

One of the fallacies about a tracheostomy is that the patient is unable to speak afterwards. This is not usually true. Once the operation site has healed, the initial tube is replaced by a silver or plastic one without a cuff. A speaking valve can then be attached: during quiet respiration, air travels back and forth through the tube, but on forced expiration the valve will shut, diverting the air up through the glottis where it can be set into vibration and used for phonation.

FURTHER READING

Corbridge R, Steventon N 2009 Oxford handbook of ENT and head and neck surgery, 2nd edn. Oxford University Press, Oxford

Clarke R, Bull PD 2007 Diseases of the ear, nose and throat (Lecture Notes Series), 10th edn. Wiley-Blackwell, Chichester

Lee K J (ed) 2008 Essential otolaryngology: Head and neck surgery, 9th edn. McGraw-Hill Medical, New York

15 Ear and nose

THE EAR

Anatomy

External ear

This is merely the pinna and the auditory meatus (Fig. 15.1).

Middle ear (tympanic cavity)

The tympanic membrane separates the external from the middle ear. The middle ear cleft comprises the Eustachian (auditory) tube and middle ear cavity which communicates with the mastoid air cells. The bony roof of the attic of the middle ear separates it from the middle cranial fossa. The middle ear cavity is in contact with the external atmosphere through the Eustachian tube, which opens into the postnasal space and contains three articulating ossicles (Fig. 15.1) – the malleus, incus and stapes – which are supported by ligaments. The annular ligament surrounds the footplate of the stapes (3.5mm^2 in area) and restrains this to movement in the oval window. The second, round window, below the oval window, is covered only with a membrane, which allows the transmission of pressure and movement of fluids in the inner ear.

There are two muscles in the middle ear: tensor tympani and stapedius; these pull in opposite directions and modify the motion of the ossicles, increasing their stiffness and protecting the delicate inner ear from excessive oscillation of the chain of small bones.

Inner ear

There are three parts to the inner ear:

- anteriorly, the cochlea with the organ of Corti, for hearing
- in the middle, the vestibule with the utricle and saccule, which are concerned with static balance and linear acceleration
- posteriorly, three semicircular canals in different planes – the organ of balance, which is concerned with angular acceleration.

The otic capsule of the inner ear contains perilymph and has connection with the subarachnoid space. Inside the capsule is the membranous labyrinth with sensory cells and containing the endolymph, which is produced by stria vascularis. Endolymph is absorbed mainly by the endolymphatic sac which lies in the posterior cranial fossa between the petrous bone and the dura. The cochlear and vestibular divisions of the VIIIth nerve join and travel through the internal auditory meatus to the brainstem. The VIIth (facial) nerve also travels through the internal auditory canal and traverses the medial and posterior walls of the middle ear cavity to emerge through the stylomastoid foramen.

Physiology

Hearing

The eardrum and the ossicles amplify sound waves through the lever effect of the ossicles and because the area of the eardrum is more than 20 times that of the footplate of the stapes. This allows reduction of acoustic impedance when sound energy is passed from air into liquid in the labyrinth.

Micromechanical oscillations of the stapes result in movement of liquid in the cochlea and motion of the basilar membrane with the sensory hair cells. The point of maximum movement of the basilar membrane is determined by the frequency of the introduced tone: high-frequency tones correspond to a place in the basal turn of the cochlea; and low-frequency tones to one in the apical turn. The movement of the cilia of the receptor hair cells generates electric impulses in the cells, and bioelectric events then follow in the auditory nerve.

Sound frequency is measured in hertz (Hz) where 1 Hz is equal to 1 cycle per second. The range of frequencies which can be appreciated as sound by humans is approximately 20 to 18 000 Hz. The ear can discriminate an enormous intensity range of 100 000 : 1, and for practical measurement it can be compressed into a logarithmic decibel scale of 0–120 dB.

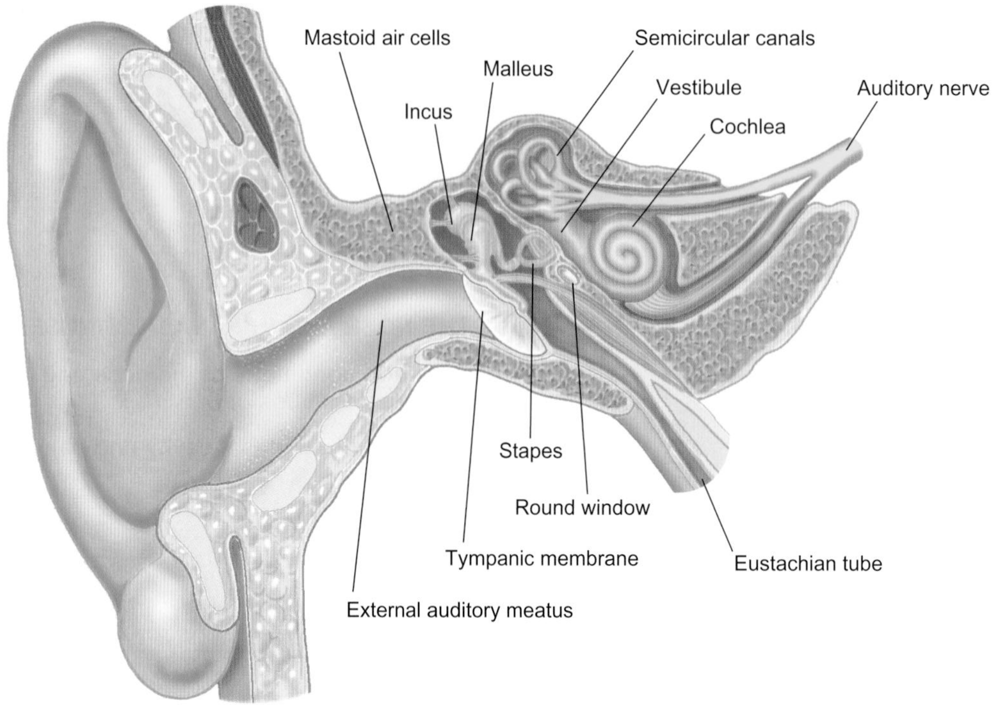

Fig. 15.1 Anatomy of the ear.

Balance

Movement and acceleration in any of the three planes of the semicircular canals cause movement of the endolymph with deviation of the gelatinous cupola with the embedded sensory hair cells in the semicircular canals. In the saccule and utricle, there is displacement of the sensory hair cells, which are embedded in the gelatinous otolith membrane containing particles of calcium carbonate, and respond to changes in linear acceleration or gravity force. The stimulus triggers the action potential of the vestibular nerve. All of the inputs from the labyrinth, the eyes and somatosensors relay to the brain. Central processing takes place, and responses return to the muscles to maintain posture and eye position, with the cerebellum ensuring a smooth, coordinated response. An alteration in vestibular response on one side as opposed to the other, results in imbalance in the central response which affects control of the eyes, causing them to oscillate – vestibular nystagmus.

Common symptoms

Common symptoms are:

- hearing loss – congenital or acquired (sudden or progressive)
- aural discharge
- otalgia – pain in the ear
- tinnitus – variable noises in the ear
- vertigo.

Otalgia

Pain in the ear may arise from pain receptors supplied by the afferent fibres of:

- the Vth and Xth cranial nerves
- C2 and C3, which supply the external ear
- the IXth, supplying the middle ear.

When otalgia is a presenting symptom and no local disease is found in the ear, a referred otalgia is possible from a distant area innervated by any of the above nerves. Usual causes are:

- dental disease
- temporomandibular joint disorders
- maxillary sinusitis
- inflammatory and malignant lesions of the pharynx, posterior tongue and larynx
- conditions in the back of the neck and cervical spine.

Tinnitus

The subjective perception of tinnitus, which is characterised by rushing, hissing or ringing sounds of varying intensity in the ear or head, may be associated with dysfunction in the cochlea and the auditory pathway. A rhythmic pulsatile tinnitus is suggestive of vascular lesions such as:

- arteriovenous malformations
- arterial aneurysms
- glomus tumour in the middle ear
- sound transmission from major vessels in the neck.

Tinnitus can sometimes be detected objectively on auscultation of the ear and the mastoid. Crackling sounds can be associated with dysfunction of the Eustachian tube and rhythmic myoclonus of the muscles attached to it.

Vertigo

Vertigo associated with a peripheral vestibular lesion is most commonly rotatory but can be experienced as a swaying or tilting of either the patient or the surroundings. Movement and positional changes tend to make the vertigo worse. Central vestibular lesions tend to produce less intense vertigo, positional changes have less effect and the patient may experience disturbance of gait and other neurological symptoms and signs.

Clinical examination

Examination of the auricle and the mastoid precedes otoscopic examination. Wax should be removed if it obstructs the view, but this should not be done by syringing if a perforation of the tympanic membrane is suspected, because of a risk of introducing infection. The normal tympanic membrane reflects the directed light in the shape of a cone which is seen in the antero-inferior part of the membrane. The prominent landmark is the handle of the malleus (Fig. 15.2). The tympanic membrane is divided into the pars tensa and the pars flaccida (the upper area). It is very useful to use examination with a microscope to evaluate scars, retractions and types of perforation. The presence of perforation may allow damage to the ossicles, granulations and cholesteatoma to be seen. The nasal cavities and posterior nasal space must be examined in order to exclude infection or tumour which may cause Eustachian tube insufficiency or blockage and consequent failure of air circulation to the middle ear. A full assessment of the head and neck is performed to exclude referred otalgia.

Investigations

Auditory function

There are different types of hearing loss, as follows:

- conductive – from lesions in the external auditory meatus and the middle ear
- sensorineural – from cochlear and retrocochlear lesions
- mixed – when both types of hearing loss are present.

Tuning fork tests

Rinne test. A vibrating tuning fork which generates sound at 512 Hz is placed near the external meatus (air conduction, AC) and then firmly on the mastoid process (bone conduction [BC], a measure of sensorineural function of the cochlea). Normally sound is detected better by AC than by BC. Conductive loss means that sound conduction through the middle ear apparatus is reduced. The convention is as follows:

- normal – AC better than BC → Rinne test positive
- conductive loss – BC better than AC → Rinne test negative
- sensorineural loss – AC better than BC but both reduced compared with normal → Rinne test positive and reduced.

Weber test. A vibrating tuning fork is placed either on the vertex of the skull or on the forehead midway between the ears. The patient indicates on which side the sound is better lateralised by bone conduction. The interpretation is as follows:

- conductive loss – sound lateralised to the affected side
- sensorineural loss – sound lateralised to the side with better cochlear function.

Pure tone audiometry

The hearing threshold can be measured in decibels of hearing level (dBHL) for air and bone conduction at each frequency between 250 and 8000 Hz (Fig. 15.3).

Impedance audiometry

The middle ear compliance (i.e. how much of the applied sound energy is reflected from the tympanic membrane) and middle ear pressure (the difference, if any, between pressure externally and in the cavity) can be measured with an instrument applied to the ear canal. A very low compliance could be the result of a middle ear effusion. A lower or negative

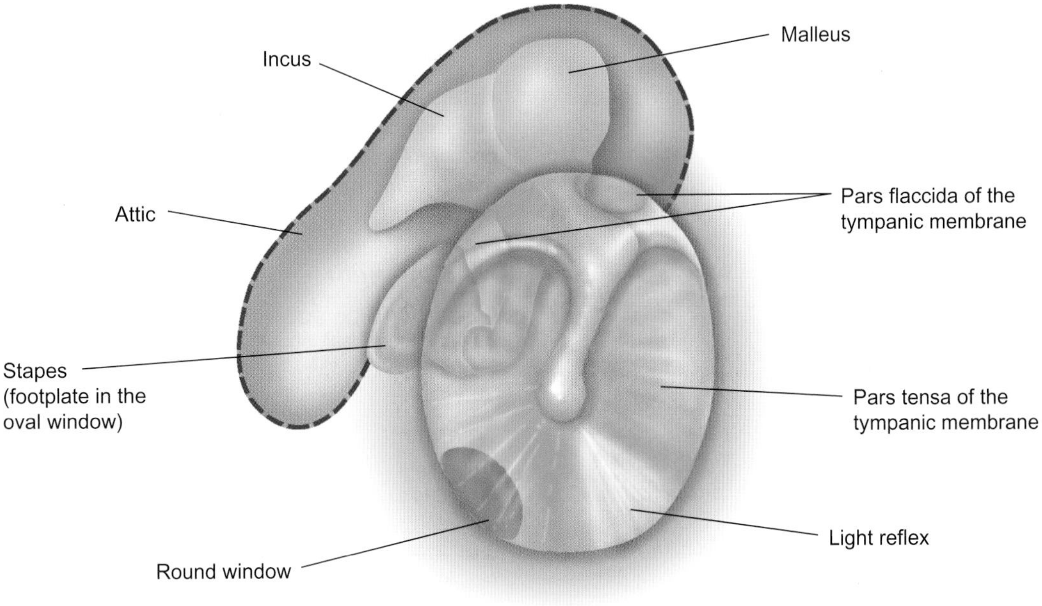

Fig. 15.2 The external aspect of the tympanic membrane.

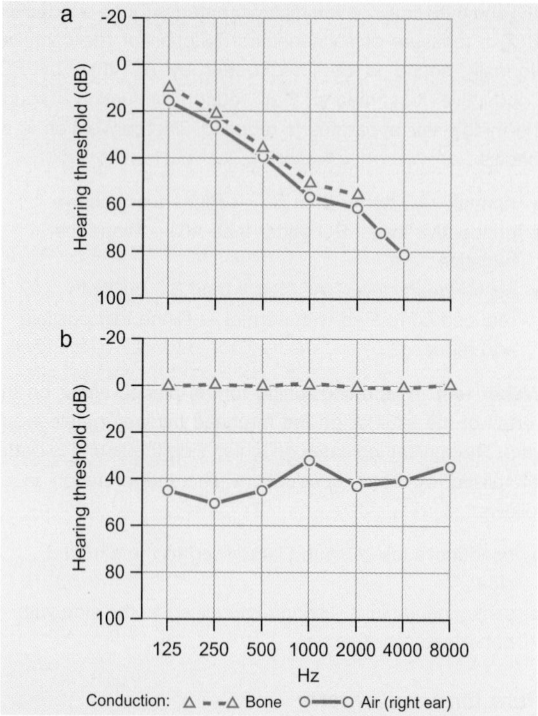

Fig. 15.3 An audiogram. (a) Sensorineural loss with reduced hearing levels by both air and bone conduction. (b) Conductive hearing loss with reduced hearing level by air conduction and normal bone conduction.

pressure within the middle ear than without indicates insufficiency of the Eustachian tube.

Electric response audiometry

Electrical responses to sound stimuli can be recorded from the cochlea, brainstem and cortex. Auditory-evoked potentials of a few microvolts can be recorded from the scalp as the 'auditory brainstem response' which occurs within 10 ms. This has become a useful objective test in children and in patients in whom reliability of subjective audiometric tests is doubtful. It also has wide-ranging application in neuro-otological diagnosis and detection of acoustic tumours.

Vestibular function

Clinical

Spontaneous and positional nystagmus, eye movements, stance, gait and limbs are all tested.

Nystagmus. This condition is defined as involuntary (usually rapid) rhythmic, transverse (although occasionally vertical – see below) eye movements:

- Vestibular nystagmus is a rhythmic oscillating movement of the eyes resulting from either induced stimulation of the labyrinth or vestibular disease; it has a slow vestibular and a fast cerebral correcting component trying to restore the eye position in the direction of gaze.
- Labyrinthine nystagmus is always horizontal-rotatory or horizontal.
- Vertical nystagmus and multiple other forms occur only in central vestibular lesions.

Head positional testing

This can induce benign positional vertigo (BPV) and nystagmus when the defect is thought to be in the labyrinth and the detached otolith floats in the semicircular canal of balance. BPV occurs with a short latency, lasts a few seconds and fatigues on repetition; usually it is a self-limiting condition which resolves within a few months.

Electronystagmography

The velocity of nystagmus can be assessed by graphic recording. Labyrinthine nystagmus is enhanced when visual input is abolished by closing the eyes or by darkness.

Caloric test

This test is based on the principle of cooling or heating the labyrinth by a flow of water in the external ear canal. A convection current is set up in the semicircular canal which in turn induces vertigo and nystagmus. In vestibular hypofunction these may be reduced or absent.

DISEASES OF THE EXTERNAL EAR

Foreign bodies

In these cases, there is always a danger of forcing the foreign body further into the ear canal where it may damage the drum and the middle ear. Extraction of foreign bodies should therefore be done by skilled ear, nose and throat (ENT) personnel.

Trauma to the auricle

Aetiology and pathological features

Haematoma of the auricle occurs in boxers and those who take part in other contact sports such as rugby football. The blood extravasates between the cartilage and perichondrium. If untreated, the blood becomes organised, causing a cauliflower deformity composed of fibrous tissues. Perichondritis and abscess may develop as a consequence of secondary infection. The cartilage deprived of vascular supply may undergo necrosis, leading to marked deformity of the auricle.

Management

Prevention

Suitable headgear should be worn by those engaged in contact sports.

Treatment

The haematoma is evacuated through a wide-bore needle or by incision of the skin. A firm dressing must be applied in order to prevent further bleeding. If a subperichondrial abscess forms, it should be incised and drained. *Pseudomonas aeruginosa* is not uncommonly cultured in these patients, and broad-spectrum antibiotics are indicated.

Furuncle

Aetiology and pathological features

This is an infection of hair follicles and is usually caused by *Staphylococcus aureus*. Recurrent infection may have diabetes as the underlying cause.

Clinical features

There may be severe earache, and any movement of the auricle (and thus of the auditory canal) or pressure on the tragus causes considerable pain. Mild hearing deficit may occur in cases of complete obturation of the ear canal. The external canal will be oedematous, with swelling in front of or behind the auricle.

Management

Furuncle is treated by a combination of the insertion of an antiseptic wick and systemic antibiotics.

Otitis externa

Aetiology and pathological features

Environmental factors which predispose to otitis externa are:

- heat
- humidity
- swimming
- any irritation which predisposes to scratching.

Specific causes are:

- infection – bacterial, fungal, viral
- reactive inflammation – eczema, seborrhoeic dermatitis, neurodermatitis.

A spreading necrotising type with osteomyelitis of the base of the skull may develop in immunocompromised or elderly diabetic patients. *Pseudomonas aeruginosa* and anaerobic organisms are often found.

Clinical features

In the common irritative type, discharge from the ear and, sometimes, mild pain are present. In the spreading, necrotising variant, there is systemic disturbance, more severe local symptoms and signs of spread which may include the development of a VIIth nerve palsy.

Management

In the mild type, treatment is by a combination of topical antiseptics or antibiotics incorporated into steroid-containing ear drops; if the condition is particularly troublesome, this is supplemented by systemic antibiotics after culture has been obtained. Aural toilet is essential, and infected debris is removed by mopping with a cotton wool carrier or by microsuction. Fungal infection may follow after prolonged treatment with antibacterial drops. In the severe necrotising form, therapy should consist of intensive local treatment with excision of dead tissue, the administration of systemic antibiotics and control of diabetes if this is present.

DISEASES OF THE MIDDLE EAR

Acute otitis media

Aetiology and pathological features

The incidence is highest in the first 5 years of life and thereafter it becomes infrequent. Most children have a history of preceding viral upper respiratory tract infection. Inflammation of the postnasal space and adenoids may spread via the Eustachian tube to the middle ear. Oedematous mucosa in the tube causes blockage and, if secondary bacterial infection spreads along the tube, a middle ear abscess will result. Under the age of 5 years, *Haemophilus influenzae* is isolated in about 30% of cases.

As tension rises, rupture of the tympanic membrane occurs usually in the pars tensa. In the majority, the inflammation resolves and the tympanic membrane heals without any sequelae. However, in a small proportion, complications develop and there is loss of hearing. Other problems are:

- a chronic middle ear effusion in about 5%
- scarring of the tympanic membrane and the middle ear (tympanosclerosis)
- chronic suppurative otitis media consequent to a non-healing perforation
- progression to acute mastoiditis.

Clinical features

Symptoms

Pain and hearing loss are early symptoms; if the drum perforates, a purulent discharge develops and the pain usually subsides.

Signs

There is malaise and pyrexia. The drum is reddened and tense. A perforation may be visible with discharge emerging through it.

Management

Amoxicillin is the preferred drug in children and should be administered for 10 days.

Acute mastoiditis

Aetiology and pathological features

Mastoiditis is the consequence of a preceding otitis media, and with the advent of powerful antibiotics the incidence has diminished considerably. Nevertheless, silent or masked mastoiditis can develop. There is cellulitis and osteitis in the air spaces which may go on to abscess formation. Spread can take place through the temporal bone to cause subperiosteal abscess or intracranial complications – an extradural abscess.

Clinical features

Symptoms

Symptoms are:

- pain
- fever
- aural discharge
- hearing loss.

Signs
Signs are:

- erythematous swollen mastoid and external canal
- the ear is pushed outward and forward if subperiosteal abscess develops.

Investigation
Sometimes, because of swelling in the canal, it is difficult to visualise the inflamed drum. Mastoid X-ray shows clouding of the air cells and sometimes formation of an abscess with erosion of bone.

Management
Very early stages are treated with intensive parenteral antibiotics. If resolution fails to occur, the inflammatory process is decompressed by a simple cortical mastoidectomy, preserving the posterior meatal wall and the middle ear ossicles.

Otitis media with effusion

The alternative names for this condition are chronic serous otitis media and glue ear.

Aetiology and pathogenesis
Accumulation of non-purulent fluid in the middle ear is common in children aged between 2 and 6 years. Many causative factors have been suggested, but the most probable is low-grade inflammation with partial block and dysfunction of the Eustachian tube and interference with the free flow of air in and out of the middle ear so that negative pressure develops in the middle ear.

Clinical features
Symptoms
Symptoms are:

- impaired hearing
- delay in learning to speak and acquiring a vocabulary
- other learning difficulties
- inattentiveness
- recurrent earaches.

Signs
Many children with this condition are discovered during routine audiometric screening. Otoscopic examination reveals a lustreless immobile tympanic membrane. Sometimes fluid levels can be seen in the middle ear. In long-standing disease the drum may become thin, atrophic and retracted.

Management
In many instances, reassessment after 3 months is advisable because in more than 90% the effusion will resolve spontaneously. Unresolved middle ear effusion with hearing loss requires anterior–inferior myringotomy, aspiration of the liquid and a ventilation tube (grommet) inserted into the tympanic membrane (Fig. 15.4). If there are associated features of nasal obstruction, the adenoids are curetted. The ventilation tube remains in the tympanic membrane for about 12 months, helping to restore to normal the mucus-producing mucosa of the middle ear, and is then spontaneously extruded from the tympanic membrane.

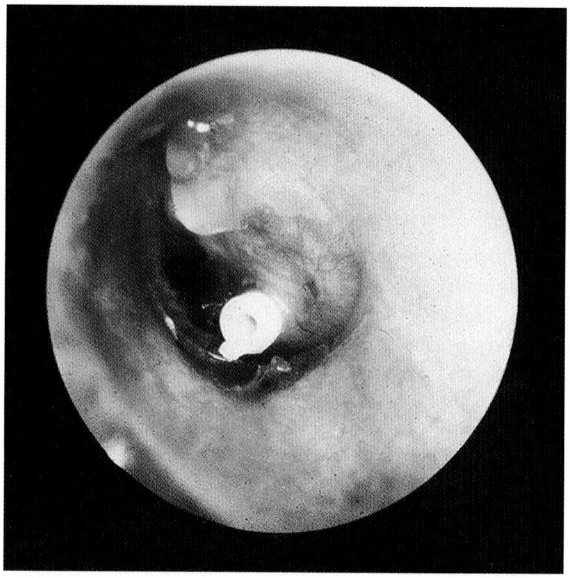

Fig. 15.4 A grommet inserted into the anterior inferior quadrant of the left tympanic membrane.

Middle ear effusion in adults
Aetiology and pathogenesis
Serous middle ear effusion may develop after:

- an upper respiratory tract infection
- allergic or vasomotor rhinitis
- exposure to changes in ambient pressure such as flying or diving (barotrauma) when the Eustachian tube does not equalise pressure.

In adults, carcinoma of the postnasal space invading the Eustachian tube is a rare precipitating cause.

Chronic suppurative otitis media
Aetiology and pathological features
This condition usually follows acute otitis media and has the same underlying causes. However, it may be chronic from the outset. There are two types:

- tubotympanic suppuration, which is limited to inflammation of the mucosa
- attico-antral disease with destruction involving the mastoid bone.

In the former, complications are unlikely, while the latter is unsafe.

Clinical features
Tubotympanic disease
The discharge is mucopurulent but it may cease and reappear after an upper respiratory tract infection or if water passes through the perforation in the tympanic membrane. This opening is central in the pars tensa and does not involve the bony margins (Fig. 15.5a). An audiogram shows conductive hearing loss.

Attico-antral disease

This presents as suppuration with or without cholesteatoma. The latter is a mass of keratinised squamous epithelium which increases in size as skin desquamates. Initially it forms in the developed retraction pocket of a perforated tympanic membrane in the attic. Spread then occurs, so destroying the middle ear ossicles and the temporal bone and eroding the bony canal of the facial nerve. Hearing loss can be marked. Vertigo may be present if the cholesteatoma has eroded the bony wall of the most prominent lateral semicircular canal, causing a fistula. Otoscopy reveals a superior perforation leading into the attic or a posterior marginal-type perforation involving the bony margin Fig. 15.5b. With bony involvement, granulations are common. Flakes of cholesteatoma can be seen in the area of the attic. CT may sometimes be helpful to reveal the extent of the bony erosion and the fistula of the lateral semicircular canal of balance.

a

b

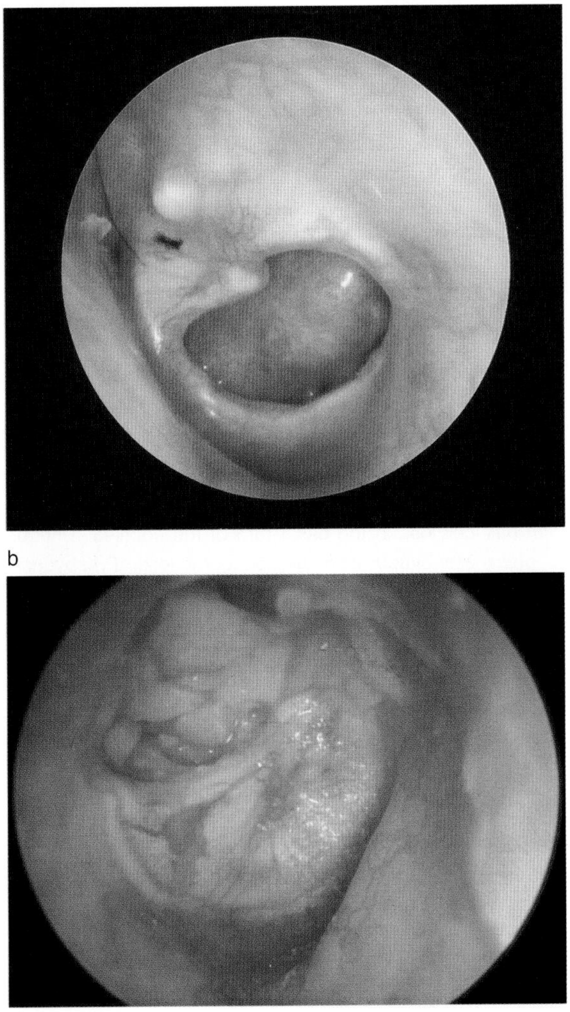

Fig. 15.5 (a) Large perforation of the tympanic membrane in the pars tensa. (b) Chronic otitis media with cholesteatoma and granulations in the attic.

Management

Tubotympanic disease

Active suppurative tubotympanic disease is treated with combined antibiotic and corticosteroid ear drops. For those who do not wish to wear a hearing aid or who want to swim, repair of the tympanic membrane (myringoplasty) can be done when the perforation is dry. The tympanic membrane can be supplemented by a graft of fascia from the temporalis muscle.

Attico-antral disease

Conservative treatment is ineffective in the presence of cholesteatoma. Classical radical mastoidectomy lays open the mastoid and excises the posterior meatal wall and the contents of the tympanic cavity (apart from the stapes) to create one safe cavity. Reconstruction of the tympanic membrane with a fascial graft and artificial ossicles (tympanoplasty), with the aim of improving hearing, may then be considered.

Complications of otitis media

Pathological features

The infective process in both acute and chronic otitis media may cause bone destruction and may also spread along veins, so leading to intracranial sepsis and the complications listed in Box 15.1. Figure 15.6 illustrates the complications that can arise.

Clinical features

In chronic otitis media, the development of pain in the ear and headache are a warning of a possible intracranial complication. Vertigo occurs in labyrinthitis, and suppuration will lead to complete destruction of the hearing and balance organs. In developed intracranial complications the symptoms and signs are those of:

- systemic infection
- meningitis
- raised intracranial pressure (Ch. 30)
- focal neurological abnormalities.

CT and MRI of the head are essential for accurate diagnosis.

Management

Joint management with the neurosurgeon is essential. The underlying disease in the mastoid is explored as described above.

Box 15.1 Complications of otitis media

Intratemporal
- Mastoiditis
- Labyrinthitis
- Facial nerve palsy

Intracranial
- Extradural abscess
- Meningitis
- Lateral sinus thrombosis
- Temporal lobe abscess
- Cerebellar abscess

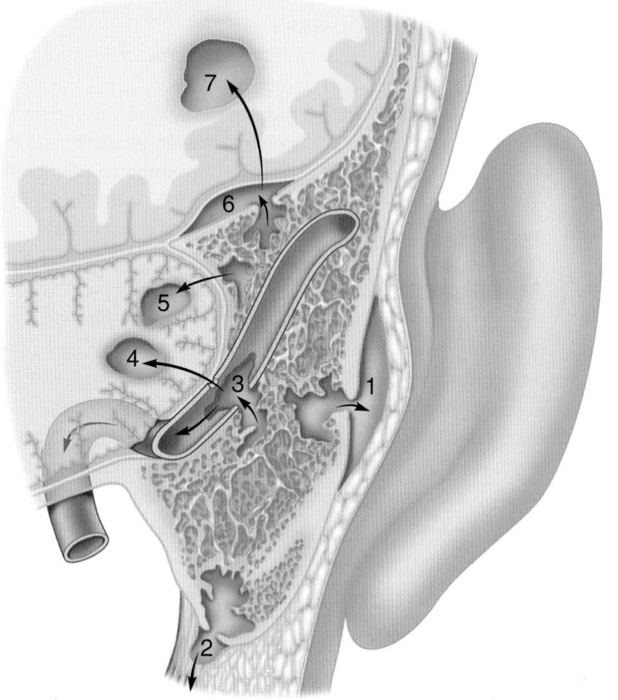

Fig. 15.6 Complications of otitis media. 1. Mastoiditis with subperiosteal abscess. 2. Mastoiditis with pus from the air cells of the tip of the mastoid spreading into the neck. 3. Sigmoid sinus thrombosis. 4, 5 Cerebellar abscess. 6. Epidural abscess. 7. Brain abscess in the temporal lobe.

Otosclerosis

Aetiology and pathological features

Otosclerosis is a localised disease of bone which affects the otic capsule. It is inherited as an autosomal dominant trait with incomplete penetrance. New spongy bone forms and, if this is in the area of the stapes, there may be ankylosis and conductive deafness.

Clinical features

History

There is a strong family history and both ears are affected in 90% of patients. The first manifestations are in the second decade and are progressive. Pregnancy and lactation aggravate the condition.

Physical findings

The tympanic membrane is normal and mobile in the presence of conductive hearing loss on an audiogram.

Management

If the patient does not wish to have a hearing aid, then stapedectomy is advised. The operation restores the mobility of the ossicular chain by perforating the stapes footplate, removing the arch of the stapes and replacing this with a piston prosthesis.

DISEASES OF THE INNER EAR

Sensorineural hearing loss

The causes of this kind of loss are:

- genetic abnormalities of the cochlea
- maternal infections during pregnancy – rubella, cytomegalovirus, syphilis
- perinatal hypoxia
- viral and bacterial labyrinthitis
- meningitis
- ototoxic drugs – gentamicin, neomycin, furosemide (frusemide), salicylates
- sudden idiopathic hearing loss (possibly viral or vascular)
- noise-induced hearing loss
- fracture of the temporal bone and trauma to the ear
- barotrauma, rupture of the round window membrane, perilymph leak.

In acquired hearing loss, the high audiometric frequencies are usually affected first, and this type of loss is associated with hair cell loss in the basal turn of the cochlea. Tinnitus is often associated with sensorineural loss. Presbycusis is sensorineural hearing loss with ageing; an audiogram reveals bilateral symmetrical high-frequency loss. Exposure to high-intensity noise causes characteristic bilateral hearing loss on the audiogram with a dip at 4000 Hz as the earliest change with depletion of hair cells at the basal turn of the cochlea.

Management

Hearing aids

Normal speech is at an intensity of 40–70 dB, and some form of amplification is required if the audiogram shows a hearing loss of more than 40 dB. An aid may also have a masking effect on tinnitus, which is often associated with sensorineural hearing loss.

Air conduction aids consist of a miniature microphone, an amplifier and a receiver which feed the sound into the ear, and a mould in the auditory canal. The apparatus is usually mounted behind the ear, but the advent of microelectronics means that a more cosmetically acceptable aid can, in mild to moderate loss, be placed entirely within the auditory canal. Improved signal processing and programmable digital multichannel aids work more selectively to amplify various speech frequencies and reduce interference from ambient noise.

Bone conduction aids are used when there is a congenital absence of the pinna and atresia of the canal. The aid is anchored to a titanium screw in the mastoid that has become osseo-integrated by ingrowth of bone. Sound waves are transferred into the cochlea by bone conduction.

Cochlear implant

Those who do not benefit from even the most powerful hearing aid and have profound bilateral deafness usually have a destroyed receptor organ and may be considered for a cochlear implant. In this procedure, electrodes are inserted into the spiral of the cochlea to stimulate the surviving neurons electrically (Fig. 15.7). Speech is coded in a small

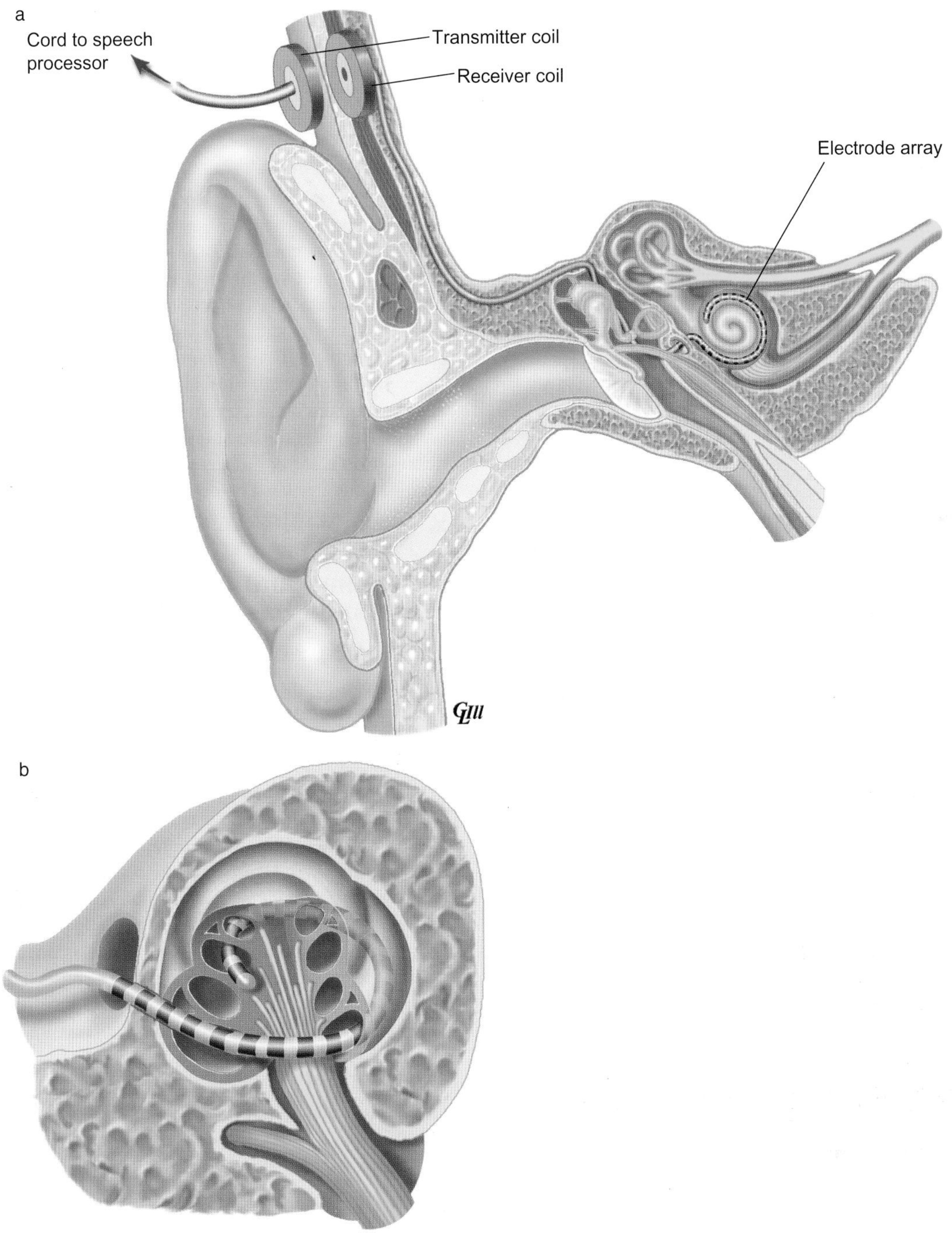

Fig. 15.7 The electrodes of the cochlear implant are inserted and stimulate the surviving nerve endings. (Adapted from H.G. Hirsch. Intelligibility improvement of noisy speech for people with cochlear implants. Speech Communication 12 (1993) 261–266. Reproduced by permission of Cochlear™.)

speech processor worn externally and transmitted across the skin behind the ear into the implant. The patient hears the sound (about 50% can discriminate speech without having to lip read), and their speech production improves.

Acoustic neuroma

Clinical features

The early symptoms are unilateral or markedly asymmetric sensorineural hearing loss and tinnitus. Such patients should be suspected of having an acoustic tumour unless there is a clear association with trauma or acute infection. Vertigo is rare, but patients with large tumours may have ataxia. Numbness of the side of the face (Vth nerve) follows.

Investigation

The audiogram reveals unilateral sensorineural hearing loss. MRI scan of the internal auditory meatus and the posterior cranial fossa reveals even the smallest tumour (Fig. 15.8).

Management

The tumour is removed by neurosurgery. The smaller the tumour, the easier is the operation and the less the likelihood of damage to the facial nerve. A proportion of tumours may not grow further and the patient may be followed up by monitoring the tumour size at 6-monthly intervals on MRI. Another option is gamma knife radiosurgery to arrest the growth of the tumour; this may be considered in particular for elderly patients.

Ménière's disease

Pathological features

Endolymphatic hydrops, which causes distension of the membranous labyrinthine spaces, is thought to be a pathological feature of Ménière's disease, but the reason for this is unknown.

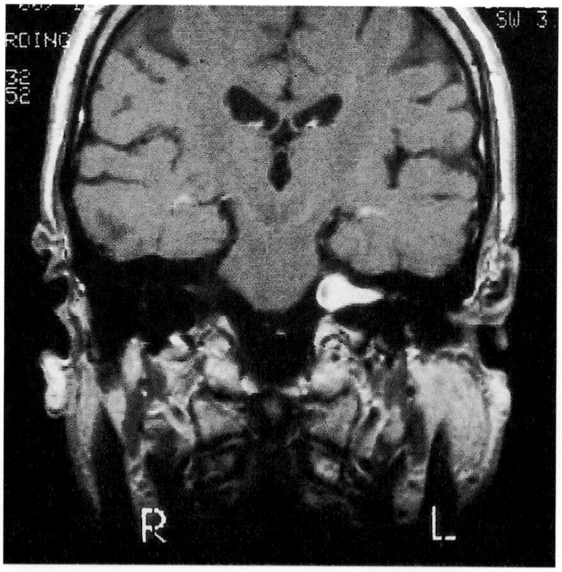

Fig. 15.8 MRI scan showing small left acoustic tumour.

Clinical features

Symptoms

There is a characteristic triad of symptoms which recur:

- attacks of vertigo
- fluctuating sensory hearing loss at low audiometric frequencies
- tinnitus.

Some patients also experience a sensation of fullness and pressure in the ear during the attack. Over years the hearing gradually deteriorates in the affected ear, and occasionally the disease is bilateral.

Signs

There are no specific physical findings.

Management

Attacks of vertigo are treated with vestibular sedatives (diazepam, cinnarizine, prochlorperazine). A salt-restricted diet is advised in an endeavour to reduce the frequency of attacks. It is thought that betahistine may have a positive prophylactic effect on the microcirculation in the cochlea, and it also has a positive effect on balance by reducing vestibular receptor resting firing rate. Surgery is indicated if medical treatment fails. Decompression of the endolymphatic sac and vestibular neurectomy does not destroy hearing and therefore is preferred to labyrinthectomy, which destroys the inner ear completely. Injections of gentamicin into the middle ear and delivery to the membranous round window through which it diffuses into the inner ear are effective in alleviating vertigo by reducing vestibular function.

Ear trauma and fracture of the skull base

Pathological and clinical features

Fractures of the temporal bone are associated with a severe head injury. Haematoma over the mastoid and blood in the external canal are important signs easily detected on simple clinical examination. A leak of cerebrospinal fluid (CSF) into the middle ear and through the auditory canal is a complication of fracture of the middle cranial fossa. CSF may also escape from the middle ear through the Eustachian tube – CSF rhinorrhoea. Conductive hearing loss is the result of blood in the middle ear (haemotympanum) or disruption of the ossicular chain. Vertigo or imbalance may suggest rupture of the round or oval windows. Profound deafness occurs if the fracture extends into the inner ear and may be associated with the above symptoms and also tinnitus. Fractures which involve the facial canal may produce a VIIth nerve palsy.

Management

The ear canal should not be syringed, nor should drops be instilled, because of the risk of introducing infection. Antibiotics are given and any CSF leak usually settles spontaneously. At a later stage, reconstruction of the ossicle chain (ossiculoplasty) may be needed to improve hearing. Very occasionally, exploration of the facial nerve is indicated with neural repair. Compensation for vestibular dysfunction can take several months.

THE NOSE AND PARANASAL SINUSES

Anatomy

A central septum divides the nasal cavity into two halves and supports the cartilaginous part of the nose. The anterior part is cartilage and the posterior bone. The lateral wall has three turbinates – inferior, middle and superior – with a corresponding meatus under each turbinate (Fig. 15.9). The anterior ethmoidal cells and the maxillary and frontal sinuses open into the middle meatus, and their ostia, which are close together, form the ostiomeatal complex. The posterior ethmoidal cells and the sphenoid sinus open into the superior meatus. The nasolacrimal duct opens into the inferior meatus.

The relationships between the sinuses and other structures have clinical importance in the spread of infection and tumours and in trauma. The maxillary, ethmoidal and frontal sinuses are related to the orbit, and the ethmoidal and frontal sinuses to the anterior cranial fossa. The sphenoid sinus is concealed by its position. On the lateral sides of the sinus lie the cavernous venous sinus, the internal carotid artery and the IIIrd, IVth and Vth cranial nerves. The pituitary fossa intrudes into the roof.

The arterial supply of the nose is provided from branches of both external and internal carotid arteries. The venous drainage is extracranial, but there are intracranial communications. The nerve supply to the nose and its sinuses is from the trigeminal nerve. The olfactory epithelium is in the branches of the superior part of the nose, and the filaments of the olfactory nerve pass through the cribriform plate. Autonomic sympathetic and parasympathetic fibres provide vasomotor innervation to the cavernous tissue in the nasal mucosa and also secretomotor control. The parasympathetic fibres relay in the pterygopalatine ganglion, and their stimulation causes swelling and increased secretion from the mucosa.

Physiology

The functions of the nose and sinuses are:

- air passage to and from the lungs
- warming, humidification and cleaning of incoming air (air conditioning)
- protection by mucociliary transport and immunological factors
- sense of smell
- resonators for speech production
- initiation of nasal reflexes – sneezing.

General features of nasal and sinus disease

Clinical features

Symptoms

These include:

- nasal obstruction – which can be unilateral or bilateral, intermittent or permanent
- mouth breathing – because of nasal obstruction, which in turn leads to dryness in the throat
- discharge and postnasal drip – clear serous discharge is common in allergic conditions and mucous or purulent discharge is associated with rhinosinusitis.

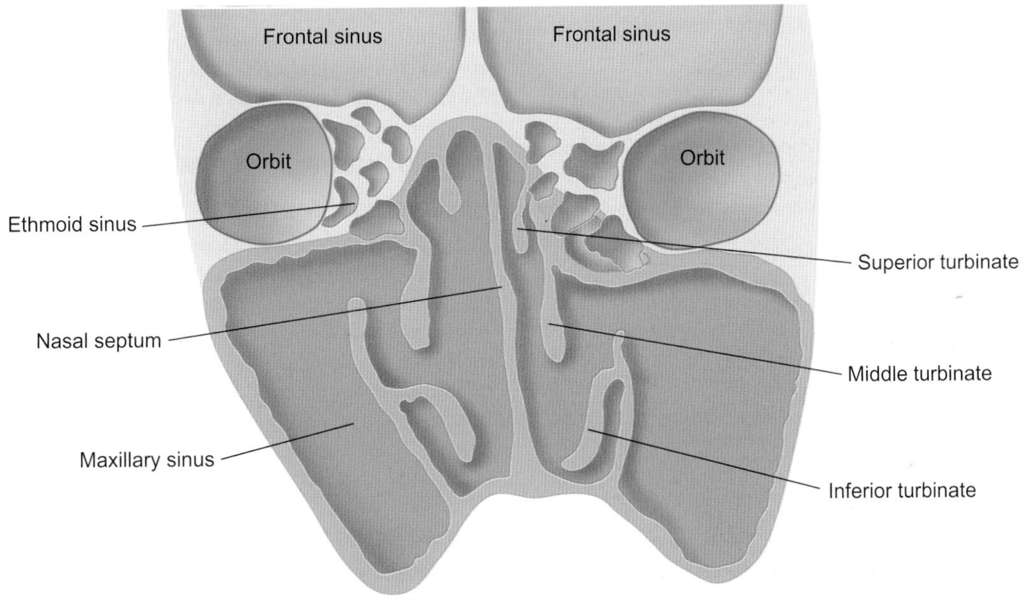

Fig. 15.9 Coronal section to show the sinuses and particularly the ethmoid air cells.

A unilateral discharge in a child probably originates from a foreign body. A bloodstained discharge with unilateral symptoms may be associated with tumour. Unilateral copious watery discharge suggests CSF rhinorrhoea
- facial pain – dull and well-localised, although it sometimes may radiate into the teeth and around the eyes or ear
- headaches, especially in sphenoiditis
- loss of smell
- bleeding
- cosmetic nasal deformity.

It is important to distinguish sinus pain from neuralgia, and referred pain from the teeth, temporomandibular joint or cervical spine.

Signs

The anterior part of the nose can be examined using a nasal speculum and a head light. Deformities of the septum, mucosal changes, prominent vessels and inferior and middle turbinates can be seen. Nasal polyps, tumours, ulcerations and foreign bodies can be identified. The posterior nasal space with the choanae and openings of the Eustachian tubes can be examined through the mouth by introducing a small mirror behind the soft palate.

Application of decongestant drops or 10% cocaine spray causes vasoconstriction and, by reducing the swelling of the mucosa, improves visibility. Cocaine also has a topical anaesthetic effect, and rigid or flexible nasal endoscopes can be used to examine the ostiomeatal complex and the posterior part of the nose and the postnasal space.

Investigation

Imaging

Plain X-ray will show if there is gross disease. CT scanning of the sinuses gives precise images and shows mucosal swelling, fluid levels or opacity as well as bony erosion by tumours. MRI is especially useful for delineating tumour spread.

Rhinomanometry

Nasal resistance to airflow can be calculated from measurements of flow and transnasal pressure. However, the results do not always correspond to the subjective feeling of nasal obstruction.

Immunological

Skin prick tests may identify a possible allergen. A weal of at least 2 mm diameter and greater than the reaction to the control solution is considered positive. The serum-specific IgE and the radio allergosorbent test (RAST) quantify an allergic response.

Mucociliary clearance

Saccharin is placed in the front of the nose and the time (normally 20 minutes) is measured for a sensation of sweetness to be recognised as the substance reaches the pharynx on the mucous blanket.

Smell

A short exposure to various bottles containing pungent substances establishes whether smell is reduced or distorted.

COMMON CONDITIONS OF THE NOSE AND PARANASAL SINUSES

Nasal foreign bodies

It is not unusual for children to insert foreign bodies into a nostril. The object may go undetected for some time, and presentation is with symptoms of unilateral purulent and sometimes offensive discharge. A radio-opaque concealed foreign body may be seen on X-ray. It should be removed with forceps or a hook, a procedure which may require a general anaesthetic.

Fractures of the nose

A nasal injury may be associated with other fractures of the face, including those of the zygoma, bony orbit and middle third of the face.

Clinical features

The symptoms are:

- nasal deformity
- obstruction
- bleeding.

Examination of the nasal cavity may reveal:

- deviated septum
- septal haematoma.

Management

Displaced nasal fractures may be reduced immediately or in 7–10 days after swelling has subsided. For old nasal injuries, the nasal deformity may be corrected by mobilising the external nasal pyramid by performing osteotomies of the nasal bones and rhinoplasty. A plaster of Paris splint is applied for 2 weeks to stabilise the nasal bones.

Septal haematoma and abscess

Pathological features

After nasal trauma a haematoma may develop between the mucoperichondrial flaps of the septum. The outcome may be that the septal cartilage is deprived of its blood supply. Secondary infection can develop, and an abscess may form. If untreated, the cartilage may undergo necrosis and the nasal bridge loses its support, leading to a saddle-type nasal deformity.

Upon examination, the septum will be very swollen and fluctuant to palpation with a probe.

Management

The haematoma must be incised and drained. Nasal packing should be applied so as to allow the perichondrium to adhere to the cartilage. Antibiotics should be given.

Deviated nasal septum

A septal deviation can be either traumatic or developmental. In either event, nasal obstruction results. The patient will complain of such obstruction, and the deviation will be apparent on clinical examination.

Management

Submucous resection (SMR) of the septum is done by elevating the mucoperichondrial flaps and resecting the deviated part of the septal cartilage and bone. In septoplasty, the cartilage is mobilised and the excision is more conservative. Excessive resection of the cartilage may lead to collapse of the nasal dorsum and tip. A septal perforation may occur if the mucoperichondrial flaps are perforated on both sides.

Epistaxis

Pathological features

Bleeding from the anterior part of the nose is more common and less severe than that from the posterior part, where the arteries are larger and have undergone degenerative change in older patients. Several vessels anastomose in the anterior septum, known as Little's area, which is a frequent site of origin of bleeding.

Bleeding can be the consequence of local or systemic causes, which include:

- trauma – nose-picking, fracture, surgery
- tumours – angioma, angiofibroma of postnasal space, carcinoma of the nose, postnasal space or sinuses
- local infection with ulceration
- prominent vessels in Little's area
- atherosclerotic degeneration of greater nasal arteries
- haematological – blood disease, bleeding diatheses, hereditary telangiectasia, coagulation defects, treatment with anticoagulants.

Management

The nose is anaesthetised and decongested with lidocaine and phenylephrine. The bleeding vessel can be cauterised chemically with silver nitrate or by electrocautery. More accurate cauterisation of the bleeding vessels may be achieved by using a fibreoptic naso-endoscope, particularly in the posterior aspect of the nasal cavity. If the bleeding point cannot be identified or is not controlled with cautery, a Merocel expandable nasal tampon or ribbon gauze impregnated in bismuth iodoform paraffin paste (BIPP) is packed into the anterior nasal cavity. When the bleeding is from the back of the nose and anterior packing is ineffective, an epistaxis balloon is introduced through the nose into the postnasal space to occlude the posterior nares and choanae; it is then drawn forward through the nose and secured.

When even a balloon is ineffective, re-insertion of a postnasal pack through the mouth and securing this in front of the nose is required and is combined with anterior packing usually under general anaesthesia. The packs remain for 48 hours, during which time antibiotics are necessary. Frequently, repeated haemorrhage may require ligation of the appropriate vessel. The external carotid artery can be ligated in the neck or, alternatively, the sphenopalantine artery, which is the branch of the maxillary artery in the back of the nose, can be clipped by an endoscopic intranasal approach. If the bleeding arises from the upper part, the ethmoidal arteries are ligated by gaining access through the medial wall of the orbit.

Rhinosinusitis

Aetiology and pathological features

Pathological changes in the nasal cavities are usually accompanied by similar mucosal changes in the sinuses. The causes are:

- allergy
- infective
- non-allergic
- autonomic

In allergic rhinitis, inhaled substances are the most common allergens. Pollens from grass, trees and flowers are responsible for seasonal symptoms. House dust, the house dust mite, and dog and cat fur cause more-perennial symptoms.

Autonomic rhinitis is a disorder of the autonomic nervous system in which a predominance of parasympathetic stimulation causes swelling of the nasal mucosa and hypersecretion.

Acute infective rhinitis is that which occurs in the common cold as a result of viral infection. Secondary bacterial infection may supervene, and the common microorganisms are *Haemophilus influenzae* and *Streptococcus pneumoniae*. Sinusitis is usually an extension from the nasal infection. Any condition which interferes with mucociliary transport, drainage and ventilation, including mechanical factors such as a deviated septum, polyps, hypertrophy of the turbinates and swollen mucosa, especially around the ostiomeatal complex, predisposes to the development of infective sinusitis. Swollen mucosa blocks the natural ostia of the sinuses. Pus reduces the activity of cilia, thus leading to stasis in the sinuses. In chronic infection, the mucosa may be damaged and granulations may develop. Infections of the maxillary sinus can also develop from a dental abscess. Mycotic infections occasionally occur in immunosuppressed and diabetic patients.

Clinical features

Allergic rhinitis

Symptoms

Symptoms include:

- nasal itching
- bouts of sneezing
- profuse watery discharge
- postnasal drip.

In chronic allergic rhinitis, nasal stuffiness is a prominent symptom.

Signs

The mucosa will look oedematous and wet and the turbinates can become hypertrophic.

Infective rhinosinusitis

Symptoms

Symptoms are usually unilateral and include:

- pain over the affected sinus and around the eye
- headache
- mucopurulent discharge
- nasal obstruction
- loss of smell.

In chronic infection, pain may not be present.

Signs

The mucosa will be congested and the turbinates swollen with muco-pus in the nasal cavity. The sinus can be tender to palpation.

Sinus X-ray and CT may reveal opaque sinuses or a fluid level (Fig. 15.10). Bacteriological studies should be carried out on the muco-pus.

Management

Allergic rhinitis

Once the allergen is known, appropriate advice should be offered on how best to avoid it, although there is no evidence of benefit from attempts at eradication of the house dust mite. Desensitisation is possible, but carries a small risk of anaphylaxis.

Antimuscarinic ipratropium bromide is sometimes helpful in autonomic rhinitis. The prophylactic use of a mast cell stabiliser (sodium cromoglicate) and steroid sprays is effective in allergic rhinitis, and they do not seem to have any adverse systemic effects. If the symptoms are not controlled by sprays, non-sedating oral antihistamines can be added. If medical treatment fails to relieve the nasal obstruction, the enlarged hypertrophic turbinates can be reduced by diathermy to the inferior turbinates.

Infective rhinosinusitis

Initially, acute sinusitis is treated with antibiotics (amoxicillin) and decongestant drops (0.5% ephedrine, xylometazoline) which reduce the swelling of the mucosa and may improve ventilation and drainage through the natural ostia. Surgery of varying extent is required to re-establish air flow, drainage and mucociliary clearance when medical treatment has proved ineffective.

Sinus washout is done under local anaesthesia with lidocaine and phenylephrine in acute sinusitis if the pain and infection do not resolve. A trocar and cannula are passed through the thin medial wall of the sinus under the inferior turbinate. The washout is examined bacteriologically.

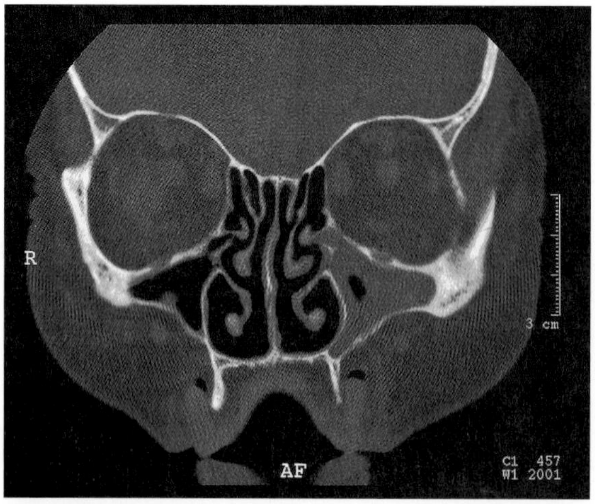

Fig. 15.10 CT scan of the sinuses showing opaque left maxillary sinus due to sinusitis.

Intranasal antrostomy is a permanent large opening made under the inferior turbinate or usually by expanding the natural ostium in the middle meatus.

Radical antrostomy (Caldwell–Luc operation) removes the anterior wall of the maxillary sinus above the gum. The irreversibly changed granulating mucosa is then removed.

Operations on the ostiomeatal complex open the maxillary ostia, the ethmoidal air cells and fronto-ethmoidal duct, and the maxillary and sphenoid ostia, so enabling their ostia to be expanded intranasally under direct vision using a fibreoptic endoscope – endoscopic sinus surgery.

External ethmoidectomy decompresses the orbit where there are orbital complications due to unresolving ethmoiditis and abscess formation. The incision is made between the medial canthus of the eye and the bridge of the nose, and after it has healed the scar is invisible.

Frontal sinus trephine is indicated when the frontonasal duct remains blocked and serious complications are imminent. The incision is made below the lower margin of the eyebrow and a hole drilled through the orbital wall of the sinus. A plastic tube is left in situ to permit irrigation of the sinus.

Fronto-ethmoidectomy is carried out for complications of sinus infection and when there is permanent change to the mucosa which requires its removal. It is also undertaken for mucoceles of the sinus. A large frontonasal opening is created for drainage and a plastic tube left in for several months.

Complications of infective sinusitis

The following may occur in acute or chronic sinusitis:

- orbital complications – periorbital cellulitis, subperiosteal abscess, blindness, suppuration of orbital contents
- osteomyelitis complications – in the frontal bone and maxilla; a discharging sinus may follow
- intracranial complications – meningitis, extradural, subdural and brain abscesses, cavernous sinus thrombosis.

Orbital and intracranial complications more often follow infection in the adjacent ethmoidal, frontal and sphenoid sinuses.

Infection spreads:

- along veins
- by rupture of an abscess through eroded thin bone and then periosteum
- through a bony defect after injury.

Clinical features

Orbital complications

Symptoms

Symptoms are:

- diplopia and restricted eye movement
- reduction of visual acuity.

Signs

Signs are:

- swollen eyelids
- proptosis with displacement of the orbit outwards and downwards.

Intracranial complications

Symptoms

Symptoms are:

- headache
- drowsiness
- photophobia.

Signs

Signs are:

- pyrexia and rigors
- personality changes (frontal abscess)
- fits and neurological localising signs.

Cavernous sinus thrombosis occurs rarely and is characterised by:

- proptosis
- swelling of the eyelids and conjunctiva
- ophthalmoplegia.

Investigation of complications

CT scan demonstrates opaque sinuses, bony defect, abscess formation in the ethmoidal and orbital areas with displacement of the eye, and brain abscess.

Nasal polyps

Aetiology and pathological features

Nasal polyps are pale greyish pedunculated oedematous mucosal tissue masses which project into the nasal cavity. Usually they originate in the region of the ethmoids but can arise from any part of the nose or sinuses, and usually they are multiple and bilateral. Their cause is not fully understood. They are rare in children and, if found, the possibility of mucoviscoidosis should be considered. Confusion may also occur with a congenital meningocele. In about 25% of cases, they are associated with asthma and in 8% there is a linkage with both asthma and aspirin sensitivity. Polyps have a tendency to recur following treatment.

Clinical features

Symptoms

Nasal obstruction is the main complaint. Loss of smell and sneezing are common. Nasal polyps may block the ostia of a sinus and predispose to development of secondary sinus infection and a mucopurulent discharge.

Signs

The lesions are visible on endonasal examination, although a polyp may develop in the maxillary sinus and protrude through the ostium into the back of the nasal cavity and the postnasal space (antrochoanal polyp).

Investigation

A sinus X-ray may show swollen mucosa but is not of particular help.

Unilateral nasal polypoidal swellings should always be subject to biopsy and histological examination to exclude a tumour.

Management

Medical treatment with topical steroid sprays can be employed if the symptoms are not severe, the polyps are small and there is no associated infection. However, in the majority, surgical removal is required. A snare or forceps is used close to the stalk, and sometimes the ethmoidal air cells are also cleared. The postoperative use of a steroid spray can reduce recurrence. A short course of systemic steroids could be considered in severe recurrent polyposis.

TUMOURS OF THE NASAL CAVITY AND SINUSES

Both benign and malignant tumours in the nasal cavity and sinuses are rare.

Benign tumours

Inverting papilloma

The presentation is with unilateral nasal symptoms, usually of obstruction. The examination will reveal a unilateral polypoidal swelling, biopsy or removal of which will reveal the benign nature of the tumour. It has a tendency to recur and there is a small risk of malignant change. A CT scan indicates the extent of the tumour.

The tumour is removed using the lateral rhinotomy approach, with the incision on the side of the nose.

Osteomas

An osteoma may be an accidental finding on sinus X-ray and is more common in the frontal sinus. The frontonasal duct may be obstructed and be responsible for sinusitis or mucocele. Sometimes osteomas expand in all directions, causing pressure erosion of the bony walls of a sinus. In the presence of symptoms, they are removed using a frontoethmoidectomy or sometimes an osteoplastic frontal flap operation which lifts the anterior wall of the sinus.

Angiofibroma

Found only in adolescent males, this tumour occurs in the posterior part of the nose and the postnasal space and expands towards the base of the skull. Patients present with frequent severe nose bleeds. Embolisation to reduce vascularity is carried out before removal by surgery. Radiotherapy is used in some centres.

Malignant tumours

The majority of malignant tumours are of squamous cell origin. An increased occurrence of adenocarcinoma has been described in workers with wood.

Tumours arising in the nasal cavity and the ethmoids present with nasal and eye symptoms when they expand towards the orbit. Maxillary tumours present late with dental, orbital and nasal symptoms and facial swelling. Sometimes the first feature is a lymph node in the neck.

Treatment in most cases is by a combination of radiotherapy and surgery. Maxillectomy may need to be combined with exenteration of the orbital contents. Craniofacial resection may be required when there is an extension of tumour into the anterior cranial fossa.

FURTHER READING

Behrbohm H, Kaschke O, Nawka T, Swift A 2009 Ear, nose, and throat diseases: with head and neck surgery, 3rd edn. Thieme, Stuttgart

Clarke R, Bull PD 2007 Diseases of the ear, nose and throat (Lecture Notes Series), 10th edn. Blackwell Publishing, Oxford

Lalwani A 2007 Current diagnosis and treatment in otolaryngology – head and neck surgery, 2nd edn. McGraw-Hill Medical, New York

16 Chest and lungs

LUNG CANCER

Epidemiology

Lung cancer was rare in the 19th century. Carcinoma of the lung is now the most common cause of cancer death in the world (almost one million deaths per year) and the third most common cause of death overall. The incidence is rising in women, and lung cancer is now the leading malignant cause of death for this group too, ahead of breast cancer. Approximately 1% of the USA's gross national product is spent on the management of lung cancer patients.

Lung cancer is strongly associated with smoking. Smoking is also often responsible for most cases of chronic obstructive pulmonary disease (COPD), but there is no direct correlation between COPD and lung cancer. As discussed below, this has important therapeutic consequences.

Aetiology

Tobacco

There is a very clear association between lung cancer and tobacco, often with a latent period of 10–30 years. The risk factors are the number of cigarettes consumed per day, the age of onset of smoking (those who start smoking before 16 have the greatest damage to DNA), the length of time of smoking, the type of tobacco – unfiltered, high-tar and nicotine cigarettes give the highest risk. Cigar and pipe smoking are also associated with an increased risk of lung cancer, but this is of a lesser magnitude than with cigarette smoking. Passive exposure to tobacco smoke is also a risk. Following smoking cessation the risk of developing lung cancer slowly decreases, but never reaches the level of lifelong non-smokers.

Other factors

Exposure to asbestos and certain chemicals, toxic metals and radioactive compounds and byproducts (radon) also increase the risk of developing lung cancer.

Pathological features

Lung cancers are commonly divided into small-cell carcinoma (SCC), derived from neuroendocrine cells, and non-small-cell lung cancer (NSCLC), of epithelial origin (Box 16.1). The figures quoted below are US data, but similar figures are seen in western Europe.

Non-small-cell carcinoma

Squamous-cell carcinoma

This used to be the commonest type, accounting for 60% of lung tumours. It now represents around 30% of lung cancers in the USA. They tend to be fairly central lesions, and can be slow growing with later development of metastases. The growth starts as squamous metaplasia and progresses first to carcinoma in situ and then invasive carcinoma. Although usually solitary, there may be more than one area of primary squamous carcinoma occurring both in the lung and elsewhere in the upper aerodigestive tract at one time. Continuing to smoke after treatment encourages further de novo development of squamous carcinoma in any of these locations.

Adenocarcinoma

This is now the most frequent type of lung cancer, accounting for around 40% of lung cancers in the USA. It has a tendency to be more peripheral, arising in the small bronchial glands, because of deeper inhalation of the smoke from filtered low-tar and low-nicotine cigarettes (which is the way the smoker extracts the same amount of nicotine from them). These do have a tendency to metastasise earlier.

Bronchoalveolar carcinoma is a subtype of adenocarcinoma which respects the normal lung architecture. It can be multifocal and bilateral.

Large-cell carcinoma

These are poorly differentiated epithelial tumours which do not meet the criteria to be classified as either squamous-cell

Box 16.1 Pathological classification of lung tumours

Lung cancer
- Small-cell carcinoma
- Non-small-cell carcinoma
  - Squamous-cell carcinoma
  - Adenocarcinoma
  - Large-cell (undifferentiated) carcinoma

Neuroendocrine tumours
- Benign – typical carcinoid
- Intermediate – atypical carcinoid (= well-differentiated neuroendocrine carcinoma)
- Malignant
  - Large-cell neuroendocrine carcinoma
  - Small-cell carcinoma

carcinoma or adenocarcinoma. They represent 10–20% of lung tumours. They have no distinguishing distribution or macroscopic appearance.

Small-cell carcinoma and neuroendocrine tumours

Small-cell carcinoma represents around 20% of lung tumours. Histologically the cells are very small and round. This is an anaplastic tumour which may occur in multiple lung sites and is highly malignant. Hormone production is common because its cells produce amine precursors. This causes paraneoplastic symptoms in about 15% of patients: hyponatraemia, Cushing's syndrome, neurological syndromes such as the Eaton–Lambert syndrome (a myasthenic syndrome). The typical presentation of SCC is 'small tumour, huge nodes'. Metastases are frequently present at the time of initial diagnosis.

There is a spectrum of neuroendocrine tumours which runs from the benign typical carcinoid tumours to well-differentiated neuroendocrine carcinoma (also known as atypical carcinoids), to large-cell type neuroendocrine carcinoma and ultimately to small-cell carcinoma. These tumours are of increasing aggressiveness–typical carcinoids, are benign lesions and small-cell carcinoma is a highly aggressive and lethal lesion.

Clinical features of lung cancer

Symptoms

General. Weight loss, malaise and fatigue are common, especially with more advanced disease.

Respiratory. *Cough* is the most common symptom, occurring in nearly half of patients. *Sputum production* is variable. *Haemoptysis* on at least one occasion is frequent but is usually not massive. This symptom must never be trivialised. *Dyspnoea* can be caused by intrinsic or extrinsic airway obstruction and by pleural effusion with loss of function of part of the lung. Occasionally, pulmonary embolism (an expression of paraneoplastic thrombophlebitis, or Trousseau's syndrome) can be responsible.

Other chest or local symptoms. *Non-specific chest pain*, usually heaviness, is often described; *specific local pain* may be associated with invasion of the chest wall by tumour or involvement of the skeleton by metastases. *Pain or numbness in the arm* occurs from brachial plexus invasion by a superior sulcus tumour (Pancoast tumour). Hoarseness can occur due to involvement of a recurrent laryngeal nerve by the tumour or metastatic lymph nodes. *Dysphagia* is the consequence of compression or invasion of the oesophagus in the same way.

Signs

General. Clubbing of the fingers may occur in 30% and hypertrophic pulmonary osteoarthropathy in 3% with painful swelling of the wrists and ankles. These regress rapidly with complete tumour resection. A marked increase in jugular venous pressure occurs with superior vena cava obstruction, and distended veins may be visible over the upper arms and chest along with swelling of the upper body from the level of the heart up.

Respiratory. Localised wheezing can indicate a partially obstructed bronchus. Inspiratory stridor indicates significant narrowing of the airway and mandates urgent referral to a specialist centre. An area of decreased air entry and/or bronchial breathing may occur due to an obstructed bronchus or pleural effusion. Percussion with dullness and associated decreased fremitus indicate an effusion.

Signs of metastases. Any new neurological complaint or sign such as headache, blurred vision, hallucinations, syncope, convulsions, imbalance can indicate CNS involvement. New bone or joint pain may be the sign of metastases. Enlarged scalene or supraclavicular nodes may be locoregional palpable metastases; subcutaneous nodules may be skin metastases. An enlarged liver may indicate diffuse involvement. Laboratory investigations may reveal anaemia, hypercalcaemia and elevated alkaline phosphatase levels.

Staging of lung cancer

The TNM staging of lung cancer was modified in 2009 (Boxes 16.2 and 16.3).

This staging system can also be used for SCC, but more commonly SCC is staged as limited- or extensive-stage disease. Limited disease is when the disease is limited to one hemithorax with hilar or mediastinal disease which can be encompassed in a tolerable radiotherapy portal. The precise definition of limited/extensive disease therefore varies somewhat from centre to centre.

Evaluation of the lung cancer patient

The evaluation of the lung cancer patient is a three-step process:

- What is the stage of the disease?
- What extent of resection is necessary to completely resect the lesion (i.e. segmentectomy, lobectomy, pneumonectomy)?
- Can the patient tolerate this resection?

The process is outlined in Box 16.4 and described below.

Determination of the stage of the disease

Rule out the presence of distant metastases

The four most common sites are brain (if any new neurological symptoms are present a brain MRI is mandatory), adrenals and liver (CT chest and upper abdomen and/or PET scan and/or liver ultrasound) and bone (bone scan or PET scan with additional conventional X-rays and/or CT or MRI as indicated). The CT chest scan will also evaluate the chest for

Box 16.2 TNM staging of lung cancer (2009)

Tumour (T)

- T1a – the tumour is contained within the lung and is smaller than 2 cm across.
- T1b – the tumour is contained within the lung and is between 2 and 3 cm across.
- T2 – the tumour is between 3 and 7 cm across **or** has grown into the the main bronchus more than 2 cm below the part where it divides to go into each lung **or** the tumour has grown into the visceral pleura **or** the tumour has made part of the lung collapse. T2 tumours that are 5 cm or smaller are classed as T2a and those larger than 5 cm are T2b.
- T3 – the tumour is larger than 7 cm **or** has grown into one of the following structures – the chest wall, the mediastinal pleura, the diaphragm, the phrenic nerve, or the pericardium **or** the tumour has made the whole lung collapse **or** there is more than one tumour nodule in the same lobe of the lung.
- T4 – the tumour has grown into one of the following structures – the mediastinum, the heart, a major blood vessel, the trachea, the carina, the oesophagus, the vertebral column, the recurrent laryngeal nerve **or** there are tumour nodules in more than one lobe of the same lung.

Nodes (N)

- N0 – there is no cancer in any lymph nodes.
- N1 – there is cancer in the lymph nodes nearest the affected lung (ipsilateral peribronchial and hilar).
- N2 – there is cancer in lymph nodes in the mediastinum but on the same side as the affected lung or there is cancer in subcarinal lymph nodes.
- N3 – there is cancer in lymph nodes on the opposite side of the chest from the affected lung or in the supraclavicular or scalene lymph nodes.

Metastases (M)

- M0 – there are no signs that the cancer has spread to another lobe of the lung or any other part of the body.
- M1a – there are tumours in both lungs or a malignant pleural effusion or pericardial effusion.
- M1b – there are lung cancer cells in distant parts of the body, such as the liver or bones.

Box 16.3 Staging of lung cancer by TNM subsets

Stage 1 lung cancer	
1A	T1a or T1b, N0, M0
1B	T2a, N0, M0
Stage 2 lung cancer	
2A	T1a, N1, M0
	T1b, N1, M0
	T2a, N1, M0
	T2b, N0, M0
2B	T2b, N1, M0
	T3, N0, M0
Stage 3 lung cancer	
3A	T1a, N2, M0
	T1b, N2, M0
	T2a, N2, M0
	T2b, N2, M0
	T3, N1, M0
	T3, N2, M0
	T4, N0, M0
	T4, N1, M0
3B	Any T, N3, M0
	T4, N2, M0
	T4, N3, M0
Stage 4 lung cancer	
4	Any T, any N, with M1a or M1b

Box 16.4 Management of non-small-cell lung cancer (NSCLC)

Surgery provides the best chance of cure for stages I and II NCSLC. Some very highly selected stage III patients are surgical candidates (see text)

Staging of disease

- Clinical signs/symptoms
- CT chest and upper abdomen
- Bronchoscopy
- Other as dictated by clinical/biochemical findings

Determination of the extent of resection required

- CT chest
- Bronchoscopy
- FDG-PET scan

Fitness of the patient

- Pulmonary function
- Determination of residual postoperative function
- General well-being/fitness
- Other comorbidities

Operable patients – i.e. those with a meaningful chance of being cured and who are fit for the necessary resection – are offered surgery. All others (the majority of lung cancer patients) are referred either to the oncologist for chemotherapy and/or radiotherapy or to the palliative care specialist

the presence of an effusion or other lung lesions which could be secondary lesions.

Determine the intrathoracic stage of the disease

- The CT often cannot distinguish between approximation and invasion of adjacent structures. This may require surgical evaluation. However, it is often possible to determine the T stage of the tumour by CT. Standard X-rays can be helpful to localise the tumour by lobe, to investigate the skeleton and to ascertain a raised hemidiaphragm (this can indicate phrenic nerve involvement).
- CT is notoriously unreliable to determine N stage. PET scan has around 80–85% sensitivity but its specificity is around 95%. Every effort therefore should be made to obtain tissue confirmation of mediastinal lymph node involvement before ruling out surgery. This can be done by fine-needle transtracheal aspiration biopsy at bronchoscopy, by mediastinoscopy (or on occasion anterior mediastinotomy or VATS, video-assisted thoracic surgery) or at thoracotomy. Mediastinoscopy is performed through a small cervical incision and allows all the lymph nodes around the central airway to be identified and biopsied. However stations 5 and 6 are the subaortic and aortopulmonary nodes. They are on lateral side of the aorta and are therefore not accessible with mediastinoscopy. They can be biopsied by an anterior mediastinotomy or using VATS.
- MRI is superior to CT to determine vascular, vertebral and nerve (brachial plexus) involvement by the tumour. Otherwise it offers no advantage over CT.
- Bronchoscopy will determine the intrabronchial extension of the tumour if it is visible, allow detection of other intrabronchial lesions and may permit biopsies to be taken from the lesion for histological diagnosis.

Secretions can also be taken for sensitivity studies. The yield from bronchoscopy is much higher in central lesions than with peripheral ones. Tissue diagnosis from peripheral lesions is often more readily obtained by CT or fluoroscopy-guided transthoracic needle biopsy. At some point in their work-up all lung cancer patients should undergo bronchoscopy.

- If there is an effusion it is mandatory to absolutely rule out pleural involvement. If cytological analysis of the fluid is negative, pleuroscopy should be performed to examine and biopsy the pleura. Cytology has a 15–20% false-negative rate even after 2–3 aspirations of pleural fluid.

Determination of the required resection

The objective of a resection for lung cancer is to completely resect the lesion, with clear margins throughout, as well as the regional lymph nodes. This is why the 'standard' resection for lung cancer is an anatomic lobectomy with resection of the intrafissural lymph nodes and a complete mediastinal lymph node dissection. Lesser resections are reserved for exceptional patients with a small, peripheral, node-negative cancer which can be completely resected with negative margins via segmentectomy or wedge resection but who do not have sufficient functional reserve to undergo a lobectomy. The local recurrence rate is certainly higher with lesser resections, and this probably has a negative impact on survival. More-extensive resections are necessary when the tumour involves more than one lobe or the central airway in the lung. On the right side these are bilobectomies (either upper and middle lobes or middle and lower lobes) and pneumonectomy. On the left side this entails a pneumonectomy.

A 'sleeve resection' entails a pulmonary resection with a segment of bronchus and re-anastomosis of the airway (Fig. 16.1).

The extent of resection can usually be determined from the bronchoscopy and CT findings. However, in some cases it is only at the time of surgical exploration that this can be ascertained. It is therefore mandatory that the extent of resection that is physiologically tolerable by the patient be determined prior to surgery so as to allow this decision to be made safely intraoperatively.

Determination of the extent of resection that is tolerable by the patient

Whenever considering surgery it is absolutely essential to obtain a careful and very complete history. The precise functional capacity of the patient must be determined (unlimited, strenuous activity; can climb 3, 2, 1 or only so many stairs; limited in activities of daily living by breathlessness). Other important points are cough and sputum production as well as other comorbid conditions. Most lung cancer patients are smokers and therefore at high risk of having coexistent coronary artery disease. This must be ruled out by history and, if necessary, other non-invasive and invasive tests to allow surgery to be performed safely. Likewise it is imperative to examine the carotids for pulse, murmurs and bruits. Finally, right heart failure after pulmonary resection can be a devastating complication with fatal outcome. There is no reliable test to predict its onset but preoperative pulmonary hypertension is a predisposing factor and this should be ruled out if there is any suspicion.

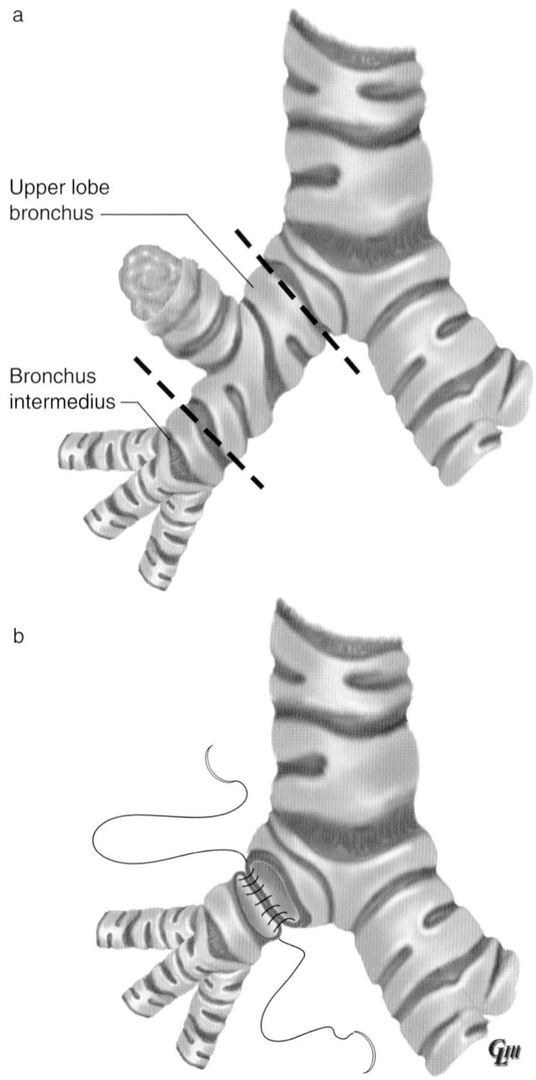

Fig. 16.1 A prototypical 'sleeve resection' – that is, a right upper lobectomy. (a) The right main bronchus is divided above the takeoff of the upper lobe bronchus, and the bronchus intermedius is cut below it. This allows the airway to be resected in such a way as to ensure adequate resection margins. (b) The bronchus intermedius is then anastomosed to the right main bronchus with a running non-resorbable suture. Some surgeons use slowly resorbable sutures, others interrupted sutures.

Careful physical examination is also important. The supraclavicular fossae and the base of the neck must be carefully and attentively examined for lymphadenopathy. If present the enlarged lymph nodes should be aspirated for cytology to rule out N3 disease.

Pulmonary function results are always expressed as absolute and relative values. The relative values are expressed as the percent of predicted values based on the patient's sex, age, height and weight. It is important to refer to these relative values rather than to absolute figures. It is obvious that a FEV_1 (forced expiratory volume in one second) of one litre is quite adequate for a very small, light woman but equally inadequate for a very large, heavy man. Furthermore it is the predicted postoperative value that is the true determinant of residual function (and therefore operability) rather than the crude preoperative value. Let us take the case of a patient with adequate clinical function who has 'very poor numbers which rule out pneumonectomy'. If the involved lung is still doing 50% of the patient's breathing, then these values indeed rule out performing a pneumonectomy. If on the other hand the tumour has obstructed the main bronchus and the pulmonary artery and the preoperative function is equal to what the postoperative function will be, then the patient is operable. If only the airway is obstructed and the artery is permeable and there is a physiological shunt through this lung then resection could actually improve oxygenation. The decision that a patient is physiologically inoperable should only be made by a specialist unit after careful evaluation of the patient, as this is quite a complex decision process.

The two strongest predictors of cardiopulmonary morbidity and mortality after pulmonary resection are the FEV_1 and the DLCO (transfer factor for CO). When the predicted postoperative FEV_1 and DLCO are both less than 40% of the predicted value the risk of significant morbidity and mortality become unacceptably high. There is also a risk of turning the patient who survives into a respiratory cripple. This is also an unacceptable outcome. In borderline patients the aerobic capacity is also a strong predictor of unfavourable outcomes. This is assessed by ergospirometry with measurement of the VO_2 max.

When pulmonary function is well preserved, no further tests are required and major resections including pneumonectomy can be performed. When there is doubt, the V/Q scan will allow the regional perfusion and ventilation to be assessed. This is then used to calculate the predicted postoperative function.

Smoking cessation prior to surgery seems intuitively to be desirable. In fact it takes 2 months for there to be a true benefit in terms of sputum reduction and full restitution of mucociliary function. Nonetheless, active smoking immediately prior to surgery does increase the operative risk. In a borderline patient it can be beneficial to defer surgery for 6–8 weeks for pulmonary rehabilitation combined with smoking cessation.

In current smokers undergoing 'curative' treatment every effort should be made to help the patient quit smoking. Smoking cessation slows the accelerated loss of lung function in COPD patients. This is important, as surgery has just deprived the patient of functional lung tissue, and respiratory failure is one of the mid- to long-term causes of death in patients who have indeed undergone a curative resection of lung cancer. Furthermore it significantly reduces the risk of developing a second primary lung cancer.

Treatment of lung cancer

Non-small-cell lung cancer

Unfortunately, most patients present initially with advanced disease that will not be curable with any modality. In these cases they must be referred to an oncologist so that palliative chemotherapy can be discussed. When there is pain or obstruction, palliative radiotherapy is also often a valid option. Palliative treatment is an active treatment option that seeks optimal symptom relief. The value of this treatment must not be underestimated to maintain quality of life, and every effort must be made to obtain it for all inoperable patients, especially when they become symptomatic. Surgery should not be offered to patients with minimal chance of cure. It submits them needlessly to the risks (morbidity/mortality) of the procedure without the benefit (chance of cure). Shields has defined a futile thoracotomy as one where the chance of cure is less than the chance of suffering major morbidity or death. Appropriate staging will ensure an exploratory thoracotomy ('open and shut') rate of less than 5%. There are patients in whom only exploratory thoracotomy can assess resectability, so the rate of this procedure should not be 0%.

Surgery offers the best chance of cure in stage I and II lung cancer, so radiation and chemotherapy are usually reserved for patients who are unfit for surgery (or who refuse surgery). If it is the general condition of the patient that precludes surgery, radical radiotherapy may still be an option but these patients are often poor candidates for chemotherapy. If this is contraindicated, then palliative care is often the only reasonable option. If it is the patient's poor respiratory reserve that rules out surgery, then radical radiotherapy may not be tolerable (because of radiation injury to the adjacent lung), but highly focused radiotherapy may be applicable. In this case palliative chemotherapy should be discussed.

Some very highly selected stage IIIa patients can be surgical candidates. Other stage IIIa patients may be considered for inclusion in neo-adjuvant (or induction) therapy protocols. It now seems that if the mediastinal lymph nodes can be cleared of tumour by neo-adjuvant therapy, surgery remains a valid treatment option for these patients. Otherwise most surgeons would refer patients with stage IIIa disease for radical radiotherapy and/or chemotherapy.

Occasional very highly selected stage IIIb patients might be appropriate candidates for inclusion in prospective trials of surgery or induction therapy (with the same caveats as for stage IIIa disease as above). This is however only exceptionally the case. These patients are usually treated with chemo- and/or radiotherapy.

Patients with stage IV disease because of a single, completely resectable brain metastasis and who do not have locally advanced disease can be considered for resection of the brain lesion followed by resection of the primary lesion with a 20–25% chance of 5-year survival. All other stage IV patients are usually treated with palliative chemotherapy or palliative radiotherapy.

Palliative chemotherapy has a modest effect on overall survival, but its proponents believe that it can improve quality of life significantly. This is not universally accepted. Palliative radiotherapy can obtain good relief of symptoms when there is pain from invasion into the chest wall or at the site of bone metastases. It can offer relief of superior vena cava syndrome (endovascular stenting is also a useful palliative procedure in this condition). It can also be very helpful when there is symptomatic bronchial obstruction or haemoptysis.

Small-cell lung cancer

The treatment of SCC is typically combination chemotherapy. Etoposide/cisplatin in combination with radiotherapy can induce complete response in around 80% of patients with limited disease. Patients with a complete response should receive prophylactic cranial irradiation. Radiotherapy for extensive disease is palliative. The treatment of stages I and II SCC is controversial, but it does seem that surgery followed by chemotherapy can offer up to 35–40% 5-year survival. Occasionally isolated secondary deposits are resected.

Prognosis

Overall, the prognosis of NSCLC is relatively poor. The 5-year survival for stage I NSCLC is around 70%. With stage II disease this falls to 40–50%. In the very highly selected stage III patients who are considered surgical candidates the 5-year survival is only around 25–30%. Otherwise it is at best 10–15%, more often much less. The median survival for stage IV disease is around 12 months, with minimal 5-year survival. Less than 20–25% of patients present with operable disease, so the overall 5-year survival for men with lung cancer in the UK is only 5–7%. Equally depressing is the very small progress in overall survival that has been made over the last 25 years and the fact that survivors develop a second primary lung cancer at a rate of 1–2% per year.

The prognosis of SCC is worse, with only 3–17% of patients with limited disease surviving 5 years (and only 30–40% of patients present with limited disease). The 5-year survival for extensive disease is 2–8%. New chemotherapy treatments may improve the prognosis.

Furthermore the survivors present with new second aerodigestive cancers at a rate of 2–10% per patient per year. Thus the mortality of survivors is 10 times greater than age- and sex-matched cohorts.

OTHER LUNG TUMOURS

Neuroendocrine tumours

The spectrum of neuroendocrine tumours spans a range starting with the benign **typical carcinoids**, which have an essentially normal 5- and 10-year survival following their complete resection. They are slow-growing lesions. The majority (70%) are central lesions. Up to 31% are asymptomatic. They can cause multiple symptoms over many years; some are due to obstruction such as wheezing, shortness of breath, cough and infection. Others are haemoptysis (frequent) or chest pain. An associated carcinoid syndrome is very rare (around 2%), as is Cushing's syndrome. Complete resection is curative. Resection should always spare as much lung parenchyma as possible. Because of their central location these tumours often lend themselves to sleeve resections (see Fig. 16.1). Endoscopic resection (whatever the technique) should be reserved for frail, high-risk patients who are poor operative candidates because of the high risk of incomplete resection and recurrence. The other indication for endoscopic resection is to allow a distal pneumonitis to clear so as to permit a safe parenchyma-sparing limited resection.

Atypical carcinoids tend to be more aggressive with much more frequent lymph node metastases (30–50%). The 5-year survival is poorer at 40–76%. **Large-cell neuroendocrine carcinomas** are uncommon lesions with a poor prognosis. **Small-cell carcinoma** is discussed above.

Other rare primary pulmonary tumours

There is a long list of these very rare lesions which are beyond the scope of this chapter, and the reader is referred to the excellent review chapters in the textbooks on thoracic surgery edited by Shields et al (2009) and by Patterson et al (2008).

Immunosuppressed patients have an increased risk of presenting with solid organ **lymphomas**, and this includes the lungs. HIV-infected patients may also present with pulmonary **Kaposi sarcoma**.

Hamartomas account for around three-quarters of all benign lung tumours. The definition of a hamartoma is an excessive focal overgrowth of mature normal cells and tissues in an organ, composed of identical cellular components. The majority are asymptomatic peripheral lung lesions which are discovered incidentally, and the obvious problem is distinguishing them from a small, early stage lung cancer. They often contain fat and cartilage. Chondrohamartomas are purely cartilaginous, as their name indicates. Central lesions can cause symptoms of obstruction. The diagnosis of hamartoma can be made on the basis of the radiological findings and the presence of fat and/or cartilage in a biopsy specimen. The usual indication for surgery is the uncertainty as to diagnosis. Simple excision is curative. Symptomatic lesions should be resected with as much of a parenchyma-sparing technique as feasible. Asymptomatic peripheral lesions only need to be resected if large, or growing in a young, fit patient.

PRINCIPLES OF CHEST DRAINAGE

The object of chest drainage is to obtain complete evacuation of all fluid and air from the pleural space so as to allow complete re-expansion of the underlying lung. Indications for insertion of a chest drain are given in Box 16.5 and the technique described in Chapter 11. If the lung cannot re-expand despite adequate drainage then it is a **trapped lung**, and this condition can only be resolved surgically if clinically indicated. If drainage cannot result in evacuation of all abnormal pleural contents, either because of their loculation or coagulation, then again only surgery will resolve the condition. In many cases thoracoscopy (also called VATS, video-assisted thoracic surgery) will be all that is needed.

It is often said that whenever there is a hole in the chest wall the lung will collapse. On this basis suction had routinely been applied to chest drains. In actual fact the lung will re-expand and occupy the entire pleural space unless there is a condition which prevents this – air or fluid trapped in the pleural space, for example. There is now some evidence that

Box 16.5 When to insert a chest drain

Absolute indications
- Pneumothorax (PNO) in ventilated patient
- PNO in trauma patient who requires surgery
- Haemothorax in trauma patient
- Symptomatic PNO in patient with limited pulmonary reserve
- PNO of any size prior to transfer of patient by air
- PNO in stable patient prior to ambulance transfer if no doctor in attendance
- Bilateral PNO
- Obtunded patient with PNO

Relative indications
- PNO prior to ambulance transfer with doctor in attendance (provide equipment if no drainage!)
- Small to moderate PNO in stable patient (other options are observation or aspiration)
- Pleural effusions

suction may not be required for chest drains in the majority of cases and indeed that air leaks and chest drainage might resolve faster without suction.

However, it is mandatory that all chest drains be attached to a device that allows air and fluid to escape freely from the pleural space without allowing air to enter into it. The most commonly used device is the **underwater seal**, which is illustrated in the single-bottle drainage system seen in Figure 16.2. This figure also illustrates double- and triple-bottle systems. Commercially available chest drain collection systems are commonly three-bottle systems.

To understand how the underwater seal works, imagine yourself with a drink and a straw. As long as the straw is in the drink and you are sucking on the straw the only way you can get air into your mouth is to either drink the glass dry or to remove the straw from the drink. So this underwater seal is a very simple, cheap and safe system as long as the drainage bottle is well below the patient (so as to prevent negative pleural pressure from 'drinking the glass dry') and the tube from the patient is below the level of the fluid (to 'keep the straw in the drink'). If the tube entering the bottle is only 2 cm below the surface of the water, the resistance to air and fluid escaping from the chest into the drainage system is negligible and easily overcome during forced expiration and coughing.

Another system of one-way valve that is commonly used is the Heimlich valve, illustrated in Figure 16.3. The inner tubing is made of very soft rubber (or some similar substance) so that it completely collapses and becomes airtight on inspiration but opens with almost no resistance to allow the free passage of air or fluid. It is imperative to ensure that a **Heimlich valve** is mounted correctly or it will rapidly produce a tension pneumothorax (see below).

The standard chest drain should be placed in the 4th or 5th intercostal space in the midaxillary line and directed up to the apex of the chest along the posterior chest wall (see Ch. 11). Most drains placed by interventional radiologists are pigtail catheters. These can be remarkably effective, but in the author's experience it is important to maintain their patency by irrigating them 1–2 times per day with 10–15 mL of sterile 0.9% saline solution.

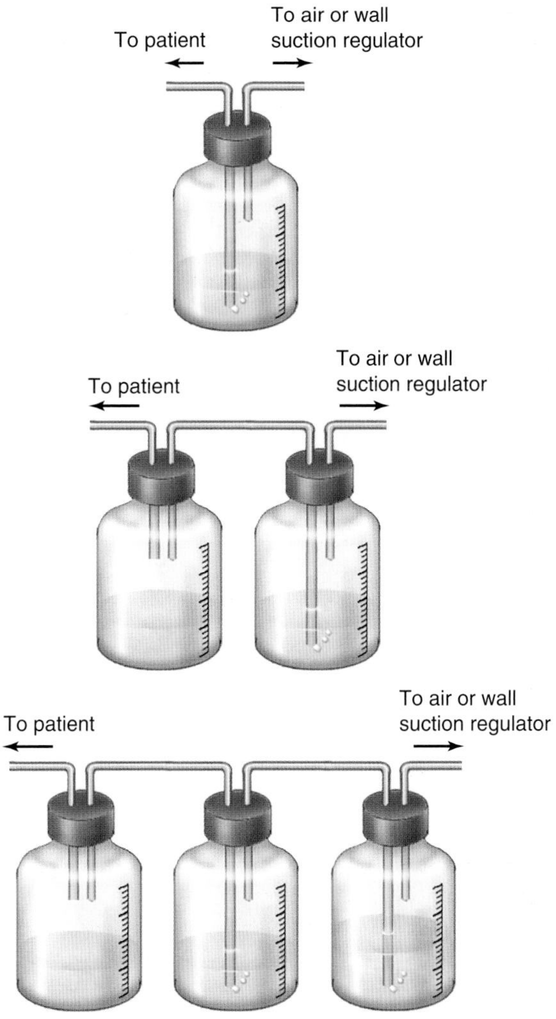

Fig. 16.2 One-, two- and three-bottle drainage systems. In the one-bottle system the single bottle is both the collection chamber and the underwater seal. The drawback of this system is that the resistance to fluid and air escaping the chest increases as the bottle fills. Two-bottle systems have the collection chamber upstream from the underwater seal chamber. If suction is applied to the one- and two-bottle systems a wall-mounted suction regulator is required. In three-bottle systems a suction-regulating chamber is placed between the underwater seal chamber and the source of suction. Most commercially available drainage systems are three-bottle systems.

Criteria for drain removal – there is much variance in local custom. The common criteria to remove a drain are no air leak for 24 hours and drainage of less than 200 mL in 24 h.

PNEUMOTHORAX

The definition of a pneumothorax (PNO) is when the pleural space contains air which separates the parietal and visceral pleura, preventing the lung from occupying its normal place in the pleural space.

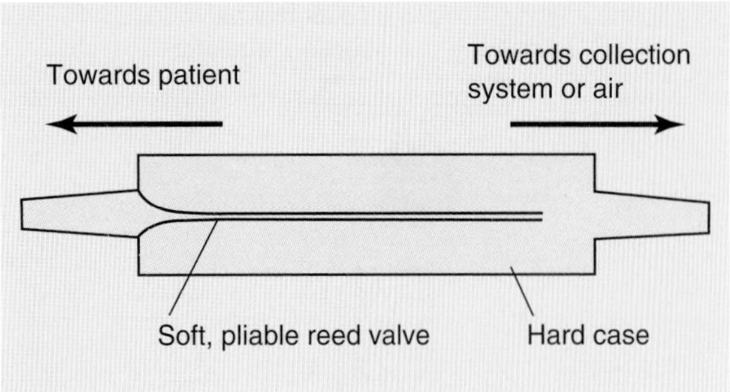

Fig. 16.3 The Heimlich valve is a simple one-way valve device. A soft, pliable reed valve is placed in a rigid container. There is virtually no resistance to air and/or fluid escaping, but any relative depression on the patient side of the valve will cause the inner reed valve to collapse and seal off the passage through the valve.

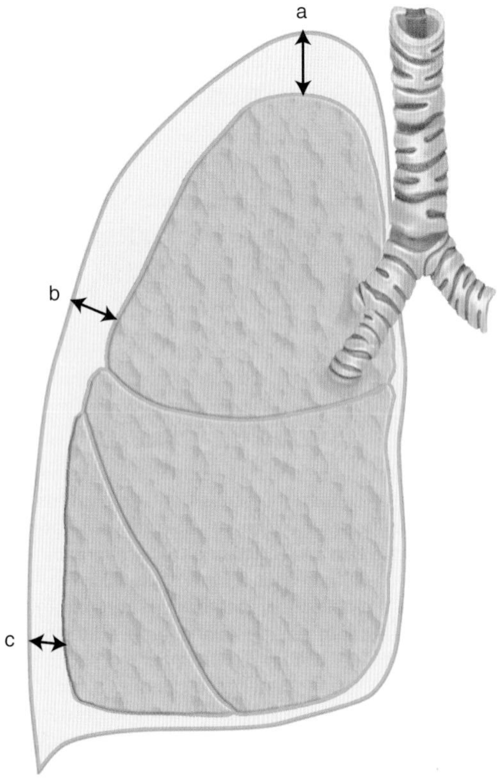

Fig. 16.4 Parameters used to calculate the percentage of a pneumothorax. See text for details of calculation.

The importance of the PNO is often expressed as a percent. The conventional way of calculating this is to measure the distance in cm by which the lung is off the chest wall at the apex (*a*), mid-way down the chest (*b*) and at the base of the chest (*c*) (Fig. 16.4). Then:

$(a + b + c) / 3 = d$; and d 10 = percent PNO

An example: on the upright PA chest film taken in inspiration, the lung is off the chest wall by 3 cm at the apex, 2 cm mid-way down the chest and 1 cm at the base of the chest;

$(3 + 2 + 1) / 3 = 6 / 3 = 2; 2 \times 10 = 20$

so this is a 20% pneumothorax.

Flying is contraindicated with a PNO because aeroplanes are only pressurised to around the equivalent of 2000 m in altitude. As pressure times volume equals a constant, the volume of the PNO will increase by ⅓ at this altitude with the attendant risk of tension.

Treatment

There are three options: observation, aspiration and drainage. Small PNOs (<10–20%) require only observation in an otherwise stable patient. They usually resolve spontaneously. If increasing in size, treatment is required. Aspiration of PNOs is very popular in the UK (less so elsewhere). This should be done with a wide-bore i.v. plastic cannula (with the needle removed), a three-way stopcock and a 50 mL syringe. This is a valid treatment option, but subsequent patient management requires common sense. *No patient with a small PNO or who has just had a PNO aspirated should be discharged home if prompt return to medical care is not possible (for example the patient is intoxicated or lives alone in an isolated home with no transportation).* Complete or increasing PNOs should be drained. It is the responsibility of the physician who initially treats the patient to ensure that there is appropriate follow-up and management of the patient.

Tension pneumothorax

This occurs when pressure builds up in the pleural space, compressing the lung and collapsing it, then causing mediastinal shift to the opposite side. This progressively causes kinking of the vena cava, which becomes obstructed. At this point there is no venous return to the heart and the cardiac output drops, causing death (Fig. 16.5).

Signs and symptoms

Features are: shortness of breath; tachypnoea; tracheal deviation to opposite side; absent breath sounds over the involved hemithorax, with hyper-resonance to percussion; cyanosis; tachycardia; pulsus paradoxus.

Treatment

This is obviously a true medical emergency which requires immediate action (Emergency Box 16.1 and Chapter 11) – drainage of the pleural space by whatever means are at hand without the customary regard to aseptic technique and pain management. In a medical setting do not wait for X-ray confirmation of the diagnosis. First insert one or two large-bore i.v. catheters into the chest in the midclavicular line a little above the nipple, then insert a chest drain using controlled, aseptic technique. In the field, use literally whatever is available. Items such as a ballpoint pen with the cartridge removed have saved lives in this circumstance.

Spontaneous primary pneumothorax

This is when a PNO occurs without an identifiable cause, which rules out any trauma or underlying lung disease. Although an obvious slight misnomer, this corresponds to a clear-cut clinical entity which occurs frequently. It occurs

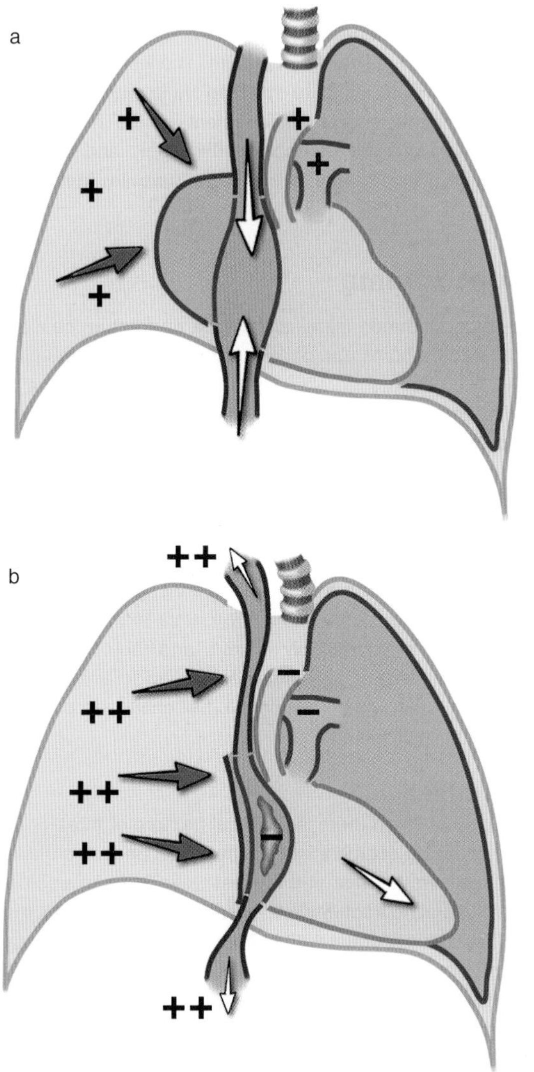

Fig. 16.5 In a tension pneumothorax the mediastinum is pushed over toward the opposite side. As the pressure increases, the superior (and inferior) venae cavae are progressively kinked and pinched off where the relatively fixed and mobile parts move. As this happens the venous return to the heart drops off and cardiac output is reduced. When this is severe enough the patient will die.

most commonly in tall, thin, young, healthy individuals – more frequently men than woman and more commonly in smokers than in non-smokers. It is caused by the spontaneous rupture of a bleb or bulla. These are small constitutional lesions which are most commonly found at the apex of the lung. Other locations are the apex of the lower lobe. Very occasionally they can occur anywhere on the lung. The PNO can occur at any time, including at complete rest. Most commonly the patient complains of sudden chest pain or discomfort. Shortness of breath is very variable, often absent. Examination shows decreased breath sounds and hyperresonance. Treatment depends on the importance of the PNO. A 10–20% PNO will often resolve without treatment. Larger or increasing pneumothoraces require drainage. Aspiration can also be attempted. Hospital admission is required

Emergency Box 16.1

Tension pneumothorax: This is a true life-threatening medical emergency

Signs and symptoms

- Anxiety, agitation
- Shortness of breath
- Tachypnoea
- Pulsus paradoxus or rapid, thready pulse (↓ BP)
- Distended jugular veins
- Tracheal deviation to opposite side
- Hyperinflated hemithorax with hyper-resonance to percussion and decreased or absent breath sounds

NB: These signs can be unreliable in a trauma patient who is bleeding

Treatment

- DO NOT AWAIT X-RAY CONFIRMATION OF DIAGNOSIS
- Insert a first large-bore i.v. cannula in anterior chest wall in midclavicular line 1–2 rib spaces above nipple. Repeat with one or two more cannulae then insert definitive chest drain under aseptic technique and remove i.v. cannulae
- Obtain chest X-ray

Differential diagnosis

The principal DD of distended jugulars and pulsus paradoxus in a trauma patient is cardiac tamponade. If insertion of cannulae does not relieve symptoms very rapidly, this diagnosis must be ruled out immediately

Any unstable trauma or ventilated patient who has had a cannula inserted for suspected tension pneumothorax must have a chest drain inserted to prevent subsequent tension pneumothorax

if there is any doubt about the PNO increasing or if the patient cannot rapidly and readily return for care if necessary, for whatever reason.

When the episode of PNO is resolved the risk of recurrence is around 20% following a first episode, 50% following a second episode and 80% after the third.

Surgical treatment

This consists in the resection of the causative bulla or bleb associated with some sort of pleurodesis procedure (a procedure which causes the visceral pleura to adhere to the parietal pleura). This is usually done by pleurectomy or pleural abrasion. (Talc pleuredesis should not be performed in these patients, because of risk of restriction.) This can be done with VATS or through a mini-axillary thoracotomy. The risk of recurrence following surgery is 2–4%. Surgery is indicated after two (or some say three) episodes, when the current episode will not resolve despite drainage, or if there is an associated haemothorax. Many authors consider bilaterality and tension to be an indication for surgery. Surgery is also indicated following a first episode for people who fly in aeroplanes professionally and for deep-sea divers.

Secondary pneumothorax

Trauma

If there is a lesion which causes a hole in the chest cavity the lung may collapse. Usually trauma causes a hole in the lung, and air escapes into the chest cavity. This can be a penetrating injury into the lung or blunt trauma with a rib fracture which punctures or lacerates the lung. If the injury constitutes a one-way valve mechanism a **tension pneumothorax** can ensue. If there is a gaping hole in this chest wall, this is an **open pneumothorax**. In this case there can be respiratory failure because more ventilation occurs through the hole than through the airway. It is important to dress these wounds so as to be occlusive during inspiration but not during expiration, so as to avoid the risk of causing a tension PNO. This is done by using an airtight dressing which is secured with tape on three sides only. This way during inspiration the dressing is sucked onto the chest wall and air cannot enter the chest. During expiration air can exit through the un-taped side.

Another frequent cause of traumatic PNO is the various invasive diagnostic and therapeutic interventions done by doctors, including placement of central venous lines and biopsies of thoracic lesions (including lung lesions).

Underlying lung disease

The most common cause of a secondary PNO is the rupture of an emphysematous bulla. Other causes are diseases such as cystic fibrosis, lymphangioleiomyomatosis, interstitial lung disease, rupture of tumours or abscesses. An uncommon cause is catamenial PNO, which is PNO that occurs at the time of menstruation. Its precise cause is unknown.

The treatment of secondary pneumothoraces is often complex and is beyond the scope of this chapter. The reader is referred to the relevant chapters in the thoracic surgery textbooks.

CHEST TRAUMA AND HAEMOPTYSIS

Penetrating trauma

The most common causes of penetrating trauma are stab wounds and gunshot wounds. In civilian disputes the weapons often have low muzzle velocity, and the injury is primarily the hole made by the bullet, which can be large due to tumbling. Military weapons are now designed to be of smaller calibre with high muzzle velocity so as to cause more indirect trauma by cavitation effects. The injuries can thus be extensive well beyond the hole itself.

There are two golden rules in penetrating trauma. The first is that by definition the intracavitary trajectory of the wounding agent is unknown, even when there is an entrance and an exit wound. A bullet can ricochet off of the spine, for example, and a knife blade can swing through an arc before exiting. The second is that any wound that is below the nipple line in front or the tip of the scapula in back is a thoraco-abdominal wound until proven otherwise.

If the heart or the great vessels are injured the wounds are usually too rapidly fatal for the patient to reach the hospital. This is why the vast majority of chest wounds are managed with chest drains and do not require surgery. The majority of chest trauma requiring surgery involves the heart and the great vessels.

The management of injuries to the chest must follow standard ATLS guidelines – the a, b, c, d, e of airway, breathing, circulation, disability, exposure. The lesion which represents the most immediate threat to life is managed first.

The diagnosis and management of the myriad chest injuries is beyond the scope of this book, and the reader is referred to the appropriate chapters in the thoracic textbooks.

Blunt trauma

The most common injury is a simple rib fracture caused by a fall. Rib fractures can occur without excessive trauma and have even been seen after vigorous coughing, but the possibility of a pathological fracture should always be considered. The treatment of simple rib fractures consists in the appropriate prescription of adequate analgesia, which must be taken as long as required. This can be for weeks. An initial chest X-ray should be obtained to rule out complications, but rib views are not recommended.

Motor vehicle accidents and injuries to pedestrians are among the main causes of blunt trauma to the chest. Such patients are often multiply injured, and their management follows the same ATLS guidelines alluded to above.

Two injuries will be discussed: flail chest and pulmonary contusion.

Flail chest

This occurs when there is a bifocal fracture of three or more ribs, so that a segment of the chest wall becomes unstable and free from the rest of the chest wall. This can also occur with bilateral rib fractures and associated sternal fractures so that the anterior chest wall is free to move independently of the rest of the chest. In this condition this segment of the chest wall will move in during inspiration and out during expiration – so-called paradoxical breathing. This reduces the efficiency of breathing and can lead to respiratory failure. The treatment is either intubation and mechanical ventilation or surgical stabilisation of the chest wall. This is a controversial procedure with strong proponents and equally strong opponents but can yield very good results in carefully selected patients.

Pulmonary contusion

The lung is a fragile organ, and violent blows can cause contusion. This will cause bleeding into the lung parenchyma. This can spill over into the airway and the clots can obstruct more or less large airways. This in itself can cause respiratory failure. There can also be an inflammatory response with development of ARDS (adult respiratory distress syndrome). Fortunately it is usually a limited lesion with spontaneous resolution. Bronchoscopy can be required to clear the airway. It can also be associated with lung laceration or injury leading to a PNO or a haemo-pneumothorax.

Haemothorax

This is the accumulation of blood in the pleural space, whatever the cause. Treatment is usually insertion of a chest drain. If the drain yields more than 1500 mL initially or more than 300–400 mL/hour, intervention will usually be required.

This may be surgery or interventional radiology to embolise a bleeding vessel. If the blood becomes clotted, surgery (often VATS) will be necessary to evacuate the clots. Haemothoraces should be evacuated to prevent the occurrence of a chronic haemothorax which will require formal decortication for treatment.

Rupture of the diaphragm

This is usually due to sudden blunt trauma to the abdomen, which causes a rapid increase in intra-abdominal pressure that tears the diaphragm. It is more common on the left side because the liver protects the right hemidiaphragm to a large degree. It is most often seen in patients with multiple injuries. The management of these patients must follow the ATLS guidelines, as alluded to above.

The diagnosis can be quite straightforward, on the basis of an elevation of the involved hemidiaphragm and the obvious presence of bowel contents in the chest. If in doubt a nasogastric tube should be inserted, and this will be seen to go down into the belly and back up into the chest. Lesions on the right side tend to be much more subtle in their presentation and can be difficult to diagnose. The rupture can be initially occult and only become evident over several days as the abdominal viscera slowly migrate into the chest. Also in intubated patients positive-pressure ventilation can artificially maintain the normal position of the abdominal organs, which subsequently migrate into the chest when the physiological transdiaphragmatic pressure is restored. It is not uncommon for the diagnosis to be delayed months or even years, especially on the right side.

Associated injuries are common. These include head, CNS and limb trauma. The most common directly related injuries are intra-abdominal and include splenic and hepatic laceration, bowel rupture, pancreatic injury and tears of the mesentery.

Repair is usually straightforward. In acute cases the trans-abdominal approach must be preferred except where there is a simultaneous intrathoracic lesion which requires immediate surgical care, which is very rare. This is because of the high incidence of simultaneous intra-abdominal injury requiring surgical care. In the chronic setting the transthoracic approach is usually preferred because at that stage there are often intrathoracic adhesions which are difficult to deal with through a laparotomy incision.

Haemoptysis

This is the expectoration of blood. The origin can infrequently be the pulmonary circulation, for example after penetrating trauma to the chest or rupture of a branch of the pulmonary artery by a Swan–Ganz catheter. However, the cause is most commonly the rupture of a dilated bronchial artery in an area of chronic inflammation or infection (such as bronchiectasis, tuberculosis, or *Aspergillus* involvement of an old tuberculous cavern).

Haemoptysis can be a very limited, self-resolving event or it can be a life-threatening catastrophe. In lung cancer there is usually just a little blood on an intermittent basis. The treatment of the lung cancer (including palliative radiotherapy) will usually resolve the problem. In the other conditions this is never a symptom to be trivialised. There can be sentinel bleeds which in themselves are not serious, but that can be the precursor to a fatal bleeding episode.

Diagnosis of the source of bleeding can be very straightforward or extremely difficult. Bronchoscopy can show a trickle of blood coming from a well-defined airway where a lesion which is bleeding can be identified. It can also demonstrate an airway with blood throughout and no identifiable source. Angiography of the bronchial arteries can be relatively straightforward in some cases and impossible to realise in others. The bleeding can have stopped at the time of the examination.

Treatment

Haemoptysis kills by drowning the patient in his/her own blood rather than from hypovolaemia. Intravenous fluids should only be administered as required, and blood only if there is hypovolaemia. Thus the first step must always be to protect the uninvolved lung. In the first instance, if the side that is bleeding is known, lay the patient on his/her side with the bleeding lung down. If the patient requires intubation the bleeding lung must be isolated either by selectively intubating the left lung with a somewhat smaller endotracheal tube than usual (if the right lung is bleeding) or with a double-lumen tube.

At the time of diagnostic angiography the bleeding vessel can be embolised. This will allow the patient to be stabilised. Angiographic embolisation often does not definitively resolve the problem, so, if the patient is fit for surgery, resection of the causative lesion should be organised once the patient has been stabilised. When the anatomic source of bleeding is known, emergency resection is the alternative to angiography. Surgery is obviously reserved for those cases where the origin of the bleeding is known. This is not always the case, however. Occasionally it can be quite difficult to localise the source of the bleeding.

THE PLEURA

Effusions

Pleural effusions are common. The causes are multiple, including tumour, infection, pulmonary disease, cardiac, renal, hepatic and pancreatic disease. The common diseases which require surgical management will be discussed.

The diagnosis of the cause of a pleural effusion can be difficult, and surgery can play an important role. Cytology has a false-negative rate of around 15–20% even after 2–3 attempts. Cultures and blind biopsies can be negative in up to 50% of cases of pleural tuberculosis. Biochemical fluid analysis can give indications but is often not helpful. In these cases inspection of the pleura with appropriate biopsies is essential.

If a pleural effusion is symptomatic, recurrent and/or persistent and there is no satisfactory treatment of the underlying cause then symptomatic relief can be obtained by pleurodesis. This is the obliteration of the pleural space by mechanical (pleurectomy or pleural abrasion) or chemical means which cause the lung to adhere to the chest wall. The most effective chemical agent is talc. Five grams of sterile asbestos-free talc is either insufflated into the pleural space at the time of surgery or it is instilled into the pleural space through a drain in the form of slurry. The success rate is 90–95%. The other commonly used agents are *tetracycline* and *bleomycin*, but they have a poorer success rate. The pleurodesis induces an intense inflammatory response (which is what will cause the lung to adhere to the chest wall) and it is not uncommon for the patients to have a fever and elevated white cell count and CRP levels after the procedure. If the cause of the effusion is not known then the surgery required combines a diagnostic procedure (pleuroscopy and pleural biopsies) with a therapeutic one (pleurodesis).

Pleural tumours

Primary

Malignant pleural mesothelioma is the main primary pleural malignancy. It is most often associated with prior asbestos exposure, with a lag time of 40 years in many cases, rarely less than 15. As asbestos was widely used as insulation in the building industry, the shipping industry and in brake linings with a peak in imports in the 1970s, it is expected that the current epidemic will peak in the year 2020. The patients are commonly in the sixth decade at the time of diagnosis. Histologically there are three subtypes: epithelioid, mixed and sarcomatous. The purely epithelioid lesions tend to be slightly less aggressive.

The typical clinical presentation is chest pain, shortness of breath and weight loss. There is a blood-tinged pleural effusion and more or less diffuse and bulky pleural involvement. The disease has a relentless downward course leading to death in an average of 8–10 months. Palliative chemotherapy can improve quality of life, and radiotherapy can alleviate pain in 50% of cases. The role of surgery is usually to confirm the diagnosis and to perform pleurodesis at the same time, if possible (see below – treatment of malignant pleural effusions). Debulking surgery (pleurectomy and decortication) can offer valid palliation in highly selected cases but does not prolong survival. In very highly selected patients with early-stage purely epithelioid lesions, aggressive surgical resection (extrapleural pneumonectomy followed by radiotherapy) is advocated by some authors; however, there are no randomised trials which demonstrate that it offers any survival advantage over conventional therapy.

Secondary

Pleural effusions due to secondary tumour involvement are a common problem. In 25–50% of cases it is the first clinical manifestation of the underlying malignancy. Symptoms are often a dry cough, shortness of breath, and a feeling of fullness within the chest and pain. Physical examination shows dullness to percussion and decreased air entry.

The tumours most commonly responsible for the condition are lung, breast, lymphoma/leukaemia, and adenocarcinoma of unknown origin, genitourinary and other.

Surgery is often required for diagnosis, as discussed above. Treatment can be chemotherapy for highly chemosensitive tumours involving the pleura. In most other cases palliative pleurodesis is indicated provided the lung is capable of re-expanding and occupying the entire pleural space. However, if there is a rim of tumour tissue trapping the lung and preventing its re-expansion, pleurodesis is doomed to fail. If the effusion is only moderately symptomatic, in other words if draining the effusion only marginally improves the patient's clinical condition, then nothing should be done. If the effusion is causing symptoms then a pleuroperitoneal shunt may be inserted. This allows the fluid to drain into the peritoneal cavity, where it is re-absorbed. The success rate is around 85%, and there does not seem to be a problem with peritoneal seeding of the tumour. The other option is to insert a permanent drainage catheter such as a Tenkoff shunt or a PleurX® drain. These allow the effusion to be drained on an 'as needed' basis in an ambulatory setting and are designed to minimise the risk of infecting the pleural space (their design is similar to that of a peritoneal dialysis catheter).

Empyema

An empyema is the infection of the pleural space. The most common cause by far is the infection of a para-pneumonic effusion. About 40% of patients with a pneumonia develop at some time an effusion that usually resolves at the same time as the lung infection resolves. Occasionally this effusion becomes infected. This explains the commonly seen clinical course. The typical patient is either elderly or frail because of underlying disease. Young, healthy patients sometimes also acquire an empyema, but this is unusual in the absence of drug abuse, immunosuppression or some other predisposing condition. The prototypical clinical presentation is that the patient develops a pneumonia, antibiotics are prescribed and after a very brief period of improvement the patient again becomes febrile and feels unwell. Often a new course of different antibiotics is prescribed. The patient continues to be unwell, has very poor appetite, and at this point radiology demonstrates a loculated effusion. Empyema can be a profoundly debilitating disease. The clinical presentation can be very non-specific and the laboratory findings inconclusive (indeed in chronified empyemas the white cell count and CRP level can be remarkably normal), so the early diagnosis of empyema relies heavily on a strong clinical suspicion.

Other causes of empyema are the infection of the pleural space during or following thoracic surgery or some other intrathoracic medical intervention, primary infection of the pleura such as sometimes seen with tuberculosis, trauma, secondary to the development of a bronchopleural fistula, rupture of an abscess into the pleura, or rupture or perforation of the oesophagus.

Microbiology: tuberculosis is an unusual cause but must be considered and ruled out in every case. In 40% of cases the offending organism is never identified. This is readily understandable from the usual course of the development of the disease process as described above. A variety of Gram-positive and Gram-negative organisms and various anaerobes can cause empyema. These include *Streptococcus pneumoniae*, *Strep. pyogenes* and *Staphylococcus aureus*.

Treatment at the different stages of disease

There are three stages in the disease process. They have distinct clinical features, and the treatment is different in each stage. The first two stages are transient in nature, lasting only a few days for each stage. It has become more and more common to see patients only when they have reached the third stage.

The exudative or acute phase

This first stage is characterised by a fairly large free-flowing effusion which is clearly an exudate. The simplest way to demonstrate the free-flowing nature of the effusion is to get a lateral decubitus film which will show that the fluid layers out along the lateral chest wall. At this stage the lactate dehydrogenase (LDH) level in the fluid is moderately elevated and the pH is only slightly low. Therefore diagnosis is not clear-cut, but this is the stage where treatment is straightforward: complete evacuation of all the pleural fluid with some sort of drain and appropriate antibiotics will resolve the infection. The drain should remain in situ until the drainage has dropped to less than around 70 mL per day (without reaccumulation of the effusion).

The fibrinopurulent or transitional stage

This second stage of the disease is when the effusion starts to become loculated. At this stage the loculations are very soft and friable, being entirely fibrinous. The lateral decubitus film will no longer demonstrate layering out of the fluid along the lateral chest wall. Analysis of the pleural fluid shows increasing LDH and decreasing pH levels, but these findings often remain non-specific. Ultrasound is often recommended, as this is the imaging modality that best demonstrates the loculations. However, CT has the advantage of showing the distribution of fluid throughout the entire pleural space and serves as a 'road map' if surgery is planned. There are two treatment options for this stage:

- The first is to insert a drain in the dominant collection (or two separate drains if there are two large, non-communicating pockets of fluid) and to instil fibrinolytic substances (urokinase or streptokinase) into the pleural space.
- The second is surgery, which at this stage will be a VATS procedure. The surgery itself is best described as a 'spring clean' of the entire pleural space, removing entirely all infected fibrinous material from within the chest. It is rather a fussy process, but it is essential that a thorough job be done.

In fit patients the author recommends surgery – at this stage the patient will have limited surgery with relatively rapid recovery and a short hospital stay, and the risk is avoided of having several days of medical therapy, failure and more extensive surgery. In higher-risk patients one naturally tends to prefer the less invasive fibrinolytic therapy.

The organising or chronic phase

In this third stage of an empyema there is fibroblast deposition and neovascularisation of the fibrinous septae forming the loculations, and a similar deposit of developing scar tissue is progressively laid down on the surface of the lung. A CT scan with i.v. contrast will show a thin layer of enhancement of the visceral and parietal pleura. This is another advantage of CT over ultrasound in the evaluation of an empyema – it allows the distinction between the transitional and chronic phases of the disease in many instances. At this stage LDH levels in the pleural fluid are usually quite high (over 1000 IU/L) and the pH is commonly <7.0. The treatment of a chronic empyema is surgical decortication of all the infected material. This operation consists of the removal of all infected material from the chest cavity as well as the meticulous removal of the peel of scar tissue and inflammatory exudate from the visceral pleura. Areas of grossly abnormal parietal pleura which restrict the chest wall should also be resected. The entire lung must be thoroughly decorticated so that it can re-expand and occupy the entire pleural space. If there is an underlying lung abscess which has ruptured into the pleural space it should usually be resected at the same time. These are fairly lengthy operations that can cause significant blood loss but they are often remarkably well tolerated even by fairly frail patients, as they remove infected tissue and restore function. However, the timing of the surgery is very important. In debilitated patients it is better to spend 10–15 days re-nourishing them and getting them as fit as possible to reduce the risk of serious morbidity and mortality. Also if there is extensive consolidation of the underlying lung due to unresolved pneumonia the lung will not be able to re-expand. Again it is essential to await good partial recovery of the lung prior to surgery. Patients unfit for decortication can undergo a more limited drainage procedure.

Chylothorax

This is the abnormal accumulation of lymph in the chest. The most common cause is iatrogenic – direct injury of the thoracic duct during an oesophagectomy, for example. The most common cause of spontaneous chylothorax is blockage of the thoracic duct by tumour in the mediastinum. Tuberculosis can also cause chylothorax.

The diagnosis of a chylothorax is usually very straightforward if the patient is being fed orally – the drainage from the chest drain is a characteristic milky white fluid, and no laboratory confirmation is required. If the patient is not being fed then the fluid appears to be serous. This is because the lymph drains the fat which is absorbed by the gut except for medium-chain triglycerides (MCTs), which are resorbed directly into the bloodstream. Laboratory analysis will show abundant lymphocytes and an elevated triglyceride level (higher than the plasma levels).

If the chylothorax is iatrogenic (for example due to direct injury during a thoracotomy for any reason) then early reoperation with ligation of the thoracic duct above and below the injury should be considered if the volume of chyle loss is high. Otherwise the first line of treatment is often medical with dietary manipulation. The patient must be placed on a strict diet containing fat only in the form of MCTs. This diet is totally unpalatable and requires a nasogastric feeding tube. If this does not resolve the problem, a trial of total parenteral nutrition should be started. If this fails (within around 2 weeks) then surgery should be considered because persistent chyle leaks lead to immunosuppression (chyle is rich in lymphocytes) and substantial protein depletion. Surgery will consist either in ligation of the thoracic duct at the diaphragm or in pleurodesis, usually by pleurectomy.

INFECTIOUS LUNG CONDITIONS REQUIRING SURGERY

There are a variety of infectious conditions of the lung which can require surgery. These are usually complex medical problems which are beyond the scope of this chapter, and the reader is referred to the appropriate chapters in the thoracic surgical textbooks. This section will outline the guiding features of these conditions and very briefly summarise some of the conditions.

All chronic septic conditions in the lung which lead to surgery can often be very debilitating diseases. Before considering surgical treatment, in the absence of a life-threatening complication, it is of primordial importance to prepare the patient for surgery. This requires a very thorough nutritional assessment and excellent nutritional support which recognises the patient's particular requirements, such as religious dietary constraints. A programme of respiratory rehabilitation with intensive chest physiotherapy is at least equally important. Complete smoking cessation is essential. Pulmonary rehabilitation programmes always include an element of general reconditioning. The patient must be made fit for surgery and optimised from a pulmonary prospective – operations for septic conditions tend often to be long, difficult and bloody procedures. These patients often have borderline pulmonary reserve, and therefore these procedures can be a major physiological insult. Some, such as thoracoplasty, are also extensive and, to a degree, mutilating procedures. The preoperative preparation is by nature a lengthy process, and the patient must be aware of the time element and demonstrate patience and fortitude. This sounds like a platitude, but is stressed by authors with extensive experience in these cases, underlying the possibly vital importance of adequate preparation, and this cannot be obtained without the patient's very active participation.

Destroyed lung

Whatever the aetiology, the lung can be destroyed by infection in part or in whole. At times all that is left is the scarred, destroyed lung, and the cause can no longer be ascertained. Often, however, the cause is known. The lung can then be the source of recurrent infection with resistant organisms which put the healthy remaining lung at risk from 'spill over' contamination and infection. These areas of destroyed lung can also be the source of recurrent haemoptysis. Pneumonectomy for sepsis or for destroyed lung is one of the most technically challenging and dangerous operations in thoracic surgery.

Tuberculosis

Tuberculosis is far from being eradicated; it is again increasing throughout the world and particularly in the developed nations such as the UK. There is also a growing problem with multiresistant organisms. This increase is due to population migrations, travel and the extent of the problem in developing countries. It is also due to a large indigenous population of people below the poverty line, often drug abusers and homeless people. Tuberculosis is also one of the defining infections in AIDS. *Mycobacterium* is a very slow-growing organism, and improper or inadequate treatment leads to the emergence of resistant organisms. Treatment requires months of multiple-agent administration. The infection is more common in precisely the populations which tend to have the poorest medical treatment and compliance with therapy. Finally, tuberculosis is a very infectious disease, but most healthy, well-nourished people with an adequate immune system will not develop active disease.

The indications for surgery for tuberculosis are a localised, resectable area of active infection with a resistant organism that will not be eradicated with medical therapy or the resection of an area of past infection, which has become complicated and a source of other problems such as superinfection by *Aspergillus*, troublesome bronchiectasis or haemoptysis. When there is infection with lung destruction that merits resection the patient should be treated medically until the sputum is completely smear negative.

Aspergillus spp.

There are principally two aspects of *Aspergillus* disease. The first is the superinfection of a pre-existing cavity (whatever the origin). The fungus grows inside the cavity, forming a fungus ball. There is no invasive infection of the surrounding lung tissue. The principal complication of this condition is haemoptysis. Invasive aspergillosis occurs in immunocompromised patients such as those undergoing aggressive chemotherapy. Surgery is indicated for aspergilloma when there are complications or in otherwise fit patients to prevent them. Surgery for invasive aspergillosis is a more complex issue. Basically if the disease is technically resectable and resistant to therapy then surgery is indicated. It can also be required to allow chemotherapy to proceed according to schedule so as to protect the patient from life-threatening disease progression during the period of bone marrow suppression.

Bronchiectasis

This is the abnormal and permanent dilatation of the airways. It can be cylindrical, varicose or saccular (cystic). The common causes are infectious – previous tuberculosis tends to involve the upper lobes, prior bacterial or viral infection the lower lobes. Other causes are ciliary dysfunction, immunoglobulin deficient states, cystic fibrosis and toxic damage to the lungs. The principal consequences are chronic inflammation of the surrounding lung and the development of hypertrophied bronchial arteries (with the attendant risk of haemoptysis), increased sputum production, superinfection of the sputum by a variety of bacteria including *Pseudomonas* spp., and airway hyperreactivity. The mainstay of treatment of bronchiectasis is medical with optimal chest physiotherapy and broad-spectrum antibiotic treatment of exacerbations. Surgery is reserved for the resection of localised disease when medical therapy has failed or for the management of serious complications such as haemoptysis. When the disease involves both lungs the indications for surgery should be very restrictive.

Lung abscesses

These are caused by infections with a bacterium which causes destruction of the underlying lung, such as *Staphylococcus aureus*, or a variety of other Gram-positive or Gram-negative organisms. The treatment of most lung abscesses is medical with antibiotics for a prolonged period of time (often 1–2 weeks i.v. followed by 4–8 weeks of oral therapy). If larger than a few centimetres in diameter, percutaneous drainage will aid resolution. The indications for surgery are the lack of response to adequate therapy after 2 weeks, rupture into the airway with contamination of the contralateral lung, rupture into the pleura causing empyema and massive haemoptysis. The results of treatment are excellent, but this can still be a fatal condition, especially when it occurs in a debilitated host, as is often the case.

THE MEDIASTINUM

Mediastinal pathology is fascinating but in reality affects very few patients. The reader is advised to refer to the chapters in the thoracic surgery textbooks for a more complete description. Below, the highlights are summarised.

Anatomy

The mediastinum is the part of the chest between the two pleural cavities. It is commonly divided into the *anterior mediastinum (*or *pre-vascular compartment)*, which is in front of the heart and the great vessels and behind the sternum. It contains the thymus and lymph nodes. The *middle mediastinum (*or *visceral compartment)* contains the heart, the great vessels, the oesophagus, the central airway, the hila of the lungs, some nerves and lymph nodes. Its posterior boundary is the front of the spine. The *posterior mediastinum (*the *retrovisceral zone)* is all that is posterior to the middle mediastinum. It contains mainly nerves.

Pathology

Masses arising in the mediastinum are principally tumours, cysts and vascular lesions such as aneurysms. The most common tumours arising in the anterior mediastinum are encompassed by the mnemonic four Ts: Thymoma, Thyroid (intrathoracic goitre), T-cells (lymphoma) and Teratoma (all the primary mediastinal germ cell tumours). A variety of rare other tumours can arise in the anterior mediastinum, such as thymic carcinoids, thymolipomas and thymoliposarcomas. Ectopic parathyroid glands can be found in the thymus or within the middle mediastinum amongst the great vessels. The tumours arising in the middle mediastinum are those associated with the organs it contains, such as carcinoma of the trachea or oesophagus as well as lymphomas. In the posterior mediastinum, neurogenic tumours and lymphomas are the most common neoplastic lesions.

Signs and symptoms

These lesions usually cause symptoms due to compression of adjacent structures. Thus stridor is heard with tracheal compression, and obstruction of the superior vena cava causes facial swelling and headaches (which worsen in the recumbent position). Cough and pain or discomfort often occur too. Occasional trichoptysis (coughing up hair) has been seen with benign teratomas.

Tumours

Thymomas are tumours of the thymus. Histologically they are divided into medullary, mixed and cortical lesions according to the Müller–Hermelink classification. They can be well capsulated, indolent, benign lesions or more-aggressive, invasive and/or metastatic lesions. They can be associated with a paraneoplastic syndrome: myasthenia gravis – see below. Treatment is surgical resection for the well-localised lesions. Multimodality therapy including combinations of surgery, chemotherapy and radiotherapy is indicated for the invasive and/or metastatic lesions. Thymomas tend to have a prolonged course even when invasive and/or metastatic. Thymic carcinoma is an aggressive lesion with a poor prognosis despite equally aggressive treatment.

Primary malignant and benign germ cell tumours can arise primarily in the thymus. The pathology of these lesions is identical to that of their gonadal counterparts. Around 15% do not have elevated tumour markers. With seminomas there are elevated β-hCG levels, but never elevated alphafetoprotein (AFP). Elevated AFP levels always indicate mixed histology or non-seminomatous germ cell histology. Treatment of seminomas is by radiotherapy, chemotherapy or both depending on the extent of the disease at the time of diagnosis. Surgery is only indicated in exceptional cases. Non-seminomatous germ cell tumours are treated with chemotherapy until normalisation of the tumour markers. If at this point there is a residual mass greater than 3 cm in diameter this should be resected. The prognosis of mediastinal germ cell tumours tends to be worse than that of their gonadal counterparts, mainly because they tend to be more extensive at the time of diagnosis.

Benign cystic lesions

These are predominantly bronchogenic cysts and digestive duplication cysts. They can arise anywhere in the middle mediastinum. The enteric cysts can communicate with the abdominal viscera. The distinction can at times be impossible to make. If they are symptomatic, resection is indicated. In young, healthy individuals surgery is usually indicated to prevent infection, which is the principal complication of these lesions apart from compression of adjacent structure.

Myasthenia gravis

Myasthenia gravis (MG) is an autoimmune disease of neuromuscular transmission. Commonly it is due to the production of auto-antibodies directed against the acetylcholine receptor. The principal symptom is weakness. Ocular MG affects the eyelids and extrinsic muscles of the eyes.

Generalised MG affects all muscle groups. Bulbar MG affects the muscles of swallowing and breathing. Medical treatment includes pyridostigmine (an acetylcholine esterase inhibitor), prednisolone and plasmapheresis. Thymectomy is often beneficial – the earlier in the course of the disease it is performed, the better the results. It can take several years for the full benefit of surgery to be reached. The results do not really depend on pathology of the thymus (normal or hypertrophied). There is much debate on the best surgical approach and whether a simple thymectomy or an extended, radical thymectomy should be performed, and as yet there is no compelling evidence of the superiority of any approach that allows complete resection of the entire thymus. Approximately 40% of patients will have complete remission of their MG following surgery, a further 30–40% will be improved, whereas the rest will be unchanged or worse after surgery. When there is a thymoma, the complete resection of the tumour principally determines the result.

SURGERY FOR EMPHYSEMA

This is an old subject that has recently been revisited with considerable media interest and hype. Now that this new wave of interest has had time to subside, the benefits and risks of the procedure are better defined. The procedure is less dangerous than when pioneered in the late 1950s, but the nature of the disease is the same, and the benefits of surgery do not last any longer. This is why there is again some drop off in interest in the procedure. The procedure is now commonly called lung volume reduction surgery (LVRS). It is also occasionally called reduction pneumoplasty.

In end-stage emphysema the lung is grossly distended by air-trapping, and this pushes the chest wall out close to its anatomic limit of motion. Thus the range of motion of the entire chest wall (including the diaphragm) is extremely limited and the 'bellows' of breathing can no longer function. Indeed in extreme cases the diaphragm is inverted and its contraction actually decreases the intrathoracic volume. If part of the grossly overdistended lung is resected the chest wall can fall back to a more physiological position and the bellows can function again because it can move back and forth to a much greater extent. In patients with a very uneven distribution of emphysema this can be done by resecting the much more destroyed part of the lung. Thus practically none of their precious residual functional lung is resected. These highly selected patients can derive terrific functional benefit from the procedure. In patients with more homogeneous disease the results tend to be disappointing because the trade-off for better mechanics of breathing is the loss of functional tissue, of which they have too little. In the patients with the best results, these can last for several years. However, many patients deteriorate to roughly their pre-LVRS function by 1–2 years after surgery. So LVRS is a purely palliative procedure. It does not prolong life. In this context it must also be said that transplantation for emphysema is also a palliative procedure that does not prolong life.

TRANSPLANTATION

After many previous attempts, the first truly successful single lung transplantation was done in Toronto in 1983. The first successful bilateral transplantation was done by the same team in 1986 – and the patient was one of the longest lung transplant survivors. Lung transplantation is usually not indicated for malignancy. Single or bilateral transplantation can be done for emphysema, intrinsic fibrosing lung disease, sarcoidosis, lymphangioleiomyomatosis and pulmonary hypertension. Lung transplantation must always be bilateral for septic lung disease such as cystic fibrosis and bronchiectasis.

Patients must have reached end-stage disease to justify the risks of the procedure and the obligatory immunosuppressive treatment. The overall survival is around 50% at 5 years, literally restoring the breath of life to these patients. Death is caused by chronic rejection, infection, lymphoproliferative disease and a variety of other causes.

STANDARD THORACIC INCISIONS

These are commonly grouped into:

- incisions giving access to one hemithorax (or one pleural space)
- those that lend access to both hemithoraces
- thoracoabdominal incisions.

Incisions giving access to one pleural cavity

The most commonly used thoracotomy is the **posterolateral thoracotomy**. The patient is placed in the full lateral position and the incision swings around the tip of the scapula through the latissimus dorsi muscle onto the chest wall which is opened in the 5th interspace (i.e. between ribs 5 and 6). This is the universal incision because it gives adequate access to virtually all parts of the hemithorax. Various **muscle-sparing** variants exist. They usually are sufficient but all do somewhat limit vision and access.

The **anterolateral thoracotomy** is performed with the patient in a dorsal decubitus position. This is why it is preferred in unstable trauma patients, for example. The incision is under the breast (which is aesthetically advantageous in women, for example) and the pectoralis major is cut or split, the seratus anterior is split and the chest is entered in the 4th interspace. Access is somewhat more limited, especially to the hilum of the left lower lobe. True **axillary mini-thoracotomies** are made through the axilla into the chest via the 2nd or 3rd interspace. These are useful for the management of spontaneous primary pneumothoraces.

Video-assisted thoracoscopic surgery (VATS) is a minimally invasive approach to the pleural space via 1–4 ports or incisions. In malignant conditions all instruments should be passed through ports to avoid seeding the chest wall. Contrary to laparoscopic surgery, free passage of air into the chest is desirable to maintain the lung in a deflated condition which is a sine qua non for vision as the chest wall is inelastic (as distinct from the abdominal wall, where inflation creates the work space). Recovery from surgery is swifter, and immediate postoperative pain is less than with thoracotomy, but the incidence of residual troublesome pain is the same with both techniques. Hospital stays are often similar with open and VATS techniques, so the advantages are somewhat less clear-cut than in abdominal surgery, especially since the cost of disposable instruments is high. However, there are clearly procedures where VATS is the preferred approach, such as the management of many pleural diseases and limited peripheral lung biopsies. Certain mediastinal procedures can also be performed using VATS.

Incisions giving access to both pleural cavities

The **median sternotomy** gives good access to the anterior mediastinum, the heart and great vessels and both pleural spaces. The middle and posterior mediastinum as well as the left lower lobe are hard to reach. The **bilateral anterolateral thoracotomy with transverse sternotomy** (an incision across the sternum joining the two thoracotomies) is also known as the 'clamshell' incision. It gives fair to very good access to all parts of the thorax.

Thoracoabdominal incisions

There are a variety of thoracoabdominal incisions. The simplest is the **median sternotomy–median laparotomy**. Many other combinations joining thoracotomies with laparotomies exist, and the reader is referred to the appropriate chapters in the textbooks for their description.

POSTOPERATIVE CARE

As in all fields of surgery good outcomes rely on optimal postoperative care. Some aspects of care of the thoracic patient are no different from those of any other surgical patient. Thoracic surgery does not represent a special risk for deep vein thrombosis and pulmonary embolism (DVT and PE), and standard prophylaxis is adequate. Some surgeons do, however, anticoagulate patients who have undergone pneumonectomy for 3 months, because a PE will be poorly tolerated.

A thoracotomy without lung resection reduces the forced vital capacity (FVC) by about 25% due to diaphragmatic dysfunction (just as does an upper abdominal incision). It is important to mobilise patients aggressively from the day of surgery – this will help overcome the dysfunction of the diaphragm, promotes lung expansion, improves ventilation-perfusion matching, is beneficial to reduce the risk of DVT and PE and promotes general well-being. Mobilisation also mandates hyperpnoea, chiefly through an increase in tidal volume. Thus mobilisation is also one of the useful techniques of chest physiotherapy.

Postoperative pneumonia in a patient who has just undergone a lung resection can be a devastating complication. Aggressive chest physiotherapy is the cornerstone of prevention. Most lung cancer patients have altered lung function – there is a direct correlation between the degree of lung destruction by cigarette smoking and the risk of developing lung cancer. Also the peak in incidence in lung cancer is in the 70s. Finally smokers have abolished mucociliary clearance of secretions and an increase in the amount of secretions to clear. The discomfort (or pain) from the thoracotomy discourages efforts to clear these secretions. It follows that pain management must be optimised.

Pain management

There are a variety of techniques to control pain, and good teamwork between the anaesthetist, the surgeon and the pain control team is essential. Every technique has its indications, contraindications and limitations. The most commonly used techniques in thoracic surgery are epidural analgesia, patient-controlled analgesia (PCA) using i.v. morphine and paravertebral catheters with an infusion of local anaesthetic agents together with PCA. Once good analgesia is ensured, do not try to convert to oral pain medications until it is clear that the drains are about to come out, as there is no benefit from this conversion at this early stage after surgery. Beware of over-zealous prescriptions of non-steroidal anti-inflammatory agents in elderly patients with impaired renal function, especially because thoracic patients are kept 'dry' to prevent pulmonary oedema and lung injury. The key in preventing troublesome post-surgery pain (which occurs with equal frequency after VATS and open surgery) is optimal early pain control, and this must be the goal for every single patient. Likewise patients must be prescribed adequate pain medication on discharge and encouraged to take it regularly until the first follow-up visit, which is customarily 3–4 weeks after discharge.

Physiotherapy

The common techniques of chest physiotherapy are first and foremost the hands-on work that is done by the patient with the physiotherapist's help to prevent and relieve atelectasis. Techniques which promote deep breathing and slow, steady expiration (sometimes against moderate resistance) help mobilise secretions to a more central position where they can be removed by coughing. As said, mobilisation is an essential part of this process. All active (by the patient) means of physiotherapy are to be preferred to passive ones. However, when the patient requires extra assistance, CPAP (continuous positive airway pressure) devices can help prevent or relieve atelectasis. If the patient is having difficulty clearing copious secretions a mini-tracheostomy device can be inserted under local anaesthetic to aspirate them.

Examinations and antibiotic therapy

A thoracic patient's chest must be examined (including careful auscultation) twice daily. Initially, daily chest X-rays should be obtained. If there is any suspicion of pneumonia (fever, increased sputum production, lung infiltrate on the X-ray) this should be treated aggressively with i.v. antibiotics which have adequate Gram-positive and Gram-negative coverage, until sensitivity studies of the offending organisms allow the spectrum to be narrowed. Chest physiotherapy should be intensified.

Drains

Almost all patients who have undergone thoracotomy have one or two chest drains. The management of chest drains owes more to local custom and habits than to evidence-based medicine. Most surgeons routinely apply suction (5–10 kPa) to drains. There is however some evidence that no suction might decrease the time drains are required to stay in, both in terms of volume of drainage and duration of air leaks. The common criteria for drain removal are no air leak for 24–36 hours and drainage of less than 150–200 mL over the last 24 hours. Again these criteria are variable from surgeon to surgeon, and the reader is advised to conform to surgeon preference.

Post-pneumonectomy

After pneumonectomy the space can be managed in several ways. Some surgeons do not insert a drain, some put in a drain which is put to underwater seal and removed the next day, some use so-called balanced drainage systems, and some clamp the drain but with intermittent periods when the drainage system is elevated to the level of the heart and unclamped for a few minutes around three times per day. The object is to ascertain the quality of the drainage fluid (serous or blood) and to 'balance' the mediastinum. The mediastinum should be very slightly shifted towards the operative side to allow optimal expansion of the remaining lung. Exaggerated shift can be equivalent to tension PNO and is to be avoided. Daily chest X-rays should be obtained, and the air–fluid level in the post-pneumonectomy space must be seen to rise every day. Drop in this level can be the sign of a breakdown of the bronchial stump with the development of a bronchopleural fistula. In this case the fluid in the chest will drain into the remaining lung, causing an aspiration pneumonia. This can be a rapidly lethal complication. If the air–fluid level in the post-pneumonectomy space drops, the patient should be immediately laid down with the operated side down to prevent spillage of the fluid into the airway, and the operating surgeon must be notified immediately.

Activity

There are per se no restrictions in activity providing reasonable care is exercised. Patients are encouraged to mobilise and go for walks after discharge. They should use the arm on the side of the surgery freely without straining to maintain shoulder mobility. The usual time to recovery for a fairly fit patient from a simple VATS procedure is 2–3 weeks. This rises to 6–8 weeks following thoracotomy and lung resection. Obviously this is dependent on comorbidities and postoperative complications as well as on interpatient variability.

FURTHER READING

Patterson GA, Pearson FG, Cooper JD, et al 2008 Pearson's thoracic and oesophageal surgery: expert consult, 3rd edn. Churchill Livingstone, New York

Shields T W, LoCicero J, Reed CE, Feins RH (eds) 2009 General thoracic surgery, 5th edn. Lippincott Williams & Wilkins, Philadelphia

17 Cardiac surgery

Cardiac surgery in the broadest sense involves all the surgical procedures of the heart and the intrathoracic aorta, including transplantation of intrathoracic organs and surgery for congenital heart diseases. However, surgery for coronary artery disease and valvular diseases predominates in the daily work undertaken in every cardiac unit.

The modern history of cardiac surgery identifies the first direct operations on the heart to relieve obstruction of the pulmonary and mitral valves; these procedures were done on the beating heart and were essentially blind, in the sense that the surgeon was unable to see the valve and had to rely on tactile sensation only – a closed valvotomy. In order to carry out open-heart surgery, the function of the heart has to be taken over temporarily. In the 1950s, two strategies were developed to overcome this problem. First came the use of hypothermia to prolong the tolerance of the brain to ischaemia and, secondly, the development of a safe extracorporeal circulation, commonly called cardiopulmonary bypass (CPB). With these tools, and the development of techniques to protect the isolated heart, surgeons have been able to design operations for congenital abnormalities, valve disease and coronary artery disease. In the UK, about 35 000 heart operations are performed each year. A brief review of these concepts is essential in order to understand this specialty.

BASIC CONCEPTS

Cardiopulmonary bypass

The CPB takes over the function of the heart and lungs for the duration of the cardiac operations. In essence it consists of:

- a venous line draining the venous blood from the patient, usually from the right atrium to the venous reservoir by gravity
- a heat exchanger to regulate the temperature of the blood and therefore the temperature of the patient
- an oxygenator for gas exchange, in which the blood is separated from a gas mixture by a system of membranes
- an arterial pump to pump the blood back to the patient
- an arterial line filter to filter the debris from the blood flowing back to the patient, usually to the aorta.

A typical circuit is shown in Figure 17.1. The flow is determined by an estimate of the body surface area and is usually set at around 2.4 L/min/m^2. Reduction of the core temperature by 5 to 10°C is common practice, but there are unresolved debates about the ideal pressure limits and the optimum temperature.

Whilst modern CPB is extremely safe and results of open-heart procedures are excellent, the CPB circuit remains far from perfect. The blood is exposed to the artificial surface of the CPB circuit for over 2 hours, and a series of inflammatory cascades – complement and neutrophil activation, cytokine generation, free-radical activity and (more recently discovered) early gene activation – with increasing severity is triggered and affects the end organs (the brain, lungs, kidneys, liver, and the coagulation and fibrinolytic systems).

Technological advances continue in this field, making CPB ever safer. Recent advances include miniaturised cardiopulmonary circuit (to minimise the artificial surface in contact with blood component) and coating the inner surface of cardiopulmonary circuits with biocompatible agents to minimise the activation of inflammatory cascades. Microemboli are an important source of complications, especially neurological, from the cardiopulmonary circuit. Shed blood within the operative field is now recognised as an important source of these microemboli. The usual practice of using a pump sucker to collect the shed blood has been modified of

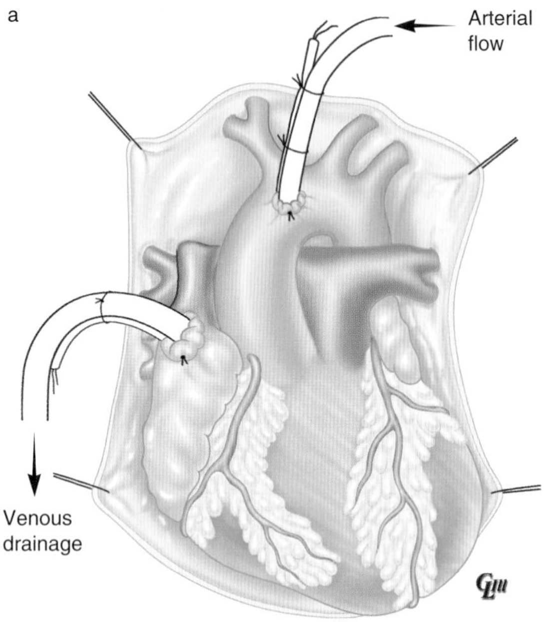

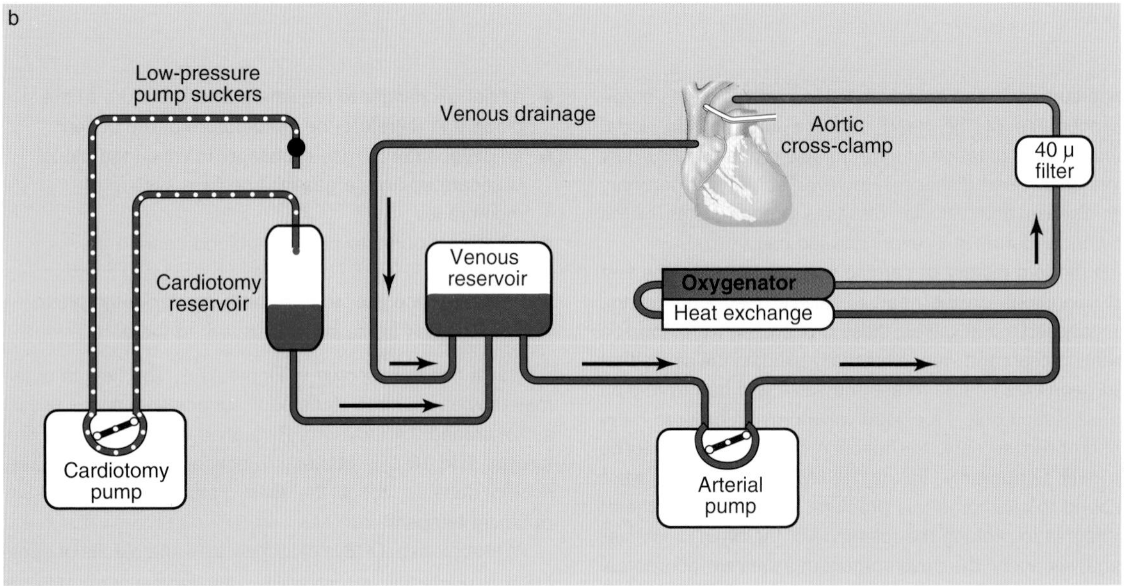

Fig. 17.1 Cardiopulmonary bypass (CPB). (a) Venous blood is most commonly drained from the right atrium under gravity, and artificially oxygenated blood is returned to the ascending aorta, thus bypassing the heart and lungs. An aortic cross-clamp isolates the heart from the systemic circulation. (b) In a typical CPB circuit, blood passes from a venous reservoir, through a roller pump, a heat exchanger, an oxygenator and a micropore filter before being returned to the aorta. Blood spilled into the pericardium is recovered by a cardiotomy system.

late by processing the blood through a cell salvaging system or through filters to minimise the microemboli being introduced in the circulation.

Use of hypothermia

The protective effect of cooling is largely due to a reduction in the oxygen requirement of the brain. This knowledge was used to allow the earliest successful open-heart surgery, and hypothermia is now used in conjunction with CPB. Profound hypothermia with circulatory arrest was developed in the 1970s to allow repair of complex congenital abnormalities and later applied to aortic arch surgery. The technique allows up to about 40 minutes of circulatory arrest if the core temperature is below 20°C. Neural tissue, particularly the CNS (brain and spinal cord) is the most sensitive organ to ischaemic injury. Lately, selective antegrade perfusion of the cerebral vessels has been used as an adjunct to minimise the adverse effects of hypothermic circulatory arrest during aortic arch surgery. Although at such low temperatures little oxygen is delivered to the tissues, nonetheless being perfused with cold blood has a protective effect by cooling and minimising the embolic load. This is an area of great interest to the surgeon undertaking aortic surgery.

Myocardial management

In the current era nearly all open-heart surgery mandates the heart to be stopped while the operations are being conducted. Surgery for coronary artery disease, i.e. coronary artery bypass grafting (CABG), is surgery on the epicardial surface. It can be therefore performed with the heart stopped using cardiopulmonary bypass or with an off-pump technique whilst the heart continues beating. The details of the operative techniques for the two approaches will be discussed later. In the UK some 80–85% of the CABG operations are performed using cardiopulmonary bypass with the heart stopped.

Whilst the cardiac surgical procedures are being conducted, the heart is deprived of any blood supply by cross-clamping the aorta beyond the origin of the coronary arteries in the ascending aorta. Operating on a perfused beating heart is possible but it is not usually desirable for the vast majority of procedures and is only utilised for open-heart surgery in very rare situations in conjunction with cardiopulmonary bypass with selective cannulation of the coronary ostia to perfuse the heart.

The early days of cardiac surgery were marred by failure to 'wean' from CPB, and by the end of the 1960s it was apparent that this was due to subendo-cardial infarction resulting from a period of global ischaemia associated with aortic cross-clamping. Subsequently the issue of myocardial protection has been addressed by the introduction of cardioplegia. The chemical composition of fluid injected to induce cardioplegia is close to that of extracellular fluid but with a potassium content as high as 20 mmol/L in order to arrest the heart in diastole. Numerous cardioplegic techniques are used in clinical practice, but the essential components depend upon the manipulation of the chemical composition and temperature of the coronary perfusion. In the absence of aortic regurgitation, the cardioplegic agent is delivered directly into the ascending aorta after cross-clamping the aorta and can be supplemented by retrograde delivery into the coronary sinus if necessary. Alternatively, the cardioplegic agent can be delivered via specially designed cannulae directly into the coronary ostia after opening the aorta.

ANATOMY

The heart

The heart is enclosed within the pericardial cavity, consisting of outer parietal layer and an inner visceral layer. It consists of four chambers: two on the right side and two on the left. The deoxygenated blood enters the heart by the superior and the inferior vena cava into the right atrium and passes through the tricuspid valve to the right ventricle. From here it is actively pumped through the pulmonary valve to the pulmonary arteries and to the lungs. Oxygenated blood from the lungs is returned to the heart by four pulmonary veins to the left atrium. It then passes through the mitral valve to the left ventricle and is pumped to the aorta via the aortic valve.

Conduction system

The heart has an intrinsic rhythm, and impulses are conducted by specialised cardiac muscle fibres. The essential components are:

- the sinoatrial (SA) node, located at the junction of the superior vena cava and right atrium
- the atrioventricular (AV) node, located at the superior aspect of the interventricular septum
- the AV bundle arising from the AV node and descending in the interventricular septum.

Sinus rhythm is generated in the SA node, conducted through the atrial wall to the AV node, and impulses subsequently pass through the bundle to initiate the ventricular contraction. However, the generation and conduction of impulses are altered in many diseases affecting the heart, and these are evident on 12-lead ECG.

Coronary anatomy

The normal heart is supplied by a left coronary artery (LCA) arising from the sinus of the left aortic cusp, located posteriorly on the aorta, and by a right coronary artery (RCA) arising from the sinus of the right cusp, located anteriorly on the aorta. There is considerable variation in the location of the coronary ostia within the sinuses.

The LCA has a main stem 1 cm in length and then divides into the left anterior descending (LAD) or the anterior interventricular artery and the circumflex artery. The LAD then descends over the anterior part of the heart between the right and the left ventricles to supply the anterior part of both ventricles as well as the anterior part of the septum. It is considered to be the most important of the three major coronary arteries because of its additional supply of the interventricular septum. The main branch of the left anterior descending is called the diagonal. The circumflex artery runs around the back of the heart between the left atrium and the left ventricle in the atrioventricular groove and supplies the lateral and posterior walls of the left ventricle and gives branches to the obtuse marginal (OM) surface of the heart.

The RCA supplies both the right and left ventricles. It runs anteriorly between the right atrium and right ventricle in the atrioventricular groove and divides at the lower border of the right ventricle into two branches: the posterior descending artery (PDA), or the posterior interventricular artery, and the left ventricular (LV) branch of the RCA. The PDA runs along the posterior interventricular groove, between the right and left ventricles, and supplies the posterior part of the septum and inferior parts of both right and left ventricles. The LV branch of the RCA, or right posterolateral artery, supplies the inferior aspect of the left ventricle.

The other small branches of the LCA and RCA are shown in Figure 17.2 and listed in Box 17.1.

For the purposes of describing the severity of coronary artery disease, i.e. single-, double- or triple-vessel disease, the LAD, the circumflex artery and the RCA are each considered individually as a single artery.

DIAGNOSTIC PROCEDURES

For the most part, the diagnosis and assessment of cardiac disease is the province of the cardiac physician, and the surgeon is asked to see the patient only when the diagnosis is established. Most units work cohesively with a high level of shared responsibility and mutual reliance. Nonetheless, cardiac surgeons need to understand and interpret the plethora of investigations relating not only to the heart but also relating to many other organ systems at risk during cardiac operations such as the lungs, cerebral circulation and the renal tract at large.

Basic concepts
Anatomy
Diagnostic procedures

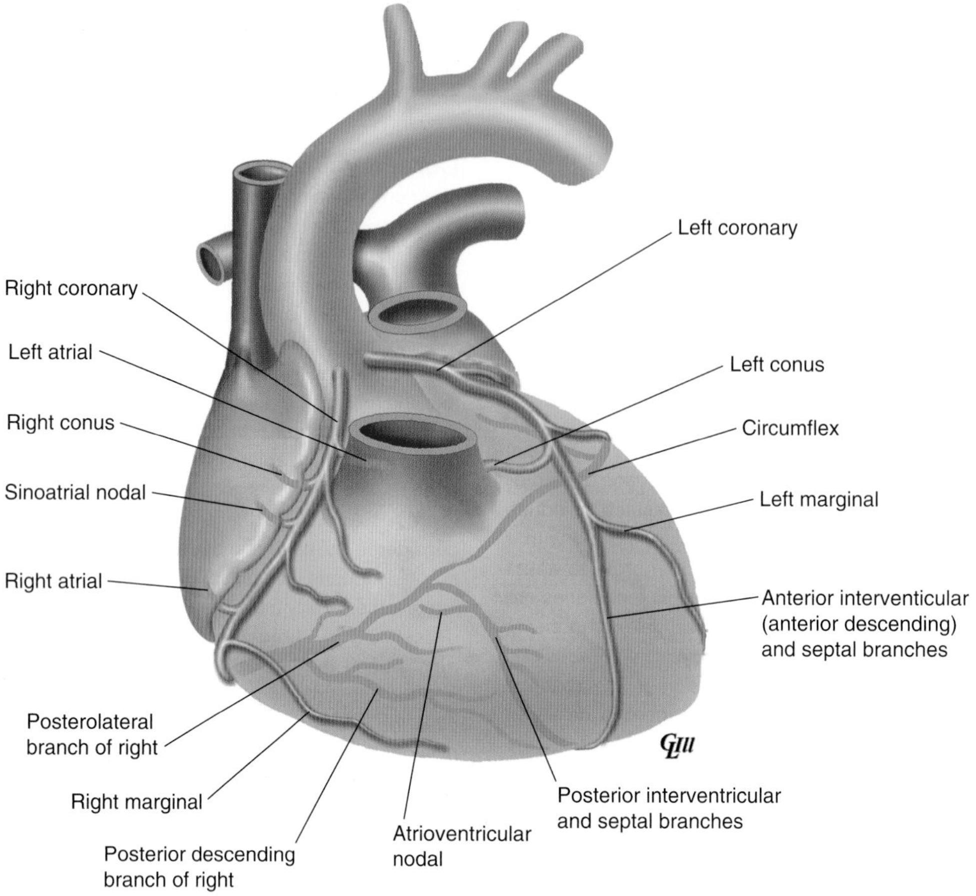

Fig. 17.2 The coronary arteries.

Box 17.1 Branches of the coronary arteries

Right coronary artery
Left atrial
Right conus
Sinoatrial nodal (60% of people)
Right atrial
Acute marginal
Posterior interventricular (posterior descending) (90% of people)
  Ventricular branches
  Septal branches
Atrioventricular nodal (90% of people)

Left coronary artery
Sinoatrial nodal (40% of people)
Circumflex artery
Obtuse marginal
Posterior interventricular (posterior descending) (10% of people)
  Ventricular branches
  Septal branches
Atrioventricular nodal (10% of people)
Anterior interventricular (left anterior descending)
  Left conus
  Diagonal
  Ventricular and septal branches

Haematological

Haematological changes are relevant in valve disease. Anaemia accentuates or creates systolic murmurs. Haemolysis, created by flow at high velocity through a small orifice in or around a valve, is associated with a high reticulocyte count.

Chest radiograph

The plain chest radiograph can give a great deal of information about the size and position of the chambers of the heart and the size of the great vessels. The cardiac shadow on a chest radiograph is a combination of both the atrial and the ventricular chambers. In mitral stenosis, the double outline of the left and right atrium can be separated along the right heart border. Other features of the X-ray which are typical of mitral stenosis are: splayed left bronchus with enlargement of the left atrium, distended lymphatics at the lung bases, pulmonary calcification, pleural effusion and increase in vascularity (plethora). The pulmonary artery knuckle is a reflection of the size of the pulmonary artery; size is increased in pulmonary valve stenosis with post-stenotic dilatation, in atrial or ventricular septal defects and in pulmonary hypertension. The aortic knuckle may be wide in aortic valve stenosis with post-stenotic dilatation and in degenerative or collagen conditions which cause aortic regurgitation. A double aortic knuckle is seen in coarctation.

The status of the lung fields is also ascertained, and this may reflect changes secondary to cardiac disorders. For example, upper lobe venous diversion, particularly in the right upper lobe, is a sign of high pulmonary blood flow or congestion from high left atrial pressure.

Electrocardiogram

Diagnostic ECG is crucial in the investigation and management of coronary artery disease. Exercise ECG performed on a treadmill according to the Bruce protocol checks the state of myocardial perfusion under demand. This is especially useful in patients who are asymptomatic or who have atypical symptoms. The exercise ECG can be a useful screening test for patients recovering from a myocardial infarction, to decide who should proceed to coronary arteriography. During operation the ECG is continually displayed, and the surgeon needs to recognise the plethora of common arrhythmias and ST changes indicative of ischaemia. ECG remains the commonest method of detecting a perioperative myocardial infarction. Left ventricular hypertrophy is commonly present in significant aortic valve disease and coarctation of the aorta. Preoperative rhythm needs to be recognised as there are options for addressing atrial fibrillation during the operation with ablation procedures. Conduction anomalies may predispose patients to postoperative pacemaker requirement. Optimising postoperative rhythm and rate is needed and often requires temporary pacing through epicardial pacing wires placed at the end of the operation and therefore it is vital that cardiac surgeons have a detailed understanding of the rhythm disturbance and solutions to the problems posed by them.

Echocardiography

Echocardiography is vital in the assessment of valve disease and can be done by either a surface probe (transthoracic) or one passed into the oesophagus (transoesophageal). Both approaches show ventricular movement and left ventricular function. Echocardiographic study may be in two-dimensional mode, M-mode or duplex colour. M-mode provides a single beam and identifies movement (M for motion) towards and away from the ultrasound source. It requires considerable skill to obtain and interpret the images and is therefore largely dependent on the skill of the operator. Two-dimensional echocardiography provides a more readily interpretable image of the heart and it has emerged as the most powerful tool in the investigation of congenital heart disease, permitting repeated non-invasive observation of anatomy and function. Transoesophageal echocardiography (TOE) produces even better views, especially of the aortic valve, the mitral valve and the descending aorta. Doppler flow mode coordinated with ECG waveforms allows measurement of blood transit times through valves, from which pressure gradients can be measured. Echocardiography alone may be sufficient for the diagnosis of many valve conditions, and angiography is only required for the exclusion of coronary artery disease.

The field of echocardiography is an ever-growing area of interest as it offers noninvasive modality for investigating the cardiac muscle and the valves and the pathologies to which they are prone. Recent advances include real-time 3-D echocardiography that gives excellent anatomical and functional detail of the heart, particularly the mitral valve. Stress echocardiography is becoming increasing popular in assessing the myocardial contractility, functional reserve and the borderline valve stenosis. Contrast echocardiography has greatly increased the ability to define the epicardial and endocardial surfaces and therefore improved the image acquisition in difficult cases and is now well established in clinical practice.

Radionuclide investigation

In myocardial perfusion scintigraphy a gamma camera detects the distribution of intravenously injected thallium-201. This isotope behaves like potassium, entering the cells, and its distribution is proportional to blood flow. It thus provides important information about viability and, if repeated after a rest period, can detect the presence of hibernating myocardium. The radiation dose of a thallium scan is approximately 25 mSv, equivalent to 250 chest X-rays, and it therefore carries a small but definite increased risk of cancer development. In the diagnosis of myocardial infarction, technetium pyrophosphate enters infarcted cells and binds to intracellular calcium. For left ventricular studies the technique of ECG gating is employed. The red cells are labelled with technetium-99. At any given moment the scintillation counts over the heart cannot usefully be distinguished from the background. The counts from many cardiac cycles are therefore stored and divided into 16 subdivisions of the R–R interval gated from the ECG. The cumulative counts provide a series of measurements of the volume of the heart in systole and diastole, and from these measurements the ejection fraction can be calculated.

Computed tomographic scanning

This technique is familiar in other fields of surgery. It can be useful in the diagnosis of aortic dissection to demonstrate the presence of a flap, haematoma or pleural effusion. It is probably the best method for identifying a calcified pericardium as seen in pericarditis. If there is concern about a retrosternal haematoma or infection in this area a CT scan can be very helpful in detecting any retrosternal collections. Improvements in technology with multiscan CT images have now enabled coronary arteries to be imaged. Scoring systems that stratify the calcification of the proximal coronary arteries have been developed, which are excellent at detecting coronary artery disease. CT images can now be processed using the latest software to generate 3D images of the aorta and the heart and are very helpful in aortic surgery.

Magnetic resonance imaging

The detection of the spin of hydrogen atoms, which in turn depends upon the water content of different tissues, forms the underlying principle of this technique. It is particularly useful in the diagnosis of complex congenital heart disease in adults, often altered by previous surgery. It provides 3D images of the aorta and is an essential investigation prior to elective surgery for aortic aneurysms. The diagnosis of infective endocarditis involving the aortic root can be difficult, and MRI can be very helpful. Recently, in combination with gadolinium, MRI scans are being used to detect and distinguish viable from necrotic myocardium. A major advantage of this imaging method is that it does not involve radiation.

Positron emission tomography

PET scanning is not widely available but has become the gold standard for the detection of hibernating myocardium. By using ^{13}N-ammonia and ^{18}F-deoxyglucose, it can give simultaneous information about regional myocardial perfusion and glucose utilisation. Regions of hibernation can be identified by preservation of glucose utilisation in regions of diminished perfusion. Regions of infarction are revealed by a concordant reduction in regional perfusion and glucose utilisation. This is of great assistance in the planning of coronary artery operations for heart failure.

Cardiac catheterisation

Cardiac catheterisation remains the diagnostic tool of choice for demonstrating coronary anatomy. **Coronary angiography** is performed by passing a catheter into a major artery (usually the femoral but also the brachial or radial), advancing it to the ascending aorta. Right-sided chambers are usually accessed via the femoral veins. Contrast medium is injected into the aortic root and selectively into each of the coronary ostia, and X-ray images are obtained. Coronary narrowings are termed haemodynamically significant if there is reduction in diameter of 50% or more in a vessel as shown on two different projections (preferably at 90° to each other). Haemodynamic implications of the narrowings are defined by Poiseuille's formula, which states that the reduction of flow through a narrowed vessel is proportional to the length of narrowing and to the fourth power of the radius at the point of narrowing. **Intra-vascular ultrasound scan** (IVUS) probe catheters are a new device available to clarify the significance of stenosis when the angiograms are difficult to interpret as it provides excellent cross-sectional anatomical images along the length of the vessel. IVUS provides excellent anatomical detail of the coronary artery lesions. Pressure wires have also become increasing popular in assessing the functional significance of a lesion in the coronary artery by simultaneously measuring the pressures on either side of a coronary lesion in pharmacologically simulated hyperaemic state and expressing it as a fraction, referred to as fractional flow reserve (FFR). Data from IVUS and FFR are vital in clarifying the significance of borderline coronary lesions.

Left main stem disease is the presence of a significant narrowing in the first common part of the LCA before it divides into the anterior descending and the circumflex. Three-vessel coronary disease is significant narrowing in all three major coronary vessels: RCA, LAD and circumflex coronary artery. Single-vessel disease is significant narrowing in just one of the three vessels, excluding the main stem. It should be noted that these radiological classifications are used as a basis for defining treatment options based on prognosis, as will be discussed later. They do not limit the actual revascularisation procedures to just three vessels, as each of these carries important branches which may themselves require attention individually. Thus it is possible and common for patients to have four or five coronary bypass grafts.

The exponential growth of interventional cardiology involving balloons, stents and coils is having a major impact on the practice of cardiac surgery and will be discussed later. In addition to imaging with radio-opaque contrast media, cardiac catheterisation remains the most reliable method for obtaining intracardiac pressures and saturations in the different cardiac chambers. Complete information can be obtained about obstruction or regurgitant valves, and abnormal shunts between the left and right heart can not only be demonstrated but also quantified.

Ventricular function

Angiography, echocardiography and the use of an isotope scan can be used to assess the ventricular function. The movement of each of several segments of the ventricle is quantified (regional wall motion) to determine the ejection fraction. The normal value is 70%. Ejection fraction is an invaluable tool to categorise the preoperative ventricular function, as it determines the operative risk and long-term prognosis.

Left ventricular pressure is directly measured by catheterisation. Pressure at the end of diastole reflects tension in the cardiac muscle. The higher this end-diastolic pressure (LVEDP) the poorer is ventricular function. Normal values are 8–12 mmHg, and these rise to 25–35 mmHg in left ventricular failure. The rise is reflected back through the left atrium, pulmonary veins and capillaries, ultimately to cause a rise in pulmonary artery pressure.

Pathological effects of occlusion

The effects of obstruction of any individual artery are determined by the degree of collateral circulation between it and other vessels. However, occlusions generally cause the following:

- LAD – an anterior or anterolateral infarction of the left ventricle
- circumflex artery – a posterolateral infarction
- RCA – likely to produce inferior myocardial infarction.

CORONARY ARTERY DISEASE

Coronary artery disease (CAD) is the commonest cause of death in the Western world, accounting for about 150 000 deaths in the UK annually and over 500 000 deaths per annum in the USA. CAD is the term used to describe all aspects of narrowing or occlusion of the coronary arteries by the process of atherosclerosis. Coronary artery bypass grafting (CABG) for CAD is a commonly performed procedure which involves restoring flow around narrowed segments of coronary artery by using a bypass graft.

The first coronary artery bypass was performed by Sabiston in 1962, but the patient died of a stroke. Much of the pioneering work was done by Favorolo and Effler at the Cleveland Clinic in 1967 and by Johnson and Lepley in Milwaukee. In the 1970s and 1980s there was an enormous rise in the number of CABG operations performed in the developed countries. However, more recently the number of procedures performed has levelled off because of an increase in angioplasty and perhaps because of plateauing of the disease in the population at large. Since 1997 the number of coronary operations in the UK has been around 25 000 per year. The requirement for surgery in the UK and similar Western countries is based on epidemiological studies which suggest around 450 operations per million of the population per year, though there is evidence that the surgical revascularisation rate in the USA is much higher. The current male : female ratio of both incidence and procedures is 4 : 1, but the number of operations in women is rising. CABG is now complemented by percutaneous transluminal coronary angioplasty (PTCA) in which the stenosis is dilated by a balloon at the tip of a catheter and a stent implanted at the site of the lesion. Changes of late that are noteworthy are the great impact of the introduction of statins and the reduction of smoking in many countries on the epidemiology of coronary artery disease. Preventative aspects and plaque remodelling benefits of statins on the population at risk has had a great impact in terms of reducing the incidence and deaths from coronary artery disease.

Epidemiology

CAD is widespread throughout the developed world, including the USA, most of Europe, the Middle East and the Indian subcontinent. There is a low incidence in China and Japan as well as in most of Africa. It is less common in France than in most other European countries.

Aetiology and pathology

Atherosclerotic disease in the coronary arteries is only a manifestation of systemic atherosclerosis. Lipid and cholesterol accumulate in the media of the arterial wall. Inflammatory changes lead to fibrosis. The intima overlying the lesions in the media may become elevated, forming plaques, or may become ulcerated. Turbulent blood flow in these areas predisposes to platelet deposition and thrombosis. Clinical manifestation includes narrowing (stenosis) or occlusion of the artery or its branches. Both may lead to insufficient blood supply to the myocardium, which in turn produces:

- exercise-induced myocardial pain (angina)
- infarction of the area of myocardium supplied – usually secondary to coronary artery occlusion by thrombosis
- ischaemia and consequent malfunction of the neural conduction system, with arrhythmias
- reduction in the efficiency of ventricular contraction
- attenuation of the ventricular wall with the development of an aneurysm.

Risk factors

- *Age*. The incidence of CAD increases with age.
- *Genetic*. There is a strong genetic component to CAD, though individual genes have not been delineated.
- *Cholesterol and triglyceride levels*. Familial hyperlipidaemia results in a higher and earlier incidence of CAD and accounts for some of the patients with a positive family history. Apart from this, epidemiological studies suggest that populations with elevated cholesterol and triglyceride have a higher incidence of atherosclerotic disease, and, conversely, populations with low lipid levels have low incidences of CAD. Recent evidence suggests that reduction in cholesterol levels slows the rate of advance of coronary atheroma.
- *Smoking*. Smoking is the single most important risk factor.
- *Hypertension*. High blood pressure and CAD are related, as hypertension increases the risks of all atherosclerotic diseases.
- *Diabetes*. There is an increased incidence of coronary artery and peripheral vascular disease in both insulin-dependent and non-insulin-dependent diabetics.

Management

The initial management strategy for patients with ischaemic heart disease secondary to CAD is medical therapy aimed at reducing the myocardial oxygen requirements. However, as the disease progresses, most patients require a more active approach. The role of surgery for CAD was established by three prospective randomised landmark trials in the 1970s that compared best medical management with CABG. Current indications for CABG are listed in Box 17.2.

However, with the recent exponential growth in percutaneous interventions in the form of angioplasty and stenting of narrowed coronary arteries, the boundaries between surgical revascularisation by CABG, angioplasty and stenting have become less clear. Indeed, several prospective randomised trials have evaluated the role of angioplasty alone, and more recently stenting has been compared with CABG in the setting of multivessel CAD.

It is important to appreciate that prognostic and symptomatic benefit represent different end-points when assessing the outcome of all the trials comparing CABG with either medical management, angioplasty or a stenting approach. The trials initiated in the 1970s compared medical treatment with CABG, trials in the late 1980s compared CABG with angioplasty PTCA, and most recently trials have compared CABG with stenting.

Evidence for CABG

CABG vs medical management

Three large landmark trials and three smaller trials have compared CABG with medical management of CAD (Table 17.1). In the 1970s, clinicians were not in doubt about the efficacy of CABG in relieving angina; the question was, did it improve

Box 17.2 Indications for coronary artery bypass surgery

- Failure of medical therapy with chronic stable angina
- Unstable angina
- Left main stem disease
- Symptomatic three-vessel disease
- Post-infarct angina
- Acute myocardial infarction with cardiogenic shock
- Failed PTCA
- Reoperation for recurrent symptoms
- Congenital anomalies, e.g. anomalous origin of any coronary artery
- Kawasaki disease
- Coronary disease concomitant with other cardiac procedures

PTCA, percutaneous transluminal coronary angioplasty.

Table 17.1 Survival at 5, 7 and 10 years in the trials comparing CABG and medical management of coronary artery disease

	Number of patients randomised		5-year survival (%)		7-year survival (%)		10-year survival (%)	
	CABG	Medical	CABG	Medical	CABG	Medical	CABG	Medical
Trials								
European	394	373	92	83	87	80	77	71
VA	332	354	83	78	78	70	64	60
CASS	390	390	95	92	89	86	81	69
Texas	56	60	82	79	73	70	59	58
Oregon	51	49	92	84	86	78	73	71
New Zealand	51	49	90	86	86	75	71	67
New Zealand	50	50	84	84	80	78	66	68
Total	1324	1325						
Mean survival			90	84	84	78	74	69

CABG, coronary artery bypass grafting; CASS, Coronary Artery Surgery Study; VA, Veterans Affairs.

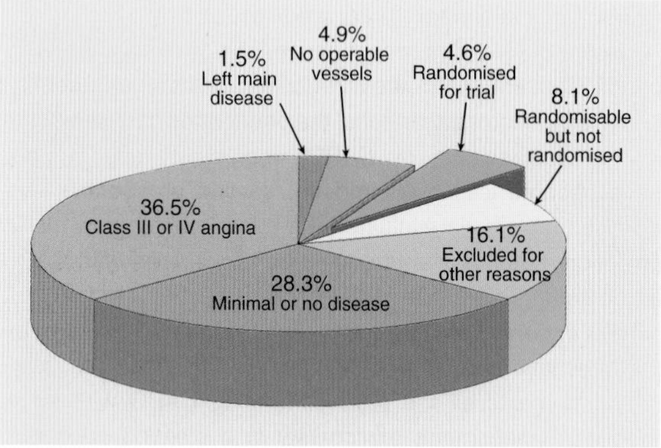

Fig. 17.3 Allocation of patients in the Coronary Artery Surgery Study registry, and reasons for exclusion from trial.

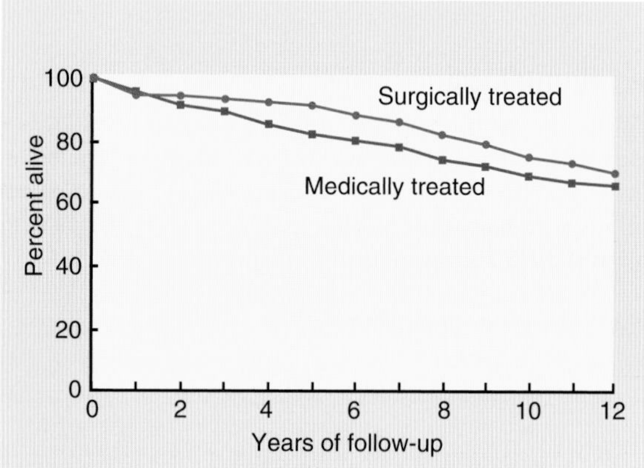

Fig. 17.4 12-year follow-up survival data from the European study comparing medically and surgically treated coronary artery disease patients.

prognosis? The patient populations of the trials differ, with various exclusions including age greater than 65 years, impaired ventricular function and previous infarction, and the patients randomised were a very small proportion of the cases considered (Fig. 17.3). The primary end-point of these trials was mortality. Survival data are available for up to 10 years of follow-up. Inspection of the data (Table 17.1) and of the overall shape of the survival plots (Fig. 17.4) shows a survival advantage for surgery over medicine which is evident beyond 1 year, probably maximal at 5 years, and then the curves tend to converge again.

In terms of symptoms, the Coronary Artery Surgery Study (CASS) trial reported a detailed analysis of symptomatic benefit in the two limbs of the trial. After a mean follow-up of 5.5 years, the surgical group had significantly less chest pain and fewer activity limitations, and a greater proportion were in NYHA class I and II. Treadmill exercise tests performed at 6, 12 and 60 months demonstrated significantly longer treadmill time, less exercise-induced angina and less ST segment depression in the surgical group. They had lower use of long-acting nitrates and beta-blockers. The results of all these trials now need to be interpreted cautiously as both medical therapy and surgical techniques have changed considerably since they were performed.

CABG vs PTCA

The practice of angioplasty was growing rapidly as these trials of surgery versus medicine were being reported. The trials of surgery versus angioplasty focused on the relief of angina comparable to that with surgery, but at lower morbidity. To date there have been nine randomised trials comparing PTCA and CABG (Table 17.2). Again it is imperative to note that, of the patients screened, only a small proportion (2.5–7.7%) were randomised, and the results cannot be generalised to all patients with CAD.

In all the trials, the prevalence of angina (grade II or more) and use of antianginal drugs at 1 year after PTCA was almost twice that following CABG (Table 17.3). At 1 month after intervention, employment status and exercise tolerance were better after angioplasty than after bypass surgery, which is hardly surprising. Thereafter, the physical activity of the CABG group improves significantly, and at 1 year there is no difference in employment status, breathlessness or physical activity. Quality of life data in the RITA trial were almost completely determined by the extent to which angina was relieved.

Table 17.2 Trials comparing PTCA and CABG for ischaemic heart disease

Trials (country)	Single- or multivessel	Number screened for trial	% randomised	Number of patients		Follow-up (years)
				CABG	PTCA	
RITA (UK)	single & multi	33 359	3.2	501	510	4.7
EAST (USA)	multi	5118	7.7	194	198	3
GABI (Germany)	multi	8981	4.0	177	182	1+
CABRI (Europe)	multi	42 580	2.5	513	541	1
Toulouse (France)	multi	NK	NK	76	76	2.8
Laussane (Switzerland)	single	NK	NK	66	68	3.2
MASS (Brazil)	single	NK	NK	70	72	3.2
ERACI (Argentina)	multi	NK	NK	64	63	3.8
BARI (USA)	multi	25 200	7.3	914	915	NK

BARI, Bypass Angioplasty Revascularisation Investigation; CABRI, Coronary Angioplasty versus Bypass Revascularisation Investigation; EAST, Emory Angioplasty versus Surgery Trial; ERACI Argentine randomised trial of PTCA versus CABG in multivessel disease; GABI, German Angioplasty Bypass Surgery Investigation; MASS, Medicine Angioplasty or Surgery study; RITA, Randomised Intervention Treatment of Angina.
CABG, coronary artery bypass grafting; NK, not known; PTCA, percutaneous transluminal coronary angioplasty.

Table 17.3 The prevalence of angina (grade II or more) in trials of CAGB vs PTCA 1 and 3 years after randomisation

Trial	1-year follow-up		3-year follow-up	
	CABG	PTCA	CABG	PTCA
CABRI	11	16	no data	
RITA	11	21	16	18
EAST	9	18	11	19
GABI	25	28	no data	
Four other trials	5	8	7	9

Prognosis. The 1-year mortality rate for all the trials combined is 2.3% for CABG and 2.9% for PTCA (not statistically different). The trials with longer follow-up also fail to show any significant difference. However for certain subgroups, this may not be the case. In the BARI trial, the 5-year mortality for diabetic patients is significantly higher in the PTCA group. This raises questions about other subgroups, such as women and older patients.

Further procedures. There was a striking difference in the need for additional, later interventions. In all trials combined, 34% of patients randomised initially to the PTCA limb required at least one additional procedure: PTCA and/or CABG. Only 3% of the CABG group required an additional procedure in the first year. Furthermore, 18% of the patients in the PTCA limbs of the trials needed CABG in the first year after the initial PTCA, whereas only 1% of the patients in the CABG limb of the trials needed a repeat CABG.

CABG vs stenting

More recently, three prospective randomised trials have compared the outcome of CABG with that of coronary stenting. The results of these trials are similar to those comparing CABG with angioplasty alone. However the re-intervention rates for the stenting group are lower than the previous re-intervention rates for angioplasty alone, although they remain significantly higher than in the CABG group. This finding suggests that the gap between CABG and percutaneous revascularisation together with stenting continues to narrow; however, there are important differences in the patient population being offered coronary angioplasty and stenting when compared with CABG. Modern stents contain elutable antimitotic agents which inhibit fibroblastic proliferation and reduce early restenosis rates even further.

Shortcomings and limitations of the trials

Before attempting to generalise the information, we should remember the many patients who were excluded and for whom the conclusions are therefore not necessarily applicable. These are:

- left main stem stenosis
- severe three-vessel disease
- impaired left ventricular function.

These are significant factors in the decision to operate, as these are the patients who have most to gain from CABG. Another limitation is that it has been usual to randomise lowest-risk patients. The ventricular function of the patients recruited in all the trials is well preserved, and a significant proportion of the patients randomised to the CABG group in the trials had two-vessel disease. These two factors in combination make it unlikely that these patients would gain prognostically from revascularisation of any form.

Clinical practice changes with time. The benefits of CABG in the trials comparing CABG with medical management tended to be attenuated after 5 years. This is primarily due to venous graft occlusion. Left internal mammary artery (LIMA) graft was used in less than 10% of the cases in the CASS, VA and European studies. The increasing use of arterial conduits for bypass grafting has significantly improved the long-term outlook for CABG patients. The practice of angioplasty is also changing rapidly, particularly with the increasing use of coronary stents and now drug-eluting stents that are likely to reduce the restenosis rates even further.

Key messages from CABG trials to date are summarised in Box 17.3 and Figure 17.5.

Conduits for CABG

A plethora of conduits have been tried for CABG, as detailed in Table 17.4. In general terms the arterial conduits have a

Box 17.3 Key messages from CABG trials data are available for CABG vs medical management, angioplasty and stenting

- CABG improves prognosis in selected groups:
  - left main stem disease
  - three-vessel disease
  - two-vessel disease involving the proximal LAD
  - poor left ventricular function
- CABG and angioplasty are equally safe in low-risk cases
- Angioplasty carries the penalty of higher recurrence and re-intervention rates
- CABG-treated patients are more likely to be free of angina
- CABG and angioplasty have similar outcomes for employment status and activity level
- Angioplasty is more cost-effective in the short term, but with time there is little difference (because of more repeated procedures with angioplasty)
- Re-intervention after angioplasty has been reduced further by stenting but remains significantly higher than for CABG

LAD, left anterior descending coronary artery.

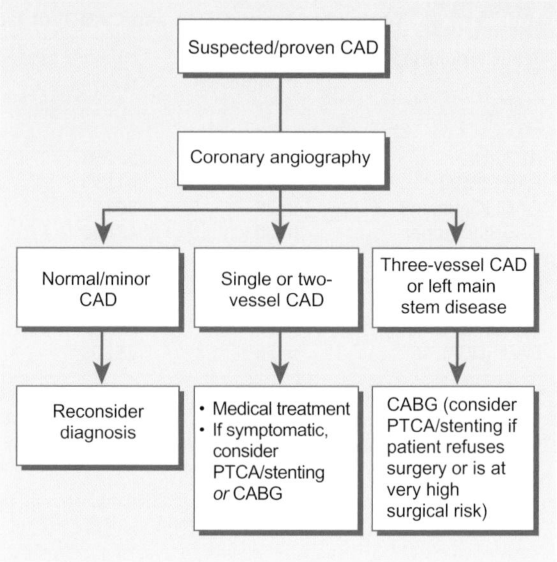

Fig. 17.5 An algorithm for the management of patients with suspected CAD.

Table 17.4 Conduits used for CABG

Conduits	1-year patency	Late patency	Comments
Arterial			
Internal mammary artery (IMA)	98%	90% at 10 years	Gold standard conduit with best long-term patency
Radial artery	90%	–	Renewed interest recently; long-term data lacking
Gastroepiploic artery	95%	90% at 3 years	Arterial conduit in routine use after IMA & radial
Inferior epigastric artery	75–85%	–	Better patency as a composite graft
Subscapular artery	?	–	Limited experience
Lateral costal artery	?	–	Limited experience
Splenic artery	?	–	Limited experience
Venous			
Long saphenous vein	80–90%	50% at 10 years	Readily available; prone to graft atherosclerosis
Short saphenous vein	75%	–	
Cephalic vein	60%	–	Thin wall
Umbilical vein	50%	–	Limited experience
Others			
Cryopreserved saphenous vein	40%	–	Poor patency; only used in emergency with no native conduits
Bovine internal mammary artery	16%	–	Poor patency
Polytetrafluorethylene	64%	14% at 4 years	Poor patency

better long-term patency. Venous conduits are prone to late graft occlusion by three mechanisms: graft thrombosis, intimal hyperplasia and graft atherosclerosis. Use of anti-platelet agents such as aspirin has greatly improved the long-term patency of grafts. Venous conduits are technically somewhat more user friendly. The use of bilateral IMA, especially in diabetes and obese patients, may be associated with a higher incidence of chest wound complications.

Conduct of CABG

In the UK over 80% of CABG operations are performed using the cardiopulmonary bypass (CPB) machine. The principles of CPB are outlined above. The patient is placed on bypass with a degree of systemic hypothermia. The aorta is cross-clamped, and cardioplegia solution is infused in the aortic root to arrest and protect the heart.

Diseased coronary arteries are then identified, and bypass grafts are constructed using the conduits prepared. Regular doses of cardioplegia are necessary every 15–20 minutes. At the completion of the operation the heart is reperfused, the patient is weaned from CPB, and the heart takes over the circulation.

Recent advances in technology have allowed coronary artery grafting to be carried out without the use of the CPB machine. This method is called off-pump or beating-heart surgery and uses a mechanical stabiliser to lift and stabilise a portion of the heart where the coronary anastomoses are being carried out, with the rest of the heart beating and maintaining a good blood pressure and circulation. In Figure 17.6, the operative set-up for a beating-heart CABG case is shown. In some units over 90% of CABG operations are being performed by this approach. Early results indicate

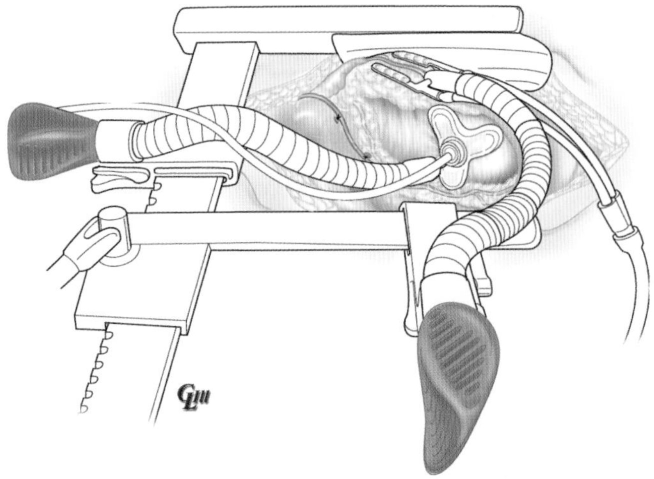

Fig. 17.6 Operative set-up for beating-heart coronary artery bypass grafting. The coronary artery is stabilised by a two-pronged platform containing suckers (Octopus) seen to the right of the figure. The apex of the heart can be manipulated via a 'Star-Fish' sucker seen to the left of the figure.

Table 17.5 Causes of stroke in open-heart surgery

Event	Origin
Solid emboli	From any left-sided site where thrombosis may have occurred – left atrial appendage, suture lines Disruption of atheromatous plaques
Air emboli	Technical in cardiopulmonary bypass
Hypoxic infarction	Low bypass pressure or flow
Hypertension	Uncontrolled during operation or soon thereafter Both hypoxic and hypertensive events may have intra- or extracranial atherosclerosis as coexistent and associated cause
Intracranial haemorrhage (rare)	Poorly controlled anticoagulation Rupture of a cerebral aneurysm

similar outcome to conventional CABG, but the exact role of beating-heart surgery remains to be defined. However, in certain high-risk groups (diseased aorta, impaired respiratory function, renal impairment, carotid disease) this approach may be preferable.

Results of CABG operation

The national operative mortality is around 2% for all patients undergoing CABG. For elective male cases the true risk can be as low as 1% or less. Morbidity includes a small risk of major stroke (about 1%) and a larger risk of transient focal neurological deficit, probably embolic in origin (2–4%). A high proportion of all patients who undergo cardiopulmonary bypass have transient neuropsychological impairment which is usually subclinical but can be detected with sensitive tests. Significant wound infection complicates 2–3% of operations. Causes of neurological deficit after cardiac surgery, and other common complications of open-heart surgery, are listed in Tables 17.5 and 17.6, respectively.

Most patients have complete relief of angina, but 10–15% have some residual symptoms, and a small minority (about 2%) are no better. Failure to relieve angina is associated with failure to bypass all diseased vessels or early graft occlusion. Most patients leave hospital 6–7 days after surgery, but convalescence can take several weeks. The 1-year patency rate for vein grafts is about 80–90%, with an attrition rate of 4% per year thereafter; a similar proportion of patients develop recurrent angina, either due to graft occlusion or progression of disease in native vessels. There is evidence that treatment to reduce platelet adherence may improve graft patency; this is now usually achieved with low-dose aspirin.

Table 17.6 Complications of open-heart surgery

Nature	Manifestations
Low cardiac output	Low blood pressure, cold periphery, poor urine output, metabolic acidosis
Arrhythmias	Atrial fibrillation Supraventricular tachycardia Multiple ectopics Ventricular tachycardia Ventricular fibrillation Asystole
Intrathoracic haemorrhage	Shock Cardiac tamponade
Respiratory	Hypoxia from lung congestion/collapse Carbon dioxide retention (underventilation) Sputum retention and infection Pulmonary embolus (very rare)
Neurological impairment	Stroke Transient ischaemic attack Cognitive impairment
Renal	Renal failure from low cardiac output
Abdominal	Pancreatitis (rare) Bowel infarction
Wound	Sternal dehiscence Mediastinitis Infected closure wires Osteomyelitis of the sternum Infected/ulcerated leg wound
Graft	Occlusion with recurrence of angina or infarction

Complications of CABG

- Preoperative – myocardial infarction from stress/anxiety or critical ischaemia.

- Intraoperative:
  - myocardial failure and lack of adequate myocardial contraction at the end of bypass, which requires additional cardiac support: (i) catecholamine infusion; (ii) intra-aortic balloon pumping; (iii) ventricular assist devices; (iv) even transplantation
  - embolic infarction from detached fragments released by manipulation of a thrombosed graft during a repeat CABG.
- Postoperative specific complications of CABG are:
  - myocardial failure – infarction, inadequate myocardial protection or excess fluid load
  - stroke, which may have occurred intraoperatively or become manifest some hours later; causes are listed in Table 17.5.

COMPLICATIONS OF ISCHAEMIC HEART DISEASE

Surgical procedures for other common complications of ischaemic heart disease include the following, with or without CABG:

- repair of left ventricular aneurysm
- repair of post-infarction ventricular septal defect
- acute ischaemic mitral regurgitation
- surgery for ischaemic ventricular arrhythmias, which may require electrical mapping at open surgery and treatment by destruction of the focus
- transplantation and ventricular assist devices (see separate section).

VALVULAR HEART DISEASE

The nature of valve surgery has changed markedly over the last 40 years. In the developed world, improved living conditions and the prompt treatment of streptococcal infections has led to a marked decline in the prevalence of rheumatic heart disease. In contrast it remains a major problem in much of Asia and sub-Saharan Africa. An ageing population is associated with a rising incidence of degenerative valve disease, and this represents the main workload for surgeons in northern Europe and North America. No ideal heart valve prosthesis exists, so if the native valve can be repaired and made to work properly this is often the best solution. There are few randomised trials in valve surgery but very many case studies. The 10-year survival studies show little difference between biological and mechanical valve prostheses and so the controversy between these two main groups remains unsettled. Preoperative left ventricular function is an important predictor of operative and long-term outcome following valvular surgery. Therefore, in modern cardiac valve surgery the objectives should be:

- to operate before irreversible myocardial damage has occurred
- to ensure that the performance of the valve, whether repaired or replaced, is durable, halting or reversing the abnormal pathophysiological processes in the left or right ventricle
- to seek to improve suboptimal results in patients where left ventricular function is poor.

Aetiology and pathology

Infective endocarditis

This is common and usually affects the aortic or mitral valves. The tricuspid is often involved in patients that are intravenous drug users. Valves affected are often not normal, though structurally normal valves are also susceptible in patients who are immunosuppressed or intravenous drug abusers; often there is a congenital or acquired abnormality, or the valve is a prosthetic one (Table 17.7). The organisms responsible are indicated in Table 17.8.

The pathological findings are destruction of the valve and clumps of infected fibrin and platelets (vegetations), particularly on the underside of the valve cusps, which may go on to cause circular erosions or abscess formation at the valve annulus. There is accompanying bacteraemia.

Rheumatic fever

This usually occurs in childhood between the ages of 5 and 12. The cause is thought to be an autoimmune reaction set in motion by an upper respiratory tract infection with group A streptococcus.

The manifestations of acute rheumatic fever include involvement of several of the large joints in sequence, the

Table 17.7 Abnormalities associated with infective endocarditis

Site	Abnormality
Aortic valve	Congenital bicuspid Rheumatic disease Degenerative disease
Mitral valve	Rheumatic disease
Prosthetic valve	Clot formation
Cardiac abnormalities	Patent ductus arteriosus Ventricular septal defect

Table 17.8 Organisms involved in infective endocarditis

Bacterium	Antecedents	Pathological features
Streptococcus viridans	Dental extraction	Often congenital abnormality of valve
Enterococcus	Prostatic disease Pelvic surgery	Older patients
Staphylococcus aureus	Intravenous prostheses Drug addicts	Acute ulcerative disease Abscess formation
Streptococcus epidermidis	Intravenous prostheses Drug addicts Artificial heart valves	Low-grade disease
Fungal infection	Immunosuppression	Indolent disease

basal ganglia, and the heart, including valves, muscle, conducting tissue and pericardium. The cardiac effects are infiltration of the myocardium with *Aschoff bodies* – granulomatous lesions with central necrosis – which progress to fibrosis. The valves develop sterile vegetations which interfere with their function, and as fibrosis progresses they may become incompetent or fibrotic. Severe damage to the valve may occur within 10 years, but, more commonly, changes sufficient to require surgery do not occur until patients are between 30 and 50 years old.

Degenerative

Degenerative valve disease is age-related in the aortic valve, may be associated with hypertension and produces aortic stenosis. Myxomatous degeneration of the mitral valve is common, and 3% of the population have mild asymptomatic prolapse. Clinically significant prolapse with significant mitral regurgitation is less common, although excessive valve tissue, such as seen in Barlow syndrome, may lead to regurgitation. More common is simple degeneration and elongation of the papillary cords, which is associated with cusp prolapse, annular dilatation and eventual chord rupture with staged increases in the amount of regurgitation and therefore worsening symptoms.

Connective tissue disorders associated with degenerative valve disease are listed in Table 17.9.

Ischaemic

Chronic ischaemia may affect the papillary muscles and their support from the ventricular wall and may cause mitral regurgitation.

Haemodynamic effects

Stenosis and/or regurgitation at any valve create a haemodynamic effect on the adjacent heart chambers and the lungs, according to the position and nature of the lesion. Stenosis produces a proximal pressure overload. A simple example is aortic stenosis with left ventricular hypertrophy. The heart is very sensitive to abnormal loading conditions and responds to an obstructed valve by hypertrophy and to a regurgitant valve by dilatation and hypertrophy. Stenosis and regurgitation in combination cause both volume and pressure overload and may lead to secondary effects. On the left side, these are pulmonary congestion and hypertension. The latter causes irreversible damage to the pulmonary arterioles (similar in nature to the effect of arterial hypertension on the systemic arterioles), and tertiary effects follow. Pulmonary hypertension leads to right ventricular hypertrophy and distension with tricuspid regurgitation and ultimately congestion of the liver and periphery. The response to significant stenosis gives rise to symptoms quite quickly, within a year or two, whereas a regurgitant valve is tolerated for a long time before symptoms occur. Thus clinical features provide a useful guide for the timing of operation on stenotic valves, but for leaking valves a reliance on symptoms alone will result in undue delay and a poor postoperative result.

Clinical features

Symptoms

Symptoms are a result of the haemodynamic effects:

- Low cardiac output is associated with fatigue and lethargy.
- In aortic stenosis, syncope and angina may occur because of low output, the latter even if the coronary arteries are normal.
- Pulmonary congestion in any combination of disease of the left side of the heart, but particularly from mitral stenosis or mitral regurgitation, gives rise to breathlessness on exertion, orthopnoea, paroxysmal nocturnal dyspnoea, cough, frothy sputum and haemoptysis. A combination of the last two implies that congestion is severe.
- Right-sided congestion causes fatigue, headaches, high skin colour, right hypochondrial pain (from liver enlargement), abdominal swelling (ascites) and ankle swelling (peripheral oedema).

Examination and physical findings

Examination should be methodical; attention to detail greatly facilitates the task of reaching the correct diagnosis.

General examination can reveal some of the systemic features of heart disease, particularly of right heart failure (Table 17.10). The visible and palpable aspects of the peripheral circulation also provide provisional diagnostic information (Table 17.11).

Jugular venous pulsation is best seen with the patient at 45°, but it may be necessary to change this to 90° to detect gross elevation of the jugular venous waveform. Observation of movement as high as the lobes of the ear may be required. The A, C and V aspects of the waveform should be assessed (Fig. 17.7). The jugular venous pressure (JVP) normally falls

Table 17.9 Connective tissue disorders and degenerative cardiovascular disease

Disease	Pathological effects	Outcome
Marfan's syndrome	Cystic medial necrosis	Mitral and aortic valve degeneration Aortic dilatation with aortic regurgitation
Ankylosing spondylitis	Inflammatory infiltration	Dilated aortic root Aortic regurgitation

Table 17.10 Systemic signs of right heart failure

Site	Finding	Significance
Skin colour	Dusky; blue	Pulmonary congestion CCF
Liver	Smooth general enlargement	Right heart failure
	Pulsation	Tricuspid incompetence
Ankles	Bilateral pitting oedema	Possible right heart failure
Lungs	Pleural effusion	Possible left heart failure
	Crackles	Pulmonary oedema

CCF, congestive cardiac failure.

Table 17.11 Features of physical examination of peripheral circulation in heart disease

Feature	Findings	Significance
Fingers and hands	Cool	Low cardiac output
	Capillary pulsation	Aortic regurgitation
	Splinter haemorrhages	Bacterial endocarditis
	Clubbing	Cyanotic heart disease
Arm pulse	Low amplitude	Low cardiac output
	High amplitude	Aortic regurgitation
		Aortopulmonary shunt
		CO_2 retention
	Jerking	Cardiomyopathy
	Double pulse	Mixed aortic stenosis / aortic regurgitation
	Locomotor brachialis	Hypertension
Carotid pulse	Slow rising; low amplitude	Aortic stenosis
	Bouncing full	Aortic regurgitation
	Head nods	Aortic regurgitation
	Systolic murmur	Referred from aortic stenosis
		Carotid artery stenosis
	Systolic thrill	Carotid artery stenosis
Neck veins	High jugular pressure (JVP)	Congestive heart failure
		Right ventricular failure
		Tricuspid regurgitation
		Tamponade (JVP rises on inspiration)
		Constrictive pericarditis

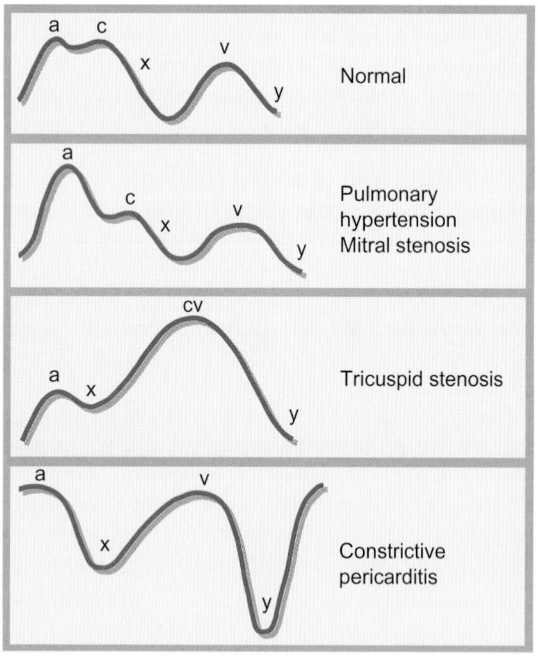

Fig. 17.7 Jugular venous waveforms.

during inspiration; the opposite indicates cardiac tamponade (Fig. 17.8).

Examination of the precordium is summarised in Table 17.12.

Auscultation

It is necessary to concentrate on each area separately. Ejection systolic murmurs in the *aortic area* indicate aortic stenosis but may also occur in subaortic stenosis and sclerosis of the ascending aorta. In aortic regurgitation, a soft systolic murmur can result from mild thickening of the aortic valve but does not imply aortic stenosis. Aortic regurgitation can only be excluded when the patient is sitting forward with the breath held in expiration, while auscultating at the left sternal edge at the level of the third or fourth costal cartilages where an early diastolic murmur is best heard.

Auscultation at the *pulmonary area* in pulmonary hypertension reveals a loud pulmonary second sound and in the presence of an atrial septal defect a fixed, widely split, second sound. In both these disorders there may be an associated pulmonary flow murmur.

The *lower left sternal edge* is a good site to hear the heart sounds, and when they are present, the third and fourth sounds are best heard here. The opening snap of mitral valve disease can be as well heard at the left sternal edge as at the apex, and as well or better with the diaphragm of the stethoscope as with the bell. The opening snap is a medium-pitched noise, similar to a very widely split second sound. The apex is the best site to hear the mid-diastolic rumble of mitral stenosis, which is low-pitched and best heard with the bell and with the patient turned towards the left. The pansystolic murmur of mitral regurgitation is loudest at the apex and radiates widely laterally as well as across the midline, occasionally reaching up to the aortic area.

With these principles in mind, specific valve disorders are discussed below.

Aortic stenosis

A bicuspid aortic valve occurs in 1% of the general population, but it rarely causes problems until middle age. Most commonly the intercoronary commissure is fused, and for reasons that are not clear this abnormal valve becomes fibrotic and heavily calcified, eventually causing severe obstruction to flow. A normal tricuspid aortic valve may become stenotic due to rheumatic heart disease or

Mechanism of cardiac tamponade

- Blood and thrombus accumulate in pericardium
- Pressure is exerted on venae cavae, right atrium and on the ventricles
- Venous return is reduced, diastolic filling of ventricles is reduced
- Cardiac input is reduced by both mechanisms
- Venous pressure outside the pericardium rises, heart rate rises, cardiac output falls, urine output falls, blood pressure falls
- No cardiac input = no cardiac output

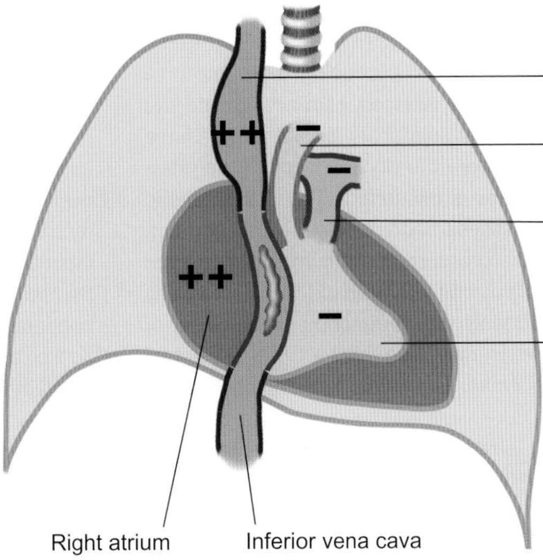

Fig. 17.8 Sequence of events in cardiac tamponade. An effusion develops, both atria and ventricles are compressed. Inflow pressure in the superior and inferior venae cavae and right atrium rises, but, despite this, ventricular volume falls and arterial pressure is reduced.

Table 17.12 Precordial examination

Site	Finding	Significance
General	Thrills	Aortic area: aortic stenosis LSE 3: VSD Apex: mitral regurgitation
Apex	Heavy displacement	Large hypertrophied or dilated left ventricle
Apex	Local tap not displaced	Mitral stenosis
Sternum	Lifting	Right ventricular hypertrophy and dilatation

LSE 3: left sternal edge, 3rd intercostal space: VSD, ventricular septal defect.

degenerative calcification associated with fibrosis and lipid absorption. This latter condition is more common over the age of 70. The classical symptoms of aortic stenosis are syncope, shortness of breath and angina, which are all closely related to exertion. Many patients are discovered because a systolic murmur is heard on incidental examination.

Once again the key investigation is transthoracic echocardiography to confirm the diagnosis, estimate the transvalvular pressure gradient, and determine the degree of left ventricular hypertrophy. A peak systolic gradient of 50 mmHg is generally taken as an indication for operation. In the presence of poor left ventricular function, overdue reliance on the pressure gradient can be misleading, as the value depends on both the cross-sectional area of the valve and the cardiac output. In borderline cases, the gradient can be measured at cardiac catheterisation, and a coronary arteriogram can be performed at the same session.

Operation is indicated to prevent sudden death and is the only effective treatment for this condition. Surgery improves symptoms and prognosis by reducing the pressure gradient and by causing a reduction in left ventricular mass. Current mortality for this operation is 2–3%.

Aortic regurgitation

The commonest cause of a leaking aortic valve in current practice is disease of the aortic root and annulus which prevents apposition of the leaflets. The cause of this disease is cystic medial necrosis, which is commonly associated with hypertension. Other aetiologies include a bicuspid valve, infective endocarditis, rheumatic disease, Marfan's syndrome, ankylosing spondylitis, Reiter's syndrome, and other rarities including syphilis. Progress is insidious and patients may remain apparently well until the heart is grossly enlarged and the left ventricle is irreversibly damaged. Symptoms include breathlessness, and some patients have a sensation like angina, particularly on lying down. The timing of operation is difficult, but as with mitral regurgitation there are criteria based on echocardiographically derived left ventricular dimensions which can help in the decision-making.

The standard operation is to replace the valve, and the factors which govern the choice of prosthesis are discussed below. Some regurgitant aortic valves can be repaired and may be a treatment option in the young patient where anticoagulation is not desired. In recent years, building on the experience of surgery for ascending aortic dissection, there has been growing enthusiasm for operations which preserve or spare the aortic valve while replacing the entire root and re-implanting the coronary arteries; this operation has been applied to annulo-aortic ectasia and more controversially to Marfan's syndrome. These valve-sparing operations are difficult and are generally done by experienced enthusiasts in specialised centres.

The operative mortality for aortic regurgitation is 3–4%, slightly higher than for aortic stenosis, reflecting impaired left ventricular function.

Mitral stenosis

Virtually all cases of mitral stenosis in the adult population result from rheumatic fever. Affected women outnumber men by 3:1. In rheumatic mitral stenosis, there is fusion of commissures, the cusps are thickened and the chordae shortened. There is obstruction to left ventricular filling, and the left atrial pressure rises, producing the symptoms of tiredness as a result of a reduced cardiac output, and shortness of breath as the pulmonary capillary pressures reach the critical point where the drying effect of the intravascular oncotic pressure is exceeded. The characteristic feature is that breathlessness becomes worse on lying flat, due to alterations in the pressure and volume relationships of the pulmonary circulation. Symptoms may progress steadily or appear suddenly with pregnancy or the onset of atrial fibrillation. Patients may also present with systemic embolisation, e.g. a stroke, ischaemic limb or mesenteric ischaemia.

The natural history is of steady deterioration, with 40% of patients dying within 10 years of first presentation and only 20% surviving for 20 years, but sometimes deterioration is very slow.

The diagnosis of mitral stenosis is made clinically, and investigations are aimed at quantifying other factors such as left ventricular function, pulmonary hypertension, and the presence of concomitant aortic valve and coronary artery disease. Coronary arteriography is required if the patient is over 40 years old or if there are risk factors for coronary artery disease. The echocardiogram is the crucial investigation, because it can confirm the aetiology and give a clear indication as to whether the valve can be repaired or will need to be replaced. Factors which would make repair (valvotomy) unlikely are severe calcification and rigidity of the anterior leaflet. At operation these aspects can be reassessed using transoesophageal echocardiography (TOE) and the effectiveness of the repair checked.

Mitral valvotomy is nowadays performed by an open technique employing cardiopulmonary bypass. The objective is to widen the orifice by sharp dissection of the commissures and if necessary to mobilise the valve by separating the chordae. Small amounts of calcium can be removed, but great care is required to avoid embolism. The left atrial appendage is carefully inspected for thrombus, which should be removed, and some surgeons routinely excise the appendage to prevent future thrombus formation.

The original mitral valvotomy was performed as a closed procedure via a left thoracotomy and in the 1950s was an extremely effective operation, provided the patient was young, in sinus rhythm and with no other valve disease. In areas of the world where rheumatic mitral stenosis is common, this operation continues to be done with excellent results, provided the patients are carefully selected. The same selection criteria apply to the use of percutaneous balloon valvotomy, which is widely performed in experienced centres in India.

Mitral regurgitation

The most common cause of pure mitral regurgitation is mitral prolapse, where the spongiosa layer of the valve leaflet is unusually soft due to a biochemical abnormality in the mucopolysaccharides. The papillary muscles are elongated, and there is an excess of valve leaflet tissue. Differences at the molecular levels have been recognised in the expression of metalloproteins in the extracellular matrix metalloprotienases in patients presenting with significant mitral regurgitation. Other causes of mitral regurgitation are ischaemia, infective endocarditis and, occasionally, rheumatic heart disease.

The haemodynamic consequence is that the larger proportion of the stroke volume passes backwards into the left atrium, and the lungs are subjected to high pressure which eventually leads to pulmonary hypertension. There is less tension development in the wall of the left ventricle, but the chamber enlarges and becomes spherical and less efficient. Symptoms may be mild for some time while the left ventricle continues to dilate. Eventually, shortness of breath on exertion or attacks of acute pulmonary oedema occur. In cases of infective endocarditis, events move much faster: the heart does not have time to accommodate to the altered volume load, and symptoms of breathlessness occur early in the natural history of the disease.

TOE is the key to the diagnosis and management. It provides information about the degree of regurgitation, anatomical and pathological changes leading to mitral regurgitation. Continuous-wave Doppler identifies the aetiology of the regurgitation and enables the surgeon to judge the possibility of undertaking a successful mitral valve repair. Cardiac catheterisation is only required to check the status of the coronary arteries.

As discussed above, the decision to operate for chronic mitral regurgitation is not straightforward. There are established echocardiography criteria based on left ventricular dimensions in systole and diastole but these need to be applied with discretion. Patients with symptomatic mitral regurgitation require surgical intervention. Enlarging left ventricle and atria, rising pulmonary artery pressures and the onset of atrial fibrillation are also factors that indicate that the long-term outlook with surgery is better than with continued medical management, even with little in the way of symptoms. Decision-making in acute mitral regurgitation is easier, as the symptoms are severe and the patient may be on the verge of requiring artificial ventilation.

The management of significant mitral regurgitation in a totally asymptomatic patient has gone through some recent changes. It is now recognised that long-term outlook – even for these patients in terms of symptoms, onset of heart failure, onset of dysrhythmias and survival – is better with early mitral valve repair than with continued medical management until the onset of symptoms and surgery at a later stage. However, the surgeon and the cardiologist caring for this group of asymptomatic patients with significant mitral regurgitation need to be confident of the surgical expertise available within the group to undertake a successful mitral valve repair.

Other causes of mitral regurgitation include functional mitral regurgitation, ischaemic mitral regurgitation and rheumatic valvular disease.

The gold standard of surgery for mitral regurgitation remains mitral valve repair. Exact techniques of repair are beyond the scope of this chapter but it is important to recognise that mitral valve repair is very specialised surgery undertaken by a small surgical group who work closely with echocardiologists in deciding the suitability of a particular valve for repair. Fortunately, in the majority of patients with mitral prolapse, it is the posterior leaflet which is defective, and this is the simplest lesion to repair. Anterior leaflet prolapse requires greater skill and more experience, and the results are less satisfactory. The operative mortality for repair is 1–2%. Long-term outlook for mitral valve repair for mitral regurgitation is significantly better than if the mitral valve is replaced. By contrast, the operative mortality for mitral valve replacement is 5–6%. There is increasing evidence that if both leaflets and their chordae are preserved the mortality of replacement may be lower and the left ventricular function is preserved in the longer run with better survival and better functional outcome.

Tricuspid valve disease

Isolated tricuspid valve disease is rare. The tricuspid valve may be involved in rheumatic heart disease along with the mitral valve, but more commonly it leaks as a consequence of raised pressures in the right ventricle associated with pulmonary hypertension secondary to left heart pathology. Tricuspid regurgitation in this setting is referred to as functional. Tricuspid valve endocarditis is invariably seen in drug addicts. Imaging of the tricuspid valve is difficult, so decisions tend to be based on clinical findings before and during the operation.

Most tricuspid valve operations are performed at the same time as surgery on the mitral valve. The operative risk for these patients is high (20%) because of their preoperative state and the damage done to the pulmonary vasculature and the liver over many years of raised pulmonary venous pressure.

Because tricuspid regurgitation is usually functional, repair is usually recommended in order to reduce the size of the annulus and enable leaflet apposition to occur. The procedure is referred to as tricuspid valve annuloplasty and it may involve implanting an annuloplasty ring in order to reduce the size of the valve annulus.

Infective endocarditis

This term includes all infections seated on valvular, congenitally abnormal hearts and great vessels. It is subdivided into native valve endocarditis (NVE) and prosthetic valve endocarditis (PVE). Infection on normal valves is rare except in immunocompromised individuals such as critically ill patients in ICU and transplant recipients. It is common in intravenous drug abusers.

The pattern of pathological organism varies according to the type of endocarditis and in PVE according to the timing with respect to the original operation. Operation may be required in NVE and is almost always required in PVE. The indications include – presence of positive blood cultures combined with haemodynamically significant valvular regurgitation, embolic complication and continued sepsis despite appropriate antibiotic therapy and the onset of conduction abnormalities due to perivalvular extension of abscess cavity resulting in destruction of conduction tissues.

TOE is very helpful in these difficult cases. Even in the absence of valvular regurgitation, if there are vegetations on the echocardiogram or evidence of perivalvular extension of the infection, early operation should be considered. These patients are best managed jointly by cardiologist and surgeon. If the infecting organism is a *Staphylococcus*, urgent operation within 24 hours of starting appropriate intravenous antibiotics should be considered.

Prevention is of course the best policy. Dental manipulations, urological manoeuvres and bowel procedures are the commonest routes of entry for microorganisms. Patients who have artificial heart valves should carry a card outlining the prophylactic antibiotic regimen laid down in guidelines issued by the British Cardiac Society. *Furthermore, any such patient who has an unexplained fever for more than 24 hours should be assumed to have PVE until proved otherwise.*

However, recently published NICE (National Institute for Clinical Excellence) guidelines have resulted in significant confusion over the routine use of prophylactic antibiotics in the UK. Historically, patients with any anatomical anomaly of the valves or the cardiac chambers and patients with implanted heart valves were recommended prophylactic antibiotics for all invasive procedures, most importantly dental. Recent NICE guidelines have differed from this recommendation and no longer support the routine use of prophylactic antibiotics. The approach taken by NICE differs from recommendations issued by other groups, such as the American Heart Association, and has resulted in a great deal of confusion in the medical community at large and, most importantly and understandably, for the patients who have been having antibiotics for a number of years prior to dental treatment and are now being told by their dentist that antibiotics are no longer necessary. This issue remains very contentious and NICE's recommendation is not universally supported amongst the cardiological and cardiac surgical community.

Choice of procedure in valvular heart surgery

There are three options:

- replacement with a mechanical valve
- replacement with a tissue valve, either a homograft (human) or a xenograft (the bioprosthesis is usually a pig valve or bovine pericardial valve)
- repair of the damaged tissue, perhaps supplemented by prosthetic material.

Indications for the different methods are given in Table 17.13, and advantages and disadvantages are given in Table 17.14.

Mechanical valves were introduced in 1962 and have gone through many developments. The original design was a ball and cage, but in small sizes this was obstructive, and haemolysis was a problem on exercise. The next valve type was a single disc held in an ingenious hinge, which was less obstructive but was associated with a higher rate of thrombosis and thromboembolism. The mechanical valve most commonly used now is a bileaflet valve made of pyrolite carbon and housed in a titanium ring.

By the end of the 1960s glutaraldehyde was introduced as a fixative for porcine valves which preserved the cellular structure and gave rise to the so-called bioprostheses. Subsequently, the same chemical preservation was applied to bovine pericardium meticulously sewn onto a stent. These are the two types of bioprosthesis in common use – porcine and bovine. Porcine bioprosthetic valves are the actual aortic valves from pig aortas mounted on a stent whilst the bovine bioprosthetic valves are made from calf pericardium sewn on to a stent. Both the bovine and the porcine valve require the biological tissue to be fixed. Leaflet tear and calcification remain the main modes of failure of the bioprosthetic valves. Extensive research into methods of fixing the tissue has resulted in optimising the temperature and the pressure at which fixation is undertaken as well the application of anti-calcification treatment to the bioprosthesis in order to reduce the rate of calcium deposition on the leaflets and hence increase their durability.

Over the last 10 years there has been an intense interest in stentless valves, modelled on the normal aortic valve. The first tissue valve used clinically in 1962 was a human cadaveric valve, referred to as a homograft. The long-term results of these valves became known in the late 1980s and were superior to those of the existing stented bioprosthetic valves. Their haemodynamic properties were also superior, with peak transvalvular gradients below 10 mmHg, in contrast to stented bioprostheses where the comparable value is 25–30 mmHg. A new generation of porcine stentless bioprostheses appeared, but whether they offer greater freedom from structural valve deterioration remains uncertain. Shortly after the introduction of the homograft, Donald Ross introduced the pulmonary autograft, which is now referred to as the Ross operation. In this complex procedure the patient's own pulmonary valve is used to replace the diseased aortic valve and a pulmonary homograft is used to reconstruct the right ventricular outflow tract. This is a niche operation, the main advantage of which is that it is a living autologous valve which when placed in children is capable of growth. Although the pulmonary homograft will degenerate, it will last longer on the low-pressure side of the circulation, and its replacement is less complicated than that of the aortic valve.

In the absence of clear guidance from randomised trials, the decision regarding the choice of prosthesis and valvular procedure has to be made on an individual basis between the patient and the surgeon. Three aspects play a crucial role in the selection of a particular valve for a particular patient – patient-related factors, prosthesis-related factors and, finally, surgeon-related factors.

For patients over the age of 65 there is a growing consensus in favour of the biological option in order to avoid the hazards of anticoagulation, which start to rise exponentially from the age of 70 onwards. Patients who require multiple coronary artery grafts in addition to valve replacement may also be candidates for biological prostheses in view of their reduced life expectancy. If a small aortic root is encountered, then one needs to bear in mind that the smaller-sized stented bioprosthesis, i.e. 17–21 mm, has a significant gradient

Table 17.13 Choice of operation on heart valves

Technique	Indication
Mechanical valve replacement	Up to age 65
Tissue valve replacement	Beyond age 65 Women of child-bearing age
Homograft replacement	Some complex problems Other groups if freely available
Pulmonary autograft	Selective use for aortic valve replacement
Valve repair	Mitral regurgitation Tricuspid regurgitation Limited use for stenotic valves

Table 17.14 Advantages and disadvantages of different types of valve surgery

Procedure	Advantages	Disadvantages
Mechanical valve replacement	Should last for life Good haemodynamics Low incidence of infection Low incidence of reoperation Readily available	Absolute need for long-term anticoagulation Increased risk of thromboembolic complications Risk of anticoagulant-related complications
Stented bioprosthetic replacement	Anticoagulation not required after 3 months	Deterioration after 8–15 years → high reoperation rate (up to 30% at 10 years) Limited lifespan in children and young patients Increased risk of infection
Stentless bioprosthetic replacement	Readily available Better haemodynamics Limited anticoagulation (3 months)	Technically more difficult than stented bioprosthesis Limited lifespan
Homograft	Anticoagulation not required	Difficult to obtain and often in short supply Deteriorate over 20 years
Reconstruction	Most suitable for regurgitant and complex congenital problems and recurrent valve infection Low embolism incidence Long-term anticoagulation not required Low infection rate Improved ventricular contraction	Technically demanding Risk of early postoperative rupture Long-term possibility of degeneration Inadequate repair may give poor results
Pulmonary autograft (Ross procedure)	Autologous tissue grows and develops with the patient Procedure of choice for aortic valve replacement in children	Technically difficult operation Long-term problems with right ventricular outflow tract conduits

across the valve and should be implanted with caution, especially in patients with high body mass index for risk of iatrogenically introducing residual patient–prosthesis mismatch, which is associated with poor outcome. If a bioprosthetic valve is mandated in these situations then a stentless valve is the preferred choice or one may alternatively choose a mechanical valve as the transvalvular gradient across an equivalent mechanical valve is significantly lower. Finally, not all surgeons are familiar and proficient at implanting stentless valves or undertaking complex aortic root replacements.

Data from large observational studies indicate that the mean actuarial survival of a biological valve is 10 years, but for patients over the age of 70 it rises to 15 years.

The outlook for patients after valve replacement depends upon several factors: left ventricular function, the presence of coronary artery disease, heart block, repair or replacement, and the ever-present risk, albeit low, of prosthetic valve endocarditis.

Anticoagulant management

For *mechanical valves,* full anticoagulation with warfarin to an INR of 3.0 (range 2.5–3.5) is essential and must be continued for life. Aspirin and dipyridamole are not suitable substitutes for anticoagulation of mechanical valves. For dental treatment and other operations, anticoagulants must be stopped 48–72 hours before and restarted 24 hours after the procedure – or earlier if there is no bleeding.

The use of anticoagulation is not mandatory with *bioprostheses and homografts,* but some surgeons anticoagulate for the first 3 months (INR 2–2.5).

TUMOURS OF THE HEART

Primary tumours of the heart are rare. Myxoma is the most common of the primary tumours. It usually arises from the margin of the fossa ovalis in the left atrium. Their clinical behaviour and appearance at operation are sufficiently characteristic for myxomas to be recognised as a discrete pathological entity. Characteristically they present in one of three ways:

- As the tumour enlarges, it causes intermittent obstruction of the mitral valve and can therefore mimic mitral stenosis.
- Friable forms of the myxoma may lead to embolism. If the embolus is removed, it must be examined histologically.
- Finally, patients with myxoma may present with vague constitutional symptoms, associated with a high ESR and CRP.

The key to diagnosis is transthoracic echocardiography, which invariably settles the diagnosis. Operation is indicated urgently because of the ever-present risk of embolism. The particular goal of the operation is to ensure complete removal of the tumour, which may be very friable. The stalk or pedicle on the left atrial wall must be completely removed to prevent recurrence.

RISK STRATIFICATION IN CARDIAC SURGERY

The operative risks of cardiac surgical procedures have been well evaluated. Increasing media and public interest has led to widespread awareness of the outcome of cardiac surgical procedures. Several models have been independently developed that evaluate the risk of cardiac surgical procedures based on a number of preoperative parameters. This risk stratification is vital in order to inform the patient of the risks associated with a particular procedure, in reporting the outcome of procedures, and in comparing the outcome of various units. The two commonly used risk stratification systems in clinical practice are the Parsonnet score and EUROscore. The Parsonnet score was developed in the USA; the more recently devised EURO system was designed on a pan-European population and gives a better estimation of the risks of cardiac surgery in the current era. The individual components of each of these two risk stratification systems are detailed in Tables 17.15 and 17.16.

Second or subsequent operations have greater risks mainly because of technical factors, such as:

- potential damage to the heart when the incision is reopened
- difficulty with aortic cannulation for connection of the CPB machine
- technical problems with grafting
- damage to an existing patent graft
- emboli detached from partially thrombosed but patent grafts which cause occlusions in the distal coronary vessels.

AORTIC DISSECTION

Dissection is the most common aortic emergency, two to three times more common than rupture of an abdominal aortic aneurysm. Hypertension is the commonest aetiological factor. In Marfan's syndrome, there is an increased risk of aortic dissection due to a generalised abnormality in elastic tissue caused by mutations in the region of the fibrillin gene on chromosome 15. Fibrillin is the major constituent of the microfibrillar system and is associated with elastin-containing tissues such as the aorta. Both pregnancy and a bicuspid aortic valve also predispose to aortic dissection.

Pathology

In aortic dissection the intima suddenly gives way, producing a transverse or spiralling tear; blood enters the media, tracks longitudinally in the aortic wall, and slits it along a line of cleavage in the outer part of the media. There is some evidence that the intramural haematoma is the first event and that the tear is secondary. The commonest sites for the intimal entry point are in the ascending aorta, 2–3 cm distal to the aortic valve, or in the descending aorta, just beyond the origin of the left subclavian artery.

The longitudinal component, which usually involves half to two-thirds of the circumference of the aorta, may extend

Table 17.15 Parsonnet risk stratification in cardiac surgery

Factor	Definition	Score
Patient-related factor		
Gender	Female	1
Obesity	Body mass index >35	3
Diabetes	History of diabetes regardless of duration	3
Hypertension	BP >140 mmHg on two occasions	3
Left ventricular function	Good: ≥50%	0
	Fair: 30–49%	2
	Poor: <30%	4
Age	70–74 years	7
	75–79 years	12
	>80 years	20
Reoperation	Second operation	5
	Third (or more)	10
Intra-aortic balloon pump	Inserted preoperatively	2
Left ventricular aneurysm	Aneurysmectomy	5
Recently failed intervention	Within the 24 hours prior to surgery	10
	>24 hours prior to surgery but on same admission	5
Renal	Dialysis dependent	10
Catastrophic states	Acute structural defect, cardiogenic shock, acute renal failure	10–50
Other rare circumstances	Paraplegia, pacemaker, severe asthma, congenital heart disease in adult	2–10
Surgery-related factor		
Mitral valve surgery	Systolic pulmonary artery pressure < 60 mmHg	5
	Systolic pulmonary artery pressure ≥ 60 mmHg	8
Aortic valve surgery	Aortic valve gradient < 120 mmHg	5
	Aortic valve gradient ≥120 mmHg	7
CABG at the time of valve surgery		2
Cumulative score	Operative risk	Operative mortality
0–4	Low	1%
5–9	Elevated risk	5%
10–14	Significant elevated risk	9%
15–19	High risk	17%
>19	Very high risk	31%

Table 17.16 EUROscore risk stratification in cardiac surgery

Factor	Definition	Score
Patient-related factor		
Age	Per 5 years or part thereof over 60 years	1
Gender	Female	1
Chronic pulmonary disease	Chronic bronchodilator or steroid use	1
Extracardiac arteriopathy	Claudication	
	> 50% carotid stenosis	
	Previous or planned surgery to limb arteries, carotids, abdominal aorta	2
Neurological dysfunction	Affecting daily ambulation	2
Previous cardiac surgery	Pericardial cavity opened previously	3
Serum creatinine	> 200 micromol/L	2
Active endocarditis	On antibiotics at the time of surgery	3
Critical preoperative state	Ventilation before anaesthetic room	
	Preop intra-aortic balloon	
	Preop inotrope	
	Preop renal failure	3
Cardiac-related factor		
Unstable angina	Requiring intravenous nitrates	2
Left ventricular function	Moderate: ejection fraction 30–50%	1
	Poor: ejection fraction < 30%	3
Recent myocardial infarction	< 90 days	2
Pulmonary hypertension	Systolic pulmonary artery pressure ≥60 mmHg	2
Operation-related factor		
Emergency	Operated on before the next operating day	2
Other than isolated CABG	Other cardiac procedure than, or in addition to, CABG	2
Surgery on thoracic aorta	Ascending, arch or descending aorta	3
Post-infarct septal rupture		4
Cumulative EUROscore	Operative risk	
0–2	Low	
3–5	Medium	
>6	High	

Operative mortality is approximately same per cent as the EUROscore for each individual patient.

forwards or backwards. Retrograde extension goes back to the aortic valve, removing the commissural support and causing the valve to leak. It may also extend around the coronary arteries, usually the right, and thus mimic an inferior myocardial infarction. It may extend a variable distance antegradely, affecting the arch vessels, the blood supply to the spinal cord, the renal arteries, the coeliac axis and the femoral arteries. A variety of ischaemic syndromes may thus form part of the clinical presentation.

Classification

Aortic dissections are classified according to their anatomical extent. The diagnostic watershed depends on whether the ascending aorta is involved. Type A dissections involve the ascending aorta, whereas Type B dissections are confined to the descending aorta (Fig. 17.9). Dissections are further classified as acute or chronic depending on the interval from onset to diagnosis, arbitrarily placed at 2 weeks. In Type A dissection 50% of patients are dead within 24 hours and 80% in 2 weeks. In general terms, Type A dissection is managed surgically to prevent the complications discussed (bearing in mind associated risks if there is neurological involvement), whereas Type B dissection is managed medically and only considered for surgery if there are any complications related to the dissection.

Operation

Cardiopulmonary bypass is usually established with a femoral arterial cannula, but axillary artery cannulation is associated with less thromboembolism and a lower incidence of neurological damage. The patient is core-cooled on bypass, down to 18°C, and a period of circulatory arrest is needed if the aortic arch is involved. Every effort is made to conserve the aortic valve. If there is dilatation of the aortic root, as occurs in Marfan's syndrome, it is then necessary to replace the aortic root and the valve and to re-implant the coronaries. The hospital mortality for acute Type A dissections managed medically is over 90%, while the UK Cardiac Surgical Register reports a mortality of 10–15% for operated cases in the last 5 years. There is little doubt this group of patients stands the best chance of survival if the diagnosis is made promptly and they are referred for urgent surgery.

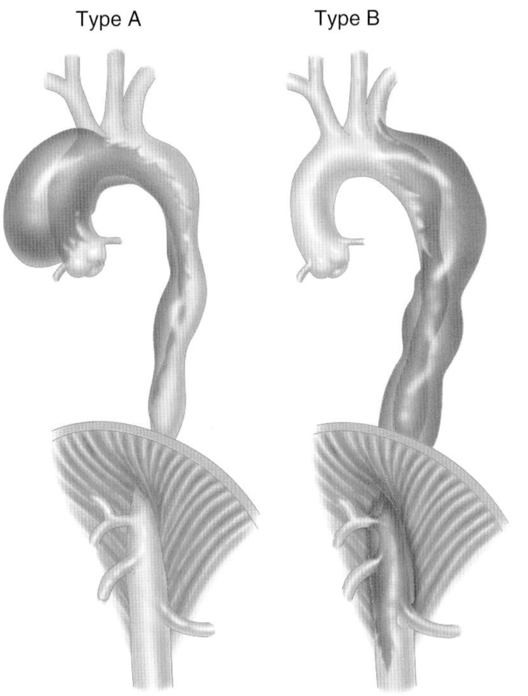

Fig. 17.9 Stanford classification of aortic dissection. Type A dissections involve the ascending aorta, whereas Type B are confined to the descending aorta.

HEART FAILURE

The number of patients with heart failure is reaching epidemic proportions in the Western world. In the UK there are approximately 100 000 new cases per year, and in the USA five times that number. Patients with end-stage heart failure may have a 1-year survival of 50%, and the figure is as low as 10% by 2 years. It is primarily a disease of the elderly and in 95% of cases is due to ischaemic heart disease. A minority of these are referred for conventional coronary artery surgery, provided a reasonable amount of viable myocardium can be demonstrated, as discussed earlier. The most effective treatment, but with limited availability, is heart transplantation.

Management

Intra-aortic balloon pump

The intra-aortic balloon pump (IABP) is a form of mechanical cardiac support. A balloon is introduced through the femoral artery and advanced to the descending aorta just beyond the origin of the subclavian artery. It is linked to an external console and is inflated in the diastolic phase of the cardiac cycle. The two principal effects of the IABP are increased coronary perfusion and reduction in the afterload for the heart during systole. The current indications for IABP use are shown in Box 17.4. A typical IABP set-up is shown in Figure 17.10a, b, and the arterial trace with the IABP counterpulsation in diastole is shown in Figure 17.10c.

Ventricular assist devices

Current devices represent the results of 25 years of dedicated research, and were brought into clinical effect in the early 1990s. Most of the devices implanted to date have been

Box 17.4 Indications for intra-aortic balloon pump

- Refractory ventricular failure
- Cardiogenic shock
- Unstable refractory angina
- Impending infarction
- Mechanical complications due to acute myocardial infarction
- Ischaemia-related intractable ventricular arrhythmias
- Cardiac support for high-risk general surgical and coronary angiography/angioplasty patients
- Weaning from cardiopulmonary bypass
- Intra-operative pulsatile flow generation
- Support for failed angioplasty and valvuloplasty

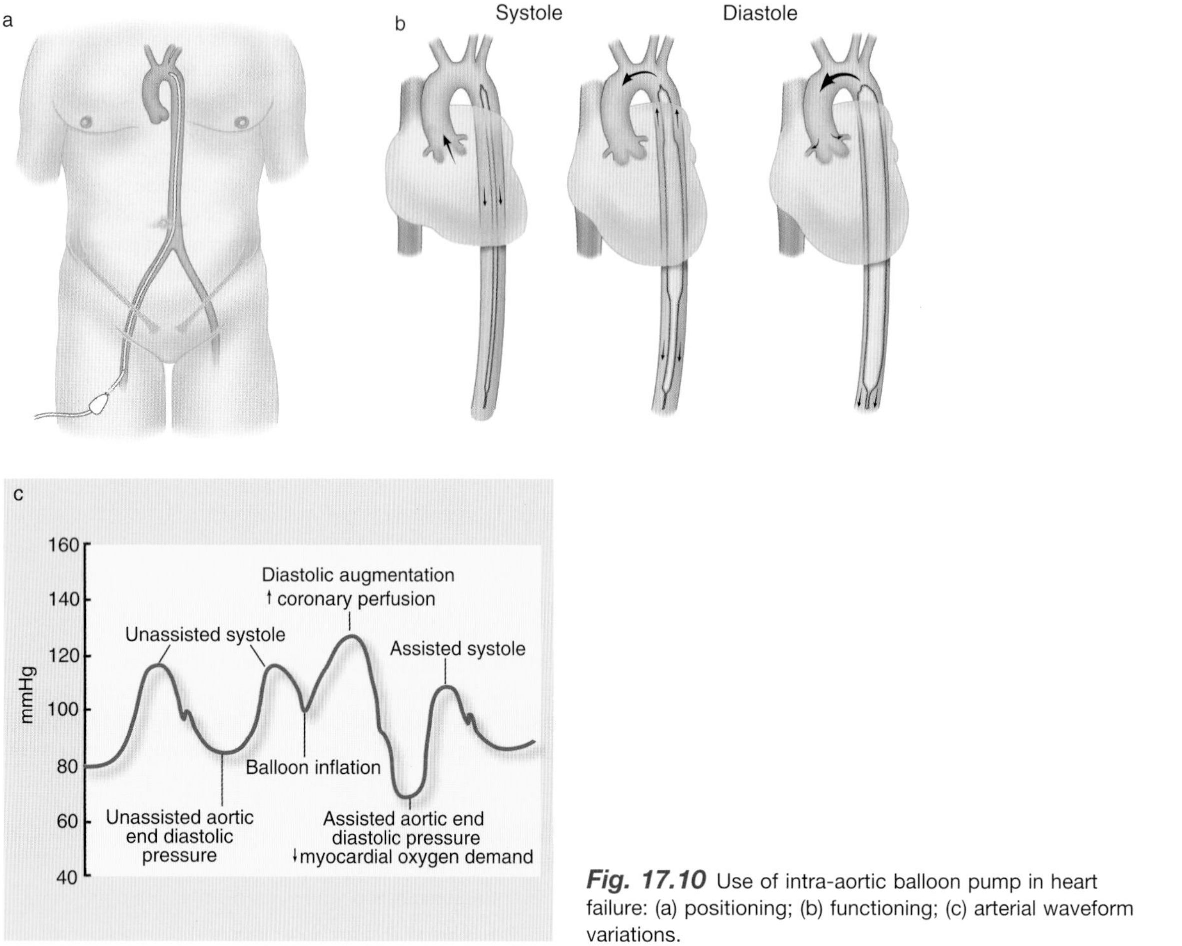

Fig. 17.10 Use of intra-aortic balloon pump in heart failure: (a) positioning; (b) functioning; (c) arterial waveform variations.

first-generation pusher-plate pumps driven either pneumatically or electrically. Although the devices are implanted in the abdomen, they require external drivelines. Nevertheless, a substantial number of patients in Europe and North America have been successfully discharged home from hospital and have pursued an active life with these devices. The majority of these patients have been 'bridged to transplantation', but a few have been successfully 'bridged to recovery'. In other words, some patients with non-ischaemic cardiomyopathy who have had a left ventricular assist device (LVAD) implanted for a number of months have, on later examination by echocardiography and intensive treadmill testing, shown remarkable recovery of their left ventricular function as a result of this prolonged period of unloading. These patients have then proceeded to have their devices removed at a subsequent operation. At the present time this is innovative treatment and the subject of intensive investigation.

Future developments

The use of implantable ventricular assist devices is in its infancy. The treatment is labour-intensive and the devices are expensive. A recent randomised trial of implantable LVAD against optimal medical treatment for patients in severe heart failure revealed a 2-year survival of 23% for the LVAD group versus 8% for the medical group. These low figures indicate how severely ill these patients were, but provide the background for future trials of chronic implantation.

Some LVADs are illustrated in Figure 17.11.

Transplantation

For details of organ retrieval and matching for transplantation see Chapter 13.

The results of cardiac transplantation are now good enough for this to be used for patients with very severe cardiac conditions for which medical management can achieve nothing further.

Indications for heart transplantation are:

- severe cardiomyopathy
- severe ischaemic heart disease, unsuitable for coronary bypass grafting or after repeated failure of that procedure
- untreatable ventricular aneurysm
- end-stage valve disease
- severe congenital cardiac abnormalities but normal lungs.

Positive criteria for recipient selection are:

- age under 50
- no evidence of renal or hepatic dysfunction
- no persistent causative problems (e.g. alcohol)

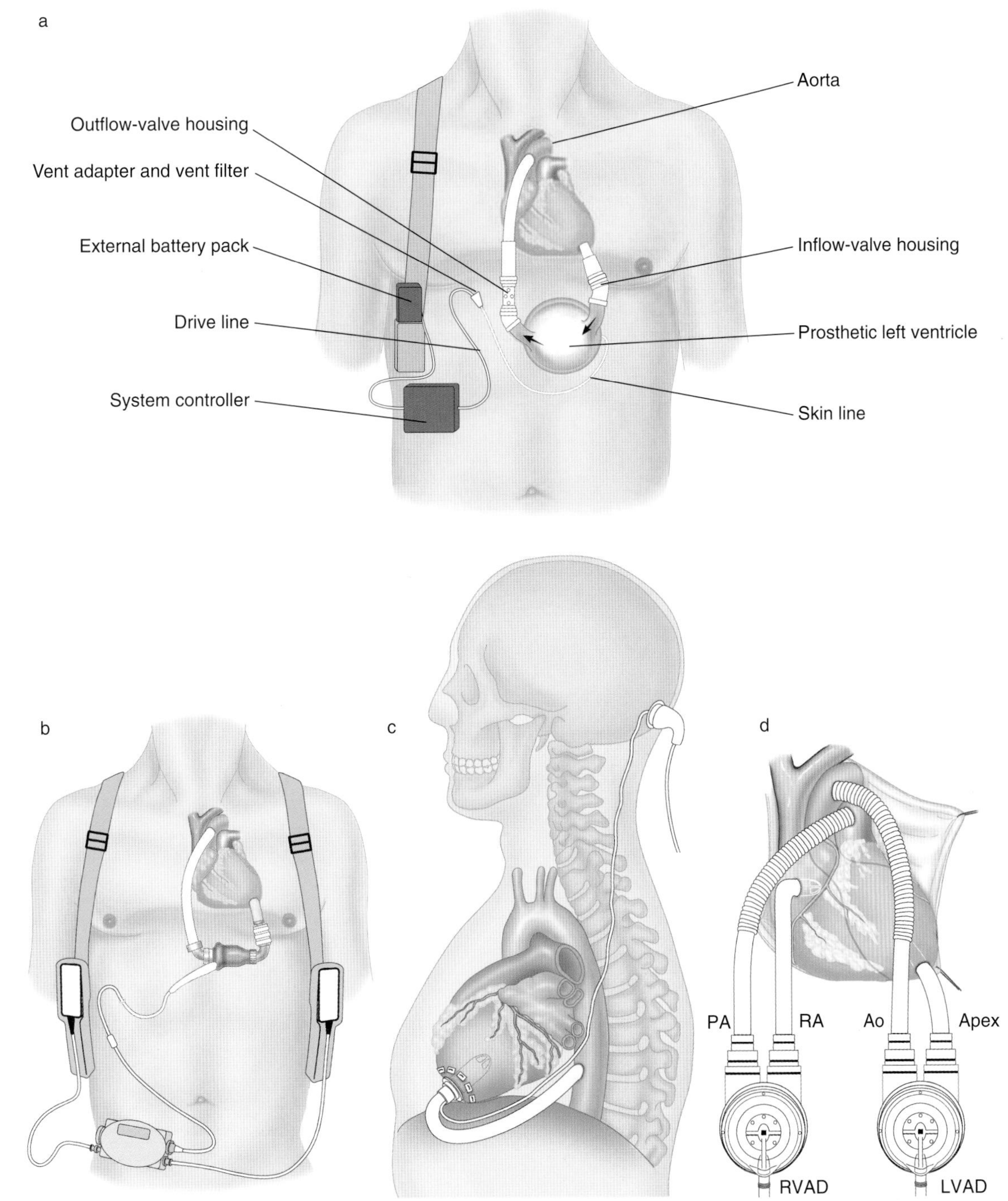

Fig. 17.11 Ventricular assist devices: (a) Vented Electric HeartMate I; (b) HeartMate II; (c) Jarvik 2000; (d) Thoratec.

- no major psychological difficulties
- no malignancy
- no evidence of sepsis.

In patients who comply with the above criteria, transplantation should be considered early. There is a significant mortality for those who have to wait for a transplant until their disease is in its end stages, with median survival of less than a year.

Operation

The heart, including the pulmonary and aortic valves, is removed, leaving atrial cuffs to which the atria of the donor heart are then anastomosed (Fig. 17.12a). The operation is completed by joining the pulmonary vessels and the supravalvular aorta of the recipient to the transplant (Fig. 17.12b). Other anastomotic techniques involving bicaval anastomosis are also used.

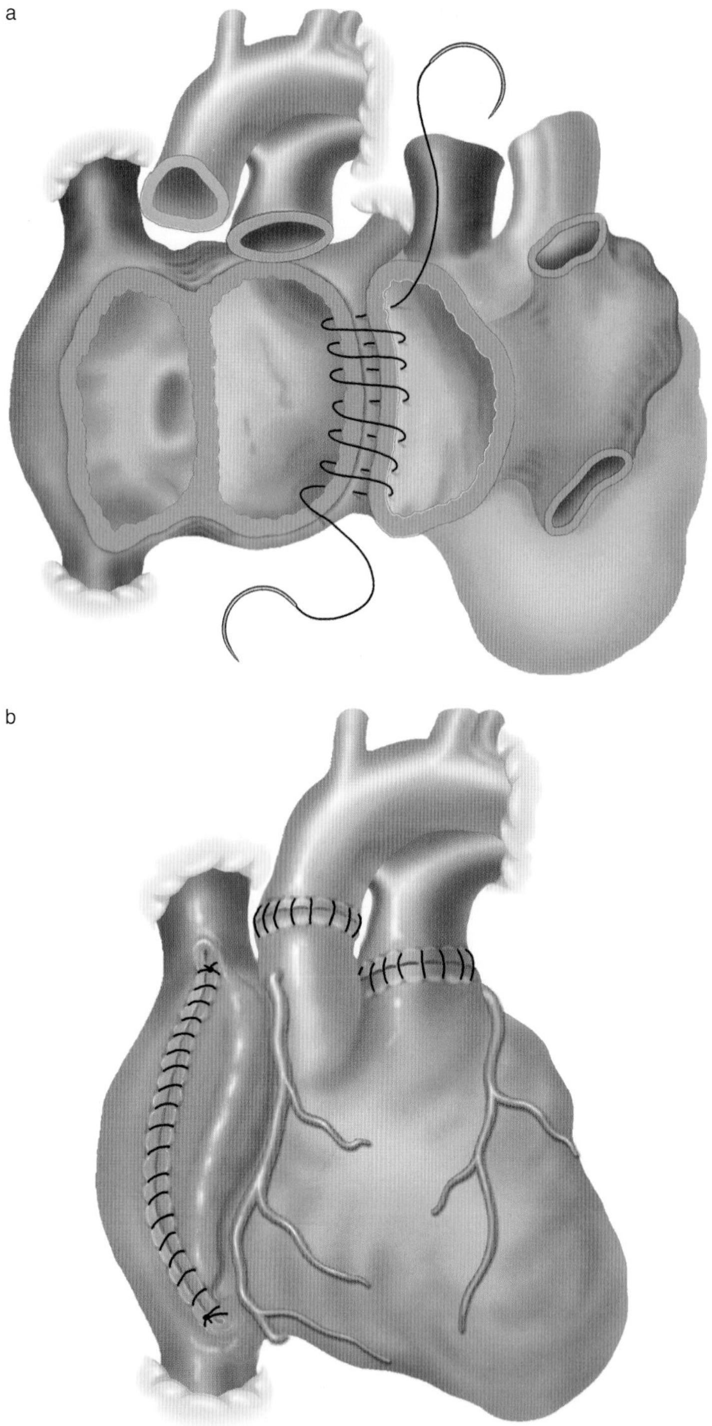

Fig. 17.12 The technique of cardiac transplantation.

Results

These vary according to the selection of both donor and recipient and also between different centres. In general in the UK, survivals are:

- 1 year – 85–90%
- 3 years – 80%
- 5 years – 70%.

Transplant activity is limited by two main factors: a shortage of donor organs and our inability to safely preserve the heart in a clinical environment for more than 4 hours. The most common source of organs is relatively young patients (males < 55 years, females < 60) who meet the criteria for death due to brainstem injury. With improving road safety, the majority of deaths are due to intracranial haemorrhage. Unfortunately many of these donors have coronary artery disease or left ventricular hypertrophy, which makes their hearts unsuitable for donation. The recipients are very symptomatic with end-stage heart failure due to idiopathic dilated cardiomyopathy or, more often, ischaemic heart disease.

TRAUMA TO THE HEART AND GREAT VESSELS

Cardiac trauma and traumatic injury of the thoracic aorta is usually seen in the context of multiple injury and is often associated with head injury. The principles of trauma care are now well formulated as per ATLS guidelines.

Blunt trauma

There are three patterns of cardiothoracic injury which may confront the trauma team:

- aortic rupture
- myocardial contusion
- rupture of a cardiac valve.

Rupture of the aorta

Aortic rupture, termed aortic transection, results from a deceleration injury. The most common site for the tear is immediately distal to the origin of the left subclavian artery. The rupture involves the intima and media, and vascular continuity is maintained by the thin adventitia supported by the surrounding mediastinal tissues. This site is favoured for such an injury because it is at the boundary of a mobile arch and a tethered descending aorta. The relevant features on clinical examination are absent or weak femoral pulses and unequal blood pressure in the arms. Fluid in the left hemithorax can be missed or underestimated. An erect posterior-anterior chest radiograph is usually impossible to obtain, and the surgeon may have to compromise with a supine antero-posterior film, which is more difficult to interpret because the cardiac shadow is enlarged and there are no fluid levels in the pleural space. In practice, if there is a haemothorax, the left pleural space may be a 'white-out' or it may have a 'ground-glass' appearance compared with the other side. However, a widened mediastinum should always raise the possibility of a transection. The diagnosis is confirmed by aortography, digital subtraction angiography or a CT scan. It is not always obvious, and there may be false-negative results.

Once the suspicion has been raised, the problem may be an extremely difficult one. The condition is likely to prove fatal and requires emergency surgery, yet the process of transfer to a cardiothoracic unit is often hazardous and attention to other associated injuries such as splenic rupture may require attention first. In some patients the aortic injury is contained and they survive to appear many years later with a calcified false aneurysm.

Operation is performed via a left thoracotomy. The mediastinum is featureless because of a spreading haematoma. Surgical options include direct suture with mobilisation of the aorta, but this requires time. However, usually an interposition graft is necessary. A shunt is inserted between the ascending and descending aorta in order to reduce the chance of spinal cord ischaemia during the period of aortic clamping. The use of a heparinised shunt avoids the need for systemic heparinisation, which may be an advantage in the presence of a head injury.

Blunt cardiac injury

The heart may be compressed between the sternum and the vertebral column. Compression forces may lead to rupture of the right ventricle, the septum or the atrio-ventricular valves. Rupture of one of the major cardiac chambers leads to tamponade and is usually fatal. Three patterns of injury are recognised amongst the survivors of cardiac compression injuries:

- myocardial contusion
- ventricular false aneurysm
- valve rupture.

If the myocardium is contused but remains intact, the consequences are similar to those of myocardial infarction. ECG changes are common and may show Q waves or a generalised ST segment abnormality. Cardiac enzymes and troponin I will be elevated. The course is similar to that of a myocardial infarct and depends on the area of damage. Echocardiogram confirms abnormal ventricular wall motion and excludes any pericardial collection.

If the myocardial injury is full-thickness, it may rupture slowly, be contained by pericardial adhesions and mature into a false aneurysm, usually of the left ventricle. This can be assessed and dealt with electively. If the rupture is sudden into the pericardium, it is likely to be fatal before the patient reaches hospital.

Rupture of a heart valve is unusual and is likely to occur at the time of the injury. It is a difficult diagnosis to make on clinical grounds in the setting of multiple injury. An echocardiogram is the diagnostic procedure of choice. Surgical repair or replacement can usually be undertaken semi-electively the following day unless there is severe haemodynamic compromise which might necessitate emergency surgery.

Penetrating injuries to the heart

Stab wounds to the heart present a wide spectrum of clinical pictures and can be a technical challenge to the emergency surgeon. Little history is available, but some idea of the length of the instrument and its direction is helpful. The site of the wound together with a relevant clinical history may enable the surgeon to anticipate the structures at risk. Two factors have to be considered: continuing haemorrhage and/or presence of cardiac tamponade. If the diagnosis of tamponade is suspected clinically the neck veins will be engorged, and a subxiphoid incision immediately inferior to the xiphoid process is the easiest route to the pericardial cavity to relieve the tamponade and can be performed quickly without having to divide the sternum or perform a thoracotomy. The pressure–volume relationship of the pericardium space demonstrates hysteresis (Fig. 17.13). Therefore aspiration of as little as 50 mL of blood from the pericardial space in acute tamponade can greatly improve cardiac filling and thus the cardiac output. In a stable situation, echocardiography will confirm the presence of significant blood in the pericardial cavity. With ongoing bleeding or uncertainty regarding the source of bleeding, a full sternotomy is needed.

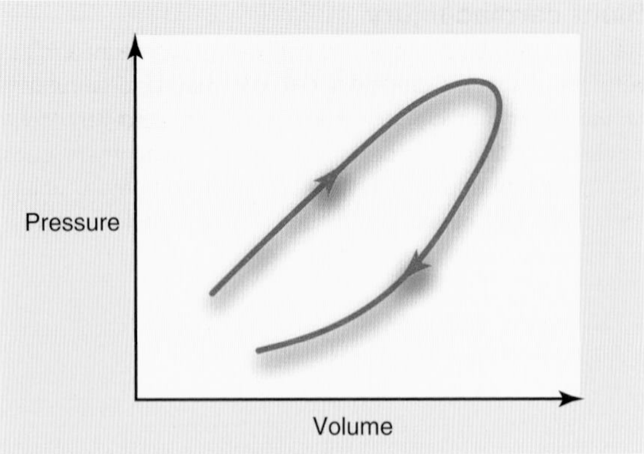

Fig. 17.13 In cardiac tamponade the pressure–volume relationship of the pericardial cavity shows hysteresis.

Bullet wounds to the heart

When a bullet penetrates the thorax and pericardium, a cardiac wound is frequently produced. High-velocity missiles produce massive through and through injuries of the heart. Occasionally, a missile may penetrate a cardiac chamber and come to lie within it. Penetrating cardiac wounds are usually accompanied by wounds involving the pleural space, internal mammary vessels, lung and wounds of the liver and other abdominal viscera.

Operative management

If there is a haemothorax, an intercostal drain should be inserted, preferably in the anterior to midaxillary line in the 4th or 5th intercostal space and definitely not below the 6th intercostal space in order to avoid passing below the diaphragm. If there is major cardiac or vascular injury, the drain will permit copious bleeding, and if the situation was previously balanced it may now become out of control and require urgent operation. Suction should not be applied to the drain, as it may lead to rapid exsanguinations.

The most effective incision is a median sternotomy because all chambers of the heart and the ascending aorta can easily be reached. If a saw is not available, a left anterior thoracotomy via the 5th intercostal space will give excellent access to the left ventricle and left atrial appendage. A right anterior thoracotomy will allow access to the right atrium, interatrial groove and right ventricle.

The left ventricle, with its thick walls, can be controlled with 3/0 atraumatic sutures, best placed as horizontal mattress sutures buttressed with autologous pericardium. As this is a semi-sterile operation it is best to avoid foreign material such as Teflon felt. The atria can be sutured directly or controlled with a side-biting clamp to allow more time. Bleeding from coronary arteries is a special problem. Small branches, well away from the interventricular and atrioventricular grooves can be oversewn. A hole in a larger branch should be controlled by taking delicate bites of epicardial fat on either side of the artery and using 5/0 or 6/0 sutures. In this way the haemorrhage can be stopped without occluding the artery. The pericardium can be left open, but drains should be placed in front of and behind the heart and connected via an underwater seal to suction.

Table 17.17 Aetiology and nature of congenital cardiac defects

Factor	Outcome
Maternal factors:	
Maternal virus infection (rubella)	Persistent ductus arteriosus Pulmonary valve stenosis Pulmonary artery stenosis
Maternal alcohol abuse	Septal defects
Maternal drug and radiation treatment	Various
Genetic abnormalities:	
Down's syndrome	Septal defects Tricuspid and mitral valve abnormalities
Turner's syndrome	Coarctation of aorta
Marfan's syndrome	Dilatation of aortic ring Aortic incompetence Aortic aneurysm
DiGeorge syndrome	Interrupted aortic arch
Williams' syndrome	Supravalvular aortic stenosis
Uncertain	Congenital aortic stenosis

CONGENITAL HEART DISEASE

The surgery of congenital heart disease requires an appreciation of disordered three-dimensional anatomy and allows little room for error. Table 17.17 summarises some of the aetiologies of the common congenital cardiac anomalies. Congenital heart surgery is in most countries performed by a relatively small number of expert surgeons working in specialised units. In recent years the care of some congenital defects has been carried out by interventional radiologists. Examples of this are valvotomy for pulmonary stenosis, the use of clam-shell devices to close an atrial septal defect and some ventricular septal defects, and the use of coils to close off large collaterals prior to corrective surgery for pulmonary atresia. There is a very close working relationship between the paediatric cardiologist and surgeon.

A functional classification is provided (Box 17.5) in which patients with congenital heart disease fall into one of four groups according to their pulmonary blood flow or vasculature. It is beyond the scope of this chapter to go into the details of individual conditions.

WORKING IN A MULTIDISCIPLINARY TEAM

Over the last decade or so, it has become increasing clear that many of the pathologies affecting the heart as well as the great vessels within the thoracic cavity, primarily the aorta, are not the sole domain of cardiac surgery. Surgical solutions remain the gold standard and alternative approaches are benchmarked against the surgical results. Changes in the treatment of aortic stenosis, aneurysms of the aorta and even coronary artery disease will be used as an example to illustrate how treatment modalities on offer has changed of late and continues to change at a rapid pace.

Box 17.5 Functional classification of congenital heart disease

Normal pulmonary vasculature
Without cyanosis
- Right-sided obstruction
  - pulmonary valve stenosis
  - pulmonary artery stenosis
- Left-sided obstruction
  - aortic stenosis
  - coarctation of aorta
- Myocardial lesions
  - endocardial fibroelastosis
  - metabolic heart disease
  - coronary artery anomalies
- Valve and vascular anomalies without shunt
  - idiopathic dilatation of pulmonary artery
  - vascular rings
  - aneurysm of sinus of Valsalva
  - Ebstein's anomaly (without shunt)

With cyanosis
- Partial systemic venous drainage to left atrium
- Ebstein's anomaly (with shunt)

Increased pulmonary vasculature
Without cyanosis
- Extracardiac left-to-right shunts
  - persistent ductus arteriosus
  - aortopulmonary window
- Intracardiac left-to-right shunts
  - atrial septal defect
  - ventricular septal defect
  - partial anomalous pulmonary venous connection
- Extracardiac to intracardiac shunts
  - ruptured sinus of Valsalva to RA or RV
  - coronary artery fistula to RA or RV

With cyanosis
- Bidirectional shunts (admixture lesions)
  - Transposition of the great vessels
  - Truncus arteriosus
  - Total anomalous pulmonary venous connection (supradiaphragmatic)
  - Double-outlet right ventricle without pulmonary stenosis
  - Atrioventricular septal defect
  - Single ventricle

Decreased pulmonary vasculature
- Tetralogy of Fallot
- Tricuspid atresia
- Transposition with pulmonary stenosis
- Double-outlet right ventricle with pulmonary stenosis
- Pulmonary atresia with ASD
- Ebstein's anomaly with ASD
- Single ventricle with pulmonary stenosis

Pulmonary venous obstruction
Without cyanosis
- Cor triatriatum
- Mitral stenosis
- Aortic stenosis
- Coarctation of aorta
- Stenosis of pulmonary veins

With cyanosis
- Hypoplastic left heart (mitral atresia, aortic atresia)
- Anomalous pulmonary venous connection (infradiaphragmatic)

ASD, atrial septal defect; RA, right atrium; RV, right ventricle.

Aortic stenosis

The pathophysiology and surgical results for the treatment of aortic stenosis have already been discussed. Without any intervention the outcome in patients with symptomatic aortic stenosis is poor, with a 50% survival at 2–3 years. The results of surgical approach for aortic stenosis have been refined to an extent that isolated aortic valve replacement can be now undertaken with a mortality of around 1–2% universally with excellent medium- and long-term outcome from a functional and survival perspective. Nonetheless, a small but not insignificant group of patients remain a very high-risk population for conventional surgery as highlighted by various risk stratification models. Quite often the operative risks in this setting are increased due to the presence of comorbidities such as impaired pulmonary function, renal impairment, cerebrovascular disease and end-stage poor cardiac function in cases of very late presentation. Risks posed result from the anaesthesia and surgery as well as from the cardiopulmonary bypass required for conventional open-heart surgery.

In an attempt to overcome these issues transcatheter aortic valve implantation (TAVI) has been developed to treat this high-risk group of patients with significant aortic stenosis. Biological valves are mounted on balloon-expandable metal stent and introduced either retrogradely through the femoral artery (exposed at the groin) or antegradely through the apex of the heart (exposed through a small anterior thoracotomy, usually in the 5th intercostal space). Once positioned in place within the stenosed native aortic valve, the stent is expanded using a balloon to enlarge the aortic orifice and has a new aortic valve implanted in place within the stent (Fig. 17.14a). TAVI has developed over the last decade or so. Initially it was reserved for use on compassionate grounds but the technology has developed to an extent and the early results have been promising such that this approach is now being used to treat patients at very high risk with conventional surgery (estimated operative mortality of the order of >20% or so). Nonetheless, there remains numerous challenges with regard to the changing stent technology, vascular access to implant the valve, and accurate positioning of the implanted valve. Despite the challenges faced, the early results are promising enough to recommend this approach to patients at very high risk with conventional open-heart surgery as general anaesthetic can be avoided if a femoral approach is taken for the TAVI and there is no need for cardiopulmonary bypass with both the transapical and the transfemoral approaches. The medium- and the long-term outlook remains uncertain at this stage and clearly only a biological valve can be implanted using this approach.

The early enthusiasm for this approach has enabled a rapid growth in transcatheter valve implantation and time will tell with regards to its durability in the longer term when compared with a conventional surgical approach. There remains quite marked scepticism amongst some in the surgical fraternity that the risk models being used to justify the use of the transcatheter approach overestimates the risk of conventional surgery. Nonetheless, as the technology evolves, there is no doubt that the transcatheter valve will be established alongside conventional surgery to address aortic stenosis, although the boundaries between different approaches will change with time and indications for each approach will be redefined over time.

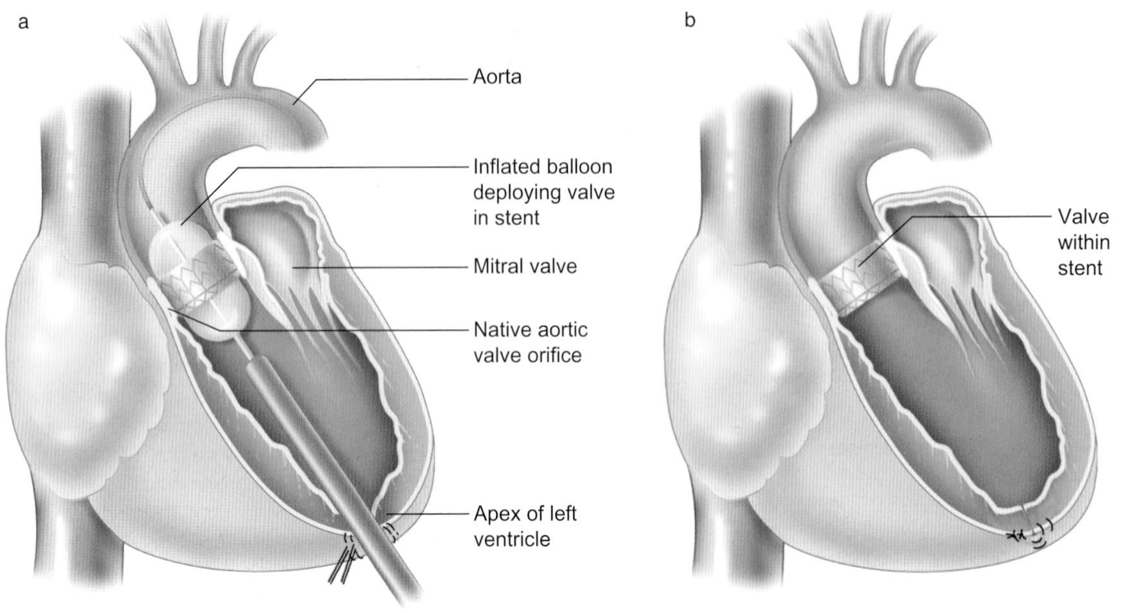

Fig. 17.14 Transapical and transfemoral catheter-based aortic valve implantation. (a) Insertion of an aortic valve prosthesis via the femoral artery. (b) Insertion of a prosthetic aortic valve via a left ventricle cardiotomy.

Aortic pathology

The three main pathologies affecting the thoracic aorta are aneurysms, dissections and traumatic aortic transaction. Conventional surgical approaches to their treatment has been discussed elsewhere. However, the approach to all three of these pathologies has been greatly redefined over the last decade to an extent that endovascular approach to the aorta has become synonymous with thoracic aortic surgery as with abdominal aortic surgery. Multidisciplinary approach here involves interventional radiologist, cardiac surgeon and cardiologist in some groups and close liaison between the expertise of the individual specialties needs to be harnessed to optimise the outcome for this challenging group of patients.

Descending thoracic aortic aneurysms can be treated relatively easily with a covered stent to exclude the aneurysmal segment of the aorta from circulation. The stents are introduced via the femoral artery and, once positioned, are expanded using a balloon. A prerequisite factor is the presence of satisfactory landing zones for the stent at either end of the aneurysmal segment of the aorta (Fig. 17.14b). The issue of excluding side branches of the aorta is rarely a major problem in addressing the descending aortic pathology. However, this approach has now been slowly expanded to address the aneurysms of the aortic arch and even the ascending aorta. The side branches in the form of arch vessels, i.e. the head and neck vessels from the aortic arch, pose a considerable challenge. However, this issue has been addressed by undertaking extra-anatomical bypasses to the cerebral and subclavian vessels prior to stenting the aneurysmal arch with a covered stent where the origins of the native arch vessels are excluded from circulation by the covered stent (Fig. 17.14b). Although conceptually this approach is very attractive and the enthusiasts continue to push back the frontiers, many challenges remain, including stent migration, strut fracture, risk of infection to this large amount of foreign material exposed to blood within the circulation and 'endoleak' (continued communication between the endolumen and space outside the stent, between it and the native aortic wall).

Similar approaches have been undertaken to address modern approaches to aortic dissection and transections, both extremely challenging surgical groups with a high operative mortality. The precise details of the treatment modalities are beyond the scope here. Suffice to say that in the setting of aortic transaction often seen in multiple injury a covered stent can be implanted across the site of injury/breach of the aortic wall often covering and excluding the left subclavian artery. This has treated some critically ill patients with excellent early results.

The approach to aortic dissection depends on the pathology. Type A aortic dissections are treated surgically because of the risk of proximal extension toward the aortic root, leading to aortic incompetence and coronary insufficiency. Type B aortic dissections only require intervention if there is malperfusion of the side branch, bleeding in the thoracic cavity or late aneurysm formation. In the cases where malperfusion is identified, there may be a role for a percutaneous approach to fenestrate the dissection flap to perfuse the true and the false lumens. Lately there has been some interest in treating the dissection of the descending aorta with a covered stent at the site of the entry point of the dissection flap in order to reduce the risk of future aneurysm formation. Long-term data on this approach are lacking at present.

Coronary artery disease

The surgical approach to coronary artery disease has already been discussed. However, the advent of drug eluting stents with significantly lower rates of restenosis compared with earlier bare metal stents or simple angioplasty alone has resulted in further challenges to surgery for coronary artery disease. Superiority of pedicled arterial grafts, i.e. pedicled left internal mammary artery grafted to the left anterior descending artery (LIMA to LAD), is well recognised with a >90–95% patency even after 20 years and remains the gold standard. Total arterial grafting is technically challenging and is not desirable in many patients. Therefore, what is in question is the continued use of vein grafts with a 50% patency at 10 years. The challenge posed by cardiologists to the surgical group has therefore been to address the problem of coronary artery disease in a 'hybrid' approach with LIMA to LAD performed surgically and to address other coronary lesions using a percutaneous approach using a drug eluting stent. The strengths of this argument are difficult to deny – especially as LIMA to LAD can be performed with a beating heart 'off-pump' technique, thereby avoiding the deleterious effects of the cardiopulmonary bypass and even more the fact that LIMA to LAD can be performed through a limited access approach using a left anterior mini thoracotomy or even totally thorasocopically. This area remains a very grey area where it is hoped that the cardiac surgeon and the interventional cardiologist continue to use evolving technology to look for better ways to advance the treatment of coronary artery disease, hopefully in collaboration with each other!

MINIMALLY INVASIVE CARDIAC SURGERY

As with all other branches of surgery there is great enthusiasm for developing minimally invasive cardiac surgical procedures. For example, transcatheter stenting of thoracic aortic aneurysms (Fig. 17.15) avoids major open surgery. However, there are two aspects that need to be considered. First, there is the issue of anatomical invasiveness, i.e. size of the incision and the resultant trauma to the chest wall, and, secondly, the concept of physiological insult of the cardiopulmonary bypass. Each of these aspects will be considered below.

Using coronary artery bypass surgery as a model procedure one can think of a conventional approach through full median sternotomy cardiopulmonary bypass with the heart arrested as the most invasive, gradually proceeding to a stage when the entire procedure could be undertaken thoracoscopically with the heart beating using an off-pump technique. Clearly there are several intermediate stages that are involved here and for all intracardiac procedures, i.e. the vast majority of valvular cases, cardiopulmonary bypass and arresting the heart are mandatory and hence the only scope for improvement is in the size of the incision.

The vast majority of cardiac surgical operations are performed through a median sternotomy approach. The extensive size of the incision and the resulting trauma to the chest wall is not only undesirable for cosmetic reasons but also has a deleterious effect on the respiratory function, postoperative pain, recovery time and possibly even blood loss. Upper partial sternotomy can be used for approaches to the aortic valve and ascending aorta and the mitral valve. Lower partial sternotomy is used for approaches to the mitral valve. Right anterior thoracotomy can be used for approaches to the aortic and the mitral valve and incisions can sometimes be kept very small (down to 4–5 cm in video-assisted cases). Employing a small incision has been shown to have improved functional outcome (cosmesis, quicker recovery time, less blood transfusion, reduced postoperative pain, reduced requirements for analgesia and improved patient satisfaction), although it is believed that the overall outcome in terms of mortality is no different to a conventional approach through a sternotomy. As a result, minimal access cardiac surgery has only been accepted in a limited way.

The physiological insult of the cardiopulmonary bypass circuit must not be underestimated. The physiological response to the bypass circuit has already been discussed elsewhere. Although it is desirable to avoid the cardiopulmonary bypass circuit altogether, this is only really an option for coronary artery bypass surgery. Beating-heart off-pump coronary artery surgery has already been discussed. Suffice to say at present, except for certain indications, i.e. diseased ascending aorta, it is considered to be an equivalent mode of conducting CABG operations. It is recognised that technically it represents a higher level of complexity to undertake CABG in this manner with the resultant concerns over the quality and patency of the anastomosis. For intracardiac procedures, cardiopulmonary bypass is mandatory. Therefore improvements to the cardiopulmonary bypass circuit is highly desired by all cardiac surgeons to minimise the physiological insult to the patient. Improvements in the conduct and design of cardiopulmonary circuit have been alluded to earlier in the chapter and remain an area of great research interest.

GENERAL COMMENTS

Access

For cardiac surgery and transplantation, access is nearly always by a median sternotomy, although more limited (minimal access) approaches are being developed for all types of cardiac procedures. Clear benefits other than cosmesis remain to be proven when compared with conventional access through a full sternotomy and these have been highlighted elsewhere in the chapter.

Preoperative patient briefing

Patients should be introduced to the recovery or intensive care unit and have its environment made familiar. Any special problems relating to individual operations should, as far as possible, be explained. Physiotherapy is begun, and the need for cooperation is emphasised.

ICU/recovery

Most cardiac surgical patients now go through a specialised recovery/ICU area, requiring a stay of up to 24 hours. The

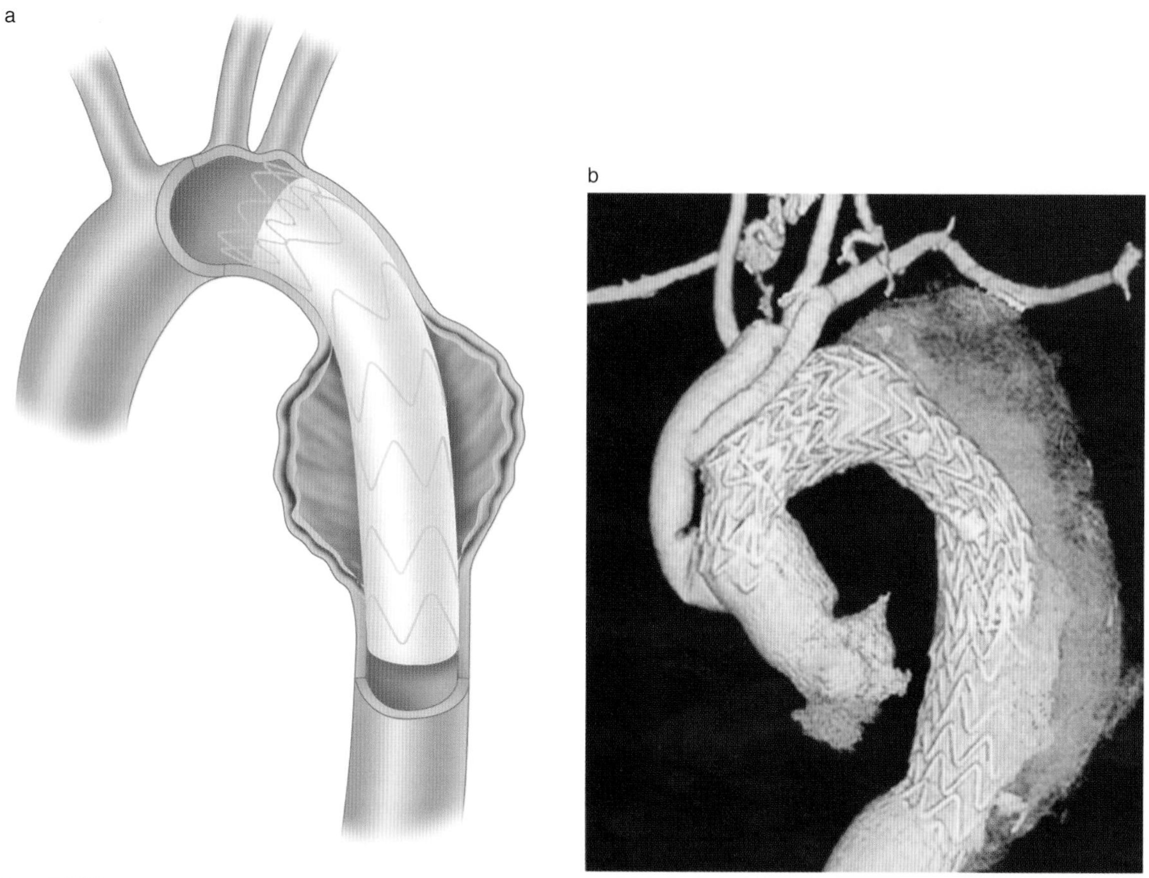

Fig. 17.15 Stenting of descending and aortic arch aneurysms.

most complex patients may still require general ICU stay, as the recovery times are longer. On return to the ward, all patients are further monitored in a high-dependency area, and early mobilisation and physiotherapy are essential in helping patients become able to be discharged home within 1 week of operation.

ICU/recovery monitoring involves:

- continuous ECG, pulse and arterial and central venous pressure monitoring
- digital oxygenation saturation probe
- hourly measure of urine output (patient catheterised)
- hourly measure of peripheral and central temperature
- quarter-hourly, later hourly, measure of blood loss from chest drains
- frequent arterial blood gas measurements for P_{O_2}, P_{CO_2}, pH and acid–base balance
- controlled infusion pumps for fluid and drug administration
- general neurological assessment.

Ventilation

Cardiac patients are ventilated until they are stable, rewarmed and are making good respiratory efforts with appropriately good arterial gases (usually 4–6 hours postoperatively). Thoracic patients are extubated in theatre and sat up early to encourage better respiratory mechanics. They are usually managed in a general recovery area rather than fast-track or ICU.

Pain control

Effective prevention of pain is of importance in all cardiothoracic surgery because it lessens the risk of postoperative myocardial events, improves postoperative respiratory movements and increases the value of physiotherapy.

Epidural analgesia and continuous opioid infusion controlled by the patient (PCA) are common methods which may be combined with local analgesia block of intercostal nerves at the time of thoracotomy.

Chest drainage

All cardiac drains are connected to a closed underwater system to prevent an open pneumothorax occurring and to allow the lungs to maintain the normal negative intrathoracic pressure. Additionally, low-pressure suction is applied to encourage the release of air or blood from the operated site; this is particularly valuable after lung resection as suction helps the lung to seal its leaks by adhering to the chest wall.

Antithrombotic therapy

For CABG, aspirin is commenced on day 1 and continued long term. For valve patients, warfarin is commenced on day 1, and INR is monitored daily until stabilised.

Long-term antithrombotic treatment depends on the procedure. After CABG with vein grafts, low-dose aspirin is necessary.

Long-term secondary preventative strategy involves the use of cholesterol-lowering agents.

Return to full activities

Most patients are able to return to work or full activities 2–3 months after a CABG. Convalescence after thoracic procedures may be shorter, but this depends on the degree of respiratory reserve available.

Secondary control of coronary risk factors is important in the long term. A statin drug is given to all hyperlipidaemic patients; hypertension and diabetes medication should be continued. Smoking must cease.

18 Oesophagus, stomach and duodenum

OESOPHAGUS

Anatomical and physiological considerations

The oesophagus is a muscular tube connecting the pharynx to the stomach, lined predominantly by squamous epithelium and guarded at both ends by sphincters. It lies anterior to the cervical vertebrae in the neck and in the posterior mediastinum in the chest and enters the abdomen through the oesophageal hiatus in the diaphragm. The last 2–3 cm are within the abdomen above the gastro-oesophageal junction with the stomach. The anatomical relationships between the oesophagus and the other mediastinal structures are illustrated in Figure 18.1. The mucosal lining of the oesophagus is pale grey and consists of squamous epithelium. The musculature of the upper two-thirds of the oesophagus is striated (though not under voluntary control) and that of the distal third is smooth. In contrast to most of the intraperitoneal gastrointestinal tract, the oesophagus is devoid of a serosal layer – a matter of some importance to the spread of malignant disease. For descriptive purposes, tumours are usually classifed as occurring in the upper, middle and lower thirds.

The two sphincters are at the pharyngo-oesophageal junction (upper) and in the region of the oesophageal opening (hiatus) in the diaphragm. Both have intrinsic and extrinsic components. The upper intrinsic sphincter has the main function of preventing access of air to the oesophagus and working in conjunction with laryngeal closure during swallowing. It relaxes on initiation of the swallowing reflex, and the superior constrictor extrinsic component contracts to expel food or liquid into the oesophagus where a wave of peristalsis carries it downwards. Disorders of the upper sphincter are considered in Chapter 10.

The lower intrinsic sphincter is the circular smooth muscle of the oesophagus, although anatomical as distinct from physiological identification of a specific sphincter zone has proved difficult. Its role is to prevent gastro-oesophageal regurgitation, and it is normally closed but relaxes in response to the swallowing wave. Relaxation may fail in oesophageal motility disorders and low resting sphincter pressures are often seen in gastro-oesophageal reflux disease (GORD). The intrinsic sphincter is supplemented by the striated muscle of the right crus, which splits to embrace the lower end of the oesophagus, but it is probably involved only in keeping the gastro-oesophageal junction closed when intra-abdominal pressure is significantly increased as in straining. Another factor which prevents reflux from the stomach is the acute angle of insertion of the oesophagus into the stomach which brings the gastric and oesophageal walls in contact when intra-abdominal pressure rises. Anatomical disorders at the diaphragmatic hiatus reduce the efficacy of the intrinsic sphincter (see 'Hiatus hernia').

Clinical features of oesophageal disease

Symptoms

Dysphagia

Difficulty in swallowing may be:

- progressive when a lesion such as a malignant growth or a stricture reduces the size of the oesophageal lumen
- non-progressive in disorders of function either of the whole oesophagus or at the lower sphincter.

Progressive difficulty eventually goes on to total dysphagia when neither food, liquid nor the patient's own saliva can be swallowed. This circumstance is an emergency.

High grades of dysphagia are often associated with regurgitation into the pharynx and upper air passages and therefore with respiratory infection.

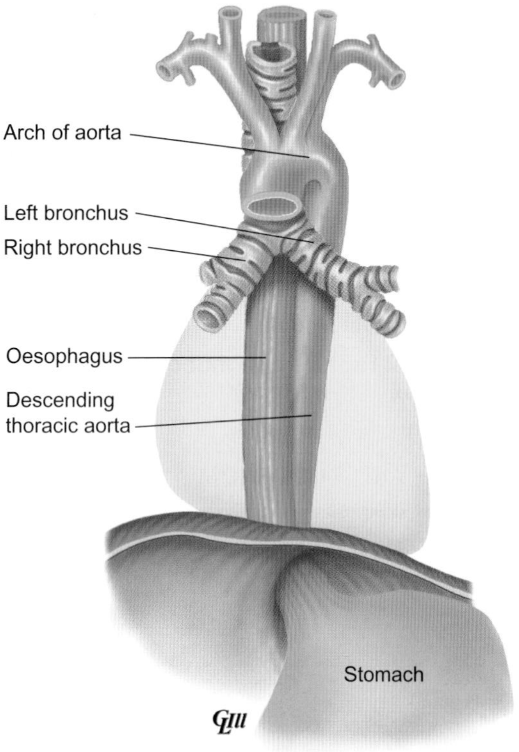

Fig. 18.1 Anatomical relationships of the oesophagus.

Pain

Pain is ill-localised in the chest (often called substernal but more correctly retrosternal) and may accompany partial dysphagia from obstruction. It also occurs in motility disorders. Confusion with pain originating in heart muscle is common.

Heartburn

Heartburn is a retrosternal sensation of discomfort and burning and may be a minor form of pain. It is the consequence of regurgitation from the stomach into the normally empty oesophagus. If there is considerable reflux, the patient may be conscious of the presence of liquid in the pharynx.

Signs

The deep situation of the oesophagus usually makes specific clinical features entirely absent. Those which may accompany individual disorders are considered below.

Investigation

Radiology

- Anteroposterior plain X-ray may occasionally show a broadening of the mediastinal shadow by a dilated oesophagus, but the finding is non-specific. An air–fluid level may be seen behind the heart if there is distal oesophageal obstruction.
- Contrast radiology, usually with barium sulphate but in special circumstances with a water-soluble contrast medium, is the standard method of establishing both anatomical and functional abnormality.
- CT scanning (and increasingly MRI) is used to assess tumours of the oesophagus giving information on the stage (T, N, M).

Endoscopy

The flexible oesophago-gastroduodenoscope (see Ch. 4) is now often used as an alternative or complement to contrast radiology to achieve a diagnosis and has the advantage of being able to take tissue for histological examination. Endoscopic ultrasound is used to assess the T and N stage of oesophageal cancers.

Manometry and oesophageal pH studies and impedence monitoring

This investigation has an important role in the analysis of disorders of motility. In addition, similar equipment can be used for monitoring the acid level in the oesophagus in patients with suspected reflux. The technique is to place a pH sensor at the end of a tube in the lower oesophagus and to make continuous recordings over 24 hours. In normals there should be little change; however, in those with reflux of acid contents, the pH falls sporadically, particularly at night.

The introduction of a capsule that can be temporarily fixed to the oesophageal mucosa at endoscopy (Bravo capsule) allows the measurement of oesophageal pH for up to 48 hours without the need for naso-oesophageal catheters. Measurements are transmitted wirelessly to an external receiver.

Oesophageal impedence monitoring measures fluid and gas flows through the oesophagus by measuring electrical impedence using a catheter with multiple electrodes. In oesophageal transit tests this can be used to measure the clearance of a swallowed bolus, while in patients with suspected gastroesophageal reflux it can be used to measure reflux independent of its acidity.

MOTILITY DISORDERS

Much has still to be learnt about these disorders, but a working classification is into those which involve:

- Hypermotility – chiefly diffuse spasm.
- Hypomotility – usually secondary to systemic sclerosis (scleroderma).
- Sphincter dysfunction – especially the inability of the lower sphincter to relax (achalasia).

HYPERMOTILITY

Diffuse oesophageal spasm

Aetiology

The cause is unknown and the condition is rare – or at least rarely recognised. There may well be a physiological link between this condition and achalasia (see below).

Clinical features

The combination of intermittent, often quite severe, chest pain with dysphagia is characteristic. The condition may lead to investigation under a provisional diagnosis of angina pectoris.

Investigation and management

A contrast study shows exaggerated oesophageal contractions which may outline the gullet as a corkscrew. Oesophagoscopy is usually normal, but manometry shows exaggerated contractions.

Drugs that reduce smooth muscle contraction (nitrates and calcium channel blockers such as nifedipine) occasionally help. Balloon dilatation is also an option, but in those with severe symptoms a long oesophageal myotomy in which all layers of muscle down to mucosa are divided may be required.

Nutcracker (super-squeeze) oesophagus

It is uncertain whether this condition is a distinct entity. It is a common manometric finding in patients who present with chest pain which is of non-cardiac origin. The symptoms are the same as those for diffuse spasm, as is the management. However, surgical treatment is rarely required.

HYPOMOTILITY

The only well-recognised disorder that causes hypomotility is systemic sclerosis – a condition of unknown cause. The muscle layer is replaced by fibrous tissue. The presence of the disease may be suspected from other features such as loss of mobility of the face and microvascular features, e.g. digital ischaemia.

Investigation and management

Contrast radiology shows diminished peristalsis, and this can be confirmed by manometry. The treatment of hypomotility is that of the complications such as gastro-oesophageal reflux (see 'Hiatus hernia').

ACHALASIA

This is commonly known as cardiospasm.

Aetiology

In the great majority of patients the cause is unknown, but a similar clinical condition is found in South America as a result of infection with a protozoan organism *Trypanosoma cruzi*. The lower sphincter fails to relax in response to the peristaltic wave, and the bolus is partially retained in the oesophagus.

Clinicopathological features

Dilatation and muscular hypertrophy occur above the lower sphincter. Histological examination shows loss of ganglion cells (see also 'Hirschsprung's disease'). In long-standing cases the oesophagus becomes elongated and its mucosa inflamed from stasis of food. The latter finding is a probable cause of the increased risk of the development of malignant change.

There is not initially frank dysphagia but rather a slowing down of the normal rate of ingestion of food, so that at a meal the patient gets 'left behind'. Obvious dysphagia ultimately develops with retrosternal discomfort, regurgitation and weight loss. Onset of these symptoms in later life may lead to confusion between achalasia and carcinoma.

Investigation

Endoscopy is essential and in older patients may show a secondary cause such as infiltration of the distal oesophagus by malignant disease. Contrast study confirms delay at the lower sphincter, although in early symptomatic patients the abnormality may be difficult to identify. Manometry shows incomplete relaxation of the lower sphincter in response to a swallow.

Management

Medical treatment with muscle relaxants is usually unrewarding. The three effective methods are:

- Balloon dilatation, which leads to resolution of symptoms in 80% although it may have to be repeated and carries a small risk of oesophageal perforation.
- Longitudinal myotomy of the gastro-oesophageal junction (known to surgeons as Heller's operation) which can be done either at open operation or via a laparoscope or thoracoscope; some surgeons combine myotomy with an anti-reflux procedure. Surgical myotomy is associated with the risk of gastro-oesophageal reflux but is otherwise a very satisfactory procedure.
- Endoscopic injection of botulinum toxin into the oesophageal wall to paralyse the lower oesophageal sphincter is effective but lasts only for a few months. Repeated injections are possible.

GASTRO-OESOPHAGEAL REFLUX DISORDERS

Features of reflux occur in association with many different oesophageal conditions, including most of the motility disturbances described above. However, reflux is particularly a symptom of abnormalities at the diaphragmatic hiatus.

Pathophysiological features

If either acid or strongly alkaline (as may occur if there are large amounts of reflux from the duodenum) secretions reach the lower oesophagus, mucosal inflammation follows. Although this is mostly a superficial oesophagitis, there may be two consequences:

- *Stricture* – this is usually predominantly an inflammatory reaction in the mucosa and submucosa, but it can, if inflammation takes place, become a fibrous narrowing.
- *Metaplastic change* – this leads to the development of gastric-type columnar epithelium in the lower oesophagus. This was first described by the British surgeon Norman Barrett and is, in consequence, often known as 'Barrett's oesophagus'. Its significance is that it is a remalignant lesion; adenocarcinoma of the lower oesophagus may develop at an estimated incidence of 0.5% per patient year.

Clinical syndromes

There are two main causes:

- hiatus hernia with reflux
- reflux without abnormal anatomy.

HIATUS HERNIA

There are two types of hiatus hernia: sliding and para-oesophageal. Occasionally these can be mixed (so-called type III). Although only the first is usually associated with reflux, both will be considered here.

Sliding hernia

The proximal stomach ascends into the chest through a lax or enlarged diaphragmatic opening, taking a circumferential cuff of peritoneum with it. The normally acute oesophagogastric angle is reduced, so that reflux is common even though the intrinsic lower sphincter is normal (Fig. 18.2a).

Aetiology

Some examples of sliding hernia may be congenital but in most the cause is not established. Obesity, increase in abdominal contents (pregnancy) and ageing may be contributory factors.

Clinical features

There is postural reflux, heartburn and occasionally some lower left chest pain. However, the latter should only be ascribed to a postulated or actual hiatus hernia with caution. Vague indigestion is rarely caused by a sliding hernia and must be explored clinically and by investigation for an underlying cause.

Investigation

Patients with the recent onset of symptoms, particularly if they are elderly, should be investigated for possible oesophagogastric cancer.

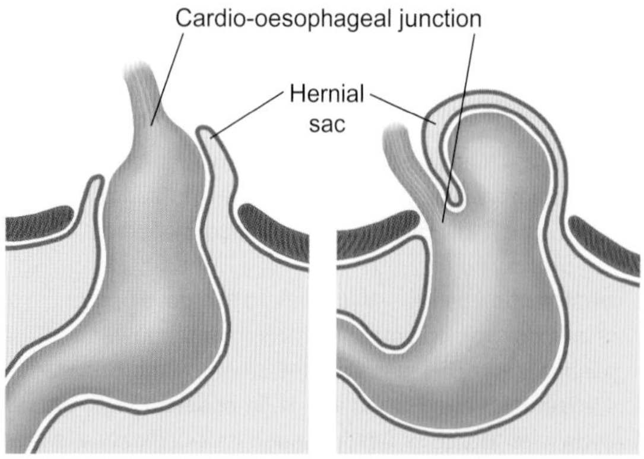

Fig. 18.2 (a) The oesophagogastric anatomy in a sliding hiatus hernia. (b) The anatomy in a para-oesophageal hernia.

Contrast radiography

The standard method of making the diagnosis is by barium swallow and meal (although some cynics say that a determined radiologist can identify a hiatus hernia in almost anyone). More often patients are now investigated by endoscopy.

Endoscopy

Although it is not always easy to identify the oesophagogastric junction, this examination allows assessment of the severity of oesophagitis, and a tissue diagnosis by examination of a biopsy may be made in patients with Barrett's oesophagus.

pH monitoring and impedence studies

Oesophageal pH and, in some patients, impedence studies are useful in cases of diagnostic uncertainty and as a baseline measurement before surgical treatment.

Management

The great majority of patients can be managed by medical measures for the control of reflux, including:

- weight loss in the obese
- sleeping with the head of the bed raised to avoid nocturnal reflux
- alginate-containing antacids which are thought to reduce free liquid in the stomach and thus reduce the volume of reflux
- acid reduction by H_2-receptor antagonists (e.g. cimetidine or ranitidine) or proton pump inhibitors (e.g. omeprazole or lansoprazole).

If these measures fail to control symptoms or the patient is not keen on long-term medication, then operation should be considered. However, it must be absolutely clear that the symptoms of which the patient complains are the consequence of the presence of gastro-oesophageal reflux, otherwise a dissatisfied patient will be the outcome. A surgical repair is now almost always carried out at laparoscopy. This involves:

- reduction of the herniated stomach below the diaphragm
- removal of the circumferential peritoneal sac
- re-establishment of the oesophagogastric angle
- reduction of the intercrural space by suturing the crura together behind the oesophagus
- an anti-reflux procedure – often loosely called a fundoplication.

The fundus of the stomach is wrapped around the terminal oesophagus so that, as intra-abdominal pressure rises, the oesophagus is compressed (Fig. 18.3). One complication of such a procedure may occasionally be the inability to belch and, in consequence, bloating – a sensation of unrelieved fullness of the stomach. In addition, some patients experience postoperative dysphagia, which is usually transient. However, the outcome is usually good, and surgery should not be withheld provided the surgeon is satisfied with the relationship between the symptoms and the hernia – particularly given evidence from oesophageal pH monitoring.

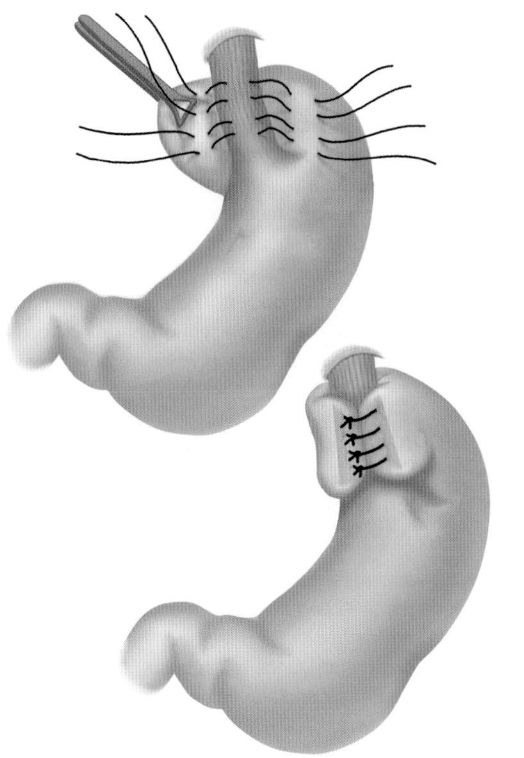

Fig. 18.3 A fundoplication operation. The gastric fundus is wrapped around the abdominal oesophagus.

Para-oesophageal hernia

Aetiology

A discrete peritoneal sac occurs at the left lateral border of the oesophagus, and the fundus of the stomach rolls into this, sometimes carrying the oesophagogastric junction into the chest (Fig. 18.2b). More complicated examples may cause a twist of the whole stomach – a gastric volvulus.

Clinical features

These patients are usually asymptomatic, although vague upper abdominal pain may occur. Incarceration going on to strangulation is not common but causes acute upper abdominal pain and what appears to be vomiting but is in fact total dysphagia. This occurrence – usually in elderly frail individuals – is a surgical emergency.

Management

Unless the patient is unfit, para-oesophageal hernias should be repaired surgically because of the risk of strangulation. Usually this is done laparoscopically.

REFLUX WITHOUT ABNORMAL ANATOMY

Aetiology and clinical features

Many patients have symptoms of reflux without any demonstrable anatomical abnormality. In some, obesity is a factor; others may have hyperchlorhydria with or without a demonstrable peptic ulcer. In the majority a definite cause is not identified.

Features of heartburn and dyspepsia are universal, with regurgitation of gastric contents in some.

Investigation

Many patients are probably treated symptomatically in general practice without investigation. However, those with troublesome features should have a barium swallow and/or endoscopy. Ambulatory monitoring of lower oesophageal pH may establish that there is persistent reflux, and oesophageal manometry identifies those with a motility disorder.

Management

Medical management as described above is often sufficient. For those with oesophagitis which is unresponsive to treatment (rare) and for patients who are not keen on long-term acid supression therapy, an anti-reflux operation should be considered.

OESOPHAGEAL DIVERTICULA

Hypopharyngeal pouch is the most common of these. Other diverticula in lower parts of the oesophagus are rare.

OESOPHAGEAL RUPTURE AND MUCOSAL TEAR (MALLORY–WEISS SYNDROME)

Aetiology

Vomiting is usually a coordinated event. The stomach and diaphragm contract so that intragastric pressure is raised; the oesophageal sphincters then relax, as does the oesophagus as a whole, and the stomach content is ejected. However, this orderly course may not take place if:

- vomiting is artificially induced, or
- the individual is confused – usually from excessive consumption of alcohol.

In such circumstances, intragastric pressure forces stomach contents into the distal oesophagus, dilating it. The oesophagus may rupture with emptying of stomach contents into the left pleural cavity. Because the relatively elastic muscle in the oesophageal wall has a greater capacity for stretch than does the folded mucosa and submucosa, quite often only these are split to produce a longitudinal mucosal tear at the oesophagogastric junction (Mallory–Weiss syndrome).

Oesophageal rupture

Clinical features

History

Forceful vomiting may be recalled, but if there has been much intake of alcohol it is sometimes forgotten. Vomiting may also have been induced either in a glutton or in someone who is mentally disturbed with a history of excessive eating but with the paradoxical desire not to gain weight (bulimia). There will be sharp left-sided pleuritic pain.

Physical findings

The effect of gastric content within the chest is to rapidly produce signs of severe sepsis with fever and circulatory disturbance. A left pleural effusion is present. The course is downhill with all the features of systemic inflammatory response syndrome. Occasionally, however, the rupture is localised and the patient is less ill with localised pleural signs and features of sepsis which are less severe.

Management

In early rupture, the oesophagus is exposed surgically and repaired. The area is drained and a gastrostomy is often done to drain gastric secretions, although whether this is effective is not established. Parenteral or enteral (jejunostomy) nutrition is used until healing is assured.

Mucosal tear (Mallory–Weiss syndrome)

The presentation of this condition is with haematemesis, and it is therefore considered in Chapter 23.

CANCER OF THE OESOPHAGUS

Epidemiology

This condition is relatively rare in the Western world. However, studies have revealed a wide geographical variation with pockets of high incidence. For example, although the incidence in Europe overall is between 2 and 8 cases per 100 000 population, in some areas of northern France this figure may be as high as 30/100 000. In the Far East the incidence is in general much higher and may be between 100 and 150/100 000 in some provinces of China. Such a level warrants screening programmes within populations at high risk. Overall, the incidence is rising worldwide.

Aetiology

Squamous carcinoma

The wide geographical variation in incidence has been attributed to social and environmental factors. There appears to be a strong association between cigarette and alcohol consumption and the incidence of the disease. However, diet is probably of greatest importance. Three factors are recognised:

- high intake of nitrosamines derived from nitrates used in food preservatives
- low intake of both vitamin A and nicotinic acid
- iron deficiency anaemia, a known associate of hypopharyngeal cancer but probably also a factor in cancer of the body of the oesophagus.

Long-standing achalasia may lead to cancer, presumably because of stasis and mucosal irritation. The reported incidence is highly variable but may reach 2%.

Adenocarcinoma

Cases of adenocarcinoma of the oesophagus now exceed those of squamous carcinoma in a ratio of 2 : 1, whereas 30 years ago the ratio was in the reverse direction. Metaplastic change in the oesophageal mucosa from squamous to columnar epithelium as a result of gastro-oesophageal reflux (Barrett's oesophagus) predisposes to the development of adenocarcinoma. Endoscopic screening of all patients with significant reflux symptoms has been recommended to identify those with Barrett's oesophagus. The magnitude of this risk varies, with dysplastic mucosal changes, intestinal metaplasia and length of Barrett's mucosa all being factors which increase the chance of malignant change. Regular endoscopic surveillance with biopsy is indicated in such patients, particularly if risk factors are present, in an effort to detect early malignant change at a stage when curative treatment is possible.

Pathological features

Nearly all lesions are a combination of narrowing and ulceration, although the extent of each varies. Spread takes place by:

- *direct invasion* first through the full thickness of the oesophageal wall and thence into adjacent structures such as the trachea or bronchi, the pericardium, chest wall and diaphragm. Once a fistula into the air passages has occurred, the condition is incurable and life expectation is short
- *submucosal infiltration* both proximally and distally so that, if mucosal destruction is used as an indication of the extent of spread, there may be an underestimate of the extent of the growth
- *lymph node involvement* in the mediastinum and, in distal lesions, around the stomach – the pattern is often not sequential. Upward spread in the mediastinum may produce a sentinel node in the supraclavicular fossa
- *the bloodstream* – this is unusual in the early stages, but by the time of death up to 90% of patients may have distant metastases (liver, lung and brain).

Clinical features

Symptoms

In early disease, for example those detected by endoscopic surveillance of patients with Barrett's oesophagus, there may no symptoms. For others the mean duration of symptoms is 4–6 months but may be up to 3 years. To compound this, as is explained below, the average delay in presentation after their onset is 3–4 months.

Early ill-defined symptoms. The lack of well-defined symptoms while the disease is developing is one reason why so few cases of oesophageal cancer are diagnosed while the condition is still in a pathologically early stage. There may be a feeling of something stuck in the oesophagus, although not necessarily after eating. Retrosternal discomfort, belching and dyspepsia are often elicited on detailed questioning but may have been discounted by the patient.

Progressive dysphagia is the most common and important presenting symptom but may not be noticed until the oesophageal diameter is reduced by two-thirds. In the early stages, dysphagia is for solids only – particularly bulky foods such as meat and bread; only later is there difficulty with liquids. In the interim, most patients have simply accommodated to their symptoms by dietary alteration such as avoiding solids. Regurgitation after eating may be misinterpreted as vomiting, and in consequence there may be delay until dysphagia is total (inability to swallow saliva).

Weight loss. As dysphagia develops there is usually an associated dramatic decline in weight. More than 10–15% of the pre-illness weight may be lost over 4–6 weeks.

Acute obstruction. A sudden acute obstruction may occasionally be precipitated in a symptomless patient by the impaction of a large (usually inadequately chewed) food bolus.

For those patients who have developed an adenocarcinoma in an area of columnar metaplasia, a long history of heartburn suggestive of acid reflux may be elicited but is rarely volunteered. Pain is ominous and may indicate penetration of the tumour outside the wall of the oesophagus. Productive cough, particularly at night, may be produced either by aspiration of retained material into the respiratory tract or by the development of a malignant oesophagotracheal fistula. Hoarseness may mean involvement of the recurrent laryngeal nerve. Features of distant metastases can be the cause of presentation of a few patients.

Signs

Clinical examination of a patient with localised oesophageal cancer usually does not reveal any abnormalities other than evidence of recent weight loss. Total dysphagia is associated with signs of lack of water – reduced skin turgor and a coated furred tongue. A quarter of patients have palpable lymphadenopathy, which is usually in the supraclavicular region and is an indication of metastatic disease. Other signs of dissemination include hepatomegaly, jaundice, ascites, cardiac arrhythmias and features of pulmonary consolidation. Although the last may indicate advanced disease, respiratory infection may develop because of aspiration of oesophageal content.

Investigation

Radiography

Barium swallow has the advantages of:

- simplicity
- relative lack of expense
- high sensitivity in diagnosis of a stricture, although this does not necessarily indicate that it is malignant
- accurate determination of the anatomical site
- definition of the anatomy of the stomach and duodenum – important for surgical planning
- creation of a ‘road map’ for endoscopy and thus a reduction in the risk of perforation, as well as indicating the level at which a lesion is likely to be found.

However, this investigation is often now omitted in favour of endoscopy.

Endoscopy

This procedure is now usually done with a flexible instrument under local anaesthesia or sedation. It allows:

- biopsy and brush cytology for pathological confirmation of the type of cancer
- assessment (partial) of the extent of the lesion
- concurrent dilatation and temporary relief of obstruction, although this is not usually performed.

However, it has some dangers, such as:

- perforation of a malignant or fibrotic stricture or diverticulum – flexible instruments make this unlikely unless dilatation of a stricture is undertaken
- failure to detect a small lesion – though in experienced hands this is rare.

Further investigation

Once the diagnosis is confirmed, further study is required to assess the stage of the disease and to determine the suitability of the patient for operative treatment.

Endoscopic ultrasound scanning (EUS)

It is possible to obtain images from an ultrasound probe attached to an endoscope within the oesophagus which can accurately measure the depth of penetration of the growth into the oesophageal wall and assess involvement of mediastinal and perigastric lymph nodes.

Computed tomography

CT scan of both chest and abdomen may also detect metastases but is also helpful in determining the size of the primary and whether it is attached to surrounding structures. A fistula into the air passages may also be detected.

PET scanning

PET scanning (FDG) is increasingly used to exclude distant metastatic disease in patients being considered for radical treatment (surgical resection or chemoradiotherapy). It may identify metastases not seen on other imaging modalities.

Screening

The relative rarity of the condition in Western societies makes routine screening economically inappropriate, although it is indicated in high-risk groups such as those with Barrett's oesophagus. However, in places where the incidence is high (such as China and Japan), routine flexible oesophagoscopy and/or obtaining oesophageal specimens for cytology are increasingly being recommended to detect early asymptomatic disease.

Management

Endoscopic treatment

For very early cancers (mucosal/submucosal involvement only) endoscopic therapy by submucosal resection (EMR) or radiofrequency ablation (RFA) may be considered, particularly in patients at high risk for operative treatment. Careful endoscopic follow-up is required because of the risk of local recurrence of cancer. These techniques and photodynamic ablative therapy (PDT) are also used for patients with high-grade dysplastic change within a Barrett's oesophagus.

Surgical resection

Surgical resection of oesophageal cancer is confined to patients with ‘operable’ disease – locally removable cancer and no detectable distant metastatic disease – who are considered fit enough for the major operation required.

There is good evidence now that neoadjuvant chemotherapy, sometimes combined with radiotherapy, increases the frequency of complete cancer excision and significantly improves overall survival rates and disease-free interval. Such multimodal treatment is now standard practice apart from patients with very early stage disease (T1,N0,M0).

Contraindications to surgery include:

- poor cardiovascular, pulmonary or renal function
- tracheo-oesophageal fistula
- other evidence of advanced local disease
- distant metastatic disease.

The principles of resection with cure in mind are:

- wide resection margins
- radical lymph node clearance within the chest and for distal growths at the oesophagogastric junction also in the upper abdomen.

The conventional method of resection is by open operation which may involve opening both the abdomen and thorax. However, two alternatives are now available:

Trans-hiatal removal. The abdomen alone is opened and the oesophagus freed in the chest by blunt dissection through the diaphragmatic hiatus. Stomach (or colon) for reconstruction is then passed through the posterior mediastinum to the neck where it is anastomosed to the upper oesophagus through a cervical incision. This procedure is used by some surgeons for patients with Barrett's oesophagus containing high-grade dysplasia and thus having a very high risk of developing adenocarcinoma.

Minimal access surgical removal. The whole procedure can now be done by minimal access dissection within the chest (thorascopy) and abdomen (laparoscopy), although there is little current evidence that this method is better than open operation.

Other methods of restoring swallowing

In patients unsuitable for surgical treatment, other methods can be used to relieve dysphagia, as follows.

Chemotherapy (e.g. with 5-fluorouracil [5-FU] and cisplatin), either alone or preferably in combination with radiotherapy, may lead to total disappearance of the local tumour in 30% of patients.

Combined radiochemotherapy is used in some centres as primary radical treatment for squamous carcinoma. Resection in these cases is reserved for local recurrent or residual cancer.

Endoscopic insertion of self-expanding metal endoprostheses – some of which are covered with a plastic membrane through the area of tumour stricturing and may provide palliation by improving swallowing. Covered stents can also be used to close fistulas between oesophagus and trachea.

Local endoscopic destruction of the tumour by laser or argon-beam diathermy, which can be repeated.

Prognosis

The outcome of resection depends on the stage of the growth. When tumour is confined to the mucosa, a 5-year survival of 80–90% is possible, but any further spread means a fall-off to less than 5% for growths that have penetrated the full thickness of the gullet. Combined regimens of resection and neoadjuvant combinations of radiotherapy and/or chemotherapy are producing improved results.

STOMACH AND DUODENUM

PEPTIC ULCER DISEASE

Surgeons are now mainly called on to treat the complications of this condition (Box 18.1), but to do so they require some understanding of the causative mechanisms responsible, the pathological changes and their effects.

Epidemiology

Helicobacter pylori infection is now recognised as the main cause of peptic ulceration. There is a close association between peptic ulcer disease and poor socio-economic conditions and their consequences. Hence the condition is more common in the developing rather than the developed world. Relevant factors may be tobacco and alcohol consumption, which tend to be higher amongst the poor and deprived.

In duodenal ulcer, males outnumber females by a factor of 4, but gastric ulcer is equally distributed and its incidence increases with age.

Box 18.1 Indications for surgical intervention in peptic ulcer

- Urgent complications
  - Bleeding (Ch. 23)
  - Perforation (Ch. 23)
- Obstruction – usually by inflammation and fibrosis at the outflow of the stomach
- Malignancy – gastric 'ulcer' (always a primary cancer which has been partially digested)

Aetiology

The discovery of *Helicobacter pylori* as a strong associate of peptic ulceration in both the stomach and duodenum, and the additional observation that its eradication can lead to cure, has made it clear that infection with this bacterium is the cause of peptic ulceration in most case. The mechanisms by which the organism exerts it effects, and particularly the way in which it causes the acid hypersecretion commonly seen in duodenal ulcer, are still uncertain. Moreover, there must be an idiosyncratic component to the *H. pylori*–ulcer diathesis because many people have *H. pylori* present without suffering a peptic ulcer.

A relationship is also apparent between acute peptic ulceration and the consumption of non-steroidal anti-inflammatory agents (NSAIDs). Patients, particularly the elderly, are increasingly being prescribed these drugs, and there is therefore a rising incidence of acute ulceration with complications such as perforation and haemorrhage. It is not clear whether the relationship implies a cause of peptic ulceration, but it seems more likely that NSAIDs upset the balance between mucosal regeneration and repair and therefore present a hazard for anyone who also has a peptic ulcer.

Other antecedents of peptic ulcer which can have a bearing on management are shown in Table 18.1.

Anatomical and pathological features

These features are of mucosal loss accompanied by chronic inflammation with varying amounts of fibrosis. An ulcer penetrates to a varying depth in the gastric or duodenal wall and may involve neighbouring organs such as the pancreas. Free perforation into the peritoneal cavity takes place when the rate of ulceration exceeds that of repair, and the final event is that the base of the ulcer becomes necrotic and gives way. An artery in the base may undergo fibrinoid necrosis of its media so that it becomes rigid and therefore more difficult for natural processes to close should bleeding take place; this is a more likely explanation of continued bleeding than the presence of atherosclerosis in the arteries of the gastric or duodenal wall, which is almost unknown.

Gastric ulcers can occur anywhere but are most commonly found on the lesser curvature at the junction of antral and acid-secreting mucosa. It used to be thought that a benign gastric ulcer could undergo malignant change, but what appear to be instances of this are merely partial peptic digestion of a primary malignant tumour.

Clinical features

Symptoms

Both gastric and duodenal ulcers cause epigastric pain, and it is often difficult to distinguish one from the other, although it is often stated that patients with gastric ulcer have pain on eating and those with duodenal ulcer complain when they are hungry. Pain felt in or going through to the back can mean that the ulcer has penetrated into retroperitoneal structures such as the pancreas. Indigestion is often associated with the pain. Heartburn from acid-peptic reflux is common. Symptomatic episodes with temporary remissions which can last weeks or months are more characteristic of duodenal than gastric ulcer. In both, the symptoms are relieved by antacids.

Vomiting is seen in gastric outflow obstruction (usually from a duodenal ulcer, although a pyloric channel gastric ulcer can also be the cause). Obstruction is the consequence of inflammatory oedema and/or fibrosis. In the first it subsides with effective anti-ulcer treatment; in the second it persists. The vomitus is usually free from bile and may contain partially digested food, recognisable as a meal taken a day or more before. Patients with gastric outflow obstruction often lose weight, but unless the obstruction is complete and vomiting profuse, they do not become dehydrated in that absorption of water and electrolyte still takes place across the gastric wall.

Signs

In uncomplicated peptic ulcer, epigastric tenderness is the only feature, and even this is non-specific since a mild degree of tenderness can be present in normal people. Obstruction is associated with a succussion splash – a splashing sound heard upon gently rocking the patient's abdomen to and fro. When obstruction is present, there may be signs of weight loss and of extracellular fluid volume deficiency with a lax dry skin and empty collapsed veins. Features of hypokalaemia such as drowsiness are the consequence of:

- loss of hydrogen ions from the stomach
- compensatory renal excretion, first of sodium ions but later, and more importantly, of potassium ions.

Investigation

Endoscopy

The current initial investigation of the patient with indigestion which suggests peptic ulceration is by endoscopy, although, if this is the first episode, young patients (<40 years) may be treated symptomatically in the first instance. The whole of the upper GI tract, from the oesophagus to at least the junction of the first and second parts of the duodenum, is examined. All gastric ulcers are subjected to biopsy and brush cytological examination. Biopsy from the antrum may be taken for urease testing – an indication of *Helicobacter pylori* infection. Duodenal ulcers are assessed for their depth and degree of obstruction and for any stigmata which suggest bleeding. Repeat endoscopy is essential for those with a gastric ulcer.

Contrast radiography

Before the development of flexible endoscopy, a double-contrast barium meal was the usual method of investigation in suspected ulcer disease, and it is still occasionally used.

Table 18.1 Contributing factors in the cause of peptic ulcer

Factor	Site of ulcer	Presumed mechanism
Helicobacter pylori infection	Duodenum and stomach	Hypergastrinaemia, mucosal injury
Non-steroidal anti-inflammatory drugs (NSAIDs)	Stomach and duodenum (usually acute)	Imbalance between mucosal regeneration and acid-pepsin digestion (speculative)
Genetic susceptibility	Duodenum	Non-secretors of blood group O into gastric secretions
Hyperchlorhydria	Duodenum	Increased number of acid-secreting cells in stomach (increased parietal cell mass – ?also genetic)
Hyperparathyroidism	Duodenum	Hypercalcaemic stimulation of acid secretion
Benign or malignant gastrinoma (Zollinger–Ellison syndrome)	Stomach and duodenum	Unchecked gastrin hypersecretion

Ulcers are identified as craters which retain a fleck of barium, and the surrounding mucosal oedema can also often be shown.

Ultrasound and CT scanning

These investigations may be indicated if there is gastric outlet obstruction or concern about malignancy or perforation.

Biochemical investigations

Measurement of gastric acid secretion is no longer done routinely, although in those with duodenal ulcer, acid output is usually raised. Such investigation may have a small place in assessment of:

- suspected gastrin-induced hyperchlorhydria (Zollinger–Ellison syndrome)
- peptic ulcer recurrence after surgical treatment (see below).

Gastric outflow obstruction. If this is suspected, serum concentrations of sodium, potassium and chloride and the arterial $P\text{CO}_2$ level should be measured, especially if operation is contemplated.

Helicobacter infection

Evidence of *H. pylori* infection can be obtained by breath test following urea ingestion (containing ^{13}C), serum antibodies (not necessarily indicative of current infection) and faecal antigen testing.

Management

Uncomplicated peptic ulcer is treated by:

- *Regimens to eradicate H. pylori* if present using antibiotics such as amoxicillin and metronidazole or clarithromycin in combination with acid-reducing proton pump inhibitors (e.g. omeprazole, lansoprazole).
- *Reduction of acid secretion* with H_2-receptor antagonists such as cimetidine and ranitidine; or with proton pump inhibitors, which block the hydrogen–potassium–ATP enzyme system in the gastric (parietal) cells that secrete acid.

After successful *H. pylori* eradication, no further treatment should be required. In patients with recurrent peptic ulcer disease in the absence of *H. pylori* infection, maintenance acid supression therapy may be required.

The place of surgery

There is no doubt that surgical procedures can reduce acid output and, because the final common pathway to peptic ulcer is the action of acid-pepsin on the gastroduodenal mucosa, they may prevent ulceration. However, as more effective agents for treatment have been developed, and particularly as the elimination of *H. pylori* seems to be able to produce permanent cure, elective operation is no longer used.

Complications

Anatomical relationships determine that posterior wall ulcers penetrate the regions of the gastroduodenal artery and thus bleed, whereas anterior wall ulcers penetrate the peritoneum and thus perforate into the peritoneal cavity. For the management of perforation and bleeding, see Chapter 23.

Gastric outflow obstruction. A trial of non-operative treatment is undertaken because the features of obstruction may stem from inflammation and oedema. If this fails, then fibrosis is present and a pyloroplasty or bypass (gastroenterostomy) is necessary. Rarely the anatomy at the pyloroduodenal junction necessitates a partial gastrectomy.

Gastrocolic fistula. In Zollinger–Ellison syndrome and, in the past, after simple gastroenterostomy, an ulcer may penetrate from stomach to colon and cause faecal contamination of the stomach and small bowel. The result is intractable diarrhoea. Complicated surgical revision is then required after acid secretion has been brought under control.

GASTRODUODENAL TUMOURS

The only common tumour of the stomach is cancer. Occasionally, gastrointestinal stromal tumours (GIST) are found in the stomach or duodenum, as are polyps. Cancer arising in the duodenum is very rare and usually originates from the periampullary mucosa at the lower end of the common bile duct.

Gastric cancer

Epidemiology

After cancer of the colon, rectum and pancreas, carcinoma of the stomach is the most common cause of death from gastrointestinal cancer, and also the third most common cause of cancer death in men and the fourth in women. However, in the Western world, the incidence of this condition has diminished: in England and Wales in 1960 there were around 14 000 recorded deaths compared with just over 10 000 in the mid-1980s. However, over the last decade there has been a marked rise in the incidence of adenocarcinoma around the oesophagogastric junction, including the gastric cardia.

As with oesophageal cancer, there is a worldwide variation in incidence: more common in the East (China and Japan) than the West. Even in the West, racial differences occur: proximal tumours are more commonly seen in whites. The peak age distribution is 50–70 years, but the disease can occur at any age from early adulthood; 5% of patients are less than 35 years of age. Gastric cancer is predominantly a male disease (M : F ratio = 3 : 1).

Aetiology

The cause is largely unknown. The most likely proximate pathological event is gastric atrophy which causes hypochlorhydria and is a consequence of:

- prolonged *H. pylori* infection after initial active chronic gastritis
- pernicious anaemia
- gastric operations for peptic ulcer, particularly partial gastrectomy; the lead time is long – up to 25 years – but the widespread use of this type of operation in the 1950s and 1960s has led to the suggestion that those

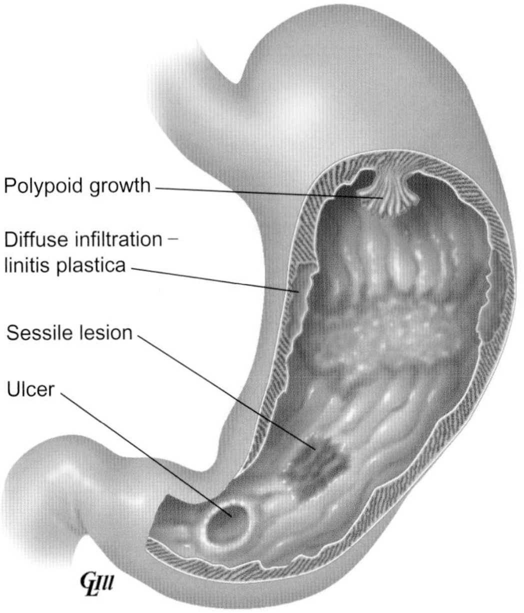

Fig. 18.4 Macroscopic types of gastric carcinoma.

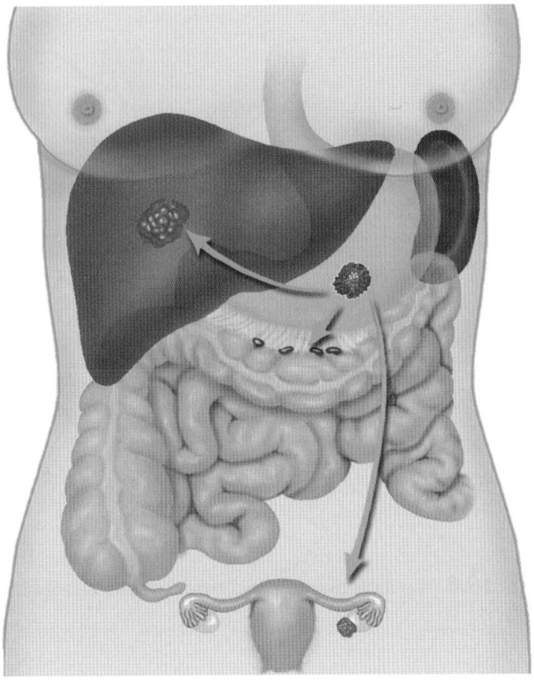

Fig. 18.5 Routes of spread of gastric carcinoma: portal venous to liver; lymphatic to local nodes; transcoelomic to pelvis.

who have been subjected to it should have routine endoscopic follow-up (see 'Screening').

Contributory factors may be:

- nitrate intake (see 'Cancer of the oesophagus')
- smoking.

A few tumours may originate in adenomatous polyps or dysplastic mucosa, but this is rare in contrast to the colon (see Ch. 12).

Pathological features

At the time of clinical presentation, most cancers of the stomach are microscopically if not macroscopically advanced. The gross disease is of four types (Fig. 18.4). Microscopically, the great majority of tumours are adenocarcinomas of columnar or cuboidal type, but classifications based on cellular patterns are not of value in prognosis. Adenocarcinoma is a locally invasive tumour which directly infiltrates the full thickness of the gastric wall to involve the serosal layer and contiguous structures such as the pancreas, transverse mesocolon, or left lobe of the liver (free perforation into the peritoneal cavity occurs in only 1%). Peritoneal seeding (transcoelomic spread) may take place with either diffuse nodules and ascites or deposits on the ovaries in the female (Krukenburg tumours) or in the rectovesical or rectovaginal pouch (Fig. 18.5). In addition gastric cancer is a good example of a tumour which spreads via lymphatic channels to local and regional lymph nodes (Fig. 18.6). These two features – serosal and lymphatic involvement – are the most important determinants of long-term survival following surgical resection. Liver metastases are usually a late feature.

Staging

Rather than histological classification of the primary tumour, pathological staging (see Ch. 5) is a more useful indicator of prognosis. A number of staging systems have been devised, the most popular of which are the Union Internationale Contre le Cancer (UICC) stage and the TNM system. Comparison of the two for gastric cancer is given in Table 18.2 together with 5-year survivals after radical resection. UICC stage I (T1 N0 M0) is often called 'early gastric cancer' and implies that the disease has not spread beyond the submucosa. At this stage, there is a high possibility of a cure (see 'Prognosis', below).

Clinical features

Failure to recognise the early features (chiefly symptoms) and to submit the patient to appropriate investigation and biopsy as soon as possible is an all too common occurrence in patients with gastric cancer. As with all gastrointestinal cancer, it cannot be overemphasised that early diagnosis is the key to cure.

Symptoms

Early tumours are usually without symptoms and are only detected by screening endoscopy. The nature and frequency of symptoms are shown in Box 18.2 and lead to some general principles:

- Any feature of dyspepsia in a previously asymptomatic individual over the age of 40 should always be viewed with the gravest suspicion and presumed to be caused by carcinoma of the stomach until proven otherwise.

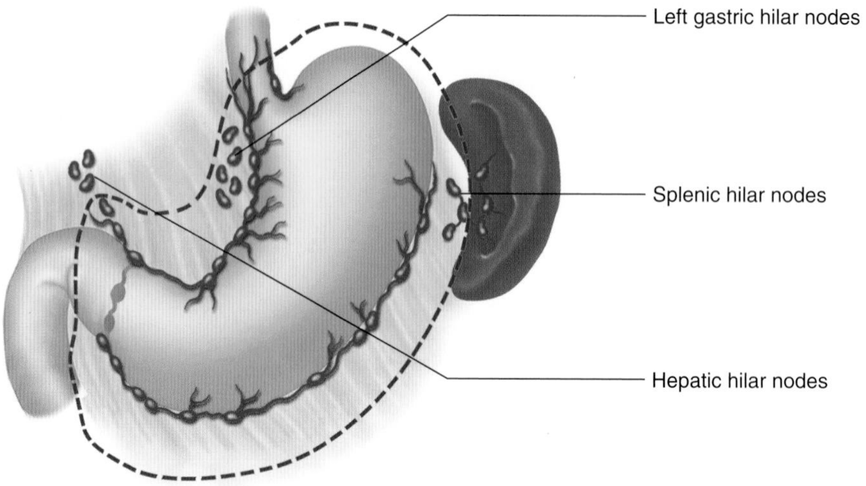

Fig. 18.6 The local and regional lymph nodes surrounding the stomach to which a carcinoma may spread.

Table 18.2 Staging, treatment and survival in carcinoma of the stomach

UICC stage	TNM stage	Method of treatment	5-year survival (%)
I	T1 N0 M0	Radical resection	70
II	T2 N0 M0	Radical resection	30
III	T0–4 N1–3 M0	Radical resection	10
IV	T4 N3 M0–1	Palliation	1–2

Box 18.2 Symptoms and signs of carcinoma of the stomach

Symptoms
- Weight loss (72%)
- Pain (51%)
- Nausea/vomiting (40%)
- Anorexia (35%)
- Abdominal discomfort (22%)
- Dysphagia (22%)
- Melaena (20%)
- Upper gastrointestinal bleeding (11%)

Signs
- Weight loss (26%)
- Abdominal mass (17%)
- Abdominal tenderness (15%)
- Hepatomegaly (13%)
- Rectal 'shelf' (4%)
- Cervical lymphadenopathy (4%)
- Ascites (3%)

- Anorexia is common and rarely is the only symptom of an early lesion.
- Dysphagia is usually associated with proximal lesions.
- Weight loss and abdominal pain are the most common symptoms, and the frequent occurrence of the first is a reflection of the advanced nature of the majority of tumours.
- Significant bleeding – haematemesis and/or melaena – is not all that common, but all gastric cancers cause some oozing and this may be sufficient to produce microcytic hypochromic anaemia with the non-specific symptoms of lassitude and fatigue (see below).
- Tumours within the antrum and pylorus present with the symptoms of gastric outflow obstruction – fullness, nausea and vomiting.

Physical findings

The best circumstance is not to find any abnormalities. The frequency of occurrence of individual signs is given in Box 18.2. Signs of gastric outflow obstruction may be present. The presence of metastatic spread is indicated clinically by:

- a hard lymph node in the left supraclavicular fossa at the junction of the thoracic duct with the subclavian and internal jugular veins
- ascites
- irregular hepatomegaly
- a hard 'shelf' anteriorly on rectal examination.

Screening

Routine endoscopic screening has been widely adopted in Japan, where the disease is much more common than in Europe. Because the disease occurs less frequently in the West, screening is not cost-effective. Screening of those at high risk (pernicious anaemia and after gastric surgery) has also been suggested but not uniformly applied, and in consequence there is little information on its value.

Investigation

In a patient suspected of having a carcinoma of the stomach, the following investigations are appropriate.

Oesophagogastroscopy

This is the most sensitive procedure for determining the presence or absence of a gastric neoplasm. It provides information on the anatomical site and enables multiple biopsies and brush cytology to be taken. However, if the histological and cytological reports on a gastric ulcer fail to show malignant cells, this must not be taken as absolute proof that the condition is benign. A short period (6–8 weeks at the most) of appropriate treatment for peptic ulcer is given and the examination repeated. Even if there are signs of healing, this does not mean the lesion is benign, and careful examination of further biopsies from the ulcer or healed area are necessary.

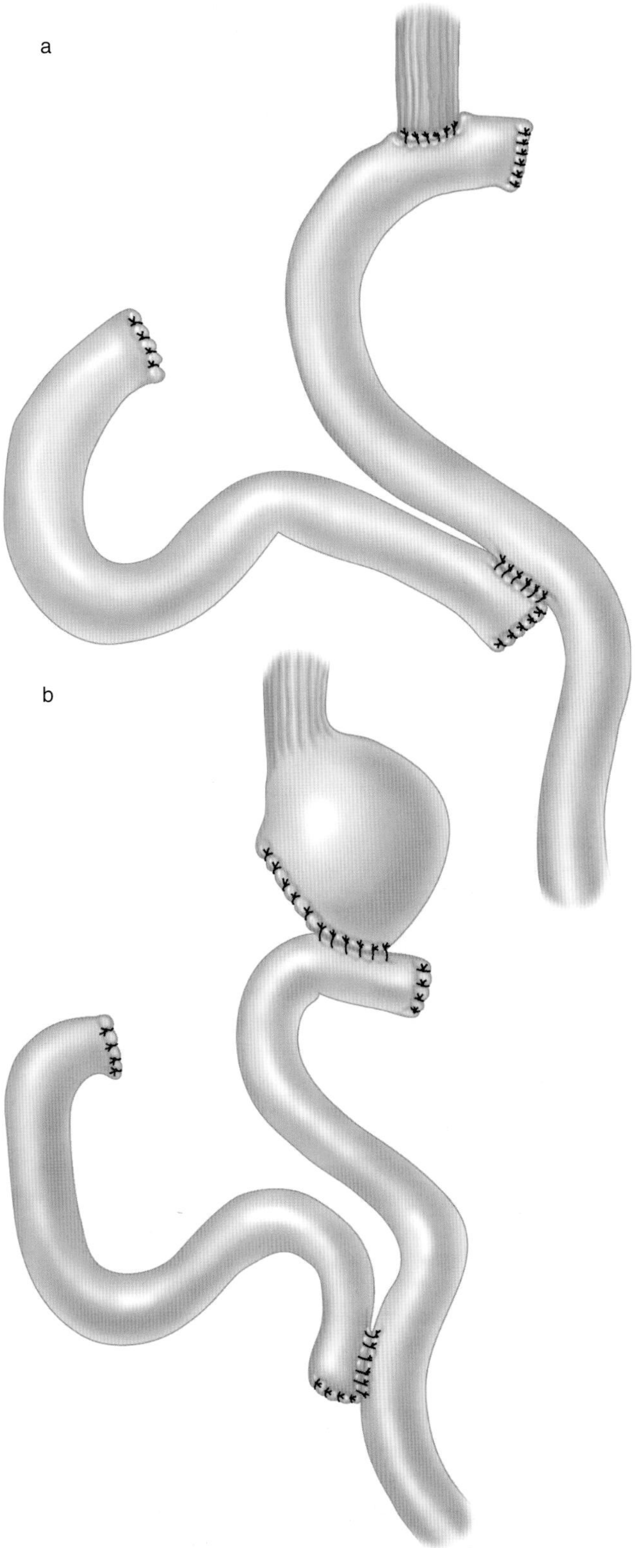

Fig. 18.7 Types of reconstruction after gastrectomy: (a) oesophagus anastomosed to a Roux-en-Y jejunal loop; (b) proximal stomach remnant anastomosed to a Roux-en-Y loop of jejunum (subtotal gastrectomy).

Imaging

Double-contrast barium meal. This examination can provide similar information to that of endoscopy but cannot reliably detect early cancer or give pathological confirmation of the disease.

Computed axial tomography, ultrasound and PET scanning are helpful by their ability to demonstrate the presence of unsuspected liver or other distant metastases and lymph node metastases. Both may also help to decide on resectability (sometimes called 'operability', which is distinct from 'curability').

Endoscopic ultrasound is being increasingly used to determine nodal status, depth of penetration of the primary tumour and also the extent of submucosal tumour spread. The extent of submucoal spread is particularly important for planning the extent of resection required for cancers near the pylorus and oesophagogastric junction.

Haemoglobin level and red cell morphology

It is important to recognise that to discover microcytic hypochromic anaemia in a patient with gastrointestinal symptoms is not to have made a diagnosis which initiates a course of treatment but only to have elicited a sign, which should lead to an urgent search for a source of blood loss within the GI tract.

Almost half of those with gastric cancer are anaemic, and this may require correction by transfusion. In some with unresectable tumours, repeated blood transfusions may be the only palliative procedure possible.

Laparoscopy

This procedure has contributed considerably to identifying irresectability, particularly by the detection of small liver or peritoneal metastases. Laparoscopy is now usually done before a laparotomy for resection is undertaken.

Management

Cure

The only curative treatment is surgical resection. In the UK, only 30–40% of patients are suitable for an attempt to cure, although up to 70% of growths may be resectable. Resection for cure means removal of the growth, the stomach or a large proportion of it and the regional lymph nodes as a single anatomical block. The extent of resection is a subject of debate. In Japan, where the best results are obtained, the stomach is removed together with the nodes within 3 cm of the tumour (N1) and the regional nodes (N2), sometimes with even more radical node resections (N3). In the West, many surgeons question the use of such radical resections because of a higher operative mortality and morbidity and because randomised controlled trials do not show a survival benefit; they prefer partial resections of the stomach and the N1/N2 nodes only. Two methods of reconstruction after total gastric resection are shown in Figure 18.7.

There is increasing evidence that neoadjuvant chemotherapy improves survival in patients undergoing resection for stomach cancer and standard treatment in the UK now includes pre- and postoperative chemotherapy. In some centres, particularly in the USA, postoperative adjuvant radiotherapy is used to reduce loco-regional recurrence.

Preoperative total parenteral nutrition (TPN) is indicated only in those patients with objective criteria of malnutrition. In this group, postoperative infections are diminished by nutritional support, but TPN has no other impact on mortality and morbidity.

Palliation

Surgical resection. This may be done in spite of nodal or metastatic disease that makes cure impossible. Such treatment may alleviate troublesome symptoms such as abdominal pain, dysphagia, blood loss and vomiting. However, because of late diagnosis and advanced disease, bypass of an obstructing lesion in the distal part of the stomach may be all that is possible.

Laser ablation. For unresectable tumours at the cardia, considerable improvement in swallowing may be obtained by the use of a laser through the endoscope so as to core out a passage through an obstruction. Repeated treatments throughout the remaining life of the individual are required. Endoscopic insertion of a stent across the malignant stricture is increasingly used as an alternative to bypass surgery.

Chemotherapy. A considerable proportion of patients respond to chemotherapy with carboplatin-based regimens, and this should be offered to patients with a good performance status and low comorbidity. Measurement of tumour markers such as plasma CEA or CA 50 may be useful in assessing response. Occasionally, after chemotherapy, it is possible to resect a gastric carcinoma previously deemed unresectable on CT scanning.

Prognosis

The relationship between stage and prognosis has been given in Table 18.2. In consequence, in the West the outlook for most patients is poor and is rather worse for patients with tumours of the cardia and fundus than for those with antral lesions. Increasing the public and general practitioner awareness of the importance of prompt investigation of new dyspeptic symptoms should result in more patients being identified who are suitable for curative resection.

FURTHER READING

Deaver JB, Ashurst APC 2007 Surgery of the upper abdomen. VI: Surgery of the stomach and duodenum. Kessinger Publishing, Whitefish

Griffin SM, Raines SA 2009 Oesophagogastric surgery: a companion to specialist surgical practice, 4th edn. Elsevier, Edinburgh

Patterson GA, Pearson FG, Cooper JD, et al 2008 Pearson's thoracic and esophageal surgery, 3rd edn. Churchill Livingstone, New York

19 Bariatric surgery

DEFINITION AND AETIOLOGY

Obesity is a chronic multifactorial disease related to genetic and environmental factors. In the vast majority of cases, the ultimate cause of obesity is unknown and therefore no specific therapy is currently available although dieting and other behavioural therapies are widely used. In less than 5% of cases a secondary cause of obesity can be recognised, such as hypothyroidism, Cushing's syndrome, steroid treatment or psychiatric conditions.

Obesity reduces life expectancy and is associated with increased risk of developing several associated diseases including type 2 diabetes, cardiovascular disease, hypertension and sleep apnoea (Box 19.1). The clustering of such comorbidity has been described as the 'metabolic syndrome.'

The degree of obesity is classified according to the Body Mass Index (BMI) (Table 19.1). The BMI is calculated by dividing the weight in kilograms by the square of the height in metres:

$$\text{BMI (kg/m}^2\text{)} = \text{weight (kg)/height (m)}^2$$

A person is defined as being obese if the BMI is greater than 30 kg/m^2. Morbid obesity is defined as a BMI over 40 kg/m^2. In addition to BMI, other measurements (anthropometric), such as the waist circumference and the fat/muscle body composition and distribution, may be considered.

EPIDEMIOLOGY

Obesity has reached epidemic proportions and has been recognised as a global public health problem. In the last few decades, obesity has risen at alarming rates worldwide, especially in developed countries. The prevalence of obesity in the United States and in Europe has been estimated to be approximately 50% and 15–20%, respectively.

MANAGEMENT OF OBESITY

The non-surgical management of obesity includes diet, exercise programmes, pharmacotherapy and behavioural modification. It has been estimated that over 95% of morbidly obese patients subjected to medical weight-reduction programmes regain all of their lost weight within two years of the onset of therapy.

Surgery for the treatment of obesity, also known as bariatric surgery, is recommended as a treatment option for people with morbid obesity when specific selection criteria are fulfilled, including failure of non-surgical measures to achieve or maintain adequate, clinically beneficial weight loss for at least six months (Box 19.2).

Surgery for obesity has resulted in substantial weight loss, long-term maintenance of weight loss, improvement or cure of associated diseases including type 2 diabetes, hypertension, and increase in life expectancy. Improvements of quality of life, social interaction and psychological well-being have also been demonstrated. Comprehensive evaluation and appropriate selection by a multidisciplinary team specialised in the management of obesity are essential to warrant the optimal care of the morbidly obese population (Box 19.3).

SURGICAL OPTIONS

Traditionally, there are two types of operations for morbid obesity: gastric *restrictive* operations (where food intake is restricted) and *malabsorptive* operations (where nutrients are diverted from absorption through a gastrointestinal shortcut). Recently, several gut hormonal changes (e.g. increase in GLP-1 levels, decrease in ghrelin production) have been demonstrated following bariatric surgery and these may contribute to appetite reduction and improvement of metabolic parameters seen postoperatively. Both types of obesity surgery can be performed laparoscopically utilising minimally invasive techniques; these confer significant advantages in terms of access and wound-associated morbidity (infection, incisional hernia).

Box 19.1 Obesity-related comorbidities

Cardiovascular disease
Type 2 diabetes mellitus
Hypertension
Sleep apnoea
Dyslipidaemia
Gastroesophageal reflux disease
Osteoarthritis
Polycystic ovarian syndrome
Urinary incontinence
Lower extremities venous insufficiency
Hypercoagulability
Malignant tumours (e.g. breast, uterus, colon)
Depression

Box 19.2 Indications for bariatric surgery

BMI ≥ 40 kg/m^2
BMI ≥ 35 kg/m^2 with major obesity-related comorbidity
Failure of non-surgical measures
Exclusion of secondary causes of obesity
Reasonable risk for anaesthesia and surgery
Commitment to long-term follow-up care

Box 19.3 Multidisciplinary management of morbid obesity

Endocrinologist/diabetologist
Dietician/nutritionist
Psychologist/psychiatrist
Respiratory physician
Bariatric surgeon
Anaesthetist

Table 19.1 Classification of obesity according to Body Mass Index

Classification	BMI (kg/m^2)
Healthy weight	18.5–24.9
Overweight	25–29.9
Obesity class I	30–34.9
Obesity class II	35–39.9
Obesity class III	40 or more
Super obesity	>50

RESTRICTIVE PROCEDURES

The laparoscopic adjustable gastric band

The adjustable gastric banding is a purely restrictive procedure consisting of the placement of an inflatable prosthetic ring just below the gastroesophageal junction to create a small proximal gastric pouch (Fig. 19.1). The objective is to reduce food intake and to induce an early feeling of satiety. The band should therefore help to prevent overeating and decrease the overall daily calorie intake. The gastric band can be adjusted postoperatively by injecting or removing fluid from the band via a subcutaneous injection port. The first injection normally takes place 6 weeks after the band has been placed. The number of injections required varies between patients. Studies have shown that average weight loss achieved is approximately 50–60% of excess body weight. There is, however, a large variation in results and adherence to dietary instructions and behavioural modification is necessary to achieve good results. The specific complications of gastric banding include gastric pouch dilatation, band slippage, gastric erosion, prosthesis infection, patient intolerance and subcutaneous port complications. The procedure is performed laparoscopically in the vast majority of cases.

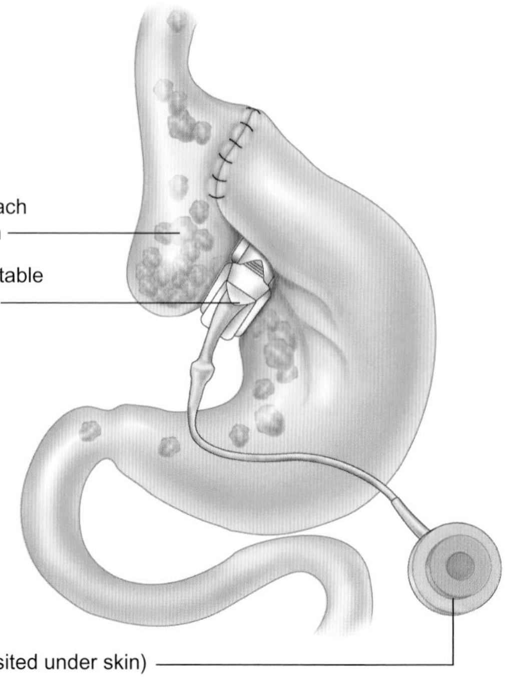

Fig. 19.1 Adjustable gastric banding.

The laparoscopic sleeve gastrectomy

The sleeve gastrectomy (Fig. 19.2) is a restrictive operation that is increasingly used in super-obese patients (BMI > 50 kg/m^2). It involves resection of the greater curve of the stomach, which is permanently removed. It has the advantage of being technically easier than malabsorptive procedures and avoids complications associated with foreign prostheses and anastomoses which may be more hazardous in super-obese patients. It also avoids malabsorptive complications such as 'dumping syndrome.' Patients may still be considered for later conversion to a malabsorptive procedure if adequate weight loss is not achieved, though recent evidence suggests it may offer an effective standalone procedure. Specific complications include leakage from the gastric staple line, bleeding and gastric tube stricture.

COMBINED RESTRICTIVE/MALABSORPTIVE PROCEDURES

The laparoscopic gastric bypass

The gastric bypass produces a restriction of food intake by creating a small gastric pouch and mild malabsorption by

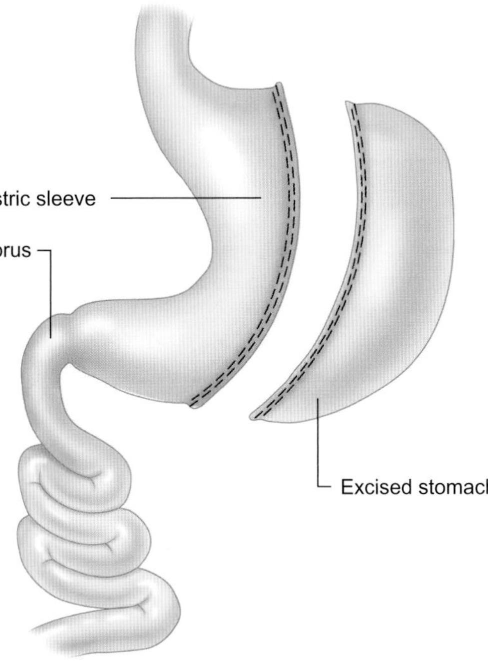

Fig. 19.2 Sleeve gastrectomy.

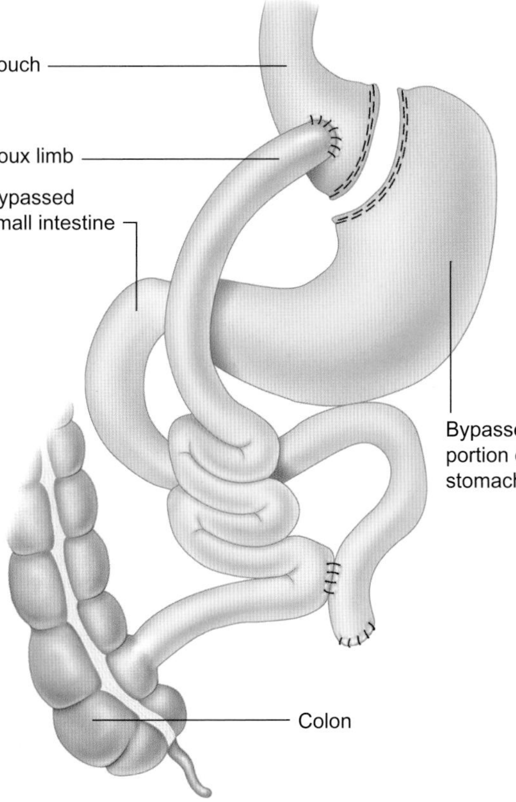

Fig. 19.3 Roux-en-Y gastric bypass.

bypassing the duodenum and the proximal jejunum (Fig. 19.3). After the stomach has been divided, the distal jejunum is connected to the gastric pouch. Food will travel from the pouch through this new connection called a Roux limb, bypassing the gastric remnant, the duodenum and the

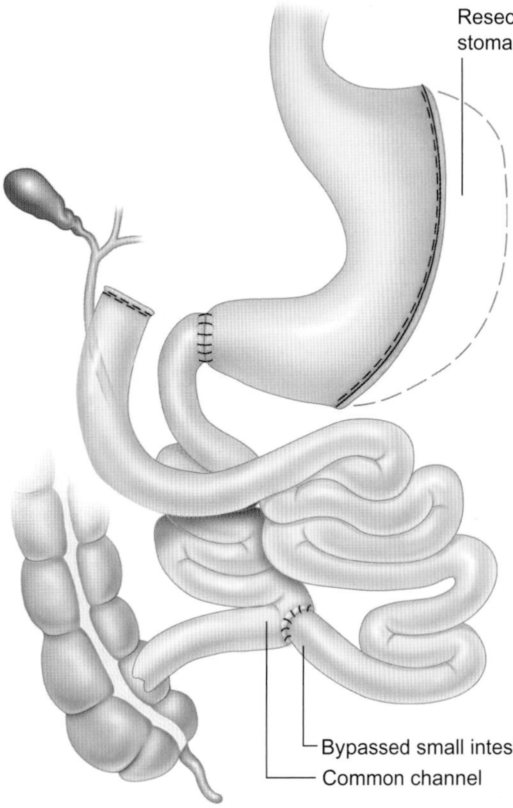

Fig. 19.4 Biliopancreatic diversion with duodenal switch.

proximal jejunum. The base of the Roux limb is reconnected to the remaining portion of the small intestine forming a Y-shape. Reduced absorption of vitamins and minerals may be experienced. The gastric bypass is considered to be major surgery and involves making permanent changes to the digestive system. Specific complications of the gastric bypass include anastomotic leaks, internal hernias, and pernicious anaemia. Weight loss is rapid in the first year and maximum weight loss is achieved at 18 months to 2 years. Expected weight loss is approximately 65–70% of excess body weight. The procedure is performed laparoscopically in the majority of centres.

The biliopancreatic diversion with duodenal switch

The biliopancreatic diversion with duodenal switch is a malabsorptive procedure consisting of a vertical subtotal gastrectomy (sleeve gastrectomy) associated with a consistent reduction of the absorbing intestine (Fig. 19.4). The bile and pancreatic juice mix with the food in the distal small bowel segment called the common limb. The length of this common limb (usually between 50 and 100 cm) is critical in the absorption of sufficient protein, fat and fat-soluble vitamins. Specific complications include anastomotic leaks and malnutrition, with diarrhoea and foul-smelling stools as frequent side-effects. Though the weight loss is substantial (70–75% of excess body weight), this procedure carries the highest mortality (1%) and is now the least commonly performed.

SUMMARY

Bariatric surgery is a discipline that requires not only specialised surgical skills but also specific expertise in managing the morbidly obese patient. Obese patients are often complex, high-risk surgical candidates because of their underlying comorbidities. A comprehensive and structured programme is required to provide the safe and effective delivery of bariatric surgery. Surgery for obesity produces sustained significant weight loss for severely obese patients with consequent improvement or elimination of their obesity-related comorbidities. The weight loss following bariatric surgery varies between patients and procedures. In contrast to medical therapies, weight loss is usually maintained for many years. Plastic surgery may be later required to remove excess skin and recontour the body after successful weight loss (e.g. abdominoplasty).

FURTHER READING

National Institute for Clinical Excellence 2006 Obesity: guidance on the prevention, identification, assessment and management of overweight and obesity in adults and children. Clinical Guidance n.43

Schauer PR, Shirmer, BD, Brethauer SA (eds) 2007 Minimally invasive bariatric surgery. Springer, New York

Sjöström L, Narbro K, Sjöström CD et al 2007 Effects of bariatric surgery on mortality in Swedish obese subjects. New England Journal of Medicine 357:741–752

20 Liver and biliary tree

HEPATIC AND BILIARY EMBRYOLOGY AND ANATOMY

Embryology

The hepatic diverticulum and hepatic primordia appear as an outgrowth of the distal foregut endothelium at stage 11 and grow into the septum transversum. Growth and proliferation lead to formation of the hepatic parenchyma, the biliary tree, gallbladder and extrahepatic bile ducts.

Clinical anatomy

The liver lies below the diaphragm and extends across the upper abdomen. The liver is adherent to the under-surface of the diaphragm where the peritoneal covering of the liver reflects to form the coronary and triangular ligaments (Fig. 20.1). Ventrally the covering reflects to form the falciform ligament and in this runs the ligamentum teres hepatis which is the fibrosed remains of the fetal umbilical vein – which in intra-uterine life carries oxygenated blood from the placenta to the fetus. The vein runs along the undersurface of the liver to drain into the ductus venosus, between the caudate lobe and the left lateral section, to reach the inferior vena cava. Following birth, the umbilical vein fibroses and forms the round ligament lying in the falciform ligament. Recanalisation can occur in adult life if there is severe portal hypertension.

The liver is unique in being nourished by a dual blood supply (Fig. 20.2). Blood flows to the liver from both the portal vein (80%) and the hepatic artery (20%). The portal vein carries blood returning from the GI tract and forms behind the head of the pancreas as a continuation of the superior mesenteric vein and confluence with the splenic vein and then passes in the free edge of the lesser omentum to the liver hilum where it divides into a left and right branch. The hepatic artery usually arises from the celiac artery on the ventral surface of the aorta and passes to the right along the superior border of the pancreas to ascend in the free edge of the lesser omentum to the liver hilum where it divides into left and right branches. The bile duct also lies in the free edge of the lesser omentum.

The triad of the bile duct, the portal vein branches and the arterial branches are enclosed in a fibrous (Glisson's) sheath, which is a continuation of Glisson's capsule that covers the liver.

Venous drainage of the liver is through three central hepatic veins, right, middle and left, that have a very short extrahepatic length before reaching the IVC just below the diaphragm. There are a variable number of short veins draining directly into the retrohepatic IVC. The caudate lobe of the liver drains separately and directly into the IVC. In the Budd–Chiari syndrome, where there is thrombosis of the main hepatic veins, the caudate lobe can remain functional while the remaining liver undergoes necrosis. The caudate lobe may undergo compensatory hypertrophy.

Anatomical sectors

Although the internal anatomy of the liver has been well known for many years the anatomic description of the internal structure of the liver has been confused for some time, partly because of the language used and partly because of two descriptive systems. In 2000 a single nomenclature was agreed. This anatomic description is based on the divisions of the artery and bile ducts and on this basis the liver is divided into two hemilivers, each supplied by a branch of the

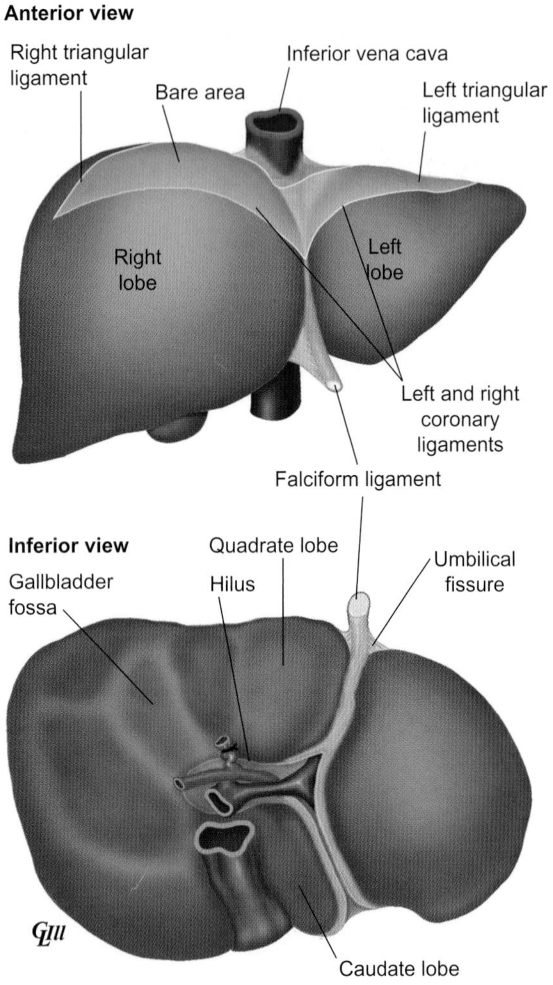

Fig. 20.1 The anatomy of the liver. Anterior and inferior surface views.

hepatic artery and the plane of separation between the right and left hemilivers lies along a virtual line (Cantlie's line) drawn between the tip of the gallbladder fossa and the IVC (Fig. 20.3). Although this plane cannot be seen clinically, it is demonstrated on vascular cast studies. Thereafter, each hemiliver is subdivided into a medial and lateral section. In the right liver the medial and lateral sections are separated in the plane of the right hepatic vein and in the left liver the medial and lateral sections by the plane of the left hepatic vein. The arterial divisions further divide the liver into eight functional units called segments (of Couinaud), where segments 1–4 comprise the left hemiliver and 5–8 the right liver (Fig. 20.4). Segment 1 is also referred to as the caudate lobe. The arterial divisions allow each segment to be resected separately, if desired. Anatomically based resections derive their names from this description as hemihepatectomies, sectionectomies or segmentectomies. A non-anatomic resection is one that is performed across boundaries without regard for the segmental anatomy.

Bile collecting system – ducts and gallbladder

The biliary collecting system and extrahepatic bile ducts

The bile caniliculi around the hepatocytes unite to form intralobular bile ductules, then interlobular ducts, and eventually converge to form the right and left hepatic ducts. The union of the left and right hepatic ducts forms the common hepatic duct and from the insertion point of the cystic duct the common bile duct lying in the free edge of the lesser omentum (Fig. 20.5). The common bile duct terminates at the ampulla of Vater adjacent to the termination of the pancreatic duct. The termination of each is guarded by a circular muscle forming the sphincter of Oddi. Although often described in illustrations, convergence of the ducts to form a single ostium in the ampulla of Vater is very unusual. A single common channel may lead to reflux of pancreatic juice into

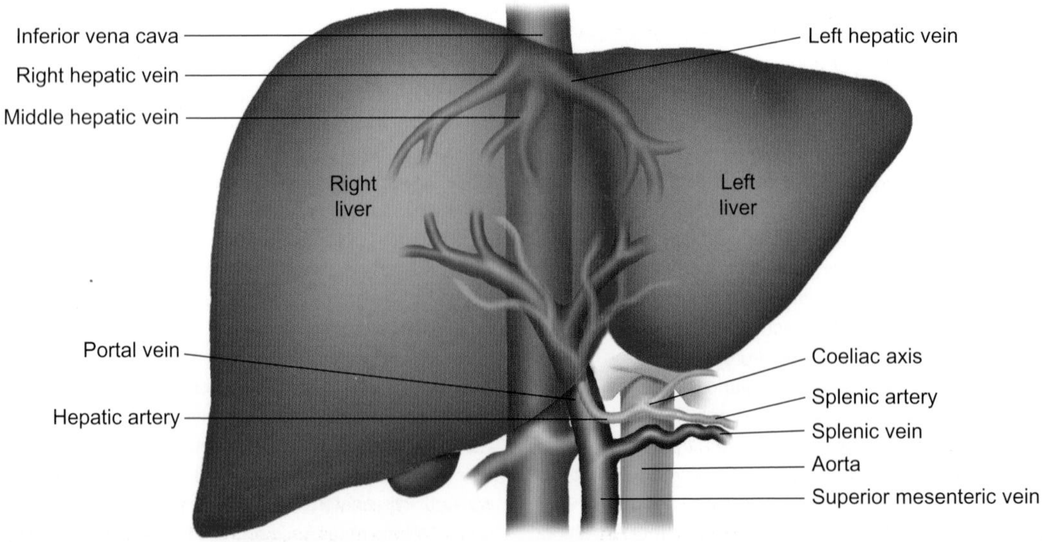

Fig. 20.2 The blood supply to and drainage from the liver.

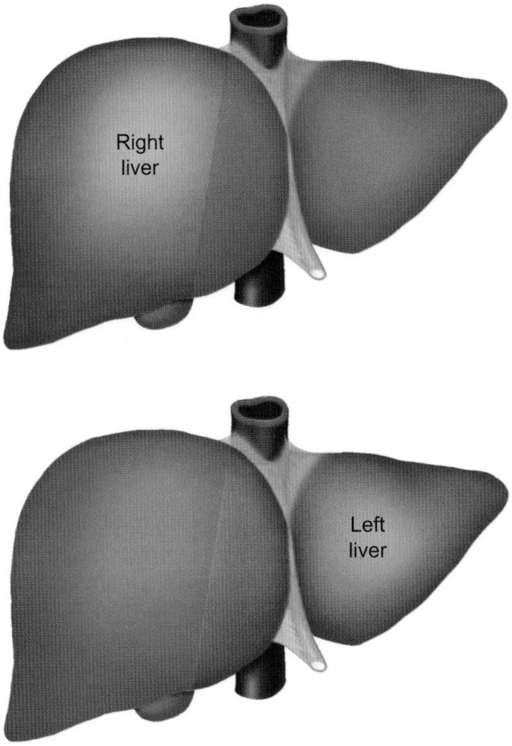

Fig. 20.3 The right and left liver.

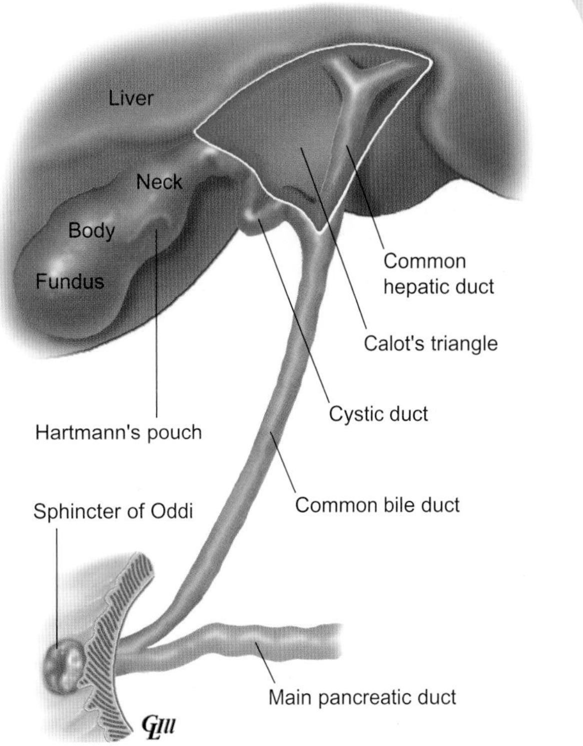

Fig. 20.5 The anatomy of the gallbladder and biliary tract with Calot's 'triangle' shown in blue.

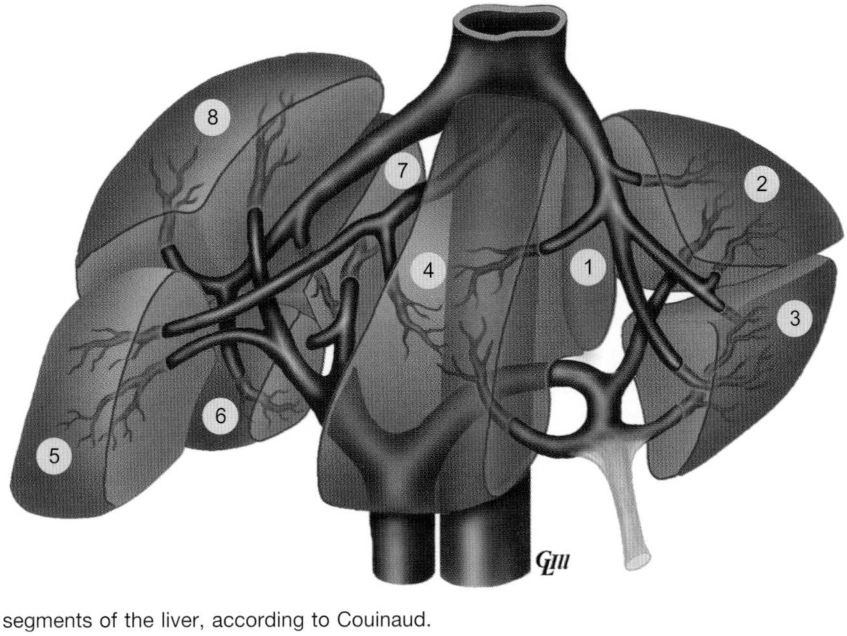

Fig. 20.4 The segments of the liver, according to Couinaud.

the bile duct and of bile into the pancreatic duct. The former is thought to be a cause of choledochal cysts and the latter the cause of gallstone-induced pancreatitis (see below and 'Pancreatitis', Ch. 22). Unlike the liver parenchyma, the biliary system throughout is supplied only with arterial blood.

The gallbladder

The gallbladder is a pear-shaped structure and variable in size but typically is the size of a small pear, although it can swell to enormous proportions in disease. The gallbladder sits on the underside of the liver in the gallbladder fossa and

Box 20.1 Congenital abnormalities of the biliary tree

Gallbladder
- Absence
- Reduplication
- Mesentery (floating gallbladder)
- Phrygian cap (fundus of gallbladder folded or kinked upon body)

Bile ducts
- Obliteration
- Low or otherwise abnormal entry of cystic duct into the common bile duct
- Low junction of a right sectoral duct with common hepatic duct
- Direct drainage of a bile duct into the gallbladder via the liver bed

thus between segments 4 and 5 (Fig. 20.5). Calot's triangle marks the important landmarks in surgery of the gallbladder (Fig. 20.5). Sometimes it hangs off the underside of the liver on a mesentery and may undergo torsion. The gallbladder is described as having a fundus, body and neck and derives blood from the cystic artery, which is usually a branch of the right hepatic artery.

Anatomical variations

As result of its complex development the biliary and arterial anatomy is highly variable and gives rise to difficulties and complications in surgery of the liver, gallbladder and bile ducts (Box 20.1). Injury to the bile duct during laparoscopic cholecystectomy remains a problem, with an incidence of about 1/500–1/1000 and is frequently due to misunderstanding of the anatomy at the time of operation. A major bile duct injury is a serious complication of this operation and requires specialist surgery to repair.

HEPATOBILIARY PHYSIOLOGY

Hepatocellular functions are listed in Table 20.1.

Reticuloendothelial function

Sixty-five percent of the reticuloendothelial system is within the liver, and it is responsible for filtering and destroying bacteria and their products that have been absorbed from the gut and for the removal of debris that results from the breakdown of intestinal cells. The hepatic reticuloendothelial cells also have similar functions in filtering blood that reaches them via the hepatic artery, but in this they are of less quantitative importance than the spleen (see Ch. 21).

Detoxification

The liver detoxifies a variety of endogenous and exogenous substances (chiefly drugs) mainly by conjugating them into less active forms.

Intermediary metabolism

Hepatocytes play a dominant role in metabolism and storage of basic foodstuffs:

Table 20.1 Hepatocellular functions

	Function
Hepatocellular component	
Nucleus	Double contour, exchange with surrounding cytoplasm
Mitochondria	Energy provider from oxidative phosphorylation: ATP–ADP
Rough endoplasmic reticulum (RER)	Synthesis of albumin, other proteins, glycogenesis
Smooth endoplasmic reticulum (SER)	Detoxification, synthesis of bile acids and steroids (cholesterol)
Peroxisomes	Catabolism and biosynthesis
Lysosomes	Lytic function and deposit
Golgi apparatus	'Packing' site of ingestion to be excreted
Cytoskeleton	Support of hepatocytes
Sinusoidal cells	
Endothelial cells	Barrier between sinusoids and space of Disse
Kupffer cells	Highly mobile macrophage
Hepatic stellate cells (Ito cells)	Storage of retinoids and fat
Pit cells	Highly mobile, liver-specific natural killer lymphocytes

- Carbohydrates are stored as glycogen and released in response to changes in blood sugar concentration to meet urgent energy needs.
- Fats are metabolised – to ketone bodies – for energy transfer and release. Some special products, such as cholesterol, are synthesised.
- Fat-soluble vitamins (A, D and K) are principally or exclusively stored in the liver.
- The liver is the only source of albumin and alpha-globulin. Many other specialised proteins, such as clotting factors, are synthesised there. Operations on patients with liver disease and defective protein synthesis require management of deficiency states.

Excretory function

The production, storage and release of bile into the duodenum is a fundamental function of the liver and has an impact on surgical practice because of:

- gallstone formation
- the enterohepatic circulation of bile acids, which is of importance in the digestion and absorption of fat.

Bilirubin is a breakdown product of the cleavage of haem from red blood cells by the reticuloendothelial system. On release into the circulation it is unconjugated (fat-soluble) and transported in the plasma bound to albumin. On extraction from the plasma by the hepatocyte it is conjugated with glucuronide by the enzyme glucuronyl transferase to become water-soluble and is excreted continuously in the bile. Bacterial deconjugation in the colon produces stercobilin, which colours the faeces brown. If there is infection in the biliary tree, deconjugation may take place within it, and the bilirubin may aggregate to form stones (see 'Oriental cholangiohepatitis').

Although bile is secreted continuously by the liver cells, one of its main functions is assisting in digestion. Under physiological circumstances bile is intermittently released into the duodenum. Between meals, the gallbladder acts as a reservoir in which bile is concentrated from 5 to 20 times by removal of sodium and water. Release of bile into the duodenum begins shortly after the ingestion of food – in response to stimulation of the vagus. The main flow, which is accompanied by gallbladder contraction and relaxation of the sphincter of Oddi, takes place as the result of the secretion of cholecystokinin from the duodenal wall in response to the presence of fat in the lumen. Contraction of the gallbladder in this manner against an obstructing stone causes pain (biliary colic).

In addition to concentrating bile, mucin is secreted from the gallbladder mucosa and this is believed to have a role in preventing stone formation.

JAUNDICE

Jaundice is the clinical manifestation of an increased concentration of bilirubin in plasma, the normal upper limit of which is 17 μmol/L. When hepatic uptake and excretion are decreased, the excess bilirubin in plasma spills over into the interstitial space so that the tissues become stained yellow. A symptom that often accompanies jaundice is itching, but this is probably caused by bile salts rather than bilirubin. Jaundice is usually first detectable in the sclerae when the bilirubin levels in the plasma reach >35 μmol/L. As the hyperbilirubinaemia worsens the skin and mucous membranes also become stained yellow. It is important to distinguish between jaundice that occurs because of increased bilirubin production or because of a block to excretion at the hepatocyte or canaliculus (which usually requires medical management) and that caused by extrahepatic obstruction to bile drainage (which may need endoscopic, surgical or radiological intervention). Close cooperation between gastroenterological physicians, surgeons and radiologists is required to effectively manage such patients.

Classification of jaundice

The classification of jaundice is outlined in Box 20.2.

Prehepatic

This is a sequel to increased breakdown of red cells – haemolysis. The rate of production of bilirubin is sufficiently fast to saturate the uptake – conjugation mechanisms in the liver. The bilirubin in plasma is unconjugated and therefore is not excreted by the kidney, resulting in acholuric jaundice.

Box 20.2 Classification of jaundice

- Prehepatic – haemolytic
- Hepatic
  - congenital defect of hepatocyte function
  - hepatocellular injury or infection
- Posthepatic – obstruction to bile duct

Hepatic (or hepatocellular)

This, as its name implies, is caused by some disorder of the liver cell at the stages of uptake, conjugation or secretion of bilirubin, including also malfunction of the cells which line the bile canaliculi. Intrahepatic cholestasis occurs when there is a failure to excrete conjugated bilirubin into the cannuliculi within the liver, and it is a common occurrence in patients with hepatocellular jaundice. Jaundice may be caused by:

- Defective uptake occurs with mild intermittent jaundice in otherwise healthy individuals (Gilbert's syndrome).
- Congenital absence of glucuronyl transferase is associated with severe jaundice and early death (Crigler–Najjar syndrome).
- Congenital impairment of excretion of conjugated bilirubin into the bile is known as the Dubin–Johnson–Rotor syndrome.

All the above conditions are rare, apart from Gilbert's syndrome.

The common causes of hepatocellular jaundice are:

- viral diseases of the liver cell – hepatitis A, B, C, D and E
- other hepatic infections
- alcoholic liver disease
- hepatotoxic drugs, such as the phenothiazines, which act mainly on the canalicular cells, but include many others with varied actions within cells.

Posthepatic

This type of jaundice is often called obstructive or 'surgical' jaundice, which implies that the cause is a mechanical obstruction in the extrahepatic biliary tree (extrahepatic cholestasis). The term identifies those patients whose jaundice may be capable of relief by some form of mechanical intervention – either by surgery, endoscopy or interventional radiology. In these patients, the relatively intact hepatocyte conjugates bilirubin which is then released back into the plasma and excreted by the kidney so that the urine is dark and the stools pale. The same phenomenon occurs in patients with intrahepatic cholestasis caused by cannicular obstruction within the liver. Causes of extrahepatic cholestasis include:

- obstruction in the lumen of the biliary tree – gallstones
- obstruction in the wall of the ducts – biliary atresia; bile duct carcinoma (cholangiocarcinoma); postoperative stricture
- extrinsic compression – pancreatitis; pancreatic tumour; secondary deposits in the hilar lymph nodes of the liver.

Investigation

Biochemical

The three most useful measurements are the serum concentration of bilirubin, alkaline phosphatase and the transferases:

- **Bilirubin.** A raised level of plasma bilirubin indicates disruption of its normal passage from blood, through the hepatocyte and down the biliary collecting system into the duodenum. Serial measurements are helpful in following the course of hepatic or biliary disease.

- **Alkaline phosphatase.** This substance is secreted predominantly from the cells of the collecting system, which proliferate in the presence of obstruction. A raised serum level in the presence of jaundice is therefore a good indicator of cholestasis – either extrahepatic or intrahepatic. The latter being caused by some drugs such as chlorpromazine and also seen in the later stages of viral hepatitis.
- **Transferases.** These enzymes are constituents of the hepatocyte. If their serum levels are raised, the implication is that there is hepatocellular damage. Usually this is primary, within the hepatocyte, but, in long-standing extrahepatic obstruction, secondary interference with hepatocellular function may take place.

The biochemical patterns of jaundice in hepatocellular and cholestasis including extrahepatic obstruction are shown in Table 20.2, although there can often be some overlap. Other measurements that may be of value in jaundice are:

- **Albumin concentration.** This gives a guide to the synthetic capacity of the liver and the nutritional state of the patient.
- **Clotting factors.** These are synthesised in the liver. The most easily assessed is prothrombin. Vitamin K is a cofactor in its synthesis. Because the vitamin is fat-soluble and is therefore not well absorbed from the intestine in the absence of bile, its limited hepatic stores soon become exhausted. The hypoprothrombinaemia of jaundice responds to the administration of parenteral vitamin K provided hepatocyte function is preserved, as is nearly always the case when the jaundice is caused by obstruction. Measurement of the prothrombin time is therefore an essential preliminary before operation in a jaundiced patient.
- **Alpha-fetoprotein (AFP).** See hepatocellular carcinoma, below.
- **Hepatitis virus markers.**

Imaging

Ultrasound

Ultrasound scanning reliably detects a dilated ductal system and so helps to distinguish parenchymal liver disease from extrahepatic bile duct obstruction. The characteristic texture of the cirrhotic liver can also be identified. In addition, cysts, abscesses and tumours can be delineated, and guided fine-needle aspiration and biopsy (Ch. 4) are possible.

Table 20.2 Biochemical patterns of jaundice

	Alkaline phosphatase	Aspartate and alanine transferases
Hepatocellular damage	↑	↑↑↑
Cholestasis including extrahepatic biliary obstruction	↑↑↑	↑

CT scanning

CT scan has the advantage over ultrasound of providing more precise anatomical information and, unlike ultrasound, is unaffected by the presence of obesity or bowel gas. The image is enhanced with oral contrast medium to delineate the bowel and with an intravenous contrast agent to show vascular structures.

Cholecystography/cholangiography

Magnetic resonance cholangiopancreatography (MRCP) now provides good images of the biliary and pancreatic ductal system, and this non-invasive method has replaced diagnostic ERCP and PTC.

Percutaneous transhepatic cholangiography (PTC – Fig. 20.6) is achieved by introducing a fine needle (usually called a skinny or Chiba needle) through the substance of the liver into a bile duct. Success rates are reduced if the biliary system is not dilated. PTC is of particular value in determining the anatomical level and the nature of obstructing hilar lesions.

Endoscopic retrograde cholangiopancreatography (ERCP – Fig. 20.7) similarly delineates the biliary tract but also can show the pancreatic ductal system.

At both ERCP and PTC, bile may be aspirated for microbiological examination and cells may also be obtained for cytological assessment. Both procedures are usually now performed only for therapy, such as the placement of biliary stents to relieve obstruction or the removal of biliary stones by endoscopic sphincterotomy or dilatation of the sphincter of Oddi.

Arteriography

Selective coeliac and superior mesenteric angiograms can show the abnormal circulation of a tumour (tumour blush – Fig. 20.8). The late-phase images of an angiogram

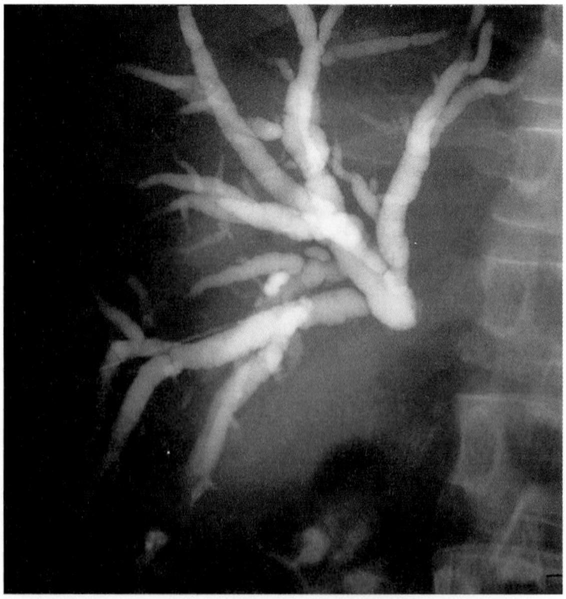

Fig. 20.6 A percutaneous transhepatic cholangiogram. The needle is seen coming from the patient's right side. The common hepatic duct is obstructed by a tumour.

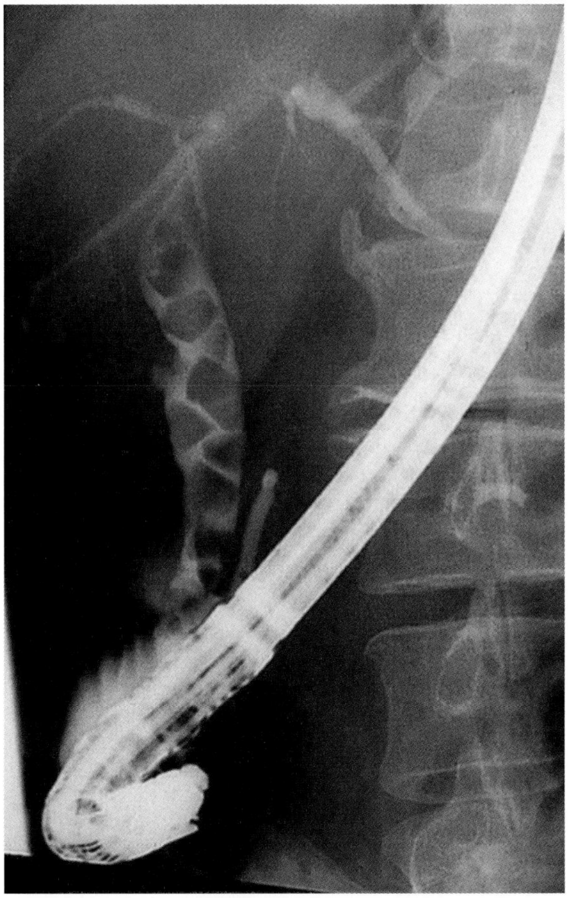

Fig. 20.7 An endoscopic retrograde cholangiopancreatogram showing the biliary ductal system with multiple bile duct stones.

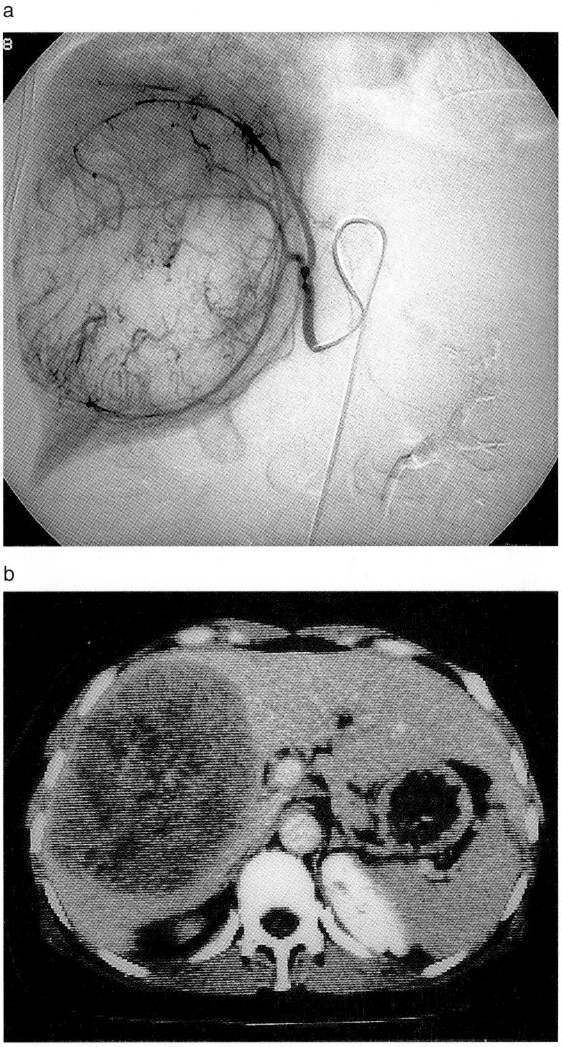

Fig. 20.8 (a) A tumour blush seen on hepatic angiography, and (b) the corresponding CT scan. Note that the arteries are displaced around the tumour.

demonstrate the portal vein, and therefore neoplastic involvement of both arterial and venous vessels can be assessed. However, vascular reconstruction using CT or MRI images is comparable to direct angiography. Invasive angiography is now usually performed only as a precursor to embolisation.

Laparoscopy

Laparoscopy permits direct visualisation of the liver and may be combined with laparoscopic ultrasound to provide both accurate staging and biopsy of diseased liver tissue. Because of the accuracy of modern staging imaging many surgeons do not use laparoscopy prior to resection. If laparoscopy is used it is normally performed immediately before planned laparotomy for liver resection.

Biopsy

Percutaneous liver biopsy is an invasive procedure which is used in the diagnosis of diffuse liver disease or for confirmation of metastatic malignancy. Accuracy is increased when insertion of the needle for biopsy or liver cytology is guided by ultrasound, CT or at laparoscopy.

General management

Preparation for liver surgery

Surgical operations are usually major, and the preparations outlined in Chapter 5 must be followed in detail. Major resections may require specialised support for abnormalities in the clotting system and for postoperative nutrition by either the enteral or parenteral route (see Ch. 5).

The jaundiced patient

Clotting

The most likely problem is vitamin K deficiency, which can be corrected by parenteral administration of the synthetic derivatives menadione or phytomenadione (K1). The synthesis of prothrombin, set in motion by restoring supplies of vitamin K, takes some hours, so the prothrombin time must, except in dire emergencies, be rechecked before operation is undertaken. In emergency cases fresh frozen plasma may be used to correct clotting.

Antibiotic prophylaxis

Sepsis from organisms that originate in the GI tract is a major cause of death in the surgical management of jaundice, partly because of interference with hepatic reticuloendothelial function. Prophylactic antibiotics against enteric organisms, such as cefuroxime or ciprofloxacin, are used routinely at the time of surgery or invasive procedures such as PTC and ERCP.

Preliminary biliary decompression

In a patient who will subsequently require an operation, liver function may be improved by biliary decompression which is done by one of the following methods:

- passing a catheter percutaneously into the liver substance and then into a bile duct at PTC
- ERCP with or without dilatation of an obstructing lesion and insertion of biliary stent (plastic or expanding metal) or occasionally a nasobiliary drainage catheter (Fig. 20.9).

Hepatorenal syndrome

This condition is probably one variant of the systemic inflammatory response syndrome (SIRS) in which renal and hepatic failure develop in response to severe injury or sepsis, especially if there is depression of the immune system. A patient with jaundice is particularly liable to develop acute kidney injury, and measures to prevent this include:

- adequate preoperative hydration
- avoidance of intraoperative hypotension
- maintenance of high urine flow by the use of an osmotic diuretic (mannitol) which opposes the action of increased secretion of antidiuretic hormone on the distal tubule after operation; and also by administration of a low dose of inotrope which increases renal plasma flow and glomerular filtration rate.

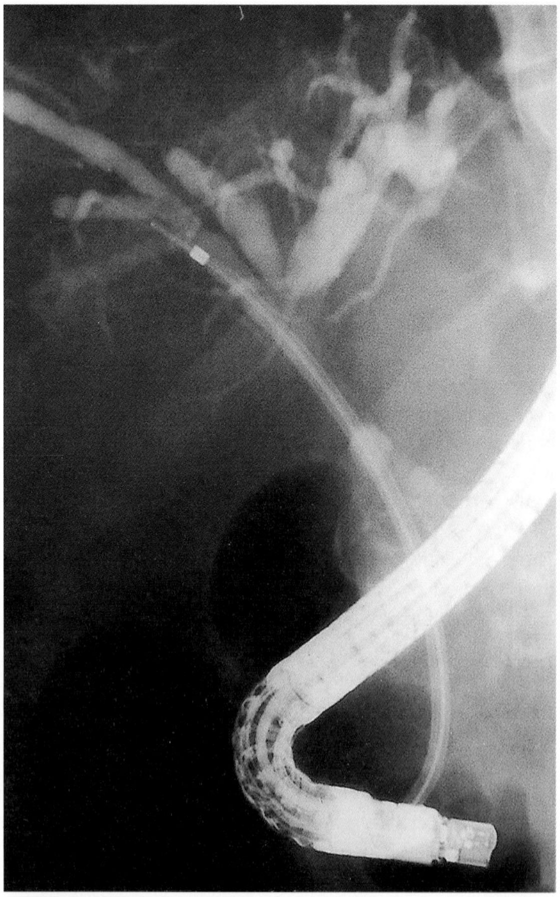

Fig. 20.9 Endoscopic insertion of a biliary stent over a guide wire.

NON-NEOPLASTIC CONDITIONS OF THE LIVER

CONGENITAL CONDITIONS

Biliary atresia

Aetiology and pathological features

The commonest cause of prolonged neonatal jaundice is extrahepatic biliary atresia. The cause is not known. There may be single or multiple points of obstruction, and the proximal ducts may dilate considerably. If not relieved, liver failure ultimately ensues with death in the first year of life, only a few infants surviving beyond 6 months.

Clinical features

Mild jaundice is not uncommon in the neonatal period. However, persistence and progression beyond 2 weeks is definitely abnormal and then the distinction has to be made between obstruction and hepatitis. This can usually be achieved by the biochemical profile (Ch. 4) and ultrasound scanning.

Management

There are two management options:

- For the majority, hepatic portoenterostomy (Kasai operation – Fig. 20.10) should be attempted within 60 days of birth; delay beyond this time is associated with the rapid development of intrahepatic fibrosis and a reduced chance of success.
- When evidence of deteriorating liver function is apparent, liver transplantation should be considered (see Ch. 13).

Congenital cystic disease

Cysts may be solitary or multiple. Multiple cysts are frequently associated with polycystic disease of the kidney (see Ch. 32).

Clinical features

The cysts are often small, asymptomatic and found only incidentally either at laparotomy, during investigation of other problems, or at postmortem examination. Large cysts may present with pain in the right upper abdomen, which may radiate to the right shoulder and is believed to be caused by stretching of the liver capsule.

Management

In a few instances, percutaneous aspiration under image control is used but refilling of the cyst after needle aspiration Is common and so, occasionally, surgical decompression by fenestration or 'de-roofing' is required for the relief of

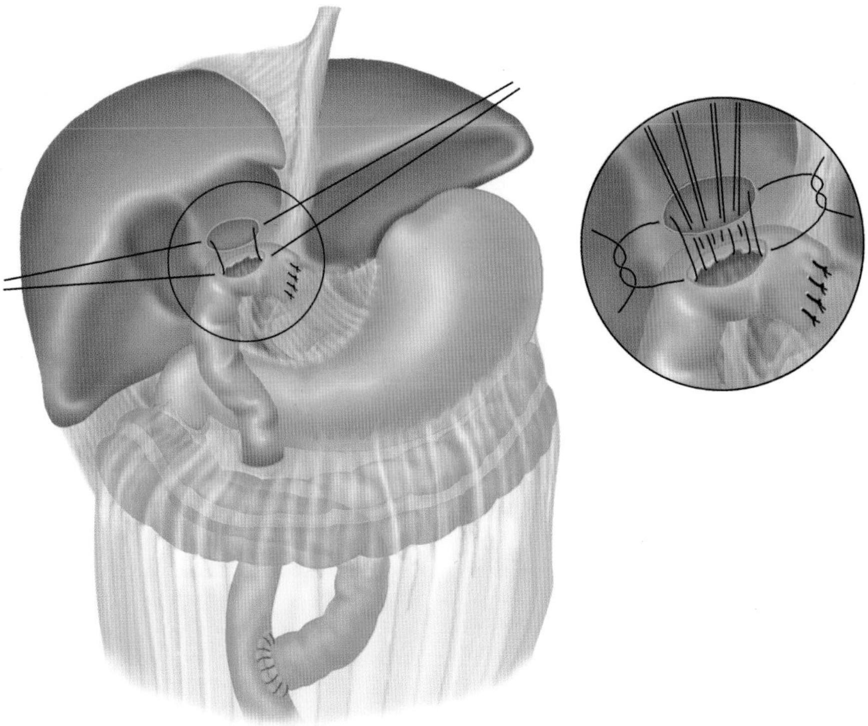

Fig. 20.10 The Kasai operation. A Roux-en-Y loop of jejunum is sutured to the hepatic hilum.

symptoms. Rarely, in cases of multiple cysts located in the right or left liver, resection may be indicated. In patients showing multiple bilateral cysts with compromise of the quality of life and reduced functioning liver parenchyma, liver transplantation should be considered. In cases of polycystic liver and kidney disease associated with terminal renal insufficiency the therapy of choice is a combined liver and renal transplant.

Congenital cystic dilatation of the intrahepatic ducts (Caroli's syndrome)

This is a rare congenital but non-familial disorder with saccular dilatation of the intrahepatic ducts. The cause is not known.

The syndrome is usually diffuse but is occasionally confined to one liver segment or lobe. In some cases there is associated renal tubular ectasia. Clinical features are of recurrent upper abdominal pain and cholangitis in childhood or early adult life. Cholangitis is treated with systemic antibiotics. Localised disease is susceptible to resection. Chronic cholangitis may lead to a secondary biliary cirrhosis. Bile duct carcinoma is described in some cases. Liver transplantation should be considered in patients presenting with a secondary biliary cirrhosis.

Choledochal cyst

This term is used to describe dilatation of all or part of the extrahepatic biliary tree with or without associated cystic change of the intrahepatic bile ducts. Choledochal cysts are classified as follows:

- Type I: cystic (Ia), segmental (Ib), or fusiform (Ic) dilatation of the extrahepatic bile duct
- Type II: the cyst forms a diverticulum from the extrahepatic bile duct
- Type III: cystic dilatation (choledochocele) of the distal common bile duct lying mostly within the duodenal wall
- Type IV: type I associated with intrahepatic bile duct cysts.

Types I and IV are usually associated with an anomalous biliary–pancreatic ductal junction which allows pancreatic juice to flow retrogradely into the biliary tree. These types of choledochal cyst in particular are associated with a much increased risk of cholangiocarcinoma (see below) development. Patients may present with upper abdominal pain and raised liver enzymes and amylase. Others are found incidentally on ultrasound scanning. Surgical excision of the cyst with hepaticojejunostomy Roux-en-Y is normally recommended.

INBORN ERRORS OF METABOLISM

These are discussed in detail in Chapter 13 (see 'Liver transplantation').

HEPATIC TRAUMA

The liver may be injured either by blunt or penetrating injury to the abdomen or chest. The commonest causes are road traffic accident (RTA), sporting injury, falls and violent aggression. In all cases there is a high probability of concomitant serious injury at other sites. Most liver injuries in the UK arise from blunt rather than penetrating trauma and this is in contrast to countries where gun crime is common.

Clinical features

In blunt trauma the liver is the second most common site of injury within the abdomen, after the spleen, and is involved in about 50% of deaths from blunt abdominal trauma. Liver trauma complicates about 15–20% of blunt injuries to the abdomen and of these about half will have splenic trauma. The mechanism of the injury, a sudden compression of the liver between the ribs and the spine, disrupts the hepatic substance and results in a diversity of injury from contusions, subcapsular (contained beneath an intact Glissonian capsule) haematomas or lacerations. The surgical right side of the liver is far more likely to be injured and most blunt injuries involve segments 4, 6, 7 and 8. Associated gallbladder injury or portal triad injury is uncommon and occurs in about 5% of blunt injuries to the liver but is more common in penetrating injuries. Massive haemorrhage, bile leaks, and fistulae are not uncommon in portal triad injury and early mortality or long-term complications are more likely to occur. The risk of mortality from blunt abdominal trauma rises with the severity of the liver injury and with an increase in the number of other organs involved.

Small injuries may not manifest any clinical signs. Larger injuries may show signs of volume loss but it is possible that even an extensive injury may be undetected clinically unless a complication results later.

Management

While the clinical history and diligent clinical examination remain important in the management of abdominal trauma there is little evidence to support decision making based simply only clinical examination.

The type of institution, the haemodynamic status of the patient and the availability of imaging are likely to determine whether imaging is useful in the individual management of blunt abdominal trauma. Immediate focused abdominal ultrasound and CT are both helpful. The sensitivity and specificity of CT imaging has been demonstrated to be high and CT can be used to classify the severity of injury (see Table 20.3), but is not necessarily a guide to management. The decision to operate is complex and includes an assessment of other intra-abdominal injuries. Surgeons have moved increasingly to a non-operative strategy in the management of both blunt and penetrating liver trauma. Most cases of grade I–III are likely to be haemodynamically stable and can be managed by a trauma service without a specialised liver unit. The survival should approach 100% in this setting. The more severe injuries should be transferred to the care of a specialist unit depending of course on the stability of the patient and other concomitant injuries that might take precedence. Even some high-grade injuries in stable patients can be managed non-operatively but complications such as re-bleeding, biloma, abscess, compartment syndrome or other event requiring intervention occur in about 15%. While re-bleeding tends to occur in the early days after injury, infective or biliary complications may not manifest themselves for weeks or months after injury. Injury grade IV or V and requirement for blood transfusion is predictive for a complication in the non-operatively managed patient. In the unstable patient or where laparotomy is performed for other reasons, the initial management of liver trauma, especially by a non-specialist, is simply to control the damage by perihepatic packing using gauze rolls in anticipation of resuscitation and radiological re-evaluation of the liver with possible arterial embolization if required.

The involvement of more than one hepatic vein or a portal triad injury increases the probability that operative management will be required. Immediate vascular or biliary reconstructions are really only for the specialist unit and bile injuries should be controlled by peritoneal drainage and, if possible, bile duct intubation. Massive haemorrhage from a portal vein injury might be controlled by ligation but the resulting liver and bowel ischaemia leads to a very high mortality. Arterial ligation in the presence of intact portal venous inflow is unlikely to cause mortality.

Table 20.3 Classification of liver injury

Grade	Injury	Description
I	Haematoma	Subcapsular <10% surface area
	Laceration	Capsular tear <1 cm parenchymal depth
II	Haematoma	Subcapsular, <10–15% surface area. Intraparenchymal <10 cm diameter
	Laceration	1–3 cm parenchymal depth, <10 cm length
III	Haematoma	Subcapsular >50% surface area. Intraparenchymal >10 cm diameter
	Laceration	More than 3 cm depth
IV	Laceration	Parenchymal disruption involving more than 75% of hepatic lobe
		More than 3 segments within a lobe
V	Vascular	Juxtavenous injuries; i.e. IVC or central hepatic veins

Modified version of AAST liver trauma scoring system, after Moore EE, Cogbill TH, Jurkovich MD, et al: Organ injury scaling: spleen and liver (1994 revision). J Trauma 38:323, 1995

LIVER INFECTIONS

Pyogenic liver abscess

Aetiology

This condition is uncommon in the UK, usually affecting the elderly or debilitated. In 25–50% of sufferers the abscess is cryptogenic, i.e. the primary site of infection remains undiscovered. Biliary infection (cholangitis) is the commonest source; the other main cause is bacterial seeding via the portal vein (portal pyaemia) from an intra-abdominal site – an abscess related to appendicitis, pancreatitis, diverticular disease or perforation of the GI tract. The condition must be distinguished from amoebic abscess (see below).

Pathological features

About half of all liver abscesses are multiple. Solitary abscesses are usually found in the right lobe of the liver, directly under the diaphragm. Common organisms are: *Streptococcus milleri*, *Escherichia coli*, *Streptococcus enterococcus*, *Staphylococcus aureus* and anaerobes such as *Bacteroides* spp.

Liver infections
Neoplasms of the liver
Benign tumours

Clinical features

Presenting symptoms are variable but there is often fever, malaise, anorexia and upper abdominal pain. Jaundice is rare.

Investigation

Laboratory investigation

There may be a neutrophil leucocytosis, secondary anaemia and hypoalbuminaemia.

Imaging

Abdominal and chest X-rays may show a raised right hemidiaphragm, right basal pleural effusion, or an air–fluid level within the liver.

Ultrasound, CT and MRI are the best methods with which to establish the diagnosis and, with prophylactic antibiotics, may be used to guide aspiration to obtain pus for microbiological analysis, often combined with percutaneous drain insertion.

Management

All patients are treated with systemic antibiotics which, in multiple abscesses, may be the only form of treatment feasible. Those large enough to be readily detected on imaging rarely respond to antibiotics alone and require drainage. The morbidity and mortality are high if abscesses are multiple or inadequately drained; in such cases either multiple drains should be placed percutaneously or a surgical procedure will be required.

Hydatid disease

This condition is described in Chapter 9. Liver disease may present with hepatomegaly, which, if the cyst is active or infected, is associated with tenderness. Ultrasound and CT (Fig. 20.11) will show whether a cyst is single or multiple. Both also detect calcification. Calcified cysts are usually dead and therefore do not require treatment. Obstructive jaundice or cholangitis by daughter cysts obstructing the common bile duct is managed initially by endoscopic sphincterotomy. Large, superficially placed and symptomatic cysts may require surgical evacuation with special precautions being taken to kill the brood capsules before the contents are released.

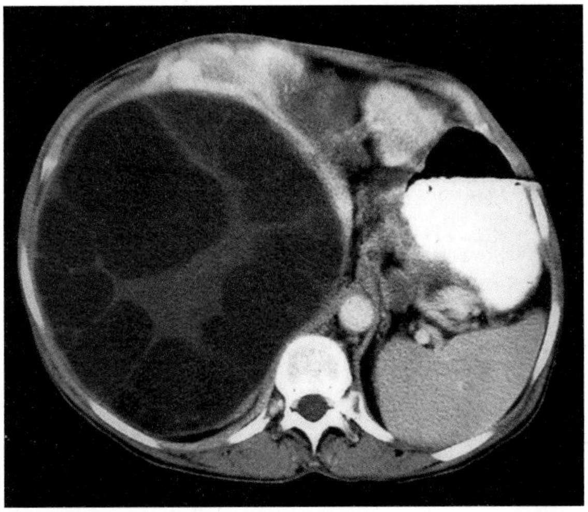

Fig. 20.11 CT scan of a right-sided hepatic hydatid cyst. The daughter cysts can be easily seen.

Amoebic liver abscess

Amoebic liver infection and abscess is a complication of *Entamoeba histolytica* colitis (Ch. 25). The amoebae enter the portal circulation through an ulcer in the colonic mucosa.

Pathological features

The amoebae establish a colony which first leads to hepatitis and then to necrosis and abscess formation most commonly in the upper part of the liver. Extension of the focus may lead to pleural effusion, bronchopleural fistula and lung abscess. Rupture into the peritoneal cavity may also occur.

Clinical features

History

There may or may not have been a background of colitis. There is progressive painful right upper-quadrant pain with sweating, rigors and a swinging pyrexia. Involvement of diaphragm and lung may lead to respiratory symptoms. Shoulder pain is not uncommon.

Physical findings

Right upper-quadrant tenderness, hepatomegaly and jaundice are common findings.

Investigation

Ultrasound or CT delineates the abscess and may be used for image-guided aspiration to obtain a specimen for microscopy and bacteriological culture when secondary contamination is suspected.

Stool examination is routine.

Serology: the amoebic fluorescent antibody titre is raised in 90% of patients.

Management

Metronidazole is specific for amoebic infection, although resistance is increasing. If the patient's condition does not rapidly improve, antibiotic effective against enteric organisms should be prescribed, because of the frequency of secondary infection. Abscesses may need to be aspirated percutaneously under ultrasound/CT guidance, but only occasionally is open operation required.

NEOPLASMS OF THE LIVER

BENIGN TUMOURS

These are common incidental findings and the majority do not cause any symptoms. Larger lesions might cause discomfort depending on size and location or present as biliary disease.

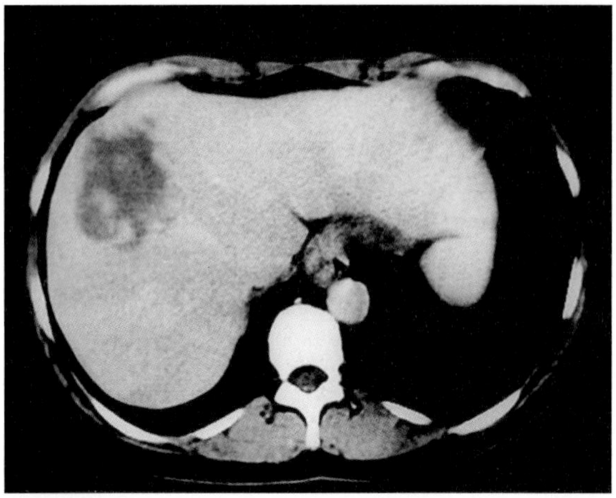

Fig. 20.12 CT scan of the liver, showing a haemangioma.

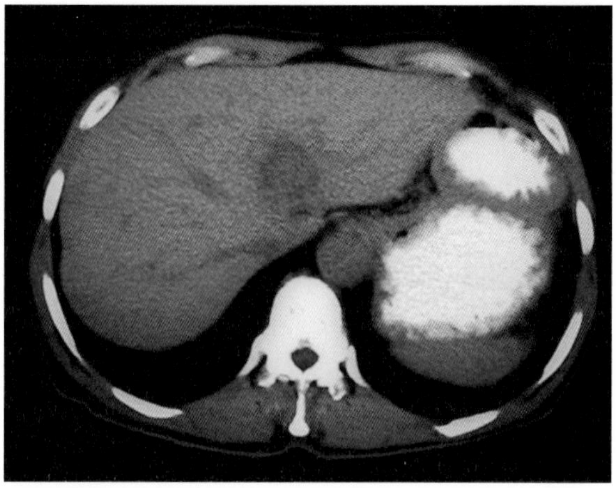

Fig. 20.13 A hepatic adenoma seen on CT scanning.

Haemangioma

The most common benign tumour is cavernous haemangioma. These are composed of thin-walled dilated vessels (Fig. 20.12). The autopsy incidence is up to 20% and small haemangiomata are common in liver imaging. In children the sex distribution is said to be equal but in adults the female : male ratio is 5 : 1.

Usually there are no symptoms but compression of adjacent structures may cause discomfort. Compression of hepatic venous outflow can be a cause of Budd–Chiari syndrome. In large or giant haemangioma rupture or a consumptive coagulopathy (Kasabach–Merritt syndrome) may occur, but thankfully these are rare events.

Imaging by ultrasound shows acoustic enhancement behind the lesion due to improved transmission through the blood within. Ultrasound with contrast can be useful in distinguishing small haemangiomata from malignant tumours. Triple-phase CT has a high sensitivity and specificity for haemangioma and characteristically shows hypo-attenuation in the unenhanced phase, intense enhancement in the arterial phase and pooling of contrast in the venous phase. MRI has a higher degree of sensitivity and specificity for haemangioma. T1-weighted images show hypoattenuation while T2-weighted images are very bright. Use of contrast agents shows peripheral nodular enhancement with centripetal filling. Angiography is seldom helpful over and above non-invasive imaging and is not normally used.

The specificity of imaging does not reach 100% and confusion with other hypervascular lesions such as hepatoma, focal nodular hyperlasia (see below), and hypervascular adenomas and metastases is possible.

Focal nodular hyperplasia (FNH)

This is a benign tumour nearly always in women in the 3rd or 4th decade. FNH is composed of all the normal elements of liver tissue but they are present in a disorganised way. Large malformed blood vessels sit in a fibrous stroma forming a well-defined mass surrounded by normal liver. FNH is usually solitary and asymptomatic. Diagnosis is usually incidental on scanning and confirmed either by CT or MRI to demonstrate the central scar which is present in 80% of FNH. However, diagnostic overlap can occur with well-differentiated HCC or fibrolamellar HCC. A sulphur colloid scan may help. In some cases excision or needle biopsy may be considered or the patient can be reimaged at a suitable interval to assess for growth.

Adenoma

Hepatic adenomas (Fig. 20.13) are composed of normal liver tissues. They may comprise biliary elements and these are common, usually <1 cm, and are called biliary hamartomas.

Adenomas composed of hepatocytes are rare but more common in females, 1/100 000. There is a strong association with oestrogen exposure through contraceptive pill use and which raises the incidence to 4/100 000. Hepatic adenoma can complicate pregnancy and is also linked to glycogen storage disease and diabetes.

Large adenomas can cause discomfort or rupture and cause haemorrhage. Malignant transformation is recorded but very uncommon in small lesions <5 cm.

Distinguishing benign adenoma from malignant lesions is very difficult and no test is specific. A smooth border, intralesional fat or bleeding, and a pseudocapsule suggest, but are not diagnostic of, adenoma. Adenoma do not normally enhance on FDG-PET scan. In some cases excision or needle biopsy may be considered. Alternatively, if the clinical history and imaging do not suggest malignancy, the background liver is normal and the AFP is not elevated these patients can be observed with imaging and AFP monitoring and cessation of oral contraceptives. Larger tumours should be considered for resection not only because of the risk of malignant transformation but also because of the hazard of rupture.

Management

Accurate differentiation from malignant tumours and between the benign tumours is necessary. Haemangioma and FNH are generally observed unless there appears to be tumour growth, symptoms or diagnostic uncertainty. Adenoma can be observed but larger lesions require excision to mitigate the risk of rupture and/or malignant transformation.

MALIGNANT TUMOURS

Malignant tumours of the liver are listed in Box 20.3.

Hepatocellular carcinoma (HCC)

In the West the incidence is 2–5/100 000 but increasing due to the rise in the prevalence of viral hepatitis, mostly hepatitis C. In Africa and the Far East it is far more common with an incidence ten-fold greater than Western populations; the main cause of cirrhosis is hepatitis B in China and South-east Asia but hepatitis C in Japan. Viral hepatitis increases the risk of developing HCC by about 100-fold over the non-infected person. Hepatitis B virus immunization has been shown to reduce the incidence of HCC in Taiwan.

HCC is uncommon in a normal liver and most HCC (80%) occur in the cirrhotic liver.

Clinical features

The patient with HCC is typically in the 5th or 6th decade with a strong male preponderance. The presentation can be very varied and vague especially if superimposed upon the general malaise of chronic liver disease. Patients at risk because of known cirrhosis or viral hepatitis may be under regular follow-up within a liver clinic and HCC diagnosed by routine investigations (AFP or scanning). Pain, weight loss, jaundice and ascites signify advanced disease. Physical examination might reveal hepatomegaly and the signs of chronic liver disease. Features of metastatic disease such as pleural effusion, bone pain, pulmonary embolism or neurological symptoms may be present and indicate disseminated disease.

Diagnosis

Imaging initially is likely to consist of ultrasound scan and about 75% of tumours are multifocal. CT is likely to be more reproducible and precise while MRI more likely to show up smaller lesions not demonstrated on CT and also tumour thrombus in the portal vein, a feature of HCC. AFP is elevated in about 80% of cases and the presence of an enlarging mass >2 cm with radiological characteristics of HCC on two modalities or an enlarging mass >2 cm on one imaging modality but with AFP elevation <500 ng/mL is sufficient to be certain of the diagnosis. Confirmation by percutaneous needle biopsy needs to be carefully considered as there is a risk of tumour seeding into the abdomen and along the needle track.

Box 20.3 Primary malignant tumours of the liver

Hepatocellular
- Hepatocellular carcinoma
- Fibrolamellar variant hepatocellular carcinoma

Biliary system
- Cholangiocarcinoma
- Klatskin tumour (hilar extrahepatic cholangiocarcinoma involving junction of left and right hepatic ducts)

Mesodermal
- Haemangiosarcoma

Predisposing factors are:

- chronic liver disease from viral hepatitis (hepatitis B or C infection)
- alcoholic cirrhosis
- aflatoxin exposure from *Aspergillus flavus*
- hereditary haemochromotosis
- alpha-1 antitrypsin deficiency
- glycogen storage disease
- HIV infection.

Management

The initial principles are management of liver dysfunction – most of these patients will have cirrhosis – and associated complications such as varices, jaundice, coagulopathy and nutritional failure.

The only curative modalities are resection or transplantation. The treatment of HCC remains a difficult area. Benefit from resection is seen only in patients with small tumours <5 cm and well-preserved liver function; such patients are few. Selection for transplantation in HCC is based on the Milan criteria which suggest good results can be obtained in patients transplanted for solitary tumours <5 cm or up to 3 tumours all <3 cm.

Other treatments include:

- Embolisation of the hepatic artery – most malignant tumours in the liver derive their blood supply from the hepatic artery.
- Transcatheter arterial chemo-embolization (TACE) through the hepatic artery based on the same principle to deliver targeted drug, usually doxorubicin, to the tumours. The drug is usually bound to lipiodol which binds to the tumour hepatocytes thus keeping the drug within the tumours. TACE leads to a modest benefit over supportive care alone.
- Local tumour ablation by direct alcohol injection or thermoablation using RFA or microwave, cryotherapy, and more recently yttrium-90 labelled glass microsphere embolisation (TheraSphere®).
- Systemic therapies in various cytotoxic regimens sometimes in combination with immunomodulatory agents such as interferon-alpha have been studied but as yet the only agent to show statistically significant benefit in Phase III studies is the multi-targetted tyrosine kinase inhibitor sorafenib.

Fibrolamellar HCC

This variant of HCC has its own characteristics and natural history that distinguish it from the common HCC. Fibrolamellar HCC occurs in a much younger population (2nd or 3rd decade) and usually on the background of a normal liver. The clinical presentation may be with pain, mass or cachexia. The liver function tests are usually abnormal but the AFP is not elevated and patients do not usually have hepatitis or cirrhosis. Distant disease is not common although regional nodal disease occurs.

Prognosis is said to be better than HCC and if possible aggressive resection is indicated. However, recurrence within 2 years is common.

Diagnosis can be made confidently on CT scan but diagnostic confusion between fibrolamellar HCC and FNH can occur as fibrolamellar HCC can have a central scar in some cases. Calcification within the tumour is seen in about 40% of cases. Secretion of neuroendocrine hormones such as pancreatic polypeptide, gastrin, C-peptide and calcitonin may cause paraneoplastic phenomena.

Non-epithelial cancers such as haemangiosarcoma and carcinoids of the liver are very uncommon.

Intrahepatic cholangiocarcinoma

Aetiology and pathological features

Cholangiocarcinoma may be either intra- or extrahepatic. Primary sclerosing cholangitis, exposure to thorotrast and infection with liver fluke increase the incidence of cholangiocarcinomas. Extrahepatic cholangiocarcinoma are strongly associated with smoking and the tumour causes a fibrous stricturing of the bile ducts and almost always the presentation is with features of biliary obstruction. These are more fully discussed below. The incidence of intrahepatic cholangiocarcinoma is said to be higher in patients with viral hepatitis or HIV infection.

Clinical features

The symptoms of intrahepatic cholangiocarcinoma may be vague with upper abdominal discomfort, malaise or a right upper quadrant mass. Pain, weight loss, jaundice or ascites are features of late disease. The tumour marker CA19.9 is sometimes elevated .

Investigation

A combination of ultrasonography and CT or MRI may provide the diagnosis and location but distinguishing intrahepatic cholangiocarcinoma from hepatocellular carcinoma on cross-sectional imaging may be difficult.

Needle liver biopsy

In cases of irresectable tumour or in patients unsuitable for radical surgical treatment, the diagnosis may be confirmed by needle biopsy. The needle is directed into the tumour under ultrasound or CT scan guidance. It is obviously easier to obtain cells from larger, more accessible tumours. It should be noted that it is not always possible to diagnose the tumour on the basis of needle biopsy, and that biopsy carries a small risk of seeding tumour along the needle track.

Management

Resection is the best therapy as these tumours are poorly reponsive to chemotherapy. Transplantation is proposed as eventual therapy in some cases.

Metastatic cancer

Epidemiology

Metastatic disease to the liver commonly arises from primary cancers in the colon, pancreas, stomach, breast, lung and small intestine. In Western countries a solid mass in the liver is much more likely to be metastatic disease than a primary liver cancer. Autopsy data show that liver metastases are present in about 50% of all patients dying of cancer.

Clinical features

Liver metastases seldom cause symptoms and are either an incidental findings in the investigation of other tumour-related symptoms or are detected during the staging process of known primary cancers.

Investigation

The detection of metastatic disease involves the use of the extracorporeal imaging modalities of MRI and CT-PET scanning. CT-PET is best for detection of extrahepatic metastases. MRI is best for intrahepatic metastatic disease and is used for surgical planning. The majority of livers with metastatic disease will have multiple lesions and only about 10% are solitary metastases. Bilobar disease is not uncommon.

Management

The presence of liver metastases is a poor prognostic feature and, untreated, these patients are unlikely to survive more than a few months. Liver resection can be considered if all disease can be removed (or ablated) whilst leaving adequate functioning liver tissue. This is usually only done in the absence of extrahepatic metastatic disease, and is most often performed for patients with treated colorectal primary adenocarcinomas.

Results of surgery

There are a number of important observations:

- The treatment of metastatic colorectal cancer has improved vastly in the past decade and is now commonly treated by surgery. Data accumulated from many large prospective and retrospective cohort studies all suggest that long-term cure following the surgical removal of liver-only metastases in patients with otherwise curable colorectal cancer is possible in about 50–60% of cases. A prospective randomised study has never been conducted and it is most unlikely that such a study containing a 'no treatment' arm will ever be performed.
- The results from resection are superior to other means of treatment such as systemic chemotherapy, embolisation, radiation or regional intra-arterial infusion of chemotherapy, all of which are now considered only in palliative cases not suitable for radical surgical resection. Even in those patients achieving complete radiological response from systemic chemotherapy, the recurrence or reappearance rate of treated metastases is about 80%.
- About 25% of new cases of colorectal cancer will have liver metastases at initial presentation (synchronous disease) and about 50% of cases will develop liver metastases some time later (metachronous disease).
- Only about 25–30% of liver metastases from colorectal cancer are resectable at presentation. The use of systemic chemotherapy to downsize bulky disease increases the resectable population and adjuvant chemotherapy following complete resection of liver metastases appears to reduce the risk of relapse in the liver and has been shown to improve long-term survival.
- Direct regional infusion of chemotherapy into the hepatic artery is also effective in downsizing disease

and preventing future relapse in the liver but the advantages of this method over systemic delivery of combination chemotherapy are uncertain.

Patient and treatment selection

In the surgical approach to liver metastases the surgeon needs to consider the principles of liver surgery and oncologic integrity.

- The post-resection liver should have adequate inflow and outflow and with adequate parenchymal mass to maintain life until liver regeneration has taken place. As yet no easy and reliable method exists to predict the liver's capacity to regenerate and its residual liver function. Surgeons should take into account the quality of the liver parenchyma, the age of the patient, the size of the liver remnant, exposure to neoadjuvant chemotherapy and comorbid factors such as obesity and diabetes.
- In the past it was felt that a wide margin of tumour clearance >1 cm was necessary for good local control but this view is now altered such that a histologically clear margin in the resected specimen yields equivalent results. Positive margins at resection lead to a high local recurrence rate.
- Where a single resection cannot adequately clear all evaluable disease the liver surgeon might seek to combine the surgical approach with thermoablation techniques such as cryotherapy or more commonly radiofrequency ablation (RFA) either at the time of operation or separately by a radiologically guided percutaneous approach. In some cases a staged approach involving a second operation following liver regeneration might be the most appropriate strategy.
- Combining the various techniques of surgery, RFA, portal vein embolisation (used to produce regeneration of the non-embolised lobe preoperatively) and staged resections with the use of neoadjuvant chemotherapy allows a greater number of patients to be treated and potentially cured. This multidisciplinary approach allows about 50% of patients with metastatic colorectal cancer to be treated with operative mortality of <5%.
- RFA is probably equivalent to surgery in small tumours <2 cm and can probably be substituted for surgery in livers with a small number of small metastases. Since the morbidity is much less, RFA is an ideal modality for the fragile patient. The limitation of RFA to adequately treat liver tumours means that at present surgical removal of tumours is still the accepted 'gold standard'. Difficulties with RFA relate to tumours located close to major vessels where cooling from blood flow may impair thermoablation or lesional size at either extreme – small tumours are difficult to target accurately and larger tumours cannot be heated adequately to ensure good tumour necrosis.
- In inoperable patients regional infusion of chemotherapy by intra-arterial catheter carries a significant morbidity and while the reduction in tumour size and progression-free interval of such patients is improved, this does not translate into an increase in overall survival over and above that which might be achieved with systemic chemotherapy.
- Prognostic factors that predicate a poor prognosis following liver resection of metastases from colorectal cancer are a short disease-free interval, multiple large metastases, bilaterality, positive margins following resection, extra-hepatic disease, poor response to systemic chemotherapy, very high preoperative CEA, and synchronous presentation.
- Other tumour types where liver resection for metastases has an important role are neuroendorine tumours of the GI tract. The presence of liver metastases often gives rise to physical symptoms or functional syndromes from hormone production. Complete surgical removal or debulking of metastatic disease in selected cases can be a most useful treatment.

Complications of surgery

Liver surgery for metastatic disease is not without complication. Major complications such as bile leak, abscess and haemorrhage occur with a frequency of about 2–5% and liver failure in about 2–3% of resections. Preoperative chemotherapy has a significant damaging effect on the liver, causing steatosis and fibrosis, and increases the risk of complications.

Liver transplantation

This is discussed in Chapter 13.

GALLSTONES (CHOLELITHIASIS)

Epidemiology

Gallstones are very common, with a prevalence of 10–15%. Although the aphorism that gallstones arise in 'fair, fat and fertile females in their fifties' often holds true, stones can affect patients of all ages and both sexes. However, they are 2–4 times more common in women. Cholesterol is the principal constituent of the great majority of stones, either as a pure cholesterol stone (20%) or as a mixed one combined with deconjugated bile pigment, especially bilirubin (75%). Stones composed of pigment alone account for the remaining 5%. Types of gallstone are described in Table 20.4.

Aetiology

The following three factors predispose to gallstone formation.

Table 20.4 Gallstones – type and classification

	Constituents	Consistency	Radio-opaque on CT scanning (%)
Cholesterol	Cholesterol	Crystalline hard	15–20
Black pigment	Bilirubin	Hard	60–70
Brown pigment	Calcium bilirubinate	Soft	0

Cholesterol supersaturation

Although cholesterol is insoluble in water, in bile it is normally solubilised in lecithin–bile acid aggregates (known as micelles). If the concentration of cholesterol in bile is high, the capacity of this mechanism may be exceeded – cholesterol supersaturation. Cholesterol supersaturation occurs when:

- plasma oestrogen levels are increased – e.g. obesity, pregnancy and in women taking oral contraceptives
- there is depletion of the bile acid pool – e.g. in resection or disease of the terminal ileum which interrupts the enterohepatic circulation.

Stasis of bile

Stone formation is enhanced by a reduced rate of bile flow (stasis), which occurs particularly in:

- fasting – lack of food stimulus to gallbladder emptying
- total parenteral nutrition – for the same reason as fasting
- truncal vagotomy – loss of neural stimulus to gallbladder emptying.

Increased bilirubin secretion in bile, or deconjugation

Bilirubin is kept in solution in bile by conjugation with glucuronide. Pigment stones are encountered when there is:

- increased breakdown of red blood cells – haemolytic disorders such as spherocytosis, sickle cell disease and malaria
- failure of conjugation – hepatocyte insufficiency in the formation of glucuronide, or excess glucuronidase; the latter may be the consequence of bacterial activity, but the role of infection in stone formation remains uncertain and bacteria may be a consequence of stones rather than their cause.

Clinical features

Asymptomatic stones

Gallstones anywhere in the biliary tree may remain asymptomatic (silent) and therefore undetected for many years. Ultrasound scanning done on patients with vague abdominal symptoms has resulted in more frequent discovery of such incidental stones.

Symptomatic stones

Stones become clinically evident by the complications they cause, which are classified according to their anatomical site (Box 20.4).

Box 20.4 Complications of gallstones

Gallbladder
- Biliary colic
- Acute cholecystitis
- Empyema
- Mucocele
- Cancer

Common bile duct
- Obstructive jaundice
- Cholangitis
- Pancreatitis

Small intestine
- Gallstone ileus

STONES IN THE GALLBLADDER: URGENT MANAGEMENT

Biliary colic

Clinical features

History

A stone impacted within the gallbladder – usually in Hartmann's pouch or the cystic duct – causes pain. Although often referred to as colic, the pain is usually constant in the epigastrium and right upper quadrant and may radiate through to the back in the region of the inferior angle of the scapula. Such pain is better called obstructive (see also 'Renal colic', Ch. 32). Attacks last for a few minutes to half an hour and may be exacerbated by ingestion of fatty food which stimulates the release of cholecystokinin (CCK) and consequent gallbladder contraction. Vomiting is common. Fever is absent. The pain spontaneously settles when the stone either becomes disimpacted or, less commonly, is passed into the common bile duct. Recurrent attacks are common and often of variable duration and severity.

Physical findings

The patient is apyrexial. Abdominal tenderness is usually absent.

Investigation

Blood examination

The white cell count, serum amylase and C-reactive protein are usually normal. There may be mild elevation of alkaline phosphatase and/or aspartate transferase.

Imaging (Table 20.5)

Ultrasound reliably detects 98% of gallbladder stones (Fig. 20.14) but is less reliable in identifying those that are within the bile ducts. In addition, ultrasound can also provide information about the:

- thickness of the gallbladder wall, an increase above normal being indicative of past or present inflammation
- diameter of the common bile duct
- architecture of the liver and pancreas.

Should stones be detected in a bile duct, the choice of management lies between ERCP with sphincterotomy and ductal stone extraction and laparoscopic cholecystectomy with bile duct clearance (see below).

Management

The initial administration of a parenteral analgesic such as morphine or pethidine relieves the acute exacerbations of pain, and over a few hours the condition nearly always resolves. If the diagnosis is confirmed by imaging, subsequent cholecystectomy is usually indicated. Chronic cholecystitis is the usual pathological finding on histology. This entity is the outcome of recurrent attacks of obstruction and

Stones in the gallbladder: urgent management

Table 20.5 Imaging in gallstone disease

Investigation	Information	Comments
Plain X-ray	10% of gallbladder stones	Not a useful investigation
Ultrasound (external)	98% of gallbladder stones	Unreliable for duct stones
Endoscopic ultrasound	99% gallbladder stones	Operator dependent Useful for small stones
MRCP	Shows gallbladder + duct	Best non-invasive method for ductal stones
HIDA, hepatic iminodiacetic acid – radionuclide scan	Shows bilary excretory function	Occasionally useful for assessing possible biliary tract obstruction, e.g. ductal stricture

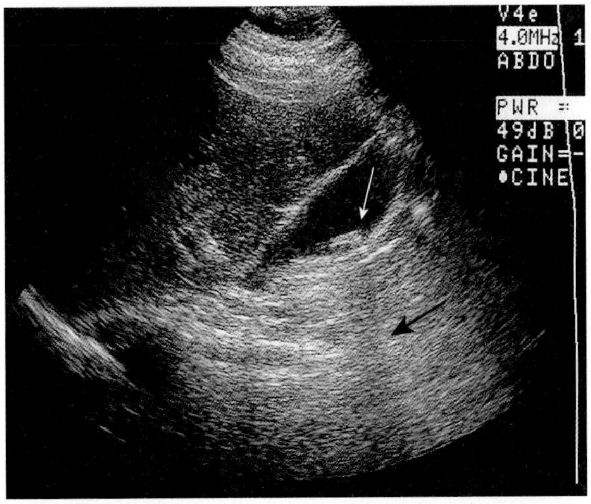

Fig. 20.14 Gallbladder stones (white arrow) detected with ultrasound – note 'acoustic shadow' (black arrow).

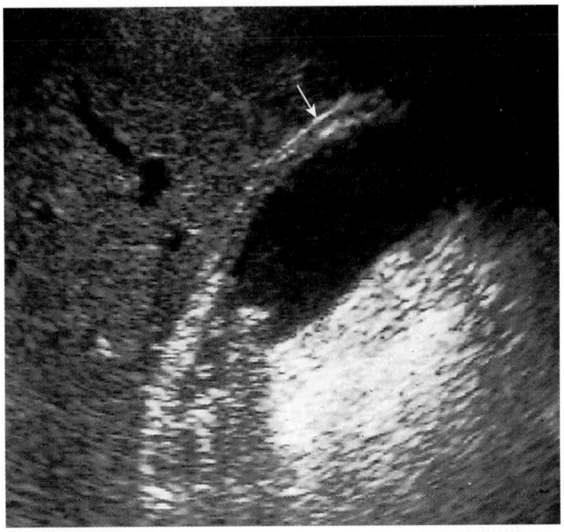

Fig. 20.15 Acute calculous cholecystitis confirmed on ultrasound scanning. Note thickened (oedematous) wall – white arrow.

inflammation which result in the changes of chronic inflammation in the gallbladder wall.

Acute cholecystitis

When a stone impacts at the outlet of the gallbladder, water continues to be absorbed through the gallbladder wall, and the concentrated bile can initiate a chemical cholecystitis. Secondary infection superimposed on this generates acute bacterial cholecystitis.

Clinical features

History

The symptoms are similar to those of biliary colic, but the pain is more severe and persistent. Nausea and vomiting are not uncommon, and fever is usually present.

Physical findings

Tenderness and guarding are often present in the right upper quadrant. In less severe instances, laying the hand lightly on the upper right abdomen and asking the patient to take a deep breath cause a catch in breath because of pain when the inflamed gallbladder impacts on the examining hand – Murphy's sign. Hyperaesthesia of skin over the right ribs 9–11 posteriorly (Boas's sign) may also be present. If inflammation spreads beyond the gallbladder, a mass, composed of the enlarged gallbladder and adherent omentum and bowel, may be palpated under the right costal margin.

Investigation

Blood examination

There is leucocytosis and the bilirubin concentration and liver enzymes may be mildly raised either as a result of partial obstruction of the common hepatic duct by a stone lodged in Hartmann's pouch or because of local inflammation. The serum amylase concentration may be moderately elevated but not to the levels seen in acute pancreatitis (Ch. 22).

Imaging

Ultrasound shows the enlarged gallbladder with stone(s), a thickened wall and a surrounding rim of pericholecystic fluid from local oedema (Fig. 20.15).

Management

Initial treatment is non-operative, with pain relief and systemic antibiotics. Intravenous fluids may be required. Most attacks resolve, and definitive treatment by cholecystectomy is done during the initial hospital admission. Interval surgery (4–6 weeks) is now less common; it is inconvenient for the patient and carries no advantage over operation early in the course of the episode.

In a few patients the initial attack does not resolve with antibiotic treatment because a perforation of the gallbladder or the formation of an empyema occurs. If progression is thought to be taking place despite antibiotic treatment, as judged by failure of symptoms to subside and the persistence of local signs, the gallbladder should be drained percutaneously by ultrasound-guided cholecystostomy or laparoscopy (or laparotomy) performed with a view to cholecystectomy or gallbladder drainage.

Free perforation

This is caused by a progressive rise in tension in the gallbladder; the blood supply of the wall is reduced, and gangrene occurs, usually at the fundus. Abdominal pain becomes increasingly severe and more generalised. Perforation may lead to diffuse peritonitis or a pericholecystic abscess which demands urgent exploration, peritoneal lavage and a cholecystectomy.

Mucocele

A stone may impact in the neck of the gallbladder without causing inflammation either from the concentrated bile or from secondary infection. The result is a mucocele – a distended gallbladder full of clear mucus. Cholecystectomy is indicated.

COMMON BILE DUCT STONES (CHOLEDOCHOLITHIASIS): URGENT MANAGEMENT

Obstructive jaundice

Impaction of a stone in the common bile duct, usually at the duodenal papilla, causes obstructive jaundice. There may have been preceding biliary colic, but the main presenting complaints are jaundice, pruritis, dark urine and pale bulky stools. Little is to be found on clinical examination, and in particular the gallbladder is impalpable because it is likely to have undergone inflammation and fibrosis and is thus unable to distend.

Investigation

Ultrasound usually shows dilatation of the bile ducts and may identify ductal stones. MRCP or ERCP confirms the diagnosis and differentiates a stone and other causes of obstructive jaundice.

Management

There is a choice for management of bile duct stones – either endoscopic (ERCP) or laparoscopic (or occasionally open) surgery. ERCP with sphincterotomy of the lower bile duct sphincter of Oddi (or balloon sphincter dilatation) and extraction of the ductal stone(s) is commonly used. Subsequently, if it has not already been done, the gallbladder should be removed unless the patient is elderly or at high operative risk. The alternative, particularly if the gallbladder has not been removed previously and the patient is fit, is laparoscopic cholecystectomy with bile duct clearance using either a transcystic (via the cystic duct) or choledochotomy (incision into the common bile duct) technique. Occasionally open operation is indicated or becomes necessary during a laparoscopic procedure. Both approaches are currently used.

Acute cholangitis

Aetiology and pathological features

Organisms enter the biliary tree either from the gastrointestinal tract via the duodenal papilla or by excretion in the bile after reaching the liver via the bloodstream. In the bile they multiply in the presence of obstruction to cause inflammation. Ductal stones are the cause in the Western world. On the Pacific rim, parasitic infection with liver flukes (*Clonorchis sinensis*) and ascariasis are associated with secondary bacterial cholangitis. The causative organism is usually a Gram-negative enteric bacterium, typically *Escherichia coli*.

Infected bile in the biliary tree is potentially fatal because it may lead to septicaemia and hepatorenal failure. Long-term sequelae of repeated attacks of cholangitis include liver abscesses, secondary biliary cirrhosis, liver failure and portal hypertension.

Clinical features

A past history of biliary disease may be obtained. Presentation is with abdominal pain, high fever with rigors and jaundice (sometimes termed Charcot's triad). In addition, elderly patients are often confused and hypotensive (Reynold's pentad). The liver may be somewhat enlarged and tender. The gallbladder is impalpable.

Investigation

The white cell count will usually reveal leucocytosis, while liver function tests will show cholestasis. There is a positive blood culture in most instances.

Ultrasound or CT scanning may show gallbladder stones, a dilated duct and sometimes a ductal stone.

Management

Resuscitation with intravenous fluids and parenteral antibiotics is begun on a best-guess basis. A prompt response will result in relief of symptoms, resolution of fever and rapid reduction in jaundice. Failure to achieve this indicates the need for bile duct drainage by urgent ERCP or PTC. If possible, stones should be extracted, but effective biliary drainage is the first essential requirement. Definitive treatment of cholelithiasis can be deferred until the acute episode has settled.

STONES IN THE SMALL INTESTINE: URGENT MANAGEMENT

Gallstone ileus

Aetiology

A gallbladder which contains stones may erode into adjacent small bowel, usually the duodenum. Stones can then be shed through this cholecystenteric fistula into the gut. A large stone that has a diameter greater than the narrowest part of the small bowel (terminal ileum) may impact to produce lower small-bowel obstruction (Ch. 24).

Clinical features

The biliary tract disorder is usually silent, particularly, as is often so, when the patient is elderly. Vague attacks of colic may have occurred as the stone passes down the gut. Eventually the history is of low small-bowel obstruction.

Physical findings are discussed in Chapter 24.

Investigation

In addition to the characteristic features of small-bowel obstruction on a plain radiograph or CT scanning, it may be possible to see:

- air in the biliary tract (aerobilia)
- a calcified gallstone in the right lower quadrant.

Management

The condition is usually found at operation for small-bowel obstruction without a clear cause. A soft stone is crushed from without; a harder one is milked retrogradely and extracted via a small enterotomy. The small bowel proximal to the obstruction is carefully examined to exclude other stones. Treatment of the fistula should be deferred and may not be required.

GENERAL MANAGEMENT OF GALLSTONES

Stones in the gallbladder

The approach in the case of the patient with silent or with relatively uncomplicated gallstones which cause symptoms such as recurrent biliary colic is still subject to some controversy.

Asymptomatic stones

Only about a third of patients will become symptomatic, with an annual incidence of symptom development of approximately 1%. Therefore, for most patients, operation is not advised. Operation may be considered in the following cases:

- There is a non-functioning gallbladder which is thought to render an attack of acute cholecystitis more likely.
- In diabetics, because this condition carries a greater risk of complications following the development of such features as biliary colic or cholecystitis; elective operations for silent stones may pre-empt this risk.
- A cholecystenteric fistula has been identified.
- The patient is young.

Symptomatic stones

The common presentation is with acute episodes of biliary colic or acute cholecystitis. Occurrence of one of these is an indication for operation unless:

- the patient refuses, or
- there are strong medical contraindications such as cardiorespiratory disease, although it must be remembered that a further acute attack may lead to disastrous decompensation.

Surgical management

Cholecystectomy constitutes the treatment of choice in patients who have had biliary colic, acute cholecystitis or a previous episode of obstructive jaundice caused by a stone. However, it is unwise to remove the gallbladder for vague upper abdominal pain or doubtful findings on ultrasound, because symptoms often persist postoperatively.

Before operation, consideration should always be given to the possibility of choledocholithiasis. Common bile duct stones may be detected by ultrasound, CT, MRCP or operative cholangiography. There are many permutations and combinations regarding the diagnosis, timing and method of extraction of common bile duct stones. Some surgeons perform operative cholangiography on all patients, others opt for a selective policy and some surgeons never use this technique relying instead on other imaging modalities. Factors which alert the surgeon to the possibility of choledocholithiasis include:

- history of jaundice or pancreatitis in the preceding 6 months
- elevation of serum bilirubin or alkaline phosphatase concentrations
- dilatation of the common bile duct beyond 10 mm on ultrasound scanning.

Cholecystectomy is a procedure now almost always done by laparoscopic means (see Ch. 5) and with a mortality well below 1%. In acute cholecystitis, cholecystectomy is done early (within 48 hours of the onset of symptoms) either as a standard policy to avoid recurrent attacks of cholecystitis or because symptoms and signs have failed to resolve.

Complications include:

- leak of bile from the gallbladder bed, the stump of the cystic duct or injured bile duct, which leads to an intraperitoneal accumulation and possible biliary peritonitis
- bleeding from a ligature that has slipped off the cystic artery
- operative damage to the bile ducts.

The last of these is the most serious, and its occurrence temporarily increased after the introduction of laparoscopic cholecystectomy. It is prevented by a sound understanding of the possible ductal anatomical variations and by careful operative technique. If it occurs, it may be recognised at once and repaired (although a stricture may still subsequently result) or it may present postoperatively with a bile leak, recurrent attacks of cholangitis or obstructive jaundice.

Late complications of damage to the bile ducts are best dealt with at specialised hepatobiliary centres by dissection and anastomosis of the dilated ducts above the site of obstruction to the small intestine usually via an isolated loop (hepaticojejunostomy Roux-en-Y).

Stones in the bile ducts

These may be the prime cause of symptoms or be present along with gallbladder stones and identified either preoperatively or by cholangiography during operation. In either event they should be removed. The choice for ductal stone extraction lies between the following:

- pre- or postoperative ERCP in combination with laparoscopic cholecystectomy
- cholecystectomy and exploration of the common bile duct either at open operation or laparoscopically.

Each approach has advantages and potential problems.

Common bile duct stones (choledocholithiasis): urgent management
Stones in the small intestine: urgent management
General management of gallstones

ACALCULOUS CHOLECYSTITIS

Aetiology and pathological features

Acute cholecystitis may develop in the absence of gallstones. This primary (or acalculous) cholecystitis usually afflicts very ill, often diabetic, patients in an intensive care unit, suffering from burns or the septic complications of major surgery. The condition is a severe form of acute cholecystitis which often progresses to gangrene and perforation. The mortality may approach 15%.

Clinical features

The coexistence of other serious illnesses in a patient who may be unconscious often masks the diagnosis. It is important to remember the possibility in a critically ill patient who develops signs of an acute abdomen.

Investigation

Diagnostic features on ultrasound or CT scanning are those of gallbladder dilatation with oedema in the wall.

Management

Percutaneous cholecystostomy under ultrasound guidance with gallbladder drainage and parenteral antibiotics may suffice unless perforation has occurred, in which case cholecystectomy is required.

GALLBLADDER TUMOURS

Benign

Adenoma

This is an uncommon tumour which predisposes to gallbladder carcinoma. It is usually an incidental finding on ultrasound scanning. Adenomas less than 1 cm in diameter can be observed, but larger ones should be removed by cholecystectomy as there is an elevated risk of malignancy.

Three other conditions can mimic the appearance of an adenoma on ultrasound:

- **Cholesterosis,** in which plaques of cholesterol are laid down in the gallbladder mucosa and cause a thickened irregular mucosal appearance which is sometimes known as strawberry gallbladder. Cholecystectomy is indicated in patients with symptoms provided these are clearly related to the biliary tree.
- **Soft adherent non-calcified stones** which may be difficult to distinguish from adenomas on scanning.
- **Adenomyoma** is a localised collection of cystic spaces in the gallbladder wall; it is a benign condition and, in its generalised form, is known as adenomyomatosis.

Malignant

Epidemiology, aetiology and clinical presentation

Cancer of the gallbladder is rare and the peak incidence is in the 60–80 year age range. There is a wide geographic variation of incidence. The highest incidence is among women in India, South America and the Far East. The lowest incidence is in the countries of North-West Europe. In the United States about 10 000 new diagnoses of gallbladder cancer are made every year.

Ninety-five percent are associated with gallstones, and this is reflected in the male:female ratio of 3:7 in the UK. Other risk factors include previous cholecystitis, a family history of gallbladder cancer or gallstones, a porcelain gallbladder (calcification of the gallbladder wall), smoking, obesity and the presence of a gallbladder adenoma (see above). Ninety percent of the growths are adenocarcinomas, and the remaining 10% are squamous carcinomas which are believed to arise from areas of mucosal squamous metaplasia. The presentation might be with vague symptoms of malaise, upper abdominal discomfort and nausea. Pain, jaundice or a palpable right upper quadrant mass imply advanced disease. Careful examination of routine cholecystectomy specimens where gallbladder cancer was not suspected preoperatively suggests an incidence of 1%.

Pathological features

Gallbladder cancers tend to invade locally into the adjacent liver. They have a dismal prognosis because the great majority have invaded the liver beyond resectability at the time of presentation. The overall 5-year survival is 2–5%. The only tumours with a favourable prognosis are those early cancers found during pathological examination of a gallbladder removed for biliary symptoms.

Surgical management

The standard operation for gallbladder carcinoma is the ‘en bloc’ cholecystectomy, which means cholecystectomy with resection of liver segments V–IV. In some cases lymphadenectomy of the hepatoduodenal ligament extended to the hepatic artery is done. Patients having a diagnosis of an incidental carcinoma found on histopathology after routine cholecystectomy should be considered for radical surgery depending on the stage and site of the tumour. Many early cancers are cured by cholecystectomy alone.

Cholangiocarcinoma

Cancers of the bile ducts are not common, comprising about 2% of all GI tract malignancy with an incidence of 1/100 000. Cholangiocarcinomas may arise anywhere in the biliary system and for surgical purposes are divided into intrahepatic or extrahepatic. The extrahepatic sites include the upper end of the extraheptatic bile duct (hilar tumours) and the distal end of the bile duct. The tumours show a submucosal growth pattern and microscopic examination shows the cancer spreading 10–20 mm either side of the visible disease. Lymphotropic and neurotropic metastases are common and the presence of nodal disease is a strong predictor of poor outcome. Only about 20% of patients are surgical candidates. The proximity of the bile duct to other structures in the hepatic ligament such as the portal vein and hepatic artery means that invasion of these occurs early and often the local extent of disease prevents curative surgery or distant metastatic disease is already evident. All cholangiocarcinomas are poorly sensitive to chemotherapy and the only curative modality is radical surgical resection. These are aggressive cancers and prognosis is poor except for cancers detected and operated for early-stage disease. The histologic type is adenocarcinoma in nearly all cases although squamous cell and neuroendocrine types are occasionally seen.

Extrahepatic cholangiocarcinoma

The presentation is usually (>90%) with painless jaundice as the tumour obstructs the bile duct. Other non-specific symptoms such as itching, weight loss and anorexia are each seen in about a quarter of cases. The patient undergoes evaluation of the site of obstruction by invasive investigations such as ERCP or PTC or more commonly now by non-invasive investigations such as CT and MRI. Distal bile duct cholangiocarcinomas may show as a mass in the periampullary region while a hilar cholangiocarcinoma may produce a mass in the liver hilum. Distal cholangiocarcinoma are managed as for head of pancreas cancer (Ch. 22) and comprise about 40% of all extrahepatic cholangiocarcinoma. Hilar cholangiocarcinomas, or as they are sometimes called Klatskin tumours, involve the upper end of the bile duct at the biliary confluence and comprise about 60% of extrahepatic cholangiosarcomas.

Choledochal cyst, primary sclerosing cholangitis and infestation with parasites such as *Clonorchis sinensis* and *Opisthorchis viverrin* are recognised predisposing conditions. Other risk factors are smoking and oriental cholangiohepatitis.

The Bismuth-Corlette classification divides these tumours into 4 groups according to site (Box 20.5). Involvement of the local vessels, the portal vein and hepatic artery are particularly important in the surgical evaluation of hilar cholangiocarcinoma. This can usually be satisfactorily be achieved by CT angiography or MR angiography. The use of PET scan in the staging of hilar cholangiocarcinoma identifies a further 20% or so of patients that have disease not identified on conventional anatomic imaging.

The Type IV hilar cholangiocarcinoma is often regarded as being irresectable. Surgery usually involves resection of the extrahepatic biliary system combined with partial hepatectomy. It is thought important to resect the caudate lobe when dealing with a hilar cholangiocarcinoma.

Box 20.5 Bismuth-Corlette classification of hilar cholangiocarcinoma

Type I – Below the confluence
Type II – Confined to confluence
Type IIIa – Extension into right hepatic duct
Type IIIb – Extension into left hepatic duct
Type IV – Extension into right and left hepatic ducts

Preoperative cytological or histological confirmation is difficult to obtain and the decision to treat surgically is based on the clinical history and imaging findings. Inoperable patients are treated by relief of the jaundice by biliary stenting with endoprosthesis. Biliary stents can be deployed either at ERCP or by percutaneous approach, PTC. A plastic stent might last 3–4 months before becoming occluded by biliary debris and then the patient becomes jaundiced again requiring re-stenting. Metallic expanding biliary stents although more costly, have prolonged patency.

Palliative therapies such as chemotherapy, radiotherapy or photodynamic therapy are usually contingent upon obtaining histological or cytological proof of malignancy. Liver transplant has occasionally been employed in hilar cholangiocarcinoma, but its use is currently very limited. Data from the Mayo Clinic suggests that good results can be obtained in carefully selected patients using a combination of high-dose radiotherapy followed by liver transplantation.

FURTHER READING

Blumgart LH 2006 Surgery of the liver and biliary tract and pancreas, 2 volume set, 4th edn. Saunders, Philadelphia

Garden OJ 2009 Hepatobiliary and pancreatic surgery: a companion to specialist surgical practice, 4th edn. Saunders, Edinburgh

Garden OJ, Rees M, Poston GJ et al 2006 Guidelines for resection of colorectal liver metastases. Gut. Online. Available: www.gutbmj.com

21 The spleen

STRUCTURE AND FUNCTION OF THE SPLEEN

Anatomy

The spleen lies in the left hypochondrium within the protection of the rib cage, weighs 75–250 g in the adult and is impalpable; threefold enlargement is required for the organ to become palpable. Its surface marking is the left 9th, 10th and 11th ribs in the midaxillary line. The organ is friable and highly vascular, being supplied primarily by the splenic artery. Ligation of the splenic artery away from the hilum does not usually cause infarction, because of collateral flow via the left gastroepiploic and short gastric arteries. The artery usually divides before it enters the spleen so that each major branch supplies a segment. Thus the organ can be divided into transverse segments each supplied by an end artery, with relatively little blood flow between them; partial resection is thus possible, particularly in trauma. Blood enters the red pulp of the spleen, percolates along the splenic cords and is then filtered through tiny pores into the venous sinuses. Segmental veins leave the hilum and unite to form the splenic vein behind the tail of the pancreas. The vein contributes up to 40% of portal venous blood flow.

The spleen lies against the undersurface of the diaphragm, and in certain pathological states adhesions can develop between the diaphragmatic peritoneum and the splenic capsule. Embryologically the organ grows within the dorsal mesogastrium. Thus in adult life it is connected to the greater curvature of the stomach and to the left kidney by double peritoneal folds usually known (loosely) as ligaments: the gastrosplenic ligament contains the short gastric vessels (vasa brevia), but the lienorenal ligament is relatively bloodless. The medial or visceral surface of the spleen is related to the greater curve and fundus of the stomach, tail of pancreas and colon at the left colic (splenic) flexure and to the left kidney and adrenal gland. Because of these arrangements, the stomach or pancreatic tail may be injured during splenectomy, and the spleen can also be damaged during mobilisation of the stomach or left colon, operations on the distal pancreas or sometimes during a transabdominal approach to the left kidney and adrenal gland.

The spleen contains a higher proportion of fibrous tissue in the young and appears to become softer with age; this feature has a bearing on attempts to conserve the spleen after injury.

Physiological considerations

Haematological functions

Haematopoiesis

In fetal life the spleen makes red cells, but in adults this function is reactivated only in myeloproliferative disorders that impair the ability of the bone marrow to produce sufficient red blood cells. Adult splenic haematopoiesis leads to the production of abnormal red cell forms.

Red cell maturation and destruction

The spleen moulds reticulocytes into biconcave discs and also removes effete and damaged red cells from the circulation. After splenectomy, abnormal erythrocytes, which would have been destroyed by the organ, appear in the peripheral blood. They include target cells and some which contain intracellular inclusions such as Howell–Jolly bodies (nuclear remnants), Heinz bodies (denatured haemoglobin) and Pappenheimer bodies (iron granules). Although the human spleen has little or no function as a red cell reservoir, it is a major storage site for iron and holds a proportion of the platelets and macrophages that are available to the circulation.

Immunological functions

An increased susceptibility to severe infection after splenectomy (overwhelming postsplenectomy infection, OPSI) was reported 70 years ago but remained virtually unknown until 1952. It is now realised that the spleen plays a major role in both humoral and cell-mediated immunity.

Antigens are filtered by the dendritic cells in the white pulp and are presented to immunocompetent cells in the germinal centres of the follicles. Immunoglobulins, in particular IgM, are subsequently produced by plasma cells, resulting in hyperplastic germinal centres. The spleen is a crucial site for production of the non-specific opsonins tuftsin and properdin. These antibodies are of both B- and T-cell origin and react with encapsulated bacteria and fungi, making them more susceptible to phagocytosis.

DISORDERS OF THE SPLEEN

Hyposplenism

The causes and effects of hyposplenism are summarised in Box 21.1.

Splenic agenesis is occasionally seen as a congenital anomaly, and splenic atrophy can develop in conditions such as coeliac disease and sickle cell anaemia. However, most patients become hyposplenic as an outcome of splenectomy. The haematological consequences are mostly short-lived. Persistence of abnormal red blood cells is accompanied by leucocytosis and thrombocytosis, with peak values 1–2 weeks after operation; the platelet count can remain elevated for months or years. The raised count usually does not mean a greater tendency to thrombosis.

Box 21.1 Causes and effects of hyposplenism

Causes

Congenital
- Asplenia (usually associated with other anomalies)
- Splenic hypoplasia in Fanconi's syndrome

Acquired
- Coeliac disease
- Dermatitis herpetiformis
- Sickle cell disease
- Systemic lupus erythematosus
- Ulcerative colitis
- Crohn's disease
- Lymphangiectasia

Iatrogenic
- Splenectomy
- Partial splenectomy and splenic artery ligation

Effects

Red cell abnormalities
- Abnormalities of shape (e.g. target cells)
- Abnormalities of surface (e.g. craters and pits)
- Cytoplasmic inclusions (e.g. Howell–Jolly bodies)

Platelet abnormalities
- Increased number (thrombocytosis)
- Abnormal function (thrombocytopathia)

White cell abnormalities
- Increased number (leucocytosis)
- Abnormal function (postsplenectomy sepsis)

Immunological consequences of splenectomy

Such consequences depend on the age of the patient and are greatest in infants. Reduced ability to opsonise and then phagocytose encapsulated bacteria leads to an increased incidence of infection by *Streptococcus pneumoniae* (pneumococcus) but also by *Neisseria meningitidis*, *Haemophilus influenzae* and *Escherichia coli*. The lifetime risk of developing OPSI is estimated at 2–4% and is higher in children than in adults; the risk is also greater if the spleen is removed because of a haematological disease (thalassaemia, lymphoma) rather than for trauma.

Hypersplenism and splenomegaly

Hypersplenism is defined as overactivity of the spleen in one or more of its functions in relation to destruction of formed elements in the blood, with or without splenomegaly. The consequences may be anaemia, leucopenia, thrombocytopenia or a combination of all three: pancytopenia. In spite of increased production of cells in the bone marrow, pooling and increased destruction in the spleen explains the pancytopenia. Causes of hypersplenism are listed in Table 21.1. If hypersplenism is severe and poorly responsive to non-operative treatment splenectomy is indicated.

Splenomegaly is enlargement of the spleen and can be either primary (of unknown cause) or secondary to other splenic disorders. Hypersplenism and splenomegaly may occur together or separately.

Aetiology

Infections

Mild enlargement may be seen with any acute and prolonged infection. Infectious causes of more serious enlargement include viruses (such as Epstein–Barr, cytomegalovirus and HIV), tuberculosis, brucellosis and syphilis.

Tropical diseases

Diseases such as malaria, kala-azar (leishmaniasis) and schistosomiasis can lead to massive enlargement of the spleen, which is then susceptible to minor trauma. There is also an idiopathic form of tropical splenomegaly.

Table 21.1 Causes of hypersplenism

Condition	Mechanism	Blood disorder	Splenomegaly
Inherited haemolytic anaemias – Spherocytosis – Elliptocytosis	Increased red cell fragility	Anaemia	Variable but rarely large
Autoimmune haemolytic anaemias	Antibodies to red cells	Anaemia	Usual
Thalassaemia Sickle cell disease	Abnormal haemoglobins	Anaemia	Variable
Immune thrombocytopenic purpura (primary or secondary)	Antibodies to platelets	Thrombocytopenia	Rare
Portal hypertension	Raised splenic venous pressure with delayed transit of blood	Pancytopenia	Always
Rheumatoid arthritis (Felty's syndrome)	Uncertain	Leucopenia or pancytopenia	Always

Splenic abscess
This is an uncommon lesion usually associated with severe systemic infection and a high mortality rate. Sources of metastatic abscess of the spleen are typhoid and paratyphoid fever, osteomyelitis, otitis media and puerperal sepsis.

Portal hypertension
Whatever the underlying cause, the spleen enlarges but seldom to a great extent. Features of liver disease and of hypersplenism may be present. Splenic vein thrombosis without occlusion of the portal vein may produce segmental or left-sided portal hypertension with splenomegaly and oesophageal varices, for which splenectomy alone is curative.

Blood disorders
Haemolytic anaemias
Haemolytic anaemias of all types increase the workload of the spleen in removing defective red cells. The organ progressively enlarges and may eventually become too active in red cell destruction and exacerbate the anaemia.

Hereditary spherocytosis is the commonest type of congenital haemolytic anaemia. The critical lesion is an increase in permeability of the erythrocyte membrane to sodium. Sodium leaks into the erythrocyte, increasing its osmotic pressure. It swells, giving a typical spherical shape on a peripheral blood film and increasing osmotic fragility; periodic crises of anaemia occur, especially if the patient develops a viral illness. Hereditary elliptocytosis is a rare variant.

Acquired haemolytic anaemia is an autoimmune disease, which occurs either in a primary (idiopathic) form or secondary to an underlying disorder such as systemic lupus erythematosus or to the administration of certain drugs (e.g. penicillin); it is commonest in older women. Splenomegaly occurs in 50% and is generally associated with mild fever and jaundice. The Coombs' test is positive because the red cells are coated with immunoglobulins or complement; the reaction occurs at different temperatures according to the presence of warm or cold antibodies.

Thalassaemia
Thalassaemia, common in those from the Mediterranean littoral and sub-Saharan Africa, is the result of a defect in haemoglobin peptide synthesis which is transmitted as a dominant trait. The disease is a group of related disorders – alpha and beta – depending on which haemoglobin peptide chain has reduced synthesis. Heterozygotes have a mild form of anaemia, whereas homozygotes have severe chronic anaemia and retardation of growth (thalassaemia major). The characteristic malar hypertrophy is due to overactive haematopoiesis in the upper jaw.

Sickle cell disease
Sickle cell disease is another common haemoglobinopathy in which normal haemoglobin A is replaced by haemoglobin S. Sickle cell disease is more likely, because of repeated minor splenic infarctions, to cause hypo- rather than hypersplenism.

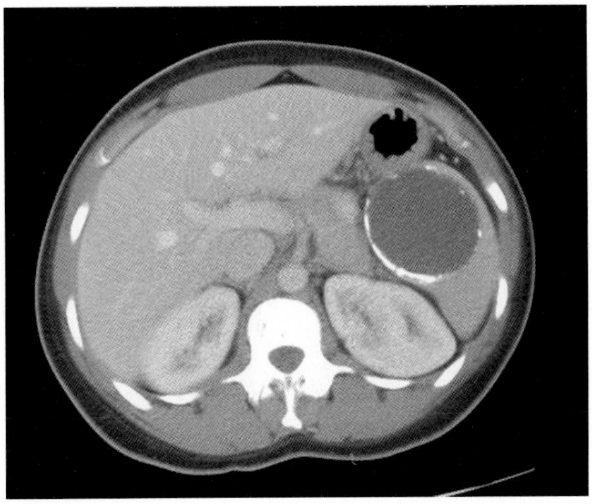

Fig. 21.1 Abdominal CT showing a traumatic splenic pseudocyst resulting from liquefaction of a previous haematoma.

Immune thrombocytopenic purpura (ITP)
Although this disorder involves splenic destruction of platelets, the organ is rarely enlarged. Splenomegaly can, however, be a feature of the secondary type that develops as a consequence of lymphoproliferative disease, infection or drugs. Both types of ITP are associated with circulating antiplatelet antibodies. ITP can develop acutely in children, often after a viral illness. The chronic form tends to be seen in adult females and is characterised by a history of heavy periods.

Splenic cyst
This is a rare condition. Cysts can be either congenital in origin (dermoid and mesenchymal inclusion cysts) or parasitic from echinococcal (hydatid) infestation. Occasionally a traumatic pseudocyst results from liquefaction of a previous splenic haematoma (Fig. 21.1). Splenic cysts need to be distinguished from pancreatic pseudocysts formed in the lesser sac following severe acute pancreatitis and from neoplastic cysts arising from the pancreatic tail.

Myeloproliferative diseases
Many types of myeloproliferative disease are characterised by splenomegaly, including:

- myeloid and lymphocytic leukaemia
- polycythaemia rubra vera
- myelofibrosis (also called myelosclerosis).

In myeloid leukaemia there is enlargement of the red pulp, whereas in myelofibrosis extramedullary haematopoiesis develops in the liver and spleen as a result of obliteration of the bone marrow by fibrous tissue. Massive splenomegaly and secondary hypersplenism may result. The huge spleen causes dragging abdominal discomfort, which may be exacerbated by the pain of recurrent splenic infarcts. Hypersplenism predisposes to fatigue and dyspnoea (because of anaemia), spontaneous bleeding (thrombocytopenia) and opportunist infection (neutropenia).

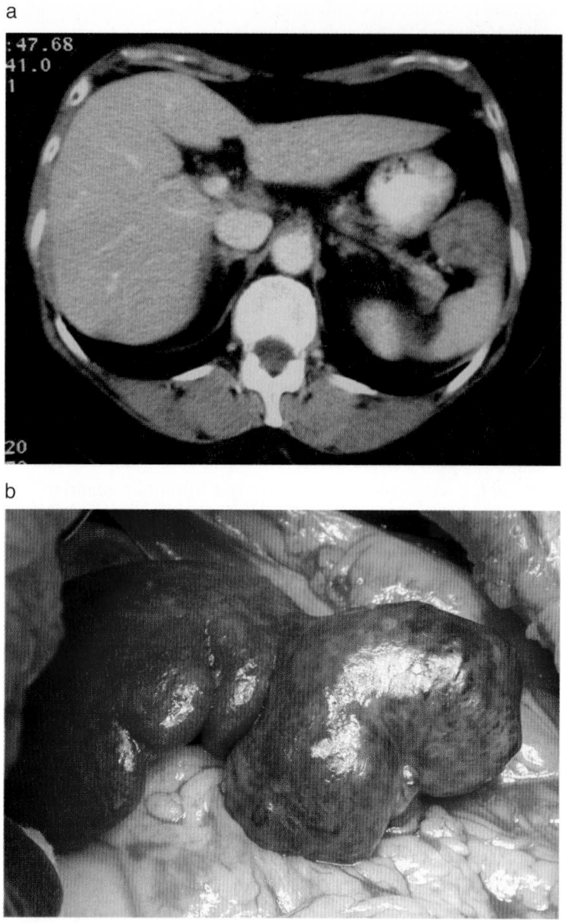

Fig. 21.2 (a) Abdominal CT and (b) intraoperative picture showing an ovarian metastasis on the inferior pole of the spleen.

Lymphatic malignancy

The spleen is very frequently enlarged in patients with tumours of the lymphoid system, e.g. lymphoma, Hodgkin's disease and other, rarer disorders which are more difficult to classify.

Metastatic disease

The spleen is occasionally the site of metastatic disease (Fig. 21.2).

Metabolic

Porphyria is a hereditary error of catabolism of haemoglobin resulting in porphyrinuria, abdominal crises precipitated by barbiturates, anaemia, photosensitivity and neurological or mental symptoms in advanced stages. Splenomegaly is often present. In Gaucher's disease, the spleen actively stores the abnormal lipoid glucocerebroside, leading to enormous enlargement of the spleen. There is associated anaemia, brown discoloration of the skin of the hands and face and conjunctival thickening (pinguecula).

Clinical features

History

Splenomegaly is generally painless unless the organ undergoes patchy infarction, as can occur in chronic myeloid leukaemia, vascular occlusions produced by sickle cell disease or from an embolus in bacterial endocarditis. There may be both pleuritic and shoulder pain. Otherwise the history is that of the disease causing the splenic enlargement or hypersplenism.

Features include recurrent anaemia, purpura and respiratory infections, which are the consequences of the neutropenia. Specific symptoms related to the underlying condition may be present.

Physical findings

These vary with the cause. Splenomegaly is frequent but, as indicated in Table 21.1, may not be present when the condition involves destruction of only one cellular element of the blood. Thrombocytopenia is associated with purpuric skin lesions and a risk of intracranial haemorrhage. Leucopenia occurs, with a variable increase in bacterial infections.

There can be mild tenderness if the spleen is enlarged secondary to an acute infection. A mass in the left upper quadrant of splenic origin has the following characteristics:

- It is dull on percussion.
- It moves downwards and medially with respiration (unlike the kidney which moves downwards only).
- A notch may be felt.
- It cannot have its upper margin defined on palpation.

In addition, care must be taken to ensure that the examining hand can get below a very large spleen; palpation is begun low down in the right iliac fossa. Difficulty may be experienced in differentiating splenomegaly from the following:

- an enlarged left kidney, which also moves on respiration but should be palpable in the loin and have a band of resonant gas-containing colon in front of it
- gastric or colonic tumours – these scarcely move on respiration, and the examining hand can generally interpose between the mass and the costal margin
- mass arising from the pancreatic tail, such as a large pseudocyst; this is typically deeply placed and less discrete on palpation.

Ultrasonography, computed tomography (CT) scan, or magnetic resonance image (MRI) scanning shows the size of the spleen and whether it is indeed the cause of the mass.

Investigation of hypersplenism

Blood tests

Peripheral blood films may demonstrate malarial parasites; infectious mononucleosis gives rise to atypical lymphocytes, and serological tests are positive (Paul–Bunnell, Epstein–Barr virus titres).

Bone marrow function

A precise diagnosis is essential before proceeding to splenectomy because splenomegaly may, in such circumstances as infiltration of the bone marrow (malignancy, myelofibrosis), indicate that the spleen has taken over the marrow's function in producing formed elements of the blood. Bone marrow biopsy should therefore be performed to confirm that the marrow is still active.

Red cell dynamics

Production can be studied by giving radiolabelled iron, and destruction by ^{51}Cr labelling. External scanning over the spleen demonstrates its activity in each regard. If splenectomy is undertaken for hypersplenism, a preoperative search by imaging, supplemented by a wide exploration at operation, must be made for accessory spleens (splenunculi) which could otherwise enlarge and lead to recurrence of the original condition.

Management

Indications for splenectomy are summarised in Box 21.2.

Infections

Splenomegaly during the course of an acute infectious illness is treated with the appropriate antimicrobial agents. The massive enlargements seen in the tropics because of specific infections may require splenectomy because of pain and/or secondary hypersplenism. Splenic abscesses are drained as part of the overall management of severe septic states. The drainage may be performed percutaneously under ultrasonic or CT guidance.

Blood disorders

Many of the congenital red cell and haemoglobin disorders respond to splenectomy (which must include the removal of any accessory spleens), especially if there is a high rate of haemolysis. In diminishing order, the operation is indicated for:

- spherocytosis
- thalassaemia major
- sickle cell anaemia
- elliptocytosis.

In ITP, corticosteroid therapy will often (75%) improve the platelet count. Splenectomy is indicated for patients who fail to respond to steroids and immunosuppressive agents (e.g. azathioprine) or who relapse when therapy is withdrawn. Steroids have a similar response rate in acquired haemolytic anaemia, but again splenectomy is indicated for treatment failures; generally only those patients with warm antibodies respond to the operation.

Box 21.2 Indications for splenectomy

Traumatic or spontaneous rupture (when preservation is not possible)
Iatrogenic injury (e.g. at left hemicolectomy) if haemostasis cannot be achieved
Immune thrombocytopenic purpura unresponsive to medical therapy
Hereditary spherocytosis or elliptocytosis
Autoimmune haemolytic anaemia unreponsive to medical therapy
Myeloproliferative disorders with painful splenomegaly
Thalassaemia major with hypersplenism
Splenic marginal zone lymphoma
Gastrectomy for cancer with splenic hilar invasion
Distal pancreatectomy – if splenic preservation is contraindicated or not possible
Bleeding gastro-oesophageal varices secondary to splenic vein thrombosis
Splenic abscess
Splenic artery aneurysm
Hydatid cyst (rare)
Non-parasitic splenic cyst (rare and usually deroofed)
Secondary carcinoma (rare)
Massive haemangioma (rare)

Lymphatic malignancy

The role of operative treatment in these disorders is:

- establishment of the diagnosis by lymph node biopsy, usually from the neck but occasionally from the axilla
- very occasionally to remove a massive spleen that is causing symptoms or hypersplenism.

Ruptured spleen

Aetiology

In blunt abdominal trauma, the spleen is the most vulnerable organ despite its relatively protected site. The mechanism is a direct blow or fall. Road traffic accidents and sports injuries are common causes. Rupture is often associated with fractures of the overlying ribs. Other injuries – particularly to the head – may also occur and appear to dominate the damage profile. In most patients the spleen is healthy and of normal size, but if there is splenomegaly, relatively minor trauma can cause bleeding (e.g. infectious mononucleosis and malaria). Spontaneous rupture can occasionally occur (Fig. 21.3), although in such circumstances very minor trauma may have been forgotten. The spleen can also be damaged inadvertently during the course of an abdominal operation which involves procedures in the left upper quadrant, when a relatively minor capsular tear may cause persistent bleeding.

Pathological features

Elaborate classification of the extent and nature of splenic rupture has been devised and can assist the surgeon in deciding whether to attempt splenic conservation.

The important practical distinction is between immediate and delayed rupture. In the first, the capsule and, to a greater or lesser extent, the underlying organ are torn and bruised,

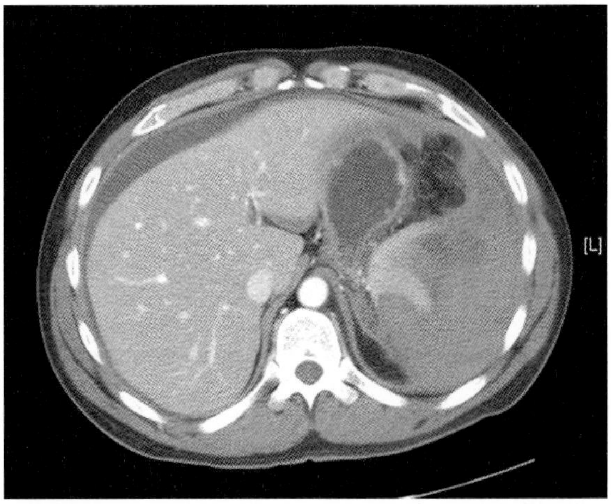

Fig. 21.3 Abdominal CT showing a spontaneous splenic rupture in a patient with acute pancreatitis secondary to alcohol. Haemodynamic instability and anaemia led to laparotomy and splenectomy.

bleeding is extensive and the clinical presentation is prompt. The most extreme example is when the spleen is completely avulsed from its artery or vein. In delayed rupture, the capsule remains initially intact or, on occasion, the leak of blood is local and only into the left upper quadrant. Presentation may then be delayed for hours, days or even weeks.

Clinical features

History

An obvious injury to the left chest wall or the abdomen may have been sustained. Conscious patients complain of abdominal pain that is generalised but usually most severe in the left upper quadrant. Pain may also be felt in the tip of the left shoulder because irritation of the undersurface of the diaphragm stimulates the phrenic nerve (C4 dermatome: Kehr's sign). An unconscious patient cannot report these symptoms, and there is danger that the abdominal condition may be overlooked unless very careful attention is paid to the clinical findings. Head injuries do not cause circulatory collapse.

Physical findings

Hypovolaemia In frank rupture there is considerable rapid blood loss into the peritoneal cavity, and pallor, low blood pressure, rapid pulse and restlessness develop.

Abdominal signs There may be external bruising and tenderness over the upper left abdomen and lower left ribs – the latter suggesting fracture. Typically there is abdominal tenderness, guarding and rigidity. Occasionally a splenic mass is felt if there is pre-existing splenomegaly or a large subcapsular haematoma.

Delayed rupture has an insidious presentation with anaemia, vague left upper quadrant and left shoulder pain and mild tenderness in the left upper quadrant. The signs may become acute if free rupture eventually takes place.

Investigation

Few tests are required when frank rupture of the spleen causes a haemoperitoneum. In other patients, imaging may be required to confirm the diagnosis of rupture or a subcapsular haematoma.

Blood examination

Haematocrit is normal at first until haemodilution occurs over some hours. Leucocyte count is raised (as in other forms of trauma).

Imaging

X-ray Chest X-ray often shows fractured ribs, and the left hemidiaphragm may be elevated by the underlying haematoma. Abdominal X-ray is not usually indicated, but if done may show splenomegaly or a subdiaphragmatic soft-tissue mass.

Ultrasound (see FAST scanning Ch. 3) and CT may demonstrate the rupture of the splenic capsule and show free blood in the peritoneal cavity. A subcapsular haematoma can be demonstrated. In a haemodynamically stable patient, the progress or resolution of a haematoma may be assessed by repeated scanning (see below).

Management

Until recently, any but the most trivial splenic injury was regarded as an indication for splenectomy. Nowadays, because of better recognition of the risk of postsplenectomy sepsis, an attempt is made to preserve splenic tissue. Splenic salvage is particularly desirable in children, who are at greater risk. However, the prime goal is to save the patient's life, and attempts at splenic preservation should not be continued if there is continuous bleeding.

Management may follow three main courses (Fig. 21.4):

- Non-operative – splenic injury is suspected, but there are few clinical signs, and imaging shows a limited haematoma; the patient is admitted for a few days to ensure that the haematocrit does not decrease and repeated imaging shows either no enlargement or resolution.
- Initial non-operative followed by operation – indicated by increasing physical findings and decline in haematocrit which imply continued bleeding. As a rough guide, the need for more than two units of blood to be transfused indicates laparotomy.
- Emergency operation – a patient in hypovolaemic shock is, if possible, resuscitated immediately and then proceeds to laparotomy; sometimes it may be necessary to operate in the presence of hypotension in order to control bleeding.

At operation, a rapid search is made for other sites of bleeding, notably from the liver and tears in the mesentery. Unless the organ is extensively shattered or bleeding is uncontrollable, an attempt is made to preserve it. Simple manoeuvres may suffice, such as topical haemostatic agents (e.g. oxidised regenerated cellulose: Surgicel®) applied with gentle pressure over a swab. Alternatively, the organ is mobilised and accurate suture is performed with or without ligation of the splenic artery to reduce blood flow. Enclosing the spleen in a bag of absorbable mesh may also control bleeding. Finally segmental resection may be feasible, especially with modern haemostatic technologies such as ultrasonic dissection and topical haemostatic agents are available (see Ch. 8). If splenectomy proves unavoidable, some surgeons leave splenic tissue behind within an omental pocket, but the function of such autotransplants is doubtful.

Operation is also indicated for a delayed rupture that presents with late haemoperitoneum or (rarely) drainage for an infected splenic haematoma.

SPLENECTOMY

Preoperative management and postoperative complications are summarised in Box 21.3.

Preoperative management

Hypersplenism

Before removing the spleen, it is necessary to show that there is excessive destruction of blood elements in the spleen and that there is adequate bone marrow function to

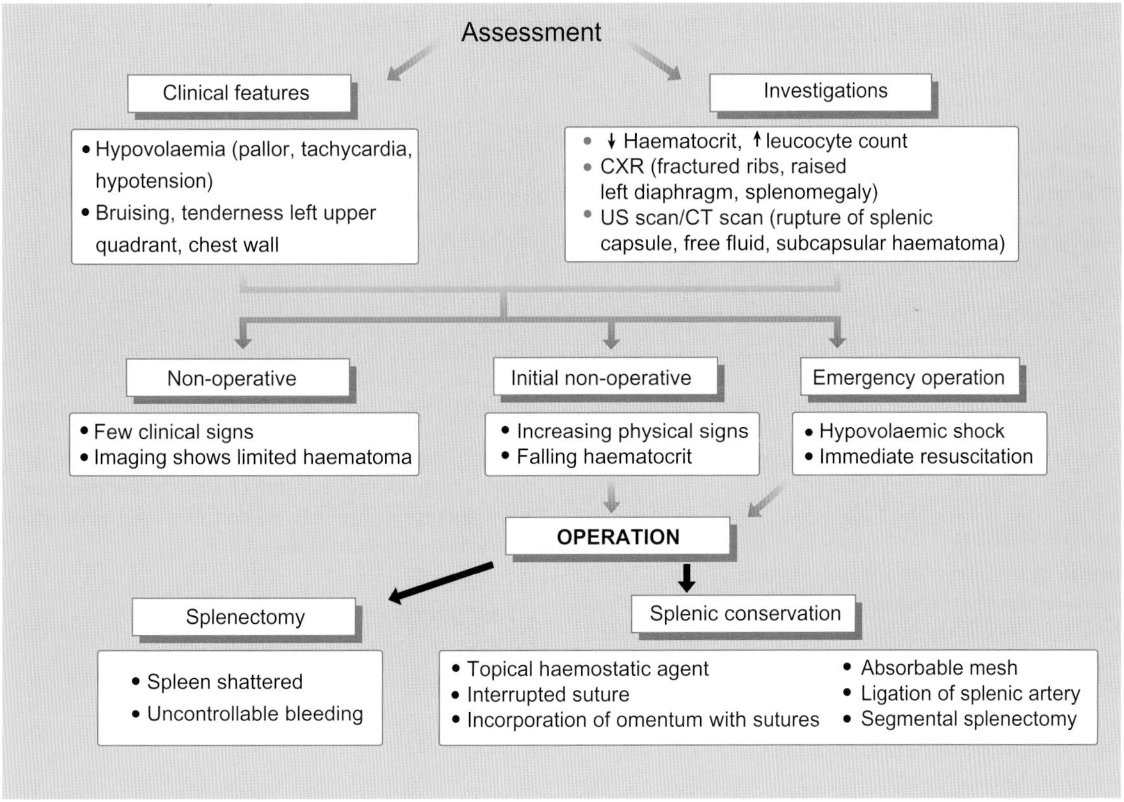

Fig. 21.4 Management of the ruptured spleen.

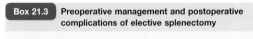

Box 21.3 Preoperative management and postoperative complications of elective splenectomy

Preoperative management
- Demonstrate excessive destruction of blood elements (anaemia, leucopenia, thrombocytopenia, pancytopenia)
- Demonstrate adequate bone marrow function (bone marrow aspirate)
- Correction of anaemia and thrombocytopenia (steroid therapy and platelet transfusion)
- Prophylaxis against OPSI (see Table 21.2)

Postoperative complications
- Haemorrhage
- Gastric dilatation, haematemesis and gastric fistula
- Left basal atelectasis
- Pancreatic fistula
- Thrombocytosis
- OPSI (overwhelming postsplenectomy infection)

cope should the spleen have become an important site of erythropoiesis.

Prophylaxis against OPSI

This should be undertaken in all patients who are to undergo an elective operation that could involve splenectomy. Immunisation is required not only when splenectomy is planned but also in operations on adjacent organs in which the spleen may form part of the dissection – e.g. total gastrectomy and operations on the distal pancreas. The regimen is considered in Table 21.2.

Correction of cytopenia

Specific correction includes that of anaemia and occasionally of thrombocytopenia (steroid therapy and platelet transfusion, although platelets are better infused only after the spleen has been isolated by ligation of its artery).

Risk of infection

Patients with leucopenia should receive antibiotic prophylaxis against Gram-positive organisms. Immunoglobulin therapy may also have a role.

Operation

The spleen can be safely removed via a left subcostal or midline laparotomy, but extension into the chest is occasionally needed if the organ is massive. Laparoscopic splenectomy is widely used for small or moderate-sized spleens, notably for ITP. A preoperative ultrasound scan should be made for (pigment) gallstones in patients with haemolytic anaemia and, if found, cholecystectomy considered at the same time as splenectomy. Accessory spleens, which can cause recurrence of haemolytic and thrombocytopenic disorders, should be removed if found in such patients. If the organ is large and adherent, it may be advisable to expose and ligate the splenic artery at an early stage: indeed, some surgeons do this in all cases. Adhesions to the diaphragm and mesocolon need to be divided before the peritoneal attachments of the spleen are incised and the organ is mobilised into the wound. Care must be taken when dividing the short gastric vessels not to injure the stomach and, when the

Table 21.2 Prophylaxis of overwhelming postsplenectomy infection (OPSI)

Method	Duration	Problems
Oral penicillin/erythromycin	Up to age 16 ? indefinitely	Compliance Resistant strains
Vaccination: ■ Pneumococcal ■ Meningococcal group C ■ *Haemophilus influenzae* type B (Hib) ■ Influenza ■ Additional meningococcal groups A, C, W and Y	Repeated 5–10-yearly On travel abroad Every year	Wide variety of strains, not all covered Efficacy uncertain
Education: ■ Avoidance of malaria and tick bites (babesiosis) ■ Medalert bracelet or other document		Compliance

splenic vessels are ligated, to avoid injury to the tail of the pancreas.

Complications

Bleeding

This may result from persistent oozing in the splenic bed and is the commonest cause of subphrenic haematoma and abscess. These complications are more frequent in patients with preoperative thrombocytopenia.

Gastric and pancreatic fistulae

These may follow ischaemic injury to the stomach following too close ligation of the short gastric blood vessels or trauma to the tail of the pancreas in the splenic hilum. They can be avoided with careful technique.

Thrombocytosis

This is the rule after splenectomy, but venous thromboembolism is not especially common; antiplatelet agents or subcutaneous heparin may be given if the platelet count rises above 1000 x 10^9/L.

Overwhelming postsplenectomy infection

OPSI is the most serious late complication of splenectomy.

Pathological features

The functional role of the spleen in protection from infection has been discussed above, and, although much remains to be discovered, it is apparent that it plays a major part in dealing with bloodstream invasion by encapsulated organisms such as pneumococci and meningococci. The commonest form of OPSI is therefore pneumococcal or meningococcal septicaemia. Adrenal haemorrhage may occur and contribute to death by adding an element of acute adrenal insufficiency. In addition, infections with *H. influenzae* are an important risk. In tropical regions, tick-borne infections and malaria are also common.

Clinical features

Postsplenectomy sepsis often starts insidiously but can rapidly develop into a fulminant infection. There is fever, vomiting, dehydration and circulatory collapse often without specific features that alert the clinician to the diagnosis. An upper abdominal scar may be indicative even in the absence of a definite history of splenectomy.

Investigation

Evidence of acute infection should be sought by:

- white blood cell count for leucocytosis
- blood smear examination for organisms
- blood culture
- CSF examination and culture in the presence of neurological clinical features.

Management

The intravenous administration of fluids and antibiotics should be started on a best-guess basis without waiting for the results of culture and organism sensitivities. The mortality rate is at least 50%, which emphasises the need for prophylaxis.

Prophylaxis

The occurrence of OPSI could be much reduced (although exactly by how much is not known) if vigorous preventative measures were used in those at risk. Although the condition was originally thought to be limited to infants and children, it is now known to occur at all ages, which justifies universal prophylaxis after splenectomy.

There is no absolute agreement on regimens, but guidelines have been issued and are summarised in Table 21.2. Patients should not leave hospital without prophylaxis having begun.

FURTHER READING

Bland KI 2010 Surgery of the pancreas and spleen: handbooks in general surgery. Springer, New York

Williamson RCN 2006 Spleen. In: Kirk R M (ed) General surgical operations, 5th edn. Churchill Livingstone, Edinburgh

22 The pancreas

ANATOMY AND PHYSIOLOGY

Embryology

The pancreas begins in fetal life as ventral and dorsal buds of the foregut, each with its own drainage duct. As the foregut rotates and develops, the two buds fuse to partially surround the superior mesenteric vessels. The larger dorsal pancreas forms the body, tail and upper part of the head, and the ventral pancreas forms the rest of the head and the uncinate process. Fusion of the duct systems results in the duct of the ventral bud becoming the main duct (of Wirsung) which drains into the duodenum through a shared opening with the common bile duct at the major papilla (ampulla of Vater). The duct of the dorsal bud persists as the smaller accessory duct of Santorini, which drains into the duodenum through the minor papilla.

Anatomy

The pancreas lies across the posterior abdominal wall at the level of L1. The head is surrounded by the concavity of the duodenum. The uncinate process and lower part of the head (ventral duct derivatives) pass posteriorly and to the left of the superior mesenteric vessels. The body of the pancreas forms the main bulk of the gland and extends across the midline, ending in a tail lying close to the splenic hilum (Fig. 22.1). The main pancreatic duct leads from the tail to the head of the organ, gradually increasing in size as it drains ductules from the pancreatic substance. It usually joins the common bile duct to open into the second part of the duodenum through a common channel and single orifice. This opening is visible from the luminal surface of the duodenum as a small nipple – the major papilla.

Developmental anomalies of the pancreas

Pancreas divisum is a relatively common (5%) anatomical variation in which most of the pancreas drains into the duodenum through the duct of Santorini and the minor papilla, which is situated about 2 cm proximal to the major papilla.

Annular pancreas is a rare cause of extrinsic compression of the second part of the duodenum from failure of the two developing pancreatic buds to fuse. A cuff of pancreatic tissue surrounds the duodenum.

Both pancreas divisum and annular pancreas may be associated with drainage abnormalities and pancreatitis.

Heterotopic pancreas Accessory budding of the primitive duodenum results in nodules of pancreatic tissue in abnormal positions such as the stomach, duodenal wall, jejunum or in a Meckel's diverticulum. Heterotopic nodules are present in 20% of the population.

Physiology

The human pancreas is both an endocrine and an exocrine organ, and these two functions are performed by different cell populations. By far the majority of the gland (up to 98% by weight) consists of acinar cells which synthesise the exocrine pancreatic enzymes and drain into the intraglandular ductules which are tributaries of the main pancreatic duct. The principal hormones that control release of exocrine secretions are secretin and cholecystokinin (CCK), which are produced from the APUD group of cells in the duodenum and upper jejunum.

Secretin is released into the bloodstream when acidic gastric contents enter the first part of the duodenum. It stimulates secretion of a watery, alkaline pancreatic juice rich in electrolytes.

CCK is released when fatty acids and amino acids enter the duodenum; it stimulates contraction of the gallbladder and relaxation of the distal bile/pancreatic duct sphincter (of Oddi) as well as secretion of a pancreatic juice rich in enzymes. These enzymes are involved in the breakdown of carbohydrates, fats and proteins, the most important of which are amylase, lipase, colipase, phospholipase and a family of proteases: trypsinogen, chymotrypsinogen and elastase. The proteases are secreted in inactive forms (proenzymes: zymogens) that are subsequently activated in the lumen of the duodenum by enterokinase, which is probably secreted from the same source as secretin and CCK. Intrapancreatic enzyme activation can cause autolysis of the pancreas and may be one of the pathophysiological mechanisms of pancreatitis.

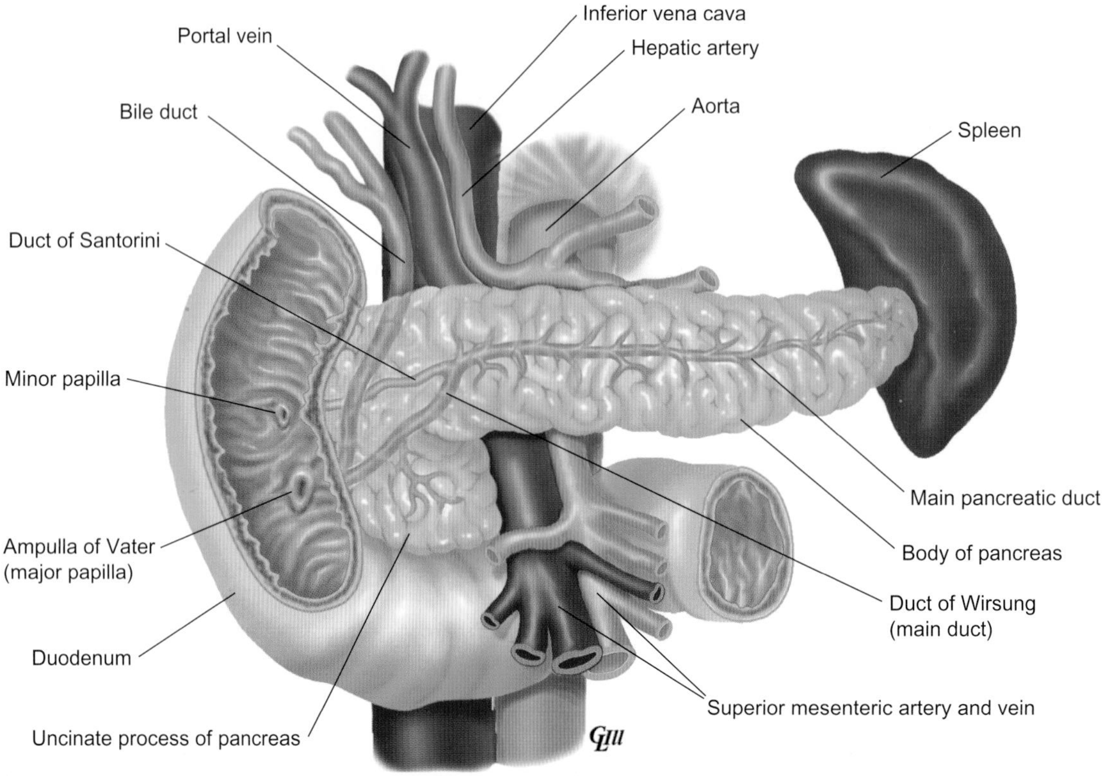

Fig. 22.1 Important surgical relations of the pancreas. Note the intimate relationship of the uncinate process and neck of the pancreas with the superior mesenteric vessels and portal vein (not shown – formed behind neck by junction of superior mesenteric and splenic veins).

Box 22.1 Investigation of pancreatic function

Exocrine
- Serum amylase and lipase concentration
- Duodenal enzyme concentrations after:
  - stimulation with CCK and/or secretin
  - food stimulation (Lundh meal)
- PABA test
- Faecal elastase measurement
- $^{14}CO_2$ breath test
- fluorescein dilaurate test

Endocrine
- Glucose tolerance test
- Plasma levels of:
  - insulin
  - glucagon
  - pancreatic polypeptide

CCK, cholecystokinin; PABA, *p*-aminobenzoic acid.

The endocrine portion of the human pancreas is arranged as islands of endocrine tissue (the islets of Langerhans) within the exocrine gland. The islets have a rich vascular supply, and the endocrine cells secrete hormones directly into the portal blood.

Measurement of function

A large number of physiological tests have been devised to measure both the exocrine and endocrine functions of the pancreas. Some of the most important are shown in Box 22.1.

Exocrine function

Direct tests

Direct tests of exocrine function rely on measurements of secreted enzymes into the gut. The Lundh meal and its variants involve the collection of pancreatic secretion through a nasogastric tube first at rest and then after the administration of a standard meal. Bicarbonate concentration and trypsin and lipase levels are the most common measurements made. Pancreatic insufficiency results in low post-stimulation secretion of enzymes. However, enzyme secretion has a large reserve capacity, and measurement of secretion in this manner is rarely helpful in the diagnosis of mild to moderate insufficiency such as may occur in the early stages of chronic pancreatitis.

Indirect tests

Indirect tests that may be of value include:

- the PABA test
- faecal elastase test
- $^{14}CO_2$ breath test
- fluorescein dilaurate test.

PABA test N-benzoyl-L-tryosyl *p*-aminobenzoic acid is a synthetic peptide which is hydrolysed by pancreatic chymotrypsin to release free *p*-aminobenzoic acid (PABA), which is absorbed, metabolised and excreted in the urine. Reduction in the absorption of PABA occurs if pancreatic chymotrypsin secretion is low.

Table 22.1 Methods of visualisation of the pancreas

Technique	Purpose
Ultrasound	Gland size Presence of gallstones Cysts Calcification Tumour Duct dilatation Venous encasement/obstruction
CT	As for ultrasound and may better define vascular involvement in malignant disease and pancreatic necrosis and inflammatory collections in severe acute pancreatitis
MR	MRI similar to CT but MRCP can also give good images of the bile and pancreatic ducts
Endoscopic ultrasound	May give additional information and permit guided biopsy
PET scanning	May demonstrate undetected metastatic disease
Laparoscopy	Valuable for detection of small liver and peritoneal metastases

The faecal elastase test measures the concentration of the pancreatic elastase-1 enzyme found in a stool specimen using an enzyme-linked immunosorbent assay (ELISA). Results of this test give a good indication of exocrine pancreatic status. Levels of faecal elastase lower than 200 μg/g of stool indicate an exocrine insufficiency.

$^{14}CO_2$ breath test The amount of $^{14}CO_2$ in expired air is measured following oral ingestion of a ^{14}C-labelled fatty acid (^{14}C-oleic acid) compared with that after ingestion of labelled triglyceride (^{14}C-itrolein). Impaired triglyceride absorption with normal fatty acid absorption indicates that pancreatic disease is the cause of the steatorrhoea.

Fluorescein dilaurate test In the fluorescein dilaurate test fluorescein dilaurate is cleaved by the pancreas-specific cholesterol ester hydrolase activity and the liberated fluorescein is absorbed and excreted in the urine. Fluorescein recovery is a reflection of exocrine pancreatic function.

Endocrine function

Measurement of pancreatic endocrine function may be required if a functioning endocrine tumour is suspected (see Ch. 32).

Imaging (see also Table 22.1)

Plain X-ray

Plain abdominal X-ray may show small bowel ileus in acute pancreatitis and calcification in chronic disease.

Ultrasound

Ultrasound is commonly used as a first-line investigation because it is cheaper, non-invasive and relatively easy to perform. Imaging may be impaired by overlying bowel gas. Ultrasound can be used to detect abnormalities of pancreatic size and shape and the presence of cysts or tumours. Guided needle aspiration cytology and fine core needle biopsy may be performed under ultrasound control – although a decision about needle aspiration or biopsy should be agreed at a multidisciplinary meeting beforehand.

Computed tomography (CT) scanning

CT gives more precise anatomical definition and is not affected by bowel gas. Rapid sequence spiral or helical CT (Ch. 4) accompanied by intravenous injection of contrast can now provide high-definition images of pancreatic tumours and show their relationship to major vessels such as the superior mesenteric and portal veins and the superior mesenteric artery. CT-guided aspiration and core needle biopsy may be obtained.

Magnetic resonance imaging

MRI scanning provides additional information to ultrasound and CT, especially in cystic tumours or disease. MRI can be used to generate impressive images of the pancreatic and biliary ductal systems – magnetic resonance cholangiopancreatography (MRCP). MRCP is now preferred to diagnostic ERCP (see below), which carries the risk of inducing acute pancreatitis or cholangitis.

Endoscopic ultrasonography (EUS)

Endoscopic ultrasound (EUS – an ultrasound probe attached to the end of a flexible endoscope) is increasingly used to assess pancreatic disease. The body of the gland is well visualised because of its close proximity to the posterior aspect of the stomach, and the head is within the duodenal loop and also easily seen. Vascular invasion may be assessed and guided needle biopsies taken through the endoscope. Cyst fluid may be aspirated for cytology, amylase and CEA concentrations, which can be used to discrimate between the inflammatory and neoplastic cystic disease. EUS is also good at detecting very small gallbladder or bile duct stones not seen on other non-invasive imaging.

Endoscopic retrograde cholangiopancreatography (ERCP)

ERCP involves passage of a flexible, side-viewing endoscope into the duodenum and cannulation of the major (and sometimes the minor) duodenal papilla. Contrast medium is injected to outline the pancreatic duct (pancreatography) and the bile ducts (cholangiography). The procedure is described as retrograde because the contrast medium flows in the opposite direction to normal biliary and pancreatic juices. The technique produces good images of the pancreatic duct and is useful in the diagnosis of pancreatic duct strictures and their cause, for the identification of bile duct and pancreatic duct stones and for defining congenital abnormalities and leaks from the biliary or pancreatic ductal systems. Transient asymptomatic hyperamylasaemia after ERCP is common. Complications of diagnostic ERCP occur in 2–3% of patients and include acute pancreatitis and cholangitis; for this reason and the recent improvements in non-invasive imaging, diagnostic ERCP has been more or less abandoned.

ERCP is, however, used widely for treatment, e.g. the removal of bile duct stones after diathermy cutting of the sphincter at the major papilla (sphincterotomy) or balloon dilatation. Plastic or expanding metal tubes (stents) can be placed through strictures of the bile and pancreatic ducts to relieve obstruction and brushings taken from strictures for cytology. Additional complications of therapeutic ERCP include bleeding and duodenal perforation.

Visceral angiography

Visceral angiography is no longer used to assess resectability as equivalent information is now available from contrast enhanced CT or MRI scans. Rarely, therapeutic angiographic embolisation is used to stop bleeding from an artery involved in complicated pancreatitis or following pancreatic surgery.

PET scanning

FDG-PET scanning is increasingly used to detect metastatic cancer. The scan detects metabolically active tissue and may show secondary deposits not seen on other imaging modalities.

Laparoscopy

Laparoscopy is useful as a final staging investigation in those under consideration for resection of a pancreatic tumour, particularly tumours over 2 cm, and is often performed immediately before a planned resectional operation. Small, undetected liver or peritoneal metastases are discovered in perhaps 20% of patients.

Diagnosis of a pancreatic mass

A common clinical situation is a mass in the pancreas, which may or may not be causing jaundice. Differentiation between a benign and malignant condition is vital, the likely diagnosis being pancreatic cancer or chronic pancreatitis. Any combination of the above imaging techniques may be used but none is error-free. Elevated levels of tumour markers in the blood, particularly CA 19-9, suggest malignancy, but raised levels also occur in inflammatory conditions. Percutaneous needle aspiration for cytology (or core needle biopsy) under ultrasound (conventional or endoscopic) or CT guidance or at laparoscopy may confirm malignancy, but this may be technically demanding and the lesion may not be accurately targeted. False-negative results are common. There is also a risk of cancer dissemination along the needle track. For these reasons, biopsy is not usually recommended before surgery in patients with a potentially resectable tumour.

PANCREATITIS

Classification

Pancreatitis is by far the most important benign condition of the pancreas. It is important to distinguish between acute and chronic pancreatitis. In acute disease, endocrine and exocrine function, as well as the gross structure of the gland, return to normal after resolution of the attack unless complications occur. In chronic pancreatitis, there are permanent structural changes which can lead to a small, fibrotic gland with either exocrine or endocrine functional impairment or both. Recurrent attacks of acute pancreatitis may lead to the changes of chronic pancreatitis.

Box 22.2 Acute pancreatitis

- Gallstones and alcohol cause 70–80% of cases
- Presents with acute upper abdominal/back pain and vomiting
- Serum amylase (>1000 IU/L) is diagnostic
- Serum lipase >5 × upper limit of normal is diagnostic
- 70% of cases are 'mild', 30% 'severe'
- Complications may be systemic (SIRS, multi-organ failure, hypocalcaemia, hyperglycaemia) or local (pancreatic necrosis, pseudocyst or abscess)
- 5–10% hospital mortality

Acute pancreatitis

Acute pancreatitis exhibits a broad spectrum of clinical severity, ranging from mild and self-limiting (in most cases), to a rapidly fatal disorder associated with multi-organ failure and death. Characteristics are outlined in Box 22.2.

Aetiology

A number of conditions are known to predispose to pancreatitis (Table 22.2). The most common (60–70%) are gallstone disease and alcohol consumption. The mechanism by which these aetiological factors trigger pancreatitis is not clear and may differ between patients. Intraglandular activation of pancreatic juice, obstruction to drainage of secretions, metabolic intralobular changes and ischaemia have all been implicated.

Gallstones

The mechanisms by which gallstones cause acute pancreatitis are not fully understood. However, it is known that patients with multiple small stones in the gallbladder are more likely to develop pancreatitis than those with large or solitary stones; small gallstones can be detected in the faeces of patients soon after an attack of stone-related pancreatitis. It has therefore been postulated that acute pancreatitis may follow passage of a stone through the major papilla; less commonly, a stone may be identified impacted in the papilla during an attack. In either circumstance, reflux of bile or duodenal contents along the pancreatic duct may follow with intraductal activation of pro-enzymes by enterokinase or possibly infected bile. Autodigestion of the pancreas (particularly by trypsin and phospholipase A) then occurs. Once enzymes are activated, cell membranes are digested, and oedema, proteolysis, vascular damage and necrosis may follow. Gallstones rarely lead to chronic pancreatitis but are often associated with recurrent attacks of acute pancreatic inflammation unless they are surgically removed.

Alcohol

Alcohol alone can damage the pancreas, and excessive drinking can precipitate an acute episode of pancreatitis. Recurrent episodes of acute pancreatitis may occur in heavy consumers of alcohol, and may lead to chronic pancreatitis (see below). The precise mechanism of action is not known.

Pathological features

The mildest form of pancreatitis is characterised by interstitial oedema with inflammatory exudate (oedematous pancreatitis). In more severe forms, there is glandular necrosis

Table 22.2 Known and suspected causes of pancreatitis

Cause	Possible mechanism
Gallstones	Duodenopancreatic reflux Ampullary obstruction with infected bile reflux into pancreatic duct
Alcohol	Unknown
Iatrogenic:	
- ERCP	? Hypertonic contrast injury ? High-pressure injury
- Operation at or around the major papilla	? Obstruction to duct
Neoplasm	Obstruction
Pancreas divisum	
Choledochocele	
Duodenal cysts	
Viral infection:	Pancreatic cell infection
- Coxsackie B	
- Mumps	
- Epstein–Barr	
- Cytomegalovirus	
Bacterial infection:	Pancreatic infection
- *Mycoplasma pneumoniae*	
Trauma – usually ruptured duct in body of gland (over vertebral column)	Direct trauma ± ductal obstruction
Hyperparathyroidism	Hypercalcaemia
Sarcoidosis	
Malignancy	
Hyperlipidaemia	Unknown but occurs in Fredrickson's types I, III, IV, V
Drugs:	Unknown
- Corticosteroids	
- Azathioprine	
- Thiazides	
- Tetracycline	
- Antiretroviral agents	
- Valproate	
- Furosemide (frusemide)	
- Sulphonamides	
Cushing's syndrome	Unknown
Hypothermia	Unknown
Hereditary – trypsinogen gene mutations	Presumed enzyme activation within pancreas
Pregnancy	Unknown

(necrotising pancreatitis) which results from microcirculatory stasis within the gland leading to infarction. Surrounding peripancreatic tissues may also develop necrotic changes (peripancreatic necrosis). Infection may supervene in necrotic tissue (infected necrosis) possibly by translocation of organisms from adjacent bowel.

Clinical features

These vary with the severity of the attack.

History

The principal symptom is abdominal pain, usually localised to the epigastrium or upper abdomen but which may radiate to the back in the upper lumbar region or between the scapulae. Pain ranges from mild discomfort to an excruciating level in severe cases. Rarely, acute pancreatitis can occur in the absence of pain. Nausea and repeated vomiting are present in most instances.

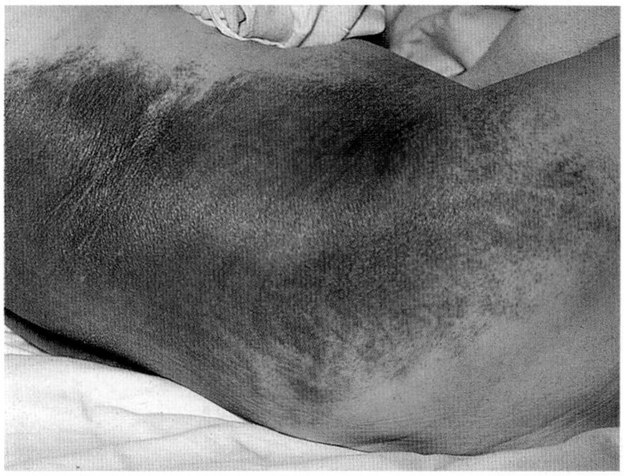

Fig. 22.2 Extensive flank bruising in acute pancreatitis – Grey Turner's sign.

Physical findings

General findings may be of an acutely ill patient with signs of circulatory insufficiency. In the abdomen, the degree of tenderness, guarding and rigidity found depends on the amount and nature of the inflammatory process. Rarely, body wall ecchymoses occur, around the umbilicus (Cullen's sign) or in the flanks (Grey Turner's sign – Fig. 22.2). Both are a consequence of haemorrhagic fluid tracking from the retroperitoneum. The remaining clinical features depend on the local and systemic complications that occur.

Diagnosis

The clinical manifestations of acute pancreatitis are so varied that the condition must be considered in the differential diagnosis of all instances of upper abdominal pain until the serum amylase concentration (see below) has been demonstrated to be within the normal range. Hyperamylasaemia, however, cannot be relied upon alone and must be evaluated in conjunction with the history and physical signs.

Investigation

Serum amylase concentration

Elevation of the serum amylase level occurs in a number of acute abdominal emergencies such as acute cholecystitis, bowel ischaemia and perforated peptic ulcer, but a concentration in excess of 1000 IU/L (or >4 times the upper limit of normal) is highly suggestive of acute pancreatitis. Very rarely, other causes of hyperamylasaemia (such as macroamylasaemia – a benign condition associated with amylase molecules of abnormally large molecular weight which are not adequately cleared by the renal tubules) may confuse the diagnosis.

Serum lipase concentration

Elevated serum lipase levels are also seen in acute pancreatitis (2–5 times normal values), the level rising within 4 hours of the attack and remaining elevated for 4–7 days. The elevation of serum lipase lasts longer than amylase and this test is therefore particularly useful in patients with delayed presentation of abdominal pain.

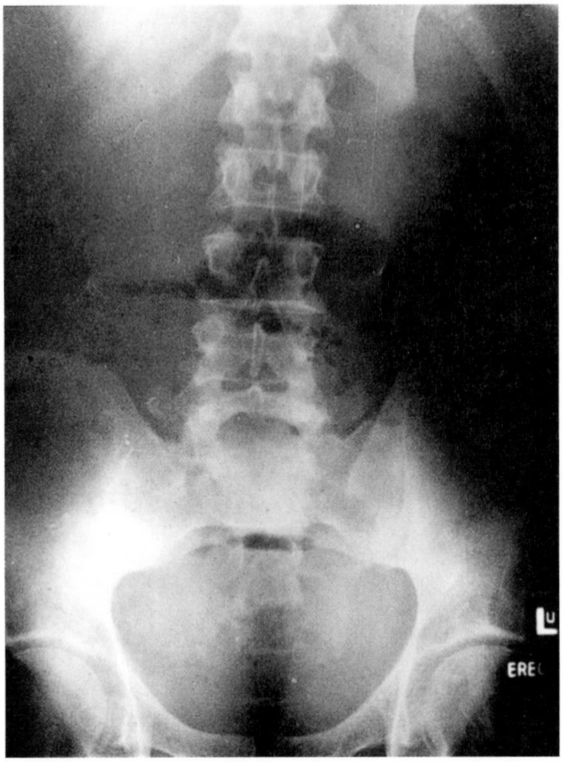

Fig. 22.3 Plain abdominal X-ray showing a dilated loop of small bowel in the epigastrium in acute pancreatitis – the sentinel loop.

Liver function tests

Significant elevation of liver enzymes, especially the transferases, at presentation is highly suggestive of gallstone aetiology. Jaundice raises the possibility of a persisting, obstructing common duct stone, and should raise concern about possible concurrent acute cholangitis.

Imaging

If an upright chest X-ray shows air under the diaphragm, then the cause of the acute abdomen is not pancreatitis but a gastrointestinal perforation, even if the serum amylase is elevated. A plain abdominal X-ray is not required in patients with a diagnosis of acute pancreatitis, but has often been performed and may show a sentinel dilated loop of small bowel overlying the pancreatic region (Fig. 22.3). Either X-ray may occasionally show calcified gallstones (15% of cases).

CT may be useful in clinching the diagnosis by demonstrating a swollen gland with inflammatory changes in the surrounding tissues (Fig. 22.4) and identifying the underlying cause, particularly gallbladder stones, although these are better seen on ultrasound. Contrast enhanced CT scanning is also used at a later stage (usually after 72 hours) to assess the extent of pancreatic necrosis and the development of other complications (see below). It is indicated in patients with persisting organ failure, signs of sepsis or clinical deterioration – typically occurring 6–10 days after onset of acute pancreatitis.

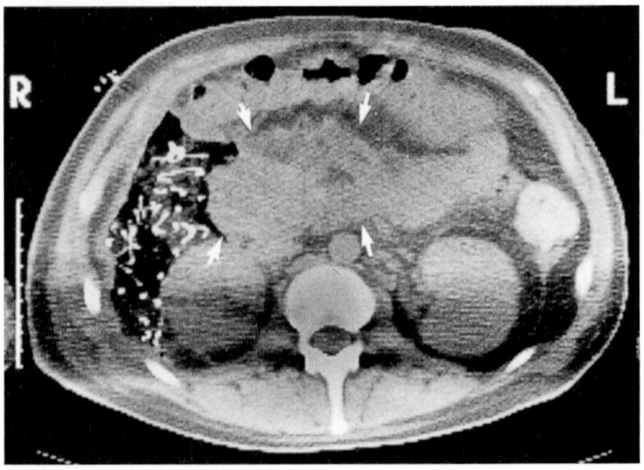

Fig. 22.4 CT image of acute pancreatitis.

Table 22.3	Features that may predict a severe attack present within 48 hours of admission to hospital (taken from the UK Guidelines for the management of acute pancreatitis – see Further Reading)

Initial assessment:
Clinical impression of severity
Body mass index >30
Pleural effusion on chest radiograph
APACHE II score >8

24 h after admission:
Clinical impression of severity
APACHE II score >8
Glasgow score 3 or more
Persisting organ failure, especially if multiple
C-reactive protein >150 mg/L

48 h after admission:
Clinical impression of severity
Glasgow score 3 or more
C-reactive protein >150 mg/L
Persisting organ failure for 48 h
Multiple or progressive organ failure

Prognosis

The severity of an attack of acute pancreatitis can be assessed in a number of ways (Table 22.3). These include:

- initial clinical condition
- single prognostic factor measurements such as CRP
- multiple prognostic factor scoring systems.

The Glasgow scoring system is widely used (Table 22.4). Measurements are made at presentation or within 48 hours of admission. The presence of three or more positive factors indicates a severe attack of acute pancreatitis; mortality is correlated with the number of positive factors. It is worth emphasising that hyperamylasaemia is not one of the predictive criteria. More recently the APACHE II score has been applied and gives a semi-continuous assessment of severity of pancreatitis, as it does of any acute surgical illness.

Mortality rates

The overall mortality is 5–10%. Most patients (70%) have a mild attack with less than three positive prognostic criteria

Table 22.4 Factors which predict the severity of pancreatitis (Glasgow system)

Factor	Level
Age	>55 years
Leucocytosis	>15 × 10^9/L
Blood urea concentration	>16 mmol/L (no response to fluid administration)
Blood glucose concentration	>10 mmol/L in the non-diabetic
Serum albumin concentration	<32 g/L
Serum calcium concentration	<2.0 mmol/L
Lactate dehydrogenase	>600 IU/L
Aspartate aminotransferase	>100 IU/L
Arterial $P\text{O}_2$	<60 mmHg (8.0 kPa)

If more than three of the above are positive, the attack is severe.

Emergency Box 22.1

Management of acute pancreatitis

In all cases

- Intravenous fluids – large volumes of crystalloid and colloid may be necessary
- Nil by mouth ± nasogastric drainage
- Analgesia – pethidine ± epidural
- Prediction of disease severity

May be needed in severe cases

- Antibiotics
- Urgent ERCP + sphincterotomy (for gallstone pancreatitis only)
- Respiratory support ± endotracheal ventilation
- Cardiovascular support with inotropes
- Renal support – haemofiltration/dialysis
- Correction of metabolic abnormalities (calcium, glucose, etc.)
- Nasojejunal (enteric) or intravenous nutrition
- Surgical debridement of infected pancreatic necrosis

and a low mortality (0–2%). A severe attack carries a higher mortality (20–30%). Death occurs for three principal reasons:

- early – from multisystem organ failure in fulminant attacks
- from co-morbid conditions – mainly cardiorespiratory problems, particularly in the aged
- late – from local complications, mainly infected necrosis but more rarely colonic necrosis or haemorrhage from eroded retroperitoneal vessels.

Management (Emergency Box 22.1)

Therapy is, in general, supportive, with management of complications if and when they develop. Mild pancreatitis usually resolves with parenteral fluid replacement, bowel rest (nothing by mouth and nasogastric intubation and drainage because of ileus and abdominal distension) and analgesia. Opiate analgesia is often necessary, but morphine is avoided because it is associated with contraction of the sphincter of Oddi. A severe episode requires more intensive support, ideally in a high-dependency or intensive care unit (see Ch. 10). Treatment includes intravenous replacement of large amounts of fluid lost into the retroperitoneum, respiratory support, which may include endotracheal ventilation, the treatment of renal failure and often antibiotics – either prophylactic or as a result of bacterial culture. Paralytic ileus may be prolonged and intravenous nutrition is then necessary. Fluid balance requires careful monitoring; normal saline, plasma substitutes (colloids) and blood may all be required. Cardiovascular observations, including central venous pressure measurements, and urine output are helpful guides (see Ch. 10). Urgent ERCP with sphincterotomy and stone extraction is indicated in severe gallstone-related pancreatitis, particularly if there is concern about an associated acute cholangitis. In many patients nutrition can be adequately achieved by naso-jejunal tube enteral feeding until oral intake is resumed.

Table 22.5 Complications of acute pancreatitis

System or site	Nature and cause
Cardiovascular	Circulatory failure – Hypovolaemia – Cytokine release
Respiratory	Hypoxia and respiratory failure (ARDS) – Abdominal distension – Cytokine release – Bacterial translocation
Renal	Acute renal failure – hypovolaemia
Haematological	Disseminated intravascular coagulation
Metabolic	Hypocalcaemia – calcium deposition in areas of fat necrosis Hyperglycaemia – islet cell dysfunction Acid–base disturbance from tissue necrosis
Nutritional	Muscle wasting/catabolism SIRS Infected retroperitoneal slough – bacterial translocation Pancreatic abscess – infected fluid collection
Retroperitoneum	Fat necrosis – enzyme release
Pseudocyst	Effusion with or without duct damage
Gastrointestinal	Prolonged paralytic ileus – retroperitoneal inflammation GI bleeding – necrosis of gut wall Colonic necrosis Duodenal obstruction
Hepatobiliary	Jaundice/obstruction of common bile duct
Vascular	Portal/splenic vein thrombosis Haemorrhage from arterial rupture

ARDS, adult respiratory distress syndrome; SIRS, systemic inflammatory response syndrome.

Complications

The more severe the attack, the more likely it is that complications will develop (Table 22.5).

Systemic

Systemic complications usually occur soon after the onset of the acute attack (within 0–7 days), although they can take place after this time. They include:

- cardiovascular collapse because of hypovolaemia from massive exudation of fluid into the retroperitoneal tissues and the release of inflammatory cytokines; cardiac function may also be directly depressed

- hypoxia is common and of multifactorial origin – abdominal distension, cytokine release and bacterial translocation from the gut; ARDS (Ch. 10) may develop
- hypocalcaemia – thought to be the result of calcium deposition in areas of fat necrosis
- hyperglycaemia – from disturbances of insulin metabolism
- acute coagulopathies.

Local

Local complications usually occur more than a week after onset. Pancreatic and peripancreatic inflammation may lead to tissue necrosis and collections of inflammatory fluid. Secondary infection of these may follow, probably by bacterial translocation from the gut, and lead on to infected slough, abscess, bacteraemia and a secondary systemic response (SIRS – Ch. 9). Biliary obstruction may be caused by inflammation or fluid collections around the head of the gland. Inflammation may also cause portal or, more commonly, splenic vein thrombosis. CT changes in the early stages of the disease (multiple fluid collections, extensive pancreatic necrosis as indicated by non-enhancement of necrotic areas on contrast enhancement) may also give an early indication of local complications.

Necrosis and infection

Dead areas within the gland or surrounding tissues may, if they remain sterile, resolve over time, and whether they should be removed is a matter of controversy. However, when these areas are infected and there is a systemic response, they should usually be removed by surgical debridement. This has usually been achieved by laparotomy with full exploration of the pancreas, lesser sac and surrounding areas of fat necrosis. Necrotic tissue is debrided and large-bore drains left close to the areas of necrosis/pancreatic remnant. Postoperative retroperitoneal irrigation through the surgically placed drains is then often undertaken. More recently a laparoscopic approach to the retroperitoneum and lesser sac has been used successfully in selected cases.

Acute fluid collections/pseudocysts

Acute fluid collections are relatively common, and many will resolve spontaneously. They may mature into pseudocysts after 4–6 weeks as a wall of granulation and fibrosis is formed. They start either as 'sympathetic' inflammatory collections (usually in the lesser sac of the peritoneum) or as the consequence of rupture of the pancreatic duct or one of its tributaries. When a peripancreatic fluid collection is of the first kind, it usually resolves spontaneously and is managed expectantly. Pseudocysts larger than 6 cm diameter that persist for longer than 6 weeks are more often in communication with the duct and require internal draining by cyst gastrostomy or cyst jejunostomy. This may be performed surgically or by endoscopic drainage. Occasionally percutaneous pseudocyst drainage is used, but there is a high recurrence rate once the drain is removed, and the technique is best avoided.

Chronic pancreatitis

Aetiology and pathological features

Alcohol is the usual cause of chronic pancreatitis (80% in developed societies). Pancreatitis can also occur in other conditions where free drainage of the pancreatic duct is impeded (e.g. pancreas divisum, papillary or pancreatic tumours, biliary stents, traumatic duct stricture). In these conditions structural changes may develop, leading to chronic pancreatitis. Other causes of chronic disease include:

- familial/hereditary – trypsinogen gene mutations
- nutritional in tropical countries, probably of toxic origin.

As with acute pancreatitis, the precise underlying mechanisms leading to the development of chronic pancreatitis are not fully understood. Heavy consumption of alcohol is a common association and it is in such circumstances that the morphological changes have been most studied. The earliest change appears to be deposition of plugs of protein within the smaller pancreatic ducts. The lumen becomes obstructed, and dilatation follows. Atrophy of the acini then occurs. There may be an accompanying inflammatory infiltrate, but this is variable. Fibrosis takes place around the affected ducts. Eventually only a few acinar and islet cells remain, with widely dilated pancreatic ducts. Intraluminal calcification of the protein plugs also occurs, so that stones form. Other changes seen in chronic pancreatitis include ductal strictures and dilatation, intrapancreatic cysts and chronic pseudocysts.

Chronic pancreatitis is not reversible, but it is possible that progress can be arrested if the causative factor, such as alcohol, is withdrawn. However, this is an uncommon outcome and the disease is most often progressive.

Clinical features

History

The predominant symptom is chronic abdominal pain, mainly in the epigastrium or upper abdomen. It may radiate to the back, can be continuous, severe and relentless. An alternative course is chronic pain punctuated by acute exacerbations which resemble acute pancreatitis. Such episodes are usually mild and of brief duration; their relationship to alcohol is variable, but some seem to be precipitated by a bout of heavy alcohol consumption. Chronic pain may be accompanied by severe weight loss caused by anorexia and fat malabsorption. Regular analgesic consumption frequently leads to opiate addiction. Patients with chronic pancreatitis may have pain-free intervals and acute exacerbations of their chronic condition. Depression is common.

Steatorrhoea occurs when the secretion of pancreatic lipase is reduced by 90% and is present in about half the patients. The development of diabetes is more common. Both occur more often when the pancreas is calcified (Fig. 22.5).

A relatively short clinical presentation suggestive of chronic pancreatic inflammation should always raise the suspicion of cancer of the gland (see below). Conversely, chronic pancreatitis carries an increased risk for the development of cancer. Less commonly, chronic pancreatitis causes obstructive jaundice and occasionally cholangitis. Obstruction or thrombosis of the splenic vein can lead to segmental portal

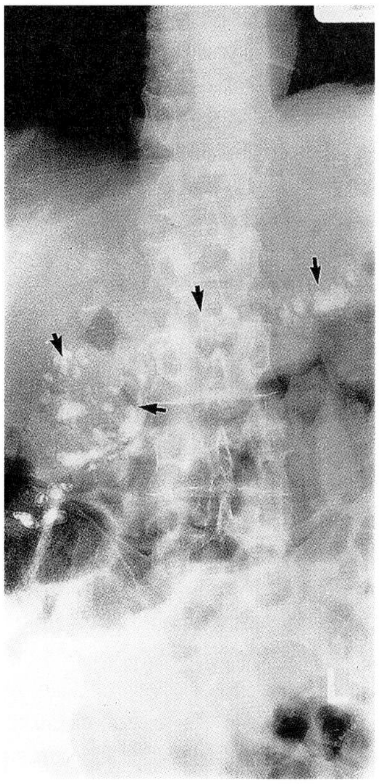

Fig. 22.5 Plain abdominal X-ray showing scattered calcification throughout the pancreas (arrowed) in a case of chronic pancreatitis.

hypertension with oesophageal varices and upper gastrointestinal bleeding.

Physical findings

Evidence of malnourishment may be obvious. Other signs may be few, but some patients show the characteristic features of alcoholic liver disease.

Investigation

Endocrine function

If frank clinical diabetes is not present, the glucose tolerance test may still be abnormal, although this is also true in pancreatic carcinoma.

Exocrine function

Tests have been outlined above but are not often used for diagnostic purposes as distinct from planning therapy.

Concentration of serum amylase

In the diagnosis of chronic disease this is not of value, although the level may be increased during an acute episode of pain.

Imaging

Plain X-ray can show a characteristic transverse outline of the calcified gland (Fig. 22.5), although this investigation is not indicated for investigation of chronic pancreatitis.

Ultrasound and CT can demonstrate both a reduction and an increase in the size of the gland, duct dilatation or the presence of calcification. They may also demonstrate intrapancreatic cysts or chronic pseudocysts.

ERCP (Fig. 22.6) and MRCP are also useful to confirm the anatomical abnormality – a dilated and/or strictured main

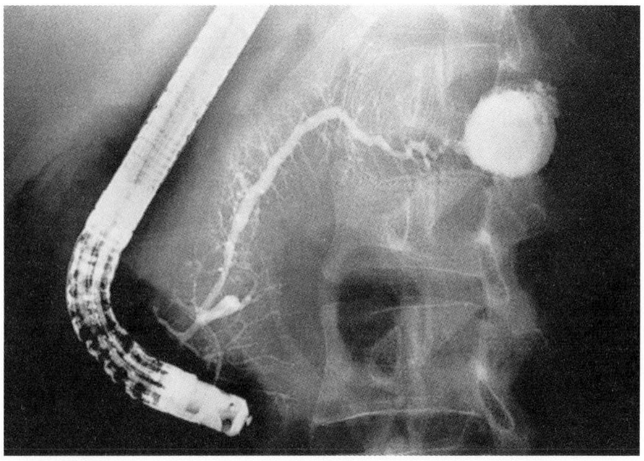

Fig. 22.6 Endoscopic retrograde pancreatogram showing a pancreatic duct of irregular calibre with blunted side branches. Distally the duct has a large cystic dilatation. The endoscope and cannula can be clearly seen.

(chain of lakes), blunted side branches and sometimes associated stones. ERCP is usually only now performed when endoscopic therapy is planned: for example, stone removal, ductal dilatation or stenting.

It is often difficult to distinguish between chronic pancreatitis and carcinoma, especially as cancer may develop on a background of chronic pancreatitis. Pancreatic imaging combined with EUS and targeted needle biopsy may be helpful. However, it must be remembered that a needle biopsy which shows chronic pancreatitis does not exclude carcinoma, as secondary (obstructive) inflammation is often found adjacent to a carcinoma. In some cases, particularly if obstructive jaundice has developed, resection of a pancreatic mass is recommended without a definite pathological diagnosis of malignancy, the final diagnosis only being made on histopathology.

Management

Measures for control

In alcohol-induced chronic pancreatitis, absolute cessation of drinking is advised but rarely achieved. Control of pain may require long-term use of opiates which, together with the misery of the disease, may lead to addiction.

Steatorrhoea is treated with pancreatic supplements, usually combined with acid suppression therapy. Diabetes mellitus may be unstable and difficult to control. The insulin requirement is often greater than in idiopathic diabetes, perhaps because pancreatic glucagon is lacking.

Surgical intervention

The indications for operation are:

- correctable anatomical complications which are considered to be associated with either pain or recurrent exacerbations of pancreatitis – e.g. an obstructed pancreatic duct, or a chronic pseudocyst
- obstructive jaundice
- rarely, intractable pain with a diffusely damaged gland
- the development of a possible malignant mass (see above).

Operation involves either drainage of a cyst or obstructed duct, or partial or complete pancreatic resection for intractable pain or a suspicious mass. If total pancreatectomy is performed, islet cell transplantation can be considered in an attempt to prevent the development of brittle diabetes mellitus. Hypoglycaemia is a not uncommon cause of death after total pancreatectomy. Surgical management for chronic pain is controversial. Good results are only obtained if other factors, such as alcohol, are controlled and patients are well motivated and carefully selected.

Complications

Pancreatic pseudocyst

This is the commonest complication found, especially if careful ultrasound examinations are performed, and they usually arise from within pancreatic tissue. Small cysts do not usually require drainage. Larger ones can give rise to localised pain, nausea and vomiting or biliary obstruction. A smooth, tender mass is occasionally palpable in the epigastrium, but a cyst can be easily identified on ultrasound or CT scan. Surgical treatment has been used for most large cysts, but a non-operative policy with aspiration and close follow-up by ultrasound examination is now advocated by some centres.

Pancreatic ascites

Alcoholic pancreatitis with a communication between the pancreatic duct and the peritoneal cavity is the usual cause of this rare complication. The amylase content of the ascitic fluid is very high. Treatment is by temporary endoscopic insertion of a stent into the pancreatic duct, operative drainage of the duct fistula into a jejunal loop or resection of the portion of the gland that contains the fistula.

PANCREATIC TUMOURS

Pancreatic carcinoma

Cancer of the exocrine pancreas is an aggressive disease with a poor prognosis; the median survival from the time of diagnosis barely exceeds 5 months. Even with recent advances in surgery, anaesthesia, intensive care, cytotoxic chemotherapy and radiotherapy, there have been only modest improvements in outcome over the last 50 years. Characteristics are outlined in Box 22.3.

Epidemiology

Pancreatic cancer has now overtaken gastric cancer to become the fourth leading cause of death from malignant disease in Western society. In the UK, this amounts to some 5000 deaths a year and is continuing to increase steadily. Across western Europe the disease causes some 30 000 deaths a year, and in North America over 27 000. The peak incidence occurs between the ages of 50 and 70 years, although it occasionally occurs in those as young as 30. Pancreatic cancer is a disease of the developed world; for example, the prevalence of the disease in Afro-Caribbeans in the Bay Area around San Francisco is twice as high as that seen in western Africa, and there is a 10-fold difference in incidence between the USA and India. Within the USA, the incidence of pancreatic cancer in blacks is five times greater than that in Japanese Americans and Hispanics from Puerto Rico.

Box 22.3 Pancreatic cancer

- 5000 deaths/year in United Kingdom
- Presenting symptoms may include upper abdominal/back pain, jaundice, weight loss, vomiting
- 95% adenocarcinoma
- 80% of patients have unresectable tumours
- Lymphatic, liver and peritoneal metastases common
- <20% 5-year survival after resection
- 6 months median survival
- Palliative treatments include analgesia, endoscopic biliary stenting, chemotherapy, surgical bypass or endoscopic enteric stenting for duodenal stenosis

Aetiology

Putative factors are shown in Box 22.4. However, their exact contribution is unclear. All studies show the disease to be commoner in men than in women, with a ratio ranging from 1.5 : 1 to 2 : 1, although there is evidence of a rising incidence in women in some countries.

There is an established link between pancreatic cancer and cigarette smoking, perhaps through nitrosamine inhalation. Smoking also raises serum lipids, which in turn may predispose to pancreatic cancer, because high-fat diets are also related to an increased incidence of the disease. Other factors include employment in chemical industries and obesity.

The role of alcohol consumption is also unclear, although chronic pancreatitis has been linked to the development of pancreatic cancer. A causal relationship with diabetes mellitus has been confused by the fact that up to 15% of patients with pancreatic cancer develop diabetes in the period before presentation.

A family history of pancreatic cancer (first-degree relative) and a number of identified cancer genetic risk factors (e.g. BRCA 1 or 2, FAP and HNPCC) all increase the risk of pancreatic cancer.

Pathological features

All but 5% of cancers are adenocarcinomas which originate from the pancreatic ducts; the remainder are of acinar origin and said to be less aggressive. Seventy percent of tumours occur in the pancreatic head. Only 1% have a cystic component (cystadenocarcinomas). The solid tumours are white in appearance and woody on palpation; at operation their gross appearance can mimic chronic pancreatitis, making histological diagnosis essential either by biopsy or by resection. Spread of the growth is by the four typical routes:

Box 22.4 Putative aetiological factors in exocrine pancreatic cancer

- 'Western' lifestyle: probably dietary factors
- Cigarette smoking
- High-fat diet
- Chronic pancreatitis
- Obesity
- Family history/genetic risk factors

- direct invasion of neighbouring tissues including perineural spread
- lymph node involvement
- blood-borne metastases to the liver and beyond
- within the peritoneal cavity – transcoelomic spread.

Direct invasion

Cancers arising in the pancreatic head invade and obstruct the lower end of the common bile duct to produce extrahepatic obstructive jaundice. The development of obstruction causes the biliary tract to dilate and if, as is usually the case, the gallbladder is not diseased, then it shares in the distension (see Courvoisier's law, below).

Further, in 15–20% of those with a carcinoma in the pancreatic head, direct invasion of the duodenum results in gastric outflow obstruction and vomiting. Local infiltration of retroperitoneal tissues – the coeliac plexus, splenic and portal veins – may be responsible for some symptoms (see below) and may also determine irresectability.

Lymphatic

The nodes adjacent to the gland, the pre-aortic coeliac glands and the nodes at the porta hepatis are all frequently involved.

Vascular

The tumour drains into the portal vein, and liver metastases are most common.

Transcoelomic

Spread across the peritoneal cavity results in peritoneal seedlings and ascites.

Perineural

This is common and may contribute to the pain often experienced by patients with pancreatic cancer.

Clinical features

History

The typical presenting history is of a middle-aged patient with obstructive jaundice and pruritus. There may be associated weight loss and epigastric pain which radiates through to the back and can sometimes be alleviated by sitting crouched forward. A recent diagnosis of diabetes mellitus may have been made. If duodenal invasion has occurred, vomiting is present and is usually indicative of an advanced tumour.

A carcinoma of the body or tail almost always presents late because of the insidious progression of the tumour before symptoms occur. However, in retrospect there is often a non-specific prodromal phase of vague symptoms of malaise, weight loss and epigastric pain radiating to the back. Very few such patients have surgically resectable tumours by the time these symptoms occur.

The major clinical diagnostic problem is that early symptoms mimic other commoner disorders such as peptic ulcer, oesophagitis with heartburn, angina and biliary colic. Many will have spent several months undergoing investigation for these disorders before the correct diagnosis is established or jaundice develops.

Physical findings

Examination may reveal only jaundice. There may be scratch marks over the trunk and limbs as a consequence of bile-salt-induced pruritus. Features of weight loss, such as ill-fitting clothes, are often present. Other possible findings include:

- a palpable enlarged gallbladder – two-thirds of those with pancreatic cancer and obstructive jaundice exemplify Courvoisier's law, which states that this finding indicates a malignant distal biliary obstruction; however, the reverse is not true, because previous gallbladder stone disease may have produced fibrosis and rendered the gallbladder non-distensible even in the presence of malignant obstruction
- occasionally a palpable mass in the epigastrium which characteristically transmits aortic pulsation
- abdominal distension and ascites
- a palpable, hard, left supraclavicular lymph node (Virchow's gland).

Diagnosis

The other condition that frequently produces a similar clinical picture is a gallstone in the common bile duct, usually impacted at the lower end and causing progressive obstructive jaundice.

Less common causes of obstructive jaundice are:

- malignant compression of the bile duct by metastases in portal lymph nodes
- drug-induced cholestatic jaundice (no intrahepatic ductal dilatation on ultrasound scanning)
- a carcinoma of the duodenum or papilla at the lower end of the common bile duct
- carcinoma of the bile duct (cholangiocarcinoma)
- Mirizzi's syndrome – cholecystitis and a gallstone in Hartmann's pouch with local inflammation and oedema causing stricturing of and sometimes erosion into the common hepatic duct
- sclerosing cholangitis.

Investigation

Biochemical

Liver function shows an obstructive pattern. The commonest difficulty is with intrahepatic cholestatic jaundice, where the pattern may overlap with extrahepatic obstruction.

Glucose tolerance is impaired in many patients.

Coagulation studies

In the presence of jaundice, prothrombin time is prolonged (see the International Normalised Ratio).

Imaging

Ultrasound may show a normal common bile duct or demonstrate a dilated intra- and extrahepatic biliary tree (in the presence of jaundice), a mass in the head of the pancreas and possible liver metastases.

A CT scan is valuable in demonstrating the relationship of the tumour to the superior mesenteric vessels and portal vein. In addition, it may show lymphatic and hepatic metastases.

Endoscopy can demonstrate a malignant mass infiltrating the medial wall of the second part of the duodenum from which a biopsy may be obtained. MRCP may indicate a malignant stricture of the common bile duct and often also the pancreatic duct ('double duct' sign). The stricture appears shouldered, abrupt and tight.

Endoscopic ultrasound is occasionally useful in the detection and evaluation of small pancreatic lesions, including endocrine tumours (see Ch. 32), ductal stones and cholangiocarcinoma of the biliary ducts. It is occasionally also helpful in assessing vascular invasion of the superior mesenteric vessels or portal vein.

PET scannning may be used in patients being considered for surgical resection to exclude metastatic disease not seen on other staging investigations.

Laparoscopy is also often used to exclude small peritoneal or liver metastases before an attempt at resection.

Specific serum tumour markers

Both carbohydrate antigen 19-9 (CA 19-9) and carcinoembryonic antigen (CEA) may be elevated in pancreatic cancer. CA 19-9 is usually elevated in patients with pancreatic cancer but is also raised in obstructive jaundice of any cause and is therefore unreliable in patients with unrelieved jaundice. Although these markers are not specific enough to be diagnostic, they often support a clinical diagnosis, particularly if there is a progressive rise on repeated estimations.

Management

The objectives and methods of intervention are:

- resection of the primary lesion for cure (feasible in less than 20% of patients)
- alleviation of obstructive jaundice
- pain control
- treatment of exocrine failure and of diabetes
- chemotherapeutic and/or radiotherapeutic palliation.

Surgical resection

Less than 20% of pancreatic cancers are resectable at the time of presentation, and these are predominantly lesions in the pancreatic head.

The most common operation performed is a pylorus-preserving pancreatoduodenectomy. The pancreatic head, lower common bile duct (and usually gallbladder), duodenum (apart from proximal section of first part of duoenum), a short length of proximal jejunum and the surrounding tissues including lymph nodes are resected. The remaining common bile (or hepatic) duct, the body and tail of the pancreas and the remaining duodenum are then anastomosed separately to the jejunum (sometimes the pancreas to the stomach). This is a major procedure but, in expert hands, the hospital mortality is less than 5%.

Tumours found at operation to be irresectable are palliatively treated by biliary and usually also duodenal bypass.

Alleviation of obstructive jaundice

Endoscopic, percutaneous radiological or surgical methods can be used to achieve this.

Endoscopic stenting at ERCP The major papilla is cannulated via the endoscope and a plastic or expanding metal stent placed through the obstructing tumour. Bile and pancreatic juice can be collected or ductal brushings or biopsy taken for cytological or histopathological analysis.

However, the procedure is not free from hazard:

- The mortality is 1–2%, usually related to the introduction of infection into an obstructed biliary system – prophylactic antibiotic cover is required.
- Plastic stents have a median survival of 14 weeks before silting up with biliary debris, and, should the patient survive beyond this time, a replacement is necessary; expanding metal inserts last longer but may occlude from tumour ingrowth.
- Duodenal obstruction may develop because of progression of the tumour – although this can now also be treated by endoscopic enteric metal stent placement.

In some patients (maybe 10%) ERCP stenting is unsuccessful. A percutaneous cholangiogram (PTC) can be performed and a plastic or metal stent inserted along the track into the biliary tree and through the bile duct stricture.

Palliative surgical decompression This can be undertaken by either anastomosis of the gallbladder to the jejunum (cholecystojejunostomy) or direct anastomosis of a loop of isolated jejunum to the dilated hepatic duct (hepaticojejunostomy). Both can be combined with a gastroenterostomy to manage duodenal obstruction – currently the most frequent indication for operative palliation, although increasingly being replaced by endoscopic duodenal stenting. Cholecystojejunostomy is quick and easy for both the patient and the surgeon; however, early failure may follow from occlusion of a low insertion of the cystic duct into the common hepatic, and the slightly more demanding hepaticojejunostomy is preferred.

Pain relief

Many patients with pancreatic cancer require strong analgesic (usually opioid) use to deal with intractable pain caused by invasion of the coeliac plexus. Relief may be achieved by a coeliac plexus nerve block with alcohol or radiofrequency ablation (RFA), either at the time of operation or under radiological control. Otherwise, analgesia can be achieved by the methods described in Chapter 6.

Treatment of exocrine and endocrine pancreatic insufficiency

The clinical features of this condition are malabsorption with weight loss and steatorrhoea. Pancreatic enzyme supplements are prescribed, and the patient is advised to take as much with each meal as is necessary to control the loose motions.

Diabetes secondary to pancreatic cancer occasionally requires insulin for control. Dietary carbohydrate restriction, sometimes supplemented by oral hypoglycaemic agents, is usually adequate.

Chemotherapy and radiotherapy

Chemotherapy regimens so far devised, either alone or in combination, are not curative. Regimens that have shown some palliative response (10–30%) are based on combination therapy using 5-fluorouracil (5-FU). Single-agent gemcitabine is also widely used, sometimes combined

Table 22.6 Pancreatic cysts

Inflammatory cysts	Non-inflammatory cysts (neoplastic)
Pseudocyst (post-pancreatitis)	Serous cystadenoma Mucinous cystadenoma/ adenocarcinoma* Intraductal papillary mucinous neoplasm (IPMN)* Solid pseudopapillary tumour of pancreas*

*Potential for malignant change.

with capecitabine (an oral form of 5-FU). Adjuvant chemotherapy following surgical resection provides a survival advantage of upto 10% at 3 years.

In addition external beam radiotherapy and more recently cyber-knife radiotherapy are used for localised but irresectable cancers, often combined with palliative chemotherapy.

Prognosis

Pancreatic cancer carries a poor prognosis, and most patients are dead within 2 years of diagnosis – more than half within 6 months. Even for those patients fortunate to present with a surgically resectable lesion, the 5-year survival after successful removal is less than 20%. Early involvement of palliative care services is important for most patients.

Pancreatic cysts

Pancreatic cysts are fluid collections in or around the pancreas. They are divided into inflammatory and non-inflammatory types (Table 22.6). They may be identified during investigation of upper abdominal pain or occasionally jaundice or acute pancreatitis. They are increasingly being found incidentally during scanning (ultrasound, MRI or CT) for other conditions.

Inflammatory cysts follow an attack of acute pancreatitis. They do not have an epithelial lining and are also known as pancreatic pseudocysts (see above). They may cause abdominal pain or occasionally obstruct the bile duct (jaundice) or duodenum (vomiting). Pseudocysts may resolve over the course of a few weeks. However, if they are connected to the pancreatic ductal system they will persist and often require drainage into the stomach (endoscopic or surgical) or small intestine (surgical). Such connecting cysts will have a high fluid amylase level if aspirated at endoscopic ultrasound or percutaneously.

Non-inflammatory cysts are neoplastic lesions that may be benign, premalignant or malignant. They are often asymptomatic or may cause abdominal pain, or occasionally jaundice or acute pancreatitis. The difficulties in management are firstly identifying the type of cystic lesion and secondly advising on whether the patient should undergo resection.

Serous cystadenomas consist of multiple small cysts and may have central calcification on imaging. They are benign and usually asymptomatic. Occasionally when large they are resected because of abdominal pain.

Mucinous cystadenomas have larger cysts and sometimes peripheral calcification. They are potentially malignant and can develop into an adenocarcinoma. For this reason resection is normally recommended for any cyst greater than 3 cm in diameter, provided the patient is fit enough for operation.

Intraductal papillary mucinous neoplasm (IPMN) is a condition associated with dilatation of the pancreatic ducts with excess mucin production. Mucous secretions may be seen at the pancreatic ductal orifice at endoscopy. IPMN is divided into main duct and side branch types, although there is overlap. Cystic components are often seen. There is a high risk of malignant change (adenocarinoma) particularly in the main duct type. Resection of the involved pancreas is normally advised.

Solid pseudopapillary tumours of the pancreas are rare neoplasms occuring mainly in young Asian and black women. They may be large and are potentially malignant. Resection is recommended with a good prognosis after complete excision.

Investigation is by a combination of ultrasound, CT, MRI and occasionally PET scanning. Cyst appearance and size, calcification on CT, the presence of pancreatic ductal dilatation and evidence of malignant change (wall thickening, positivity on PET scanning, evidence of metastatic spread) may establish a provisional diagnosis and guide management. Where there is diagnostic uncertainty endoscopic ultrasound (EUS) may be helpful, especially when combined with cyst aspiration for fluid analysis (cytology, amylase and CEA levels). A high amylase suggests IPMN (or a pseudocyst) and a high CEA is indicative of a mucinous cystadenoma/ cystadenocarcinoma.

Islet cell tumours

These tumours are discussed in detail in Chapter 32.

FURTHER READING

Blumgart LH 2006 Surgery of the liver, biliary tract and pancreas, 4th edn. Saunders Elsevier, Philadelphia

Beger HG, Matsuno S, Cameron JL 2007 Diseases of the pancreas: current surgical therapy. Springer, Berlin-Heidelberg

Garden OJ 2005 Hepatobiliary and pancreatic surgery: a companion to specialist surgical practice. Saunders Elsevier, Philadelphia

The UK Working Party on Acute Pancreatitis 2005 UK Guidelines for the management of acute pancreatitis. Gut 54: 1–9

23 Acute abdominal conditions

ACUTE ABDOMEN

Urgent abdominal conditions form the bulk of the emergency activity of general surgeons. The range of causes is very wide and management often challenging. Many of the conditions are considered elsewhere in this text: intestinal obstruction (Ch. 24); trauma (Ch. 3); vascular emergencies (Ch. 29); acute urological disorders (Ch. 33); large-bowel disorders and acute lower-bowel haemorrhage (Ch. 25).

Resuscitation by appropriate fluid management, accompanied by adequate monitoring, is fundamental to securing a successful outcome in many of these conditions, even before the definitive diagnosis has been made (see Ch. 7).

Definition

The term 'acute abdomen' is a loose one encompassing all those conditions that present with clinical features of short duration (arbitrarily less than 10 days) which might indicate a progressive intra-abdominal condition that is threatening to life or capable of causing severe morbidity. Not all patients will turn out to have such a threatening condition, but they need to be considered as being in danger until surgical evaluation has been completed. The majority of such patients have pain as their chief symptom. There are a very large number of possible causes, but most patients are found to have one of a relatively small number of common conditions.

Surgical practice has for many years observed a policy of management based on 'it is better to look and see rather than to wait and see', because of the often progressive nature of many causes of the acute abdomen. However, with the development of new technologies (e.g. laparoscopy, ultrasound and CT scanning – see below), the surgical objective has now become to reach a management decision which separates those who must have an operation to prevent dangerous progression from those who do not. Often this decision involves making an accurate diagnosis of the cause, but this is not always immediately necessary. The important matter is to classify the patient correctly into one of three categories based on the evidence available:

- operation necessary
- operation not immediately necessary; further information should be sought but may be followed by the need for surgery
- operation not necessary.

These categories span a spectrum of causes which can be graded in terms of their threat to life on a scale of 1 to 10 (1 = conditions which are never life-threatening; 10 = conditions which are associated with great risk of serious complications or death – Table 23.1). For example, a patient eventually labelled as having non-specific abdominal pain for which a cause is not identified and from which no physical adverse effect follows would be classed as 1, whereas a patient with a ruptured aortic aneurysm (Ch. 29) would be classed as 10. However, it is more difficult to allocate other conditions on the scale in such a precise way, because their severity is subject to variation between individuals (e.g. on the grounds of age and comorbidity) and also depends upon the rapidity with which management is undertaken. Because of this, the causes of the acute abdomen shown in Table 23.1 are assigned a score of <5, 5 or >5. All the standard features of history-taking and physical examination apply to the evaluation of a patient thought to have an acute abdomen.

Structured data sheets

These sheets were introduced to make sure that data entered for computer analysis were complete and uniform (Fig. 23.1); they force rigorous collection of information and have, in consequence, a power of their own to improve the analysis of the individual episode. They provide a useful reminder of the information required in any patient with a possible acute abdomen.

General clinical features

Pain

Abdominal pain has three origins:

- visceral
- parietal
- extra-abdominal.

Table 23.1 Severity scale for causes of the acute abdomen

Condition	Grade <5	Grade 5	Grade >5
Non-specific abdominal pain	•		
Ruptured abdominal aortic aneurysm			•
Ovarian cyst rupture or torsion		•	
Perforated peptic ulcer		•	
Urinary tract infection	•		
Ectopic pregnancy rupture		•	
Mesenteric adenitis	•		
Diverticulitis		•——	——•
Renal colic	•		
Appendicitis		•——	——•
Pseudo-obstruction	•		
Small-bowel obstruction		•——	——•
Fitz-Hugh–Curtis syndrome	•		
Malignancy	•		
Salpingitis	•		
Cholecystitis	•——	————	——•
Mesenteric adenitis	•		
Intestinal ischaemia		•——	——•
Terminal ileitis	•		
Intussusception		•——	——•
Gastritis/duodenitis	•		
Volvulus of the colon		•——	——•
Gastroenteritis	•		
Inflammatory bowel disease		•——	——•
Torsion of appendices		•——	——•
Meckel's diverticulum rupture			•
Testicular torsion		•——	——•
Sickle cell crisis	•		
Referred pain from chest (myocardial infarct, pneumonia)			•
Abdominal tuberculosis	•——	————	——•
Porphyria		•	
Irritable bowel syndrome	•		
Diabetes mellitus	•		
Dysmenorrhoea	•		

Visceral pain

Visceral pain is generated either because of muscular contraction (colic) in organs such as the gut or ureter or because of stretching of the wall of a hollow organ (gallbladder) or the capsule of a solid one (aching pain from an enlarged liver). Organs from which such pain arises do not have a precise surface representation, so that the sensation is not accurately localised by the patient. However, pain which arises from the embryonic foregut (down to the second part of the duodenum) is usually located to the epigastrium; from the midgut (second part of the duodenum to the midtransverse colon) to the periumbilical region; and from the hindgut to the suprapubic area. Visceral pain is often severe and, in general, is central, as in bowel obstruction (Ch. 25) or biliary colic (Ch. 20); ureteric pain is ipsilateral (Ch. 33).

In pain of visceral origin, a distinction should be made between colic, which truly comes and goes at (fairly) regular intervals, and distension, where the persistent tension on the wall or capsule of an organ produces pain of the same nature but which is more continuously present. In clinical practice the difference is often not appreciated, but it helps the clinician to think clearly about cause (see, for example, biliary pain, Ch. 20).

Parietal pain

Parietal pain has its origin in the abdominal wall at any depth from the skin through to the peritoneum. The parietes have an accurate surface representation, so that the patient can usually indicate where exactly the pain is; examples are peritonitis (see 'Appendicitis', Ch. 25) and abdominal wall bruising. Sudden onset of diffuse parietal pain, associated with physical findings of peritoneal irritation, usually means perforation of a hollow viscus, rupture of an abscess into the general peritoneal cavity or bleeding.

The combination of initial visceral pain and later local irritation is characteristically seen in acute appendicitis (Ch. 25) or acute cholecystitis (Ch. 20). The initial pain of obstruction to the lumen of the organ is manifest as central colic and then, when inflammation develops, it produces localised pain at the site where the organ is in contact with the parietal peritoneum of the anterior abdominal wall. There is a potential diagnostic trap when an area of peritoneal irritation is not in contact with the anterior abdominal wall and therefore does not produce pain (see below).

Extra-abdominal pain

Extra-abdominal pain may take two forms:

- pain that originates from sources that share innervation with the abdominal wall – approximately T9 to L1 – such as may occur in conditions which involve the spinal nerves
- pain from a wide variety of disorders where the mechanism is not well understood.

Apparent pain

To the three origins – visceral, parietal and extra-abdominal – should be added two clinical occurrences of apparent abdominal pain:

- Münchhausen's syndrome (so-called because it recalls the tales of Baron Münchhausen who invented marvellous adventures). There are certain individuals who present repeatedly with dramatic symptoms which often include pain as a prominent feature. There is usually a convincing story of an acute abdomen but without a cause. It is easy to be taken in by such patients, and they move from hospital to hospital undergoing needless investigation and surgery. However, it is important to take reported symptoms at face value in all cases unless there are clear records demonstrating previous episodes when no cause for pain has been found.
- Drug-dependent patients may feign pain to obtain analgesic drugs, although such patients may also develop acute abdominal conditions.

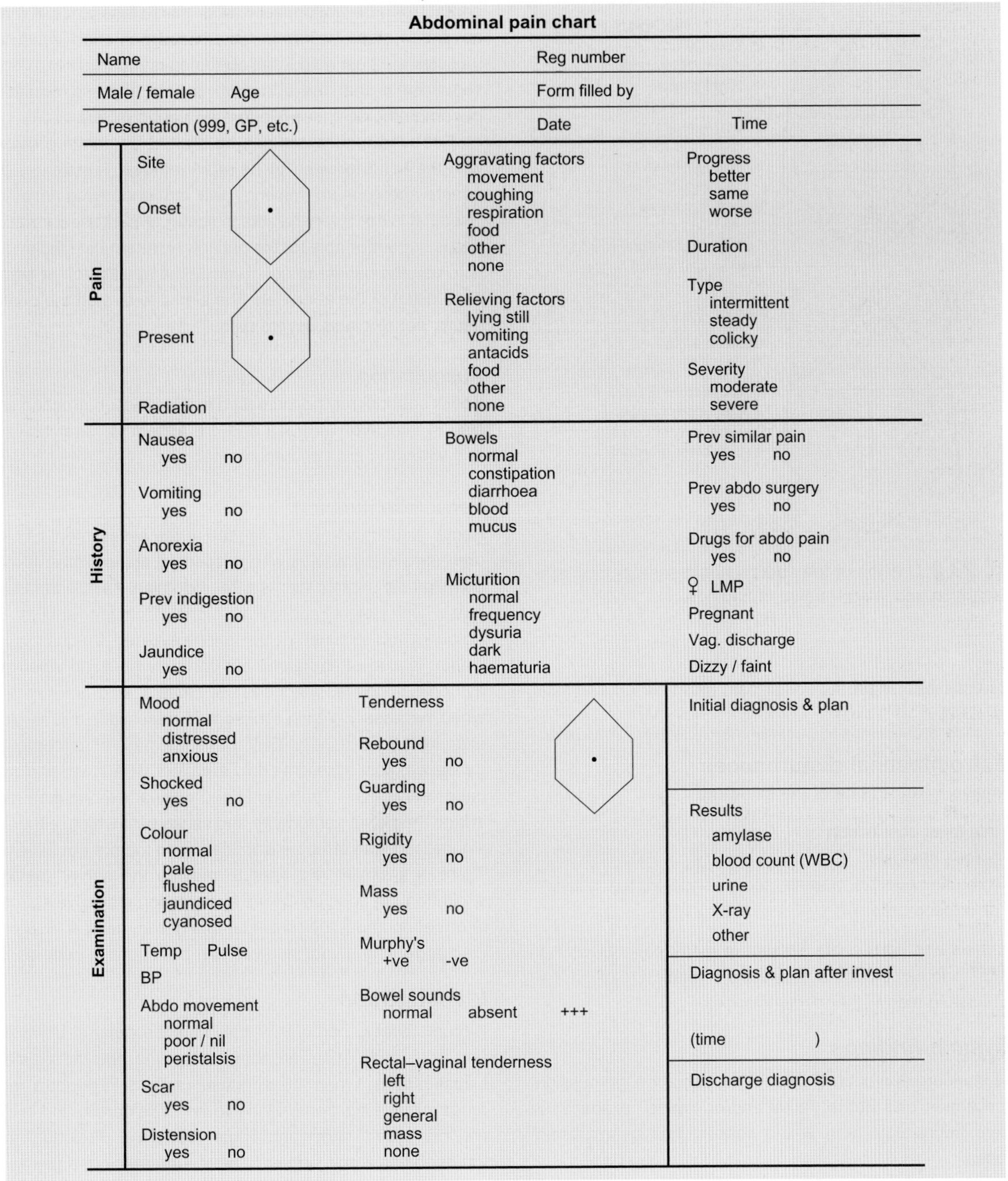

Abdominal pain chart

Name | Reg number
Male / female | Age | Form filled by
Presentation (999, GP, etc.) | Date | Time

Pain

Site
Onset
Present
Radiation

Aggravating factors: movement, coughing, respiration, food, other, none

Relieving factors: lying still, vomiting, antacids, food, other, none

Progress: better, same, worse
Duration
Type: intermittent, steady, colicky
Severity: moderate, severe

History

Nausea: yes no
Vomiting: yes no
Anorexia: yes no
Prev indigestion: yes no
Jaundice: yes no

Bowels: normal, constipation, diarrhoea, blood, mucus

Micturition: normal, frequency, dysuria, dark, haematuria

Prev similar pain: yes no
Prev abdo surgery: yes no
Drugs for abdo pain: yes no
♀ LMP
Pregnant
Vag. discharge
Dizzy / faint

Examination

Mood: normal, distressed, anxious
Shocked: yes no
Colour: normal, pale, flushed, jaundiced, cyanosed
Temp | Pulse
BP
Abdo movement: normal, poor / nil, peristalsis
Scar: yes no
Distension: yes no

Tenderness
Rebound: yes no
Guarding: yes no
Rigidity: yes no
Mass: yes no
Murphy's: +ve -ve
Bowel sounds: normal absent +++
Rectal–vaginal tenderness: left, right, general, mass, none

Initial diagnosis & plan

Results: amylase, blood count (WBC), urine, X-ray, other

Diagnosis & plan after invest
(time)

Discharge diagnosis

Fig. 23.1 Structured sheet for collection of data.

Pain patterns

The patterns of pain can often be helpful in diagnosis of the acute abdomen. Radiation is the term used when pain starts in one place and then spreads to another while the initial pain usually persists. Radiation of pain through to the back is characteristic of involvement of a retro-peritoneal structure such as the pancreas (Ch. 21) or abdominal aorta (Ch. 28), while radiation of unilateral visceral pain to the testis in the male or groin in the female suggests a ureteric origin. Shoulder-tip pain may occur with irritation of the undersurface of the diaphragm – the phrenic nerve and the skin of the shoulder have a common segmental nerve supply (C3 and 4).

Pain localisation

Visceral pain is imprecisely localised. Parietal pain is more accurately localised and, when associated with the physical signs of inflammation in the same area, is frequently used to guide both further investigation and management. For example, a patient with pain in the right iliac fossa (possible acute appendicitis) is managed differently from one with the same features in the left iliac fossa (possible colonic

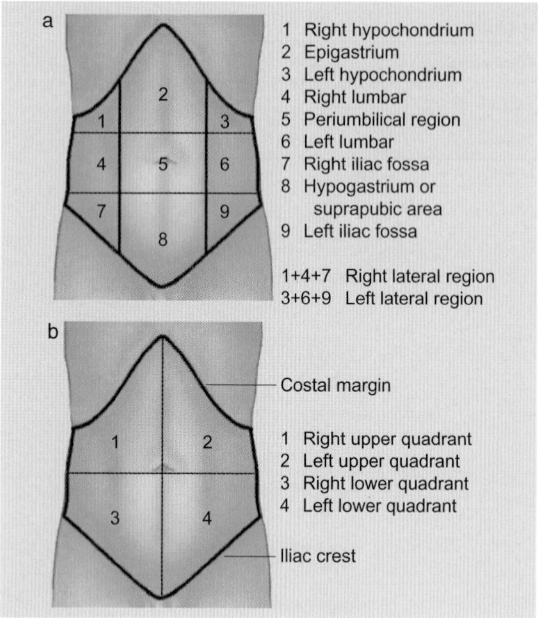

Fig. 23.2 Division of the abdomen into sectors facilitates description and interpretation of findings.

diverticulitis) or right subcostal pain (possible cholecystitis) (Fig. 23.2).

Gastrointestinal disturbances

Vomiting indicates one of the following:

- intestinal obstruction
- pyloric stenosis
- the reflex effect of another acute condition, e.g. biliary or ureteric colic.

Anorexia and nausea are present in many patients with an acute abdomen but are non-specific in relation to cause and can arise in many other circumstances.

Physical findings

The standard approach of inspection, palpation, percussion, auscultation plus pelvic (rectal and/or vaginal) examination where appropriate (and where consent has been gained) is used.

Inspection

The patient's general appearance may reveal the extent of pain and dehydration. The presence of abdominal scars may be helpful for diagnosis (e.g. previous appendicectomy or cholecystectomy) and the nature of any surgery should be confirmed with the patient if possible.

Palpation and percussion for peritoneal irritation

When pressure is applied to the anterior abdominal wall over a site of irritation of the parietal peritoneum, the clinical response is a spinal reflex which causes involuntary contraction of the overlying abdominal muscles – 'guarding' (see 'Murphy's sign', which is the involuntary catching of the breath as a consequence of peritoneal pain in a patient with acute cholecystitis). Inflamed visceral peritoneum must be in contact with the abdominal wall for this to take place. A more advanced stage occurs in generalised peritonitis when the muscles are held rigid – the abdomen is 'board-like'. A consequence is that the abdomen is held still and breathing becomes thoracic (see 'Perforated peptic ulcer').

Rebound tenderness can be elicited by gentle pressure with the hand followed by its rapid removal. It indicates the parietal peritoneum moving over an underlying inflamed viscus. It is not a very reliable indicator of peritoneal irritation and is uncomfortable for the patient. An alternative technique is to ask the patient to cough or by the application of gentle percussion of the abdomen. The aim is to stretch the peritoneum, *not* to cause severe pain.

Auscultation

Bowel sounds may be increased in intestinal obstruction and also in infective diarrhoea and are absent in paralytic ileus and when the gut has become necrotic.

Pelvic examination

Rectal examination is *not* needed in the assessment of children (and many adults) with suspected appendicitis. It may be helpful in some patients with abdominal pain, particularly those with lower abdominal signs. Consent should be obtained and repeated examinations avoided. Vaginal examination is also often helpful but can only be done when the hymen is no longer intact and even then should be used only when necessary. Again, consent is necessary and vaginal examination is usually best done as part of a complete gynaecological assessment of a patient with lower abdominal or pelvic pain. Both rectal and vaginal examination may irritate the pelvic peritoneum and cause pain which, although ill-localised, can often be identified as to the right or left side. There is a similar response to moving the cervix (cervical excitation). In addition, pelvic examination may give specific information about the presence of a pelvic mass and vaginal discharge, and a vaginal swab can be taken for culture.

Investigation

Circumstances, particularly the patient's general condition and the localisation of pain, determine the appropriate investigations. When the diagnosis remains in doubt a wide range of investigations needs to be considered, and these are discussed under individual disorders. Provided that the condition is not judged to be life-threatening, a period of observation and review after a few hours (and preferably by the same clinician) is useful.

Routine urine testing

The presence of red cells or white cells can focus attention on the urinary tract as a possible cause of the problem. Other findings, such as the presence of glucose, ketone bodies and nitrites, may help in management. A pregnancy test should be performed when a fertile woman complains of abdominal pain.

Blood

Routine blood tests for full blood count, urea and electrolytes, liver function tests and C-reactive protein are taken. It must be remembered that intra-abdominal inflammation in its early stages does not necessarily cause a raised white cell count or C-reactive protein; there is usually a delay of several hours before these acute inflammatory markers become elevated (see 'Appendicitis' below). Screening for thalassaemia and sickle cell disease should be done in Afro-Caribbean patients. Electrolyte abnormalities (such as a low potassium concentration) occur with vomiting or diarrhoea. Other blood investigations are considered under individual conditions. The serum amylase concentration must be measured in all patients with acute upper abdominal pain.

Imaging

Plain X-rays have a selective place. Abdominal X-ray should confirm the diagnosis of intestinal obstruction. An erect chest X-ray may show separation of the liver from the undersurface of the diaphragm by free air if there is a gastrointestinal perforation, although this finding is positive only in 60% of cases.

Ultrasound may be very helpful in the assessment of patients with abdominal pain. Ultrasound visualisation of the appendix almost certainly indicates a swollen organ which is inflamed, while the presence of gallstones within a distended gallbladder indicates biliary colic or acute cholecystitis. An abdominal aortic aneurysm can be outlined (Ch. 29). Intestinal masses may be seen such as intussusception in children (Ch. 36). Ultrasound also has a secondary place in management of the acute abdomen either for guided biopsy or for percutaneous drainage of ascites or an abscess.

Computed tomography (CT). CT scanning is now widely used for the investigation of acute abdominal conditions. When possible, intravenous contrast injection is used as this gives much more information by producing arterial and venous definition. CT carries a significant radiation dose and should be used with discretion in younger patients and pregnant women. CT scanning may also identify incidental but significant abnormalities. CT scanning is used for the assessment of patients with intestinal obstruction (Chs 24 and 25) and suspected ureteric colic (Ch. 33). It is the investigation of choice for seriously ill patients with acute abdominal pain in whom a diagnosis has not been made.

Laparoscopy has an important place in the assessment of patients with acute abdominal pain. It is also increasingly used for therapy (e.g. appendicectomy, closure of perforated ulcers). Laparoscopy is helpful in patients in whom the requirement for operation remains uncertain after initial assessment and investigation. For example it is particularly useful in women with lower abdominal pain in whom the diagnosis may be either appendicitis or a number of other causes which do not require operation or in which the organ involved requires a different operative approach (Box 23.1). Laparoscopy is also useful when the clinical features in a suspected acute abdomen are atypical.

Box 23.1 Causes of non-traumatic right iliac fossa pain and tenderness in young women

- Appendicitis
- Salpingitis
- Ovarian cyst (rupture or torsion)
- Mesenteric adenitis
- Terminal ileitis (Crohn's disease, *Yersinia* infection, tuberculosis)
- Right ureteric calculus
- Urinary tract infection
- Meckel's diverticulum (inflammation, perforation or torsion)
- Cholecystitis
- Perforated duodenal ulcer

ACUTE APPENDICITIS

Aetiology and pathological features

The cause of acute appendicitis is thought to be obstruction of the appendicular lumen by either a mass of inspissated faeces (faecolith) or oedema. Distal to this, bacterial multiplication takes place and tension rises. Blood supply is then compromised, and progression to gangrene is common. The appendix then ruptures and leads to a spreading peritonitis caused by enteric organisms (including *Bacteroides*). Alternatively, a severely inflamed appendix may be walled off by surrounding omentum and loops of bowel (an appendix mass) which will eventually contain pus (an appendix abscess). Appendicitis and many of the conditions that mimic it are commonest in the age range 2–40 years. Untreated, the condition threatens life and, although uncommon at the extremes of age, the highest mortality is in the very young and the elderly, mainly because the diagnosis is more difficult in these patients.

The appendix may be in a number of different positions in relation to the caecum: medial; medial and below; extending over the pelvic brim into the pelvis; retrocaecal; or retroileal. The clinical features of inflammation are modified accordingly.

Clinical features

Symptoms

The history typically begins with central abdominal pain of a visceral type – ill-localised and usually around the umbilicus – accompanied by a variable amount of anorexia, nausea and one or more episodes of vomiting. As the organ becomes inflamed, local peritoneal irritation causes parietal pain felt in the right iliac fossa. Occasionally the progression to gangrene is so rapid that these symptoms are largely absent or unrecognised by the patient, who presents with the diffuse abdominal pain of generalised peritonitis. Other variable features of the history are:

- previous similar attacks – suggestive of recurrent appendicitis
- more frequent vomiting if the appendix is retroileal
- variable urinary symptoms – frequency and dysuria – because of an inflamed appendix close to the right ureter or bladder
- mucous diarrhoea because of the formation of an appendix mass in the pelvis which irritates the wall of the rectum or sigmoid colon.

Appendicitis is most difficult to diagnose at the extremes of life, i.e. under 4 and over 70 years of age.

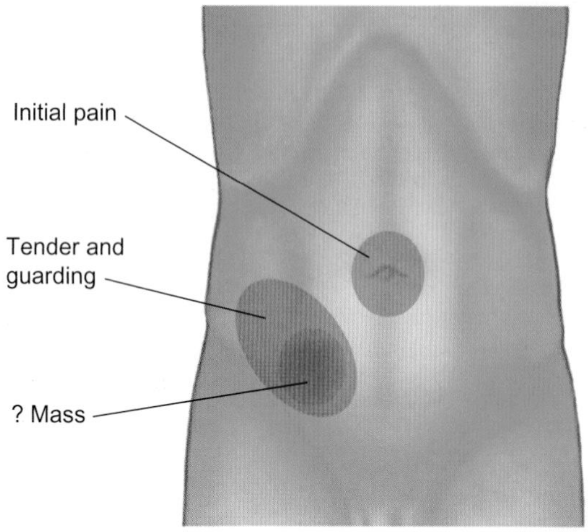

Fig. 23.3 Area of maximal tenderness in most cases of acute appendicitis.

Physical findings

General A coated tongue and foul breath accompanied by mild pyrexia are characteristic, but absence of all three does not exclude appendicitis.

Abdomen Local tenderness and guarding at McBurney's point – the junction of the middle and outer thirds of a line which joins the umbilicus to the right anterior superior iliac spine – is present when the appendix is in its most common position, medial to the caecum (Fig. 23.3). However, these abdominal signs vary in position, are often much reduced in retroileal and particularly retrocaecal appendicitis, and may be absent if the organ is in the pelvis. It is often said that pressure applied in the left iliac fossa causes increased pain in the right lower quadrant (Rovsing's sign), but this is unreliable and not recommended as a diagnostic sign.

Pelvic examination is especially helpful when the inflamed appendix is in the pelvis. Rectal examination is usually sufficient, but in women, where pelvic inflammatory disease and other gynaecological causes are possible, a vaginal examination is usually also done (see above).

Investigation

When the clinical features are typical, the diagnosis is not difficult to make, but a wide variety of conditions can mimic appendicitis; in the past, up to 25% of patients submitted to operation with a provisional diagnosis of acute appendicitis did not have the condition, and few had the need for an operation. Apart from the routine investigations indicated above, ultrasound and CT scanning and laparoscopy are all useful in diagnosis and management.

Laparoscopy is most valuable in young (15–40 years) females, who may have gynaecological disease (e.g. ruptured ovarian cyst, pelvic inflammatory disease) or acute appendicitis. Ultrasonography has a place in any patient where the diagnosis is in doubt and is particularly useful in excluding ovarian disease. The finding of an enlarged appendix is highly suggestive of appendicitis, but a negative ultrasound scan does not exclude this diagnosis. CT scanning is increasingly used for diagnosis of acute appendicitis, particularly in the elderly, patients at high operative risk or those with an atypical presentation.

Management

Acute appendicitis with or without peritonitis

Once the diagnosis has been made, the likelihood of progression (or the presence already of spreading inflammation) demands the removal of the organ – appendicectomy (USA: appendectomy) – which is now usually done laparoscopically, although it may also be done through a small transverse incision in the right iliac fossa. Prophylactic antibiotic therapy (Ch. 9) reduces the incidence of wound infection.

Appendix mass

Some doubt surrounds the choice of management, and good clinical evidence is not available to resolve the issue. The choice is between:

- non-operative management, with nothing by mouth, parenteral fluids, antibiotics and frequent reassessment of clinical state – the mass may resolve (the great majority), deterioration may occur and prompt operative treatment, or an abscess may form
- operative management, in which case the mass is explored and the appendix removed, unless an abscess is found which it is judged better to drain only.

Appendix abscess

If it is clear either on clinical examination or by the use of ultrasound that an abscess has formed, this is drained usually by an ultrasound-guided percutaneous technique, or alternatively by an incision over its most prominent point.

Elective appendicectomy

This procedure is often carried out after successful non-operative management of an appendix mass, although some surgeons do not believe this is necessary. It is also occasionally done in some patients who will be out of reach of surgical facilities should they contract appendicitis (e.g. polar scientists and technicians, astronauts). Good evidence that either of these reasons is valid is absent.

Elective appendicectomy may also be recommended after undoubted recurrent attacks of appendicitis, but this is rare. Appendicectomy should not be done for vague right iliac fossa pain; the usual result is a patient who has had a surgical procedure and still has the pain.

ACUTE UPPER-GASTROINTESTINAL BLEEDING

The usual presentation of upper-gastrointestinal (UGI) bleeding is haematemesis – the vomiting of blood – a dramatic symptom. It is an indication of bleeding into the GI tract somewhere between the lower end of the oesophagus to the duodeno-jejunal flexure. Some blood usually passes downwards through the gut and is subject to digestion. As a result, haematemesis is usually accompanied or followed by melaena – the rectal discharge of altered dark blood. Occasionally, UGI bleeding may be so rapid that bright unaltered blood is passed per rectum. Sometimes haematemesis may be absent in bleeding from the UGI tract and the only clinical feature is melaena.

Epidemiology and aetiology

In the UK, UGI bleeding leads to 50–100 hospital admissions per 100 000 population each year. There are many possible causes, but only a few are common. Peptic ulcers account for more than half, and oesophageal varices, caused by portal hypertension, account for about 5–10%. In countries where liver disease is common, oesophageal varices are much more likely to be the cause of haematemesis (up to 40%), although their incidence in the UK is on the increase. In severely ill patients with renal or hepatic failure, gastroduodenal erosions are a common source of bleeding.

Between a third and a half of patients who present with haematemesis are taking non-steroidal anti-inflammatory agents (NSAIDs), which can exacerbate peptic ulcer and also be associated with acute erosions.

In the UK, the incidence of duodenal ulcer (DU) is much higher than that of ulcers in the stomach (gastric ulcers – GU). However, more gastric than duodenal ulcers cause haematemesis (55% GU; 45% DU), and more deaths are attributable to bleeding from GU than from DU (55% GU; 45% DU). Unusual peptic ulcers which can also bleed are those in the lower end of the oesophagus and those associated with hypergastrinaemia (Zollinger-Ellison syndrome). Gastric cancer is a relatively rare cause of haematemesis, although blood may ooze from the surface of the tumour to cause anaemia.

Mortality

UGI haemorrhage is a serious condition. Mortality rates for the common causes taken over all ages are 5–30% and have not changed much over the years. Table 23.2 gives the results of a world survey of 4431 patients who presented with UGI bleeding. In this survey, the mortality was highest for those with varices. The low mortality for bleeding peptic ulcer of 4.2% is, however, not typical; figures around 10% are common. Death depends chiefly on three factors:

- age – e.g. in peptic ulcer it is very low in those under 50 years but very high in those over 80
- concomitant disease in the cardiorespiratory system
- cause of bleeding.

In some instances, bleeding is a terminal event in a patient already very ill or dying. In the UK there is evidence that bleeding increasingly occurs in the old and ill. In consequence, what are real advances in management for individual patients are not reflected in an overall fall in mortality.

Table 23.2 Mortality for haematemesis – by diagnosis

Condition	Mortality (%)
Peptic ulcer	4.3
Varices	30.7
Erosions	7.1
Cancer	14.2
Mallory–Weiss syndrome	2.0

Clinical features

Fresh blood may be present in the vomit. Alternatively, if it is retained for a short time in the stomach, it becomes darkened by the action of acid and when vomited has the appearance of coffee grounds. If acute bleeding is haemodynamically significant – in excess of a blood donation (500 mL) – the patient may feel faint and show pallor. The vomit may then contain large quantities of fresh blood or clot. The Valsalva effect of vomiting may further reduce venous return to the heart and cause a vasovagal syncope (faint). With larger losses, the classical signs of haemorrhagic shock are usually present, with sweating, tachycardia and, depending on the volume lost, hypotension and air hunger. When the bleeding is severe, melaena may be an early feature. The passage of bright red blood in large quantities from the rectum indicates either a haemorrhage from below the duodeno-jejunal flexure or massive, very rapid blood loss from the upper GI tract.

Immediate diagnosis

Unless the bleeding is clearly minor, the initial history and physical examination should be brief and focused on the features essential to urgent management. There are three components to immediate diagnosis:

- Make sure that there has been acute loss of blood.
- Assess the amount and rate of bleeding – this, along with measures to restore circulating volume, is the first priority.
- Determine the cause, which often leads on to a decision as to how the episode should be treated.

Has bleeding occurred?

It is obviously important to establish that there has actually been a haematemesis. Measures which help are:

- Eliminate swallowed blood (e.g. from a nosebleed) as a cause.
- Examine what has been vomited – if it is not obviously fresh blood and clots are absent, test for haemoglobin; intestinal obstruction can produce what looks like coffee ground vomit.
- Do a rectal examination – fresh or altered blood gives confirmation of bleeding and can also be used in assessing the rate of loss.

Amount and rate of bleeding

- Make the usual observations of the circulation (pulse, blood pressure) to assess the amount of blood lost.
- In haemodynamically significant bleeding, insert a central venous catheter for measurement of central venous pressure (CVP).

Management

A cooperative multi-disciplinary approach to management is essential because it makes key decision-making easy and rapid. A team who are specialised in the management of GI bleeding has been shown to be effective in reducing mortality. Detailed guidance on the management of GI bleeding has been issued by the Scottish Intercollegiate Guidelines Network (SIGN – see Further reading).

Table 23.3 The Rockall score for patients with upper GI bleeding

Variable	Score 0	Score 1	Score 2	Score 3
Age	<60	60–79	>80	
Shock	No shock	Pulse >100	SBP <100	
Comorbidity	Nil major		CCF, IHD, major morbidity	Renal failure, liver failure, metastatic cancer
Diagnosis	Mallory–Weiss	All other diagnoses	GI malignancy	
Evidence of bleeding	None		Blood, adherent clot, spurting vessel	

Table 23.4 Salient historical features in common causes of haematemesis

Cause	Mechanism	Historical features
Mucosal tear at cardia (Mallory–Weiss syndrome)	Forceful attempted vomiting	Acute inebriation Initial clear vomit Bright red haematemesis
Oesophageal varices	Rupture or erosion of mucosa over varix	Past liver disease Absence of peptic ulcer history Dark red haematemesis
NSAID-induced erosions	Breakdown of mucosal barrier to acid	Pain-producing associated disorder (e.g. rheumatoid arthritis) Intake of NSAID
Peptic ulcer	Peptic digestion of vessel in base of ulcer Fibrinoid necrosis of vessel holding lumen open Exacerbation of ulceration by NSAIDs	Previous episodes of dyspepsia Diagnosed ulcer Recent worsening of symptoms Blood of variable colour with or without clots
Angiodysplasias	Rupture or mucosal digestion of a surface lesion	No history on initial occurrence
Other causes to consider	Varies with cause	Examples: – History of anticoagulant intake – Haematological disorders

Initial management

Assessment of the Rockall risk score for upper GI bleeding should be undertaken in all patients and gives an indication of the risk of mortality (see Table 23.3). The first three variables (age, shock and comorbidity) form an initial score (pre-endoscopy assessment) and provide a guide to management. A total score of 0 predicts a mortality of less than 1%, whereas a total score of 2 gives a predicted mortality of 5.6%. The higher the total score, the greater the predicted mortality and rebleeding rate. Patients with a score of 0 may be considered for outpatient follow-up rather than admission to hospital. Those with an initial score of 1 or more should be admitted and have early endoscopy (within 24 hours). The methods of dealing with acute bleeding from any cause are followed. Frequent measurement of the CVP is not only valuable in monitoring the success of volume replacement (particularly in the elderly) but also may give early warning of further bleeding before changes in pulse rate or blood pressure have occurred.

Requirement for blood

The objective should be to maintain a haemoglobin level greater than 10 g/dL. The quantity of blood necessary to do this and to restore a normal level of CVP is an indicator of the volume lost in the acute phase, and in bleeding from peptic ulcer is also helpful in determining the treatment (see below). It has been shown that patients with peptic ulcer or erosive bleeding who vomit altered blood and do not have melaena and whose haemoglobin level remains above 12–10 g/dL, are unlikely to rebleed. Simple rules for the provision of blood are given in Emergency Box 23.1.

Emergency Box 23.1

Guidelines for cross-matching blood in haematemesis

Clinical state	Action
Without haemodynamic problems	None
With haemodynamic problem	4 units
Anaemic (Hb <10 g/dL)	1 unit of blood for every 1 g deficit below 10 g/dL
Continued bleeding	Guided by clinical features but at least 4 units
Rebleed if under 60 years	No action unless there is haemodynamic instability
Rebleed if over 60 years	4 units

Diagnosis of cause

Given that the patient has a stable circulation, either because the loss is small or because it has been corrected, further details can be obtained for both history and physical findings.

History The relevant features associated with different common causes are shown in Table 23.4.

Physical findings Signs of chronic liver disease should be sought, including neurological features suggestive of encephalopathy. Other findings vary with the cause, e.g. the presence of supraclavicular lymph-adenopathy in bleeding from gastric carcinoma.

Upper GI endoscopy is the key to achieving a diagnosis. If haemodynamic instability is present, it may be required as an emergency but can usually be deferred until the next scheduled endoscopy session. In the seriously ill, the procedure is not without some hazard, the main one being aspiration of regurgitated blood. Sedation should be kept to a minimum, particularly in the elderly.

To identify a lesion does not always imply that it is the cause of the haematemesis; for example, in patients with oesophageal varices because of alcoholic liver disease, up to 40% of episodes of bleeding are from peptic ulcer or acute gastric erosions. However, precise diagnosis can be achieved in nearly all instances and is the best basis of a management plan.

Definitive management

In any haematemesis from whatever cause, the initial definitive management is endoscopic. If this is unsuccessful then radiological intervention or surgical treatment are considered.

Peptic ulcer

Management

Many episodes of haematemesis from ulcers are self-limiting, and replacement of blood volume, withdrawal of precipitating factors (such as NSAIDs), testing for *Helicobacter pylori* infection and acid suppression therapy are all that is required. Proton pump inhibitor therapy should be started in all patients with ulcers, using high-dose intravenous therapy initially in patients at risk of rebleeding (active bleeding or a visible vessel on endoscopy). A course of *H. pylori* eradication therapy should be started if infection is confirmed.

However, continued bleeding or rebleeding within a few days can occur, especially in the elderly. Factors which help to predict the likely course of the patient are:

- age – those under 40 are unlikely to bleed continuously or to rebleed and, even if they do, are better able to respond satisfactorily to any haemodynamic disturbance
- ulcer size – those with a large (greater than 1.5 cm diameter) lesion are more likely to rebleed
- endoscopic stigmas (see Box 23.2).

The presence of any of these adverse factors is an indication for local control of the bleeding ulcer at the time of initial endoscopy. There are a number of methods including:

- local injection of vasoconstrictor (at least 13 mL of adrenaline in saline 1 in 10 000)
- thermal coagulation with a heater probe
- cold coagulation with a cryoprobe
- laser therapy
- application of clips onto the bleeding vessel.

Any of these techniques can achieve control in the majority of episodes. Failure immediately to stop bleeding from a visible vessel is usually regarded as an indication for immediate operation or radiological embolisation.

Rebleeding after peptic ulcer haemorrhage is most likely within the first 3–4 days and is thought to be caused by peptic digestion of the clot, which seals the mouth of the vessel. The evidence for further loss is shown in Table 23.5. Repeated control by endoscopic methods can be attempted but, particularly in elderly patients with other problems such as cardiac or respiratory disease, alternative intervention by radiological embolisation or operation should be considered. The decision for or against operation is one that has to be made for each patient by the management team. The decision can be guided by the criteria listed in Emergency Box 23.2.

Radiological embolisation

Visceral angiography is usually performed via a catheter inserted into the common femoral artery. Initial injection into

Box 23.2 Endoscopic stigmas which suggest the likelihood of further bleeding from peptic ulcer

- Actively bleeding vessel
- Visible vessel in ulcer base
- Adherent clot
- Black spot in ulcer base

Table 23.5 Rebleeding in peptic ulcer

Class of evidence	Features
Haemodynamic evidence of continued blood loss after resuscitation	Persistent – low or falling CVP; tachycardia; hypotension
Clinical evidence of continued or repeated bleeding	Further fresh haematemesis (not old blood)
Re-endoscopy	Visible fresh bleeding
Haematological	Progressive haemodilution beyond 24 hours

Emergency Box 23.2

Indications for surgery for a bleeding duodenal ulcer

Timing	Age (years)	Basis of decision
Immediate	Any	Uncontrollable spurting vessel at endoscopy Clinical exsanguination
Delayed	Over 60	More than 4 units of blood required for haemodynamic stabilisation or more than 8 units over 48 hours
	Under 60	More than 8 units necessary for stabilisation or more than 12 units needed over 48 hours
On rebleeding	Over 60	One rebleed after initial successful control but while still in hospital
	Under 60	Two rebleeds after initial successful control but while still in hospital

the coeliac axis vessels (guided by the known site of ulceration) may identify an actively bleeding site or an arterial pseudoaneurysm. If a bleeding point is found, the vessel is blocked by coils and/or haemostatic gels both proximal and distal to the bleeding point. If no definite bleeding site is seen, embolisation may be guided by the endoscopically identified ulcer.

Operations for bleeding peptic ulcer

Surgery is done first and foremost to save life. The aim is to stop the bleeding and to minimise the chance of it recurring.

Duodenal ulcer. The ulcer is exposed and the bleeding vessel under-run with a suture. Very large ulcers may require a Polya-type partial gastrectomy (Ch. 18).

Gastric ulcer. Limited excision of the stomach may be possible but other cases require partial gastrectomy – usually of the Billroth I type (Ch. 18). A gastric cancer may be found at operation in a patient thought to have a bleeding gastric ulcer and is dealt with by a more radical resection, although the distinction between peptic ulceration and cancer may not be easy.

Follow-up

Patients who have *Helicobacter pylori* infection should be checked for successful eradication after appropriate therapy. Failure to eradicate should lead to second-line eradication therapy or maintenance acid suppression treatment with a proton pump inhibitor. Patients with gastric ulcers should undergo repeat endoscopy and biopsy to ensure healing and rule out carcinoma. NSAID, aspirin and anticoagulant therapy should be avoided if possible, but if necessary is usually covered by long-term proton pump inhibitor therapy.

Bleeding oesophageal varices

These are an increasingly common cause of upper GI bleeding and usually occur in patients with known liver disease or a history of alcoholism. Variceal bleeding in childhood or adolescence is the exception.

Aetiology

The varices form at the junction of portal and systemic circulations at the lower end of the oesophagus or in the cardiac part of the stomach as a consequence of portal hypertension from any cause.

Epidemiology

About 50% of those who have varices sustain a bleed, and 70% of those who bleed will do so again within a year. The mortality for each episode may be as high as 50% and is related to:

- the amount of blood lost
- ability to control the bleeding
- the severity of liver dysfunction.

Management

The treatment of bleeding varices is complex.

Lowering portal pressure

Lowering arterial input to the portal system, and therefore portal pressure, can be achieved by the intravenous infusion of terlipressin which should be continued for at least 48 hours. In addition, octreotide or high-dose somatostatin are given for 3–5 days. Secondary prophylaxis aimed at preventing recurrent bleeding is usually undertaken with a beta-blocker such as propranolol after endoscopic variceal treatment.

Tamponade

Balloon tubes (Sengstaken–Blakemore) will nearly always arrest bleeding, but a rebleed is likely when the pressure is reduced – as it must be after 48 hours to avoid mucosal necrosis. There is a high incidence of respiratory complications. They may be used as a temporary measure to control bleeding.

Endoscopic therapy

Oesophageal varices are treated by the endoscopic application of rubber bands. Gastric varices usually found in the cardia may also bleed and are best treated by endoscopic cyanoacrylate injection.

Radiological portosystemic shunt (TIPS)

If endoscopic treatment fails patients may undergo transjugular intrahepatic portosystemic shunt (TIPS) insertion. An expanding metal stent is placed from an hepatic vein to a portal venous branch within the liver under image intensification guidance, providing an effective shunt to reduce portal hypertension. It may also be used as a prophylaxis against further variceal bleeding, particularly for gastric varices.

Gastric erosion (stress ulceration)

This cause of bleeding is associated with liver failure (multiple derangements of haematological factors affecting clotting), renal failure or other multi-organ failure, particularly following trauma or severe burns. Endoscopy in severe cases always shows gastric erosions although they do not always bleed. Bleeding from erosive gastritis may often be a terminal event in the seriously ill.

Management

Initially this is non-operative, with intravenous acid suppression agents such as omeprazole or ranitidine, blood transfusion and correction of coagulopathy. Any possible cause should be corrected. Surgical intervention is rarely necessary, but gastric resection may occasionally save a seriously ill victim.

Incomplete lower oesophageal tear (Mallory–Weiss syndrome)

The mechanism is the same as that for a complete tear (see Ch. 18). The history is typically of an initial blood-free vomit followed by bright red haematemesis later. Most episodes of bleeding from this cause are usually minor and self-limiting but are occasionally severe and persistent. Endoscopic treatment is attempted if bleeding persists or active bleeding is seen. If this is unsuccessful then operation should be considered. The stomach is exposed, opened and the tear oversewn, nearly always with good results.

Dieulafoy's lesion

A small punched-out mucosal hole erodes a vessel, usually high on the lesser curve of the stomach. The condition is uncommon and of unknown cause. Bleeding may be considerable and difficult to find either at endoscopy or at operation. Oversewing or excision at operation is the correct treatment.

Rarer causes of haematemesis

These include:

- arteriovenous malformations – these are rare. Angiodysplasia is the commonest, although it is seen much more frequently in the colon. Vascular ectasias are more diffuse and give streaky appearances at endoscopy. Vascular lesions may also be part of a diffuse syndrome such as hereditary haemorrhagic telangiectasia. Management is complex and beyond the scope of this text
- bleeding via the biliary tract (haemobilia) or pancreatic duct (haemosuccus pancreaticus)
- aorto-enteric fistula.

FURTHER READING

Black J, Thomas W, Burnand K, Browse N 2005 Browse's introduction to the symptoms and signs of surgical disease, 4th edn. Hodder Arnold, London

Britt LD, David DD, Feliciano V (eds) 2007 Acute care surgery: principles and practice. Springer, New York

Ellis H, Mahadevan V 2010 Clinical Anatomy: Applied anatomy for students and junior doctors. Wiley Blackwell, Oxford

The Scottish Intercollegiate Guidelines Network, September 2008 Management of acute upper and lower gastrointestinal bleeding: a national clinical guideline. Online. Available: http://www.sign.ac.uk

24

Small-bowel disease and intestinal obstruction

Diseases and disorders of the small bowel which may require surgical management are usually those associated with mechanical (such as obstruction), infective or bleeding problems. Clinical problems in the alimentary tract are now often dealt with by a gastroenterological team which includes physicians and surgeons working with radiologists and other specialists.

Anatomy

The length of the small bowel is on average 6 m (22 ft) in an adult. The duodenum is technically part of the small bowel but is usually considered separately. The small bowel proper begins at the duodeno-jejunal flexure to the left of the second lumbar vertebra in the root of the transverse mesocolon. Here there is a variable but usually well-developed fold of peritoneum known as the ligament of Treitz. The mesenteric root extends obliquely downwards and to the right for 12–15 cm to lie over the right sacroiliac joint. A conventional distinction is made between the proximal half (jejunum) and the distal half (ileum), but one merges smoothly into the other. The jejunum has a different pattern of vascular arcades and a wider diameter. Its wall is thicker because of the presence of prominent mucosal folds (valvulae conniventes) and, as its name implies, it usually seems to be empty. The valvulae are an important identifying feature on plain abdominal X-rays.

The turnover of intestinal mucosal cells is rapid, and they have a life of only a few days before being discarded, their contents digested and recycled. The submucosa of the distal ileum contains well-defined collections of lymphoid tissue – Peyer's patches. Their exact function is not well understood but they probably produce an immune response to intraluminal antigens derived from gut bacteria. They may be the entry point of specialised organisms such as *M. tuberculosis* (see below). Inflammatory enlargement of an area of lymphoid tissue is almost certainly involved in the genesis of intussusception (see below).

Vitello-intestinal abnormalities

Persistence of the vitello-intestinal duct takes a variety of forms:

- an open communication between the ileum and the umbilicus – vitello-intestinal fistula
- a free diverticulum of the terminal ileum (Meckel's diverticulum), about 25–30 cm from the ileocaecal valve, usually with a wide mouth; ectopic gastric mucosa may be present for reasons that are not known and may cause clinical problems
- a fibrous strand which is connected to the umbilicus and is attached either to the antimesenteric border of the ileum or to the apex of Meckel's diverticulum; acute intestinal obstruction may then occur, often with strangulation.

Physiology

Motility

There are two movements:

- peristalsis – a coordinated wave of contraction extending over some centimetres of the gut and propelling the contents forward
- segmental movements over a short distance which mix the bowel contents.

If there is an air/liquid interface, both actions produce bowel sounds. A peristaltic wave is characteristically associated with a gurgle (borborygmus) which lasts a second or more and may be quite audible to the unaided ear. Segmental movements produce fainter 'clicks' of shorter duration which are detected by auscultation anywhere on the abdominal wall (there is no need to move the bell of the stethoscope around, but it is necessary to listen for at least 1 minute to be sure that bowel sounds are absent). Both types of sounds are louder and more frequent if small-bowel activity is increased, as in obstruction (see below) or diarrhoea.

Secretion and digestion

These processes, which begin in the mouth and stomach, continue and are completed in the small bowel. The small intestine secretes the succus entericus, which has an electrolyte concentration approximately the same as that of the extracellular fluid. The overall flux of liquid in 24 hours is large, but the alimentary tract normally contains at any one moment only about 1 L of secretion. Diversion of intestinal content because of obstruction, the formation of a communication between the gut and the exterior (fistula), or diarrhoea rapidly causes extracellular fluid volume depletion.

Absorption

Water and electrolytes are absorbed throughout the whole of the small bowel with high efficiency unless normal antegrade motility is interfered with.

Glucose, simple peptides and amino acids are almost completely absorbed in the jejunum (but see 'Adaptability' below).

Fat is emulsified by bile salts and broken down into fatty acids and monoglycerides which form micelles – small molecular aggregates of bile salts, monoglycerides, fatty acids and cholesterol which can then present their components to the mucosal surface for absorption. However, bile salts are not absorbed until they are recycled by the terminal ileum, from which they are transported by the portal blood to the hepatocytes for resecretion into the bile. This enterohepatic circulation is a mechanism for preservation of molecules which require complex synthesis; removal or disease of the terminal ileum interrupts this and also reduces the reabsorption of vitamin B_{12} – intrinsic factor complex, so that a macrocytic anaemia may develop.

Adaptability

Although, as described, absorption of different substances is to a degree localised, the small bowel is adaptable, so that extensive resection can be done without obvious effects. Survival with a total length of 20 cm has been recorded, but it is a surgical principle to preserve as much healthy bowel as possible. Supplementary parenteral nutrition has been used in those with very short lengths of small bowel, but transplantation is becoming increasingly feasible (see Ch. 13).

Fistula

An external communication between the bowel and the skin may be the result of disease (for example, Crohn's disease, see below) or a complication of surgery where an anastomosis has failed to heal. The effects vary with the level in the bowel. A fistula high in the jejunum produces large losses of succus entericus and rapid extracellular fluid volume deficiency over a few days. In addition, the skin is digested by the high enzyme content of the escaping fluid. By contrast, a terminal ileostomy, say after resection of the large bowel (Ch. 25), may result in a daily output of about 500 mL and digestive action is rarely as severe. A fistula from the large bowel is usually not associated with water and electrolyte disturbance.

Microbiology

Most organisms ingested by mouth are destroyed by the action of acid and pepsin in the stomach, and the healthy small bowel is usually regarded as practically sterile. However, a large inoculum (as in gastroenteritis) or bacteria resistant to digestion (e.g. *M. tuberculosis*) may survive. Any organisms in the small bowel are confined to the lumen by the protective action of the mucosal barrier. However, obstruction of the small bowel is associated with a variable breakdown of this protection. A similar loss is also seen with reduction in blood supply to the bowel either from local effects or as a result of general reduced perfusion (see Ch. 10). Organisms, usually of faecal origin, increase in number and may penetrate the normally protective mucosal barrier and translocate into the interstitial space of the gut wall (Ch. 9). It is thought possible that they may then migrate into the portal blood. The systemic effects of bacterial endotoxins which enter the circulation in this way are thought to be a factor in the production of the systemic inflammatory response syndrome (SIRS) and multi-organ failure.

INTESTINAL OBSTRUCTION

There are a number of different ways of defining and classifying obstruction of the alimentary tract distal to the stomach. The distinction between mechanical and paralytic obstruction is important. In the first, there is a site (sometimes multiple) at which forward passage is prevented, but above this the bowel is initially normal and active; in the second, the whole bowel is inactive. The word 'ileus' merely means obstruction, but in surgical practice it is usually reserved for the paralytic forms (see below) – although surgeons still speak of gallstone ileus, which is an example of mechanical obstruction.

Mechanical obstruction

Further classification can be done in a variety of ways, all of which have their uses in individual circumstances. The clinical course may be acute, subacute or chronic. The condition may affect either the small or the large bowel. The cause may be specified – such as inflammatory adhesions or tumour – or described according to its position in relation to the bowel wall – i.e. luminal, mural or extramural (Box 24.1). The

Box 24.1 Classification of mechanical obstruction

Luminal
- Gallstone (gallstone ileus)
- Food bolus
- Meconium ileus

Mural
- Stricture
  - Congenital
  - Inflammatory
  - Ischaemic
  - Neoplastic
- Intussusception

Extramural
- Adhesions
  - Congenital
  - Inflammatory
  - Malignant
  - Ischaemic
- Hernia
  - External
  - Internal
- Volvulus (twisting)
  - Congenital
  - Acquired

obstruction may be either 'open loop' – i.e. bowel content can escape proximally – or 'closed loop', in which a segment of gut is obstructed at both ends; large-bowel obstruction is always potentially closed loop because the ileocaecal valve resists regurgitation from the caecum into the terminal ileum. Finally, the blood supply may also be obstructed – strangulation. The venous drainage is first interfered with, and later arterial obstruction leads to haemorrhagic infarction.

Pathophysiology

Proximal to an obstruction, intestinal contractions are increased in both magnitude and frequency. The bowel diameter increases and, because of this, contractions may eventually fail. The intestinal wall becomes oedematous and this, with reduced reabsorption of secretions, may cause extracellular volume deficiency. If strangulation occurs a length of small bowel becomes ischaemic with resultant SIRS and lactic acidosis. Eventually a strangulated loop will die (usually within 4–6 hours) and rupture, with the production of a severe bacterial peritonitis which is often fatal. Distension of the abdomen by the dilated loops may restrict diaphragmatic movement and so interfere with respiratory function. Vomiting may result in inhalation.

Clinical features (Box 24.2)

Symptoms

Abdominal pain is the first symptom and is central, ill-localised and characteristically colicky in nature, coming in waves with pain-free intervals of minutes. Large-bowel obstruction causes lower-abdominal colic and may eventually produce the more constant pain of distension. A strangulated loop in contact with the inner aspect of the abdominal wall – that is the parietal peritoneum – causes well-localised, often severe, pain.

Vomiting follows the pain, and the higher the level of obstruction, the earlier and more profuse it is. Initially, upper-gastrointestinal contents are produced (food residue and dark greenish fluid) but, unless the obstruction is in the upper jejunum, dark brown, bitter, foul-smelling (faeculent) material soon appears (vomiting of faeces is not a feature of intestinal obstruction but does sometimes occur in the relatively rare circumstance of an internal fistula between the large bowel and the stomach). In obstruction distal to the ileocaecal valve, vomiting may be absent because the small bowel can continue to propel its content into the distensible colon above the obstruction.

Distension is usually evident and is generally more marked the more distal the obstruction. Proximal jejunal obstruction (which is relatively uncommon) may be without distension.

Constipation. Most flatus passed per rectum is air that has been swallowed, so that complete obstruction at any level is associated with absolute constipation for both stool and gas. This occurs early in large-bowel obstruction and later in small-bowel obstruction. Incomplete obstructions, as may occur in the large bowel from a progressively encircling tumour, cause reduction in the size and frequency of bowel motions, with visible changes in the stool – and sometimes also mucus and blood (see Ch. 24).

Box 24.2 Clinical features of small-bowel obstruction

- Colicky central abdominal pain
- Vomiting
- Abdominal distension
- Constipation

Physical findings

General

Loss of water and electrolyte (and, in strangulating obstructions, blood) causes the circulatory changes that are discussed below. Temperature may be raised in a strangulating obstruction, but in simple obstruction it is usually normal.

Abdomen

Distension is present which is approximately related to the level of obstruction – the lower the obstruction in the small bowel, the greater the distension. In large-bowel obstruction, and because of the competence of the ileocaecal valve, the distension may outline the colon only, with a visible caecum. An abdominal scar suggests but does not prove that the cause of a small-bowel obstruction may be adhesions. Visible peristalsis may occasionally be seen in a thin patient and may coincide with an audible rush – see 'Auscultation' below.

Palpation may show:

- a mass anywhere in the abdomen – this suggests a specific cause for the obstruction
- an irreducible mass at a hernial orifice – a strangulated hernia
- tenderness and guarding – this is highly suggestive of strangulation in patients presenting acutely, but can be difficult to interpret in the first few days after an abdominal operation.

Percussion produces a tympanitic note because of the presence of gas-filled loops of bowel, although in a slowly developing low small-bowel obstruction, fluid may predominate.

Auscultation reveals increased frequency of the segmenting sounds, which are high pitched and tinkling and have been likened to the sound of water lapping against the side of a small boat. Loud peristaltic rushes may be heard and coincide with an attack of colic. When mechanical obstruction is indicated by other clinical findings but bowel sounds are absent, the condition is usually advanced or there is peritonitis which has resulted from perforation of an involved loop.

Rectal or vaginal examination may reveal a pelvic mass. However, in small-bowel obstruction the procedure is usually unhelpful.

Investigation

Imaging

Plain abdominal X-rays taken in the supine position is the standard and most reliable means of diagnosis. Four questions are posed:

- Is this an obstruction?
- If so, is it in the small or large bowel?
- What is the level of obstruction in the small or large bowel?
- Can a specific cause be determined?

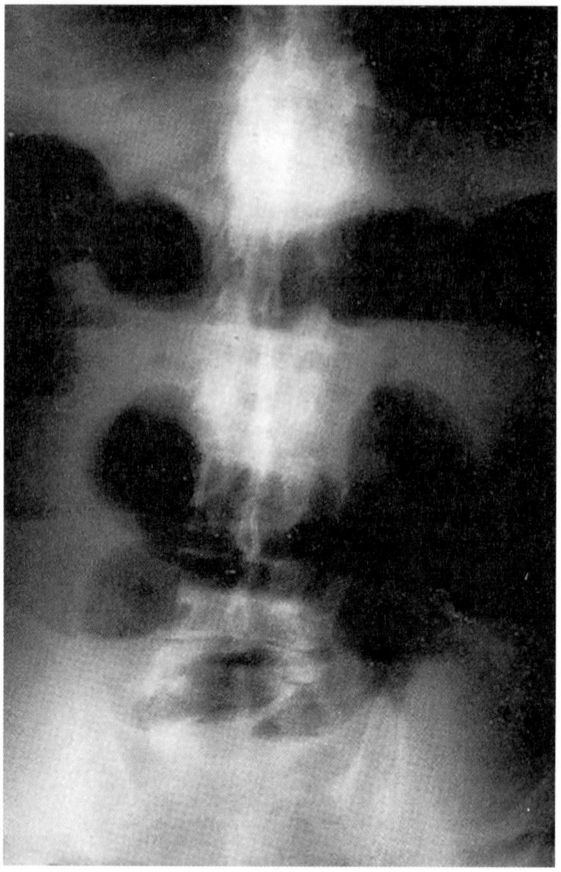

Fig. 24.1 Small-bowel obstruction – erect X-ray.

The characteristic appearance of small-bowel obstruction is of a number of distended, gas- and fluid-filled loops of bowel with, in the erect posture, fluid levels. The levels are frequently arranged in a stepladder pattern (Fig. 24.1). Particularly in the jejunum, the valvulae conniventes may be visible. Adjacent loops may be separated by a variable distance which gives an indication of the amount of oedema fluid in the bowel wall. Gas is usually absent from the large bowel.

Large-bowel obstruction causes accumulation of gas which outlines its wall proximally and which is maximal in the caecum. With a competent ileocaecal valve, the small bowel may be normal. The pattern of gas may give a nearly exact localisation of the cause, with a cut-off point between distended proximal and collapsed distal colon. A more confusing appearance may occur if the ileocaecal valve is incompetent – gas being seen in both small and large bowel.

Contrast X-rays are not usually needed, but a water-soluble contrast medium (e.g. Gastrografin) by mouth is sometimes used when there is doubt about the diagnosis. Serial exposures can be made over some hours and the progress of the contrast medium followed. Its entry into the large bowel after 1–2 hours effectively excludes complete small-bowel obstruction.

When large-bowel obstruction is clinically suspected, it may occasionally be useful to carry out a retrograde contrast study from the rectum, because experience has shown that the differential diagnosis of a truly mechanical obstruction from pseudo-obstruction – a disorder of motility which mimics it – is difficult (see 'Pseudo-obstruction', below). However, CT scanning (see below) is now commonly used to distinguish mechanical large-bowel obstruction from pseudo-obstruction.

Ultrasound is sometimes useful to elucidate the nature of a mass in the presence of intestinal obstruction.

CT scanning is now widely used in the investigation of patients with suspected bowel obstruction. The diagnosis of obstruction can be confirmed, the level identified and the cause often seen. In addition, information on strangulation and other disease (e.g. metastatic cancer in the liver) may be obtained.

Haematological and biochemical

A raised white cell count suggests either an active inflammatory cause or strangulation, as does a metabolic acidosis. The disturbance of water and electrolyte metabolism which occurs in acute obstruction – particularly of the small bowel – requires routine tests both for diagnosis and to set up baselines for subsequent therapy. The concentration of amylase in the serum may be raised in acute obstruction (although not more than four times the upper limit of normal, a level diagnostic of acute pancreatitis), so that this condition needs to be included in the differential diagnosis of acute pancreatitis (Ch. 21).

Management

Individual conditions are considered below, but there are some general principles, the first being the choice between non-operative (conservative) and operative management.

Non-operative

The indications are:

- firm evidence that there is not a threat to the viability of the bowel – strangulation or perforation, which are suggested by signs of hypovolaemia, systemic inflammatory response and peritoneal irritation
- incomplete obstruction in either the small or large bowel with features which suggest non-progression, e.g. Crohn's disease in the small bowel
- some instances of complete small-bowel obstruction – the usual most suitable example is an adhesive obstruction (see below).

Conservative management involves:

- proximal decompression by a nasogastric tube with aspiration either continuously or on a regular intermittent basis
- water and electrolyte replacement
- repeated (4–6-hourly) evaluation of the clinical state – abdominal girth, development of tenderness, changes in bowel sounds and in cardiovascular status
- in individual circumstances, repeated plain X-rays or contrast studies and haematological and biochemical reassessment of the features of strangulation.

A limit of 5 days or less is usually placed on conservative management, although this may be extended in patients with a history of multiple previous operations or significant co-morbidity.

Operative

The indications are:

- established or suspected strangulation, including those with irreducible external hernia
- complete large-bowel obstruction with tenderness in the right iliac fossa – indicative of closed-loop obstruction with possible imminent perforation of the caecum
- failure of resolution after a period of non-operative management
- a cause (e.g. carcinoma) requiring surgical removal.

Operative management is preceded by a brief period of application of the measures outlined under non-operative management – gastric suction, water and electrolyte replacement. The only indication for urgent operation is when strangulation or other causes of non-viability of the bowel are likely. At operation, the obstruction is relieved and, if possible, the underlying cause removed. Dead or damaged intestine must be excised. Occasionally an irremovable obstruction (e.g. a fixed neoplasm) is bypassed.

CAUSES OF MECHANICAL OBSTRUCTION

The causes of mechanical small-bowel obstruction can be classified as intraluminal, mural and extramural. The common causes encountered in clinical practice are listed in Box 24.3.

INTRALUMINAL

Gallstone 'ileus'

A sizeable stone in the gallbladder erodes through into adjacent duodenum and is then carried distally until it impacts, usually in the relatively narrow ileum. The condition is now rare in the developed world because of the usual early treatment of gallstones.

Clinical features

Often there is a variable history which suggests bouts of intermittent obstruction. Eventually, complete obstruction supervenes but the symptoms in a distal small-bowel obstruction are sometimes difficult to interpret.

Physical findings are of considerable distension because of the long length of small bowel involved and with largely fluid-filled loops.

Investigation and management

The radiological findings are often diagnostic because, apart from the features of intestinal obstruction, air can often be seen in the biliary tree.

The gallstone is removed through an enterotomy slightly proximal to the point of impaction, and the more proximal small bowel is examined for additional stones. A subsequent procedure may be done to deal with the disease in the biliary tree, although this is often not required.

Box 24.3 Common causes of small-bowel obstruction

- Adhesions – especially postoperative
- Hernias – external or internal

Food bolus

The common causes of food bolus are:

- poor chewing of food in an edentulous patient
- a previous gastric resection which has destroyed the pylorus
- high consumption of indigestible fibre (e.g. orange pith)
- occasionally, partial obstruction for some other reason with impaction of partially digested food at the site of narrowing.

The clinical features are similar to those of gallstone ileus – low small-bowel obstruction.

Management

Operation is usually indicated even if a confident preoperative diagnosis has been made, because there is always the risk of confusing the condition with one arising from another cause. The bolus can often be milked distally into the large intestine, and it is rarely necessary to open the bowel and risk contamination of the peritoneal cavity.

Meconium 'ileus'

This is discussed in Chapter 36.

MURAL

Neonatal obstructions and intussusception

These are discussed in Chapter 36.

Inflammatory

Crohn's disease, tuberculosis and, in the large bowel, diverticulitis may all produce obstruction by causing either inflammatory or fibrous strictures or by adherence of a loop of bowel to the inflammatory area. Diverticulosis of the large bowel causes obstruction by:

- adhesions between the inflamed colon and the small bowel
- an inflammatory mass in the colon which leads to a clinical picture of large-bowel obstruction.

In the small bowel, other causes of obstructive strictures are potassium chloride tablets (now rare because the current prescriptions are enteric-coated) and the ingestion of NSAIDs, which may be associated not only with stricture but also with bleeding.

Neoplastic

Colorectal carcinoma is a common cause of large-bowel obstruction (Ch. 25). Small-bowel neoplasms occasionally also cause obstruction (see below).

EXTRAMURAL

Adhesions

Throughout the world, these are second only to strangulated external hernia as the commonest cause of small-bowel obstruction; in developed countries, where hernias are usually treated early, they are the leading cause.

Aetiology

A small minority of adhesions are the result of developmental disturbances (congenital adhesions). The great majority are scars on the peritoneum caused by previous inflammation.

The peritoneal mesothelial cells have a potent fibrinolytic mechanism based on the tissue conversion of plasminogen to plasmin. In consequence, any fibrin produced by inflammation in the peritoneal cavity is usually broken down before it can become 'organised' into fibrous tissue. If fibrolysis fails, usually because of peritoneal inflammation, then the usual process of wound healing takes place and fibrous tissue is deposited. The small bowel, rather than moving freely within the peritoneal cavity, becomes attached to itself or to an adjacent fixed point and can therefore kink or twist (Fig. 24.1). Adhesions may be a simple isolated band that can trap the bowel and narrow it from without, or may be complex and dense involving the whole peritoneal cavity.

The time course of adhesion formation is comparable to that of the inflammation/ischaemia which are the underlying causes. Acute processes can produce adhesions in a matter of days – although this does not necessarily mean that obstruction follows, and an adhesion can lie dormant for months or years. Thus post-surgical adhesive obstruction may be manifest either within a few days of an operation – when it may be difficult to distinguish from a persistent paralytic ileus (see below) – or years or decades after the operation.

Apart from the causes shown in Table 24.1, it has often been postulated by exasperated surgeons, reoperating for the umpteenth time on a patient with adhesive obstruction, that there are patients who are 'adhesion formers'. The current evidence for this is unconvincing, and usually some underlying cause can be found.

Clinical features

There has long been controversy as to whether or not adhesions can cause pain other than that associated with intestinal obstruction. Chronic or recurrent pain is often ascribed to their presence, particularly pelvic pain in women. Although there is no strong evidence to support this association, pelvic adhesions are the commonest cause of secondary female infertility.

Management

This is on the lines outlined above. Strangulation is always a possibility that should be considered on the clinical evidence and which if suspected should prompt urgent surgery.

External hernia

This is discussed in Chapter 27.

Table 24.1 Adhesions

Classification	Underlying cause	Examples
Congenital	Abnormality or arrest of development ? Ischaemia	Duodenal obstruction Persistent vitello-intestinal duct with volvulus
Acquired	Trauma	Post-surgical obstruction
Cell damage	Irradiation	Pelvic radiotherapy for gynaecological cancer
Intraperitoneal inflammation	Inhibition of fibrinolysis	Peritonitis Focal inflamed areas, e.g. diverticulitis of the colon Peritoneal dialysis in renal failure
Ischaemia	Inhibition of fibrinolysis	Partially devascularised bowel Surgical procedures
Peritoneal loss	Lack of local fibrinolysis	Wide surgical excision
Intraperitoneal foreign materials	Foreign body inflammation	Surgical materials: implants, sutures
Abnormality of fibrous tissue	Unknown	Colectomy for polyposis coli Stromal fibrous response to malignant disease

Internal hernia

This takes place into a recess of a peritoneal fold formed either during development (e.g. around the junction of the duodenum and jejunum at the ligament of Treitz) or as a consequence of operation (e.g. lateral to a colostomy or ileostomy). They are increasingly seen after laparoscopic gastric bypass for obesity, when small bowel may herniate between the jejunal and transverse colon mesenteries (Peterson's space).

Clinical features and management

Features are of intestinal obstruction without obvious cause. The clinical trap is that a loop of bowel may be strangulated but is not in contact with the anterior parietal peritoneum and therefore does not produce symptoms and signs of peritoneal irritation. In consequence, disastrous delay may occur.

Early operation should be done on any patient who presents with acute small-bowel obstruction with no obvious cause.

Volvulus

This is the general term for a twist of the bowel around its mesenteric axis. Both obstruction and ischaemia of the involved loop can occur. For neonatal volvulus, see Chapter 36.

Aetiology

Volvulus is less common in the small than in the large bowel.

Small bowel

The apex of the loop involved is tethered by an adhesion, often to the abdominal wall or other adjacent viscera at one point, and rotation takes place around this. A rotation of more than 180° may result in strangulation.

Large bowel

Rotation occurs at two main sites:

- caecum – when there is a persistent mesentery (uncommon)
- sigmoid colon – when the existing mesentery is usually more extensive than normal; this is the commoner cause of large-bowel volvulus which, although infrequent in the UK, is more often encountered in the developing world.

Caecal volvulus can occur in adults of 30 years of age or more, but sigmoid twists are more common in older people.

Clinical features and management

Small bowel

The clinical features are those of acute small-bowel obstruction with localised abdominal pain if strangulation has developed. Involvement of a considerable length of small bowel is, if strangulation occurs, associated with marked circulatory disturbance (shock).

Operation is undertaken usually for small-bowel obstruction of unknown cause. The volvulus is untwisted, the cause relieved and, if any bowel of doubtful viability is found, this is resected.

Large bowel

The features are those of large-bowel obstruction, occasionally with a background of repeated episodes. In caecal volvulus, although obvious intestinal obstruction is present, the clinical and radiological features may be confusing. An X-ray will show a grossly dilated viscus which may be confused with gastric outflow obstruction.

Sigmoid volvulus is, in theory, easier to diagnose. The patient is elderly. The features are those of large-bowel obstruction, perhaps with previous episodes. The presentation is often acute with signs of circulatory insufficiency because of infarction. A grossly distended, drum-like abdomen is characteristic. The plain supine abdominal X-ray should be diagnostic with an Omega sign. CT scanning is usually diagnostic of both caecal and sigmoid volvulus.

In caecal volvulus there is only a limited place for non-operative management because this is a closed-loop obstruction. Particularly if signs of peritoneal irritation are present, operation is immediately undertaken, the ileum and right colon resected and the bowel reconstructed by ileotransverse anastomosis.

In sigmoid volvulus unlike caecal volvulus, non-operative treatment is the initial choice. A sigmoidoscope or colonoscope is introduced, a wide-bore flatus tube is passed along it and the sigmoid loop decompressed by careful negotiation of the obstructed loop. As one authority has remarked, 'protective clothing is recommended as the results of decompression are usually explosive'. Once decompression has been achieved, a decision on surgical excision of the mobile sigmoid colon can be taken at a later date, but this should usually be done because recurrence is common.

Failure to relieve the volvulus by these means, or signs of peritoneal irritation that suggest strangulation, require urgent operation. The colon is resected either with or without primary anastomosis.

CAUSES OF ILEUS

In cases of ileus, intestinal obstruction is present but the cause is failure of motility rather than a mechanical obstruction. Loss of forward propulsion must be recognised, but the treatment is different from that of mechanical obstruction.

'Paralytic' (dysdynamic) ileus

Aetiology

This condition predominantly affects the small bowel. The causes are either dysfunction of sympathetic outflow or peripheral inhibition of peristalsis. A summary of causes is given in Table 24.2. There are two groups:

- postoperative – from handling of the bowel at surgical exploration; this is relatively transient (18–24 hours)

Table 24.2 Adynamic and dysdynamic ileus

Underlying cause	Mechanism	Examples
Sympathetic outflow dysfunction	Reflex inhibition	Temporary postoperative ileus Spinal injury Acute disorders, e.g. renal colic
	Pelvic and retroperitoneal bleeding or effusion	Trauma Anticoagulation Acute pancreatitis
	Malignant infiltration	Ogilvie's syndrome – ileus in association with malignant disease in the retroperitoneum
Local	Peritonitis	Bacterial infection
	Advanced mechanical obstruction	Overdistension
Biochemical	Interference with normal contractility of smooth muscle	Hypoxia Potassium deficiency Uraemia Diabetes mellitus
Pharmacological	Neurological/muscular inhibition	Antimuscarinics Ganglion blockers Antidiarrhoeal agents

- secondary causes – either within or outside the peritoneal cavity.

Clinical features

The features are those of intestinal obstruction but without pain or evidence of intestinal activity, i.e. no bowel sounds. In the early postoperative period, it may be difficult to distinguish paralytic ileus from adhesive mechanical obstruction with a poorly functioning small bowel. The pain and the difficulty of examination produced by an incision may also confuse. Features that suggest 'paralytic' ileus include:

- absence of colic
- abdominal silence on auscultation
- large- and small-bowel distension on plain X-ray.

Management

Identification of the cause is basic to clinical management. If this can be eliminated or allowed to run its course, all that is needed is to keep the stomach empty by nasogastric suction or gastrostomy and to maintain water and electrolyte balance. Pharmacological methods of stimulating the gut have largely been abandoned. If the condition is prolonged in duration (more than 5 days), parenteral feeding may be required.

Pseudo-obstruction

This term is applied to a dysdynamic ileus that affects the large bowel.

Aetiology

The causes are similar to those given in Table 24.2, but the condition is more common in the elderly and in those confined to bed by another condition such as a hip fracture. Respiratory disease with hypoxia is a common accompaniment. The name Ogilvie's syndrome is sometimes used as a synonym for pseudo-obstruction but strictly should be limited to those instances which occur because of widespread retroperitoneal infiltration by malignant disease. Pseudo-obstruction is not the same as faecal impaction, where there is a failure to defecate usually with overflow incontinence of faeces but where the features of intestinal obstruction are absent.

Clinical features

The picture is of large-bowel obstruction, but increased bowel sounds are not usually present. The caecum and transverse colon dilate (and caecal rupture can occur). Plain films do not show a typical cut-off point, which is often present in mechanical large-bowel obstruction. As with paralytic ileus, the clinical problem is to distinguish between mechanical obstruction and dysdynamic pseudo-obstruction. Digital rectal examination may be diagnostic – a gush of faecal fluid and flatus occurring on withdrawal of the finger.

Investigation

To operate on a patient who turns out to have pseudo-obstruction, besides being unnecessary in most instances, carries a high mortality from accompanying or causatively associated illness. Because of this, a patient who is thought on clinical grounds to have large-bowel obstruction, and in whom either there is no obvious cause or there are aetiological predisposing factors for pseudo-obstruction, should have a water-soluble contrast enema, abdominal CT scan or colonoscopy. Twenty percent or more of such patients turn out to have pseudo-obstruction, but a smaller (though significant) number in whom a provisional diagnosis of pseudo-obstruction has been made prove to have a mechanical lesion. If the diagnosis is confirmed as pseudo-obstruction, the bowel is decompressed by passing a colonoscope, preferably leaving behind a long flatus tube to prevent re-dilatation. If identified, an underlying cause, such as hypoxia or hypokalaemia, is treated.

Neostigmine can also be used to relieve colonic pseudo-obstruction, but needs to be used with caution in patients with heart disease and cardiac monitoring is mandatory.

Box 24.4 Causes of acute vascular disturbances in the gut

Arterial
- Thrombosis on an atheromatous plaque – usually at the ostium of a main vessel such as the superior mesenteric
- Embolus
  - atrial fibrillation
  - mural thrombus after myocardial infarction
  - detached atheromatous plaques
- Reduced arterial flow – low cardiac output due to hypotension or heart failure
- Desmoplastic obliteration – carcinoid tumour

Venous
- Stasis
  - portal hypertension
  - portal venous system thrombosis
- Sepsis
- Coagulopathies – sickle cell disease

Vascular disturbances in the gut

The blood vessels of the gut have extensive anastomoses. In consequence, considerable vascular obstruction to mesenteric arteries or the portal venous system may exist without any clinical effects. Acute presentation is the rule. Relatively rarely, chronic insufficiency occurs. The causes are summarised in Box 24.4.

Severe acute ischaemia, whether from arterial or venous causes, results in haemorrhagic infarction. Blood and extracellular fluid are lost into the affected loop, so producing hypovolaemia; the haemodynamic effects are potentiated by release of cytokines. Full-thickness ischaemia leads to gangrene with perforation and peritonitis.

A more gradual (subacute or chronic) reduction in arterial input may not have effects on the resting bowel, but with the increase in flow that accompanies digestion, the bowel contracts inappropriately and absorption is interfered with. The usual cause is an atheromatous plaque with narrowing at the ostium of the superior mesenteric artery.

Acute presentation

This is often an overwhelming and highly lethal event.

Clinical features

There is severe acute colicky abdominal pain, vomiting, rectal bleeding (usually dark, altered blood) and symptoms of hypovolaemia. There may be a past history of an underlying disorder such as heart disease which could give rise to an embolus.

Clinical findings are hypovolaemia and signs of strangulation in the abdomen.

Investigation and management

Similar investigations are done as for intestinal obstruction. Contrast-enhanced CT scan may be diagnostic. Intestinal perforation is absent, but air may be seen in a swollen bowel wall. Arteriography is occasionally indicated, but the condition is usually so urgent that operation is required.

Management is by restoration of circulating blood volume and exploration of the abdomen. If possible, the gangrenous loop or loops are resected, but involvement of the whole small bowel (and often the right colon) carries a high mortality and very poor prognosis. Primary anastomosis may be done or the ends of the bowel are exteriorised until it is certain that further infarction has not taken place. If the cause is embolic, it is very occasionally possible to remove the clot and re-establish flow.

Subacute and chronic presentation

Clinical features

The history is often vague and the diagnosis is not made for some time. Features are:

- diffuse pain shortly after eating – so-called abdominal angina
- loss of weight – partly from malabsorption but also because the patient reduces intake to avoid pain
- occasionally diarrhoea.

The physical findings are non-specific. An abdominal bruit is sometimes detected on auscultation, but many abdominal bruits are not associated with vascular obstruction.

Investigation and management

If the condition is suspected on clinical grounds, contrast-enhanced CT scanning or selective angiography is done to outline the origins of the mesenteric vessels and plan treatment.

Untreated, the symptomatic patient often goes on to acute mesenteric infarction. A direct attack on the obstruction can be made either at operation or by balloon angioplasty. Alternatively, a bypass graft is sometimes feasible.

Crohn's disease (regional ileitis or enterocolitis)

Aetiology

The cause of this condition is not known, although there appear to be three interactive cofactors: genetic susceptibility, the environment and the host immune response. Various organisms have been associated with Crohn's disease and it has been suggested that it is an inflammation produced by unusual strains of mycobacteria, although this seems unlikely.

Pathological features

There is a transmural inflammation with oedema, fissures and non-caseating foci of epithelioid and giant cells (granulomas) leading on to fibrosis. Although the terminal ileum is most commonly involved, skip lesions can occur throughout the small bowel. Both oedema and fibrosis can cause intestinal obstruction but this is usually caused by a fibrous stricture. Internal fistulae may form between loops of bowel or into the retroperitoneal tissues or other structures. Healing is accompanied by fibrosis. The condition is often limited to the terminal ileum – either with or without a varying degree of involvement of the large bowel (see Ch. 25), but it can occur anywhere in the gastrointestinal tract (Fig. 24.2). Associated perianal disease is common (Ch. 26).

Clinical features

Presentation may be acute or chronic, or a combination of both.

Acute

An episode of right iliac fossa pain and tenderness takes place which may mimic appendicitis (Ch. 25) and lead to surgical exploration. If a mass in the right iliac fossa is found, care should be taken not to explore – unless the matter is thought urgent – until investigation has established the nature and extent of the process.

Alternatively, the features may be those of low small-bowel obstruction (see above).

Chronic

There are symptoms of general ill health with weight loss, colicky abdominal pain and diarrhoea. The physical findings are non-specific unless there is a mass present which is firm, irregular and often slightly tender.

Investigation

Imaging

Small-bowel disease is detected by barium meal (Fig. 24.3) and follow-through which shows:

- mucosal irregularities and ulceration
- strictures – especially the string sign of Kantor
- skip lesions with apparently normal bowel between them
- internal fistulae.

MR scanning may be used to show evidence of active disease, whilst CT or ultrasound scanning is used to

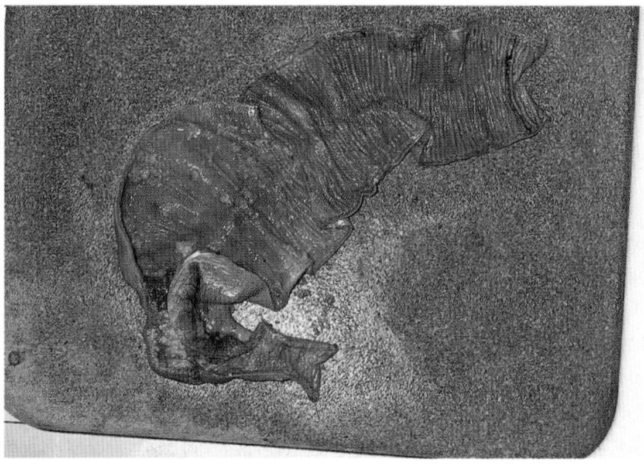

Fig. 24.2 Crohn's disease of the distal ileum – pathological specimen.

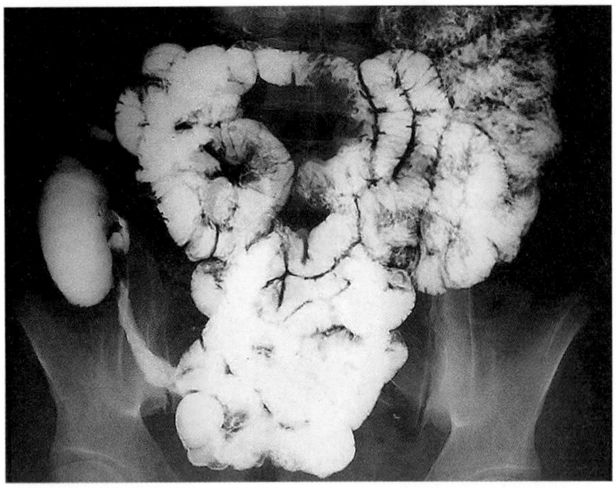

Fig. 24.3 Crohn's disease demonstrated with barium follow-through – note narrowed terminal ileum.

investigate complications, e.g. abscesses or fistula. Caspule endoscopy is widely used although there is the risk of causing small-bowel obstruction by capsule impaction at the site of a small-bowel stricture.

Biopsy

Even if symptoms of large-bowel disease are absent, the rectal mucosa may be visibly abnormal or a biopsy may show typical appearances. Biopsies may also be obtained from the mucosa of the right side of the colon and terminal ileum at colonoscopy. If a patient is clinically diagnosed as having Crohn's disease at laparotomy – which may occur if the presentation mimics appendicitis – a biopsy of the bowel is avoided because there is a risk of fistula formation. However, a lymph node biopsy may be helpful, particularly in distinguishing the condition from tuberculosis.

Management

Medical treatment of Crohn's disease is complex and the detail is beyond the scope of this book. In general the condition is managed with immunosuppressive drugs including aminosalicylates, corticosteroids, cytotoxic drugs (azathioprine and mercaptopurine) and/or cytokine modulators such as the anti-TNF alpha monoclonal antibodies infliximab and adalimumab.

Surgical management may be required when there is:

- intestinal obstruction
- abscess or fistula
- (sometimes) large-bowel disease (see Ch. 25)
- a failure to respond to medical management
- intolerance of medical therapy
- failure to thrive in children
- bleeding.

Surgery usually involves resection of a diseased segment of small bowel which may also be the cause of obstruction, but complete disease excision is not necessary. Half of all patients who have surgical treatment require further procedures within 10 years. Stricturoplasty can enlarge a narrowed fibrotic segment of small bowel provided the disease is no longer active, and it is less radical than excision. Bypass used to be done if resection was regarded as likely to be difficult but is not now used. Surgery may also be required for large-bowel disease (see Ch. 25).

Tuberculosis

Aetiology

The organism enters the gut via the lymphoid follicles found in the mucosa of the ileum. The source is either ingested or acquired from a focus of infection already present, such as an open pulmonary lesion with swallowed sputum. Both human and bovine strains of *M. tuberculosis* can be the cause, but the latter is now very uncommon in the UK. In immunodeficiency states such as AIDS, unusual strains of mycobacteria, particularly *M. avium intracellulare*, may be found.

Tubercular infection in the small bowel is now uncommon in the developed world but remains a feature of communities with poor nutrition and continuing foci of tubercular infection elsewhere.

Pathological features

A typical tubercular inflammation takes place in the wall of the ileum with:

- ulceration
- lymph node enlargement and subsequent caseation and calcification
- healing with the formation of strictures.

In addition, tuberculosis may involve the peritoneum to produce tuberculous peritonitis characterised by the presence of miliary nodules and the development of ascites.

Clinical features

Weight loss, low-grade pyrexia, anaemia, diarrhoea and vague lower-abdominal pain may be present. Ulceration causes blood loss, and a frank rectal haemorrhage may occur. Either the inflammatory mass or the development of a stricture may cause acute intestinal obstruction.

A mass in the right iliac fossa has to be distinguished from one caused by Crohn's disease, which it resembles closely. Ascites may be present. There may be low-grade or frank intestinal obstruction.

Investigation

A barium follow-through can outline the terminal ileum, and a contrast enema may show distortion of the caecum. Ultrasound and CT/MR scanning may show thickened bowel loops, intestinal obstruction, lymph node enlargement, abscess formation or ascites. The appearances may be difficult to distinguish from those of Crohn's disease. Half of patients with tuberculous ileitis also have a radiological pulmonary lesion.

Management

As with all other manifestations of tuberculosis, the primary treatment is with antituberculous drugs, although this is becoming increasingly problematic with the development of resistant strains. The surgeon's tasks are:

- to establish the diagnosis by laparoscopy or laparotomy if necessary

- to manage complications such as bleeding and obstruction if they fail to respond to medical treatment.

Radiotherapy effects

Rapidly dividing tissues – which include the mucosa of the small and, to a lesser extent, the large bowel – are sensitive to irradiation. Abdominal or pelvic radiotherapy to treat malignant disease can cause damage both to the mucosa and to the small blood vessels in the wall of the gut. Fortunately, with better radiotherapeutic techniques this is now less common.

Clinical pathological features

The major pathological changes are mucosal atrophy and intramural fibrosis. Strictures with low-grade intestinal obstruction and ulceration with bleeding may follow. Presentation is with bleeding from the gut, intestinal obstruction, occasionally perforation and internal or external fistula formation.

Management

Surgical excision of the damaged loops may be required, but reconstruction must use healthy unirradiated bowel or poor healing with stricture formation or anastomotic breakdown are common.

DIVERTICULA OF THE SMALL BOWEL

Jejunal diverticula

This uncommon problem is probably congenital but the cause is unknown. There are multiple herniated areas through the mesenteric aspect of the jejunum, usually bulging to one side.

The clinical features are:

- perforation of one diverticulum
- macrocytic anaemia thought to be the consequence of infection with small-bowel bacterial overgrowth
- enterolith formation with small-bowel obstruction.

Management

Surgical intervention is required for emergencies, and bacterial overgrowth treated with antibiotics.

Meckel's diverticulum

Anatomy and epidemiology

The embryological development and the forms the remnant may take are described earlier in the chapter. Occurrence follows a rough 'law of 2s': 2% of the population; 2 ft (60 cm) from the ileocaecal valve; 2 inches (5 cm) in length; and twice as common in males as in females (Fig. 24.4).

Clinical presentation

The diverticulum is notorious for the different ways in which it may present:

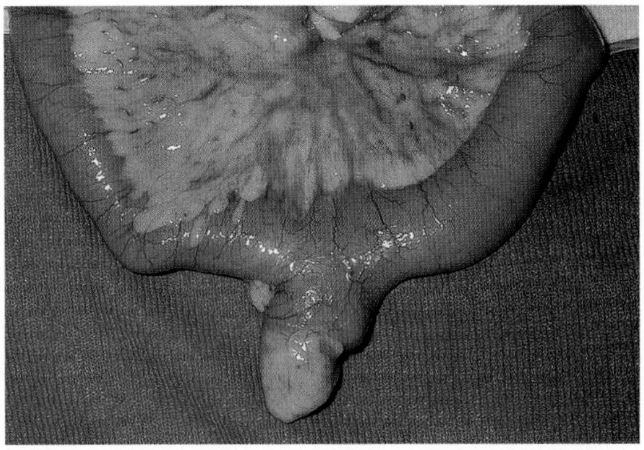

Fig. 24.4 Meckel's diverticulum.

- persistent vitello-umbilical fistula
- acute diverticulitis which mimics appendicitis (see Ch. 25)
- perforation and peritonitis as a consequence of inflammation or from a retained foreign body such as a fishbone
- intestinal obstruction when the diverticulum or an associated band is attached to the umbilicus and causes a small-bowel volvulus or internal herniation
- intestinal obstruction caused by ileo-ileal intussusception
- pain or bleeding from a peptic ulcer secondary to the presence of ectopic parietal cells.

The peptic ulcer occurs on the mesenteric border of the adjacent ileum, and the presentation is of pain and lower small-bowel bleeding (nearly always in children or young adults), which can be very heavy. Confirmation of its origin in a Meckel's diverticulum can sometimes be obtained by visceral angiography or radionuclide scanning with ^{99m}Tc sodium pertechnetate (which detects the ectopic gastric mucosa).

Management

An asymptomatic diverticulum discovered at exploration for another reason is usually removed in a child, but in an adult over 30 years old it has been established that it is innocuous and may be left. Symptomatic diverticula are dealt with according to the complications that they cause.

SMALL-BOWEL NEOPLASMS

Epidemiology and aetiology

Primary tumours of the small bowel are relatively uncommon and account for only 5% of gastrointestinal neoplasms. Aetiological factors include:

- inherited conditions
- immunocompromise – particularly Kaposi sarcoma, adenocarcinoma and lymphoma
- geographical location
- Crohn's disease

Inherited conditions

Small-bowel tumours are associated with:

- Familial adenomatous polyposis (FAP), although most of the neoplasms arise in the duodenum (see 'Familial polyposis coli'; Ch. 25)
- Peutz–Jeghers syndrome – an ill-understood inherited relationship between intestinal polyps, mainly in the jejunum, and marginal pigmentation around the buccal and anal mucosa; the usual presentation is with intussusception.

Gardner's syndrome – this is a rare disorder in which small-bowel adenomas and carcinomas are associated with skeletal abnormalities and desmoid tumours.

Immunocompromise

There are three circumstances:

- Coeliac disease in which there is gluten-sensitive enteropathy with a wide variety of other manifestations of atopy – there is an increased incidence of small-bowel cancer
- Acquired immunodeficiency, as in AIDS, which makes the patient liable to Kaposi sarcoma and lymphoma
- Immunosuppression, chiefly in transplant patients, is associated with small-bowel lymphomas.

Geographical location

There is no doubt that lymphomas are more common in the Middle East than elsewhere. The cause is unknown but may reflect an infectious agent.

Crohn's disease

Crohn's disease is associated with an increased incidence of small-bowel adenocarcinoma.

Pathological features

Benign tumours

Benign tumours – adenomas of various form – are commoner in the duodenum, particularly in association with familial polyposis coli and at the ampulla of Vater. Progression to carcinoma can occur. Other tumours are:

- Gastrointestinal stromal tumours (GIST) are intra- or extraluminal and may give rise to bleeding or obstruction, and may metastasise particularly if they are large and have a high mitotic rate.
- Lipomas are commoner in the large than in the small bowel and, because of their bulk, are liable to cause intussusception with abdominal colic and rectal bleeding.
- Neurofibromas can occur in isolation or as part of the general picture of neurofibromatosis; bleeding or obstruction may occur.

Malignant tumours

- Lymphomas are either primary or part of a more generalised disorder.
- Adenocarcinoma is more common in the duodenum but also occurs elsewhere.
- Secondary tumours are rare but occur in lung and breast cancer and also in malignant melanoma.

Management

Tumours are usually identified and staged by CT scanning. Biopsy may be possible in proximal lesions by endoscopy. Surgical resection of the involved segment of small bowel is indicated in GIST and adenocarcinoma. Adjuvant chemotherapy is often given after resection of adenocarcinoma and imatinib after resection of high-risk GIST. For benign tumours resection is only indicated if it is causing significant symptoms (e.g. obstruction, bleeding) or there is concern about possible malignant tumour formation. Lymphoma is usually treated by cytotoxic chemotherapy, although perforation may necessitate emergency resection.

25 Large bowel, including appendix

THE LARGE BOWEL

Structure

Macroscopic

The large intestine is a muscular tube approximately 135 cm long extending from the ileocaecal valve to the junction of the rectum and anal canal. It has a greater diameter than the small intestine and is recognised by fatty appendages (appendices epiploicae) and by a sacculated appearance which is the consequence of the three longitudinal strips of smooth muscle (taeniae coli), which are shorter than the colon itself. The caecum is in the right iliac fossa and normally does not have a mesentery. The base of the appendix is attached to its posteromedial aspect below the ileocaecal valve. However, the position of the appendix in relation to the caecum is very variable (see below).

The caecum extends upwards to become the ascending colon, which turns to the left below the right lobe of the liver at the hepatic flexure to pass transversely across the abdomen as a long (~50 cm) dependent loop of transverse colon with a mesentery. Its course is in front of the right kidney and second part of the duodenum; the mesocolon is attached to the inferior border of the pancreas, and the transverse colon ends at a relatively fixed splenic flexure. Here the bowel turns abruptly downwards as the descending colon in contact with the posterior abdominal wall to reach the brim of the pelvis. Below this point the bowel regains a mesentery and the loop (sigmoid colon) projects forwards into the pelvis before the colon ends retroperitoneally as the rectum.

Blood supply

Arterial supply is the consequence of the development of the first parts of the colon (caecum to splenic flexure) from the midgut and of the remainder from the hindgut (Fig. 25.1). The proximal arteries are branches of the superior mesenteric artery: the ileocolic, right and middle colic arteries. The descending colon and sigmoid are supplied by branches of the inferior mesenteric artery: left colic and sigmoid arteries. All of the colic vessels form anastomosing loops which extend from the distal ileum to the distal sigmoid and which create a continuous marginal artery about 1 cm from the bowel wall. The arrangement ensures a continued arterial input if local arterial obstruction develops. The vascular anastomosis is most tenuous in the region of splenic flexure (see 'Ischaemic colitis', below). From the marginal artery, long and short vessels penetrate the bowel wall to supply muscle and mucosa, and their sites of penetration are points of potential weakness (see 'Diverticular disease', below).

Venous drainage corresponds to the arterial input. Blood from the proximal colon enters tributaries of the superior mesenteric vein, which is joined by the splenic vein to form the portal vein, which leads directly to the liver. The distal colon drains into tributaries of the inferior mesenteric vein, which joins the splenic vein.

Physiology

Extensive or total colectomy is a frequently performed procedure (Box 25.1). Therefore, some understanding of the function of the colon (Box 25.2) is important.

Sodium and water absorption

Normally about 1.5 L of water, 200 mmol of sodium and 100 mmol of chloride pass through the ileocaecal valve every 24 hours. In transit through the colon, 95% of the sodium and water is reabsorbed across the mucosal colonocytes. In exceptional circumstances, water absorption can be increased three to four times, and this ability can be used for rehydration when other routes, such as the intravenous one, are not available.

Sodium can diffuse down a chemical gradient; however, it is usually transported from the colonic lumen across the

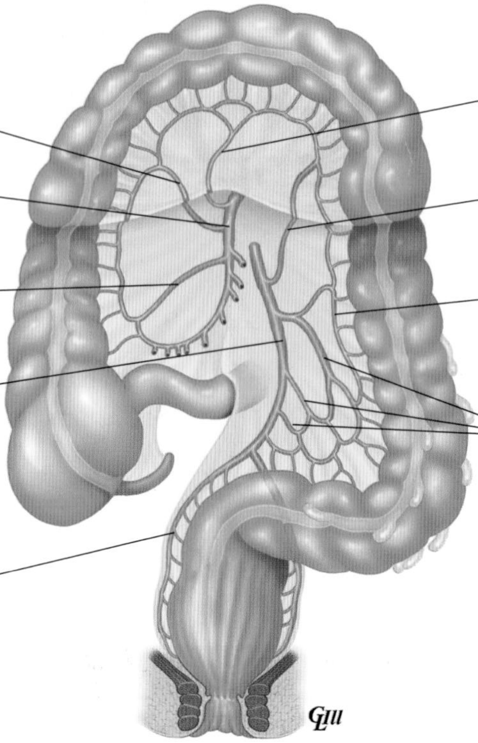

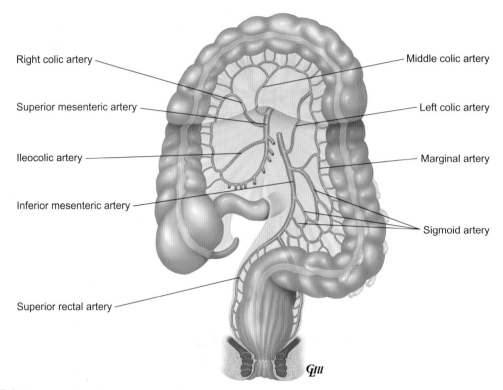

Fig. 25.1 Blood supply to the colon and rectum.

Box 25.1 Indications for colectomy

- Neoplasms of the colon
- Diverticular disease
- Ulcerative colitis
- Crohn's disease
- Volvulus
- Slow-transit constipation
- Ischaemia

Box 25.2 Functions of the colon

- Water absorption
- Sodium and chloride absorption
- Bacterial metabolism and fermentation
- Storage and evacuation of faeces

colonocyte into the plasma by two energy-dependent mechanisms:

- sodium–potassium exchange in the cell membrane
- sodium–proton exchange at the luminal surface.

Chloride absorption is down an electrical gradient and by exchange for bicarbonate.

Water moves from the lumen into the cell because the latter is at a higher osmotic pressure, due to the active transport of solutes, principally sodium, chloride and short-chain fatty acids (see below).

Bacterial metabolism and fermentation

The colon contains 99% of the organisms in the gastrointestinal tract, and more than 400 different types have been identified. Bacteria make up approximately 80% of the weight of normal faeces.

Bacteria in the colon are of surgical importance because:

- they cause fermentation (anaerobic release of energy) by breakdown of carbohydrates to produce short-chain fatty acids (SCFAs)
- they are the source of potentially lethal complications if the mucosal barrier is damaged.

Short-chain fatty acids are mainly the consequence of the action of bacteria on a substrate which is loosely called dietary fibre and which is composed of non-starch polysaccharides such as cellulose and many other plant components such as dextrin, inulin, beta-glucans and oligosaccharides. An increase in dietary fibre causes increased colonic motility and more rapid transit, partly because of the water-absorbing properties of fibre, but mostly because of increased bacterial activity and fermentation. SCFAs are reabsorbed and form part of the body's energy cycle. A byproduct of these chemical reactions is gas (flatus), a mixture of carbon dioxide, hydrogen and methane with varying amounts of other gases, such as hydrogen sulphide, depending on the substrate.

Storage and evacuation of faeces

The content changes in consistency as it traverses the large bowel, from liquid in the right colon to a firm semi-solid stool on the left. The transit time between the caecum and evacuation via the rectum is very variable but is normally about 36 hours (slightly more in the female). Faeces are propelled by a combination of mass peristalsis and segmental contractions. Factors which influence colonic motility are:

- the fibre content of the diet
- amount of fluid in the colon
- laxative use
- hormones, e.g. cholecystokinin
- psychological factors such as stress
- food in the stomach, which can initiate a reflex colonic contraction (gastrocolic reflex).

Colonic motility is also subject to the circadian rhythm in that resting tone is considerably reduced at night.

FUNCTIONAL DISORDERS

Constipation

This condition is defined as either excessive straining at stool or the passage of two or fewer stools in a week (the Rome criteria for functional bowel disorders). It is a common complaint; prescriptions for laxatives in the UK cost the NHS about £20 million a year. The common causes are listed in Box 25.3. The commonest of these is inadequate dietary fibre, and the most important is malignant disease of the left colon. When constipation occurs shortly after birth Hirschsprung's disease should be considered (see Ch. 36). Very occasionally, this disease presents for the first time in adult life.

Slow-transit constipation. A small number of patients, usually female, have chronic constipation which does not respond to increase of dietary fibre or laxatives; there is no structural abnormality but transit time is slow. The patient's complaint may be sufficiently severe to require surgical treatment; the options include the use of antegrade continence enemas (via an appendix or an ileal conduit), sacral nerve stimulators and total colectomy with anastomosis of the ileum to the rectum, but the results are not always satisfactory.

Irritable bowel syndrome (IBS)

Irritable bowel syndrome is a functional bowel disorder characterised by chronic abdominal pain, discomfort, bloating, and alteration of bowel habit. IBS is the commonest cause of abdominal pain. The symptoms may be relieved by bowel movements. Diarrhoea or constipation may predominate, or they may alternate. IBS may begin after a gastrointestinal infection or a stressful life event. Investigation including the rectum and colon is normal. Treatment is aimed at the relief of symptoms. Dietary manipulation, antispasmodic medication and psychological interventions all have a role. There is no role for surgical intervention.

Box 25.3 Causes of constipation

- Inadequate dietary fibre
- Neoplasms of the colon, rectum and anus
- Benign lesions of the anus
- Endocrine disease, e.g. myxoedema
- Drugs, e.g. codeine phosphate
- Hirschsprung's disease
- Slow-transit constipation
- Psychological and behavioural abnormalities
- Neurological causes: cerebral, e.g. stroke, spinal, e.g. multiple sclerosis, paraplegia, neoplasm

INFLAMMATORY DISEASE

Inflammation of the large bowel is known as colitis, and inflammation of the rectum is known as proctitis. Boxes 25.4 and 25.5 list the non-infective and infective causes of colitis and proctitis, respectively.

Ulcerative colitis

Epidemiology and aetiology

This condition is common in Scandinavia, the UK and North America. There is a higher incidence in rural dwellers. Current smoking may protect against ulcerative colitis, whereas it increases the risk of Crohn's disease. Females are more commonly affected than males, and the condition is prevalent in late adolescence and early adult life.

The cause is not known but the following may be involved.

Genetics

There is a higher familial incidence of ulcerative colitis than would be expected by chance. However, no clear genetic pattern of expression has been identified.

Box 25.4 Non-infective causes of colitis/proctitis

- Ulcerative colitis
- Crohn's disease
- Ischaemic colitis
- Irradiation colitis

Box 25.5 Infective causes of colitis/proctitis

Bacterial
- *Salmonella*
- *Shigella*
- *Mycobacterium tuberculosis*
- *Staphylococcus*
- *Gonococcus*
- *Campylobacter*
- *Clostridium difficile*

Viral
- Enteroviruses
- Cytomegaloviruses
- Herpes

Spirochaetal
- *Treponema pallidum*

Chlamydial
- *Lymphogranuloma pallidum*

Protozoal
- *Entamoeba histolytica*

Metazoal
- *Schistosoma mansoni*

Mycotic
- *Histoplasma capsulatum*

Transmissible agents

The histological and clinical features of the disease have some things in common with those that occur in acute bacterial infections of the colon, but in spite of intensive microbial investigation a specific organism has not been identified.

Diet

The prevalence of the disease in countries in which the diet is low in fibre and contains additives suggests that the use of highly milled flour and certain additives (e.g. carrageen) may be factors. A small number of patients with ulcerative colitis are made symptomatically worse by taking milk protein, which is the consequence of mucosal hypolactasia.

Psychodynamics

Introversion and depression are commonly seen, and the symptoms are often made worse by psychological stress. However, it is probable that these matters are secondary rather than causative.

Immunology

The failure to find any infective agent has led to the suggestion that the destructive inflammation of the colonic mucosa is autoimmune, similar to that found in, for example, thyroiditis. However, markers of autoimmune disease such as antinuclear factor are no more common in these patients than in the normal population.

Pathological features

The major feature is inflammation of the mucosa with increased vascularity and haemorrhage. In spite of the name of the disease, macroscopic ulceration is not common except in very severe and advanced disease. The changes are usually most marked in the rectum (proctitis) and spread for a varying degree proximally into the colon. Rarely, the entire large bowel is involved but the disease does not extend proximal to the ileocaecal valve although a 'backwash ileitis' may affect the terminal ileum. Box 25.6 lists the histological features; the most diagnostic of these is the crypt abscess (Fig. 25.2). Dysplastic change is thought to be a marker for the risk of malignant change (see below).

Clinical features

Symptoms

The most characteristic symptom is bloody diarrhoea with associated social embarrassment and discomfort. There are periods of remission followed by acute relapse. Disease confined to the rectum is usually mild and without systemic effects. More extensive colonic involvement leads to ill health, weight loss, symptoms of anaemia and complaints of abdominal pain.

Box 25.6 Histological features of ulcerative colitis

- Lymphocyte and neutrophil infiltration of lamina propria
- Crypt abscess formation
- Goblet cell depletion
- Destruction of surface epithelium (ulceration)
- Mucosal oedema
- Dysplasia

Physical findings

In mild disease, physical signs are few or absent. Those with a more severe or extensive condition look ill, show signs of weight loss, anaemia and dehydration. Abdominal examination may show colonic distension and tenderness.

Complications

Fulminant colitis

The severity of colitis can be assessed using the Truelove and Witts' criteria (Table 25.1). Severe attacks require admission to hospital for intensive medical management and often require urgent coloectomy.

Toxic megacolon (acute dilatation)

The medical management of severe colitis is complex and beyond the scope of this book. Severe inflammation may cause the colon (particularly the transverse part) to dilate. There is severe acute systemic disturbance with:

- toxaemia
- anaemia from bleeding

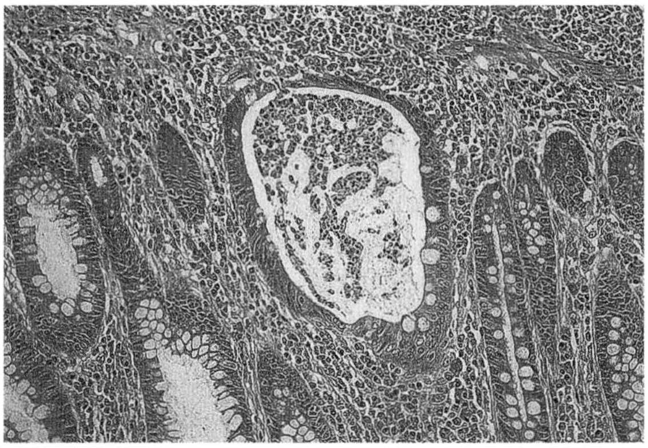

Fig. 25.2 Histological appearance of a crypt abscess in ulcerative colitis.

Table 25.1 Truelove and Witts' classification of severity of ulcerative colitis: six or more bowel motions per day associated with at least one other 'severe' criterion is indicative of a severe attack

Activity	Mild	Moderate	Severe
Number of bloody stools per day (*n*)	<4	4–6	>6
Temperature (°C)	Afebrile	Intermediate	>37.8
Heart rate (beats per minute)	Normal	Intermediate	>90
Haemoglobin (g/dL)	>11	10.5–11	<10.5
Erythrocyte sedimentation rate (mm/h)	<20	20–30	>30

After Truelove SC, Witts LJ 1955 Cortisone in ulcerative colitis: final report on a therapeutic trial. British Medical Journal ii:1041–8.

- acute loss of water and electrolyte
- progressive abdominal distension.

The last of these may lead to perforation of the colon with general peritonitis, which carries a high mortality and gives the complication its sinister reputation.

Treatment is with water and electrolyte replacement and intensive medical treatment (see below). High-dose hydrocortisone (400 mg/day) is started and antibiotics may also be given. Close monitoring of both the systemic condition (such as 12-hourly blood analysis including inflammatory markers such as C-reactive protein and white cell count) and the degree of colonic dilatation (by serial plain X-ray and measurement of the diameter of the caecum or ascending colon) is required to detect deterioration or the likelihood of perforation. Blood transfusion is required if haemoglobin is less than 10 g/dL. Parenteral nutrition is often required. The patient should be assessed jointly by an experienced physician and surgeon on a 12-hourly basis during the acute phase of colitis. Failure to respond to intensive medical therapy after 48–72 hours, or deterioration in the patient's condition during this period, is an indication for intravenous ciclosporin therapy or operation. Surgery involves urgent removal of the colon – usually leaving the rectum intact – and a diverting ileostomy may be required. Once the patient has recovered, further surgery may be considered as discussed below.

Massive haemorrhage

This is rare and usually responds to transfusion and intensive treatment of the disease.

Carcinoma

Adenocarcinoma develops as a result of dysplastic change in long-standing colitis. The risk is very small in those who have had the disease for less than 10 years. Thereafter, it increases in those who have total colitis, so that by 20 years it approaches 20%. The hazard is much less in patients with limited disease. The presence of a cancer is an absolute indication for surgery.

Complications other than in the gastrointestinal tract

Systemic complications (Box 25.7) are uncommon and are usually an indication of the severity of the colitis. If this is successfully treated, such complications usually resolve. An exception is urinary calculus after removal of the colon and ileostomy. It is thought that this is partly the result of increased water loss via the ileostomy which leads to a more concentrated urine. However, disorders of oxalate metabolism may also be involved.

Box 25.7 Non-gastrointestinal complications of ulcerative colitis

- Skin disorders, e.g. erythema nodosum, pyoderma gangrenosum
- Eye disorders, e.g. iritis, episcleritis
- Arthritis, e.g. ankylosing spondylitis, peripheral rheumatoid-type arthritis
- Liver disorders, e.g. chronic liver disease, sclerosing cholangitis
- Renal disorders, e.g. ureteric calculi following ileostomy, secondary amyloidosis, glomerulonephritis

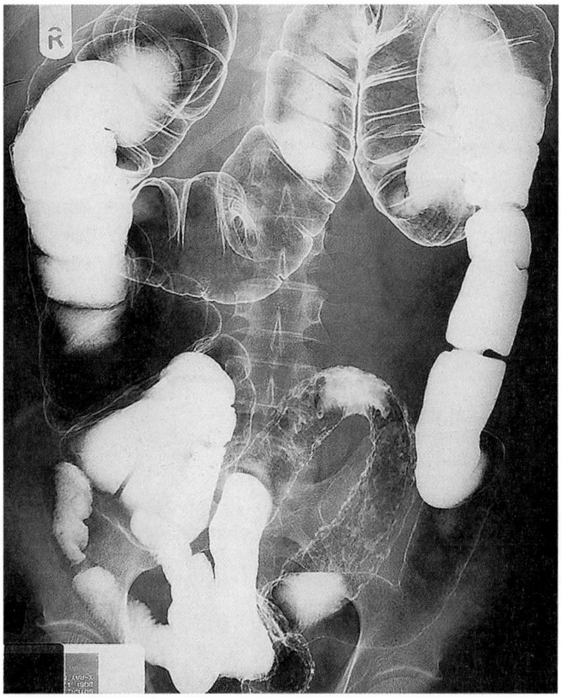

Fig. 25.3 Barium enema in a patient with ulcerative colitis.

Investigation

All patients suspected of having ulcerative colitis should have a sigmoidoscopy and biopsy of the rectal mucosa. Stool cultures are carried out to exclude an infective cause. Except in the mildest cases, in which the proximal limit of the disease can be seen at sigmoidoscopy, a barium enema (Fig. 25.3) or more commonly a colonoscopy is used to determine the extent. The latter, accompanied by multiple biopsies, is the most precise method and may also reveal an unsuspected carcinoma. Colonoscopy may be delayed until after treatment in patients with severe attacks because of the risk of perforation.

CT or MRI scanning may be useful to define the extent of disease and identify complications such as perforation.

Management

Medical

Most patients have minimal disease which can be adequately managed by a combination of 5-aminosalicylic acid (5-ASA) or prednisolone suppositories. Oral sulfasalazine or other 5-aminosalicylic acid based drugs such as mesalazine (fewer side-effects) are effective in more extensive disease. Budesonide is a steroid taken orally which is not absorbed. More extensive disease with incapacitating symptoms may require admission to hospital for systemic steroids, immunosuppression (e.g. ciclosporin, mercaptopurine, azathioprine or methotrexate) and/or the use of biological response modifiers (e.g. infliximab – a monoclonal anti-TNF alpha).

Surgical

Apart from special circumstances when a temporary diversion of the faecal stream by ileostomy alone is done, the objective of surgery is to remove all or nearly all diseased large bowel. The indications for surgery are given in Box 25.8.

When there is time, electrolyte balance, toxaemia and anaemia are corrected preoperatively. Mechanical preparation of the bowel is contraindicated because of the risk of perforation. Perioperative antibiotic prophylaxis is essential (Ch. 9). If either a temporary or a permanent stoma is contemplated (which is common – see below), a specialist in stoma care as well as the surgeon should discuss the matter with the patient.

Operative procedures

Proctocolectomy with permanent ileostomy

This is the standard procedure in elective or semi-elective cases (Fig. 25.4): all diseased or potentially diseased bowel is removed and the patient is rapidly restored to full health. However, the permanent stoma requires an appliance to be worn and can have its own complications (Box 25.9), although these can usually be avoided. In urgent cases a total colectomy with ileostomy is performed, the rectum is left in situ.

Patients usually adapt well to the alteration of body image inevitably produced, but their occasional difficulty in doing so and a natural distaste for a stoma in both themselves and their surgeons has led to the development of other techniques.

Ileorectal anastomosis after colectomy

In some patients, the rectal disease may not be severe or may resolve after colectomy and temporary diverting ileostomy; ileorectal anastomosis (Fig. 25.5) may then produce a good functional result. However, there is risk of subsequent carcinoma in the rectum, and inflammation may recur. Lifelong surveillance is necessary.

Continent ileostomy

The objective is to improve the cosmetic appearance of the stoma by avoiding a spout and to do away with the need for an appliance to be worn continuously.

The technique is to fold the distal ileum on itself to form a pouch with a valve at its end (Fig. 25.6). The pouch is emptied at the patient's convenience with a tube. The procedure is complex and has had a high incidence of complications and failure of continence.

Box 25.8 Indications for surgery in ulcerative colitis

- Severe exacerbations of colitis
- Severe exacerbations of non-gastrointestinal manifestations
- Toxic colon/acute dilatation
- Chronic colitis refractory to medical treatment
- Development of premalignant changes (dysplasia) in colon/rectum
- Development of carcinoma of colon/rectum

Box 25.9 Complications related to ileostomy

- Para-ileostomy hernia
- Protrusion/prolapse of ileostomy
- Renal calculi
- Electrolyte imbalance
- Para-stomal dermatitis
- Psychological/sexual problems

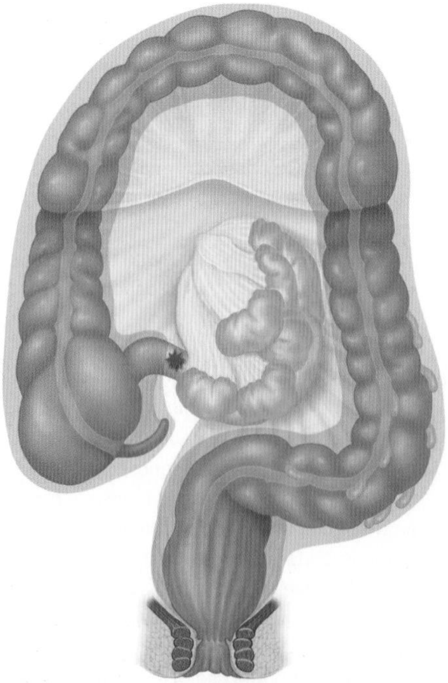

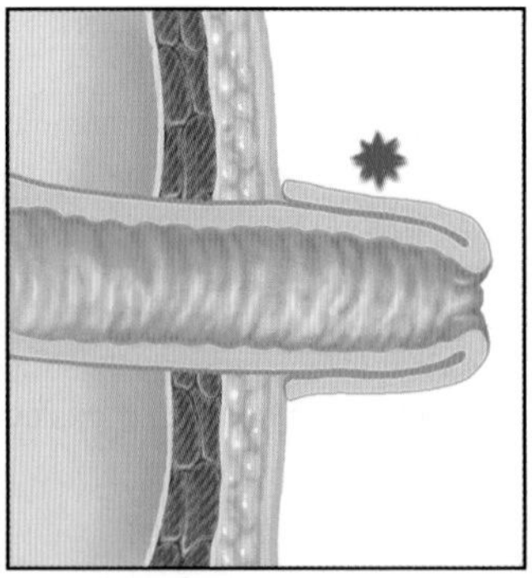

Fig. 25.4 Operation of proctocolectomy and ileostomy.

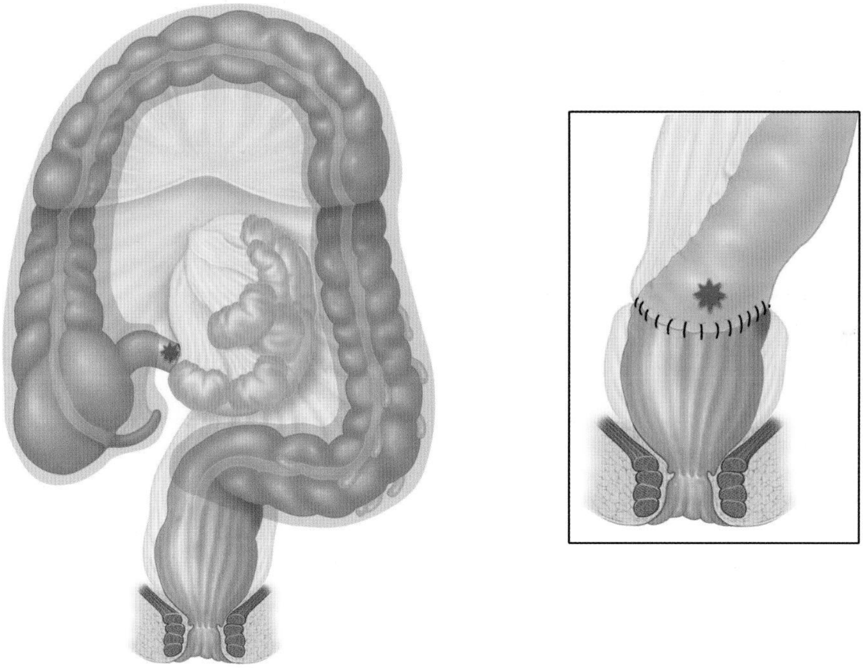

Fig. 25.5 Operation of colectomy and ileorectal anastomosis.

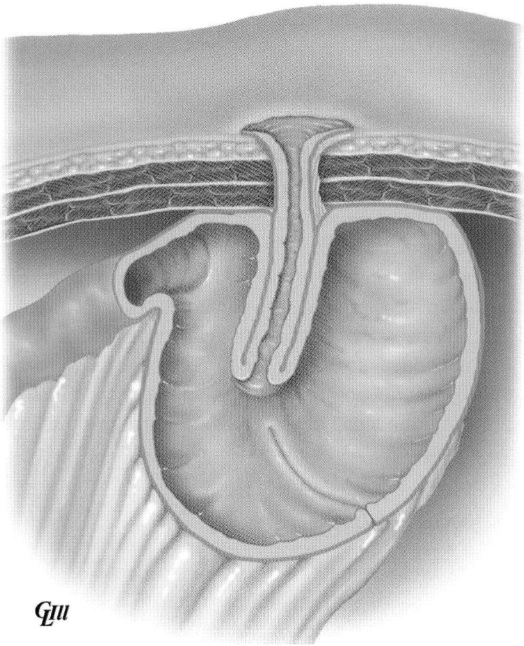

Fig. 25.6 The continent ileostomy.

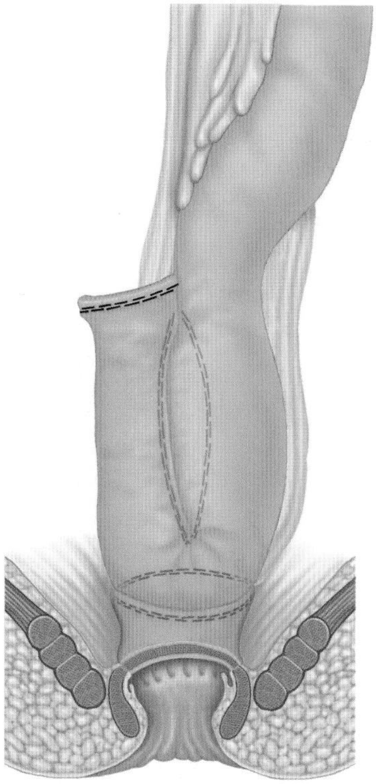

Fig. 25.7 Ileal pouch with ileo-anal anastomosis.

Ileal pouch and ileo-anal anastomosis

The technique is to form a similar pouch but to anastomose it to the anal verge after all large-bowel mucosa has been removed (Fig. 25.7). Patients usually defecate normally (although usually fairly frequently) and in some cases they need to empty the pouch by use of a per-anal tube. The operation is technically complex with a significant complication rate, but is a major advance over proctocolectomy and permanent ileostomy.

Crohn's disease of the colon

This condition characteristically affects the small intestine (for more-detailed treatment, see Ch. 24) but may involve the large bowel either in isolation (20% of cases) or in combination with small-intestinal disease (50% of cases).

Clinical features

Symptoms

The diarrhoea and other complaints are often indistinguishable from those of ulcerative colitis, and the systemic upset is the same. However, there may be associated complaints of perianal problems such as fissure and fistula (Ch. 26). Patients with ileocolic Crohn's disease usually have less diarrhoea and more abdominal pain.

Clinical findings

The abdominal findings may be non-specific, although a mass in the right iliac fossa or an abdominal wall abscess/fistula are very suggestive. There is a high incidence of anal lesions such as:

- fistula
- perianal abscess
- chronic fissure
- anal ulceration
- oedematous skin tags.

Investigation

Sigmoidoscopy or colonoscopy may not distinguish the disease from ulcerative colitis. Characteristic histopathological features may be found on biopsy including transmural inflammation, crypt abscesses and granuloma formation. Barium enema (Fig. 25.8) shows segmental and discontinuous involvement of the large bowel and the presence of fissures and fistulae in the bowel wall. Strictures are not uncommon. CT and/or MRI scanning may give additional information about the extent of disease (especially the presence of small-bowel disease which may also be demonstrated on barium follow-through examinations) and complications such as localised perforation or internal fistula. They may also be useful in the assessment of perianal disease.

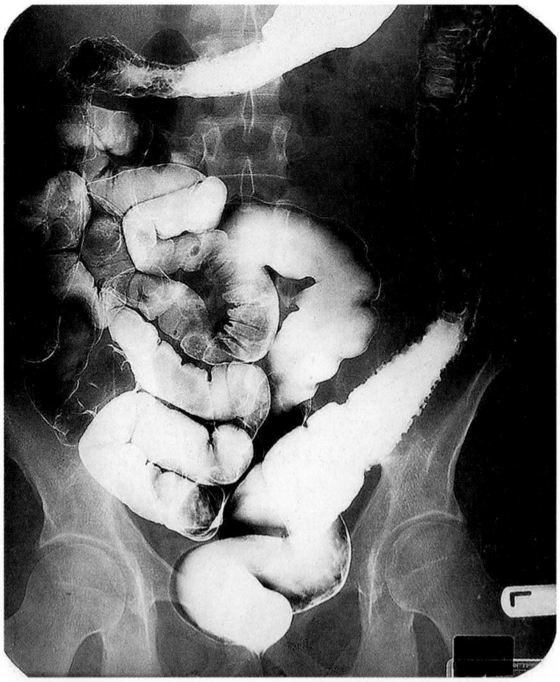

Fig. 25.8 Barium enema in a patient with Crohn's disease of the large bowel. Note deep ulcers and sparing of rectum.

Management

The medical treatment is similar to that for ulcerative colitis (see above). Colectomy may be required for severe or intractable disease. The management of the disease in the small bowel, and particularly of obstruction, is described in Chapter 24.

Ischaemic colitis

This condition is uncommon in those under the age of 50. The frequent occurrence at the splenic flexure, where the arterial anastomotic loops are least well developed, suggests that the cause is reduced arterial input, perhaps from the development of degenerative arterial disease.

Clinical features

Symptoms

Symptoms are:

- acute left-sided abdominal pain
- dark red rectal bleeding.

Clinical findings

Clinical findings are:

- fever
- hypotension
- abdominal tenderness.

Investigation and management

A plain abdominal X-ray may show a distended splenic flexure in which oedematous mucosa may be detected. This finding is confirmed by CT scanning or barium enema where the thumbprinting of the mucosa is apparent. In some cases the diagnosis may be confirmed by colonoscopic biopsy, but the risk of perforation is increased.

Spontaneous resolution is the rule. Occasionally progression leads to gangrene for which emergency surgery is required. Intermediate between these is ischaemia that leads to late stricture for which surgery is needed.

Infective diseases

There is a wide variety of organisms capable of causing colitis (see Box 25.5). They are of surgical importance only because of the need to detect treatable infective agents in patients who may at first sight seem to have ulcerative colitis or Crohn's disease.

DIVERTICULAR DISEASE

Diverticular disease is very rarely congenital, in which case the walls of the diverticula contain all layers of the normal colon. Much more commonly it is acquired and the diverticula are serosa-covered outpouchings of mucosa alone through gaps in the muscularis propria which transmit the terminal blood vessels. The diverticula are usually found in the left colon, especially the sigmoid, but quite frequently involve the entire colon.

Epidemiology and aetiology

Acquired diverticular disease is rare under the age of 35, after which there is a progressive increase in incidence, so that 50% of those in their eighth or ninth decade are affected though not necessarily symptomatic. The condition is common in Western countries but rare in China, India and Africa.

The most popular explanation of the cause is that a low-fibre diet is associated with increased intraluminal pressure, which leads to pulsion herniation of mucosa alongside blood vessels. There is some physiological evidence to support this, and the treatment of symptoms with a high-fibre diet is often successful. However, not all patients with diverticular disease consume a diet low in fibre, and some Japanese have a particular form of the disorder exclusively in the right colon, a phenomenon which cannot be explained by the low-fibre theory.

Pathological features

The anatomical features are given above. Diverticula have a narrow neck, and inspissated faeces may accumulate within them. Inflammation may follow with a number of outcomes:

- persistent inflammation in a segment of bowel wall
- local inflammation of the affected diverticulum, leading to perforation.

Perforation may in turn be:

- local into the pericolic tissues
- into the peritoneal cavity with generalised peritonitis
- into an adjacent organ such as the bladder with the formation of a fistula.

Clinical features

Symptoms

These are frequently absent and the diagnosis is made following a colonoscopy or barium enema done for other reasons, chiefly to exclude a large-bowel carcinoma. There may be mild left lower abdominal pain which accompanies a long-standing irregularity of bowel habit with episodic slight diarrhoea or more usually constipation with the passage of small quantities of hard faecal pellets.

Signs

In uncomplicated disease, signs are absent or minimal. There is occasionally tenderness over the descending colon, and this portion of the bowel may be palpable.

Investigation

Barium enema or colonoscopy is the usual method of confirming the diagnosis (Fig. 25.9), but it should be deferred in patients with complications in whom CT scanning is the investigation of choice (see below). The diverticular openings may also be seen at colonoscopy. Diverticular disease is notorious for its ability, at barium enema examination, to conceal a coexistent carcinoma. If there is any doubt colonoscopy should be performed.

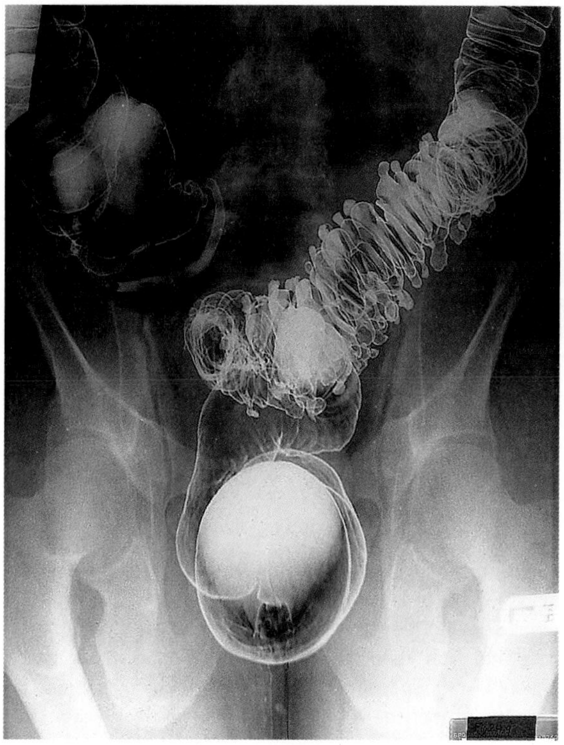

Fig. 25.9 Barium enema in a patient with diverticular disease.

Management

There is no evidence that increasing the amount of dietary fibre prevents the development of diverticula. However, in the presence of mild symptoms (such as pain) attributed to their presence, the use of added fibre or other bulking agents (e.g. ispaghula) has been conclusively shown to be of benefit. If pain is severe or unresponsive, resection of the affected segment (usually the sigmoid) may be considered.

Complications

Inflammation

Involvement of a segment of the bowel wall may cause severe abdominal pain, pyrexia and tenderness over the affected segment. Progression to local perforation may take place, with a collection of inflammatory tissue and eventually pus around the sigmoid colon – a pericolic abscess. Its presence is indicated by a mass. Confirmation can be obtained by ultrasound examination or more usually by CT scan. Although an early inflammatory process may settle with restricting oral intake and antibiotic therapy, a pericolic abscess may need to be drained. Repeated attacks may prompt surgical resection of the diseased area, either at laparoscopic or open operation.

Peritonitis

It is thought that this is the result of a process similar to that of gangrenous appendicitis – a faecolith impacts in the mouth of the diverticulum and the blood supply is obstructed. A number of sequelae may occur (Table 25.2). The diverticulum becomes gangrenous and may rupture into an unprotected cavity. If this occurs the following features will be seen:

Table 25.2 The Hinchey classification for colonic perforation due to diverticular disease

- Hinchey I – localised abscess (para-colonic)
- Hinchey II – pelvic abscess
- Hinchey III – purulent peritonitis (the presence of pus in the abdominal cavity)
- Hinchey IV – faeculent peritonitis.

After Hinchey EJ, Schaal PG, Richard GK 1978 Treatment of diverticular disease of the colon. Advances in Surgery 12:85–109.

- generalised abdominal pain often accompanied by pain in the tip of the shoulder from the extensive pneumoperitoneum
- evidence of severe sepsis – fever and circulatory collapse
- abdominal tenderness and rigidity.

This complication is a surgical emergency, and surgical management of the site of perforation is essential. This may require colonic resection, often with temporary stoma formation, and later reoperation to restore continuity. In some patients with purulent rather than faecal peritonitis it may be possible to manage the problem by peritoneal lavage and drainage, sometimes performed laparoscopically. In such cases later elective colonic resection may be required, but can be performed when the patient's condition is improved, may be possible laparoscopically, and usually avoids stoma formation.

Fistulation

The clinical features depend on the structures involved. A blind track into the pericolic tissues may only be found on barium enema. A bladder fistula is characterised by complaints of pneumaturia and recurrent bladder infection, and a fistula into the vagina is characterised by the passage of gas and faecal content per vaginam. Surgical treatment is required in both these latter cases.

Haemorrhage

Large-volume rectal haemorrhage, which is thought to be the consequence of the erosion of a vessel in the neck of a diverticulum, is a well-recognised complication of diverticular disease. Indeed diverticular disease is the commonest cause of large-volume rectal bleeding, particularly in patients over 50 years. Rapid exsanguination may be life-threatening in elderly patients. Diagnosis is usually straightforward but it is sometimes difficult to distinguish bleeding from vascular malformations (angiodysplasia) which can occur in the elderly at any site in the large bowel. Most cases are managed non-operatively, but sometimes ongoing bleeding prompts further intervention. Haemorrhage from a diverticulum may be difficult to localise in patients with anatomically extensive disease. Selective angiography of the large-bowel arteries is usually required, after which the treatment can be radiological (embolisation – although there is a risk of colonic necrosis and perforation) or surgical. Limited colonic resection is undertaken when the site of bleeding has been confirmed; otherwise a subtotal colectomy with ileostomy or ileo-rectal anastomosis may be necessary.

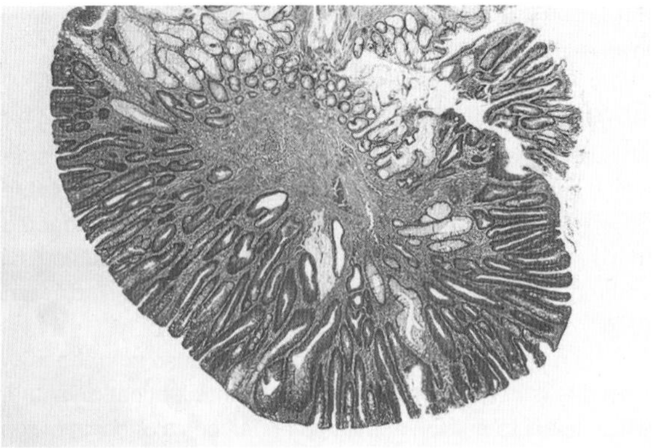

Fig. 25.10 Histological appearance of a tubular adenoma of the colon.

Volvulus of the large bowel

See Chapter 24.

NEOPLASIA

BENIGN NEOPLASMS

Adenomas

Aetiology and epidemiology

Benign large-bowel neoplasms are associated with a number of different conditions, many of which have a genetic component (see, for example, familial adenomatosis polyposis, below). The lifetime incidence in the Western world's population is 20–25%, but elsewhere the condition is much less common. Adenomas are linked to a low-fibre, high red meat, high fat diet.

Pathological features

The most common and important neoplasm is an adenoma which arises from the glandular or epithelial cells. The tumour is most often a polyp with a stalk, but flat (sessile) lesions also occur. The histological appearance is a basis for classification into tubular, villous or tubulovillous (Fig. 25.10). Tubular polyps tend to be pedunculated and spherical; the other two types are more often multifronded and sessile. They may be single or multiple, and in some hereditary syndromes many hundreds or thousands are present. The important clinicopathological correlate of an adenoma is that it is a premalignant lesion and exposure of its surface over the years to the faecal stream may initiate the development of an adenocarcinoma. This polyp–cancer sequence is most likely in lesions over 1 cm in diameter. Not all polyps are adenomas. The other causes of protrusions of mucosa that are anatomically polyps are given in Box 25.10.

Clinical features and diagnosis

Most adenomas are both asymptomatic and devoid of signs. Unless there is a family history or there are so many lesions that bleeding is obvious, the diagnosis is made either as the result of a screening programme (see below) or on incidental examination of the large bowel by colonoscopy or barium enema for unexplained iron deficiency anaemia or other symptoms.

A rare clinical syndrome is when a villous adenoma in the rectum is sufficiently large that large quantities of potassium-rich mucus are lost from it and the patient becomes hypokalaemic.

Management

The finding of an adenomatous polyp, particularly if it is larger than 1 cm, requires the following action:

Box 25.10 Classification of colorectal polyps

Neoplastic
- Adenoma
  - Tubular
  - Tubulovillous
  - Villous

Non-neoplastic
- Hamartoma
  - Juvenile
  - Peutz–Jeghers
- Inflammatory
  - Lymphoid
  - Inflamed oedematous mucosa
- Miscellaneous
  - Metaplastic
  - Connective tissue polyps

- complete examination of the large bowel by colonoscopy to exclude or identify other similar neoplasms
- removal of all lesions, which can usually be achieved endoscopically
- regular lifelong surveillance for recurrence and/or the development of large-bowel cancer in selected cases (see Fig 25.11)

Familial adenomatous polyposis (FAP)

This is an autosomal dominant condition with a high degree of penetrance.

Pathological features

Multiple adenomatous polyps develop in the colon and also sometimes in the small bowel especially the duodenum. The colonic polyps usually start between the ages of 13 and 30 years, although sometimes this does not take place until the fourth decade. Progression through the polyp–cancer sequence is inevitable. Not infrequently, there are other manifestations outwith the colon, including desmoid tumours, congenital hypertrophy of the retinal pigment epithelium (CHRPE), fibromas, osteomas, sebaceous cysts. The latter three conditions linked with FAP are known as Gardner's syndrome.

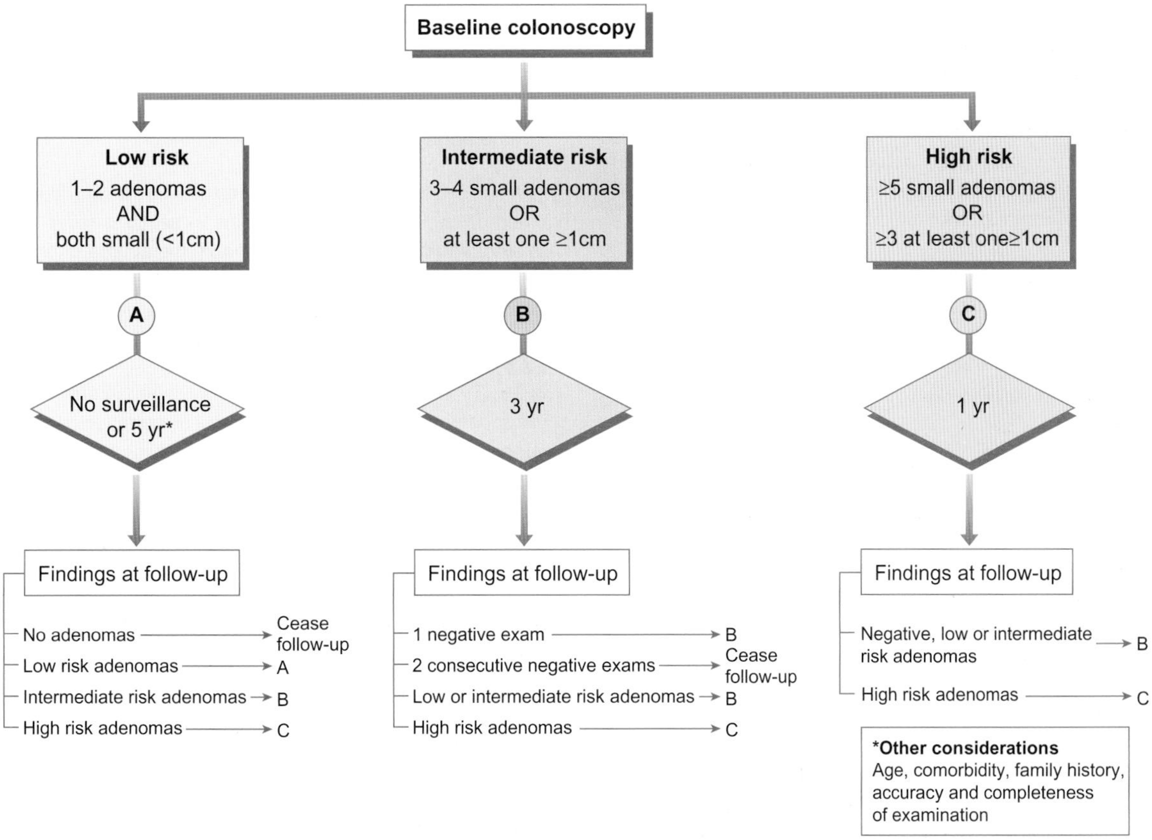

Fig. 25.11 Colonoscopic follow-up of colonic adenomas (after Atkin and Saunders, Gut 2002;51(Suppl V):v6–v9).

Clinical features

The condition is initially asymptomatic, although a family history may be present. Blood from the rectum is the most common symptom, and there may be other less specific complaints such as tenesmus and diarrhoea.

Diagnosis and management

The diagnosis is made by endoscopy. Wireless capsule endoscopy of the small bowel should be done to exclude small-bowel polyps. Siblings should be examined. Total colectomy is essential because of the universal progression to cancer. An ileo-anal pouch reconstruction is usually possible.

MALIGNANT NEOPLASMS

Epidemiology and aetiology

Malignant tumours of the large bowel are common and are the third commonest cause of cancer death in the UK at 18 000 per year. The highest incidence of adenocarcinoma, which accounts for 98% of the tumours, occurs in New Zealand, Australia, western Europe and North America. The lowest is in Asia, Africa and South America, although Argentina is an exception. The disease can develop at any age from the second decade, but the peak incidence is in the sixth and subsequent decades. The important aetiological factors are described below.

Dietary factors

Bile salt conversion There is indirect evidence that a diet rich in animal fat is a major risk factor. It is suggested that such a diet, common in the Western world, produces an environment within the gut which favours bacteria that convert bile salts to carcinogens, and work on experimental animals supports this hypothesis.

Low intake of fibre has also been claimed to predispose to neoplasia because it slows transit and thus increases the time of exposure of the mucosa to carcinogens.

Adenomatous polyps

The polyp–cancer sequence is considered above. It probably accounts for the development of the great majority of large-bowel cancers, a matter which emphasises the importance of screening (see below).

Genetic factors

Familial adenomatous polyposis (FAP) as an inevitable cause of cancer is described above. There is a 2–3 times increased risk to a first-degree relative of a patient with adenocarcinoma.

Hereditary non-polyposis colon cancer (HNPCC, also known as Lynch syndrome) is an autosomal dominant condition which has a high risk of colon cancer and other cancers including endometrium, ovary, stomach, small intestine, hepatobiliary tract, upper urinary tract, brain, and skin. The increased risk is due to inherited mutations that impair DNA mismatch repair with resultant micro-satellite instability. MLH1, MSH2 and MSH6 gene mutations account for almost all cases. HNPCC leads to between 2 and 7% of colorectal cancers.

Inflammatory bowel disease

Long-standing and total ulcerative colitis as a cause is described above. Crohn's disease is also associated with a fourfold increase in the risk of colorectal carcinoma.

Pathological features

Distribution

The anatomical distribution is shown in Figure 25.12.

Synchronous lesions

Up to 3% of patients have one or more synchronous cancers, and 75% have at least one benign adenoma.

Macroscopic classification

Tumours are classified as follows:

- polypoid
- ulcerative
- annular
- a combination of the above.

Spread

Direct extension in the transverse axis of the bowel wall eventually causes complete encirclement. Tumour cells which arise in the mucosa penetrate the submucosa and muscle to reach the serosal surface of the bowel, or, where the bowel is extraperitoneal, as in the rectum, they spread into the fascia and the structures contained in it such as the sacral plexus (posteriorly), the ureters (laterally), and the bladder in the male or the uterus and cervix in the female (anteriorly).

Lymphatic permeation and embolisation carry tumour cells initially to local (paracolic) nodes and from there to nodes which lie on the course of the blood supply to the bowel. In consequence, spread is largely upwards towards the aorta and the portal vein.

Haematogenous Malignant cells can often be seen within the lumen of capillaries and small veins in sections taken from colorectal tumours. They are probably the source of emboli which enter the tributaries of the portal vein and so reach the liver, which may be involved at the time of treatment in up to 40% of cases. Spread beyond the liver to lung, kidney and bone is uncommon at diagnosis.

Transcoelomic implantation follows penetration to the serosal surface and causes ascites. Cells may also be implanted on the ovaries.

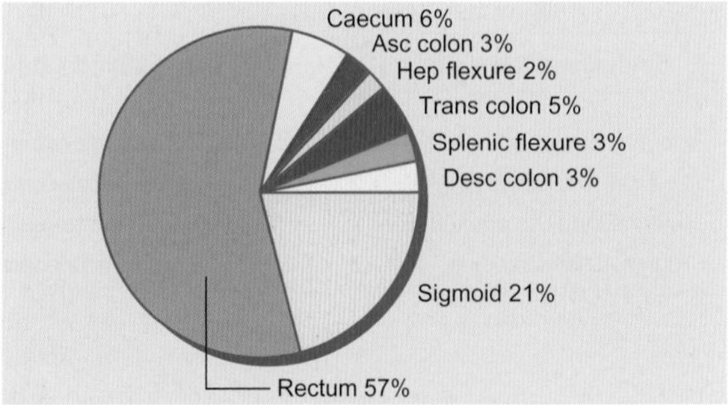

Fig. 25.12 Anatomical distribution of colonic carcinoma.

Direct implantation Exfoliated cells remain viable within the lumen of the bowel and may be implanted if the mucosa is breached – as at the site of an anastomosis or in a haemorrhoidectomy wound if that procedure is carried out in a patient with an unsuspected proximal carcinoma.

Staging

The conventional method of staging is by the Dukes classification (Fig. 25.13):

- Stage A – the neoplastic cells are confined to the mucosa. The 5-year survival is 90%.
- Stage B – the tumour has extended through all muscle layers and possibly reached the serosa; metastases to lymph nodes are absent. The 5-year survival is 75%.
- Stage C – lymph node metastasis has occurred. The 5-year survival is 50%. Stage C cases are often divided into C1 (local lymph node involvement only) and C2 (more-proximal nodes involved). C2 carries a worse prognosis than C1.
- Stage D – this was not part of the original classification but is often used to describe a patient with disseminated metastatic disease. 5-year survival is 6%.

The TNM (Table 25.3) system is also widely used.

Screening for colorectal cancer

The good results obtained in Dukes stage A cancer and the known polyp–cancer sequence encouraged the idea that attempts should be made to detect asymptomatic polyps and early cancers. A nationwide screening programme has been introduced in the UK. The population is being offered testing for faecal occult blood every 2 years from the age of 60 to 70 years. If blood is detected, individuals are invited to undergo colonoscopy. Regular screening should reduce deaths from colorectal cancer by 16%. High-risk groups (strong family history, e.g. HNPCC, those with previous adenomatous polyps, etc.) should already be included in a more intensive screening programme, and start testing at an earlier age.

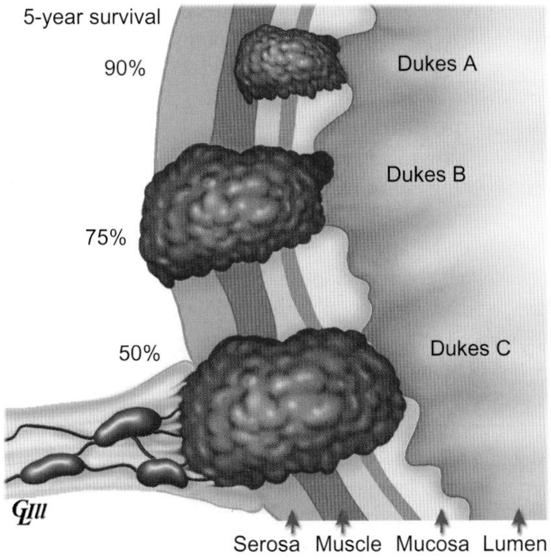

Fig. 25.13 Dukes staging of colonic carcinoma.

Clinical features

Symptoms

The most important symptoms are listed in Box 25.11.

A distinction can be drawn between the presentation of tumours in the right side, the left side and the rectum.

Right-sided tumours have non-specific complaints such as malaise, weight loss, vague abdominal pain and occasionally a self-detected mass in the abdomen. A frequent reason for the patient seeking medical advice is the development of symptoms of iron deficiency anaemia: any patient who does so and in whom the cause is not obvious should undergo urgent full investigation of the large bowel and upper GI tract, usually done by combined upper GI endoscopy and colonoscopy. The liquid nature of the contents of the right side make presentation with intestinal obstruction rare.

Left-sided tumours are more likely to present with obstructive symptoms, because the stool is semi-solid or completely solid and the calibre of the bowel is less. There is colicky abdominal pain and a change in bowel habit which may include either constipation or diarrhoea, or alternation between the two. A distal tumour may lead to the passage of mucus which is confused with a loose motion. Visible blood in the stool is rare (10%). Acute intestinal obstruction may supervene.

Rectal tumours are more likely to be associated with rectal bleeding, usually on defecation, and mucous discharge is common as is tenesmus.

A growth that has spread locally may cause:

- faecal incontinence from invasion of the anal sphincters
- back pain because of involvement of the sacral plexus
- urinary infection, a rectovesical fistula or renal failure through infiltration of the ureters.

Table 25.3 TNM staging system for colorectal cancer

Tumour
T1: Tumour invades submucosa
T2: Tumour invades muscularis propria
T3: Tumour invades through the muscularis propria into the subserosa, or into the pericolic or perirectal tissues
T4: Tumour directly invades other organs or structures, and/or perforates

Node
N0: No regional lymph node metastasis
N1: Metastasis in 1–3 regional lymph nodes
N2: Metastasis in 4 or more regional lymph nodes

Metastasis
M0: No distant metastasis
M1: Distant metastasis present.

Box 25.11 Symptoms associated with colorectal carcinoma

- Alteration in bowel habit
- Rectal bleeding and/or mucus
- Abdominal pain
- Malaise
- Weight loss
- Tenesmus

Physical findings

These are often absent. A mass may be palpable in the abdomen or on rectal examination. In advanced disease, weight loss may be obvious, there may be evidence of spread (ascites and hepatomegaly), and signs of bowel obstruction may be present.

Investigation

Sigmoidoscopy

All patients with symptoms that suggest a large-bowel carcinoma must have a digital rectal examination and colonoscopy. Any mucosal abnormality is biopsied. However, sigmoidoscopy can only see, at best, as far as the mid-sigmoid colon (about 25 cm) using the rigid instrument, or to the splenic flexure with a flexible sigmoidoscope. Full visualisation of the large bowel requires colonoscopy, barium enema or CT pneumocolon (virtual colonoscopy).

Colonoscopy

Direct visualisation of the entire colon is the investigation of choice, but the procedure is expensive in time and resources and can be technically difficult. It carries a small risk of perforation (1 in 500–1000 procedures). Even if a distal colonic or rectal cancer is found, it is important to examine the proximal colon to exclude synchronous tumours or polyps.

Barium enema

Barium enema was the traditional method of investigating the colon. It is now used as an alternative to colonoscopy or CT pneumocolon. Identified lesions require follow-up colonoscopy for biopsy or treatment (Fig. 25.14).

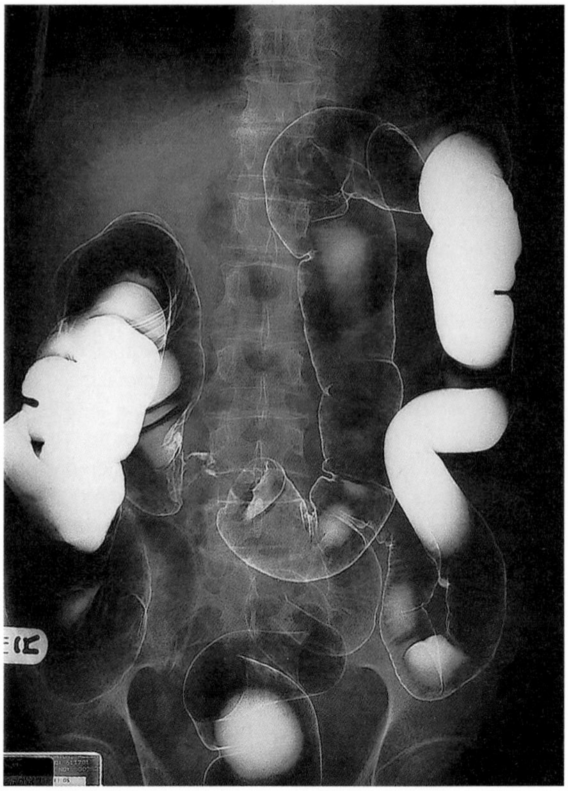

Fig. 25.14 Barium enema in a patient with colonic carcinoma.

CT pneumocolon (virtual pneumocolon)

After bowel preparation air is insufflated into the rectum and colon. Prone and supine scans are acquired and mucosal lesions readily identified. In the case of a probable cancer being seen, the scan may also be used to exclude metastatic disease. The scan also picks up incidental extra-colonic abnormalities.

Assessment of extent of disease and of spread

Carcinoembryonic antigen (CEA) does not play a part in selecting treatment but can be a useful marker of the elimination of disease and the emergence of recurrence. Therefore a pretreatment measurement is desirable.

A preoperative CT scan is required to assess the local extent of the tumour and also exclude or define metastatic disease. In some cases PET scanning may be used to better assess metastatic disease. MRI scanning is the best modality to assess the local extent of rectal cancers.

Management

The management of colorectal cancer has become a truly multispecialty programme in which the surgeon plays a vital role. Patients are discussed at a Multidisciplinary Meeting (MDM) and a treatment plan agreed.

Laparoscopic or laparoscopic assisted operations are being increasingly performed for patients with colorectal cancer. These usually result in less postoperative pain, smaller scars and a more rapid recovery compared with traditional open operations. There is good evidence that, performed in well-trained hands, laparoscopic colorectal resection does not compromise tumour clearance or lymph node harvest.

Colon carcinoma

The treatment of Dukes A to C disease is primarily by surgical removal, and this is accompanied in B and C tumours by adjuvant therapy. Right-sided tumours are removed by a right hemicolectomy and those on the left by a resection tailored to the segment of bowel involved (Fig. 25.15). The preoperative preparation and the common complications of surgery are given in Boxes 25.12 and 25.13.

Rectal carcinoma

Patients with rectal cancer, particularly the more locally advanced tumours which extend close to the proposed surgical resection margin, are usually treated preoperatively with chemoradiotherapy – a combination of radiotherapy with concomitant chemotherapy (either intravenous fluorouracil or oral capecitabine, the latter sometimes combined with irinotecan). Such treatment shrinks most tumours and reduces the risk of 'margin positive' resections and consequently also local pelvic recurrence.

A tumour in the mid- or upper rectum is removed by resecting the distal colon and involved rectum and restoring continuity by joining the large bowel to the stump of rectum – anterior resection (Fig. 25.16a). The anastomosis may be done with either sutures or staples, and the latter are particularly useful when the rectal stump is short and access

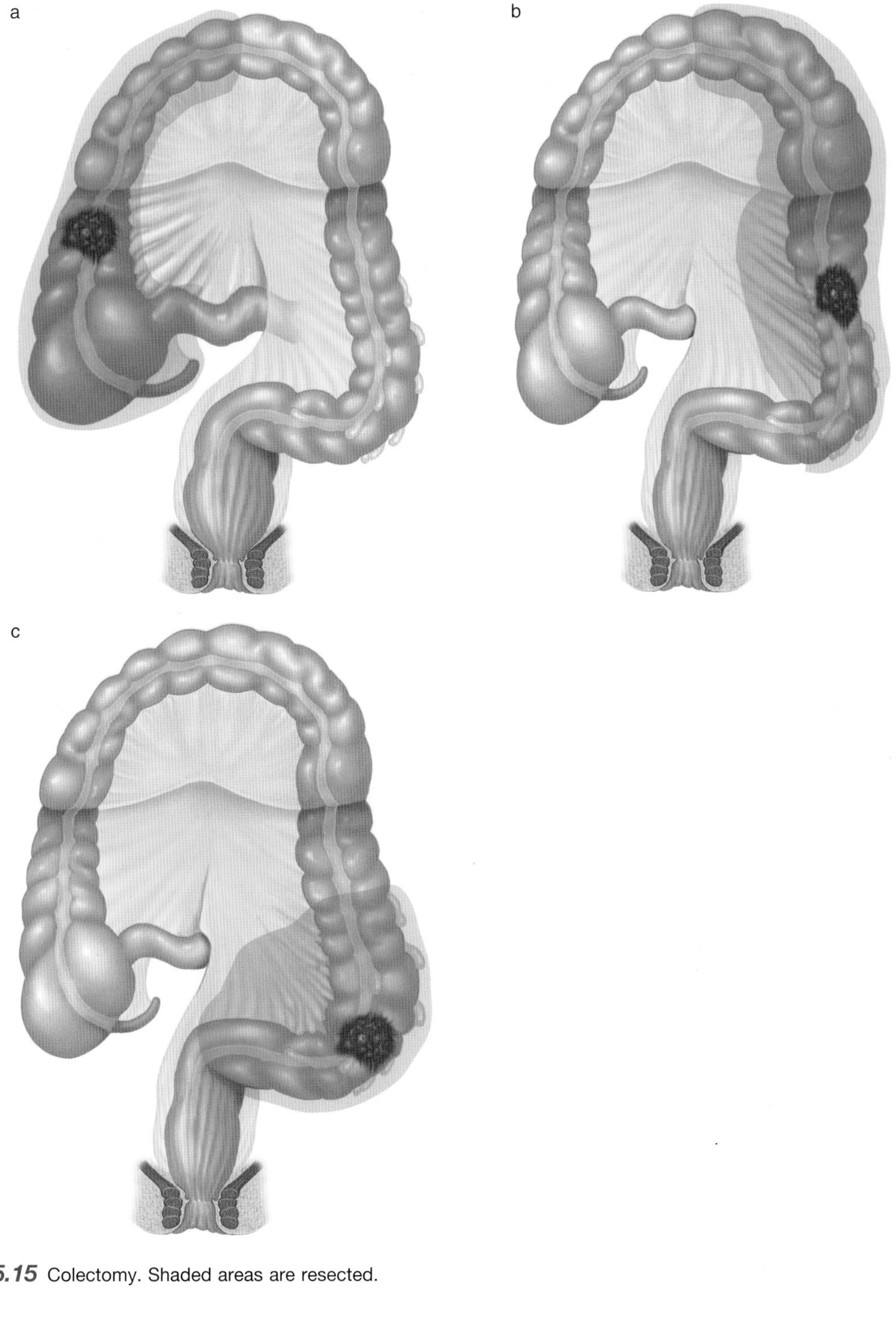

Fig. 25.15 Colectomy. Shaded areas are resected.

Box 25.12 Preoperative preparation for colectomy

- Bowel preparation by oral laxative or whole gut irrigation – not used by all surgeons
- Antibiotic chemoprophylaxis
- Thromboembolism prophylaxis
- Correct anaemia
- Correct electrolyte deficiencies

difficult. A low rectal tumour may require the removal of the whole rectum and adjacent sphincters – abdominoperineal resection and end colostomy (Fig. 25.16b).

Adjuvant therapy

Patients with lymph node metastases confirmed after colonic resection for adenocarcinoma are offered adjuvant chemotherapy with FOLFOX (a combination of folinic acid (leucovorin), fluorouracil and oxaliplatin), capecitabine (an oral

Box 25.13 Complications of colectomy and rectal excision

- Haemorrhage
- Ureteric damage
  - Urinary leakage
  - Ureteric stricture
- Damage to bladder function
  - Acute retention
  - Urinary incontinence
- Impaired sexual function – erectile dysfunction, retrograde ejaculation – nerve injury
- Damage to duodenum (right hemicolectomy)
- Damage to spleen (left hemicolectomy)
- Anastomotic complications
  - Stricture
  - Leakage
- Complications of stoma
  - Parastomal hernia
  - Prolapse
  - Electrolyte imbalance
  - Ischaemia
  - Stenosis
- Diarrhoea/constipation

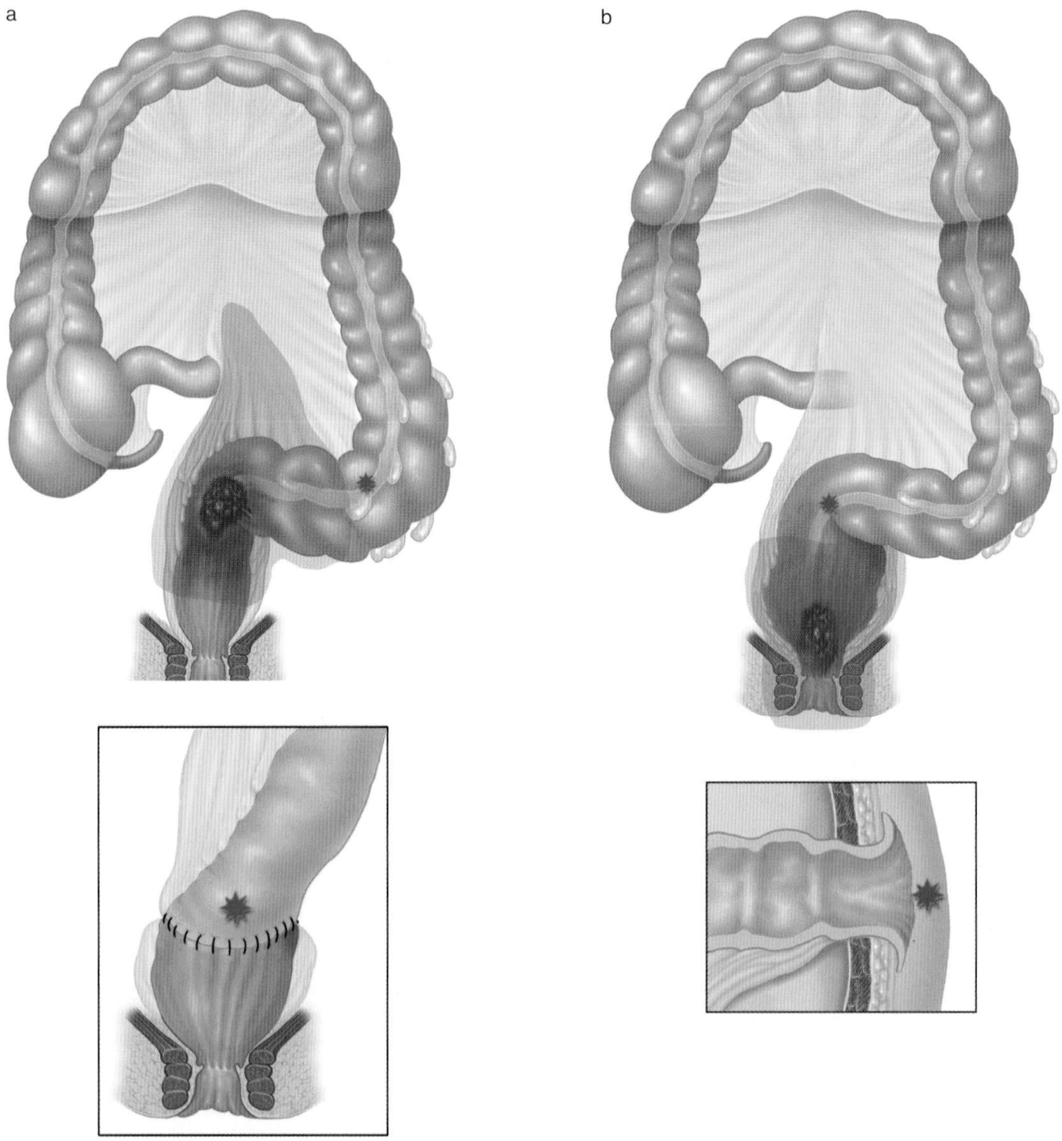

Fig. 25.16 Surgical management of rectal carcinoma. (a) Anterior resection of the rectum. Shaded area is resected. (b) Abdominoperineal excision of the rectum and anus. Shaded area is resected.

alternative to fluorouracil) or other alternative chemotherapy regimen because such treatment had been shown to reduce the risk of cancer recurrence and improve patient survival.

Radiation

Radiotherapy is used for some rectal cancers before surgery (see above). It can also be used to treat early rectal cancer – either alone or after local excision, locally advanced colon cancer after margin-positive resection, or for palliation of metastatic disease.

Chemotherapy

New combinations of chemotherapy agents are increasingly used in the management of colorectal cancer. Adjuvant chemotherapy is commonly used after colonic cancer resection and used in combination with radiotherapy before rectal cancer excision (see above). Patients with metastatic disease at presentation or developing after initial treatment are usually offered palliative chemotherapy with combinations of agents such as FOLFOX (a combination of folinic acid (leucovorin), fluorouracil and oxaliplatin) or FOLFIRI (a combination of folinic acid (leucovorin), fluorouracil and irinotecan). Cetuximab (a monoclonal epidermal growth factor inhibitor) is now also recommended in addition to these regimens for patients with metastatic disease confined to the liver.

Hepatic metastases

Liver metastases, when the only site of secondary or recurrent cancer, are increasingly being treated by liver resection (see Ch. 20) or other ablative techniques such as radiofrequency ablation (RFA), microwave treatment or cryotherapy. These alternative technologies are usually given using image guidance – ultrasound or CT scanning – either percutaneously using specially designed probes or at open operation when they may be combined with hepatic resection. In all cases patients are also treated with chemotherapy before and/or after resection or ablation using the agents described above for palliative treatment of metastatic disease. Prolonged survival is increasingly seen, even in the presence of liver secondaries, as a result of such multi-modality treatment.

Box 25.14 Causes of rectal bleeding

- Haemorrhoids
- Anal fissure
- Diverticular disease
- Colorectal cancer
- Colorectal polyps
- Arteriovenous malformations
- Ischaemia
- Trauma
- Colitis
- Solitary rectal ulcer
- Other anal conditions
  - Fistula
  - Squamous carcinoma
  - Warts

RECTAL BLEEDING

Rectal bleeding is a common symptom (Box 25.14). Usually the bleeding is of a minor nature and can be investigated on an elective basis. Rarely, bleeding is of a profuse nature requiring urgent investigation and treatment and occasionally urgent surgical intervention. In the younger patient, rectal bleeding is usually of benign origin (e.g. haemorrhoids) and can be effectively managed by non-surgical methods (see Ch. 26). In the older patient, malignancy must always be excluded. Where the patient presents with acute large-volume rectal bleeding, it may be appropriate to exclude upper-gastrointestinal causes in the first instance (see Ch. 24). Once these have been excluded, the lower-GI tract needs to be investigated by urgent colonoscopy supplemented by visceral angiography if required. In the older patient, acute bleeding is likely to be the consequence of either diverticular disease (see above) or an arteriovenous malformation. Sometimes no cause can be identified for massive haemorrhage, and a subtotal colectomy has to be performed by the surgeon.

THE APPENDIX

Anatomy

The appendix is a blind-ending tube varying from 2 to 20 cm in length (average approx. 9 cm) which arises from the posteromedial wall of the caecum and whose anatomical position in the pelvis may vary considerably:

- behind the caecum (retrocaecal) – 65%
- projects downwards into the pelvis (pelvic) – 31%
- immediately below the caecum (subcaecal) – 2%
- in front of the terminal ileum (pre-ileal) – 1%
- behind the ileum (post-ileal) – 0.4%.

The main artery is the appendicular artery, which is a branch of the ileocolic that runs behind the terminal ileum to reach the base of the appendix and extends to its tip via the mesoappendix.

Histology

The mucosa is similar to that of the colon in that it is of columnar type with crypts containing numerous mucus-secreting glands. The distinguishing feature is the presence of extensive lymphoid tissue in the lamina propria, which contains plasma cells, lymphocytes, eosinophils and macrophages embedded in a fibrocellular reticulum. In addition in this layer congregations of lymphocytes are seen, so forming lymphoid follicles. The outer layers of the appendix are formed from the inner (circular) and outer (longitudinal) layers of smooth muscle which are continuous from the caecum, and these in turn are covered by a complete serosal layer.

Function

In herbivores, the appendix and the caecum are highly developed and are recognised to be of considerable importance in the digestion of cellulose by bacteria. In humans, the appendix is generally recognised to be vestigial, but the predominance of lymphocytes suggests that the organ may play a role in defence mechanisms against bacterial infections.

THE APPENDIX AND DISEASE

Acute appendicitis

The significance of the appendix to the surgeon lies in its importance as a common cause of the acute abdomen (see Ch. 23).

Mucocele of the appendix

This is a rare condition which can be difficult to differentiate clinically from its malignant counterpart – cystadenocarcinoma (see below).

Pathology

A diffusely enlarged appendix develops as a result of a lumen filled with mucus. The latter arises secondarily from obstruction of the lumen by mucosal hyperplasia, adenoma or cystadenocarcinoma. The diagnosis of carcinoma cannot usually be made on clinical grounds and can only be based on microscopic evidence of invasion of the appendix wall by mucin. Rupture of a mucocele may result in pseudomyxoma peritonei. The latter syndrome is a consequence of coelomic spread and implantation of mucin-secreting cells with resultant mucinous ascites and later intestinal obstruction.

Clinical features and management

Most mucoceles are asymptomatic and are only discovered 'en passant' during laparotomy or at CT scanning.

Where symptoms occur, appendicectomy is curative.

TUMOURS OF THE APPENDIX

These are rare, accounting for less than 1% of all intestinal tumours, but, because of their position, they can be extremely difficult to diagnose. The pathology of these tumours is as follows:

- carcinoid – 85%
- mucinous cystadenocarcinoma – 8%
- caecal adenocarcinoma – 4%
- miscellaneous – 3%.

Carcinoid tumour

The incidence of carcinoid tumours is approximately 0.5% of appendicectomy specimens, and although the majority are benign, they have the potential to invade locally, metastasise and secrete biologically active substances.

Pathology and clinical features

These are small, well-circumscribed but non-encapsulated tumours usually located in the tip of the appendix and frequently only recognised microscopically (70% <1.0 cm diameter). The tumour is composed of nests of uniform argyrophilic cells with occasional acinic development.

The majority are asymptomatic. Metastatic spread to the liver and carcinoid syndrome are extremely rare with appendix carcinoids.

Treatment

Most authorities agree that for small (microscopic) carcinoids, appendicectomy is sufficient treatment, and such patients have a 99% 5-year survival. For more-extensive local disease, more radical excisional surgery (e.g. right hemicolectomy) is advocated. Distant metastasis has only been recorded where the tumour exceeds 2 cm in diameter.

Mucinous cystadenocarcinoma

These tumours are recognised by the presence of mucus-secreting epithelial mucosal cells. The mucin may penetrate the appendix wall and give rise to pseudomyxoma peritonei.

Clinical features

The tumour is usually asymptomatic but may, on occasions, give rise to appendicitis or present with an abdominal mass. At the time of presentation, approximately 50% of these tumours will have undergone intra-abdominal spread.

Treatment

These tumours are slow-growing; hence right hemicolectomy is usually adequate treatment and a 5-year survival of 70% can be expected. Simple appendicectomy is inadequate surgical treatment.

Caecal adenocarcinoma

Most of these tumours arise from the base of the appendix and thereby rapidly lead to occlusion of the appendix lumen and may then give rise to the pathological features of acute appendicitis.

Clinical features

Most tumours are symptomatic, presenting as acute appendicitis.

Treatment

Since the operative findings are those of acute appendicitis, the danger is one of inadequate surgery, i.e. the surgeon performs appendicectomy alone. The presence of a firm mass at the base of the appendix should alert the surgeon to the possibility of malignancy, and a radical right hemicolectomy is required. The prognosis is that of adenocarcinoma of the colon, i.e. it is dependent on histological grading and Dukes staging.

FURTHER READING

Keighley MRB, Williams NS 2007 Surgery of the anus, rectum and colon, 2 volume set, 3rd edn. Elsevier Saunders, Edinburgh

NICE technology appraisal guidance 105, August 2006 Laparoscopic surgery for colorectal cancer. [Online] Available: www.nice.org.uk

NICE technology appraisal guidance 176, August 2009. Cetuximab for the first-line treatment of metastatic colorectal cancer. [Online] Available: www.nice.org.uk

Phillips RKS 2009 Colorectal surgery: a companion to specialist surgical practice, 4th edn. Elsevier Saunders, Edinburgh

26 Anal and related disorders

The anal canal is a structure of considerable importance in that it controls two of humanity's most unsociable physiological needs: defecation and the passage of flatus. Disturbances in its function or structure result in troublesome symptoms which need careful assessment if management is to be effective. At all times it must be remembered that disorders in the rectum and colon must be excluded before treatment is begun. The possibility of sexually transmitted diseases occurring in the anal region must also be kept in mind.

GENERAL CONSIDERATIONS

Anatomy and physiology

Embryology

The anal canal – the last 3–4 cm of the alimentary tract – is derived from a fusion of the embryological hind gut (endoderm) and the proctodeum (primitive skin – ectoderm – of the posterior perineum). Thus it is made up of both visceral and somatic structures and is also, because it is a junctional area, subject to developmental abnormalities.

Epithelial lining (Fig. 26.1)

Fusion between the hind gut and skin occurs at the transitional zone, which is proximal to a ring of the so-called mucosal anal valves. Distally there is the pecten where the canal is lined with stratified squamous epithelium and has the same sensitivity as that of the rest of the body. Hair-bearing skin follows.

Muscles (Fig. 26.2)

The internal sphincter is a condensation of the lower end of the circular smooth muscle of the rectum. The external sphincter is a complex plate of striated muscle which surrounds the anal canal and part of which is attached posteriorly to the coccyx. The function of both sphincters is related to defecation and continence. The longitudinal smooth muscle of the rectum continues into the anal canal, within the intersphincteric space, traverses the internal sphincter and is attached to the epithelium and skin. It probably functions as a suspensory ligament for the epithelium of the canal.

In addition to the sphincters just described, the puborectalis sling is a specialised part of the levator ani in the floor of the pelvis. Its fibres, which run from the back of the pubis to the last two segments of the coccyx, also encircle the junction between the rectum and anus. Their contraction draws the junction anteriorly to create a 90° angle between the anal canal and the rectum. The muscular contraction and angulation bring the anterior rectal wall into contact with the posterior proximal end of the anal canal so that a flap mechanism forms to counter a rise in intra-abdominal pressure, aiding the maintenance of continence. The arrangement is analogous to the ease with which flow from a garden hose is controlled by bending it to a right angle.

The intersphincteric space (outside the longitudinal muscle) represents a plane of fusion between the internal and external sphincters. It is an important surgical landmark, being utilised in a number of surgical procedures as well as being a pathway for the spread of perianal sepsis.

Nerve supply

Sensory

The sensation of rectal distension originates from sensory receptors within the muscles of the pelvic floor contiguous with and surrounding the rectum and is conveyed by the autonomic afferents (pelvic splanchnic nerves – S2 and S3). The central nervous system can, by mechanisms that are not fully understood, distinguish between the presence of solid, liquid and flatus in the lower rectum and proximal anal canal – a property of considerable social utility. The sensation of pain is conveyed via the parasympathetic and sympathetic nervous systems from the richly innervated anal papillae and surrounding tissues. The distal anal canal (because of its derivation from the proctoderm) is supplied by the pudendal nerve and shares the same sensory characteristics as normal skin.

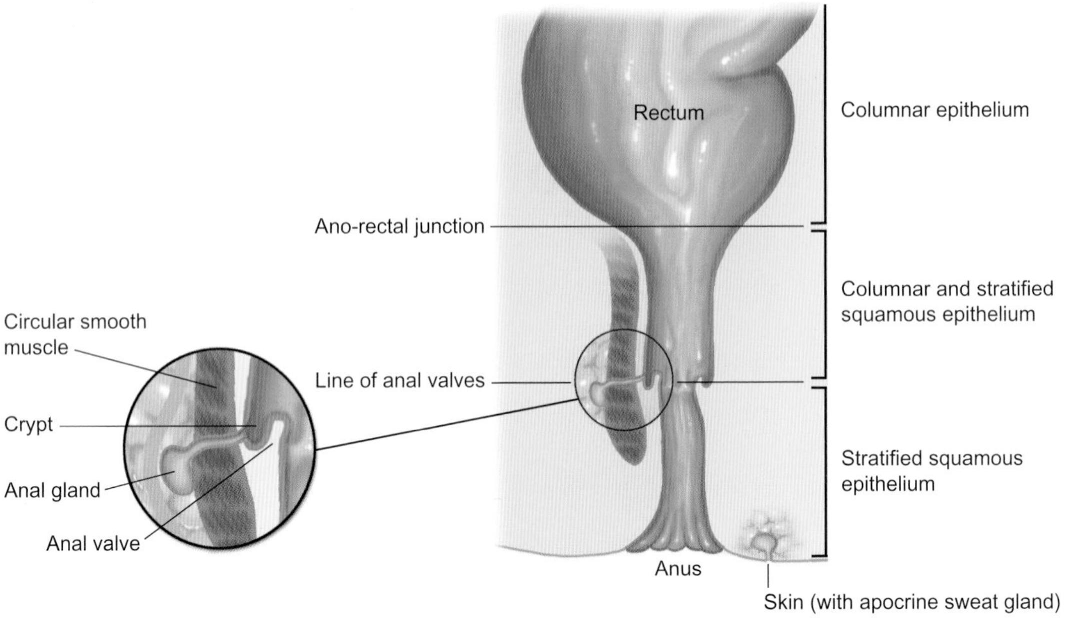

Fig. 26.1 The epithelium of the distal rectum and anal canal.

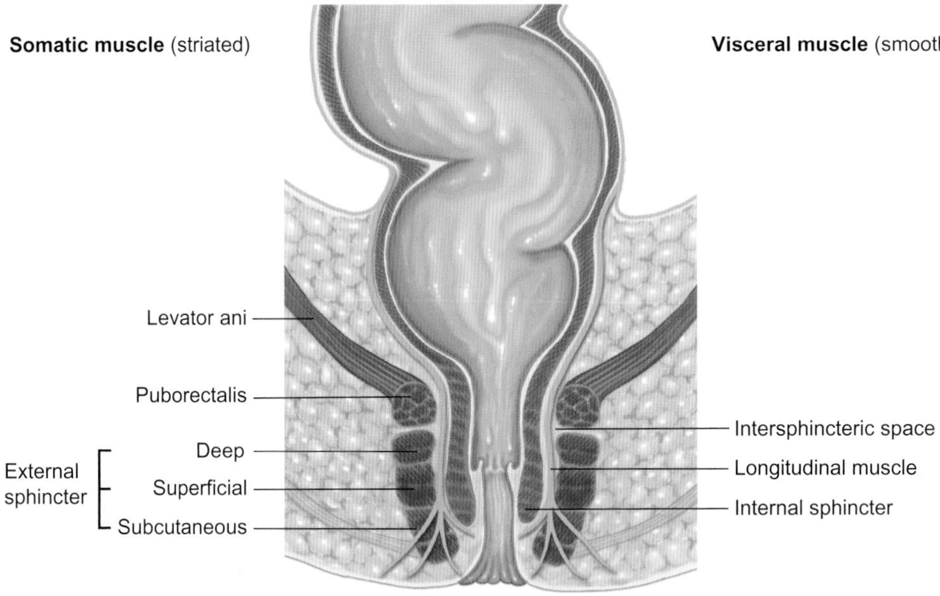

Fig. 26.2 The anal sphincters.

Motor

The levator ani muscles and the external sphincter are supplied by the pudendal nerve (S2 and S3) and the perineal branch of S4. The internal sphincter is innervated by both sympathetic and parasympathetic fibres, but it is the parasympathetic component which maintains constant contraction, so keeping the anal canal normally closed with positive intra-anal resting pressure. The external sphincter also contributes to this but can contract voluntarily to meet challenges initiated by contraction of the rectum (see 'Defecation' below).

Blood and lymphatic supply

Particular points to note are as follows:

- The anal canal is a watershed between the portal and systemic circulations, which is of special importance in relation to venous drainage.
- Venous plexuses lie in the subepithelial tissues both above and below the line of the anal valves.

In the left lateral, right posterior and right anterior positions, the venous plexuses, together with some arteriovenous anastomoses, are surrounded by smooth muscle, elastic and fibrous tissue to form three anal cushions. It is thought that their function is to complete the closure of the anal canal as sphincter tone brings them into contact with each other. An increase in the size of the cushions is the starting point of haemorrhoids.

Defecation

Defecation is the result of the interplay of many factors, not the least of which is activity within the colon and rectum.

Distension by flatus or faeces (which may be liquid or solid) causes a reflex small decrease in the contraction of the internal sphincter which allows a sample of rectal contents to enter the upper anal canal. Here they encounter sensory receptors at the dentate line which permit discrimination of their nature. At the same time muscular activity is also initiated in the rectum, and pressure within it rises. If it is socially convenient for defecation or the passage of flatus to take place, the internal sphincter and the puborectalis and external sphincter relax, the anorectal angle straightens and the bolus is passed. At the end of defecation there is increased electrical activity in the external sphincter and puborectalis, the anal canal closes and the anorectal angle is restored. By contrast, if the moment is not convenient, the external sphincter and puborectalis continue to contract, returning the bolus to the rectum. Problems with this orderly sequence (incontinence) are discussed below.

Symptoms of anal disorder

Bleeding

Loss of blood from an anal lesion occurs characteristically at the time of defecation. Traditionally, so-called 'outlet bleeding' is bright red in colour and appears separate from the stool. It is worth remembering, however, that the characteristics of the bleeding are notoriously inaccurate at predicting its cause, and proximal lesions may exist in the presence of anal pathology. Larger quantities of blood with or without the passage of a stool usually mean that the bleeding is higher in the gastrointestinal tract.

Pruritus

Itching can be either part of a generalised problem (jaundice or blood dyscrasia) or of local cause.

Pain

The embryological origin of the anal canal results in two types of pain. The mucosa of the proximal canal is insensitive to touch, gripping or cutting (hence it is possible to take a biopsy without anaesthetic). However, disorders deeper in the wall of the canal at this level may cause ill-localised pain felt in the perineum (see 'Anal sepsis'). The skin of the distal canal is sensitive, and problems at this level are associated with well-localised pain. Pain is often brought on by defecation.

Swelling or lump

The patient may complain of a swelling or lump at the anal verge. These may appear spontaneously or only on straining. Commonly, swellings are due to enlarged anal cushions (haemorrhoids), prolapsed rectal mucosa or skin tags, but care must be taken to exclude neoplasms or sexually transmitted infections such as anal warts.

Discharge

There are three types of discharge:

- faecal soiling – usually the result of either distortion of the anal anatomy, say by a tumour, or of incontinence
- mucoid – a change in the mucosa of the rectum and/or proximal anal canal which is commonly inflammatory but may imply a mucus-secreting tumour
- purulent – almost always associated with sepsis.

Alteration in bowel function

A change in consistency and frequency of the stool (e.g. loose or hard motions) is generally the manifestation of an intestinal disorder. Loss of differentiation (flatus, liquid or solid stool) and faecal incontinence may be a manifestation of intestinal disorder, but is more usually the result of injury to the sphincter complex.

Clinical examination

Anal conditions cannot be diagnosed without clinical examination, which is an essential feature in the assessment of any patient with symptoms provisionally attributed to the anal canal and its surroundings. In addition, the rectum must always be examined to make certain that the underlying cause is not more proximal. Patient consent should be obtained – verbal consent is sufficient – after the procedure has been explained. The presence of a chaperone should be offered to the patient, and is recommended for all intimate examinations. The patient's consent and presence of a chaperone should be recorded in the clinical records.

The position of the patient and adequate lighting are both important. In the UK, the left lateral position is found to be acceptable to most patients and is preferred. Should a vaginal examination be considered necessary, then the supine position is adopted.

Examination has three components – inspection, palpation and endoscopy – the last of which is by sigmoidoscopy and proctoscopy. None of these is omitted.

Inspection

After initial inspection of the skin of the anorectal verge, the buttocks are separated, which usually brings the lower part of the anal canal into view. The patient should be asked to strain to see if mucosa emerges, especially if there is a history of prolapse. It is not always possible for the patient to do this and prolapse may be more satisfactorily confirmed with the patient in the squatting position. Some measure of the external sphincter's ability to contract can be obtained by eliciting the 'anal reflex' – touching the perianal skin with an orange stick or a pin which is followed by reflex contraction of the external sphincter. The response of the voluntary muscles to a request for contraction can also be assessed.

Palpation

The index finger is covered with a suitably soft thin rubber glove which is lubricated. First, the perianal skin is palpated to feel for induration, which is an important sign of sepsis or malignancy. The finger is then passed into the anal canal superiorly and anteriorly to avoid the common sites of a painful lesion. Each quadrant is palpated to assess swelling or induration and also to get a feel for resting tone and voluntary contraction of the muscles. Finally the finger is inserted – preferably by extending the terminal digit of the examining finger – into the lower rectum. Here the contents (if any), the rectal wall and structures outside the rectum, such as those in the postrectal space, the prostate or, as far as they can be felt through the pouch of Douglas, the uterus and ovaries are all evaluated.

Endoscopic examination

There are two procedures for this: proctoscopy and sigmoidoscopy.

Proctoscopy

The proctoscope is short – less than the index of most examiners – and therefore is only of value for examination of the anal canal. It is of no use to exclude rectal disease. However, it is relatively easy to do and can give some information about anorectal conditions such as haemorrhoids.

Sigmoidoscopy

Sigmoidoscopy is done with either a rigid or a flexible instrument. The latter is able to traverse the rectosigmoid angle more effectively but requires more skill to use. The rigid sigmoidoscope is still used for initial examination in some units, although inspection is often limited to the rectum. Biopsies of the mucosa may be taken and should be correctly oriented on filter paper, before fixation in formalin to allow the best possible preparations for the histopathologist to examine (Fig. 26.3).

Investigation

Examination under anaesthesia (EUA)

Pain, discomfort and social resistance to being examined may mean that assessment of the lower bowel and anal canal can only be satisfactorily undertaken with the patient anaesthetised. Recourse to EUA should never be regarded as a sign of defeat and can often lead to a much more accurate assessment than in those who are able to tolerate a rectal examination without anaesthesia. The procedure is the same as that outlined above.

Imaging

In the knowledge that proximal pathology may coexist, flexible sigmoidoscopy or colonoscopy may be required in patients with anal disorders, simply to establish normality in the colon and rectum.

Ultrasound

Intraluminal ultrasound provides very accurate information about the structure of the anal canal. Damage to the internal and/or external sphincters can be clearly identified by ultrasound, and it can assist in localising perianal sepsis and fistulae. In addition, transrectal ultrasound can provide staging information on rectal neoplasms.

Magnetic resonance imaging

MRI is currently the most accurate way of delineating perianal sepsis. It can very accurately identify primary and secondary fistula tracts as well as localised abscess. In addition, it can provide accurate data on extraluminal spread of rectal neoplasms.

Fistulography

Rarely used, this may assist the delineation of a fistula but is of little value in management. It is, however, useful to find the origin of discharge in the perineum when the primary disease is within the pelvis (e.g. diverticular disease). Fistulography has now been superseded by MRI.

Evacuation proctography

Cinephotography of the expulsion of contrast medium from the rectum during actual or attempted defecation is used to assist in the diagnosis of obstructed defecation. Some centres are now performing dynamic MRI evacuation proctography with good results.

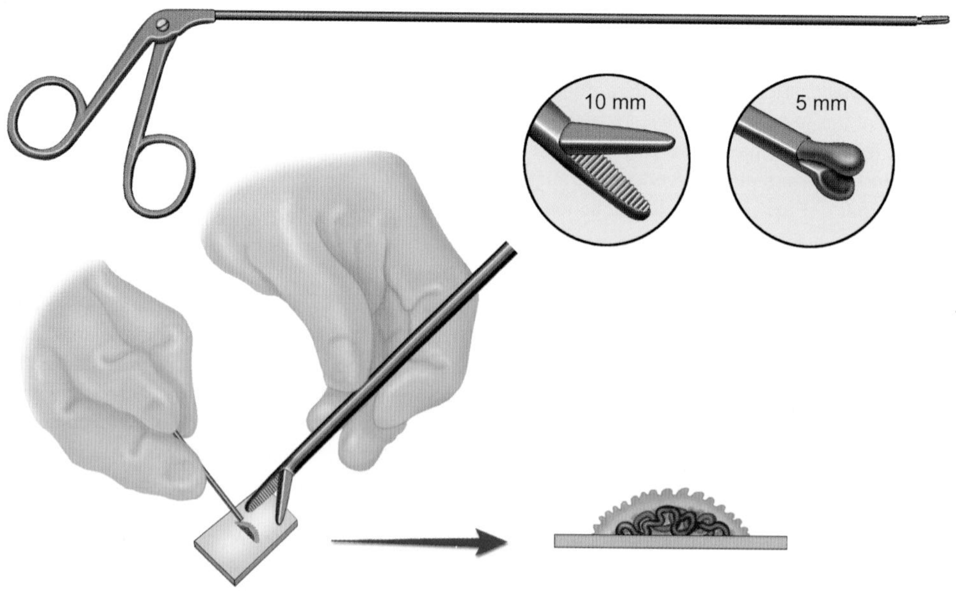

Fig. 26.3 Rectal biopsy.

Table 26.1 Bacteriological examination of anorectal material

Condition	Examination	Finding
Acute abscess	Standard cultures	Intestinal organisms – ?fistula
Gonorrhoea	Fresh swab and culture	*Neisseria gonorrhoeae*
Syphilis	Dark ground examination	Spirochaetes
Fungal infection	Direct microscopy of scrapings of perianal skin culture	Pathogenic organism
Tuberculosis	Histopathological examination	Caseating granulomas
		Organisms on Ziehl–Neelsen stain
	Culture for *Mycobacterium tuberculosis*	Organism and sensitivity

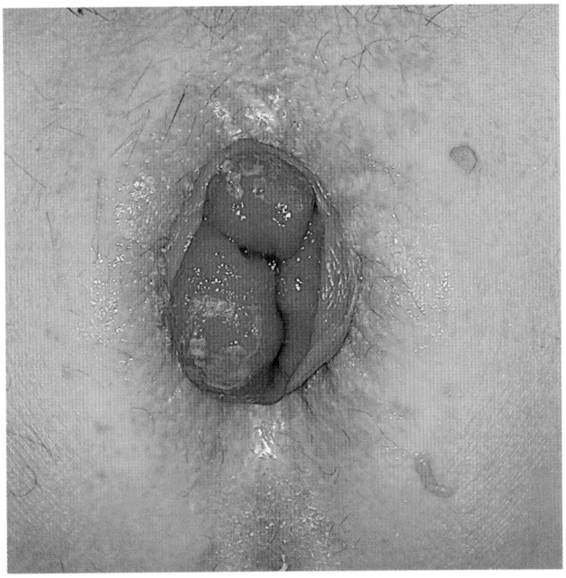

Fig. 26.4 Third-degree prolapsed haemorrhoids requiring manual reduction.

Microbiological studies (Table 26.1)

Culture of pus in patients with acute abscesses may be helpful in determining whether or not a fistula is present – the presence of gut organisms usually means this is so – but is not usually crucial to management. By contrast, the diagnosis of most sexually transmitted diseases and the uncommon fungal infections of the perianal skin are usually confirmed by nucleic acid amplification tests (NAATs).

Physiological studies

The following are widely used to evaluate patients with faecal incontinence:

- anal canal pressure – at rest, during voluntary contractions and in response to rectal distension
- electromyography of the external sphincter and its response to pudendal nerve stimulation.

HAEMORRHOIDS

Definition and classification

Most patients refer to any abnormality in the anorectal area as 'piles'. The word is, indeed, an alternative name for haemorrhoids, but to minimise confusion it is one best avoided in the description of clinical conditions.

Haemorrhoids are engorgement of the haemorrhoidal venous plexuses with redundancy of their coverings. The cushions may:

- remain in their usual position in the anal canal (internal)
- descend to involve the skin of the distal anal canal so that they prolapse on defecation (intero-external), but reduce spontaneously
- become of such a size that they are always partly outside the canal (external; Fig. 26.4).

The alternative terms used are first-, second- and third-degree haemorrhoids.

Although they develop from the three cushions, and therefore have the positions of left lateral, right posterior and right anterior (the primary haemorrhoids), secondary haemorrhoids do occur in between these, and in consequence the abnormality may become circumferential.

Aetiology

Most patients with haemorrhoids do not have an obvious predisposing cause, although there may be a family history. In women, pregnancy may lead on to haemorrhoids as may pelvic tumours (ovarian and uterine). Constipation and straining at the time of defecation may also be a factor. It has been suggested that patients with haemorrhoids have an increased resting anal canal pressure and the effort required to overcome this may be the underlying reason for straining at defecation. The evidence to support this view is conflicting but it has provided the basis for one form of treatment.

It is sometimes suggested that carcinoma of the rectum may be an antecedent. This presumed relationship is probably coincidental because both conditions are relatively common and therefore may be present together.

Clinical features

Symptoms are:

- *bleeding* – usually at defecation but, intermittent, bright red into the pan and/or on the toilet paper; spurting and dripping of blood may occur after defecation and at other times of exertion
- *discharge* – faecal soiling or a mucus leak because the haemorrhoids prevent complete anal closure
- *pruritus* – if cleaning of the perianal skin becomes difficult or there is discharge
- *discomfort* – when there is stretching of the sensitive external component
- *swelling* – in intero-external or external haemorrhoids only
- *prolapsed* – often either not reported by the patient or called a swelling

Table 26.2 Symptomatic classification of haemorrhoids

Stage	Symptoms
Internal (first degree)	Bleeding
Intero-external (second degree)	Prolapse with spontaneous reduction; bleeding present or absent
External (third degree)	Prolapse which requires replacement; bleeding present or absent

- *pain* – only when there are complications (see 'thrombosis')
- *bowel function* – many patients have a sluggish bowel function which leads to straining.

A traditional symptomatic classification of haemorrhoids based on only two of the above symptoms may give some guidance for management (Table 26.2).

Signs

The appearance of haemorrhoids varies, from a slight increase in the size of the normal anal cushions, visible only at proctoscopy, to large intero-external haemorrhoids apparent on inspection of the anal verge. It is important to identify accurately what is seen. The external component of second- and third-degree haemorrhoids comprises the perianal skin and hair and, depending on the extent of prolapse, the pecten at the junction of the skin and mucosa. There is always a groove between the external and internal components which corresponds to the line of the anal valves. In patients with a prolonged history of prolapse, the normal intermingling of columnar and squamous epithelium at the transitional zone becomes all squamous and therefore opaque.

It may not always be possible to confirm the presence of prolapse at examination in the left lateral position. Straining assists the diagnosis, especially after the passage of a proctoscope.

Conditions that are related to haemorrhoids and which may cause diagnostic confusion are summarised in Table 26.3.

Table 26.3 Conditions related to (and which may be confused with) haemorrhoids

Condition	Position
Anal skin tags	Anal margin
Fibrous anal polyps	Line of the anal valves
Prolapse of rectum	Similar to haemorrhoids but circumferential
Thrombosis in perianal skin (perianal haematoma)	Distal to mucocutaneous junction
Fissure	Primarily at the mucocutaneous junction but may have a distal skin tag
Benign tumours of the rectum	Within the rectum at sigmoidoscopy
Varices	Rare but almost impossible to distinguish
Haemangioma	Rare congenital abnormality

Management

Reassurance

Often all that is required is explanation of the symptoms to alleviate the fear of a more sinister diagnosis. It is also worth remembering that the natural history of haemorrhoidal bleeding is cyclical, and that the success of many therapeutic procedures may simply reflect the natural cycle of the disease. While sometimes alarming, rarely does the blood loss lead to significant anaemia. The patient should be informed that if their pattern of bleeding changes, further medical assessment should be sought to rule out sinister pathology.

Bowel regulation

Because of the tendency to constipation, advice about ensuring a more regular bowel habit (increased intake of fluids, fruit and vegetables and the addition of bulk by the use of fibre) and the avoidance of prolonged straining is useful.

Proprietary suppositories

Most of these contain a variety of ingredients which include topical corticosteroids, local anaesthetics and antibiotics. There is no reason why such a cocktail should influence the symptoms of uncomplicated haemorrhoids, and there is no objective evidence that they do. Their prescription is probably the outcome of ignorance about the cause of symptoms, an imprecise diagnosis and a poorly thought-out plan of management.

Treatments directed at the haemorrhoids

The various surgical treatments are considered in Table 26.4 in order of increasing severity and intervention from the patient's point of view. The various mechanisms of action are:

- submucosal vascular occlusion – produced in the main vessels to reduce bulk and fix redundant mucosa by fibrosis
- excision of redundant tissue – this is necessary for prolapse; lesser treatments may succeed unless there is symptomatic engorgement of the external venous plexus
- reduction in anal canal pressure.

Table 26.4 indicates that a given therapy may have more than one mode of action.

Injection sclerotherapy

This is usually the first treatment for those with bleeding or early prolapse. Phenol 5% in almond oil is injected into the submucosa at the anorectal junction in amounts up to 5 mL at the three primary sites. The injection must be submucosal, which can be observed by seeing the mucosa lifted from the muscle and assuming a pearly appearance (Fig. 26.5). A superficial intramucosal injection causes ulceration, and one that is too deep may result in an oleogranuloma

Table 26.4 Treatment of haemorrhoids

Method	Appropriate for	Occludes blood supply at anorectal junction	Fixes mucosa	Excises redundant tissue	Reduces anal canal pressure
Injection sclerotherapy*	First degree	•	•		
Infrared coagulation	First degree	•	•		
Band ligation*	Second degree	•	•	•	
Lateral sphincterotomy	Second degree				•
Haemorrhoidal artery ligation	Second degree	•	•		
Haemorrhoidectomy*	Second and third degree		•		

*Preferred methods.

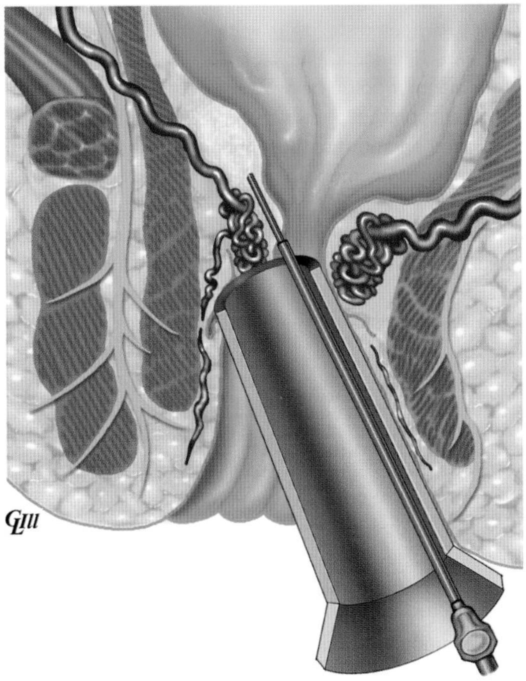

Fig. 26.5 Injection sclerotherapy.

– accumulation of the oil in the extrarectal tissues with low-grade inflammatory reaction. Too deep an anterior injection may also lead to prostatitis. Should the injection be intravascular – avoided if the needle is kept on the move – severe pain may be felt in the right hypochondrium and injection must stop immediately.

The initial results are satisfactory for the control of bleeding – although it should be remembered that symptoms may be intermittent – but injection sclerotherapy may need to be repeated. Meta-analysis suggests equivalent results are achieved by a high-fibre diet.

Infrared coagulation

A small burn is made in the mucosa and submucosa to a predetermined depth. This method, which is similar to injection sclerotherapy, is not widely practised and has secondary haemorrhage as a significant complication.

Band ligation

This technique combines excision of redundant mucosal tissue with fixation of the mucosa to the underlying muscle (Fig. 26.6). There are three major problems: pain and haemorrhage after application of the bands and urinary retention, usually secondary to pain. Care must be taken to place the bands above the dentate line to avoid incorporating the sensitive epithelium from low in the anal canal, causing severe immediate pain. Pain may occur subsequently because of necrosis of the anal epithelium distal to the point of application. Bleeding may take place at any time up to 20 days after application and may be severe. However, band ligation is effective treatment for intero-external haemorrhoids.

Haemorrhoidal artery ligation

This is a relatively recent development and is performed by ligating the distal submucosal branches of the superior rectal arteries. The placement of each ligature may be guided by a specially designed Doppler probe. It is painless and effective, but not in prolapsed haemorrhoids.

Haemorrhoidectomy

This remains the most effective therapy for large prolapsing haemorrhoids. There are various techniques:

- *ligature* – of the base of the haemorrhoid and excision of redundant tissue; the wounds heal by granulation and re-epithelialisation
- *closed* – after ligation-excision, the mucocutaneous defect is closed by suture with the objective of primary union
- *submucosal* – the enlarged cushions are dissected beneath their coverings and, as with the closed procedure, the defect is closed.

All these procedures aim to excise as much redundant epithelium and vasculature as possible. The differences lie in how this is achieved and the manner in which the wounds are left at the end of the operation. In the UK, the technique of simple ligature and excision has always enjoyed much success and has been the routine. However, the other techniques are gaining in popularity because of reputed advantages in reduction of pain and speed of healing.

Haemorrhoidectomy has an unjustified reputation for severe postoperative pain, and patients are often warned off

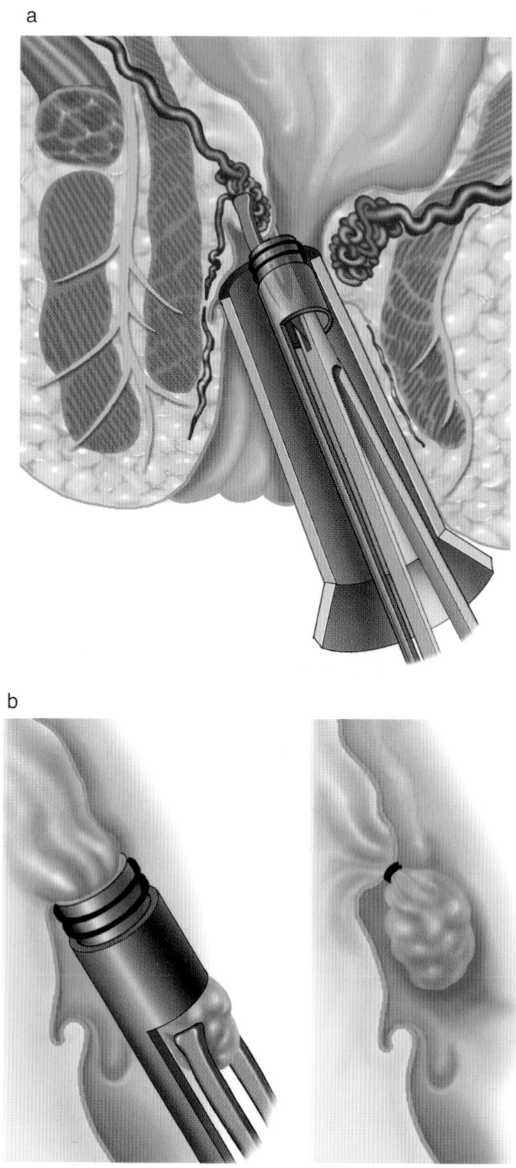

Fig. 26.6 Band ligation for haemorrhoids.

the operation by the experience of others who have undergone it. With a better understanding of postoperative pain relief (Ch. 6), use of non-adherent or non-use of dressings and the appropriate use of lubricant laxatives, the course after operation, although not without some discomfort, is coped with well by nearly all patients and is now often performed as a day-case procedure.

Stapled haemorrhoidectomy or haemorrhoidopexy. A modified circular stapling gun can be used to excise a circumferential strip of lower rectal mucosa pulling the redundant haemorrhoidal tissue back into its correct anatomical position. The remaining haemorrhoidal tissue, with its blood supply interrupted, is thus still of use for the maintenance of faecal continence. This procedure, known as the procedure for prolapsed haemorrhoids, has gained much popularity throughout mainland Europe, but has met with some controversy in the UK. Increasingly practised worldwide, it seems that it does have a place in selected patients. Care must be taken in females to avoid the uncommon but serious complication of a rectovaginal fistula. Care must also be taken in patient selection to avoid performing the proceedure on those who practice ano-receptive intercourse, as the staple line is palpable and may cause injury. Studies have suggested that postoperative pain is significantly reduced, but at the cost of a higher recurrence rate.

Complications

Skin tags and anal polyps

These often coexist with haemorrhoids and require limited excision. Anal polyps should be transfixed before removal to avoid postoperative bleeding.

Thrombosis

Established haemorrhoids may develop thrombosis within their veins. A precipitating factor is the descent of intero-external haemorrhoids below the external sphincter, and its subsequent contraction, which cuts off venous drainage. The thrombosed haemorrhoid (or more usually haemorrhoids) is covered with both mucosa and squamous epithelium. The chief complaint is of pain and circumanal discomfort.

On examination there are obvious intero-external haemorrhoids with bluish discoloration, oedema and an ooze of blood.

The episode is best managed conservatively with local application of ice, the administration of non-constipating analgesics and lubricant laxatives and, if there are significant constitutional features, bed rest. Resolution always takes place, and definitive treatment can be planned later. Occasionally the quickest relief of pain is by manual reduction of the thrombosed mass under general anaesthesia, but further prolapse may occur. Urgent haemorrhoidectomy, if carried out carefully and by an experienced operator, may well be advantageous particularly if there is concern over necrosis and sepsis in the thrombosed tissue. A very rare complication of thrombosis is infection and portal pyaemia.

PERIANAL HAEMATOMA

This condition is sometimes known as a 'thrombosed external pile' but it has nothing to do with haemorrhoids. The cause is obscure, but what happens is thrombosis in a subcutaneous vein below the transitional zone, and the precise term is a clotted venous saccule. The result is a discrete painful swelling said to look like a small blackcurrant. On examination there is a tender lump external to the anal canal which is blue or black depending on the duration of the episode.

Perianal haematomas may resolve with symptomatic management, although during this they may rupture and ulcerate (see below). If pain is severe, the haematoma is deroofed by a cruciate incision under local lidocaine anaesthesia, with immediate relief, although it must be remembered that a vein has been opened and steps should be taken to ensure that bleeding does not occur.

FISSURE IN ANO

Fissures are ulcers consequent upon tears of the mucosa at the anal margin, which extend into the pecten.

Aetiology

The cause is not always obvious, although constipation may initiate the problem both in children and in adults; however, constipation as a cause should not be confused with constipation as a result of the fear of painful defecation. Trauma at childbirth and anal intercourse or other sexual manipulations may also be responsible in some instances. There seems little doubt that most patients have sustained hypertonicity of the internal anal sphincter – sphincter spasm. Whatever the precipitating event, a vicious cycle is set up of pain → sphincter spasm → constipation → greater difficulty on defecation, which makes the local condition worse. Poor blood supply in the posterior midline may help to perpetuate a fissure which some consider to be an unhealed ulcer.

Anatomy and pathological features

The common site is posteriorly in the midline but it may be anterior or lateral. Depth may range from a simple superficial break in the epithelium to a chronic lesion with exposure of the fibres of the internal sphincter. Chronic lesions may have an associated skin tag (so-called 'sentinel pile'), an anal polyp of varying size and undermining of the edges. Sometimes sepsis may complicate a fissure with a resultant superficial fistula.

Clinical features

Symptoms

- Pain usually occurs during defecation and may be severe. It may continue for some time after defecation but has usually eased before the passage of the next stool, when the cycle is repeated. Pain is more common with an acute fissure, and some chronic, indolent lesions may be relatively pain-free.
- Constipation may be the consequence of the patient's unwillingness to defecate because of pain.
- Bleeding is not usually severe and may occur only on the toilet paper after defecation.
- Discharge of small quantities of pus is uncommon but does occur.

Signs

In a patient with a painful acute lesion, separating the buttocks and gentle palpation of the anal verge reveal tenderness at the site of the fissure, which is usually posteriorly in the midline. If a stable and satisfactory doctor–patient relationship is to be maintained, a digital examination should be avoided, but it is often possible to see the lower end of the fissure by asking the patient to strain.

In more chronic lesions, a sentinel tag occasionally draws attention to the condition, as may discharge from a superficial fistula. A digital examination can usually be done and reveals thickening at the anorectal ring and a varying amount of tenderness, although this is not usually severe. Proctoscopy shows a lesion of varying depth in which the fibres of the external sphincter may be visible; there is granulation tissue and perhaps a small amount of bleeding.

Other causes of an ulcer at the anorectal verge include:

- Crohn's disease – perianal and intra-anal which can be extensive and associated with oedematous skin tags, sepsis and a bluish discoloration of the skin
- primary syphilitic chancre – more likely in homosexual patients
- herpes simplex – more likely in those who are HIV-positive
- lymphoma and leukaemia
- neoplasms – basal and squamous cell carcinoma
- excoriation (microulceration) associated with perianal skin disorders
- ruptured perianal haematoma
- nicorandil therapy for angina.

Management

Acute fissure

This condition responds well to the application of a local anaesthetic gel (1% lidocaine) just before defecation and the use of bulk laxatives. In those with sphincter spasm, 2% diltiazem ointment applied regularly to the external anal skin relieves the spasm, allowing blood supply to the unhealed ulcer or fissure. Headache resulting from cranial venous dilatation is less common than with 0.2% GTN ointment, but may prevent the patient from completing the usual 4-week course, and some clinicians will opt for botulinum toxin. All these treatments elicit a temporary chemical sphincterotomy and will fail in approximately 30% of cases. Recurrence usually requires surgical division of the lower fibres of the internal sphincter or sphincterotomy as a more permanent solution.

Chronic fissure

Chronic fissure associated with a skin tag, anal polyp, undermining of the edges of the fissure and exposure of the fibres of the internal sphincter usually requires operative treatment. Low-pressure chronic fissures are more common in women. There maybe occult sphincter damage from childbirth and in these patients a sphincterotomy should not be performed. Anorectal physiology and endoanal ultrasound are used in the preoperative assessment and a V–Y advancement, house or rotational flap may be used to heal the fissure.

Operation

The division of the fibres of the internal sphincter distal to the line of the anal valves (partial internal sphincterotomy) is most effective and is usually done laterally within the wall of the anal canal (Fig. 26.7). It is an extremely effective procedure and relieves pain almost immediately. It does however carry a small but finite risk of passive incontinence, usually to flatus. Patients should be warned of this risk and care taken not to perform too extensive a sphincter division.

ANAL SEPSIS

A variety of problems may present with suppuration – either an acute abscess or chronic purulent discharge (Table 26.5).

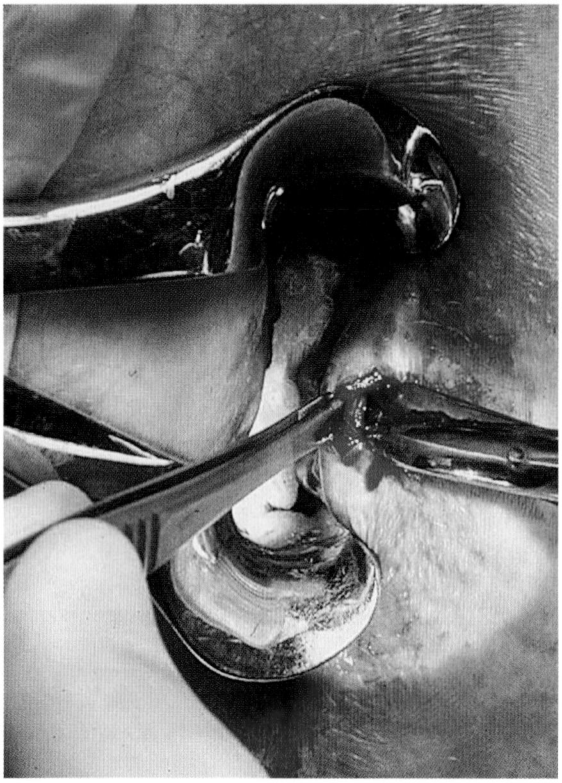

Fig. 26.7 Open lateral sphincterotomy for anal fissure. Note the fibres of internal sphincter in the base of the wound, which require division.

Table 26.5 Conditions that are associated with perianal sepsis

Condition	Usual finding
Non-specific infection	Acute abscess Fistula in ano
Tuberculosis	Chronic infection Occasionally fistula
Crohn's disease	Chronic intractable infection Complex fistula
Hydradenitis suppurativa	Skin abscesses Anal canal rarely if ever involved
Skin sepsis	Usually *Staphylococcus aureus* Abscesses are often multiple
Trauma	External: sexual intercourse; accidental injury Internal: foreign body (ingested bone)
Intrapelvic sepsis	Diverticular disease Crohn's disease
Sepsis in developmental cysts	Usually dermoid cysts
Malignant disease	Sepsis is an uncommon complication

Non-specific abscess and fistula

Infection of the anal intersphincteric glands with organisms found in the gastrointestinal tract – both aerobic (e.g. *E. coli*) and anaerobic (e.g. *Bacteroides* spp.) – is the cause of this common disorder. A variety of different anatomical abscesses and fistulae may present, an understanding of which is greatly simplified by knowledge of the routes taken by the spread of infection.

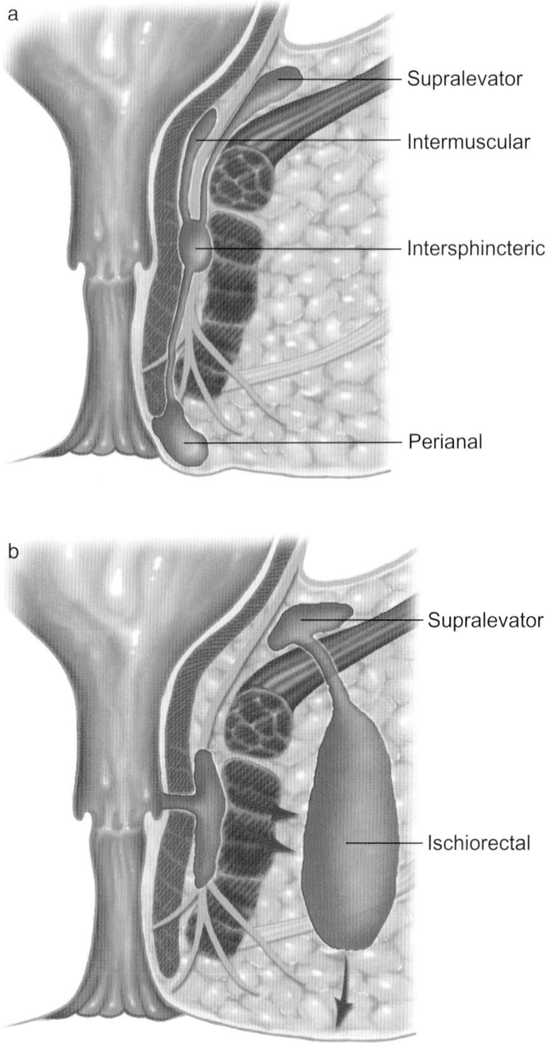

Fig. 26.8 Spread of infection: (a) vertical spread; (b) horizontal spread.

Spread of infection

Sepsis begins in the intersphincteric space and may spread in three ways:

- vertically (Fig. 26.8a)
- horizontally (Fig. 26.8b)
- circumferentially.

Anatomical sites of abscess

Typically, three named abscesses are the consequence of spread in the above directions:

- perianal – the sepsis spreading vertically downwards in the intersphincteric space presents close to the anal canal as a perianal abscess
- ischiorectal – the sepsis crosses the external sphincter and presents away from the anal canal as an ischiorectal abscess

- supralevator – the sepsis spreading vertically upwards may lead to a supralevator collection.

For any of these three routes the sepsis may also spread in a circumferential plane, leading to a horseshoe collection.

Formation of a fistula

When a fistula develops following acute non-specific inflammation, it is because pus from an abscess burrows in two directions: into and through the wall of the anorectal canal, perhaps along the anal crypt and duct from where it originated; and superficially to emerge distal to the mucocutaneous junction. Two openings are formed – internal and external – and the track that now connects them is lined with granulation tissue. One or other opening may be, at any one time, closed, and if both seal, a further abscess develops. Repeated episodes of this kind may cause further and ever more complex tracks to form.

Classification of fistula

Classification is in relation to the anal musculature (Fig. 26.9). There are two main types:

- *intersphincteric* – all the inflammatory tracks remain medial to the striated muscle or external sphincter
- *transsphincteric* – there is a primary track across the external sphincter which may be at any level from just below the puborectalis to the lowest fibres of the external sphincter. The external opening in a transsphincteric fistula is situated lateral to the pigmented perianal skin, the surface marking of the extent of the external anal sphincter.

Other types of fistula include:

- *superficial (cutaneous)* – confined to the superficial tissues with a bridge or bridges of skin between two or more openings; in effect this is a 'bridged fissure'
- *suprasphincteric* – this is very rare, and the primary track passes across the levator ani
- *extrasphincteric* – this is usually the result of intrapelvic sepsis or inappropriate surgical treatment of another type of fistula, and the track lies outside the whole sphincter complex.

a b c

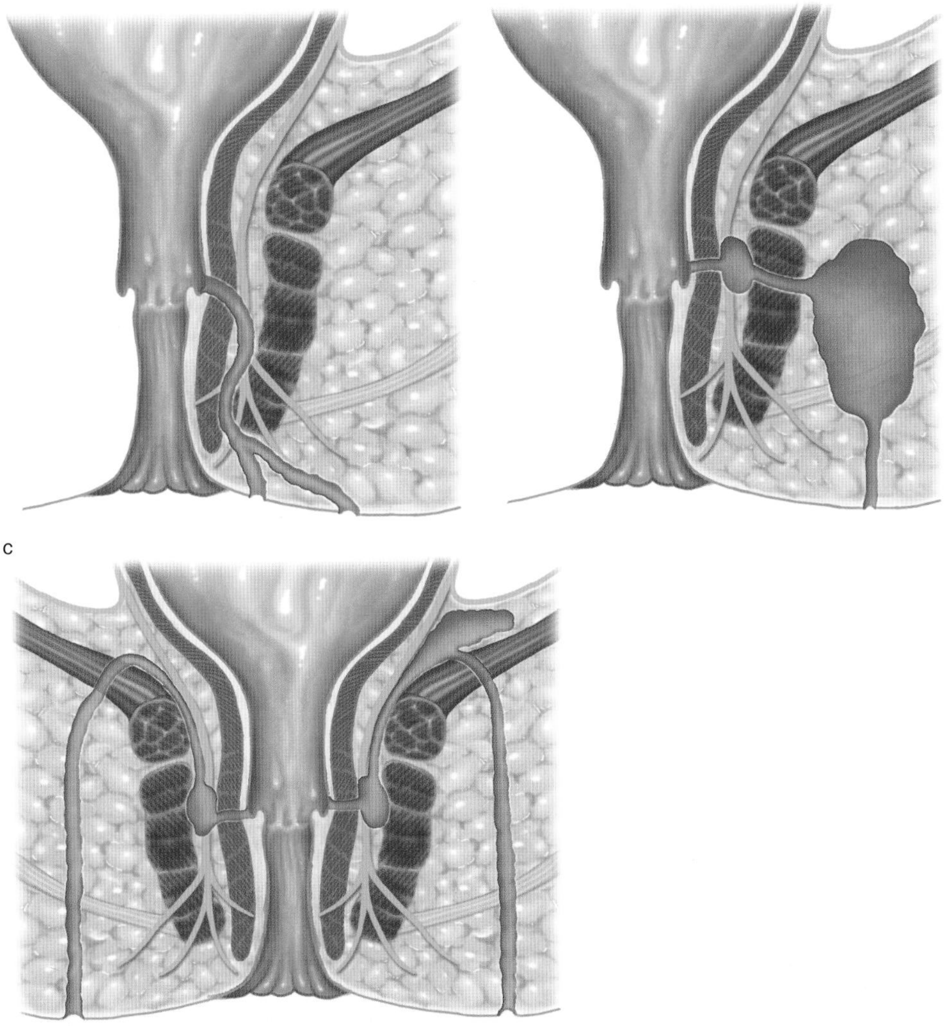

Fig. 26.9 Types of fistulae: (a) inter-sphincteric; (b) trans-sphincteric; (c) supra-sphincteric/extra-sphincteric.

Clinical features of abscess and fistula

Symptoms

There may be a past history of similar episodes or one of intermittent or continuing discharge. The chief complaint in an abscess is of pain over a period of 3–4 days accompanied by swelling and difficulty on defecation. In a fistula, discharge with or without occasional pain is usually less severe than that of an abscess.

Signs

In an abscess, signs are those of the typical features of acute inflammation, but it is unusual to find fluctuation even when the condition is of sufficient duration for pus to have formed, as there is usually marked local induration and the pus is under tension. In a fistula there may be varying degrees of inflammation around the external opening. Careful digital examination with a well-lubricated finger shows induration and is invaluable in helping to determine the course of the tract. It may be possible to express pus from either opening.

Management

Abscess

Antibiotics have little part to play – they cannot penetrate into the pus, and there is often some necrosis of surrounding adipose tissue. An acute abscess requires surgical drainage. It is unwise to do anything more even though a fistula is suspected – swelling and hyperaemia mask the precise location of the sphincters. The pus should always be sent for microbiological examination because the presence of gut organisms indicates that a fistula is likely.

Fistula

A fistula is suspected if:

- discharge persists at the site of drainage of an abscess
- gut organisms are cultured
- abscess recurs
- induration is detected either clinically or under anaesthesia.

Treatment is based on eradication of the sepsis with the preservation of maximum anal function. A fistulous track is usually laid open and allowed to heal from its base. Alternative procedures include the use of core fistulectomy, injection of fibrin glue and insertion of a collagen plug with variable results. The majority of superficial and intersphincteric fistulae (85%) are straightforward to deal with. The remainder (transsphincteric and suprasphincteric) are much more difficult and demand specialist care. Treatment is often prolonged, and laying open can be extensive; it is carried out in stages so as to minimise damage to the sphincters. A fine thread of monofilament or braided material (a seton) is often placed through the primary track around the external sphincter to act as a drain while the large wound exterior to the striated muscle of the external sphincter is allowed to heal. In the more complex fistulae in which laying open would result in an unacceptable risk of incontinence, fistula plugs can be used. These are fine cone-shaped plugs made from porcine collagen. In these complex fistulae there is a healing rate of, at best, 50%.

Failure to heal satisfactorily may be the result of:

- inadequate initial treatment
- specific (but undiagnosed) cause, e.g. Crohn's disease
- poor nutritional state
- poor wound care, e.g. epithelial bridging
- proliferation of granulation tissue which prevents epithelialisation
- ingrowth of hair.

Given the first three causes are eliminated, the success of fistula surgery depends on good postoperative care of the wound. Dressings must be applied so as to ensure that wounds heal from their depths to the surface. Cleanliness is ensured by regular bathing, especially after defecation, and by lavage with normal saline. Care is taken to ensure that bridging does not occur from the overgrowth of skin, because this causes residual pockets of sepsis. Overgrowth of granulation tissue can usually be simply managed by cauterisation with silver nitrate but may require curettage. The wound edges are shaved to prevent ingrowth of hair.

Crohn's disease (see also Ch. 25)

The anal manifestations of Crohn's disease include:

- oedematous skin tags
- bluish hue
- ulceration
- sepsis.

The last of these is managed on similar lines to that of non-specific origin, with great care not to divide muscle – any reduction in faecal control is a potential problem for patients with a major tendency to diarrhoea. However, this will only be a small, although important, part of overall management.

Tuberculosis

The possibility of tuberculous anal infection must always be remembered, and chronic granulation tissue should be examined microscopically for caseating granulomas and cultured for *Mycobacterium tuberculosis*. The appropriate antimicrobial agent is required, followed by limited surgery.

Pilonidal disease

Aetiology

The commonest site for pilonidal disease is the natal cleft. Other rarer sites include the umbilicus and the webs of the fingers in hairdressers. Hairs are found under the surface of the skin and may cause sepsis. In most instances, there is no clear explanation why this has happened, but one hypothesis is that shed hairs enter pits or crevices in the skin surface and then drill into the subcutaneous tissues. A contributory factor is puberty, with the changes in the skin that occur at this time.

Clinical features

Clinical presentation is because of sepsis, sometimes precipitated by minor repeated trauma.

Symptoms

Pain, tenderness and discharge are the cause of the patient seeking attention. Recurrent episodes may have taken place over months or years.

Signs

There are one or more openings in the midline or to either side of it, perhaps with protruding tufts of hair (all the same length). The surrounding skin shows varying degrees of inflammation, and pus is either seen escaping or can be expressed from an opening. There may be confusion with anal fistula because of an opening some distance from the natal cleft, close to or even anterior to the anus.

Management

Management options are as follows:

- No specific treatment in those who are asymptomatic.
- Laying open of the septic area with curettage of the granulation tissue – it is necessary to make certain all side tracks are fully exposed. This does, however, give rise to a wound which may take from weeks to months to heal, and is consequently falling from favour.
- Excision and primary closure. Several operations have been designed to excise the sinus and close the wound, thereby avoiding the need for prolonged postoperative nursing care, i.e. Bascom's cleft closure and the Karydakis procedure. All these aim to close the wound off the midline and minimise the risk of recurrence. Some series suggest that primary healing can be achieved in 90–94% of cases, including those for recurrent disease.

More complicated methods of surgical management involving skin flaps have been practised but, except in difficult recurrences, are no more successful than the above carefully undertaken.

Hydradenitis suppurativa

The apocrine sweat glands, which occur in the skin of the perineum, inguinal regions and the axilla, become the site of a mixed bacterial infection. Obesity, hormonal imbalance and poor hygiene are contributory factors. Varying degrees of sepsis occur, with pockets and tracks running widely in the subcutaneous tissue. The condition may be confused with anal fistula, but the anal canal proximal to the skin is not involved. The treatment is to control the contributory factors and to lay open the septic areas. Healing is slow, and plastic surgical procedures are sometimes necessary.

PRURITUS ANI

Aetiology

Pruritus ani is a symptom not a diagnosis. The key to successful management is identification of the cause, and possible causes include:

- *Post-defecatory soiling* – soft sticky stools which cannot be cleaned away from the anal verge (soiling of the underwear is often associated); a funnel-shaped anus which is difficult to clean (10% after lateral sphincterotomy – see above); or lack of good hygienic practices. It is thought that metabolites (e.g. endopeptidases) from faecal bacteria produce the itching.
- *Anal disorders* – skin tags, haemorrhoids and fissures may make cleansing difficult and so contribute to poor perianal hygiene; purulent discharge also contaminates the skin with faecal organisms.
- *Skin disorders* – dermatological diseases affecting the perianal skin include eczema, psoriasis, neurodermatitis, intertrigo, squamous cell carcinoma-in-situ (Bowen's disease) and extramammary Paget's disease (Ch. 28).
- *Infection* (rare) – bacterial (erythrasma) – infection with a *Corynebacterium* – and syphilis); viral (condylomata acuminata and molluscum contagiosum); fungal (diabetes and fungal vaginitis).
- *Infestation by parasites* (common) – lice (pediculosis) or threadworms (oxyuriasis).
- *Reactions to pharmaceuticals* – many proprietary preparations, which contain a cocktail of ingredients (local anaesthetics and steroids), are used indiscriminately and can cause contact dermatitis: prolonged application of local anaesthetics may lead to hypersensitivity reactions and steroids to skin atrophy.
- *Systemic disorders* – generalised pruritus (obstructive jaundice, reticuloses) may also affect the perineal area.
- *Sphincter dysfunction* – if a cause cannot be found, physiological assessment may reveal a sphincter defect which permits faecal leakage.
- *Psychosocial problems* – these should always be borne in mind but only sought when all other possibilities have been excluded.

Clinical features

Symptoms

Itching in the perianal skin is the initial symptom, but if the causative factor persists, then soreness and even pain, especially on walking, may occur.

Signs

The skin may be normal but more commonly shows evidence of abrasion or of the presence of one of the specific causative factors described above.

Investigation

If at all possible, a precise diagnosis should be established by investigation appropriate to the expected cause. Threadworms may be seen on the perianal skin or the rectal mucosa at sigmoidoscopy. Biopsy may rarely be required to define the nature of visible perianal disease; in the patient with no obvious cause, sphincter dysfunction should be investigated.

Management

The key to successful management is the accurate determination and treatment of the cause, which can be achieved in 90% of instances:

- Medications which may be causative are withdrawn.
- Ointments for symptomatic management should only be used when a precise diagnosis has been made and normally for a defined period only.
- Severe inflammation or excoriation usually responds to a short course of a topical steroid (betamethasone 0.1%) sparingly applied twice daily for 2 weeks.
- Threadworms – oral piperazine (all family members require treatment).
- Faecal soiling (without sphincter dysfunction) – instruction in hygiene and the use of damp cotton wool rather than toilet paper; a thin piece of cotton wool on the end of the patient's index finger may be inserted up to three or four times a day to clean a funnel-shaped anus.
- Loose motions – if a cause is not found, a small dose of codeine phosphate or loperamide facilitates cleansing by making the stool firmer.

FAECAL INCONTINENCE

Failure to have complete control of rectal contents causes considerable stress to the affected individual. A strong sense of social alienation develops together with fear of embarrassment at work or in the presence of friends, so that imprisonment within the home is common. It has long been recognised that incontinence is normal in infants and common in the very old, but the observation that there is a significant incidence in middle age is more recent. The increased awareness of the problem is the result of more concern by the caring professions such as doctors, nurses and social workers, less reluctance to discuss sensitive matters of body function, and increasing attempts to manage the condition.

Anatomy and pathophysiology

The functional anatomy and physiology of the rectum and anal canal have been described above. Disturbances in these, either locally or because of neural disorders, are the basis of all incontinence.

Definitions

Urge incontinence

This is defined as an inability to defer defecation for more than a few minutes. It is usually a sign of external sphincter injury or the result of the normal sphincter being overwhelmed, as in an acute diarrhoeal illness.

Passive incontinence

This is defined as loss of stool or flatus without the patient being immediately aware that this has occurred. This is commonly a sign of internal sphincter injury or neuropathy.

Aetiology

The causes of minor and major incontinence overlap, and the distinction is chiefly one of the severity of the clinical features and the need for treatment. Causes are categorised below, and it is clear that multifactorial obstetric events are amongst the commonest causes of faecal incontinence affecting younger women (Table 26.6).

Table 26.6 Faecal incontinence caused by obstetric events

Event	Effect
Tear during delivery	Extension backwards to involve rectal wall and internal sphincter
Too large an episiotomy	As for tear
Difficult or prolonged delivery, perhaps with forceps assistance	Pressure and ischaemic damage to motor outflow in pudendal nerves – denervation of both sphincters and of muscles of pelvic floor
Obstructed labour	Necrosis of anterior wall of rectum and posterior wall of vagina, leading to rectovaginal fistula

Inadequate closure of the internal sphincter

The sphincter may be unable to close completely because of:

- large third-degree haemorrhoids
- rectal prolapse
- large faecal mass in the rectum – impacted faeces with liquid stool leaking past and escaping through a lax sphincter
- anal canal tumour.

Damage to the sphincter complex

Damage may be caused by:

- previous surgery, usually for perianal sepsis
- overstretching – treatment of fissure; unusual sexual practices either voluntary or during sexual abuse
- obstetric injury – third-degree perineal tear extending posteriorly from the vaginal wall into the anal sphincter.

Damage to the pelvic floor

Damage may result from:

- obstetric injuries
- pelvic fractures – shearing stresses on the pelvic floor with tearing of nerves.

Loss or absence of motor innervation to the internal sphincter

This may be caused by:

- prolonged or complicated obstetric delivery – pressure on, or distraction of, the pudendal nerves
- diabetic neuropathy
- spina bifida or cauda equina tumour (both may interfere with the whole reflex arc of defecation).

Loss of cerebrospinal regulation (upper motor neuron)

Disorder or disease in the CNS interferes with higher control of defecation. Numerically these are relatively rare causes of incontinence with the exception of the central degenerative conditions of old age:

- trauma
- tumour in brain or spinal cord
- multiple sclerosis; motor neuron disease
- cerebral disease – Alzheimer's disease and other dementias; stroke.

Fistula between rectum and vagina

Developmental malformation of the anus may lead to an imperforate anus with termination of the rectum in the posterior wall of the vagina. A further cause of rectovaginal fistula, very uncommon now in the developed world but still common in developing countries, is prolonged obstructed labour with pressure of the fetal head on the posterior vaginal wall and necrosis of this and the adjacent rectum. The bladder may also be involved (see Ch. 40). In developed countries the commonest causes are Crohn's disease or as a postoperative complication following complex pelvic surgery.

Clinical features

Symptoms

There may be a relevant past history of one of the causes given above. In major incontinence, the patient recounts a life of misery and frequently brings to the clinic a map on which has been marked every known public facility they may need 'just in case'. Pads have to be worn and changed frequently, and some patients, particularly those with neurological causes, have urinary incontinence as well.

A history of recent onset of the problem and its progressive development suggests a neurological lesion.

Clinical examination

The local findings vary with the cause. There may be scarring of the perineum from surgery or obstetric intervention or other evidence of anal disease such as haemorrhoids or prolapse. On rectal examination, the anus may gape, and when a finger is inserted the resting anal pressure may be obviously reduced (weak internal sphincter). When asked to tighten the anus voluntarily, the response may be weak or absent (weak external sphincter).

The examination must include:

- full anorectal examination by sigmoidoscopy
- neurological examination, beginning with testing the sensation of the perianal skin.

Investigation

Imaging

Ultrasound. Anal ultrasound provides very accurate assessment of both internal and external sphincter. It can clearly identify damage to one or both of these structures.

Colonoscopy or barium enema should always be considered if there is a history suggestive of either a neoplasm or inflammatory disease.

Anal manometry

Direct measurement of the pressure in the anal canal at rest (internal sphincter) and on maximum voluntary contraction (external sphincter) may help to establish which muscle is at fault, although not necessarily the exact cause.

Management

Incontinence which is caused by inflammatory diarrhoea is usually manageable by treating the underlying condition. Faecal impaction is dealt with by manual removal of the faecal mass (enemas are useless) and regulation of the bowel with laxatives.

Minor incontinence from other causes (provided these are not an indication of progressive disease) may respond to a mild antimotility drug such as loperamide, an additional effect of which is to increase internal sphincter tone. Biofeedback uses the recording of the patient's own pressure trace, together with pelvic floor exercises, to encourage increased tone and increase the ability of surviving muscle fibres to undergo hypertrophy; however, controlled trials have not been undertaken.

Surgical techniques

Intervention by surgery is indicated when:

- incapacitation has failed to respond to medical management
- there is a known cause which can be corrected by anatomical reconstruction; typically this relates to obstetric or iatrogenic division of the sphincter complex and requires an overlapping anterior sphincter repair, although long-term results are disappointing.

Sacral nerve stimulation (SNS) is a relatively new technique which is gaining popularity. There is evidence of good results in patients with intact sphincters (and recently also those with sphincter defects) who have failed to improve with conservative measures. Initially, a temporary wire is placed in the 3rd sacral foramen under fluoroscopic control, and attached to an external stimulator for a trial period of 2–3 weeks. Up to 75% of patients respond to the test stimulation and they go on to have a permanent device fitted with >50% improvement in their incontinence. The stimulator is placed in a subcutaneous pocket, laterally in the buttock. Fitting of SNS requires dedicated assessment and ongoing long-term follow-up.

Problems such as neuropathy or atrophy without a demonstrable defect in the muscular ring are more difficult to manage. Traditionally they were approached by a posterior repair of the pelvic floor, but the results have been poor in some series, and this approach has lost favour. More controversial is the use of the gracilis muscle to create a neosphincter which encircles the anus or the use of an artificial sphincter. The results are uncertain in spite of the usual confident reports from early applications, and the financial costs are considerable.

In neuological conditions associated with incontinence (MS, MND), percutaneous endoscopic colostomy tubes (PEC) or ACE procedures have been performed with some success in allowing regular antegrade lavage of the distal colon and rectum, and minimising passive seepage.

When reconstructive surgery fails, a stoma to divert the faecal stream is a radical but appropriate alternative; an incontinent but manageable stoma on the anterior abdominal wall is greatly preferable to an incontinent but unmanageable opening in the perineum.

TUMOURS

Anal cancers are uncommon. They make up only about 4% of large bowel cancers. Most are squamous cell carcinomas (>80%) and arise from the squamous lining of the anal canal and perianal skin. The upper anal canal is lined by mucus-secreting epithelium, and from this adenocarcinomas may arise (<10%). Other rarer tumours have been described, including melanomas, lymphomas and sarcomas. The incidence of anal cancers and AIN (anal intraepitheial neoplasia) has increased with the increasing incidence of HIV infection.

Aetiology and pathological features

Condylomata acuminata (perianal warts). These are the consequence of infection with the human papilloma virus (HPV 16 and 18), which is most often sexually transmitted in both sexes by anal intercourse. The condition is common in patients with HIV infection.

Anal intraepitheial neoplasia. Unlike its equivalent CIN (cervical intraepithelial neoplasia), the natural history of AIN is relatively poorly understood. More than 90% of cases are associated with HPV 16 and 18 infection, HIV and immunocompromised patients. Lesions are best seen with a colposcope and staining of the perianal skin with acetic acid. Biopsies are taken to establish the degree of dysplasia (AIN I, II, or III). The management of AIN III is controversial.

Tumours arise from different parts of the anal canal. Those from the canal tend to be more poorly differentiated, whereas those from the margin are often well differentiated and keratinised.

Spread is both locally to the sphincters, perianal skin and surrounding structures and then to the regional lymph nodes (perirectal, inguinal, lateral pelvic nodes). Haematogenous spread is late and often associated with locally advanced disease.

Clinical features

The symptoms of anal cancers are not specific and have a large overlap with common parianal conditions. Rectal bleeding, perianal pain, pruritus incontinence and mucus discharge are common to a multitude of conditions resulting in anal cancers being frequently misdiagnosed as benign conditions before the true diagnosis is established. Some patients present with inguinal lymphadenopathy and it is essential that the perineum, anal canal and rectum are examined in these patients.

Management

A precise diagnosis is essential before treatment is planned. An incision biopsy may suffice, but for a small lesion a total excision biopsy is, in addition, effective treatment.

Staging prior to treatment involves CT scanning to assess for distant spread and MRI ± endoanal ultrasound to assess for local tumour spread.

Anal margin

Condylomata acuminata are managed by excision with scissors, diathermy or laser. Small-cell squamous carcinomas (<2 cm) may respond to local excision. For larger lesions, radiotherapy with or without chemotherapy is currently the treatment of choice and avoids the need for an abdominoperineal excision of the rectum.

Anal canal

Tumours of squamous cell origin are best treated with radiotherapy with or without chemotherapy. Only if there is an incomplete response should radical surgery be required, as it is for adenocarcinoma. Malignant melanomas have a very poor prognosis despite radical treatment.

FURTHER READING

Keighley MRB, Williams NS 2008 Surgery of the anus, rectum and colon, 3rd edn. Saunders Elsevier, Edinburgh

Phillips RK 2009
A companion to specialist surgical practice: colorectal surgery, 4th edn. Saunders Elsevier, Edinburgh

Zbar AP, Wexner SD 2010 Coloproctology. Springer, London

27 Hernia

No disease of the human body, belonging to the province of the surgeon, requires in its treatment a better combination of accurate, anatomical knowledge with surgical skill than hernia in all its variations.

Sir Astley Paton Cooper (1804)

GENERAL CONSIDERATIONS

A hernia is a protrusion of a viscus or other structure beyond the normal coverings of the cavity in which it is contained. It may occur between two adjacent cavities such as the abdomen and thorax or into a subcompartment of a cavity – so-called internal hernias. The most frequent hernias are external ones of the abdominal wall in the inguinal, femoral and umbilical regions, and the account that follows concentrates chiefly on these.

Epidemiology

The first record of a hernia is in the Egyptian Papyrus Ebers (1550 BC) when it was regarded as a social stigma. Abdominal hernias are common. They occur at all ages and in both sexes and account for approximately 10% of the general surgical workload. Their relative frequencies are given in Table 27.1.

Classification

Hernias are best classified as congenital or acquired.

Congenital

In congenital hernias, there is a pre-formed sac which occurs as a consequence of the ordered or disordered process of intrauterine development – the patent processus vaginalis is a good example.

Acquired

There are two types of acquired hernia:

Primary hernias occur at natural weak points, such as those where:

- structures penetrate the abdominal wall, e.g. the femoral vessels passing into the femoral canal
- muscles and aponeuroses fail to overlap normally, e.g. the lumbar region
- fibrous tissue normally develops to close a defect, e.g. at the umbilicus.

Secondary hernias develop at sites of surgical or other injury to the wall which normally constrains the contents of a body cavity (usually the abdomen), e.g. after laparotomy or penetrating injury.

Aetiology

The two main factors predisposing to hernia are increased intracavity pressure and a weakened abdominal wall. In the abdomen, the raised pressure occurs as a result of:

- heavy lifting
- cough – chronic obstructive airways disease
- straining to pass urine – benign prostatic hyperplasia or carcinoma
- straining to pass faeces – constipation or large-bowel obstruction
- abdominal distension – which may indicate the presence of an intra-abdominal disorder
- change in abdominal contents – e.g. ascites, encysted fluid, benign or malignant tumour, pregnancy, fat.

A weakened abdominal wall occurs in:

- advancing age
- malnutrition – either of macronutrients (protein, calorie) or micronutrients (e.g. vitamin C)
- damage to, or paralysis of, motor nerves
- abnormal collagen metabolism.

Often, multiple factors are involved. For example, the presence of a patent, congenitally formed sac may not cause a hernia until an acquired abdominal wall weakness or raised intra-abdominal pressure allows abdominal contents to enter the sac.

Anatomical features

A hernia consists of:

Table 27.1 Relative frequency of external abdominal hernias

Type of hernia	Incidence (%)
Epigastric	1
Umbilical	3
Incisional	10
Inguinal	78
Femoral	7
Other (rare)	1

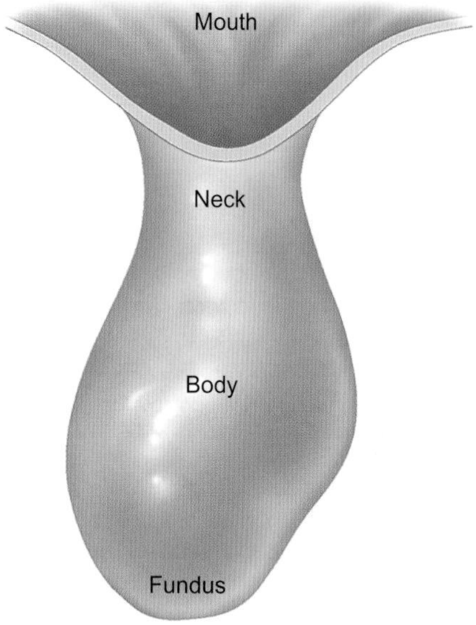

Fig. 27.1 Hernial sac.

- a sac
- its coverings
- its contents.

The sac comprises a mouth, neck, body and fundus (Fig. 27.1). The coverings of a hernia refer to the overlying layers, which are attenuated as the hernia emerges. Working from the outermost layer inwards, these are as follows:

- skin
- subcutaneous fat
- aponeurosis
- muscle
- endo-cavity fascia
- endothelial lining – peritoneum in the abdomen.

The contents of hernias vary, but most intracavity viscera have been reported. In the abdomen, the commonest contents are the small bowel and the greater omentum. Other possibilities include:

- the large bowel and appendix
- Meckel's diverticulum
- the bladder
- the ovary with or without the fallopian tube
- ascitic fluid.

Natural history and complications

The natural history of hernia development is progressive enlargement, not spontaneous regression. A notable exception is congenital umbilical hernia in neonates, where the orifice may close over the years following birth. With the passage of time, hernias enlarge and the likelihood of a life-threatening complication increases.

Hernias may be reducible, irreducible, obstructed, strangulated or inflamed.

Reducible hernia

In this type of hernia, the contents can be returned from whence they came, but the sac persists. The contents do not necessarily reappear spontaneously, but do so when assisted by gravity or raised intra-abdominal pressure.

Irreducible hernia

The contents cannot be returned to the body cavity in this type of hernia. The causes of irreducibility are:

- narrow neck with rigid margins often in association with a capacious sac (e.g. femoral, umbilical)
- adhesion formation between the contents and the sac (usually long-standing hernias).

Irreducible hernias have a greater risk of obstruction and strangulation than reducible ones.

Obstructed hernia

The obstructed hernia contains intestine in which the lumen has become occluded. Obstruction is usually at the neck of the sac but may be caused by adhesions within it. If the obstruction is at both ends of the loop, fluid accumulates within it and distension occurs (closed loop obstruction). Initially the blood supply to the obstructed loop of bowel is intact, but with time this becomes impeded and strangulation (see below) supervenes.

The term 'incarcerated' is sometimes used to describe a hernia that is irreducible but not strangulated. Thus, an irreducible, obstructed hernia can also be called an incarcerated one.

Strangulated hernia

Ten percent of groin hernias present for the first time with strangulation. The blood supply to the contents of the hernia is cut off. The pathological sequence is: venous and lymphatic occlusion; tissue fluid accumulation (oedema) causing further swelling; and a consequent increase in venous pressure. Venous haemorrhage develops, and a vicious circle is set up, with swelling eventually impeding arterial inflow. The tissues undergo ischaemic necrosis. If the contents of the sac of an abdominal hernia are not bowel, e.g. omentum, the necrosis is sterile, but strangulation of bowel is by far the most common and leads to infected necrosis (gangrene). The mucosa sloughs and the bowel wall becomes permeable to bacteria, which translocate through it and into the sac and from there to the bloodstream. The infarcted, friable intestine perforates (usually at the neck of the sac) and the bacteria-laden luminal fluid spills into the peritoneal cavity to produce peritonitis. Septic shock ensues with circulatory failure and death.

Inflamed hernia

The contents are inflamed by any process that causes this in the tissue or organ that is not normally herniated, e.g.:

- acute appendicitis
- Meckel's diverticulitis
- acute salpingitis.

It may be impossible to distinguish an inflamed hernia from one that is strangulated.

Special types of hernia

Sliding hernia (hernia en glissade)

This hernia is one in which an extraperitoneal structure forms part of the wall of the sac (Fig. 27.2). Five percent of all hernias are sliding, and indirect inguinal hernias account for the majority. On the right the caecum and ascending colon are involved, whereas on the left the sigmoid and descending colon are found in the sac. A portion of bladder may slide into a direct inguinal hernia. The incidence of sliding hernias increases with age and the duration of the hernia. Failure to recognise a sliding hernia at operation may result in damage to the structure involved.

Richter's hernia (Fig. 27.3)

In this type of hernia, only a portion of the circumference of the intestine (usually the small bowel) is trapped. The danger of this hernia is that the knuckle of bowel may become ischaemic without the development of obvious clinical features of obstruction (see 'Femoral hernia').

Hernia-en-W – Maydl's hernia

This complicated disposition of intestine in an inguinal hernia is easier to illustrate (Fig. 27.4) than to describe. If strangulation occurs, the loop affected is within the abdominal cavity.

Clinical features

Symptoms

There may be a history of factors predisposing to increased intracavity pressure (e.g. cough, heavy lifting – see 'Aetiology').

Local symptoms include:

- a lump which varies in size, may disappear when recumbent and reappear and enlarge on straining
- pain – local aching discomfort, but sometimes sharp.

Symptoms of complications may be:

- intestinal obstruction – colic, vomiting, distension and absolute constipation

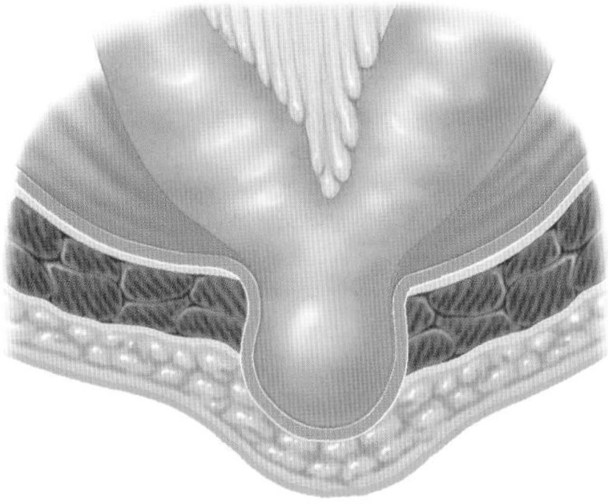

Fig. 27.3 Richter's hernia.

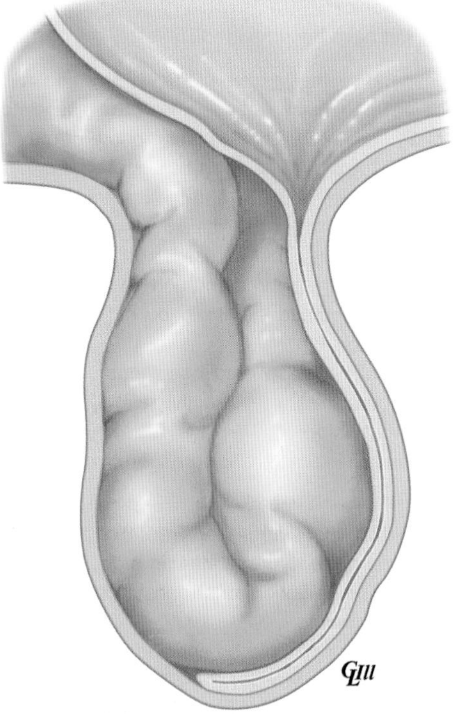

Fig. 27.2 Sliding hernia.

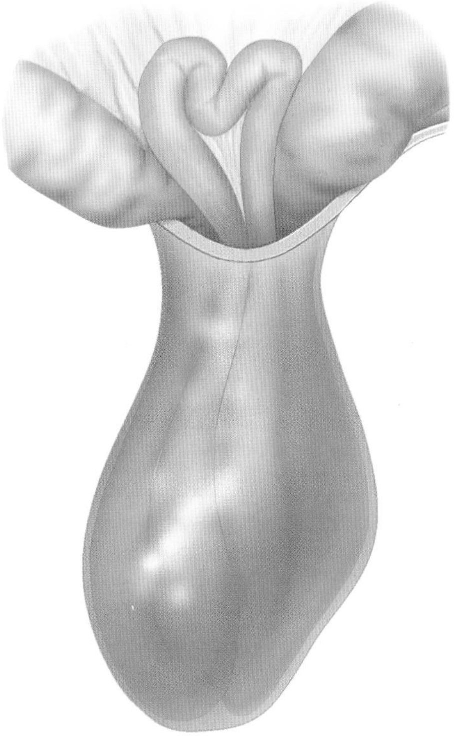

Fig. 27.4 Maydl's hernia.

- strangulation – in addition to symptoms of intestinal obstruction, constant pain over the hernia, fever, tachycardia.

Signs

The patient should first be examined in the supine position and then, in all external abdominal hernias, standing. The area of the swelling is palpated to determine the exact position and then its physical characteristics. The lump's distinguishing features are reducibility and an expansile cough impulse – the lump gets bigger and more tense. On standing, bulges become more obvious and can be made additionally prominent by coughing.

When the patient lies down, it is possible to test for reducibility – if the swelling can be returned to the abdominal cavity it is said to be reducible. Control of the hernia is the ability to prevent its reappearance by digital pressure over the point at which reduction occurred. The patient is asked to cough: if the hernia does not reappear it has been controlled and the neck of the sac accurately located.

Other hernial sites should be examined, as bilateral and simultaneous hernias are common. Other causes of a lump that may be confused with abdominal wall hernias are shown in Table 27.2. A general physical examination is essential and includes a search for predisposing causes such as benign prostatic hyperplasia and colorectal cancer.

Signs associated with complications

Irreducibility Locally there is a painless lump that does not reduce.

Obstruction The hernia is tense, tender and irreducible. There may be distension of the abdomen and the other features of intestinal obstruction.

Strangulation Signs are as for an obstructed hernia, but tenderness is more marked. The overlying skin may be warm, inflamed and indurated.

Investigation

Hernia is a clinical diagnosis.

Imaging

Ultrasound is being increasingly used to assess hernias that are difficult to define clinically, e.g. an early groin or Spigelian hernia.

Table 27.2 Other causes of lumps that must be differentiated from abdominal wall hernias

Tissue	Lump
Skin	Sebaceous or epidermoid cyst
Fat	Lipoma
Fascia	Fibroma
Muscle	Herniation through sheath; tumour
Artery	Aneurysm
Vein	Varicosity
Lymphatic	Enlarged lymph node
Gonad	Ectopic testis/ovary

CT and MRI have an occasional role in rare pelvic hernias (e.g. obturator hernia). They may also be helpful in the preoperative assessment of large incisional (or other) hernias where muliple defects may be present. In addition, CT or MRI scanning will exclude recurrent malignant disease in patients who have had previous cancer surgery.

Herniography This technique, which involves the injection of contrast medium into the peritoneal cavity and subsequent X-ray, is now rarely used in infants to identify a clinically undetectable contralateral hernia in the groin. It may occasionally be useful in confirming or refuting the presence of a hernia in a patient with chronic groin pain.

Laparoscopy

Unexpected hernias are sometimes discovered at the time of laparoscopy for undiagnosed abdominal pain.

Exploratory operation

In some infants with a convincing history from the mother, a hernia is not found on clinical examination. Exploratory operation can then be justified.

Principles of management

The natural history of a hernia is one of progressive enlargement. The risks of irreducibility, obstruction and strangulation increase with time; that of strangulation is about 10%. For these reasons, surgical opinion now is that, with very few exceptions, hernias should be operatively repaired. This serves to relieve the patient's symptoms and to eliminate the occurrence of complications, the most dangerous of which is strangulation. There is a particularly strong argument in favour of operation in those hernias that have a high incidence of this complication, i.e.:

- inguinal hernia with a narrow neck
- femoral hernia
- those that have become irreducible.

Advances in anaesthesia have made elective hernia surgery safe. A small number of patients may have associated disorders that make an operation inappropriate or may decline it; in these cases a truss (support belt) is used. For it to work the hernia must be reducible and the appliance must maintain the reduction when the patient stands and strains. It should be appreciated that a truss which does not control a hernia is a menace – by irritation and scar tissue formation it may actually increase the likelihood of incarceration and strangulation.

Presenting or predisposing conditions such as benign prostatic hyperplasia or obstructive airways disease may need treatment before the hernia is dealt with. In addition, in certain defined circumstances, preoperative preparation is necessary:

- Large hernias that warrant repair require particularly diligent preoperative preparation in order to minimise the risk of the operation and to ensure a favourable long-term outcome.
- Weight reduction should be encouraged.
- Smoking is discouraged.
- Treatment of intercurrent disease (e.g. hypertension, diabetes) is essential.

- Therapeutic pneumoperitoneum is very occasionally used for giant hernias – when viscera are in a hernia sac for long periods of time, they lose the 'right of domicile' in the abdominal cavity; replacing them suddenly into the abdomen is associated with the dangers of respiratory embarrassment, compression of the inferior vena cava and paralytic ileus. These complications may be averted by preparing the patient and the abdominal cavity by repeated intraperitoneal injections of air over the 2 weeks before operation, up to a total of 2.5 L.

Elective operations are now usually done as either day or short-stay procedures, and patients are encouraged to resume normal activities as soon as possible. Groin hernias may be repaired by a laparoscopic approach, which has marginal benefits in reduction in pain and early return to work.

Strangulation is a surgical emergency which still carries a high mortality rate, particularly if, for any reason, operation is delayed.

Surgical techniques

Herniotomy is the removal of the sac and closure of its neck. It is the first step in nearly every hernia repair and in some instances (e.g. infant inguinal hernia – see below) may be all that is required.

Herniorrhaphy involves some sort of reconstruction to:

- restore the anatomy if this is disturbed
- increase the strength of the abdominal wall
- construct a barrier to recurrence.

The first of these is usually possible by suture. The second and third may be achieved with local tissue, but the insertion of prosthetic material is also widely used. Most implants are made of non-absorbable synthetic material (e.g. polypropylene). Variant products include partly absorbable meshes (e.g. polyglactin/polypropylene), meshes with an antiadhesion surface for intraperitoneal use, and biological meshes made from processed animal tissue for use in contaminated fields or large hernial defects.

Obstruction and strangulation

The patient nearly always requires treatment of the associated obstruction of the gut.

Non-operative treatment can be considered in:

- infants
- obstructed hernia with a short history – presentation within 2 hours of onset in a hernia that was previously reducible and with no signs to suggest strangulation.

The patient is put in the head-down position and an ice pack may be applied; then an attempt is made to reduce the hernia by taxis, which consists of gentle manipulation of the swelling in the direction of the hernial orifice. Considerable experience is required. There is no place for vigorous manipulation, which carries the obvious danger of damage to the bowel or reduction en masse – reduction of the sac and its contents but with persistent trapping of the latter so that strangulation progresses.

Urgent operation is needed in the great majority of obstructed or strangulated hernias. The hernial sac and its contents are exposed and the constriction or other cause of obstruction relieved. Further surgery may be required to remove ischaemic bowel or omentum. For the reasons given above, strangulated bowel implies bacterial translocation, and antibiotics are administered.

Outcome

Mortality

For elective repair the overall mortality is less than 0.5% but increases with age to approximately 0.5–1% for those over 60 years. For emergency operations it is 10 times greater. It is a sobering observation that the mortality for strangulated obstructing hernia has remained unchanged at around the 20% for the last 50 years. Death is dependent on:

- age – older patients have a higher incidence of intercurrent disease
- contents of the sac – gangrenous intestine (present in 10% of strangulated hernias) is associated with a 40% mortality rate.

Morbidity

The overall complication rate is around 7%. Any of the complications that beset surgery can occur during or after operations for hernia. Specific to the procedure are:

- persistent wound pain – often ascribed to a neuroma which forms after damage to or division of the ilio-inguinal or other nerve
- cutaneous anaesthesia – division of a nerve
- recurrent hernia.

The rate of recurrence is between less than 1% and 10% for primary hernias (depending on the type) and 5–30% for recurrent hernias. Recurrence is associated with:

- age – the older the patient, the more likely is the hernia to recur
- presence or absence of predisposing factors
- site – high with incisional hernias; inguinal greater than femoral
- size – the larger the hernia, the more likely it is to have distorted the surrounding anatomy
- emergency or elective operation – the former being more likely to be associated with recurrence
- operation on a recurrent hernia – more difficult and more likely to fail
- experience of the surgeon.

See below for further consideration of recurrent hernias.

SPECIFIC HERNIAS

INGUINAL HERNIA

Inguinal hernias account for 80% of all external abdominal hernias. They occur at all ages, but are most common in infants and the elderly. Inguinal hernias are 20 times more common in men than in women, and more frequently occur on the right side.

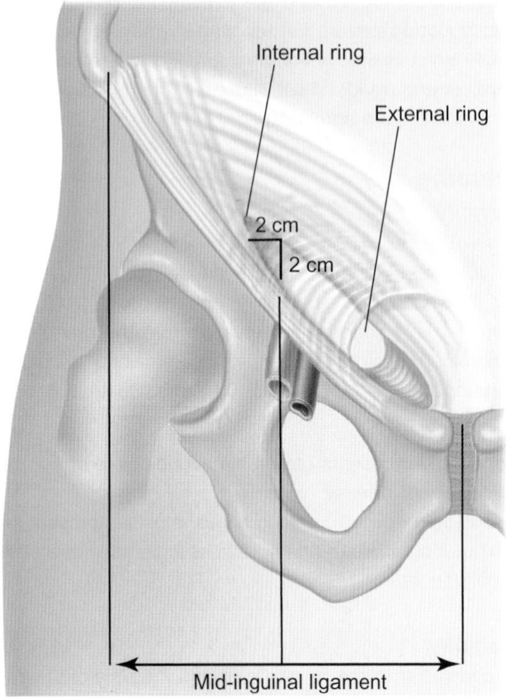

Fig. 27.5 The inguinal canal.

Anatomy

The inguinal canal (Fig. 27.5) runs in an antero-inferior direction from the internal to external inguinal rings and, in the male, is the path taken by the testis to reach the scrotum. In that sex, therefore, it contains the spermatic vessels and the vas deferens; in the female it only contains the round ligament. The internal ring lies 2 cm or slightly more above and 2 cm lateral to the mid-inguinal point – that point on the inguinal ligament midway between the anterior superior iliac spine and the symphysis pubis. To find it, the femoral artery is identified as it passes deep to the mid-inguinal point and the fingers are moved upwards and laterally. The medial aspect of the ring is bounded by the inferior epigastric branch of the femoral artery. The external ring is just above the pubic crest and tubercle to which the inguinal ligament is attached. In infants the internal and external rings are directly one behind the other but during growth they move apart.

The inguinal region and canal, particularly in the male, is a vulnerable area for the formation of hernia, but this is to some extent offset by contraction of the abdominal muscles, which compresses together the anterior and posterior walls of the canal and allows descent of the conjoint tendon to act as a partial shutter.

It is further thought that the cremaster muscle bunches the cord up into the canal, so acting as a plug.

Classification

Indirect inguinal hernia

This passes through the internal ring lateral to the inferior epigastric artery and along the canal to emerge at the external ring above the pubic crest and tubercle. Its coverings are the attenuated layers of the cord.

Table 27.3 Differences between an indirect and a direct inguinal hernia

	Indirect	Direct
Patient's age	Any age but usually young	Older
Cause	May be congenital	Acquired
Bilateral	20%	50%
Protrusion on coughing	Oblique	Straight
Appearance on standing	Does not reach full size immediately	Reaches full size immediately
Reduction on lying down	May not reduce immediately	Reduces immediately
Descent into scrotum	Common	Rare
Occlusion of internal ring	Controls	Does not control
Neck of sac	Narrow	Wide
Strangulation	Not uncommon	Unusual
Relation to inferior epigastric vessels	Lateral	Medial

Direct inguinal hernia

This hernia bulges through the posterior wall of the canal medial to the inferior epigastric artery and is therefore not covered by the layers of the cord.

Pantaloon hernia

This is a combination of both an indirect and a direct inguinal hernia.

Aetiology

Indirect hernia

In an indirect hernia, there is a congenital sac or potential sac which is the remnant of the processus vaginalis. If the processus does not close, then an indirect hernia occurs in early life, but other factors may lead to it reopening at any age. Indirect hernias are 20 times more common in men than in women. Sixty percent occur on the right (possibly contributed to by damage to the motor nerves of the abdominal muscles at open appendicectomy), 40% on the left and 20% are bilateral.

Direct hernia

This is an acquired lesion. For reasons unknown, though contributed to by accessory factors such as the wear and tear of advancing age, repeated straining and raised intra-abdominal pressure, the posterior wall of the inguinal canal becomes attenuated. Direct hernia is therefore a condition of later life and is rarely seen under the age of 40.

Clinical findings

In both indirect and direct hernias, the cough impulse that can be seen or palpated must be distinguished from normal diffuse bulging in the inguinal region, particularly in individuals of spare build. The principal differences between the two types of hernia on clinical examination are summarised in Table 27.3.

In addition to the features outlined in Table 27.3, an indirect hernia that extends beyond the external ring appears above and medial to the pubic tubercle, in contrast to a femoral hernia (see below) which is below and lateral to that bony point. The pubic tubercle can be found either by feeling laterally along the pubic crest from the upper border of the symphysis pubic or by following the adductor longus tendon from the medial side of the thigh to its origin from the body of the pubis. The tubercle is directly above.

One of the most useful methods of distinction between the two kinds of inguinal hernia is that a reducible indirect hernia can be completely controlled with a fingertip placed firmly over the internal ring.

For the clinical features and management of an infantile inguinal hernia, see Chapter 36.

Other causes of groin swelling

Although inguinal hernias are relatively easy to diagnose, there are a considerable number of other causes of swelling in this area that may require consideration when a lump is encountered. These include:

- femoral hernia
- hydrocele
- encysted hydrocele of the cord or of the peritoneovaginal canal
- undescended or ectopic testis
- lipoma of the cord
- epididymal cyst.

Management

The general principles of hernia management have been given above. Most adult inguinal hernias are repaired by open operation under local or general anaesthesia as a day-case procedure, although the number of hernia repairs performed laparoscopically is increasing, because of the perceived benefits in bilateral or recurrent cases, and also in response to patient choice. Elderly patients and those with serious medical problems require in-patient care. Open operation usually means a layered suture technique (Shouldice) or the insertion of a non-absorbable prosthetic mesh (Lichtenstein).

Open mesh repair

The mesh repair of inguinal hernia is the most common general surgical operation performed in the UK. The method involves the following steps:

- An oblique skin incision is made in the groin, 2 cm above the medial half of the inguinal ligament.
- Fat and Scarpa's fascia are divided to expose the external oblique aponeurosis, superficial ring and the inguinal ligament inferiorly.
- The aponeurosis and superficial ring are opened, avoiding damage to the ilio-inguinal nerve to allow access to the cremaster-covered cord and hernia sac. The cord is lifted off the posterior canal wall and pubic tubercle – 'dislocation'.
- The cremaster is opened to allow separation of the hernia sac from the cord structures. An indirect (lateral to inferior epigastric vessels) sac emerges through the deep inguinal ring, superior, lateral and anterior to the cord structures. A direct sac emerges through the posterior wall of the canal, medial to the inferior epigastric vessels.
- Indirect sacs are usually opened, the contents reduced, and the sac tied at its neck. Excess sac is then excised. Direct sacs are less often excised – rather they are reduced with closure of the defect with suture, or if the neck is wide, reduced with a plication stitch. Very large sacs or long inguino-scrotal sacs may be divided in the groin and transfixed at the neck, with the distal part left in situ.
- The posterior wall of the inguinal canal is then repaired by placement of a prosthetic mesh. This is placed over the whole posterior wall, with the formation of a window to transmit the cord structures without constriction. The mesh is fixed along its inferior edge to the inner part of the inguinal ligament, and to the conjoint tendon and pubic tubercle by suture.
- Closure is by repair of the external oblique aponeurosis, followed by suture of the fat and skin.

Laparoscopic repair

Mesh repair may be performed laparoscopically. This method is associated with less postoperative pain and more rapid return to normal activity. There are two main approaches to this method, TAPP (trans-abdominal pre-peritoneal) and TEP (totally extra-peritoneal):

- TAPP repair involves the insertion of a camera and instruments through all layers of the abdominal wall after insufflation of the peritoneal cavity. The hernia is then approached by incising the peritoneum from inside, creating a pocket between abdominal wall and peritoneum, reducing the hernial sac into the abdomen, and placing a mesh between the peritoneum and abdominal wall, covering the hernial orifice. The peritoneal incision is then closed to prevent contact between mesh and bowel.
- TEP repair does not involve breaching the peritoneum. Instead, a space is created between the peritoneum and the abdominal wall using a balloon which is introduced into this space. When inflated, the balloon peels the peritoneum off the abdominal wall. The balloon is then removed and the space maintained by gas insufflation. Camera and instruments may then be inserted, and the hernia sac reduced from within, and a mesh placed over the defect to prevent recurrence.

The wounds are smaller, less painful and allow earlier mobilisation compared with open repair. There is less exposure and handling of nerves and there is therefore a lower incidence of pain, paraesthesia and anaesthesia complications. The planes in which dissection and mesh placement occur make the laparoscopic method preferable in recurrent hernia repair, avoiding the need to operate on already scarred and distorted tissues. Both groins may be approached with minimal increase in the trauma of access, and therefore there is clear benefit in cases of bilateral inguinal hernia.

These procedures, however, carry a higher risk of major visceral or large vessel injury (small bowel, bladder and external iliac vessels in particular), although such injuries remain rare. The operation costs of laparoscopic procedures are higher, and general anaesthesia is required. Few surgeons would attempt laparoscopic repair in very large inguinal hernias. The recurrence rate in the laparoscopic repair is probably equivalent to open mesh repair.

Specific complications

- Urinary retention.
- A scrotal haematoma may follow extensive dissection.
- Damage to the ilio-inguinal nerve produces an area of anaesthesia over the pubic tubercle, scrotum or labia.

Outcome

Recurrence rate for inguinal hernia is one of the most hotly debated subjects in general surgery. With selection of patients only after adequate evaluation of contributing factors and with good technique, recurrence rates for groin hernias should be less than 1%. The rate is more widely quoted as 3% for primary hernias and up to 30% in the management of recurrence. However, such rates should be balanced against the population under study, the technique used and the quality of follow-up.

Recurrent inguinal hernia

Even with what seems to be optimal operative technique, hernias recur. Factors involved in recurrence include:

- predisposing causes – those with uncorrectable precipitating factors or on high-dose steroid therapy which interferes with healing
- type of hernia – indirect hernias have a 1–7% recurrence rate but direct hernias reach 4–10%
- type of operation – repairs under tension do not heal with adequate protection against recurrence
- postoperative wound infection.

Management of recurrence

Recurrent inguinal hernias should be repaired in order to avoid the same complications that occur in primary hernias, which are even more likely when recurrence has taken place. Because of scarring, the dissection can be difficult; in the male, orchidectomy is occasionally performed to allow closure of the deep ring. Recurrent hernias are best managed by the laparoscopic insertion of a mesh in the pre-peritoneal space.

FEMORAL HERNIA

With femoral, the local pain the patient may not mention, while to the tiny lump in groin she does not call attention

On strangulated femoral hernia – Zachary Cope, 1947

Femoral hernias are acquired downward protrusions of peritoneum into the potential space of the femoral canal (Fig. 27.6). They account for 7% of all hernias but, in that they are four times more common in women than in men, they constitute 33% of groin hernias in females (5% in men). They are most common in late middle age and the multiparous and, unlike inguinal hernias, are rare in children. Bilateral hernias occur in 20%.

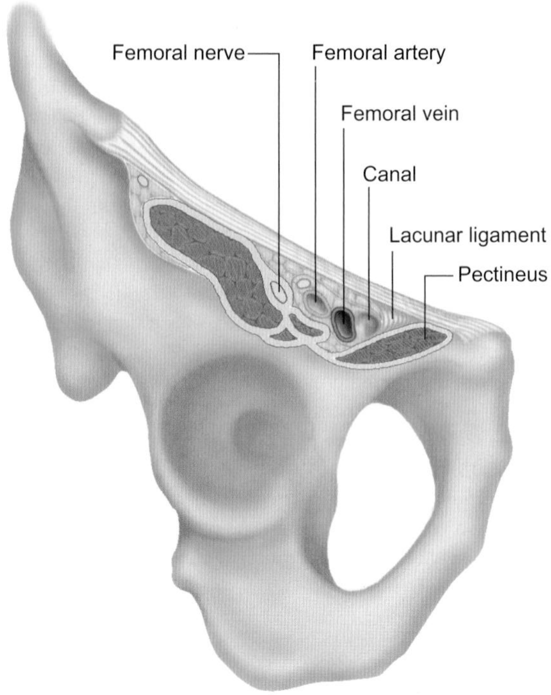

Fig. 27.6 Femoral canal.

Anatomy

The femoral canal is a 1–2 cm gap medial to the femoral sheath and femoral vein which contains a lymph node and fat. Its anterior (inguinal ligament), medial (lacunar part of the inguinal ligament) and posterior (pectineal part of the inguinal ligament) boundaries are rigid (Fig. 27.6). This narrow femoral ring produces a considerable risk of incarceration of any hernia that passes through it.

Aetiology and pathological features

As mentioned above, the hernia is acquired. The wide pelvis of the female and the laxity of ligaments after repeated pregnancy are contributory factors, as is weight loss. As the sac develops, it passes forwards through the saphenous opening whose well-defined lower edge directs it upwards to lie over the inguinal ligament in the subcutaneous plane.

The narrow canal makes a femoral hernia the one most likely to result in a Richter's hernia (30% of strangulated femoral hernias), although strangulation of an omental plug also takes place.

Clinical features

History

The patient is typically a middle-aged or elderly female, often of thin build, who complains of an intermittent lump low in the groin. However, a major problem is that she may not have noticed the lump and the first clinical presentation is with strangulation (see below), which occurs in 20%.

Signs

In a small hernia, a cough impulse is only rarely detected. A larger hernia may be seen to bulge on straining just below the medial part of the inguinal ligament. An irreducible hernia is a lump whose consistency varies according to its contents, which may extend upwards across the inguinal ligament. In consequence, it can be difficult to distinguish from an inguinal hernia, but the upper medial border of a femoral hernia is always below and lateral to the pubic tubercle. The other conditions that should be taken into consideration when a femoral hernia is diagnosed are shown in Table 27.4.

Strangulation

In contrast to a strangulated inguinal hernia, in a strangulated femoral hernia there are often no localising symptoms and signs and the lump is often small, unimpressive and overlooked by the patient (and perhaps the clinician). The classic presentation is that of small-bowel obstruction. However, the clinical features of this may be modified by the presence of a Richter's hernia which only partly obstructs the lumen of the gut so that the symptoms and signs are more like those of gastroenteritis. This, combined with the difficulty in finding the hernia, makes for a late diagnosis, sometimes only after the gut has perforated and there is spreading peritonitis.

Management

All femoral hernias should be repaired without delay because of their high risk of strangulation. A truss has no place in management because it cannot control the hernia. The principles are given above. In elective operations, repair is usually by direct incision over the hernia, excision of the sac and sutured closure of the femoral canal. For operation on a patient with obstruction or strangulation, it may be necessary to open the abdomen to find the segment of gut that has been trapped should it reduce before it can be dealt with.

UMBILICAL HERNIA

Congenital (infantile) umbilical hernia

This condition is considered in Chapter 36.

Table 27.4 Inguinal swellings which may resemble a femoral hernia

Condition	Findings
Inguinal hernia	Swelling is above and medial to the public tubercle
Saphena varix	Compressible Palpable thrill on coughing
Enlarged lymph node	Usually multiple Not fixed on deep aspect and therefore more mobile Seek cause – infection, tumour, lymphoma
Lipoma	Soft but not reducible
Femoral artery aneurysm	Expanding pulsation Bruit
Psoas abscess	Fluctuant Lateral to femoral artery Associated swelling in the iliac fossa
Ectopic testis	Empty scrotum

Adult umbilical hernia

Only a small minority of adult umbilical hernias are the outcome of the persistence of a congenital defect.

Aetiology and anatomical and pathological features

Two types of hernia occur with overlapping but different aetiological factors of clinical importance.

True umbilical hernia (Fig. 27.7)

In this condition, the protrusion is through the umbilical scar, everting the umbilicus, whose attenuated fibres are at the apex of the hernial sac. The cause is often secondary to an increase in the volume of contents of the abdominal cavity – e.g. due to obesity, ascites or large benign or malignant intra-abdominal tumours.

Para-umbilical hernia (Fig. 27.8)

The weakest area of the umbilical scar is at the superior aspect between the umbilical vein and the upper margin of the umbilical ring. It is at this point that a para-umbilical hernia develops. The emerging sac displaces the umbilical scar, which lies below and slightly to one side.

These hernias are more common than true umbilical hernias and typically are found in the obese middle-aged patient. Women are affected five times more frequently than men. Generalised inadequacy of the musculofascial layers of the abdominal wall and repeated pregnancy are important contributory factors.

The neck of the hernia is often narrow. In consequence, tissues that enter have great difficulty leaving; adhesions form and the hernia becomes irreducible. The sac progressively acquires more contents and may become very large. The contents are usually omentum, often with small bowel or transverse colon. Frequently the sac becomes loculated

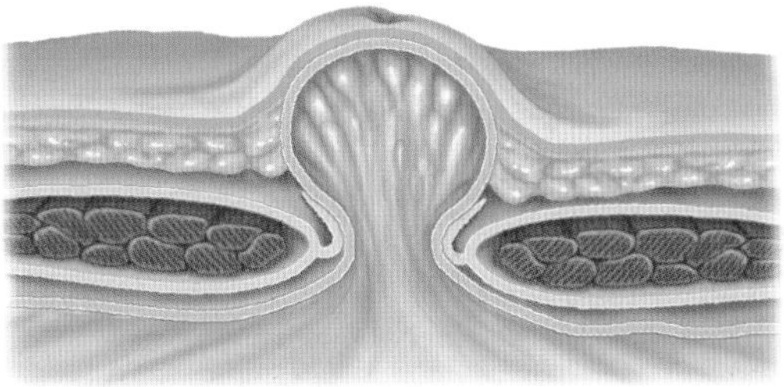

Fig. 27.7 Umbilical hernia.

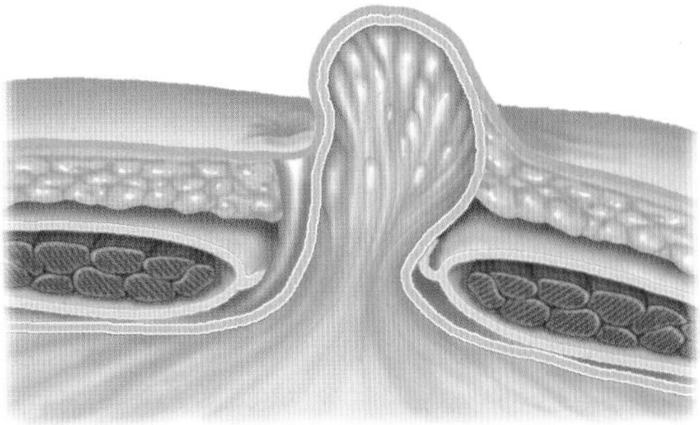

Fig. 27.8 Para-umbilical hernia.

when adhesions form between the omentum and the peritoneum. Not surprisingly, these hernias are at risk of strangulation.

Clinical features

True umbilical hernia

Symptoms

These are often present where there is an underlying cause of ascites or there may merely be gross obesity. Very rarely the patient will give a history which dates back to infancy or childhood.

Signs

Ascites may be obvious. The umbilicus is attenuated and sometimes paper-thin. Evidence of underlying malignancy should be sought both in the abdomen as a whole and at the umbilical opening, where a nodule or nodules may be palpable.

Para-umbilical hernia

Symptoms

There is local pain and a swelling at the navel. Non-specific gastrointestinal symptoms are common, and features of recurrent intestinal obstruction may have occurred.

Signs

The umbilicus assumes a crescent shape. Inspection and palpation reveal a swelling just above the umbilicus whose centre (in contrast to true umbilical hernia) is not attached to the apex of the protrusion. However, in grossly obese patients, the swelling may not be obvious to the naked eye and moreover is barely palpable. In others the hernia may be enormous. Usually it is reducible (at least in part) and there is a cough impulse. If reduction is possible, the palpable defect can be of any size, from one fingertip to admitting the fist.

Conditions that may be confused with a para-umbilical hernia include:

- cyst of the vitello-intestinal duct (rare)
- cyst of the urachus (also rare)
- metastatic tumour deposit.

Management

True umbilical hernia

Any underlying cause should be sought and dealt with. In the rare event that nothing is found and the hernia is causing symptoms, it is treated as a para-umbilical hernia.

Para-umbilical hernia

Symptomatic hernias require treatment. There is a high risk of strangulation, and repair should be advised, even in the absence of symptoms. The usual procedure is to mobilise the sac and its contents, return the latter to the abdomen, close the neck and repair the abdominal wall by overlapping its layers (Fig. 27.9).

Strangulated umbilical hernia

The patient with severe abdominal pain and vomiting and a soft non-tender umbilical hernia is a diagnostic trap. The loculated nature of the hernia allows a strangulated portion of bowel (often of the Richter's type) to go unnoticed

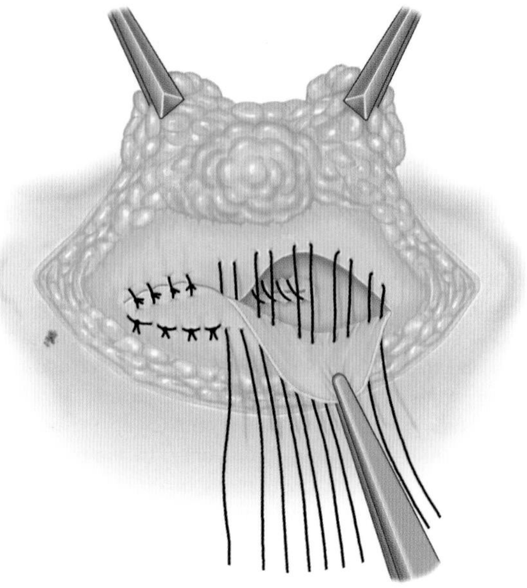

Fig. 27.9 Repair of a para-umbilical hernia.

clinically. In other instances, the local features of strangulation may be obvious. The operative approach is as for an elective case, and the strangulating contents are dealt with according to their state.

EPIGASTRIC HERNIA

Anatomy

The linea alba is the raphe formed by the junction of the rectus sheaths and the decussation of their fibres across the midline; it extends from the xiphoid process to the symphysis pubis. In its upper half, it is 1–3 cm wide and fibrous, but below the umbilicus it is a narrow cord.

Pathological features

The linea may be attenuated because of a congenital weakness in its lattice structure. Small neurovascular bundles that penetrate are also points of diminished resistance. Herniations of extraperitoneal fat through the linea usually occur in its upper half. They are found in 1% of the population from adolescence onwards. Males are three times more commonly affected than females, and the protrusions are multiple in 20% of cases. The initial extraperitoneal fat protrusion may be followed by the formation of a peritoneal sac, and omentum may enter this (intestinal contents are rare). Extraperitoneal fat or omentum is frequently incarcerated and may strangulate.

Clinical features

Symptoms

Three-quarters of epigastric hernias are asymptomatic and found incidentally on physical examination. When symptoms are present they are of two types:

- local pain – often exacerbated by physical exertion
- ill-defined pain – epigastric in site, often worse after meals (abdominal distension may strangulate the contents), and the clinical picture may mimic that of peptic ulceration.

Signs

The hernia may be visible if the patient is placed in an oblique light. The swelling is palpable in the midline and is usually tender and irreducible.

A patient who presents with vague upper-abdominal symptoms and in whom an epigastric hernia is found should be fully investigated for the possibility of peptic ulcer, gall-bladder or pancreatic disease before symptoms are attributed to the hernia.

Management

Patients with symptomatic hernias are offered repair. The herniated fat is excised. If a sac is present, the contents are reduced and the sac excised. The fascial defect is closed by suture. Any coincidental defects are similarly dealt with at the same time.

INCISIONAL HERNIA

An incisional hernia is one that occurs through the wound of a previous operation. It has the same features as a hernia that is caused by non-surgical injury to the abdominal wall.

It is realistic to expect that 1% of transparietal abdominal incisions are followed by a hernia. Such hernias comprise 10% of the total number seen.

Aetiology

Partial dehiscence of all or part of the deeper fascial layers occurs, but the skin remains intact or eventually heals. An incisional hernia is a postoperative complication and, like all such complications, its cause can be considered in terms of three factors: preoperative, operative and postoperative.

Preoperative factors

- Age – the tissues of the elderly do not heal as well as those of the young.
- Malnutrition – protein-calorie malnutrition, vitamin deficiency (vitamin C is essential for collagen maturation) and trace metal deficiency (zinc is required for epithelialisation).
- Sepsis – worsens malnutrition and delays anabolism.
- Uraemia – inhibits fibroblast division.
- Jaundice – impedes collagen maturation.
- Obesity – predisposes to wound infection, seroma and haematoma.
- Diabetes mellitus – predisposes to wound infection.
- Steroids – have a generalised proteolytic effect.
- Peritoneal contamination (peritonitis) – predisposes to wound infection.

Operative factors

- Type of incision – vertical incisions are more prone to hernia than are transverse ones.
- Technique and materials – tension in the closure impedes blood supply to the wound; badly tied knots can work loose; closure with rapidly absorbable suture material fails to support the abdominal wall for a sufficient time to permit sound union.
- Type of operation – operations involving the bowel or urinary tract are more likely to develop wound infection.
- Drains – a drain passing through the wound often results in a hernia.

Postoperative factors

- Wound infection – equal in importance with the wrong choice of suture material: there is enzymatic destruction of healing tissues; inflammatory swelling raises tissue tension and impedes blood supply; 5–20% of wound infections result in a hernia.
- Abdominal distension – postoperative ileus increases the tension on a wound; stitches may cut out.
- Coughing – generates wound tension.

An abdominal wound left open to heal by secondary intention, either planned or unplanned, will result in an incisional hernia.

Approximately 40% of incisional hernias occur with a documented episode of wound infection.

Pathological features

Most incisional hernias develop within 1 year of an operation, and it is unusual for a previously sound closure to become herniated after 3 years. Once a hernia has formed, mechanical forces ensure that it inexorably enlarges.

Incisional hernias are extremely variable. They may be wide or narrow-necked; often, as contents accumulate, adhesions develop in the sac, and just deep to the neck, so that the hernia becomes both irreducible and loculated. Incarceration and strangulation then become real dangers. The sac can assume huge proportions, eventually housing much of the normal intraperitoneal contents.

Clinical features

Symptoms

There may have been a stormy convalescence from a surgical procedure. The complaint is of a bulge in the scar. As the hernia enlarges and loculates, symptoms of subacute intestinal obstruction are common. The hernia may give rise to local discomfort. The overlying skin may become thin and atrophic; eventually ulceration and even rupture can occur. Strangulation is a surgical emergency.

Signs

Examination reveals a readily apparent, usually reducible, hernia with a cough impulse at the site of an old scar. If the hernia is complex, many fibrous bands may be felt passing between the margins of the defect. When the patient is lying flat, these hernias are deceptively small, but any manoeuvre that raises intra-abdominal pressure produces the hernia in all its glory.

Management

Even small symptomatic hernias should be repaired early. In asymptomatic hernias the risks of intestinal obstruction, strangulation and skin ulceration are such that repair, even in older patients, is often also recommended. Protracted observation simply allows the hernia to increase in size, and subsequent repair is rendered more difficult and hazardous. The surgical technique is the same as for para-umbilical hernias (see above), but larger hernias may require prosthetic mesh reconstruction of the abdominal wall.

Laparoscopic repair of incisional hernias is performed by gaining access to the peritoneal cavity to allow insufflation, followed by insertion of camera and instrument ports away from the hernia. This is not always easily achieved because of intra-abdominal adhesions. The hernia is reduced carefully by division of adhesions between contents and sac; this is the time at which injury to the bowel most easily occurs. The defect (or defects) are isolated with at least 5 cm clearance on all sides, to allow satisfactory mesh placement. Commonly, a double-sided mesh is placed with one side coated with hyaluronate facing the bowel, to minimise adhesion of bowel to mesh. The mesh is placed and secured with tacks and/or sutures intraperitoneally, with generous overlap of the edges of the defect.

Repair of very large incisional hernias involving much of the anterior abdominal wall are rarely undertaken laparoscopically because of the difficulty in securing adequate overlap of the mesh over the defect.

Outcome

The results of surgery are not as good as for primary hernias. Small incisional hernias have a recurrence rate of 2–5%, whereas in large ones it is 10–20%.

RARE BUT CLINICALLY IMPORTANT HERNIAS

The following hernias comprise only 1% of the total, but they are considered because their recognition is of clinical importance.

Interparietal hernia (Fig. 27.10)

The hernial sac lies between the layers of the abdominal wall. The cause may be congenital, when there is an associated abnormality of testicular descent, or acquired in an area of weakness in the lateral aspect of the deep inguinal ring and inguinal canal (when the sac usually communicates with a concomitant indirect inguinal hernia). The classification of such hernias is based on the anatomical location of the sac:

- properitoneal (20%)
- interstitial (60%)
- superficial (20%).

Clinical features

The properitoneal type of hernia is impalpable. The interstitial and superficial types often present with a small swelling above and lateral to the inguinal canal and deep ring. Such insignificant local features are ignored by patients, and 90% of these hernias present with intestinal obstruction that culminates in strangulation. The key to early diagnosis is to consider this type of hernia in any patient with the features of intestinal obstruction (simple or strangulating) with a palpable mass lateral to the deep ring and an abnormally placed testis.

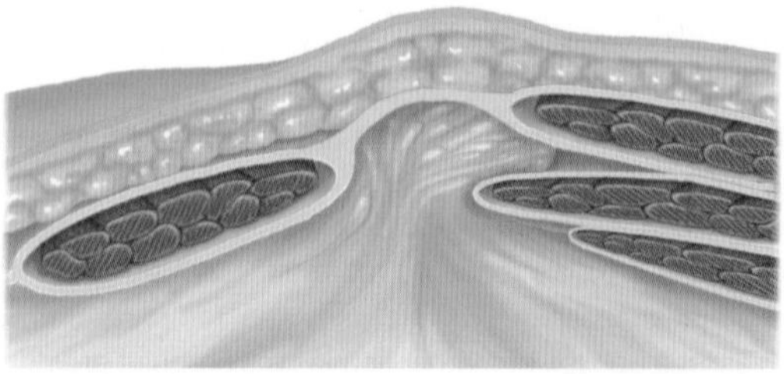

Fig. 27.10 Interparietal hernia.

Management

Operation (usually an emergency laparotomy for strangulating obstruction of unknown cause) reveals the hernial sac, which is excised and the fascial defect repaired.

Spigelian hernia

This is an interparietal hernia in the line of the linea semilunaris (the lateral margin of the rectus sheath, running from the tip of the ninth costal cartilage to the pubic crest). The hernia is usually at the level of the arcuate line, below which all aponeurotic layers are reflected anterior to the rectus muscle. The cause is related to the aponeurotic arrangement, which results in an area of weakness where fibres from the transversus aponeurosis fuse with those from the internal oblique. The hernial sac emerges and enlarges like a mushroom deep to the external oblique.

Clinical features

Symptoms

Symptoms are:

- local pain that is worse on straining
- lump
- non-specific lower-quadrant discomfort which needs to be investigated in its own right
- features of obstruction or strangulation.

Signs

Signs are:

- tenderness at the site of the hernial orifice
- lump which may be difficult or even impossible to feel.

Investigation and management

Recently, ultrasonography has proved useful in the demonstration of these hernias in patients with convincing histories but who lack clinical signs. Repair is a simple matter of excising the sac and closing the defect.

Obturator hernia

In this condition, herniation occurs along the obturator canal, which carries the obturator nerve and vessels out of the pelvis (Fig. 27.11). It is most commonly seen in frail old ladies. The hernia starts as a pre-peritoneal plug and gradually enlarges, taking a sac of peritoneum with it. A loop of bowel may enter the sac and reduce spontaneously. Eventually a knuckle fails to reduce. Further loops can then be incorporated. A Richter's strangulation is common.

Clinical features

Symptoms

Lying deep to the pectineus, these hernias are largely asymptomatic until complicated by intestinal obstruction or

Rare but clinically important hernias

strangulation. There is often a past history of intermittent symptoms of obstruction. In about 50% there may be the complaint of pain along the upper medial side of the thigh which radiates down to the knee, caused by pressure on the obturator nerve. Though present, this symptom is often not elicited.

Signs

There are rarely any signs, except those of obstruction or strangulation. The diagnosis is made in most instances at the time of laparotomy for small-bowel obstruction of unknown cause. With pressure on the obturator nerve, the patient holds the leg flexed to reduce the pain. In 20% of patients, the hernial sac protrudes medially around the pectineus and presents as a palpable swelling in the femoral triangle. Rectal and especially vaginal examination can reveal a swelling in the region of the obturator foramen.

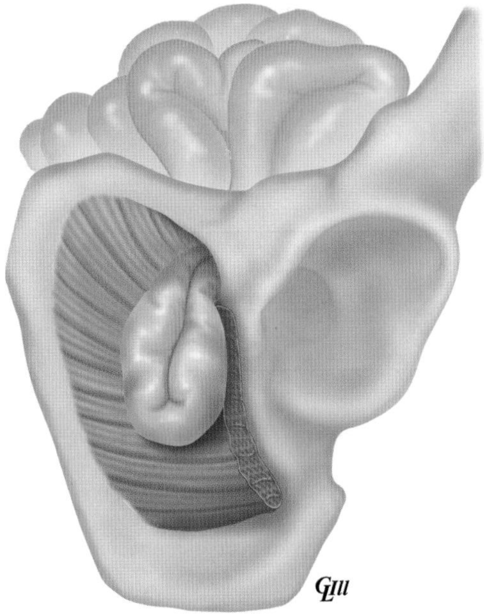

Fig. 27.11 Obturator hernia.

Management

If discovered at laparotomy, the intestine is reduced, the sac withdrawn and the defect closed. If the diagnosis is made clinically, an elective procedure by the retropubic, preperitoneal approach can be done.

Lumbar hernia

Such hernias may be:

- congenital
- acquired primary
- acquired secondary – the result of surgical incision.

Acquired hernias through an incision for lumbar approach to the kidney are not uncommon; however, with the decline in open renal surgery they are becoming less common.

Acquired primary lumbar hernia

Hernias that occur through anatomical weak points in the lumbar region – the superior and inferior lumbar triangles (Fig. 27.12) – are uncommon.

Clinical features

Most present with a bulge or lump in the flank, associated with an aching discomfort. There is usually a cough impulse and the mass is reducible. The contents are most often small and large bowel – very rarely the kidney. Some 20% become incarcerated and 10% strangulate.

An irreducible lumbar hernia must be distinguished from:

- lipoma
- soft-tissue tumour
- haematoma
- tuberculous cold abscess
- renal tumour.

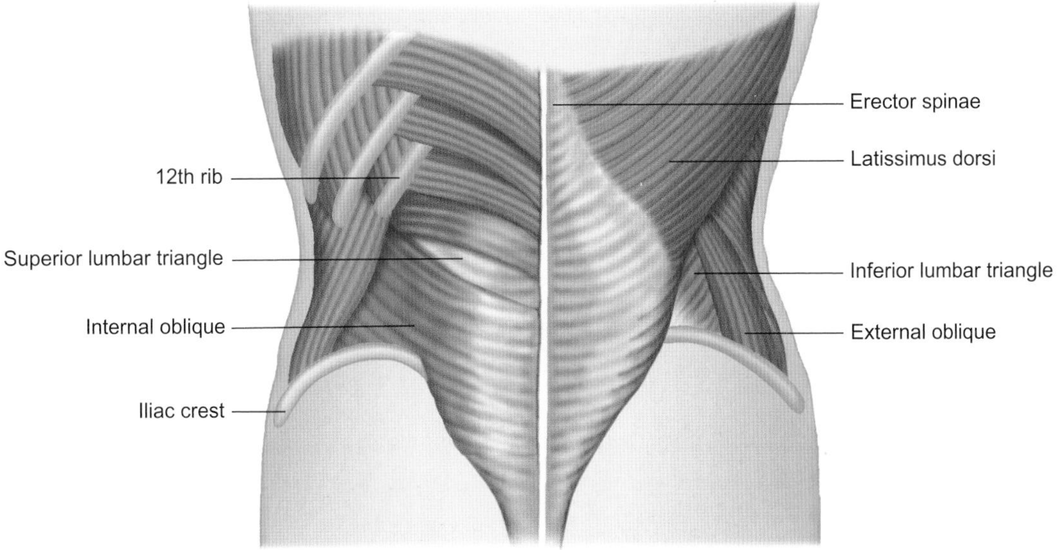

Fig. 27.12 Lumbar hernia.

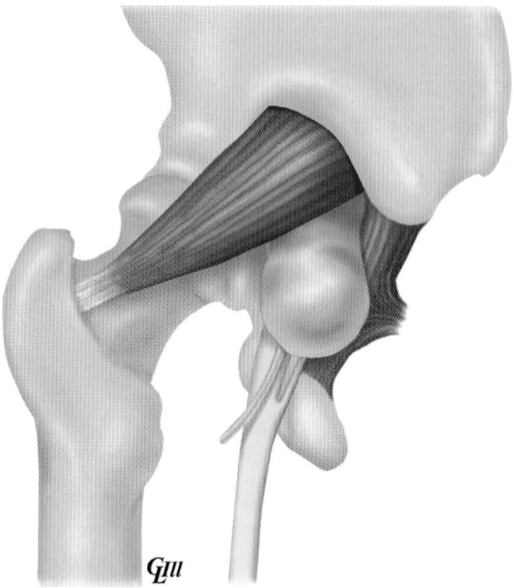

Fig. 27.13 Sciatic hernia.

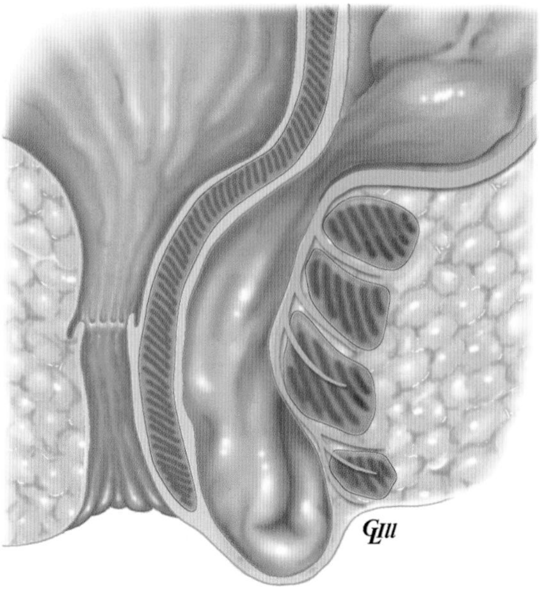

Fig. 27.14 Perineal hernia.

Management

Primary hernias are managed by direct closure of the defect. Large incisional hernias require a mesh prosthesis.

Sciatic hernia

A sciatic hernia is the protrusion of a pelvic peritoneal sac through the greater or lesser sciatic foramen (Fig. 27.13).

Clinical features

Patients present with discomfort and a swelling in the buttock, and there may be symptoms of sciatic nerve compression. If the hernia is large, there is a reducible mass in the gluteal area, made larger on standing. Herniation of the ureters can cause urinary symptoms. There is an appreciable risk of strangulation.

Management

Treatment is by excision of the sac and closure of the defect by a transabdominal or transgluteal approach.

Perineal hernia (Fig. 27.14)

These may be:

- congenital
- primary acquired
- incisional.

Primary acquired perineal hernias occur in middle-aged, multiparous women. Their broad pelvis and the muscle-weakening effect of childbirth result in herniation through the pelvic floor. Incisional perineal hernia follows 1% of combined abdominoperineal excisions of the rectum.

Clinical features

There is usually a perineal swelling and discomfort when sitting. A soft mass is found in the perineum, which is usually reducible. The wide neck has elastic margins. These hernias rarely have dangerous complications.

Management

Repair is by a combined abdominal and pelvic approach. The hernia is approached from below, the sac dissected free and reduced into the abdominal cavity. A laparotomy is performed and the pelvic floor repaired from above.

28 Breast disease

Breast symptoms are a common reason for patients to visit their doctor and many are concerned that they have breast cancer. In fact, only 1 in 10 patients referred to surgical clinics has a carcinoma – the remainder have a variety of conditions going under the general title of 'benign breast disease'. Many of the conditions that this term encompasses are not truly diseases but rather aberrations of normal development/involution of the breast that occur from puberty to old age. For this reason benign breast diseases are now referred to under the ANDI classification (Aberration of Normal Development and Involution) which highlights the relationship between normal stages of breast growth and the aberrations which represent a true disease (Table 28.1).

BENIGN BREAST DISEASE

PUBERTAL PROBLEMS

Males

One of the earliest benign problems occurs in pubertal males rather than females when hormonal stimulation of male breast buds at the time of puberty results in often embarrassing rudimentary growth – gynaecomastia. The same condition occurs in old age when certain drugs (digoxin, spironolactone, cimetidine) and conditions (cirrhosis of the liver) can, by interfering with sex hormone metabolism, induce growth of the breast buds. Very rarely the same problem can be induced by hormone-producing tumours.

Females

At puberty, excessive development is known as juvenile hypertrophy and is characterised by the growth of very large breasts which are both uncomfortable and embarrassing.

COMMON BREAST SYMPTOMS IN BENIGN DISEASE

Patients present with one or more of the following symptoms or signs:

- pain – cyclical or non-cyclical
- lumpiness and lumps
- nipple discharge
- trauma
- infection.

The common conditions underlying these symptoms are summarised in Figure 28.1.

PAIN

This is either cyclical or non-cyclical. The first follows the pattern of the menstrual cycle; the second is random in timing.

Table 28.1 Classification of benign breast disease into ANDI

Stage	Normal	Aberration	Disease
Early reproductive (15–25 years)	Lobular development Stromal development Nipple eversion	Fibroadenoma Adolescent hypertrophy Nipple inversion	Giant fibroadenoma Gigantomastia Subareolar abscess Mammary duct fistula
Mature reproductive (25–40 years)	Cyclical changes Epithelial hyperplasia of pregnancy	Cyclical mastalgia Bloody nipple discharge	Severe mastalgia
Involution (35–55 years)	Lobular involution Duct involution – dilatation–sclerosis Epithelial turnover	Macrocysts Sclerosing lesions Duct ectasia/nipple retraction Epithelial hyperplasia	Periductal mastitis/abscess With atypia

ANDI, aberration of normal development and involution.

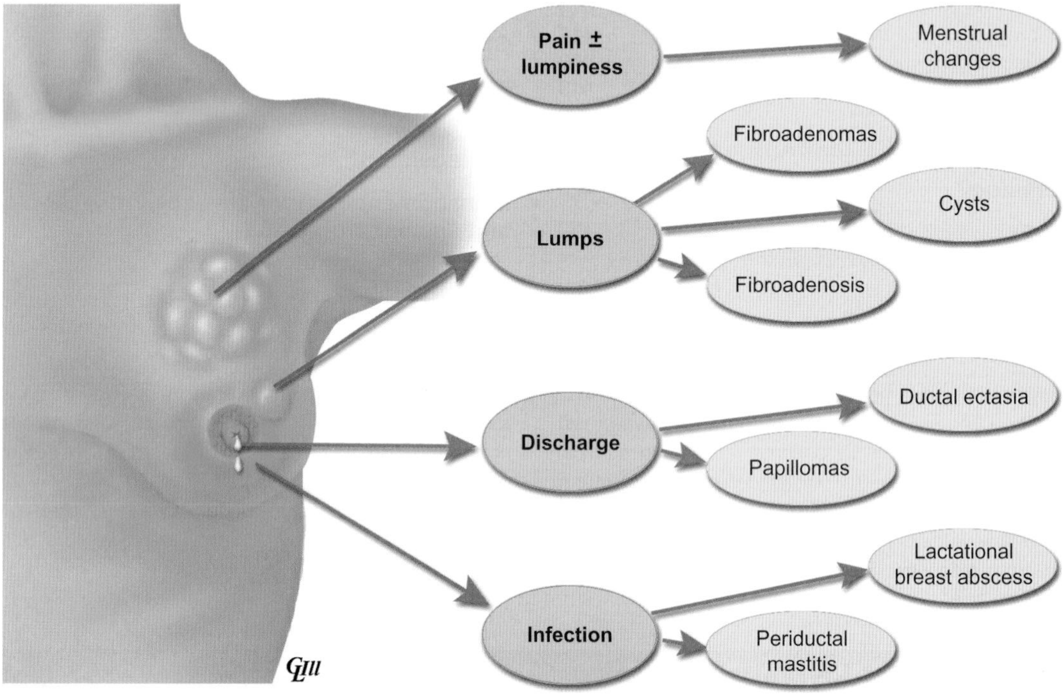

Fig. 28.1 Common causes of breast symptoms.

Cyclical pain

Onset is during the early phase of the cycle; intensity gradually worsens to reach a peak just before menstruation, easing with the start of the period. In its mildest form, the pain affects the upper outer quadrants of the breasts and causes only minor inconvenience. In more severe instances, the whole breast may feel engorged, tender and heavy; physical contact can be unbearable, which often leads to psychological distress. Some postmenopausal women get breast pain which is often related to the use of hormone replacement therapy, in that this keeps the cells of the breast active.

Not every instance follows such a clear-cut clinical pattern. Pain may be in one breast only and some may experience pain nearly all the time, although this tends to get worse as menstruation approaches. There is no clear-cut explanation for these wide variations but they are probably related to subtle differences in hormone responsiveness and sensitivity within the breast which may vary throughout life. Such variable thresholds could also account for the fact that some patients go through very bad patches which disappear as abruptly as they start.

There are few clinical findings apart from tenderness and a firm nodular feeing in the upper outer quadrants of the breast.

Investigation

In the presence of a typical history of bilateral cyclical pain, there is often little reason to embark on any investigations. Mammograms are of no diagnostic help and are difficult to interpret in women under 35, the group most frequently affected by this problem. The only value they may serve is to exclude an underlying cancer in patients whose pain is atypical or is coincidental with a lump. A pain chart in which patients record their pain and its intensity is sometimes useful in determining whether the problem is truly cyclical or non-cyclical.

Management

The most important aspect is reassurance that the condition is entirely benign and is not associated with either carcinoma or a tendency to its development in later life. Many are content to live with their discomfort if they can be reassured on both these counts.

For patients whose symptoms are severe enough for them to desire symptomatic treatment, gamma-linoleic acid, danazol and the oestrogen antagonist tamoxifen have all been shown to be effective. Gamma-linoleic acid (most easily available in the form of evening primrose oil or star flower oil) is an essential fatty acid which is thought to work by rendering breast cells less sensitive to the effects of sex hormones; 60% of sufferers experience relief, but to be of therapeutic value it needs to be taken in full dose (320 mg daily) for 3–4 months before a benefit is really experienced.

Danazol interferes with the action of oestrogen on breast tissue, and bromocriptine blocks the pituitary drive to produce follicle-stimulating hormone (FSH) and luteinising hormone (LH). Danazol is usually given in doses of 200–300 mg daily, but side-effects due to its androgenic activity occur in up to 25% of women. Tamoxifen also works by blocking the effects of oestrogen but can only be used for a short while on a named-patient basis for resistant mastalgia in view of its carcinogenic and other side-effects. Bromocriptine, a dopamine agonist, is also effective, but at the price of significant side-effects which have led to its decreasing utilisation in recent years. These treatments are effective for typical cyclical pain but are less satisfactory when the pain is not quite so typical.

Non-cyclical pain

This may be intermittent or constant and may be confined to localised areas of one breast. It can be caused by conditions both within and without the breast, including:

- mammary duct ectasia
- periductal mastitis
- trauma.

Tietze's syndrome (osteochondritis) is characterised by tenderness over the costochondral junctions.

It is often difficult to identify a specific cause of non-cyclical pain, and care must be taken not to overlook other causes of referred and localised chest wall pain.

Investigation

As with cyclical breast pain, investigation in those under the age of 35 is limited to clinical assessment with or without ultrasound as indicated. However, in older women, mammography is often a wise precaution, particularly if the pain is consistently localised to one spot or associated with a lump. A small number (10%) with such features have an underlying carcinoma.

Management

Non-cyclical pain is much more resistant to treatment than is cyclical breast pain. Hormonal manipulation is often ineffective but worth trying, as is firm support with an appropriately fitted bra. Simple NSAIDs, treatment of inflammatory conditions or an injection of lidocaine (lignocaine) and steroid into the area may all be helpful. Quite a large number find all treatment of little benefit and end up having to live with their pain until it resolves by itself, which in the great majority it eventually does.

BREAST LUMPINESS AND LUMPS

The potential diagnoses in a patient who presents with a breast lump depend on whether it is a part of a diffuse lumpiness or a single discrete isolated lump. Other features which may influence the diagnosis are whether the lump is painful and the age of the patient.

Until recently, it was axiomatic that any palpable breast abnormality should undergo excision biopsy in case a cancer, however unlikely, might be overlooked. A recent major change in management has been a shift from this approach to the use of physical examination, radiological imaging (mammography) and needle biopsy to reach a definitive diagnosis – the 'triple approach'. In consequence, there are now fewer open biopsies which lead to a diagnosis of benign disease; the current ratio of benign to malignant biopsy is 0.6 : 1.

However, mammography is of little value in women under 35 years of age because the breasts are frequently too dense for small lesions to be seen. Some radiologists feel that this is also true for women up to the age of 40 and in consequence do not recommend mammography below this age. For women unsuitable for mammography, ultrasound offers a useful tool for evaluating palpable lesions but is a very poor method of general screening of the breast to exclude malignant disease.

Lumpiness

Lumpiness can present on its own but is frequently associated with cyclical breast pain. In common with pain, it is a manifestation of the cyclical changes that go on in the female breast during the menstrual years. A variety of descriptive terms have been applied to it:

- fibroadenosis
- cystic mastopathy
- fibrocystic disease
- cystic mastitis.

All are merely descriptive of the changes seen to a varying degree on histological examination and do not give any insight into cause. Their use carries the danger that the clinical condition becomes labelled as a disease when it is in fact part of the spectrum of normal behaviour of the breast which in some individuals is more pronounced.

Discrete single lump

The common causes of a lump are:

- fibroadenoma
- cyst
- very localised fibroadenosis.

The feature uniting them all is the well-defined nature of the lump.

Fibroadenosis

Clinical features

History

The encouragement of women to undertake regular self-examination may draw attention to the possible presence of a lump or of changes in consistency. Alternatively, cyclical or non-cyclical pain may lead to the discovery of what the patient regards as a lump. Usually, the upper outer quadrants are affected but, as with pain, one side alone may be involved. The majority of women who seek medical advice are young, often in the early years after the menarche.

Physical findings

There may be single or multiple lumps in one or both breasts, which may be acutely tender, particularly premenstrually.

Investigation

Imaging

Mammography is indicated in those over the age of 35 (see also breast cancer, below). In a lumpy breast, the appearances are those of dense fibrosis with micro- or macrocystic change.

Ultrasound may be combined with mammography and is indicated as the sole initial imaging modality for those under 35.

Fine-needle aspiration cytology (FNAC)/core biopsy

Only areas of clinical or radiological concern are submitted to either needle core biopsy or FNAC. There is no place for random 'hoover' type FNAC of benign nodularity.

Management

Provided that imaging and FNAC have eliminated the diagnosis of malignancy, the essential treatment is reassurance based on the concept that the changes are part of the normal spectrum of the breast response to female sex hormones.

Fibroadenoma

These tend to affect younger women and are infrequent after about 35–40 years of age.

Pathological features

Many remain static and a small proportion either regress or increase in size.

Clinical features

Generally, the patient discovers the lump. Pain and other symptoms are absent. A rare variant, usually in older women, is known as a phyllodes tumour.

Physical findings are of a well-defined lump, nearly always in an otherwise normal breast. The consistency is rubbery to firm or hard, and there is such mobility that it may be difficult to find – hence the nickname 'breast mouse'.

Investigation and management

As with any discrete lump they should be subjected to triple assessment (clinical examination, imaging and FNAC/core biopsy). Provided all these support a diagnosis of fibroadenoma, small lesions can be left alone. However, larger lesions (>4 cm) or those in older women may be better removed. Some authorities advocate repeating the assessment at 3 months if a conservative policy has been adopted.

Cysts

Epidemiology and aetiology

Occurrence is usually at a slightly later stage of life than fibroadenoma – after 35 and through to the menopause. Cysts probably form under the same influences that cause the other cyclical breast changes.

Clinical features

The history is of a palpable and occasionally tender lump.

Physical findings are of a tense, discrete, mobile lump anywhere in the breast. Fluctuation can be difficult to elicit in a small cyst.

Investigation and management

Whenever a clinical diagnosis is made of a cyst, it should be assessed with imaging which will often be by mammography and ultrasound; this is usually followed by aspiration. It yields straw-coloured fluid and causes collapse of the cyst. Equally important, it immediately reassures the patient; however, there have to be some exceptions:

- failure of the lump completely to disappear
- bloodstained aspirate
- uncertain imaging.

Failure to disappear completely

Re-evaluation must take place within a few weeks. A persistent lump must be evaluated by mammography if not already undertaken and be subject to FNAC/core biopsy or excised for histological examination.

Bloodstained aspirate

The simple cause is a traumatic aspiration. However, this must be confirmed by cytological examination of the aspirate and by mammography. Clinical reassessment, re-aspiration if a lump is present, or excision biopsy is then the appropriate course.

In uncomplicated circumstances, follow-up is probably not necessary, but it is reassuring to both patient and doctor for a single re-examination to take place about 6 weeks later. If there has not been recurrence, the patient is discharged with the caveat that any new lump must be subject to a repeat of the initial management.

Uncertain imaging

This will usually prompt a biopsy as occasionally a carcinoma can present as an intracystic lesion which may be associated with either bloodstained aspirate or failure of the lump to disappear with aspiration but may be visible on initial imaging before aspiration is undertaken.

Multiple cysts

Some patients have multiple cysts identified at mammography or which present clinically as a lumpy breast. Danazol can be helpful in reducing the incidence of clinical recurrence. There is no benefit to routine follow-up in these patients, but they are encouraged to return with any symptomatic lumps.

NIPPLE DISCHARGE

There are three common causes:

- mammary duct ectasia
- duct papilloma
- galactorrhoea.

An important point to establish is whether the discharge is from a single or from multiple ducts. That from a single duct, particularly if bloodstained, is more likely to be associated with a papilloma. Discharges are commoner in women over 35. In younger women they may be associated with the oral contraceptive.

Mammary duct ectasia

Aetiology and pathological features

The cause, as with many breast disorders, is an exaggeration of the normal cyclical changes – a wear and tear process. The ducts adjacent to the nipple become dilated and engorged with breast secretions. Secondary infection and a retroareolar abscess may form, but even if this does not happen, fibrosis can cause nipple retraction.

Clinical features

History

The discharge can range from milky to dirty green and is often, but not always, bilateral. Occasionally it is associated with pain, usually cyclical. Acute infection causes pain and swelling.

Physical findings

The breast may have features of lumpiness (see above). The chronic inflammation often associated with the condition causes a characteristic retraction of the nipple, which gives it a slit-like appearance that may be confused with carcinoma. In acute inflammation, an abscess forms which, if not treated at an early stage, discharges at the areolar margin. A small sinus (mammary fistula) then results which can be the focus of further attacks of inflammation.

Investigation and management

If qualified by age, patients should have a mammogram to establish the general state of the breast. There is little point in sending discharge for cytological assessment unless it is obtained by ductal lavage, which is not a widely used technique.

Provided the investigations are normal, nothing further needs to be done other than to reassure the patient. If a discharge is very troublesome, excision of the duct system (Hadfield's operation) provides symptomatic relief.

Abscess

An abscess in this condition is followed, as described above, by a mammary fistula. In consequence, after drainage there is often not only a persistent discharge but also the risk of recurrence. The involved duct and its drainage area should be excised electively. The organisms involved are often a mixed culture with anaerobes that do not respond to purely anti-staphylococcal antibiotics but need drugs covering a broader spectrum such as co-amoxiclav.

Duct papilloma

This is a relatively common cause of bloodstained single duct discharge.

Clinical features

There is a serous or bloodstained discharge from a single aspect of the nipple although the patient may not realise that the discharge is localised. Other symptoms are rarely present.

The breast is normal, but there is either the spontaneous appearance of discharge from one aspect of the nipple or 'milking' of a segment produces nipple discharge from the duct draining that segment.

Investigation

The main concern, particularly if the discharge is bloodstained, is that occasionally there is an underlying malignancy although duct papilloma is benign.

Investigations are the same as for mammary duct ectasia. However, in spite of negative cytological findings, it is nearly always necessary, in a bloodstained single duct discharge, to excise the involved system to establish that a papilloma is present. The operation is known as microductectomy.

Galactorrhoea

This is a rare cause of bilateral milky discharge. It follows lactation and is caused by a persistent elevation of prolactin, although it can sometimes occur with normal hormone levels.

Management

Bromocriptine is used until the discharge subsides. Prolactinomas should be considered in long-persistent discharge but are rare.

TRAUMA

Trauma to the breast is relatively rare, although sexual encounters and love bites may be responsible for local injury. A blunt impact can interfere with local blood supply and, together with a haematoma, cause fat necrosis. Another cause is the use of therapeutic anticoagulants in patients with very large and pendulous breasts in which very minor trauma may precipitate extensive haemorrhage, which may go on to necrosis.

Clinical features

Fat necrosis causes a hard painful lump usually following a story of minor local trauma.

A hard lump is often found, with some irregularity and occasionally tethering to the overlying skin. The appearances are suggestive of a carcinoma but the condition can usually be distinguished because of the history of trauma, associated bruising and resolution of the lump with observation.

Investigation and management

Investigation is the same as for any discrete lump. The condition resolves with time, and specific treatment is not required.

INFECTION

There are two common causes of infection:

- lactational breast abscess
- periductal mastitis.

Lactational breast abscess

Aetiology and pathological features

The condition is a complication of lactation and breast-feeding; the organism involved is nearly always *Staphylococcus aureus*. It is believed that bacteria get into the breast through cracks in the nipple during feeding. A segment of breast becomes inflamed so that there is initially cellulitis; however, the nature of staphylococcal infection means that there is a rapid build-up of tension, which is further contributed to by the lobular nature of the breast and necrosis to produce an abscess after a relatively short time. The abscess may break through into neighbouring segments and thus become multilocular.

Clinical features

History

The baby may be anything from a few days to some months old. The mother may have noticed an obvious crack in the nipple, although this is unusual. Segmental pain in the affected breast rapidly becomes severe, and sleep is often lost.

Physical findings

A tender red segment in the breast is seen, perhaps with evidence of nipple damage as a crack in its surface. Fluctuation is not a feature unless the abscess is advanced and beginning to point towards the skin, which may ultimately show evidence of necrosis.

Management

If detected and treated early, acute mastitis can resolve. Anti-staphylococcal antibiotics are prescribed in full doses. If the nipple is obviously damaged, feeding on this side can be stopped but the milk must be expressed by other means. Continued pain and loss of sleep suggest that there is an abscess which in its early stages can be aspirated with a wide-bore needle under local anaesthetic. This is usually done under ultrasound control and may need to be repeated several times before the condition resolves. Skin changes of thinning and necrosis require formal drainage and breakdown of all the loculi under general anaesthetic. Such an event usually puts an end to breast-feeding.

Periductal mastitis

Aetiology and pathological features

This condition commonly affects young women in their 30s but can occur in older ladies. It is associated with smoking and is characterised histologically by a low-grade inflammatory response around the ducts adjacent to the nipple. In consequence, an alternative name is 'plasma cell mastitis'. The bacteria involved are nearly always anaerobes.

Clinical features

Tenderness develops on one aspect of the areola. There is rarely any systemic disturbance. Recurrent bouts may occur before the patient seeks medical attention.

A tender swelling at the edge of the areola is seen, which may progress to abscess formation with a periareolar sinus and discharge.

Investigation and management

Because there may be a discrete mass with only a few, if any, characteristics of inflammation, FNAC/core biopsy and mammography may be necessary to exclude an underlying carcinoma.

Inflammatory swellings may respond to antibiotics which need to cover a broader spectrum than *Staphylococcus aureus* such as co-amoxiclav; however, when an abscess has formed it requires the same treatment as a lactational abscess, which is usually drainage rather than aspiration. A complication of abscess is the formation of a mammary duct fistula, which discharges intermittently and may be associated with recurrent abscess formation. The duct segment must then be excised because, in the presence of a duct abnormality, attempts to eradicate sepsis with antibiotics are usually futile. This can prove a difficult condition to eradicate.

MALIGNANT BREAST DISEASE

EPIDEMIOLOGY

Breast cancer is the second commonest form of cancer to affect women in the developed world (lung cancer is commonest). It accounts for 18% of all cancers in women. The UK has an incidence of 2 per 1000 women per year, with a prevalence of nearly 2% in women aged 50. Whilst mortality from breast cancer continues to fall, the incidence of the disease is also increasing, with the UK having the highest worldwide standardised incidence and mortality. The probabilities of developing the disease were estimated at 1 : 13 in 1970, 1 : 11 in 1980 and 1 : 9 in 1992.

AETIOLOGY

The risk factors for breast cancer are listed in Table 28.2. The most significant factors influencing relative risk are:

- age
- country of birth
- genetic factors, particularly a history of breast cancer in a first-degree relative
- hormonal factors
- miscellaneous.

Age

Breast cancer is rare under the age of 35. Between the ages of 30 and 34 the incidence and mortality rates in the UK are 19.6 and 5.9 per 100000 women, respectively; between 50 and 54 years these rise to 145.9 and 73.7 per 100000 and they continue to increase further with age (Fig. 28.2). In general the incidence doubles every year until the menopause, when the curve starts to flatten out.

Country of birth

Generally breast cancer is less common in the Far East and more common in the West. However, migrant studies indicate that migrants assume the risk of the host community with two generations. Furthermore, although the less industrialised nations tend to have lower rates of breast cancer, this difference is diminishing. There is undoubtedly a large environmental component to breast cancer risk.

Genetic factors

Germline mutations in known and unknown breast cancer susceptibility genes account for an estimated 5–10% of cases of breast cancer (Table 28.3). Unfortunately in the majority of cases definitive markers have not been identified that would facilitate early identification of high-risk individuals. When a marker is unavailable, various statistical models of risk are available that allow the risk to individual patients to be quantified in order to plan appropriate management. Such eponymous models include the Claus and Gail models. Guidelines are available for selecting high-risk women for further investigation and treatment (Box 28.1). It should be remembered that the genes can be transmitted through

Box 28.1 Guidelines for selecting women at high risk of developing hereditary breast cancer

At least twofold relative risk
- First-degree relative who developed breast cancer at age 50 years or less
- First-degree relative who developed bilateral breast cancer
- Two or more second-degree relatives who developed breast or ovarian cancer

Fourfold or greater relative risk
- Four or more relatives affected at any age by breast or ovarian cancer
- Three relatives affected with breast or ovarian cancer with an average age of diagnosis of the breast cancer of less than 60 years
- Two relatives affected by breast cancer with an average age of less than 40 years
- One first-degree relative with both breast and ovarian cancer

Table 28.2 Factors affecting the risk of developing breast cancer

Factor	High risk	Low risk
Age (years)	Greater than 50	Less than 35
Country of birth	Northern Europe North America	Asia or Africa
First-degree relative affected	Yes	
Age at first pregnancy	>30 years	<20 years
Nulliparity	Yes	
Previous breast cancer	Yes	
History of atypical hyperplasia	Yes	

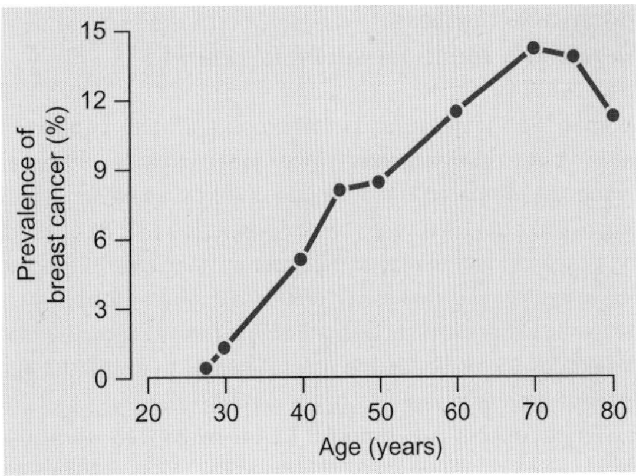

Fig. 28.2 Age and cancer of the breast.

Table 28.3 Genetic determinants of hereditary susceptibility to breast cancer

Hereditary syndromes	Gene defect	Location	Gene function	Percentage of hereditary breast cancer cases
Hereditary breast/ovary cancer	*BRCA1*	17q	Suppressor	35%
	BRCA2	13q	Suppressor	25%
	Unknown	?	?	35%
Li Fraumeni	*p53*	17p	Suppressor	rare
Cowden's	*PTEN*	10q	Suppressor	rare
Peutz–Jeghers	*LKB1*	19p	?	rare
HNPCC	*MSH2*	2p	Repair	rare
	MLH1	3p		rare

HNPCC, hereditary non-polyposis colorectal cancer.

either sex and, as penetrance is incomplete, not all carriers will develop the disease. Furthermore, as most breast cancers related to a genetic mutation occur in the younger age group, women with a strong family history who have not developed the disease by 65 are unlikely to have the mutation.

Around 60% of the 5–10% of hereditary breast cancers are now known to be related to two major breast cancer genes: *BRCA1* on chromosome 17q and *BRCA2* on chromosome 13q. They both appear to be tumour suppressor genes: *BRCA1* is associated in particular with breast and ovarian cancer, and *BRCA2* with cancer of the breast in both men and women and multiple other sites including the ovary and the pancreas. Mutations in these genes are rare in the general population, but it is now possible to offer predictive genetic testing, although the large number of associated mutations means that no reliable marker is available and, outside certain population groups, testing can only be performed if DNA is available from an index case in the family tree. Two percent of Ashkenazi Jews have characteristic *BRCA1* deletions and insertions at positions 185 (185 del AG), 6174 (6174 del T) and 5382 (5382 ins C), and *BRCA2* 999 del 5 is common in the Icelandic population. The risk of developing breast cancer associated with either gene is around 80–85% by the age of 70 years, although there are variations in penetrance associated with particular mutation subtypes. In established high-risk groups, risk-reducing mastectomy (rather than 'prophylactic' mastectomy, as risk cannot be eliminated completely) can reduce the risk of developing breast cancer by 90%.

Hormonal factors

Menarche, menopause, child-bearing and fertility

Women who undergo early menarche and late menopause suffer from approximately twice the incidence of breast cancer as compared with their peers. A woman having a child before the age of 18 years has one-third the risk of developing breast cancer than a primiparous woman over the age of 35. Infertility and nulliparity confer a higher probability of developing the disease, and a first full-term pregnancy after the age of 35 increases the risk to greater than that for nulliparous women.

These effects are thought to be related to persistent exposure to endogenous oestrogen in the absence of appropriate progesterone concentrations.

Exogenous hormones

Oral contraceptive pill There is a slightly increased risk of developing breast cancer with the use of the oral contraceptive pill and for 10 years after it has been stopped. Duration of use and type of pill are no longer thought to be important, although women who begin use before the age of 20 do have a higher relative risk. However, it should be remembered that the absolute risk in the age group is very small.

Hormone replacement therapy Oestrogen-containing hormone replacement therapy (HRT) increases the risk according to the duration of use over the age of 50. This is at least proportional to the increase seen in women whose menopause is delayed, which is a risk factor in its own right. The recent Women's Health Initiative (WHI) study from the USA has suggested that the relative risk may be even higher than this and appears to increase dramatically after a few years of use. However, relative risk must always be considered against the background of absolute risk, and the actual number of additional cancers caused is relatively small. Furthermore it appears that, although the incidence is increased, the mortality remains the same because the HRT-related cancers are generally of a good prognostic type.

Miscellaneous

Breast-feeding

Breast-feeding for a total time of greater than 36 months during a woman's reproductive years was thought to protect against the development of breast cancer. However, repeated observations have shown this to be untrue.

Diet

Dietary fat has been suggested as a risk factor, although its exact role remains controversial. The different amounts of saturated and unsaturated fat available within specific diets may be important. Omega-3 unsaturated fatty acids are found in abundance in marine food sources, and women such as Inuit and the Japanese who have a high intake of them also have a relatively low incidence of breast cancer. Furthermore, in Japan, incidence has doubled with the adoption of a more Westernised diet. Studies on immigrants confirm this trend: third-generation Japanese immigrants to the USA have almost the same risk for breast cancer as the indigenous American population.

Obesity

The information available from the epidemiological studies on diet and breast cancer is further complicated by the fact that obesity is a definite risk factor in its own right. In postmenopausal women, obesity directly correlates with an increase in breast cancer risk of up to twofold. However, these women tend to come from the more affluent Western societies where saturated animal fats in the diet are common.

Previous cancer

The risk of a second primary breast cancer is reported to be up to five times the general risk and is inversely related to age at presentation of the first. An ipsilateral second primary is more common in women with a family history. In general, about 0.5–1% of women with a previous history of breast cancer will be expected to develop a second primary each year for the next 15 years.

Women with a previous history of primary ovarian or endometrial cancer are also at an increased risk, although probably less than twice that of the general population.

Irradiation

Exposure to radiation increases risk. The effect is cumulative, and the incidence has been shown to be higher in survivors of nuclear weapon detonation and in women who have undergone multiple chest X-rays for monitoring of the progression of pulmonary tuberculosis (now uncommon).

Pregnancy

Pregnancy has been thought to be associated with a particularly aggressive form of breast cancer. Although more locally advanced cancers are diagnosed during pregnancy, there is not a higher incidence overall, and the prognosis is similar stage for stage with the normal population. In theory, a subsequent pregnancy in a patient who has had a previous oestrogen receptor-positive tumour (see below) could shorten the disease-free interval. However, evidence for this is lacking, although it is rational for such women to avoid oestrogen-containing compounds.

Previous benign disease

The relative risk of developing breast cancer in the presence of proven benign disease is outlined in Box 28.2. Benign lesions may be either proliferative or non-proliferative, with subgroups within the various types of proliferative lesions conferring varying levels of risk.

Non-proliferative lesions such as fibrocystic disease and simple cysts with or without apocrine changes in the breast do not appear to be associated with an increased risk.

Proliferative lesions are distinguished by epithelial hyperplasia that implies an increased number of cells above the basement membrane. The degree of hyperplasia is related to the number of layers found, e.g. mild hyperplasia is associated with three or more cells above the basement membrane in a lobular unit or duct. The presence of atypical cells within the hyperplasia is significant in that it confers a four- to fivefold greater risk of progressing to a carcinoma. Atypical hyperplasia may be ductal or lobular in origin. It is thought that hyperplasia forms part of a spectrum of benign disorders that have the potential for malignant transformation. Radial scars and so-called complex sclerosing lesions which are histologically similar to sclerosing adenosis are thought to have a slightly greater risk of later maligancy, although not as great as atypias. Cysts and duct ectasia do not have malignant potential.

Fibroadenomas (see above) are benign tumours. For those women with a simple fibroadenoma there is no increase in the incidence of subsequent breast cancer.

Papillomas arise from the epithelium of the large ductal network of the breast. The centrally placed papilloma tends to be single and has no proven malignant potential. However, those that occur peripherally are often multiple and can contain areas of atypical hyperplasia and even ductal carcinoma in situ (see below).

Factors without proven risk

Many possible risks have been related to breast cancer but have subsequently been disproved, although they remain a source of potential confusion (Box 28.3). Smoking is not a risk factor but, because it is related to earlier menopause, it has a popular but undeserved reputation as a protective factor. The balance of evidence supports neither a causative nor a protective role.

Gender

Male breast cancer is rare – less than 1% of all cases. It is associated with high endogenous levels of oestrogen, and is preceded by gynaecomastia in 20%. Testicular feminisation, Klinefelter's syndrome (XXY), oestrogen therapy, irradiation and trauma are all risk factors. Stage for stage, the prognosis is the same as for female breast cancer although it tends to present late. The treatment options are also similar.

NATURAL HISTORY

Tumour doubling time is the time taken for the mass of cells which make up the malignancy to double in number or the tumour to double in size. Estimates of the doubling time for a breast cancer are about 100 days and, on this basis, a growth that originated from a single cell would take 8 years to become a 1 cm diameter, clinically detectable, lump of 10^9 cells. This theoretical calculation is modified by the fact that doubling time is governed in practice by more complex factors: in the first 30 doublings the growth rate is not constant, and thereafter the rate of growth is slowed by the occurrence of cell death in the mass. A palpable breast tumour may therefore have been present for even longer than the simple calculation suggests. After 20 doublings the tumour acquires its own blood supply, and from then on cancer cells can be shed into the blood. The possibility of early spread to distant parts of the body is therefore present from an early stage and is added to by the rich lymphatic network of the breast, which can pick up cells from the intercellular spaces and transport them to the regional lymph nodes. However, successful implantation of the cells, either shed into the bloodstream or escaping from the primary

Box 28.2 Relative risk of developing breast cancer in relation to previous benign disease

No risk
- Apocrine change
- Ductal ectasia
- Mild hyperplasia (no atypia)

Slight risk
- Moderate or florid hyperplasia (no atypia)
- Sclerosing adenosis
- Papilloma

Moderate risk
- Atypical ductal or lobular hyperplasia

Box 28.3 Non-risk factors in breast cancer

- Diazepam
- Reserpine
- Cholecystectomy
- Thyroid disease
- Hair dyes
- Emotional stress
- Cigarette smoking
- Trauma to the breast with fat necrosis may distort the breast architecture but does not have malignant potential

Table 28.4 Survival in relation to axillary node status

Patient group	Survival (%) 5-year	Survival (%) 10-year
All patients	64	46
Node-negative	78	65
Node-positive	47	25

tumour via lymphatics, seldom occurs before the 27th doubling (5 cm) because, before this, natural killer cells and other macrophages of the immune system are able to cope with the malignant cell load. Systemic dissemination is critical because more than 95% of patients who die of breast cancer do so from distant metastasis. That blood-borne implanted micrometastases take place relatively early is evident from the fact that 20–25% of patients who do not have tumour in their regional lymph nodes at the time of their removal still experience relapse because of distant disease. Once tumour has also spread via the lymphatics to regional nodes, the figure rises to 50–75% (Table 28.4).

STAGING AND PROGNOSIS

It was recognised even before the concept of early micrometastases was understood that some form of staging of the disease could be helpful in assessing the likelihood of survival, although it is realised that it is blurred by the possible presence of micrometastases which will develop subsequently into distant recurrences.

TNM staging

The international TNM classification (Ch. 12 and Table 28.5) allows grouping of the disease into clinical stages. Staging allows comparison between groups of patients and also defines those unsuitable for an attempt at surgical removal but who may be suitable for the other forms of adjuvant therapy.

Node status in the axilla may be established at operation by histological examination either of an en bloc removal (axillary clearance) or by sampling nodes closest to the tumour. The technique of sentinel node sampling using blue dye and/or radioactive colloid has facilitated the identification of the lymph nodes directly draining the breast, offering the promise of more accurate lymph node staging with minimal morbidity. This is now becoming the most widely used technique to stage the axilla. The surgeon injects dye or radioactive colloid around the primary breast tumour. This drains via the lymphatic system to the axillary (or internal mammary nodes). The first node(s) to contain the dye or radioactive colloid is called the sentinel node(s). The surgeon can identify this node by inspection or a radioactive monitor. One to three of these sentinel nodes are removed and sent for histological analysis. If no cancer metastasis is identified on histology no further nodal clearance is undertaken. If the node(s) shows

Table 28.5 TNM classification of breast cancer

TNM stage	Pathological description
Tis	Carcinoma in situ (pre-invasive) Paget's disease (no palpable tumour)
T0	No clinical evidence of primary tumour
T1	Tumour less than 2 cm
T2	Tumour 2–5 cm
T3	Tumour greater than 5 cm
T4	Tumour of any size but with direct extension to chest wall or skin: (a) Fixation to chest wall (b) Oedema, lymphocytic infiltration, ulceration of skin or satellite nodes (c) Both (a) and (b)
N0	No palpable ipsilateral axillary lymph nodes
N1	Palpable nodes not fixed: (a) Inflammatory only (b) Containing tumour
N2	Fixed ipsilateral axillary nodes
N3	Ipsilateral supraclavicular or infraclavicular nodes or oedema of arm
M0	No evidence of distant metastasis
M1	Evidence of distant metastasis

Table 28.6 Stage and prognosis according to TNM classification

UICC stage	TNM	Category	5-year survival
I	T1, N0, M0	Early cancer	84%
II	T1, N1, M0 T2, N0–1, M0	Early cancer	71%
III	Any T, N2–3, M0 T3, any N, M0	LABC	48%
IV	Any T, any N, M1	Metastatic	18%

LABC, locally advanced breast cancer; UICC, International Union against Cancer.

cancer then either surgical axillary clearance or radiotherapy to the axilla is advised. Sentinel node biopsy has advantages over axillary node clearance because it carries a much reduced incidence of lymphoedema in the arm.

The presence of distant metastasis is more difficult to establish with certainty because current techniques are not sensitive enough to detect microdeposits. The outcome of TNM classification is used to define a clinical stage which can be employed as a guide to treatment and prognosis (Table 28.6).

Other prognostic indicators

As well as stage and nodal status, there are many other factors that can be used for prediction (Table 28.7).

Histological

The following favourably affect prognosis:

- low tumour grade
- high degree of elastosis

Table 28.7 Prognostic variables other than TNM in breast cancer

Biological factors	Favourable	Unfavourable
Histological type	Tubular, colloid, papillary	Scirrhous
Grade	Low	High
Necrosis	Absent	Present
Lymphocytic infiltration	Present	Absent
Oestrogen status	Positive	Negative
Reactive lymph nodes	Present	Absent
Proliferative rate	Low S phase	Aneuploid
Chromosomal defect		Deletion/alteration 1, 3, 6, 7, 9 Shortening of allele on chromosome 11
Proto-oncogenes		c-*erb*B/c-H-*ras*
Growth factors (GF)		Epidermal GF Transforming GF Platelet-derived GF Fibroblast GF Insulin-like GF

- reactive changes in the regional lymph nodes
- positive oestrogen receptor status.

Other factors have an adverse effect:

- vascular and lymphocytic invasion by tumour
- extensive angiogenesis
- expression of the proto-oncogene c-*erb*B2 (HER-2/*neu*) and loss of expression of the suppressor *p53*.

SCREENING AND PREVENTION

Screening

The relatively poor results achieved when the disease is at a later stage have led to the view that it must be detected earlier at a presymptomatic stage. Studies from New York, Scotland and Scandinavia have shown that it is likely that finding hidden cancers by proactive measures improves long-term survival by allowing lesions to be removed before micrometastases have occurred. In the UK, women between the ages of 50 and 70 years who are registered with a general practitioner are called every 3 years for a screening mammogram. There are plans for this to be extended to include women between 47 and 73 years. In the USA, screening is undertaken more frequently, with a baseline mammogram being performed between 35 and 39 years, then 1- to 2-yearly for 12–24 months and yearly from 50 years with no age limit. These intervals are aimed at reducing the chance that a cancer develops but remains undetected between mammogram episodes. In the UK this risk is thought to be low enough to warrant the 3-yearly interval.

Mammographically detected cancers are smaller, and axillary lymph node involvement is less common. A reduction of 30% in long-term mortality has been shown even if the 'lead time' is allowed for. Lead time is the difference in time between a tumour being subclinical and detectable only by screening methods, such as mammography, and when it would have become clinically apparent. If the patient still dies at the same point in time then an apparent survival advantage is gained due to the 'lead time bias' (Fig. 28.3).

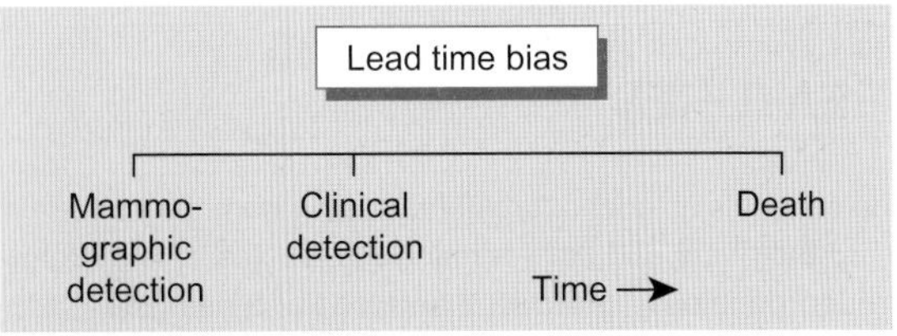

Fig. 28.3 Lead time bias spuriously suggests that screening results in a reduction in breast cancer mortality (irrespective of any real reductions achieved through screening).

Several trials are currently in progress to evaluate screening for women under the age of 50 years. Current advice is that for high-risk women under the age of 50, a specialist clinic should coordinate a personal mammography programme. If the family history is of postmenopausal cancer, mammography may be delayed until 35 years. Where the family history is of premenopausal cancer, referral at any age 10 years younger than the first presentation of the parent is thought appropriate.

Prevention

Whilst screening can reduce mortality by identifying the disease at an earlier stage, it would be far better to prevent the cancer in the first place.

It was noted that tamoxifen used in the treatment of patients with invasive disease reduced the incidence of contralateral breast cancer. It was therefore hypothesised that it could be used to prevent the disease in high-risk groups. A large trial by the US National Surgical Adjuvant Breast and Bowel Project (NSABP) recently demonstrated a 50% reduction in the relative risk of in-situ disease and a 47% reduction in the risk of invasive disease in high-risk women taking tamoxifen. However, there was an associated increase in risk of endometrial cancer and thromboembolic complications, although the tamoxifen did appear to protect against fractures. A similar compound called raloxifene, which is used to treat osteoporosis, reduces breast cancer by 54%. Unfortunately it is not clear whether this hormonal manipulation is just preventing the good-prognosis tumours and therefore having little effect on mortality. This area is still the subject of clinical trials such as the IBIS 2 trial.

It should be remembered that women who keep their weight down and exercise regularly reduce their risk of breast cancer as well as of other diseases. It is always worth pointing out to a woman who smokes that her lifetime risk of dying of breast cancer is about 1:30 whereas it is about 1:3 for a smoking-related disease.

CLINICOPATHOLOGICAL FEATURES

The cancer is an adenocarcinoma arising from the epithelium lining the ducts and acini forming the lobules. It is therefore divided principally into ductal and lobular types (see 'Carcinoma in situ', below). A feature of clinical interest is that most breast cancers are associated with fibrous tissue proliferation – they are scirrhous. The consequence is that the growth and surrounding tissue contracts so that dimpling of the skin and indrawing of the nipple may be seen.

Grade

The morphology of invasive tumours correlates with their degree of malignancy. As such the histological grade of tumour relates to the degree of differentiation. This was described many years ago by two pathologists, Bloom and Richardson. Although it has undergone some modification it is known as the Bloom and Richardson grade and classed as I, II or III, with increasing loss of differentiation the grade increases. The association with prognosis is not linear, but generally grade III is significantly worse than grade I/II. The features assessed are loss of tubule formation, increasing nuclear pleiomorphism and increasing mitotic count; these are all scored and the final value gives the grade.

Oestrogen receptor status

The majority of breast cancers are 'oestrogen dependent' tumours. As such they tend to express oestrogen receptors. The degree of expression can be measured with immunohistochemistry, and the breast cancers are labelled as either oestrogen receptor positive or negative. Oestrogen receptor positive breast cancer tends to respond to hormonal therapy and carries a better prognosis than oestrogen receptor negative tumours. Interestingly, even in the absence of oestrogen receptors, expression of progesterone receptors is also predictive of hormone responsiveness.

c-*erb*B2 receptor

This is a member of the tyrosine kinase family of receptors found on the cell membrane; it is sometimes described as HER2. It is found in about 20% of invasive cancers but a higher proportion of high grade in situ ductal cancers. Its presence is associated with a poorer prognosis. It is identified using standard immunocytochemistry or fluorescent in situ hybridisation. The receptor is the target for the newly developed drug trastuzumab. Assessment of c–*erb*B2 or HER2 receptor status is now routine in breast cancers.

Carcinoma in situ

Carcinoma in situ (CIS or TIS [tumour in situ]) refers to the period during which normal epithelial cells undergo apparent malignant transformation but do not invade through the basement membrane. There are two forms:

- lobular (LCIS)
- ductal (DCIS), representing all types of CIS that are not identified as lobular. It can be further subdivided into:
  - comedo
  - solid
  - cribriform
  - micropapillary.

More recently, as for invasive cancers, a formal grading system has been introduced for in-situ disease. However, the distinction remains primarily between LCIS and DCIS, although comedo DCIS is a particularly menacing type of CIS with reports of frequent association with microinvasive foci and lymph node metastasis. Necrosis and microcalcification are common and, because the second may be seen on mammography, the incidence may be increasing as earlier diagnosis becomes more widespread. By contrast, LCIS is not associated with any radiological markers and therefore may not be detected early.

The ratio of DCIS to LCIS is 3:1, and approximately 10–37% of those with LCIS and 30–50% of those with DCIS go on to develop invasive carcinoma.

With LCIS, future cancers may be in either breast regardless of the site of the in-situ changes. A further confounding statistic is that approximately 50–65% of future malignancies are of ductal origin, which indicates that LCIS is a marker of increased risk of diffuse bilateral disease as opposed to a true anatomic precursor of lobular cancer.

However, with DCIS, the subsequent malignancies are ductal in origin, arise in the ipsilateral breast and usually are confined to the same quadrant from which the biopsy which yielded the diagnosis was taken.

Invasive breast carcinoma

Pathological manifestations

The disease has protean pathological manifestations.

Ductal with productive fibrosis (infiltrating ductal)

This is the commonest form of cancer of the breast – approximately 80% (Table 28.8). The most common form is of nondescript but highly variable histological type. Sheets, cords, nests and trabeculae of tumour cells may be present all in varying amounts. If the main bulk of tumour is of this type then the presence of more-specific histological features in small amounts does not appear to alter the prognosis. This is ductal carcinoma of no specific type (NST).

In contrast to these tumours of no special histological type there is a group of ductal carcinomas in which the appearances more closely mirror aspects of normal tissue. They tend to be associated with a better prognosis.

Table 28.8 Relative frequency of histological types of breast cancer

Type	Frequency (%)
Ductal	80 (non-specific 50%)
Lobular/ductal combined	5
Medullary	6
Colloid	2
Other less common specific types (tubular, papillary)	2
Sarcoma and lymphoma	0.5

Medullary

This form constitutes about 6% of the total. Histologically, it has completely circumscribed borders with a syncytial sheet-like growth pattern, a diffuse infiltrate of lymphocytes and a variable number of plasma cells. Nearly 50% of these tumours are associated with intraductal carcinoma, usually at the periphery of the main tumour.

Colloid (mucinous)

Largely confined to the elderly population, this tumour accounts for approximately 2% of breast cancers. Histologically, large pools of mucin are surrounded by variable groups of tumour cells. The classical signet ring appearance of mucinous tumours in other sites is not seen in breast colloid carcinoma.

Tubular

Clinically, tubular carcinoma is found in younger than average patients, with the late 50s being the peak age, the diagnosis usually being made at mammography. In consequence, the lesion is still small (less than 1 cm), and up to a fifth of breast tumours identified at mammography may be of this type. Histologically they are well differentiated and have randomly arranged tubular elements in a loose stroma.

Papillary

This accounts for less than 2% of cases of breast carcinoma and usually presents in the seventh decade. Histologically, it is well circumscribed with marked papillary differentiation.

Other pathological types

Adenoid cystic carcinoma This type accounts for less than 0.1% of breast cancers. Similar to the tumours of the same name found in the salivary glands, it also resembles cribriform intraductal carcinoma.

Lobular carcinoma These lesions have a high propensity for bilaterality (up to 30%), multicentricity and multifocality. The age at presentation is similar to that of infiltrating ductal carcinoma, and they constitute 5–10% of breast carcinomas. Histologically, lobular carcinoma has a characteristic appearance with homogeneous small cells with small nuclei, absent nucleoli and scanty cytoplasm. They characteristically permeate a desmoplastic stroma in single file, linear fashion (Indian filing) or surround terminal ductal lobular units in a circumferential targetoid way. When abundant mucin is produced by the tumour, the nuclei are displaced laterally and the cell comes to resemble the signet ring type of gastrointestinal adenocarcinoma. Lobular carcinoma has a particular propensity for metastasising to membrane structures and forming diffusely-involved metastasis. Structures that may be concerned include the peritoneum, the pleura and the meninges as meningeal carcinomatosis.

CLINICAL FEATURES

History

In women who present symptomatically with breast cancer the main complaint is that of a solitary, non-tender breast lump of varying duration. With increasing breast awareness patients are tending to present earlier than was the case several years ago; however, there is still a group of patients where its presence has been denied for several months or years. Pain is present in fewer than 5%. Whilst it often needs investigating for reassurance, most patients with pain alone can be reassured that that it is unlikely to be breast cancer. Table 28.9 outlines the frequency of presenting symptoms and signs. It is important to note the length of time for which the mass has been present. Much less common is the patient who has a small primary and only presents when symptoms of generalised malignant disease become manifest. Finally, denial may be carried to extreme when a patient realises that she has a lump and allows it to progress to ulceration (see also 'Paget's disease' below). With extension of breast screening to include women between 50 and 70 years of age, many patients are completely asymptomatic and their first awareness that they may have a problem is when they are recalled after screening mammography. In breast units that carry out both screening and symptomatic work the screening cancers can account for 40% or more of the workload – with improvements in technology and extension of screening age this statistic may change even more.

Physical findings

Classically the mass is solitary, does not cause pain on palpation, is defined, hard and may show signs of tethering to the skin. In locally advanced disease, the lymphatic channels are obstructed and the skin becomes oedematous with thickening and the hair follicles more prominent although embedded in the rugose skin – so-called skin of the orange (peau d'orange). In practice the signs may be more subtle so that an asymmetric nodularity or diffuse thickening needs to be regarded with caution and investigated just as a solitary lump. Lobular carcinoma in particularly is notorious for producing diffuse thickening rather than a lump.

In *medullary carcinoma*, the lump may be soft, haemorrhagic and bulky, deep in the breast but characteristically mobile.

Colloid carcinoma usually presents as a bulky mass in the sixth or seventh decade.

Tubular and papillary carcinoma do not have distinctive physical findings but tend to present in older women. They are much more frequently found at screening and so are rarely detected clinically.

Table 28.9 Modes of presentation of breast cancer

Symptom/sign	Frequency (%)
Lump	76
Pain	5
Nipple retraction	4
Nipple discharge	2
Skin retraction	1
Axillary mass	1

Other malignant tumours affecting the breast

Paget's disease

This condition presents clinically as a chronic, eczematoid eruption of the nipple. Indeed the diagnosis may be confused with eczema although there are distinct differences (Table 28.10). It constitutes approximately 2% of histological types and is almost always associated with an underlying intraductal or invasive carcinoma.

Inflammatory breast carcinoma

This tumour accounts for 1% or slightly more of breast carcinomas. It is rapidly progressive and is characterised by erythema, peau d'orange and skin ridging with or without a palpable mass. Unlike other breast cancers, the commonest presenting feature is pain. The characteristic appearance of a diffusely enlarged breast is consequent upon the dissemination of tumour cells through the lymphatics of the dermis (Fig. 28.4). If the tumour cells remain within the superficial lymphatics and the blood vessels, then a condition known as telangiectatic carcinoma may arise with numerous purple papules and haemorrhagic, vesicle-like lesions covering the breast. Extensive involvement along tissue planes may produce a nodular pattern or, when associated with extensive fibrosis, a diffuse thickened lesion – a thoracic girdle (carcinoma en cuirasse).

Malignant phyllodes tumour

This accounts for about 0.5% of all breast tumours. The name is derived from its fleshy leaf-like (phylloid) appearance. There are both stromal and epithelial components, although the stromal elements predominate. On histological examination, malignant phyllodes tumours provide a spectrum of disease from frank sarcomatous malignancy to appearances almost indistinguishable from a fibroadenoma. Even with histological confirmation, its behaviour can be difficult to predict.

Table 28.10 Comparison of Paget's disease and eczema of the nipple

Paget's disease	Eczema
Unilateral	Bilateral
Progressive/continuous	Intermittent/variable
Moist or dry	Moist
Irregular/discrete	Indistinct
Nipple always involved	Nipple sparing
Pruritus absent	Pruritus present

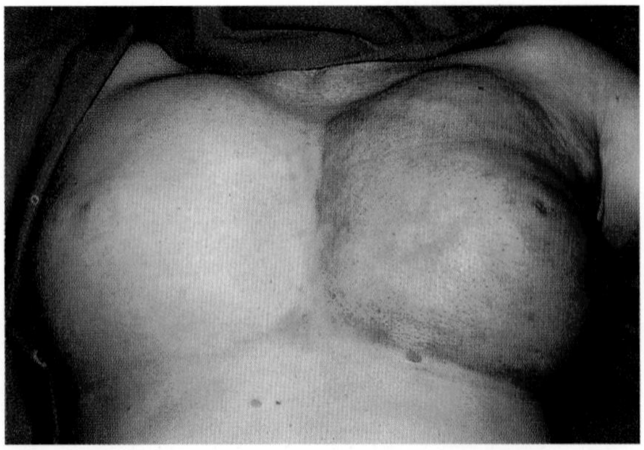

Fig. 28.4 'Peau d'orange' of cancer of the breast.

Clinical features

There is often a large, painless and nodular growth which is surprisingly mobile. With continuing enlargement of the tumour, the breast adopts a characteristic 'teardrop' appearance (Fig. 28.5). Treatment is by wide excision through normal tissues. However, as with other sarcomas, local recurrence is a feature.

Lymphoma

Primary breast lymphoma is extremely rare. The malignancy does not differ structurally from the same growth in other sites. Treatment is by mastectomy with lymph node clearance, with radiotherapy for local recurrences and chemotherapy for disseminated disease. Prognosis is favourable.

ESTABLISHING A DIAGNOSIS OF BREAST CANCER

Any palpable breast abnormality should be assessed by the process of triple assessment:

- clinical evaluation
- radiological evaluation
- cytological/histological evaluation.

A thorough history should form part of any assessment because important information can be gained on the nature of the breast mass or condition that caused the individual to ask for medical advice and also the other risk factors mentioned above: family, menstrual and reproductive history, the use of hormones and a personal history of breast cancer or breast disease.

During the course of communication with patients with possible breast cancer, it is important to convey the fact that only 20% who consult do have the disease; 50% do not have breast disease as defined pathologically; 20% have benign (fibrocystic) disease; and most of the rest have a fibroadenoma.

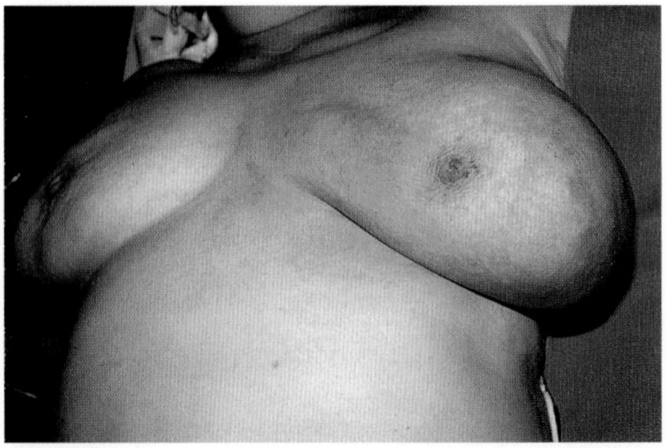

Fig. 28.5 'Tear-drop' appearance of phyllodes tumour of the breast.

Physical examination

The technique of examining the breast should involve inspection and palpation of the entire breast and lymph node-bearing areas (Fig. 28.6).

The patient must be undressed to the waist and sit facing the examiner. The breast is initially examined from the front with the arms first at the side, then raised above the head and finally placed on the hips – in this last case they should be both relaxed and pressed into the sides in order to tense the pectoralis muscle. The patient is asked to point out the supposed area of abnormality and this is examined first. However, in spite of any abnormality being discovered the following are also assessed:

- asymmetry
- visible lumps
- erythema
- cutaneous oedema (peau d'orange)
- contour flattening
- skin tethering as identified by puckering, particularly when the arms are raised
- abnormal fixation
- retraction and altered axis of the nipples; in advanced cases there may be gross ulceration of the skin overlying the lesion (Fig. 28.7).

After this, with the arms extended forwards, the patient is asked to lean forward, once again looking for skin retraction (Fig. 28.8). The breasts are then re-examined, paying particular attention to the outer border of pectoralis major. Here lymph nodes may be felt. The supraclavicular, infraclavicular and axillary lymph nodes should be examined, the examiner taking the weight of the patient's arm either on the shoulder or on the opposite arm (Fig. 28.9).

a

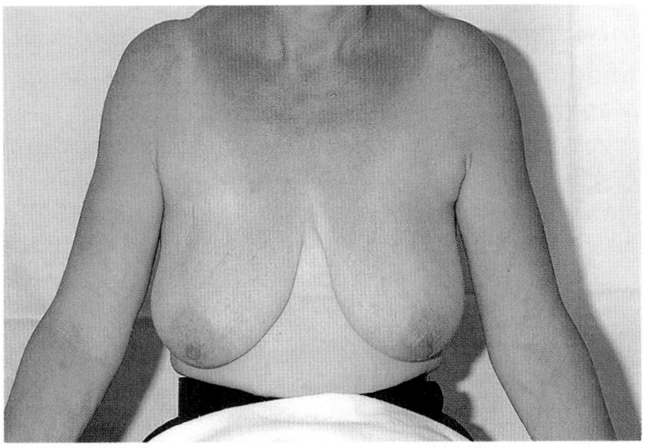

b

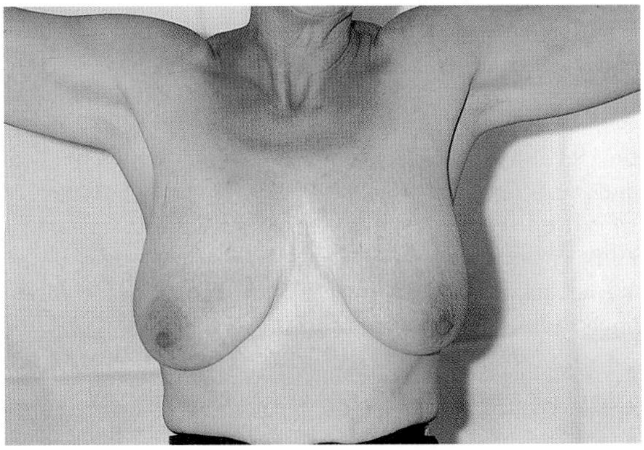

c

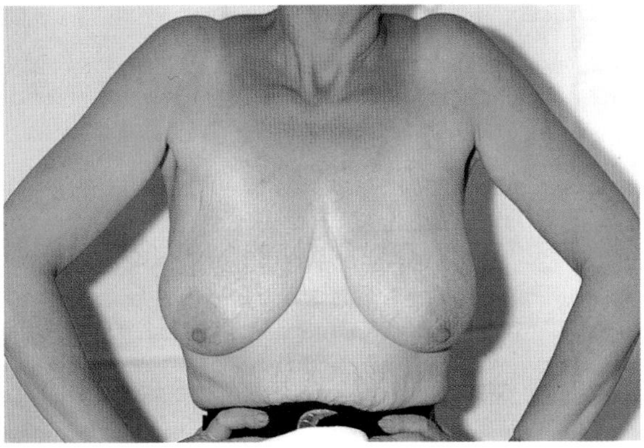

Fig. 28.6 Examination of the breast: (a) from the front; (b) with arms raised; (c) with arms pushed into the side.

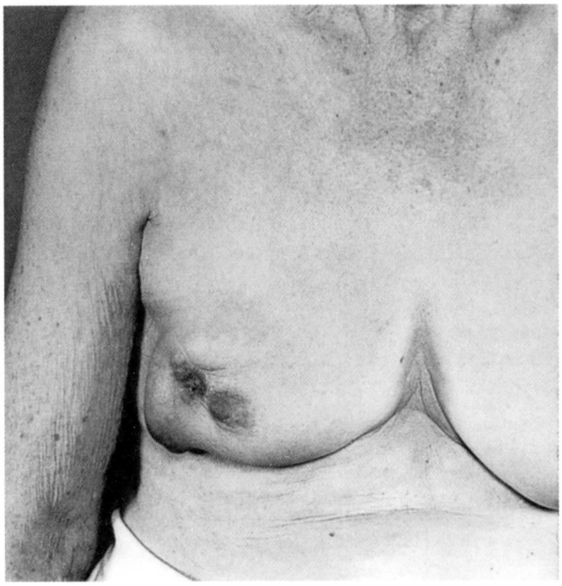

Fig. 28.7 Ulceration overlying cancer of the breast.

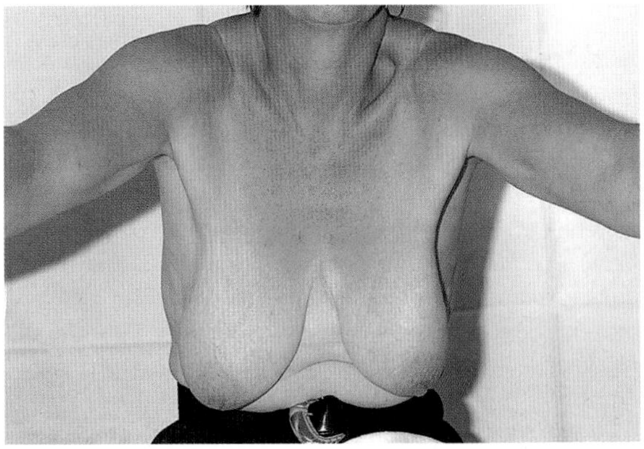

Fig. 28.8 Leaning forward to demonstrate any skin retraction.

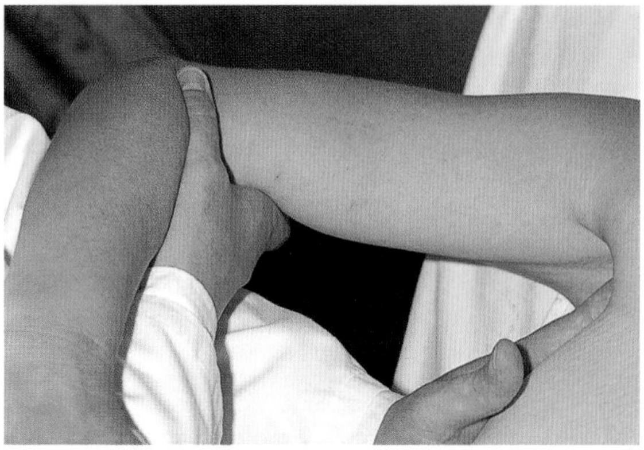

Fig. 28.9 Examination of the axillary nodes.

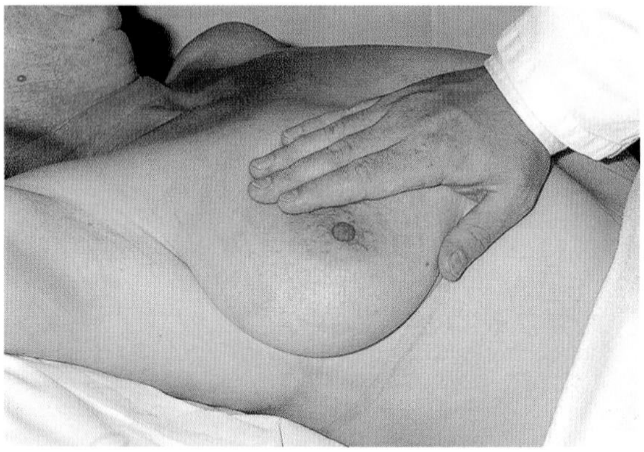

Fig. 28.10 Examination of the breast with a flat hand.

Table 28.11 Discharge from the nipple

Type	Abnormality/cause	Cancer risk
Bloody	Hyperplasia/ectasia	Yes
	Papilloma	No
Serous	Hyperplasia/ectasia	Yes
Watery	Hyperplasia	Yes
Opalescent	Ectasia/cyst	No
Milk	Hormonal	No

Further palpation of the breast is best performed in the supine position. A pillow under the shoulder of the breast allows the breast tissue to flow along the chest wall. The breast is examined initially with the patient's hand behind the head and then to the side. Care must be taken to ensure the whole breast is examined, transversely from sternum to clavicle, posteriorly to latissimus dorsi and inferiorly to the rectus sheath. In order to achieve this, the breast is examined a quadrant at a time. The examination is carried out with a flat hand (Fig. 28.10), never grasping or pinching. The nipple/areola area should be carefully inspected for epithelial changes, retroareolar masses and nipple discharge. The significance of the different types of discharge is shown in Table 28.11.

Should a mass be felt, whether related to the breast substance or in the lymph node area that drains it, its position, size, consistency and any fixation to surrounding deep or superficial structures must be carefully assessed and recorded. Fixation to skin is evaluated by pinching up the overlying skin. Mobility in relation to muscle is evaluated by palpation with the pectoralis major both contracted and relaxed. Should the patient complain of discharge, then an attempt to reproduce this should be made. Methods include 'around the clock' palpation of the areola area, quadrant by quadrant, noting any dilated ducts or nodules and, if this fails to produce the discharge, gentle compression of the subareolar tissue. The number of ducts involved and the degree of dilatation should be assessed. Any discharge that is obtained should be tested for blood using a reagent stick and be sent for cytological examination.

Many surgeons use a prepared diagram and sheet for accurate recording of information following breast examination.

Investigation

Imaging

Mammography

Mammography was first used on in-vitro specimens in 1913 by a German surgeon, Salomon. The change from xeromammography to film screening allowed a reduction in radiation dose, so that the single-view mammogram gives an average dose of 2 mGy. The estimated risk of inducing a fatal breast cancer from one such examination is 1 : 100 000 for women aged between 50 and 65 years and twice this for women aged between 30 and 49 years.

A mediolateral oblique (mlo) view taken from upper medial to lower lateral aspects is now standard and images the whole of the breast. It is usually combined with a craniocaudal (cc) view although, for screening asymptomatic women, a single mlo view is considered adequate.

Generally, mammography in women under 35 years is often not helpful because they have particularly dense breasts at this age which can mask any underlying tumours and also make interpretation very difficult. However, it should be done if there is clinical suspicion or diagnosis of malignancy.

Mammographic abnormalities that warrant further investigation include:

- radiological masses undetected on clinical examination
- microcalcifications
- stellate densities
- architectural distortion
- change from a previous mammogram.

However, even with skilled interpreters, mammography has a false-negative rate of between 10% and 15%. Therefore it is only part of the spectrum of diagnosis, and other tests must be integrated into a diagnosis.

Ultrasound

In use since the 1950s, ultrasound has been shown to be useful in discriminating solid from cystic masses and especially in the evaluation of the dense breast. Other uses include ultrasound-guided biopsy or needle localisation. In younger women, ultrasound may reveal more information than mammography, and most surgeons would perform this test first in women younger than 35. Masses smaller than 5–10 mm may not be visualised, and masses in fatty breasts are also difficult to assess. It is not a good screening tool, working most effectively when there is a palpable abnormality rather than being used to just look around; however, some younger patients, particularly with pain, are only reassured when they have had an ultrasound.

Blood flow assessment by Doppler ultrasound has been used in assessment because breast tumours have enhanced blood flow and the pattern of blood vessels is radial rather than the circumferential pattern seen in a benign lesion.

CT

This can be useful in staging the disease but does not have a role in diagnosis.

MRI

Initially, MRI mammography did not show any advantage over conventional techniques in the detection and evaluation of breast cancer. However, since the introduction of Gd-DTPA enhancement and true dynamic scanning, the results suggest a use in evaluating the indeterminate breast mass or, after surgery or neo-adjuvant chemotherapy, assessing breasts for the presence of very small satellite malignant disease, and in screening young women with a significant genetic risk. Breast tumours are noted to enhance heterogeneously and rapidly in contrast to benign tumours, which have more homogeneous and uniform enhancement. Further research is being done to evaluate the role of breast MRI in the clinical setting.

Aspiration cytology

Fine needle aspiration biopsy (FNAB) using a 21-gauge needle was a very popular means of obtaining material from a lump for diagnosis. However, it is very operator dependent, both for surgeons and histologists; consequently, it is becoming much less widely used. The major advantage was the speed of diagnosis, which could be less than 30 minutes, which when 'one stop' breast clinics started was seen as important. However, apart from very experienced cytopathologists the number of positive diagnoses can be small with being classified as suspicious or uncertain, which means another biopsy of some sort. Furthermore it is impossible in the case of a malignancy to comment on whether the cells are from an in situ or invasive lesion, which makes planning definitive surgery difficult. For that reason many centres in the UK are very selective in their use of the technique.

Wide-bore core needle biopsy

This method provides a sample of tissue for histological rather than cytological examination. The pathological diagnosis which results should be more certain because cellular architecture can be assessed. Because of this, the use of wide-bore core needle biopsy is rapidly superseding that of aspiration cytology in specialist breast clinics. Increasingly it is done using some form of guidance to improve the diagnostic yield. Although there has been criticism of the time taken to process the tissue, with new rapid processors results can be reported the same day.

Vacuum suction biopsy

This is a new technique that further develops the concept of core biopsy. Removing the sample by suction means that the needle does not need to be reinserted each time a sample is taken. This allows larger biopsy needles to be used (up to 8 gauge), and sequential cores of tissue can be taken. This means more tissue is available for analysis and, if necessary, whole lesions can be removed for diagnostic purposes. It is also used for excision of lesions such as fibroadenomas.

Open biopsy

Excision biopsy

This refers to the removal of all gross evidence of disease with a small rim of normal breast tissue. If the tumour is small enough, all macroscopic disease is removed. Incisions are made along Langer's lines (Fig. 28.11) for optimum cosmesis. Nowadays this is seen as a last resort as FNAB, core biopsy and vacuum biopsy have replaced it.

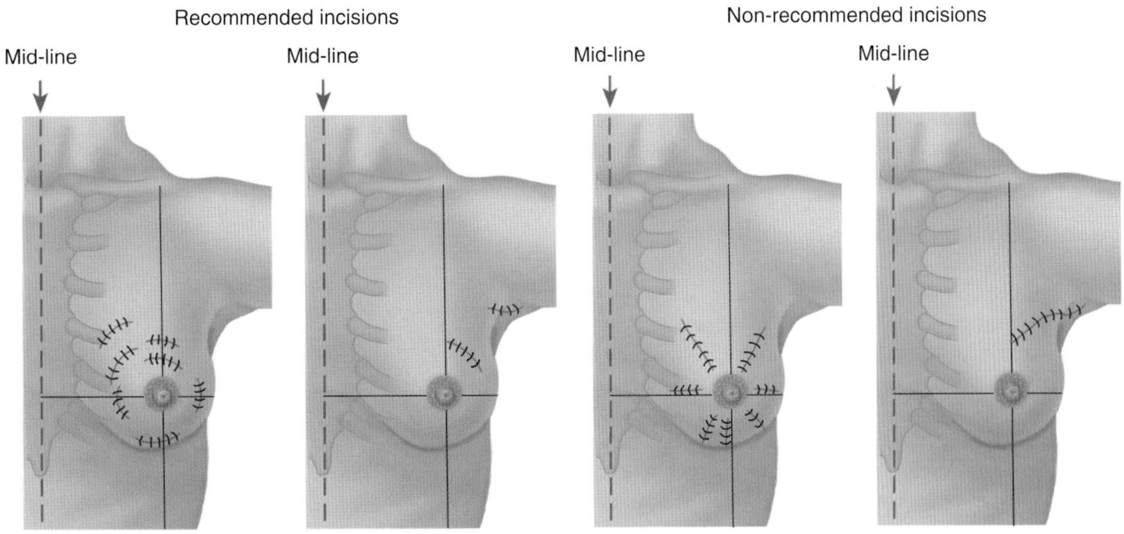

Fig. 28.11 For excision biopsy, incisions are made along Langer's lines.

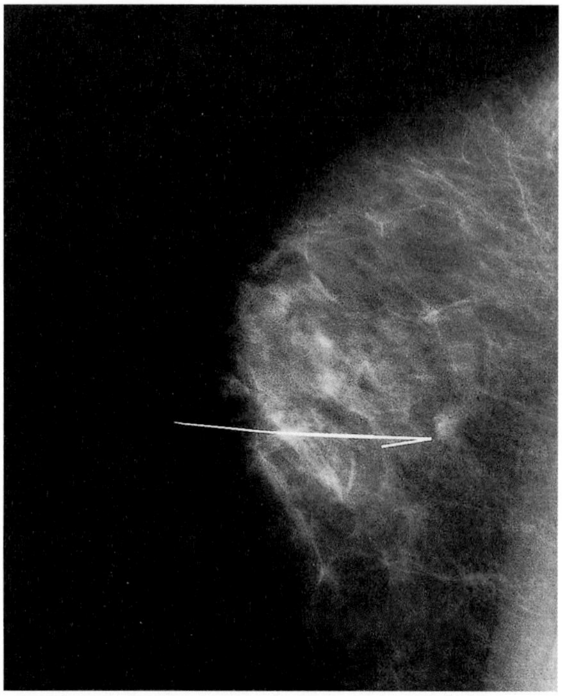

Fig. 28.12 Identification of tumour with a needle on mammogram.

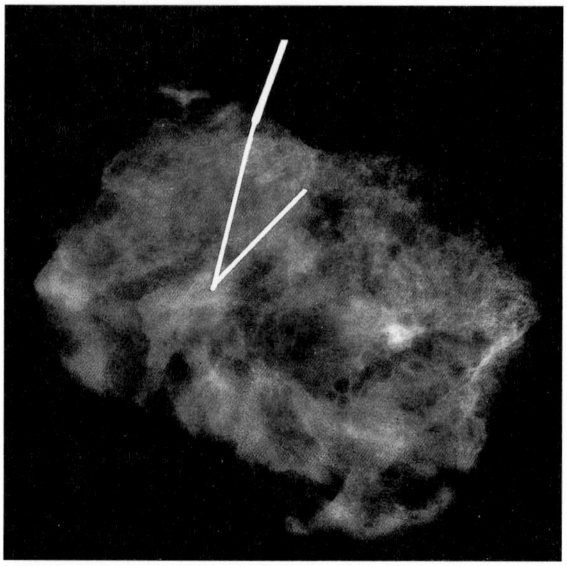

Fig. 28.13 X-ray of excised lump.

Incision biopsy

This is similar to excision biopsy except that only a part of the lump is removed. It is generally felt that this is not good surgical practice. The use of incision biopsy is therefore restricted to larger tumours, especially suspected sarcomatous lesions where the incision must be made in such a way as to facilitate later excision of the scar as part of removal of the whole lesion. The use of incision biopsy has largely been superseded by that of wide-core bore needle biopsy.

Mammographic-guided needle biopsy

Screening mammography (above) demonstrates many clinically impalpable lesions. To localise these, a marking needle is placed under mammographic guidance before surgical excision. The tissue around the needle is then excised and further imaging done to ensure that the indicated lesion has in fact been removed (Figs 28.12 and 28.13). If it is not evident in the sample, more tissue from around the site is taken until the lesion is identified.

Ultrasound-guided biopsy

Both the technique of needle-guided biopsy and real-time cyst aspiration can be used. Techniques of one or the other are dependent on the expertise available. Ultrasound can also be used to mark the site of an impalpable lesion for surgical biopsy.

Radioguided occult level localization (ROLL)

This is a very new technique to aid localisation of impalpable lesions. A radionuclide is injected at the tumour site which can then be detected in theatre using a hand-held device allowing accurate excision of the lesion.

Nipple biopsy

Conditions affecting the nipple, especially an eczema-like appearance (see 'Paget's disease', above), often warrant biopsy. A wedge of nipple–areolar complex can be excised under local anaesthetic with minimal cosmetic disruption to confirm or refute a diagnosis such as that of Paget's disease.

MANAGEMENT

Therapeutic options

The modern approach to breast cancer is multidisciplinary, with surgery, radiotherapy and chemotherapy all having important roles to play. For that reason in the UK all breast cancers are discussed at a multidisciplinary meeting at the important stages of their disease management.

The treatment afforded to patients suffering from the disease depends on the stage of the cancer at the time of presentation.

Carcinoma in situ

DCIS and LCIS have different risks for the development of invasive cancer. As yet, their natural histories have not been fully elucidated.

DCIS presents an easier problem as it generally is unilateral and is thought to be a precursor of invasive disease. Trials of segmental excision with or without radiotherapy and hormone therapy are currently underway but they must be judged against mastectomy which eliminates all the pre-invasive involved tissue. This is recommended when the disease has extensive foci and local excision margins are not clear of tumour and also for those patients who are at a high risk of developing local recurrence and reduced survival, defined as:

- size greater than 40 mm
- comedo appearances on histological examination

- high-grade tumour
- oestrogen receptor status negative.

Postoperative radiation is usually given to these patients. Breast-conserving therapy remains an option provided the patient understands the risks. The patient is followed up regularly with mammography and clinical examination, and if there is evidence of recurrent disease a mastectomy is usually done.

The treatment for LCIS is confused by the fact that it is a marker for a disease that is often bilateral, multicentric and only sometimes goes on to invasive ductal cancer. A bilateral mastectomy was once standard treatment, but it is now clear that the majority of these patients require just close follow-up.

Both DCIS and LCIS patients are considered high risk for subsequent invasive disease and are eligible for the various prevention trials which are designed to show whether the incidence and mortality from breast cancer can be reduced in high-risk groups.

Almost by definition in DCIS the lymph nodes should not be involved as this implies that the basement membrane has been breached. Therefore axillary staging has been unnecessary; however, in the case of mastectomies for multifocal disease it is recognised that small invasive cancers can be present and therefore some surgeons will carry out an axillary sample or sentinel node biopsy in order to avoid further surgery if an invasive lesion is present.

Stages I and II

Stages I and II are generally classed as early breast cancer. Although this stage of the disease is considered potentially curable by surgery the results of prospective trials, based on the hypothesis that dissemination occurs early, show that long-term survival is not enhanced by radical surgical resection as opposed to breast conservation. In consequence, the pendulum has swung towards the principle of local control and, where possible, breast conservation coupled with adjuvant systemic treatment to deal with the distant micrometastases, should they exist.

Local control is achieved by:

- complete removal of the tumour
- adjuvant local radiotherapy possibly supplemented by systemic cytotoxic therapy.

The following therapeutic approach is generally accepted for a tumour of less than 4 cm in diameter with:

- unifocal disease
- breast volume of adequate size for a satisfactory cosmetic result
- possible wide local removal of tumour – either the lump alone (wide local excision) or removal of the involved breast quadrant (quadrantectomy)
- patient willing and able to undergo local radiotherapy to reduce the risk of local recurrence from residual tumour cells
- excision margins shown to be clear on subsequent examination of the pathological specimen
- acceptability for the patient.

Breast-conserving surgery involves the removal of the tumour but leaving the majority of the breast intact, so preserving, at least in part, an important feature of the female self-image with a better cosmetic result. Within the various techniques used for conservative therapy there is considerable variation in the amount of tissue removed:

- *Wide local excision* implies the removal of the tumour with a macroscopic 1 cm margin.
- *Lumpectomy* often refers to a less radical excision but is generally an outdated term largely replaced by wide local excision (wle).
- *Quadrantectomy* involves the excision of the tumour and the associated breast quadrant and, although still classed as conservative breast surgery, a considerable amount of the surrounding breast tissue and skin is removed and the cosmetic and psychological results are not as good as for wle.

Wide local excision can be utilised for all tumours that fall into the above categories. The proponents of quadrantectomy claim a reduced local recurrence rate when compared with more local procedures.

Centrally placed lesions or diseases of the nipple are generally considered unsuitable for breast-conserving surgery although central excision including the nipple–areola complex can be considered if breast size allows.

The development of so-called 'oncoplastic' surgery has led to the introduction of breast reshaping and parenchymal replacement techniques such as breast reduction and latissimus dorsi miniflaps that have further extended the ability of the surgeon to remove larger amounts of breast tissue whilst conserving the aesthetic appearance of the breast.

In a tumour greater than 4 cm in diameter, mastectomy is more often recommended with or without local radiotherapy depending on tumour characteristics. Additional factors that would influence the decision are:

- multifocal disease
- centrally placed tumours
- small breasts precluding good cosmesis from breast conservation
- excision margins not clear after wide local excision
- patient choice.

Local radiotherapy does reduce local recurrence after mastectomy. However, there is morbidity and mortality associated with chest wall radiotherapy, because of cardiac and vascular effects. Therefore the risk of recurrence must be balanced against the overall benefit. The usual threshold is placed at 20%, and therefore women with four or more positive nodes are generally considered candidates for chest wall radiotherapy after a mastectomy and axillary clearance. If the nodes are positive on sampling then radiotherapy to the axilla is required in any case, and, as only qualitative (involved yes/no) rather than quantitative (number involved) information is obtained, radiotherapy is usually given to the chest wall if a positive sample is obtained, regardless of the number of nodes. After breast-conserving surgery, it is accepted that radiotherapy be given to the remaining breast in order to reduce the rate of local recurrence from as much as 30% to approximately 10%.

It may be possible in the future to apply selection criteria for radiotherapy after conservative breast surgery, but this is still the subject of a number of trials.

The axilla in stage I and II disease

Assessment of the pathological status of axillary lymph nodes is judged essential for future management because it has been shown that it is one of the markers for prognosis. The presence of nodal metastasis implies systemic dissemination of the cancer. Clinical assessment is of little value as 20–30% of involved nodes are impalpable clinically. The axillary nodes are at three levels according to their relation to pectoralis minor:

- level I – inferior to the lower border of the muscle
- level II – immediately behind its belly
- level III – above and adjacent to the axillary vessels.

The nodal status can be assessed by removal of soft tissue (sampling) up to level II; at least four lymph nodes should be identified at histological examination. The alternative is axillary node clearance, which is both potentially therapeutic, in that it surgically clears the axilla of any tumour-bearing nodes, and also provides the nodes needed for staging; however, it comes at a price of much greater morbidity than an axillary sample.

The concept of sentinel node biopsy has had a major impact on management. It has been demonstrated that there are usually one or two nodes that are the first nodes draining the breast. It appears that, if these nodes are identified and removed, they are predictive for the rest of the axilla. They are identified operatively by using a special blue dye and/or radioactive technetium sulphur colloid and a modified directional Geiger counter. The technique of sentinel node biopsy answers the criticism of inaccuracy that has plagued lymph node sampling. With the advance of sentinel node biopsy it is becoming common practice to assess the axilla preoperatively with ultrasound to identify any obviously involved nodes. For patients without obvious nodal metastases, a sentinel node biopsy is often carried out, whereas if involved nodes are seen the patient can go direct to axillary clearance.

If lymph node involvement is demonstrated following axillary lymph node sampling or sentinel node biopsy, axillary radiotherapy is given to help control axillary nodal metastasis, or an axillary clearance is performed. However, if an axillary clearance is performed as the primary intervention, radiotherapy for positive nodes is unnecessary – all the diseased nodes have been removed. In addition, after clearance, radiotherapy is associated with a high incidence of lymphoedema of the arm because of the combined surgical and X-ray damage to lymphatics (see 'Complications', below).

The overall concepts involved in the management of the axilla are represented in Figure 28.14.

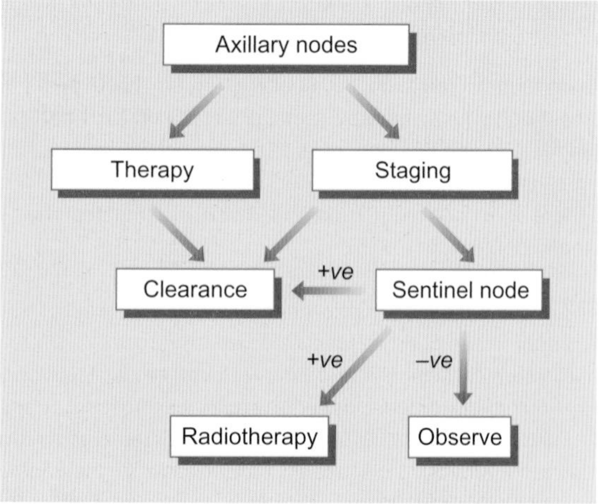

Fig. 28.14 Flow diagram showing management of axillary nodes.

Limitations of local resection (breast conservation)

There are additional limitations to those already mentioned. If the excision margins are not clear then many surgeons offer a further local excision. Histologically proven involvement of the excision margins of the second procedure results in the further offer of a mastectomy. Extensive local lymphatic and vascular invasion around the primary tumour is also an indicator of a high risk of local recurrence, and a mastectomy is considered by some to be appropriate. Those with an extensive intraductal component (EIC) are more likely to develop a recurrence, and women less than 35 years are also more likely to suffer local relapse.

Complications of local procedures

As with all surgical procedures, the complications can be divided into general and specific, and into immediate, early and late.

Specific immediate and early complications

The breast is a vascular organ with a rich blood supply. Haemorrhage during any operation on the breast can be considerable, and it is usual to make preparations for possible blood transfusion before mastectomy.

Inadequate haemostasis at the time of operation leads to the formation of a postoperative haematoma which may require evacuation under general anaesthesia. Surgical interruption of the breast lymphatics increases the possibility of the accumulation of lymph to cause a postoperative seroma which requires repeated needle aspirations over several weeks but usually settles with time.

Infection of the skin flaps can lead to skin loss and, after mastectomy, grafting may be necessary to cover the defect. Infection is more likely to develop if the skin is closed under tension, or is rendered ischaemic by a haematoma or seroma.

Complications associated with radiotherapy

Radiotherapy has specific complications, including cutaneous inflammatory reactions, photosensitisation and the development of fibrosis, and, in the long term, distortion of the breast. There have been reports of an increase in coronary artery disease in those women who have undergone irradiation to the left chest field and also of lung fibrosis. However, such complications were associated with older techniques, and modern treatment does not appear to have the same problems.

Late complications

Cosmetic

In addition to the distortion that may be caused by the fibrotic reaction initiated by the radiotherapy, surgical scarring after a breast-conserving procedure can also lead to disfiguring distortion. Reoperation may be required to produce a better appearance.

Shoulder stiffness

Surgical dissection of the axilla and radiotherapy both carry this risk. Adequate analgesia and instruction by a physiotherapist should be utilised in order to facilitate an early return to as full a range of shoulder movement as can be achieved.

Brachial plexus/intercostal nerve damage

Persistent paraesthesia or numbness in the ipsilateral arm can result from axillary radiotherapy or damage to the intercostal nerves at the time of surgery. The symptoms may decrease with time. The possibility should be raised, although not exaggerated, in the pre-treatment interview because severe symptoms are rare. True brachial plexus damage is very uncommon; more frequently seen is damage to the intercostal nerves which results in numbness on the inner aspect of the forearm. Aviodance of this problem has been one of the driving factors behind the introduction of sentinel node biopsy and sampling as staging procedures.

Lymphoedema of the arm

This is the result usually of the combination of surgical axillary lymph node clearance and radiotherapy, which are not now used together. A slight degree of temporary lymphoedema probably develops in most patients, but it may progress to massive and disfiguring swelling with loss of function. The therapeutic combination is thus not acceptable. The treatment for established lymphoedema involves the use of sequential compression bandages and dynamic sequential compression if this is available. Very rarely, if the lymphoedema is massive or in the rare occurrence of malignant lymphangiosarcoma because of impairment of local immunity, an amputation may be the only method of achieving relief.

Predicting prognosis

Because it is recognised that some breast cancers may have micrometastasised by the time of diagnosis the use of adjuvant treatments to eradicate these metastases is becoming much more common. Because these treatments vary in toxicity there is increasing use made of prognostic tools to stratify risk and better direct treatments. In the UK two tools are becoming commonly used.

Nottingham Prognostic Index (NPI)

This was described by Professor Roger Blamey and his colleagues from Nottingham. It uses the tumour size, nodal status and Bloom and Richardson grade in a mathematical formula. This allows patients to be stratified into 6 groups, ranging from extremely good prognosis to very poor prognosis, and given adjuvant treatment accordingly. It follows from this that good pathology which gives a good assessment of grade and adequate axillary surgery are very important to the prognostic process.

Adjuvant online

This system was described by an American oncologist Peter Ravden. Using a very large database of patients whose tumour characteristics and outcomes are known, an online form is produced into which a patient's details are entered. The programme then produces a report giving estimates of survival percentages based on the available adjuvant strategies suitable for the patient. Increasingly units are using this in their multidisciplinary meetings to make decisions and advise patients.

Adjuvant therapy

Both cytotoxic and hormonal therapies are used.

Cytotoxic therapy

The heterogeneous nature of breast cancer means that at any time during treatment the cancer cells contained within a metastasis may be at different stages of their cell cycle. Therefore, combination therapy that can affect the cell at different stages of its cycle is required to achieve the response rates in women with known axillary or distant metastasis.

The most effective agents are:

- the antimetabolites methotrexate, a folic acid antagonist, and 5-fluorouracil, a fluoropyrimidine
- the antimitotic anthracycline antibiotics doxorubicin and its less toxic analogue epirubicin

given intravenously. They are often combined with the alkylating agent cyclophosphamide as CMF and CAF or FEC, respectively. Response rates, as measured by objective shrinkage of metastatic deposits, vary between 20% and 70%. Complete response with eradication of tumour is very rare, less than 20%.

Chemotherapy is now considered beneficial for all women at high risk of relapse, including high-grade pre- and postmenopausal women regardless of nodal status. The maximum benefit, however, remains for premenopausal women with node-positive and oestrogen-receptor-negative disease.

Drug toxicity remains a problem, and patients should be aware of this; side-effects include lassitude, temporary alopecia, blood dyscrasias (including profound leucopenia), immunosuppression and distressing gastrointestinal symptoms including nausea, vomiting and diarrhoea. Alopecia can be managed by concealment with a wig or reduced by using a cooling cap. Upper gastrointestinal symptoms are much relieved by 5HT antagonists (ondansetron).

Hormonal manipulation

The rationale behind this method is that tumours which arise in tissue which is a target for hormones – such as the breast – may have their growth affected by either endocrine ablation or pharmacological blockade.

Hormone receptors in breast cancer

The cytosol of breast cancer cells may contain both oestrogen (ER) and progesterone (PR) receptors. Approximately 60% possess some oestrogen receptor activity, which is also a biochemical marker for the degree of differentiation and histological subtype. ER-positive tumours exhibit a 50–60% objective response rate to hormone therapies whereas only 10% of ER-negative tumours respond. The progesterone receptor is a marker of oestrogen action. Tumours which possess both ER and PR are more likely to respond to hormonal therapy than those with ER alone, and benefits are also seen in a substantial number of PR-positive ER-negative tumours. Epidermal growth factor (EGF) and the proto-oncogene c-*erb*B2 (HER-2/*neu*) are transmembrane tyrosine kinase receptors that are overexpressed in a proportion of breast cancers, these invariably being ER poor. However, when expressed in ER-positive patients there is evidence to suggest that they may predict a poor response to hormonal therapy. The situation as regards the ER receptor may even be more complex than currently understood, as a second ER receptor (ER beta) has recently been described that appears to be associated with a worse prognosis.

Pharmacological blockade

Tamoxifen is a triphenylamine anti-oestrogen that acts by binding to the oestrogen receptor and thus blocking the effect of endogenous oestrogen. Approximately 30% of all breast cancers respond to tamoxifen, with this rising to 60% if they are receptor positive. It also reduces the subsequent incidence of contralateral breast cancer in postmenopausal patients by up to 40%. The maximal benefit appears to be gained by taking 20 mg of tamoxifen for 5 years with proportional mortality reductions of 12% for 1 year, 17% for 2 years and 26% for 5 years of treatment. The absolute improvement in 10-year survival rates with 5 years of tamoxifen is 10.9% for node-positive patients and 5.6% for node-negative patients. These benefits are present in both pre- and postmenopausal women; however, the mortality reduction is not significant in ER-negative patients. Tamoxifen is associated with a 2–6-fold increase in endometrial carcinoma, but this type of malignancy is very rare and therefore a sixfold increase over the normal incidence makes little statistical impact when compared with the potential benefits. Recent interest has concentrated on the possible role of tamoxifen in prevention. Following the early publication of the NSABP prevention study P-1, it is now recommended for high-risk groups in the USA. However, the data are not fully mature, and ongoing trials in the UK are currently addressing these issues.

Some breast cancers are tamoxifen resistant or even respond unfavourably to tamoxifen. Primary resistance is usually associated with ER-negative status, and there are various postulated mechanisms for the acquisition of secondary resistance. In addition, some ER-positive breast tumours occasionally respond unfavourably to tamoxifen; it appears that these tumours are c-*erb*B2 (HER-2/*neu*) positive, and for this group chemotherapy may be more appropriate. ER beta appears to stimulate breast cancer growth and may be associated with a positive c-*erb*B2 status. The implications for the use of tamoxifen, which is a partial agonist, in this group are clear.

Alternative methods of oestrogen modulation

Adipose tissue, breast cancer tissue and the adrenal cortex can all produce oestrogen. Tamoxifen is a selective oestrogen receptor modulator (SERM) but is only a partial antagonist and has pro-oestrogenic effects on the uterus, bone and vascular endothelium in addition to the concerns over tamoxifen resistance and possible worsening of prognosis in some patients. Alternative anti-oestrogens without intrinsic oestrogenic effect have therefore been developed. These SERMs include the pure anti-oestrogen ICI 182780 (Faslodex). This has been shown to induce a response in tumours that have acquired or possessed inherent resistance to tamoxifen.

An alternative strategy is to utilise drugs that prevent the aromatisation of androgen to oestrogen. Two major types have been developed:

- *Type I inhibitors.* These are known as steroidal aromatase inhibitors; they irreversibly inhibit the attachment of the androgen substrate to the enzyme's catalytic site and include formestane and exemestane.
- *Type II inhibitors.* These are non-steroidal compounds which reversibly interfere with the cytochrome p450 moiety of the enzyme; they include anastrozole and letrozole.

These aromatase inhibitors have been shown to dramatically reduce the level of circulating oestrogen and to induce response in hormone-dependent breast cancer. Early results of a large international trial comparing anastrozole with either anastrozole plus tamoxifen or tamoxifen alone (the ATAC trial) appear to show that the aromatase inhibitor is at least equivalent and possibly superior to tamoxifen in terms of local recurrence and survival, although the data are not yet mature enough to make firm conclusions. It is possible that the steroidal aromatase inhibitors will not have the deleterious effect on bone density seen with the non-steroidal aromatase inhibitors. However, an alternative under investigation is to combine an aromatase inhibitor with a bisphosphonate to counteract the oestrogen depletion effect on bone. An additional restriction on use is that it is only of value in postmenopausal women because premenopausal women have the ovary as their main source of oestrogen so that suppression of peripheral mechanisms will have little effect on oestrogen levels.

Aromatase inhibitors are now the established second-line hormonal adjuvant therapy for breast cancer. Indeed anastrozole is licensed for use as a primary therapy if the patient is at high risk of complications from taking tamoxifen and is increasingly being used as the first-line hormonal adjuvant therapy, tamoxifen being reserved for tumours considered at very low risk of recurrence. Furthermore the aromatase inhibitors appear to confer both a response rate and survival advantage over tamoxifen when used to treat advanced disease.

The progestogen-based drug megestrol can be used as third-line hormonal therapy, but its use these days is rare.

Aminoglutethimide is a non-selective aromatase inhibitor that produces an effective chemical adrenalectomy. Steroid replacement is required, and side-effects are common. Its use has therefore largely been abandoned in favour of the new aromatase inhibitors.

Ovarian suppression and ablation

Ovarian supression and ablation can be achieved by surgical, medical or pharmacological means.

In premenopausal women, oophorectomy can be used either as a second-line therapy for recurrent disease or as a primary therapy, where it has been shown to be as effective as chemotherapy for all groups except oestrogen-receptor-negative, node-negative patients. By removing the ovaries or inactivating them with radiotherapy, the primary source of oestrogen is removed. Alternatively, a chemical oophorectomy can be performed using GnRH agonists. This effectively produces a medical castration and a resultant reduction in oestrogen release from the ovaries equivalent to surgical removal. Adrenalectomy and hypophysectomy have also been used in the past to suppress ovarian hormone production but have now been superseded by the above methods.

Trastuzumab (Herceptin)

The identification of the c-*erb*B2 receptor opened a new biological target for tumour control. The drug trastuzumab, which blocked the receptor, was developed. In clinical trials of patients with recurrent breast cancer trastuzumab proved effective in controlling disease, leading to its adoption in an adjuvant setting.

It is mainly used in patients who are strongly positive and only currently in poorer prognosis patients who receive chemotherapy first. In some patients it causes left ventricular damage so that the patient's cardiac function has to be monitored using MUGA scans.

Summary of adjuvant treatment options for early-stage breast cancer

The adjuvant treatment of early breast cancer is guided by risk of relapse and death. Table 28.12 demonstrates how risk is stratified, and Tables 28.13 and 28.14 give guidelines for adjuvant therapy according to risk stratification for node-negative and node-positive patients, respectively.

Table 28.12 Breast cancer risk stratification

Factors	Low risk	Moderate risk	High risk
Size	<1 cm	1–2 cm	>2 cm
ER status	+ve	+ve	−ve
Grade	I	I/II	III
Age (years)	>35		<35

MANAGEMENT OF MORE ADVANCED DISEASE AND SPECIAL PROBLEMS

Management of more advanced disease and special problems

Stage III disease

This stage of disease usually involves disease which is locally advanced with tumour invading local structures or extensive node involvement. It often carries a poorer prognosis.

Survival generally approaches 45% at 5 years for stage III disease. Frequently preoperative neo-adjuvant combination chemotherapy over two to six drug cycles has been used to reduce tumour size (see below) – cyclophosphamide, doxorubicin (or epirubicin) and 5-fluorouracil (the combinations being known by the acronyms CAF or FEC) is undertaken to either enable or facilitate surgery. A response rate of 60–75% is expected. The effect on the tumour cells may not only cause shrinkage but also affect the tumour cells' kinetics so that the possibility that surgery will exacerbate the progression of the disease is reduced. Invariably postoperative radiotherapy to the chest wall is undertaken following surgery.

A significant number of women can be downstaged with neo-adjuvant chemotherapy or hormonal therapy to the extent that they no longer require a mastectomy.

Table 28.14 Adjuvant treatment for node-positive patients

Patient group	Treatments
Premenopausal ER/PR +ve	(1) Chemotherapy ± tamoxifen (2) Ovarian ablation (3) Chemotherapy ± ovarian ablation ± tamoxifen
Premenopausal ER/PR −ve	Chemotherapy
Postmenopausal ER/PR +ve	Aromatase inhibitor + chemotherapy
Postmenopausal ER/PR −ve	Chemotherapy
Elderly	Aromatase inhibitor (chemotherapy if ER/PR −ve)

Table 28.13 Adjuvant treatment for node-negative patients stratified by risk[a]

Patient group	Low risk	Intermediate risk	High risk
Premenopausal ER/PR +ve	None or tamoxifen	(1) Tamoxifen ±chemotherapy (2) Ovarian ablation	(1) Chemotherapy ± tamoxifen (2) Ovarian ablation
Premenopausal ER/PR −ve	N/A	N/A	Chemotherapy
Postmenopausal ER/PR +ve	None or tamoxifen	Aromatase inhibitor ± chemotherapy	Aromatase inhibitor ± chemotherapy
Postmenopausal ER/PR −ve	N/A	N/A	Chemotherapy
Elderly	None	Chemotherapy	Chemotherapy (if ER/PR −ve)

[a]See Table 28.12.

ER, oestrogen receptor; PR, progesterone receptor. Trastuzumab added intermediate and high risk cases if strongly c-*erb*B2 positive.

Alternative presentations

Inflammatory carcinoma

As its name implies this lesion can present with all the features of an inflammatory lesion, it often comes on rapidly and may initially be treated as an abscess; however, by definition it fails to respond to antibiotics. It is important to keep the possibility of this condition in mind in ladies with apparent breast sepsis, particularly if it seems slightly atypical.

The optimum treatment regimen for inflammatory breast cancer has yet to be developed. However, the best results to date confirm that a multimodality approach is required which utilises various combinations of surgery, radiotherapy and chemotherapy. After preoperative neo-adjuvant radiotherapy and induction chemotherapy, a mastectomy with level III axillary lymph node removal is performed. Radiotherapy is administered to the wound site once this has healed and, if a favourable response to the chemotherapy has been noted, this may be continued, although the optimum duration of therapy has not been elucidated. Studies utilising combinations of chemotherapeutic agents have claimed up to 75% survival at 5 years; however, in general, survival remains at 30%.

Paget's disease

It is assumed that an underlying carcinoma is always present. A palpable growth is managed by mastectomy with either axillary clearance or sampling and, if lymph nodes are positive, local radiotherapy. The prognosis and further treatment are related to the menopausal state of the patient and the stage and grade of the primary tumour. Impalpable tumours are dealt with by mastectomy or central excision including the nipple–areola complex if breast size allows. The management of the axilla and other local treatments are guided by the final histology.

Psychological considerations in therapy

It must be stressed from the very beginning that the patient has an active role to play in the joint decision-making that necessarily accompanies successful treatment.

Mastectomy

One-third of women will suffer moderate or severe anxiety and depression after mastectomy. Concerns about body image, and effects on interpersonal relationships and family life can often lead to a dramatic withdrawal from society.

Even patients who have undergone breast-preserving procedures can have such symptoms because of persistent thoughts of recurrent or remaining disease. Counselling is required both pre- and postoperatively. It is not acceptable for a woman to be anaesthetised for a breast operation without knowing exactly what is to happen to her body. A nurse specialised in such work is a vital member of the multidisciplinary team.

Metastatic disease

Metastatic breast cancer is for the moment incurable. Despite this, the response to chemotherapy and actual survival rates are highly variable, which reflects the biological heterogeneity of the disease. There are a number of factors that are associated with the degree of aggressiveness of residual disease. Clinically, time interval between diagnosis and development of metastatic disease, organ sites involved and rate of tumour growth are indicators of aggressiveness. Biological characteristics include proliferative activity of the tumour, the hormone receptor status of the primary tumour and the amplification or overexpression of certain proto-oncogenes such as HER-2/*neu*. Host characteristics such as young age may also be important. Once the cancer has become disseminated systemically, surgery to the breast and subsequent radiotherapy are done only for local control. Combination chemotherapy can produce remission in up to 70%, with a median survival of 32 months if complete remission at initial treatment has been achieved. The most common combination in use for primary chemotherapy is the CAF or FEC regimen (cyclophosphamide, doxorubicin [adriamycin] or epirubicin, and 5-fluorouracil), with second-line chemotherapy being a taxane-containing regimen. The taxanes show great promise in the adjuvant therapy of breast cancer, but their exact role is still under investigation. Trastuzumab has been a major breakthrough in treating metastasis from tumours that express HER-2/*neu* and can be combined with chemotherapy. Currently interest is focusing on epidermal growth factor inhibitors and agents that disrupt angiogenesis.

Follow-up

Review after treatment presents some particular problems. Patients who have undergone breast-conserving surgery have a lifelong risk of local recurrence which, although a source of anxiety for the patient, can be managed with a salvage mastectomy, or even further local excision, and does not mean impending death. Patients who have undergone mastectomy have a low rate of local recurrence, but its arrival generally heralds a significant progression of the disease. In the majority of instances, local recurrence is apparent within 3 years. If breast-conserving surgery has been done, then the remaining breast tissue will be distorted by postoperative scarring and associated fibrosis; clinical examination and mammography are both very difficult to interpret, and local recurrence of the disease may be missed until it is well advanced. The detection of distant metastasis generally heralds the final phase of the disease, and both further systemic and local therapy may be required to prolong life and reduce morbidity.

Traditional follow-up is by annual mammograms and clinical examination for patients who have undergone breast-conserving surgery, and biannual or annual mammograms for patients with one remaining breast in order to detect a second primary – an assessment which continues for the rest of the patient's life. Other more specific investigations for metastases are only used if the patient complains of symptoms suggestive of secondary deposits. Indeed there is a fair amount of data to suggest that routine clinical follow-up makes no difference to the detection of recurrence or to the subsequent outcome, and it is likely that mammography alone is all that is required if combined with open access to clinic for any concerns the patient might have.

Palliation of specific problems

Bone metastases

Seventy-three percent of patients who die from the disease have skeletal metastases. However, less than half of these have symptoms, and these lesions should be managed only when recognised as a source of trouble. The exception is a lesion that threatens pathological fracture, such as one in a weight-bearing bone, which should be fixed internally and followed by radiotherapy. Palliative therapy should not be withheld, because the median survival is as high as 48 months in patients with metastases confined to bone and 17 months for those with additional deposits at other sites. Pain from osseous metastasis can be controlled with radiotherapy, NSAIDs or opiates. Bisphosphonates have recently been shown to reduce the progression and morbidity associated with bony metastases even if they are not associated with hypercalcaemia.

Transient hypercalcaemia occurs in almost half of those with bone metastasis. Levels greater than 3 mmol/L are often associated with distressing gastrointestinal and neurovascular symptoms.

Pleural and lung metastases

Pleural effusions and metastatic pleural disease are frequent problems. Up to 37% of all malignant pleural effusions are associated with metastatic breast cancer; they are nearly always the result of haematogenous metastasis, but in some locally advanced tumours, spread may be directly through the chest wall. For this reason, bilateral effusions occur in 15%. The presence of pleural metastasis is an ominous feature because it is associated with metastasis in other sites in more than half of those who present with it.

Malignant pleural effusions are initially managed by removing the pleural liquid by either needle aspiration or intercostal drainage. However, reaccumulation is inevitable, and pleurodesis is required. For this to succeed, the pleural surfaces must be in apposition, which is best achieved by intercostal drainage. An irritant such as tetracycline is successful in 70–100%. Bleomycin may also be used either initially or after failed tetracycline therapy (85% success rate).

Individual lung metastases do not generally cause problems. However, diffuse infiltration of the pulmonary lymphatics produces a stiff lung, often with bronchospasm and dyspnoea. Symptomatic relief can sometimes be obtained with bronchodilators and steroids.

Median survival is between 6 and 15 months. The median survival from diagnosis of the pleural effusion is 10 months, with half this group succumbing directly to their bronchopulmonary disease and half to distant metastasis to other sites.

CNS metastases

In autopsy series, approximately 30% of those who have died from breast cancer have been shown to have metastasis to the CNS. Of these, approximately 65% are asymptomatic, and it is rare for a brain metastasis to be the cause of death. The dura is the most common site, with the cerebellum next. Solitary metastasis occurs in approximately 40%, with the incidence of cranial dural involvement increasing threefold if vertebral body metastases are present.

Symptoms may be either of raised intracranial pressure or focal neurological problems which depend on the site of the lesion.

Untreated survival is approximately 6 weeks. With aggressive combined therapy, which, in carefully selected patients, includes surgery, radiation therapy and chemotherapy, survival may be extended to approximately 50% at 1 year.

Spinal compression

After lung cancer, breast cancer is the second most common cause of symptomatic spinal cord compression. When it has occurred, approximately one-third develop irreversible hemiparalysis, so that an early diagnosis and urgent treatment are essential. Extramedullary disease accounts for more than 97%. The metastases reach the epidural space either by direct local extension from invasion of a vertebral body or by haematogenous spread. For diagnosis, a plain X-ray is more specific than a bone scan and can accurately predict the presence or absence of metastasis in over 80%. However, if, as is rarely the case, only the intervertebral disc is involved, then plain X-ray is likely to be normal. Nevertheless, in a patient with breast cancer and back pain who has both a normal neurological examination and a normal plain film, spinal metastasis is very unlikely. CT and MRI scanning provide the diagnostic information necessary for planning treatment.

As mentioned above, treatment is a matter of urgency – with the immediate introduction of dexamethasone to reduce oedema, and subsequent radiotherapy. Approximately 50% respond to these measures. Indications for surgical decompression include:

- posteriorly placed lesions
- continued progression of disease in spite of radiotherapy
- recurrent compression after initial response to radiotherapy
- vertebral instability.

Radiotherapy is the best therapeutic option and should be given to all those treated surgically if they have not been previously irradiated at the site of compression.

Breast reconstruction following mastectomy

Reconstruction should not be considered a purely cosmetic procedure but rather a functional restoration of an important aspect of appearance and self-image.

There are five essential elements to any reconstructive procedure that also apply in breast cancer:

- coverage to allow survival of the procedure
- coverage to allow adequate tumour clearance
- repair of irradiated or scarred tissue by introduction of new blood supply, as in flap reconstruction
- recreation of the form of the lost part
- replacement of function of the lost part.

The first three relate to soft-tissue coverage and are dependent on the healing of the initial operation whatever that may have been. The last two relate to restoration of the form of the breast, which is intricately interwoven with its perceived function.

Potential candidates are likely to have a set of goals that must be achieved in order to make reconstructive breast surgery worthwhile:

- symmetry
- adequate form, consistency and size
- lasting result
- no detrimental effects on treatment and outcome.

However, each may also have their own ideas about what reconstruction, if any, is desired and what quality of cosmetic result is sought. This must be thoroughly discussed before planning the exact nature of the operation.

The reconstruction may be achieved using autogenous tissue with or without a prosthesis or by a combination of implanted expanders and a prosthesis.

In general, breast reconstruction should be offered to all women undergoing mastectomy, and facilities should allow for the reconstruction to be carried out at the same time as the mastectomy. The myocutaneous latissimus dorsi flap is particularly suitable for immediate reconstruction as it has a predominantly well-vascularised muscle-based bulk and is therefore able to withstand postoperative radiotherapy if it is deemed necessary. Flaps of this kind with an independent blood supply allow radiotherapy and chemotherapy to begin after only 10 days, in contrast to other methods of skin coverage such as free flaps that require a longer healing period.

However, some patients are either advised or prefer to wait for reconstruction until after their initial course of radiotherapy or chemotherapy has been completed. The basic shape of the breast can be achieved with a simple silicone implant provided the mastectomy flaps are not too tight (Fig. 28.15). These are now usually placed deep to the pectoralis major in order to reduce the formation of a deforming fibrous capsule – common in subcutaneous implants. Despite this advance, a prosthetic implant is often subject to deformity from scar encapsulation. Because of this, tissue expanders may be implanted at the time of mastectomy or later and expanded over a number of weeks to stimulate skin growth. Once sufficient skin is available, the expander is usually replaced with a permanent silicone implant. Scar encapsulation and subsequent deformity are much reduced. Combined prostheses that act as expanders and also contain a permanent silicone component have recently been introduced. These do not have to be replaced once expansion is satisfactory and the final shape achieved.

Autogenous tissue transfer offers the only possibility of reconstructing a breast that will match the form, shape and consistency of the opposite side. Various myocutaneous flaps are available – including the standard latissimus dorsi flap – which can be used with an implant to increase its bulk. Flaps based on the rectus abdominis (transverse rectus abdominis myocutaneous – TRAM flap) (Fig. 28.16) have become the gold standard in breast reconstruction with autologous tissue, and it is against this that all other methods must be considered. TRAM flaps can either be pedicled, drawing their blood supply from the superior epigastric vessels, or free flaps using either the internal mammary or thoracodorsal vessels for the anastomosis. In certain circumstances, microvascular techniques can be employed in order

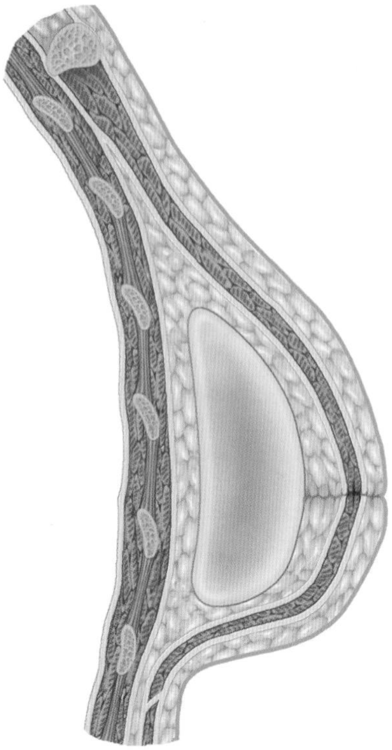

Fig. 28.15 Submuscular placement of expander/silicone implant.

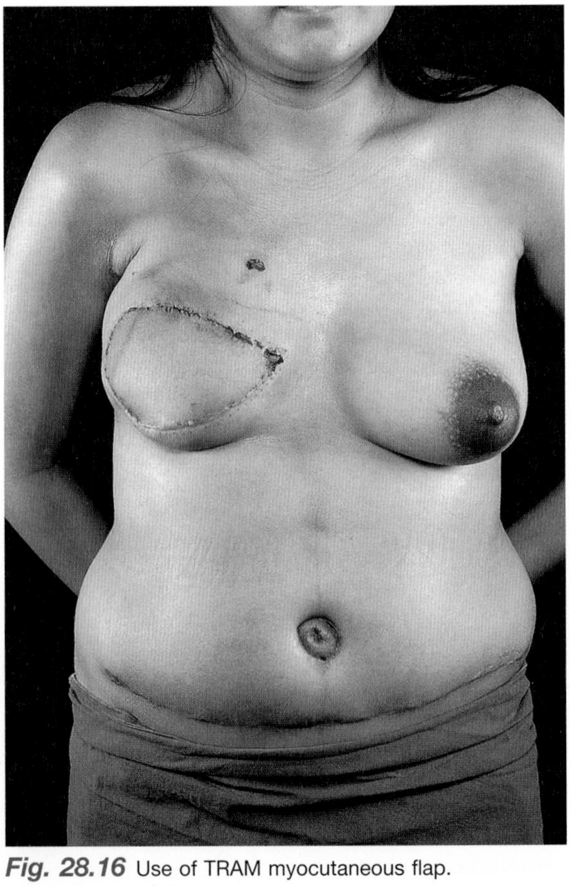

Fig. 28.16 Use of TRAM myocutaneous flap.

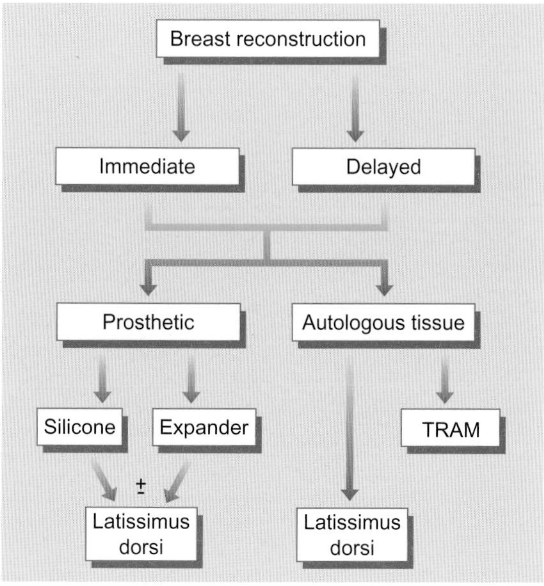

Fig. 28.17 General principles of breast reconstruction.

to facilitate the transfer of free flaps from regions such as that supplied by the gluteal vessels. The general principles involved in breast reconstruction are illustrated in Figure 28.17.

There is also renewed interest in fat stem cell breast augmentation. Fat cells from one part of the body can be transferred and grow in another, and this technique has potential for breast reconstruction after cancer surgery.

FURTHER READING

Benign breast disease

Mansel R E, Webster D, Sweetland H. 2009 Hughes, Mansel and Webster's Benign disorders and diseases of the breast: concepts and clinical management, 3rd edn. Saunders Elsevier, Philadelphia

Breast cancer

Dixon J M 2005 ABC of breast diseases, 3rd edn. Blackwell Publishing, London

Harris J R, Lippman M E, Morrow M, Osborne C K (eds) 2009 Diseases of the breast, 4th edn. Lippincott Williams & Wilkins, Philadelphia

29 Arterial disease

ARTERIAL PHYSIOLOGY AND ANATOMY

Arterial disease exerts major haemodynamic effects upon the circulation, which in turn cause the symptoms and signs of disease. Haemodynamics pervade most aspects of vascular surgery; hence in order to understand these processes, it is necessary to have a basic grasp of normal arterial physiology.

NORMAL ARTERIAL PHYSIOLOGY

Blood vessels represent a highly complex and dynamic network constructed in both parallel and series configuration. The vessel wall serves as an insulator preventing dissipation of energy and also provides capacitance, maintaining the ability to store energy during the systolic phase which is later released in the diastolic phase. This results in a more continuous flow of energy throughout the cardiac cycle.

Blood flow is governed by the following parameters:

- blood pressure, velocity and blood viscosity
- the anatomy of the arterial tree
- the mechanical characteristics of the arterial wall
- the properties of the vascular endothelium.

Blood pressure

Conventionally, blood pressure (*P*) is measured in millimetres of mercury (mmHg). It is dependent upon:

- the force of cardiac contraction
- circulatory volume
- tone – the pressure exerted by the muscular effect of the arterioles.

Blood energy

Bernoulli's theorem states that when fluid flows from one point to another, provided flow is steady and there are no frictional losses, the total energy remains constant. As blood moves away from the heart, the total cross-sectional area of the arterial tree increases so that, if total flow is to remain constant, velocity must decrease. Kinetic energy is therefore converted to potential energy and, under idealised conditions where fluid energy is conserved, this is actually associated with a small increase in blood pressure. Although the arterial system is an extremely efficient conduit, it is not frictionless and contains bends and branches. While frictional energy losses are negligible within large vessels, this becomes significant within smaller vessels. In addition, arterial flow is pulsatile rather than steady. For these reasons the Bernoulli theorem does not accurately describe events in vivo: fluid energy is dissipated, mainly as heat, through viscous and inertial losses.

Viscous energy losses

Viscosity is defined as the resistance of a fluid to flow because of intermolecular attractions; in whole blood, it is mainly determined by haematocrit and the concentration of plasma proteins. It is most conveniently expressed in relation to the value for water (relative viscosity). The relative viscosity of whole blood is approximately 3–4 and plasma is about 1.8.

Inertial energy losses

These are changes in kinetic energy as a consequence of changes in blood velocity, the pattern of flow and its direction. In-vivo inertial losses are more significant than viscous ones, especially in the presence of disease that leads to dilatation, tortuosity, narrowing or occlusion.

Resistance to flow

The diameter of peripheral vessels has the greatest effect on peripheral resistance and (given normal blood viscosity), at flow rates found within the human circulation, resistance increases markedly when vessel diameter falls below approximately 3 mm. Resistance in the human circulation is therefore from the:

- microcirculation – small arteries, arterioles and capillaries (70%)
- venous circulation (10%)
- large and medium-sized arteries (20%).

Thus, those arteries most commonly affected by atherosclerosis in health offer little resistance to flow. To summarise, as blood flows through the arterial tree, energy is lost through both viscous and inertial factors. Loss of kinetic energy is manifested by a reduction in blood velocity, and loss of potential energy by a reduction in blood pressure. In the presence of arterial disease, these losses may be excessive and may result in underperfusion of tissues and ischaemia.

Patterns of arterial flow

Three main forms are recognised:

- *laminar* – when the motion of the blood can be described by a series of concentric rings parallel to the wall of the vessel; the flow velocity is greatest in the centre and least at the vessel wall (a so-called parabolic flow profile)
- *turbulent* – a disorderly flow pattern where velocity varies randomly across the diameter of the vessel
- *disturbed* – midway between laminar and turbulent where, at certain points in the circulation, there is transient disruption of laminar flow which is re-established further downstream.

In health, the only part of the human circulation in which there is turbulent flow is the ascending aorta, although disturbed flow may occur at the origin of branches. In the presence of atherosclerosis, turbulent flow is common.

Boundary effects

The boundary layer is the blood flowing adjacent to the vessel wall. At branch points and where the lumen suddenly changes size, the layer may slow down, change or even reverse its direction. Such boundary layer separation (BLS) leads to complex local flow patterns at arterial bifurcations, anastomoses and sites of arterial disease. Atherosclerotic plaques have been observed to occur particularly at points where BLS leads to reversed or stagnant flow, e.g. at the carotid bifurcation (Fig. 29.1). The reasons for this are unknown, but may relate to mechanical changes in frictional forces (shear stress) between the blood and the vessel wall or to prolonged contact between humoral factors in the blood and the endothelium at these points.

Pulsatile nature of flow

Blood flow in vivo is pulsatile. The haemodynamic principles outlined above are useful but depend upon steady laminar flow within a straight, frictionless tube. In consequence, they do not provide a precise description of the events that occur in the human circulation. Therefore, instead of using the term vascular resistance, 'vascular impedance' better describes the opposition of the circulation to pulsatile flow and includes the effects of viscosity, bends, branches, changes in diameter, arterial elasticity (compliance) and wave reflections. In order that blood should flow, mean arterial pressure (MAP) must fall, although in health the gradient in MAP between the heart and the ankle is only of the order of 10 mmHg. Therefore, as the pressure wave moves distally, MAP and diastolic pressure fall. However, due to reflected waves from the distal circulation, systolic pressure actually increases and pulse pressure widens. For these reasons, in health the systolic ankle : brachial pressure index (ABPI) is normally greater than 1 and does not fall on exercise.

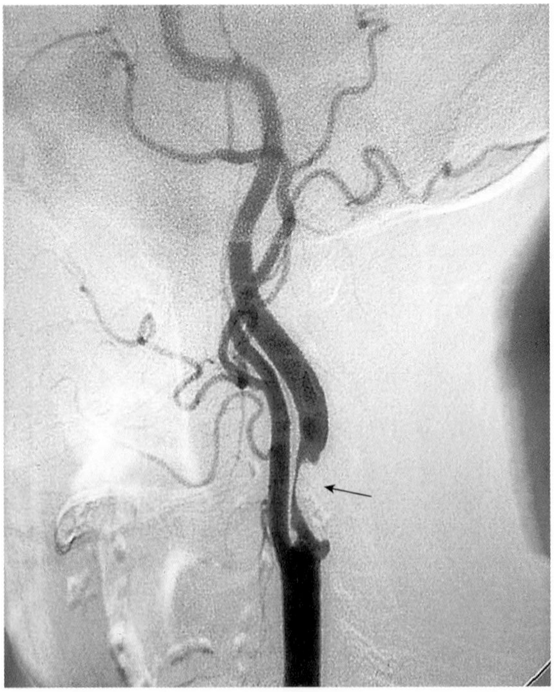

Fig. 29.1 Intra-arterial digital subtraction angiogram showing a 90% stenosis of the internal carotid artery (arrow). Note how the vessels proximal and distal to the lesion appear almost normal. This is one of the few areas of the body where arterial disease is often localised and thus amenable to endarterectomy.

Phases of arterial flow

Arterial flow is normally triphasic, consisting of:

- an initial large forward flow caused by ventricular contraction
- a short period of reverse flow in early diastole
- a third phase of forward flow in late diastole.

The duration of the reverse flow phase depends upon peripheral resistance: when this increases (vasoconstriction on exposure to cold), the reverse flow period is extended; when it decreases (exercise, exposure to heat) the opposite is the case.

Structure of the arterial tree

Arterial wall compliance

In addition to arterial geometry, blood flow is determined by the physical characteristics of the arterial wall itself, which in turn depend upon the relative amounts of collagen, elastin and smooth muscle. The compliance (elasticity) of the artery allows blood energy to be stored during systole and to be returned to the blood in diastole. As the distance from the heart increases, the elastin:collagen ratio decreases so that the more distal arteries do not store as much energy in this way and act more as passive conduits.

Law of Laplace

For a thin-walled structure, this law describes the relationship between tangential tension (T), radius (r) and intraluminal pressure (P):

$$T = Pr$$

Thus, the greater the diameter, the greater the tension in the vessel wall for a given blood pressure. This relationship also explains why blood pressure increases arterial wall stress and why hypertension is such a strong risk factor for aneurysmal dilatation, rupture and dissection (see below).

ABNORMAL ARTERIAL PHYSIOLOGY

The above account of the normal physiology indicates the complexity of the principles that govern arterial flow. The forces at work in the presence of arterial disease are even more difficult to define.

Arterial narrowing (stenosis)

This is the commonest arterial lesion. Blood flow and blood pressure begin to be reduced at about the same magnitude of narrowing; further reductions in diameter or cross-sectional area affect flow and pressure at approximately the same rate. Because flow along the length of the artery at a localised stenosis must remain constant, velocity increases. Thus, potential energy (pressure) is converted into kinetic energy and back to potential energy. If the stenosis is short, smooth, tapering and low grade, laminar flow is preserved and little energy is lost. By contrast if it is long, irregular, abrupt and high grade, turbulence is produced and energy is dissipated.

Critical arterial stenosis

This is somewhat arbitrarily defined as a stenosis which produces a reduction in flow (and usually pressure) and is normally associated with a 50% reduction in diameter (≈ 75% reduction in cross-sectional area). The greater the velocity of the blood which flows into the stenosis, the greater the inertial and viscous energy losses and so the greater the fall in pressure distal to the stenosis. Flow across a stenosis can be augmented by exercise or any other factor that results in peripheral vasodilatation and so reduces the vascular resistance of the distal circulation. Thus a stenosis may not be haemodynamically and symptomatically significant (critical) at rest but becomes so at high flow rates. This is the basis for exercise or 'stress' testing.

Atherosclerotic stenoses are frequently multiple. Because viscous energy losses are proportional to the length of the stenosis, one 4 cm stenosis is equivalent to two 2 cm stenoses of the same diameter. This is not true for inertial energy losses, because the two 2 cm stenoses cause more turbulence than a single 4 cm stenosis – a consequence of the doubling of entrance and exit effects on flow. Thus, a series of separately non-critical stenoses may act as one critical stenosis to reduce flow and pressure. When two lesions are of equal severity, both should be corrected; where they are not, the narrower one should be dealt with first. Arterial stenosis leads to loss of energy and loss of pressure. At first, only peak systolic pressure (PSP) is affected, MAP being preserved. Reduction in PSP is thus the most sensitive measure of stenosis. Stenosis also leads to changes in the normal triphasic waveform, with damping of the PSP, loss of the normal forward flow in late diastole (biphasic pattern) and then loss of normal reverse flow in early diastole (monophasic pattern). Such changes can be used to assess arterial disease by non-invasive means with ultrasound and plethysmographic techniques.

Collateral circulation

The increase in size of vessels that run parallel to a site of obstruction is a vital compensatory mechanism that affects the clinical manifestations of arterial disease and the manner of treatment. Through mechanisms that are not well understood, but which almost certainly involve a response by the endothelium to shear stress, increased flow through an artery leads to hypertrophy and dilatation. This enlargement of existing vessels provides an alternative pathway for blood flow. Effective collateral circulation is dependent upon the normal anatomy of the area involved. Disease of the superficial femoral artery with collateral flow through the profunda femoris system is perhaps the most common example of effective collateral circulation.

Collateral dilatation takes time, so that gradual development of a stenosis has a better outcome than sudden narrowing or occlusion. The formation of a collateral circulation can be augmented through exercise because the reduction in peripheral resistance on walking increases flow through the alternative pathway. A number of growth factors (such as VEGF, NO) are secreted secondary to the induced ischaemia following exercise that contributes to the formation of new collaterals. However, no matter how well a collateral circulation develops, the vessels are of lower overall diameter than that which they replace, the peripheral resistance is greater and so the blood supply to the organ or limb is poorer.

Box 29.1 Properties of the normal endothelium and arterial wall

Endothelium
- Controls microvascular permeability
- Non-thrombogenic, pro-fibrinolytic surface through production of prostacyclin, heparins and activation of fibrinolytic cascade
- Modulation of the inflammatory response through cytokine and adhesion molecule release or expression
- Modulation and initiation of thrombus formation through platelet and coagulation cascade activation
- Production of vasoactive substances such as nitric oxide, angiotensin-converting enzyme (ACE) and endothelin

Arterial wall
- Storage of blood energy
- Autoregulation – contraction and relaxation in response to myogenic and metabolic factors
- Lipid metabolism
- Production of connective tissue
- Arterial repair through migration and proliferation of smooth muscle cells

NORMAL ARTERIAL ANATOMY

Arterial wall structure

Arteries are normally distensible, compliant and have three layers:

- *intima* – a single-cell endothelial layer which rests on a basement membrane
- *media* – separated from the intima by the internal elastic lamina, composed mostly of smooth muscle cells but also, in large vessels, containing numerous elastin fibres
- *adventitia* – a meshwork of connective tissue which contains the vasa vasorum that provide blood to the media; between the media and adventitia is the external elastic lamina.

Arterial endothelium

The endothelium is not merely an inert lining (Box 29.1). The biology of the endothelial cell is complex and still imperfectly understood. Any disease process that leads to endothelial dysfunction has major effects upon arterial autoregulation, blood coagulation and fibrinolysis.

EFFECTS OF ISCHAEMIA–REPERFUSION INJURY

Ischaemic injury

All tissues rely on the circulation to deliver oxygen and nutrients and to remove the waste products of metabolism. Any pathological process that reduces the blood supply leads to the replacement of aerobic by anaerobic metabolism and the build-up of the potentially harmful products of metabolism, particularly carbon dioxide and lactic acid, with the accumulation of hydrogen ions. Through mechanisms that are poorly understood, tissues can adapt to a degree of ischaemia, especially if it develops gradually rather than acutely. However, after a certain point, cell membrane disruption and macromolecular denaturation occur, which lead to irreversible ischaemic injury and loss of function, even if normal arterial flow is eventually restored. Tissues differ widely in their tolerance of ischaemia: irreversible damage to neurons occurs after only a few minutes, but skin may survive for up to 24 hours. This variability in tissue tolerance affects the clinical manifestations of arterial disease in different parts of the body as well as the urgency and success of surgical intervention.

Reperfusion injury (RI)

The mechanisms that underlie reperfusion injury are complex and imperfectly understood. Briefly, when tissues are rendered ischaemic, the endothelium lining that vascular bed is activated. Instead of providing a smooth, non-stick surface, activated endothelial cells release pro-coagulant substances, express adhesion molecules that attract and bind leucocytes, and release cytokines that act upon the white cells to produce more cytokines and oxygen-derived free radicals. When the tissue is reperfused, leucocytes, platelets and thrombus adhere to the endothelium and imperil the microcirculation. An inflammatory response is initiated and tissues are damaged. In addition, some activated leucocytes and their products escape into the general circulation and can contribute to organ failure, such as renal failure and adult respiratory distress syndrome (ARDS, Ch. 16).

Clinical complications

Compartment syndrome (see also Ch. 35)

When severely ischaemic tissues are reperfused, the microcirculation is very permeable, and plasma leaks through the damaged capillary endothelium into the interstitial space. Ischaemic cells also swell because of membrane injury. The overall result is marked tissue swelling and oedema. Calf muscles are held within fascial compartments, which do not allow expansion. Reperfusion is therefore associated with a marked increase in intracompartmental pressure such that, despite normal arterial inflow, the microcirculation remains underperfused and cellular hypoxia persists. Clinically, the leg appears enlarged, with pain on palpation and plantar or dorsiflexion of the foot radiating to the calf. Raised plasma levels of creatine kinase (CK) and myoglobinuria are characteristic but late features of compartment syndrome. Fasciotomy is therefore necessary at the same time as revascularisation.

General metabolic effects

If a large embolus lodges at the aortic bifurcation (saddle embolus) to cause total ischaemia of the lower body, revascularisation by means of bilateral transfemoral embolectomy is usually achieved without difficulty. On reperfusion, however, deterioration rather than improvement often occurs because of the entry of metabolites, such as potassium and hydrogen ions, into the general circulation. Cardiac arrest several hours later is not uncommon.

Myoglobinuria

Irreversible damage to muscle cells causes release of myoglobin into the circulation on reperfusion. Renal tubular injury and renal failure may follow. Management comprises adequate hydration and a forced alkaline diuresis. It is important to understand that myoglobinuria may be a late phenomenon that should not delay treatment if compartment syndrome is suspected.

Reduction of reperfusion injury

Surgeons and anaesthetists take all possible measures to reduce RI by minimising the duration of ischaemia through expeditious surgery and/or the use of shunts to maintain the blood supply to the distant organ while the operation is completed. In addition, attention to fluid balance, oxygenation and certain drugs such as mannitol, allopurinol and dopamine may help to attenuate the effects of RI and protect the kidneys and the lungs from these processes.

PATHOLOGICAL FEATURES OF ARTERIAL DISEASE

A distinction is drawn between macrovascular disorders, which affect large vessels, and microvascular ones, which involve the distal parts of the arterial circulation – the smallest arteries and arterioles.

ATHEROSCLEROTIC OCCLUSIVE DISEASE

This is the commonest cause of arterial disease in developed countries. It is also known as 'arteriosclerosis' or 'atheroma' and to lay people as 'hardening of the arteries'. Atherosclerosis is found in virtually 100% of adults from developed countries and is responsible for 50% of all deaths. The prevalence of atheroma increases with age but it is not regarded as an intrinsic part of the ageing process.

Definition

The World Health Organization defines atherosclerotic occlusive disease as a variable combination of changes in the intima which include focal accumulations of lipid, complex carbohydrates, blood and blood products, fibrous deposits and calcium deposits associated with secondary changes in the media.

Development

It is still far from clear how atheroma develops. The initial lesion of atherosclerosis involves the intima and begins in childhood with the development of focal intimal thickening with an increase in smooth muscle cells and extracellular matrix known as fatty streaks. Migration of smooth muscle cells into the intima results in apoptosis and macrophage infiltration and calcification. Further accumulation of connective tissue, lipid-laden smooth muscle cells result in the formation of the fibrous plaque. More advanced lesions present with necrosis in the lipid-rich core and calcification.

In all cases the first event is probably endothelial damage caused by:

- *Mechanical injury*. At certain points in the circulation the endothelium is exposed to particularly high shearing forces, especially in the presence of hypertension. In this context, the low-pressure pulmonary circulation is very rarely affected.
- *Chemical injury*. One or more constituents of tobacco smoke almost certainly have a direct toxic effect on the endothelium. Certain lipids are also harmful.

Damaged endothelium ceases to be a functional barrier between the blood and the arterial wall, and lipoproteins, fibrinogen, leucocytes and platelets can transgress the intima. Through poorly understood mechanisms, smooth muscle cells are in turn stimulated to enter the intima from the media, take on the properties of fibroblasts and secrete collagen and matrix.

The end result is an atheromatous plaque which is elevated, pale yellow or grey, involves the intima and media, and consists of smooth muscle cells, fibroblasts, macrophages, collagen and intra- and extracellular lipid. The endothelium may be lost from the surface of the plaque to form an ulcer, with cholesterol and/or altered blood constituents (thrombus) at its base. Such a plaque is often described as 'complex'.

Aetiology

Smoking

Tobacco smoking is the single largest risk factor for arterial disease, and the risk is directly related to the number of 'pack-years' smoked. Tobacco smoke contains many hundreds of different chemicals, and it is unclear which are directly toxic to vascular endothelium. In addition, smoking increases blood viscosity and activates leucocytes to make them less deformable and more likely to become involved in inflammatory processes. Raised blood levels of carbon monoxide may also be a factor. Cessation of smoking is associated with a rapid reversal of the adverse rheological changes and a reduction in the risk of future vascular clinical events. It is not known if atheroma regresses, but certain studies suggest that it does.

Diabetes

Both insulin-dependent and non-insulin-dependent diabetes greatly increase the risk of atheroma. Lesions develop earlier in life and progress more rapidly. The distribution of atheroma may also differ from that found in non-diabetic patients (e.g. the tibial and foot vessels are more commonly affected). Both secondary increases in blood lipid levels and changes in endothelial cell metabolism may be involved.

Hyperlipidaemia

The normal plasma level of cholesterol varies between populations: in the UK, 5–6 mmol/L is usual. Many of those with arterial disease have much higher levels. The measured total cholesterol level has three main components:

- high-density lipoprotein (HDL)
- low-density lipoprotein (LDL)
- very low-density lipoprotein (VLDL)

in addition to chylomicrons. *Triglyceride* measurement forms part of the complete lipid profile.

Treatment is aimed at reducing levels of harmful LDL and increasing the proportion of beneficial HDL. Without a complete lipid profile and knowledge of the ratio of total cholesterol to HDL, a single reading of total cholesterol can be misleading.

Raised plasma levels result from:

- a high-fat diet
- a genetically determined reduction in the removal of lipid and lipoproteins from the circulation (primary hyperlipidaemia); hyperlipidaemia is one of the commonest inherited autosomal dominant conditions (approximately 1 in 500 of the UK population)
- secondary hyperlipidaemia caused by a variety of other conditions – diabetes, hypothyroidism, excessive alcohol intake and drugs (thiazide diuretics and corticosteroids).

The Heart Protection Study has clearly demonstrated that lipid-lowering therapy with statins (hydroxymethylglutaryl co-enzyme A reductase inhibitors) is indicated for all patients with peripheral arterial disease (PAD). There was a 24% reduction in myocardial infarction, stroke and revascularisation in patients randomised to statin therapy. Furthermore this effect was independent of original cholesterol levels. For patients with PAD, 5 years of statin therapy was estimated to prevent 70 major vascular events per 1000 patients treated. In summary, all patients with PAD should be treated with a statin irrespective of their age and cholesterol levels. The latest Transatlantic Intersociety Consensus Document (TASC II) recommends that all patients should aim to have levels of LDL <2.59 mmol/L and patients with disease in multiple vascular beds should aim at levels <1.81 mmol/L.

Inflammation

Humoral and cellular pathways are involved in the presence of inflammation observed in atherosclerotic lesions. Oxidised LDL enhances the secretary role of macrophages which release a variety of inflammatory molecules such as monocyte chemotactic protein (MCP-1); intercellular adhesion molecule (ICAM-1); macrophage and colony stimulating factors, soluble CD40 ligand; interleukin IL-1, IL-3, IL-8, IL-18; tumour necrosis factor alpha (TNFα). These cytokines seem to have a pivotal role in the pathogenesis of atherosclerosis by enhancing the expression of various cell surface adhesion molecules (ICAM-1, VCAM-1, CD40, CD40L), smooth muscle cells and macrophages. They also contribute to the production of reactive oxygen species, stimulate matrix metalloproteinases and induce tissue factor expression.

Infection

Chronic infection may contribute to the pathogenesis of atherosclerosis. *Chlamydophila pneumoniae*, cytomegalovirus (CMV), *Helicobacter pylori*, enterovirus, hepatitis virus A and herpes simplex virus have all been implicated.

Anatomical distribution

Although atheroma can be found throughout the circulation, it does have a predilection for certain sites – the carotid bifurcation, the coronary arteries, the infrarenal aorta and the superficial femoral artery. In any one patient, not all may be affected equally or indeed at all.

Complications

An atheromatous plaque may cause:

- narrowing or occlusion, which can result in ischaemia and infarction
- thrombosis
- athero-embolism, where fragments of plaque, cholesterol and thrombus break off and lodge in the distal circulation
- weakening of the arterial wall with aneurysmal dilatation
- periarterial inflammation.

ANEURYSMAL DISEASE

The term aneurysm denotes an abnormal localised dilatation of a blood vessel. Almost any artery may become aneurysmal, although the commonest large vessel is the infrarenal aorta, followed by the iliac and popliteal arteries. It is a chronic degenerative disease with life-threatening implications.

Classification

- Anatomical – aneurysms may be localised (saccular) or diffuse (fusiform).
- Pathological – they may be true, i.e. lined by all three layers of the normal arterial wall, or false or pseudo, i.e. formed in the adventitia or completely outside the wall.
- Aetiological – see below.

Aetiology

Atherosclerosis

There is continuing controversy over whether aneurysmal disease is just another manifestation of atherosclerosis. However, many believe it to be a separate condition – medial degenerative disease. Nevertheless, there is no doubt that aneurysmal disease shares the same risk factors as atheromatous occlusive disease (although hypertension appears a more important factor) and that aneurysmal and occlusive arterial disease often coexist. It is likely that they are caused by localised arterial wall injury superimposed on the degenerative age-related changes, haemodynamics, systemic risk factors and probably a genetically determined predisposition. In addition, there is a strong familial element in aneurysmal but not in occlusive disease. Furthermore, there are patients, some of whom have never smoked, who exhibit widespread aneurysmal dilatation (arterial ectasia or arteriomegaly) without any evidence of peripheral, cerebral or coronary occlusive disease. Risk factors associated with aneurysmal disease also include age, male sex, hypertension, smoking and chronic obstructive pulmonary disease (COPD). With the successful correction of life-threatening aneurysms, the long-term survival of such patients approximates to that of a population matched for age and sex but without aneurysmal disease. This is in sharp contrast to those with occlusive disease who have a poorer long-term prognosis because of cardiac and cerebrovascular events.

Inflammation

In some patients, atherosclerosis, whether associated with aneurysmal dilatation or not, can lead to an intense periadventitial inflammatory and fibrotic response. The reasons are unclear, but clinical problems can occur in consequence. Inflammation is a histological feature in all aneurysms.

However, approximately 10% of abdominal aortic aneurysms (AAAs) have an excessive inflammatory element: the anterior wall is extremely thick, and structures such as the ureters are often surrounded, causing obstruction and hydronephrosis or caval occlusion (peri-aortitis). There is no evidence that such aneurysms are any more or less likely to rupture, but operative repair can be technically very difficult. Patients frequently complain of abdominal or back pain, and their erythrocyte sedimentation rate (ESR) is usually raised. On computed tomography the thickened aortic wall is seen to pervade surrounding tissues. Steroid treatment has been advocated to reduce inflammation and oedema in order to relieve pain, ureteric obstruction and to make aneurysm repair more straightforward. There is no evidence that steroid treatment reduces, and it may even increase, the risk of rupture. Endovascular treatment of an inflammatory aneurysm is an attractive alternative option in aneurysms suitable for stenting.

Dissection

Weakness of the aortic wall may result in an intimomedial tear and allow blood to track under pressure through and/or outwith the various layers of the wall. Such a dissecting aneurysm usually affects the thoraco-abdominal aorta. Rupture may occur outwards (usually fatal) or inwards into the aortic lumen with the subsequent formation of a large saccular aneurysm in the weakened section. Causes of the defect include:

- atherosclerosis, usually with hypertension
- Marfan's syndrome (see below) in which there is a structural defect in the biochemical nature of the media.

Infection

The arterial wall is normally highly resistant to bacterial and other infections. However, certain organisms (see 'Arteritis' below), notably *Salmonella* and *Treponema pallidum*, have a particular ability to infect, and thus to weaken, the aortic wall, leading to the formation of a mycotic aneurysm and its rupture. In developed countries, mycotic aneurysms account for less than 1% of all aneurysms but they are still common elsewhere.

Complications

Surgeons operate on aneurysms to prevent or manage complications, the most notable of which is rupture. Other complications include thrombosis and distal embolism (e.g. popliteal and subclavian). Less frequently, aneurysms cause external compression or stretching of surrounding structures – the bronchus or recurrent laryngeal nerve (thoraco-abdominal) or the duodenum (infrarenal aorta).

ARTERITIS (VASCULITIS)

Vasculidites are defined by the presence of leucocytes in the vessel wall with reactive damage to mural structures. Although the majority of such patients do not present to surgeons, arteritis can cause macrovascular complications such as ischaemia and aneurysm. Other patients may present with Raynaud's phenomenon.

Aetiology

Vessels of any size may be infected by pyogenic bacteria, mycobacteria, fungi, viruses, protozoa, *Rickettsia*, and spirochaetes such as *Treponema pallidum*. Infection may damage the vessel wall directly through effects on the endothelium and/or vasa vasorum or indirectly through immunological mechanisms.

A range of arteritides are attributed to immunologically mediated injury. They may or may not occur in association with arthritis, myositis and myocarditis as part of a defined autoimmune connective tissue disease such as systemic lupus erythematosus (SLE). In the majority, the inducing antigen is unknown. These hypersensitivity arteritides may be further classified on the basis of the histological changes in the arterial wall.

Pathological features

Inflammation may be acute or chronic and associated with necrosis, fibrosis or granuloma formation in the vessel wall. Neutrophils, macrophages and lymphocytes are involved, as is activation of the complement system and kinins. Systemic effects are associated with the release of acute-phase proteins and lead to fever and malaise. The clinical features depend largely upon the size, type and anatomical distribution of vessel(s) affected, together with the chronicity and severity of the inflammatory process. Acute forms may have a sudden and dramatic onset, progressing to death, with all the lesions at the same stage of development. Chronic forms may have an insidious onset, a waxing and waning course, with lesions in various stages of progression and remission. Early diagnosis is important because many patients respond quickly to medical treatment but, if left untreated, have a poor prognosis (Table 29.1). Although there is no universally accepted classification of the arteritides, they may be grouped on the basis of aetiology, type of vessel affected and symptoms. There is an increasing tendency simply to use the term vasculitis.

The dominant feature may be:

- *Necrotising*. Inflammation is associated with segmental necrosis of the vessel wall, which often contains a considerable amount of fibrin (fibrinoid necrosis).
- *Acute inflammatory*. There is a short history and usually an identifiable antigen, often a drug. Small veins, arteries and capillaries are affected by an acute inflammatory response. Lesions may progress rapidly (even to death), be self-limiting in response to withdrawal of antigen or may become chronic.
- *Chronic inflammatory*. Although these are characterised by a chronic inflammatory reaction, presumably in response to repeated exposure to an antigen, often the source is unknown.
- *Granulomatous*. Inflammation is associated with the development of granulomas, with or without the presence of giant cells.
- *Fibrosis*. Excessive fibrosis is found in the vessel wall.

SURGICAL ARTERITIDES

Vasculitides are classified predominantly by the size of the vessels affected. Recently, the presence of antineutrophil

Table 29.1 Investigation of vasculitis

Investigation	Results and comments
Acute-phase proteins • C-reactive protein (CRP) • Complement factors (C)	CRP, C3 and C4 usually elevated; useful for diagnosis and monitoring treatment
ESR	Usually elevated; less responsive than CRP
Autoantibodies • Antinuclear antibody • Anti-double-stranded DNA • Anticentromere • Extractable nuclear antigen • Anticardiolipin • Antineutrophil • Anti-citrullinated protein antibodies (ACPAs)	May be of primary pathogenic significance or may simply be secondary markers of tissue injury; most helpful in the diagnosis of defined connective tissue disorders such as SLE, scleroderma and CREST syndrome
Serum electrophoresis • Cryoglobulins	Serum immunoglobulins (Ig) are usually non-specifically elevated; monoclonal Ig (paraproteins) may be present; some paraproteins (cryoglobulins) precipitate on cooling and damage skin vessels
Urinalysis	High incidence of renal involvement in arteritis mandates examination of the urine for protein, blood, casts and red cells. Plasma creatinine as well as 24-hour urinary protein and creatinine clearance should be performed
Biopsy • Renal • Temporal artery	If positive may confirm arteritis and aid more precise diagnosis; negative biopsy does not exclude arteritis because lesions are focal and can be missed
Imaging • CT • MRI	May identify vasculitic lesions in deep organs
Echocardiography	Assesses myocardial and valvular function in patients with myocarditis, endocarditis, aortitis and coronary artery aneurysms (Kawasaki disease)
Angiography	Delineates the pattern of large-vessel disease; allows planning of arterial reconstruction (Takayasu's disease)

cytoplasmic antibodies (ANCAs) can further subclassify the disease.

Large-vessel vasculitis

Giant cell or temporal arteritis

This is a chronic vasculitis affecting large and medium-size arteries. It mostly involves the cranial branches of the arteries originating from the aortic arch. The temporal and retinal arteries are frequently involved in this condition. Arm vessels may also be affected.

Clinical features

Symptoms

In retinal artery disease, blindness is the leading symptom, which may cause presentation to a vascular surgeon with the mistaken diagnosis of a transient ischaemic episode from a lesion in the carotid artery. Scalp tenderness, claudication of jaw, tongue or with deglutition can also be presenting symptoms.

Physical findings

Usual findings are:

- evidence of hypertension
- a tender, thickened temporal artery
- loss of vision.

Investigation

A markedly elevated ESR (>50 mm/h) will be found. The diagnosis is confirmed by removal of a segment of temporal artery, which shows a necrotising arteritis with a predominence of mononuclear cells or a granulomatous process with multinucleated giant cells. The condition is treated with steroids.

Takayasu's arteritis

This condition primarily affects the aortic arch (and its branches) in young women. It can affect the entire aorta or be localised.

Clinical features

Symptoms

Most patients suffer a vague prodromal illness followed, after a variable period of time, by the symptoms and signs of vascular occlusion – most commonly arm claudication, syncopal attacks and visual disturbances.

Physical findings

These will depend on the arterial bed involved. Stenosis, occlusion, thrombosis, secondary atherosclerosis and aneurysmal dilatation of affected vessels are all seen.

Investigation and management

Apart from an acute-phase response, there are no specific markers of the disease. Primary treatment is with steroids and immunosuppressants, but vascular reconstruction may be required.

Medium-sized-vessel vasculitis

Polyarteritis nodosa

This is a systemic necrotising vasculitis that affects medium and small-vessel disease and which may lead to ulceration and gangrene of the digits and abdominal pain from mesenteric ischaemia (Ch. 23).

Kawasaki disease

This occurs mainly in children, and is often associated with a mucocutaneous lymph node syndrome. It is most commonly noted in the coronary arteries.

Isolated central nervous system vasculitis

This affects medium and small arteries over a diffuse area of the central nervous system with corresponding symptoms.

Small-vessel vasculitis

Churg–Strauss arteritis

This involves mainly small arteries of the lung and skin but can also be generalised. It is often associated with vascular and extravascular granulomatosis. Patients classically present with asthma and an eosinophilia. The condition responds to steroid therapy.

A number of other small-vessel vasculitides have been described such as Wegener's granulomatosis, microscopic polyarteritis, hypersensitivity vasculitis, essential cryoglobulinaemic vasculitis and also vasculitides secondary to viral infections and connective tissue disorders.

Systemic sclerosis (scleroderma)

This condition commonly presents with Raynaud's syndrome (see below) many years before other features of the disease become apparent. It may progress to tissue loss with ulceration and gangrene of toes and fingers that may require amputation. The Calcinosis, Raynaud's, Oesophageal motility disturbances, Sclerodactyly, Telangiectasia (CREST) syndrome is a variant.

Systemic lupus erythematosus (SLE)

This condition may also present because of Raynaud's phenomenon. The reader is referred to appropriate medical textbooks for detailed description of this and other connective tissue diseases discussed in this section.

MISCELLANEOUS CONDITIONS

There are a number of other conditions that are associated with arterial disease.

Behçet's disease

This condition is characterised by orogenital ulceration and vasculitis. It is associated with venous thrombosis and thrombophlebitis as well as arterial aneurysm and occlusion.

Buerger's disease (thromboangiitis obliterans)

This may be a form of atherosclerosis or, perhaps more likely, a type of inflammatory arteritis. Small, rather than large and medium-sized, arteries are affected. Veins may also become involved and develop thrombophlebitis. Femoral and popliteal pulses are often normal, but pedal pulses are absent. Young male smokers are almost exclusively involved, and there appears to be a genetic element in that the incidence is particularly high in certain ethnic groups. Symptoms of peripheral vascular insufficiency nearly always begin before the age of 30. Complete cessation of smoking allows collaterals to form and is associated with a good prognosis, but failure to refrain almost inevitably leads to major amputation.

Marfan's syndrome

This is a familial autosomal dominant disorder in which the basic underlying defect is a mutation in the fibrillin gene (*FBN 1*) on chromosome 15. The physical manifestations are:

- long fingers
- high arched palate
- lens dislocation
- focal medial necrosis of the aorta, which may lead to aortic valve root dilatation and incompetence, dissection of the ascending aorta and the development of thoraco-abdominal aneurysm.

Ehlers–Danlos syndrome

This is a familial disorder of collagen. Patients are 'double-jointed', have wide scars and carry a high mortality from aneurysm rupture.

Fibromuscular hyperplasia

This is characterised by arterial stenoses and dilatations and results in a 'string of beads' appearance on angiography. It most often affects the renal and carotid arteries of young women and is amenable to angioplasty.

PATIENT ASSESSMENT

History

Enquire about the nature, severity, onset and duration of symptoms of the presenting complaint. Also ask about past medical history, with particular emphasis on cardiac disease (angina, myocardial infarction), hypertension (severity, duration, treatment and quality of control), cerebrovascular disease (transient ischaemic attacks [TIA], amaurosis fugax and stroke), renal disease (renal failure, requirement for dialysis) and diabetes. History of smoking, hyperlipidaemia and also diet and physical activities are important.

Systematic enquiry

Ask the patient about the following:

- a history of allergy – particularly to iodine, which may be considered as a contrast medium for arteriography
- drug therapy, past and present – particularly the use of beta-blockers, which may aggravate critical ischaemia; angiotensin-converting enzyme (ACE) inhibitors and non-steroidal anti-inflammatory drugs (NSAIDs), which may precipitate renal failure in patients with renal artery stenosis and borderline renal function
- anticoagulant therapy, in case invasive investigations and/or surgery are being contemplated
- symptoms of arterial disease elsewhere (arterial disease is nearly always multisystem) – e.g. a patient with leg ischaemia frequently has significant coronary artery and cerebrovascular disease which predispose to myocardial infarction and stroke.

Information may not be volunteered because the presenting features may supersede or mask disease elsewhere (claudication in the leg may limit exercise tolerance so that angina is not manifest, and, conversely, relief of leg pain may unmask cardiac pain).

Physical findings

General

The examination begins the moment the patient enters the consulting room. An impression of general health, vigour and mobility are important in the management of arterial disease, especially if major surgery to prolong life or to improve its quality comes to be considered. Tobacco on the breath and/or staining of the fingers suggest recent heavy cigarette smoking. Other relevant general findings are the presence of finger clubbing, anaemia, jaundice, lymphadenopathy, central cyanosis and degree of breathlessness, particularly the ability to lie flat on the examination couch (those with arterial disease often have a history of cardiorespiratory disease). Gouty tophi are infrequently found, but hyperuricaemia accelerates atheroma and is amenable to treatment. Xanthomata or xanthelasma may suggest treatable hyperlipidaemia.

Weight loss and cachexia are not usually caused by arterial disease except when the mesenteric vessels are involved. If they are a striking feature, the cause should usually be sought elsewhere.

Assess mental state and coherence. A past stroke may be evident from paralysis of a limb, hemiplegia or speech disturbance and can indicate carotid artery disease.

Walk with the patient and observe how he or she copes with a flight of stairs in order to determine the march tolerance and general level of fitness.

Cardiovascular examination

Pulse rate and rhythm, in particular the presence or absence of atrial fibrillation, are established. Blood pressure should be recorded in both arms because subclavian artery (mainly left) disease is relatively common. Although minor differences of 10–15 mmHg are not diagnostically significant, they may affect the accuracy and interpretation of future blood pressure monitoring. Subclavian artery disease may also preclude the use of an axillofemoral graft. Supra-aortic pulses (carotid, subclavian, axillary) should be gently palpated and the presence of bruits sought. A prominent carotid pulse usually signifies a tortuous vessel rather than an aneurysm.

The heart and precordium are examined in the standard way. The presence of murmurs and evidence of left ventricular hypertrophy (displacement of the apex beat) should be sought.

The abdomen must be fully uncovered from xiphisternum to the groin. Look for abnormal pulsations (Fig. 29.2). Note any scars. Palpation is gentle because both normal and aneurysmal aortas are often tender. The most important measurement in an aneurysm is width (maximal transverse diameter), not length, and allowance must be made for the thickness of the abdominal wall musculature and fat. It can be difficult to distinguish between the transmitted pulsation of an upper abdominal mass (including faeces in the transverse colon) which overlies the aorta and the expansile pulsation of an aneurysm. Positioning the patient so that the mass is no longer resting on the aorta may make the distinction obvious. Assessment of the possible presence of an aortic aneurysm, even by experts, is notoriously unreliable, and physical findings should be confirmed by ultrasound. The normal aorta bifurcates at the level of the umbilicus (L3–4), and abnormal pulsations below this area are usually iliac in origin. Aortocaval fistula is associated with a machinery murmur on auscultation, and stenoses of the aorto-iliac, mesenteric and renal arteries may produce a systolic bruit.

Lower-limb pulses should be noted together with any accompanying bruits. If there is doubt about whether it is the patient's pedal, or the examiner's own digital, pulse that is being felt, it is useful to simultaneously feel the patient's radial pulse. The femoral pulse is usually easy to feel at the mid-inguinal point (below the inguinal ligament midway between the anterior superior iliac spine and the pubic symphysis). The popliteal pulse is felt on deep palpation in the popliteal fossa with the knee flexed to relax the popliteal fascia. It is usually difficult to feel; if it is very obvious then the examiner should consider the possibility of a popliteal aneurysm. The posterior tibial pulse is felt between the medial malleolus and the Achilles tendon. The dorsalis pedis artery is a continuation of the anterior tibial and is felt on the dorsum of the foot just proximal to the groove between the first and second metatarsals, lateral to the tendon of extensor hallucis longus. In 10% of normal people it is congenitally absent, the dorsum of the foot being supplied by a

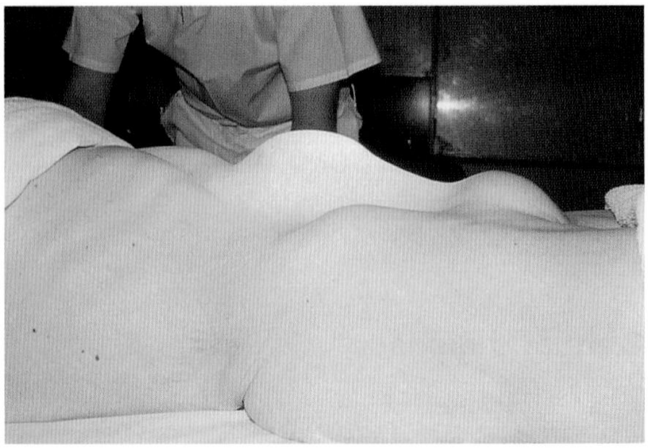

Fig. 29.2 A large abdominal aortic aneurysm is obvious on inspection of the abdomen in this thin patient.

perforating branch of the peroneal which may be felt 1 cm medial to the lateral malleolus at the ankle. Features of chronic ischaemia in the legs are loss of hair, pigmentation, ulceration, pallor or gangrene. Elevation of the severely ischaemic foot causes pallor and guttering of the veins. Dependency produces a reddish-blue appearance from the presence of desaturated blood within the skin – the sunset foot (Buerger's test). Tissue loss is usually obvious although lesions of the heel and between the toes are easily missed if examination is cursory.

Neurogenic claudication

In a small proportion of patients with intermittent claudication, pedal pulses are palpable. It is then worth asking the patient to walk until the pain comes on and to reassess pulsation. If they have disappeared, it suggests that there is an arterial stenosis but that it only becomes haemodynamically significant when the demand for flow is increased (see p. 445). However, if pulses are still present, then arterial claudication is unlikely and the diagnosis of spinal or neurogenic claudication, where pain is caused by nerve root compression, must be considered. In this condition, pain often affects the thigh and the calf equally, is present on standing not just walking, and is usually relieved only by sitting or lying down, not just by ceasing to walk. Straight leg raising may be impaired, and there may be subjective and objective neurosensory loss. There may be muscle wasting or reduced reflexes, and the femoral nerve stretch test may be positive.

Venous claudication

Obstruction to venous outflow (Ch. 30) produces a bursting pain in the calf on walking which is called venous claudication. Unlike arterial and neurogenic claudication, the pain is usually only relieved by elevation, the leg is chronically swollen and there is usually a clear history of previous deep-vein thrombosis. Arterial pulses are almost always present even though it may be difficult to feel due to oedema.

INVESTIGATIONS

An experienced vascular surgeon can often make the diagnosis of arterial disease and determine its severity and anatomical extent by a careful history and examination alone. The surgeon will also usually have at this point a fairly clear idea of the treatment options available.

Investigation must consider how to obtain the most information, in the safest and most suitable way for the patient and for the least cost. There must also be a clear idea how the results of any particular test will affect the management. A significant proportion of patients do not require surgical intervention, either because their symptoms are not vascular (or if vascular they are very mild) or because their general condition renders surgery too hazardous. In such patients, complex investigations are rarely indicated unless it is thought desirable to establish a baseline against which progression can be measured.

Although arteriography gives excellent anatomical information about the arterial circulation of the lower limb (the one which brings most patients for investigation), it is expensive, not without hazard and should not be requested in every patient who presents with symptoms and signs of lower-limb ischaemia. In addition, although intra-arterial pressures can be measured at angiography, the investigation provides little haemodynamic information. There is, therefore, a place for non-invasive studies that can be performed routinely and safely and which provide functional information through measurement of blood pressure, limb volume and flow velocity (see Ch. 4).

Risk-factor assessment

A major role of the vascular surgeon is to identify risk factors for arterial disease that influence primary and secondary prevention (Box 29.2). For example, up to a fifth of patients with arterial occlusive disease are diabetic, although in up to half of these the diagnosis may not have been made before the onset of vascular symptoms. A third to a half of vascular patients may have hyperlipidaemia requiring control with diet and/or medication. Other risk factors include hypertension, smoking, lack of exercise and obesity.

Before investigations specific to the symptomatic part of the body are conducted, it is necessary to view the patient with arterial disease as a whole and to correct risk factors as far as is possible. Many large studies show that this is a highly worthwhile exercise. For example, reduction in blood cholesterol concentrations in patients with hyperlipidaemia and coronary artery disease can reduce death from myocardial infarction by up to a third. There is increasing evidence that careful glycaemic control in diabetics reduces the vascular complications of the disease, and treatment of even mild hypertension markedly reduces the risk of stroke. Cessation of smoking is associated with a reduction in vascular events and with increased long-term patency of arterial reconstruction. The approach to vascular disease should be adopting a healthier lifestyle change, including individual risk-factor control and also exercise. Most vascular centres offer risk-factor and lifestyle management clinics providing a more holistic approach in an effort to reduce complications and improve quality of life.

Ultrasound

The principles of ultrasound investigation are discussed in Chapter 4.

Box 29.2 Risk factors for peripheral vascular disease

Causative
- Smoking
- Diabetes mellitus
- Hypertension
- Hyperlipidaemia

Associated
- Ischaemic heart disease
- Cerebrovascular disease
- Family history

Rare (consider especially in young patients)
- Thrombophilia
- Buerger's disease
- Hyperhomocysteinaemia

Ankle : brachial pressure index

Atherosclerotic stenoses cause a pressure drop between the arm and most commonly in the foot. This can be measured by detection of pulsation at the elbow and ankle with a Doppler probe while the pressure is gradually reduced in cuffs on the upper arm and just above the ankle. Normal pedal pressure is usually 10–20 mmHg higher than brachial pressure, and the normal ABPI is around 1.1. An ABPI of less than 0.9 normally indicates a haemodynamically significant lesion (which may be asymptomatic); 0.5–0.8 is associated with claudication; 0.25–0.5 with rest pain; and less than 0.25 with tissue loss – ulceration or gangrene. There is considerable variation between patients, with proximal lesions and multilevel disease having a greater effect on the ABPI than isolated distal disease. For an individual, the trend in ABPI over time is more important than the absolute value. ABPI can also be used to assess the success or otherwise of intervention. After successful surgery or angioplasty, the ABPI should rise by at least 0.15; a subsequent similar fall suggests that re-occlusion has taken place.

Non-compressible vessels

Calcified crural vessels, most commonly but not exclusively found in diabetics, may not be compressible, and the ABPI is then falsely elevated. In these cases toe pressures (using appropriate cuffs) can be obtained. Digital arteries tend to be affected less by calcification and therefore are more reliable.

Post-exercise ABPI

Inertial energy losses across a stenosis are proportional to blood velocity. In low-flow states, lesser degrees of stenosis may not produce a pressure drop, so that, at rest, the ABPI may approach normal. After exercise, increased cardiac output and reduced peripheral resistance raise flow velocity to the point where pressure across the stenosis begins to fall. A reduction in ABPI after exercise may therefore unmask mild to moderate disease. Reactive hyperaemia may be used as an alternative to exercise when the general state precludes treadmill exercise. A cuff is placed on the thigh, inflated above systolic pressure for 5 minutes and then released. The temporary ischaemia distal to the cuff causes reactive vasodilatation which leads to a phase of hyperaemic flow when the cuff is removed. The fall in ABPI on reactive hyperaemia correlates well with that found after exercise, but treadmill testing has the advantage that it gives a better impression of the patient's overall disability and of cardiorespiratory function. For example, it is important to know whether walking is actually limited by angina or osteoarthritis rather than by claudication.

Segmental pressures

By placing cuffs around the upper thigh, lower thigh and calf, the level of lesions causing significant falls in pressure can be determined.

B-mode ultrasound

This procedure is principally used in vascular surgical practice to screen for, assess the size of and follow the time course of aneurysms, particularly in the abdominal aorta (Fig. 29.3).

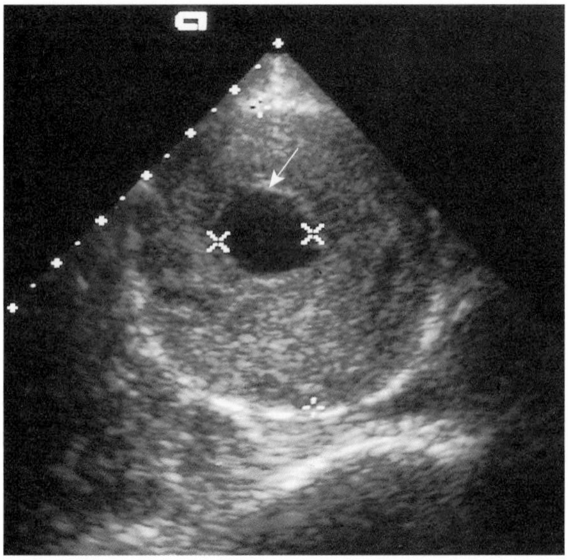

Fig. 29.3 A B-mode ultrasound scan which demonstrates a transverse cross-sectional image of a large abdominal aortic aneurysm. The appearance has been likened to that of a fried egg. The bright circular band around the egg is the aneurysm wall; the white of the egg is the laminated thrombus within the aneurysm sac; and the yolk is the channel through the centre of the aneurysm where blood still flows (arrow).

Duplex ultrasound

This has revolutionised vascular surgery and yields simultaneous anatomical and physiological information on flow in a variety of arteries safely, non-invasively and, if necessary, repeatedly. Duplex is used in many areas affected by occlusive and aneurysmal arterial disease (Fig. 29.4). Disadvantages are that the equipment is expensive and the production and interpretation of the scans require considerable experience.

Assessment of stenosis

When blood flows through an arterial stenosis, velocity increases. The high-speed jet can be localised on B-mode ultrasound with the aid of colour flow mapping, and the precise velocity of the jet can be measured. The increase in velocity is proportional to the degree of stenosis and so, by comparing the velocities proximal (V_1) and distal (V_2) to the stenosis (V_1/V_2 ratio), an estimate of the degree of stenosis can be made. For example, in the internal carotid artery, a V_1/V_2 ratio greater than 4 together with a peak systolic velocity greater than 120 cm/s and a peak diastolic velocity greater than 40 cm/s suggests a stenosis of greater than 70%. Similar assessments can be made at any other site where the artery lies superficially and can thus be insonated by the ultrasound beam. In thin patients, reliable information can even be obtained from the aorto-iliac segments. Duplex can also be used to look for stenoses within arterial (vein) bypasses – graft surveillance. Care should be taken when reporting internal carotid artery stenosis as currently there are two most commonly used methods of measuring NASCET and ECST. These do not correlate to each other. It is important then to determine which method has been used, especially when comparing different scans.

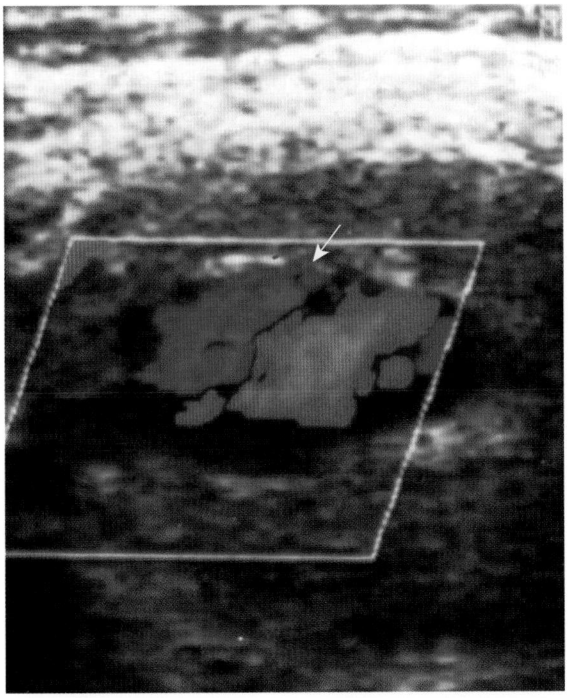

Fig. 29.4 A colour flow duplex scan of a longitudinal cross-sectional image of an aneurysm. The B-mode facility demonstrates the aneurysmal wall (arrow), while the colour Doppler indicates flow within the lumen: red, flow towards the ultrasound probe; blue, flow away from the probe. The appearance of red and blue flow within the aneurysm is indicative of turbulence.

Plaque morphology

Duplex ultrasound also provides useful information about the composition of a plaque. In the carotid artery this may relate to a plaque's propensity to cause a stroke. Thus, the more lipid-rich and the less fibrous a carotid plaque, the more likely it is to be a source of atheromatous emboli which lodge distally to cause a stroke, TIA or amaurosis fugax (transient unilateral loss of vision secondary to occlusion of the retinal artery or its branches).

Plethysmography

This is the measurement of volume change: during systole the limb expands with arterial inflow and during diastole it contracts with venous outflow. Several types of instrument are available, but the simplest to use is the air plethysmograph (APG), also known as the pulse volume recorder.

Pneumatic cuffs are placed around the thigh, calf and ankle, and the cuff at the site to be assessed is inflated with air to a pressure of 60 mmHg so that the cuff is brought in to light contact with the underlying leg. Any change in limb volume at that point produces changes in volume within the cuff such that the volume trace obtained closely resembles that of the arterial pressure wave. Air plethysmography is now more commonly used in the research assessment of the venous circulation.

Computed tomography

In vascular practice, CT is most commonly used to examine the brain in patients who present with carotid artery disease and the aorta in those with aneurysmal disease and/or dissection (Fig. 29.5). CT can be performed with and without

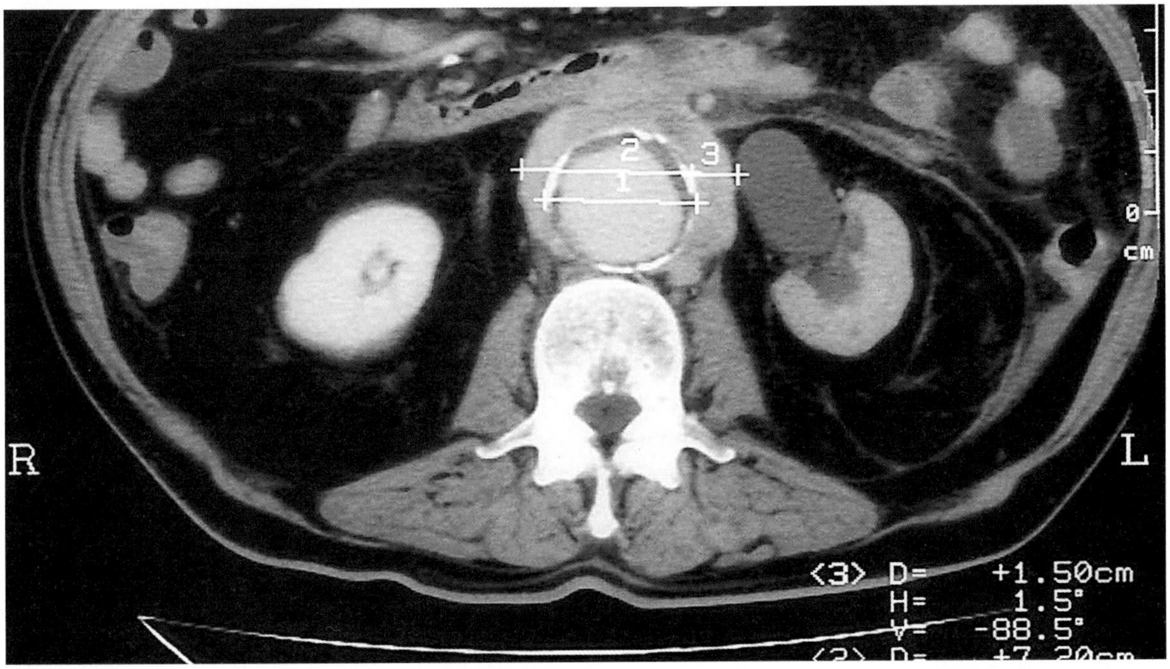

Fig. 29.5 Computed tomography (CT) scan showing a transverse cross-sectional image of a large abdominal aortic aneurysm. The examination has been performed with contrast so that the blood in the aneurysm appears white. The aneurysm is lined with a thin rim of thrombus. This particular aneurysm is an inflammatory one, as indicated by the marked thickening of the aortic wall. On the left-hand side the ureter has become involved in the periaortic inflammatory processes, and there is a hydronephrosis.

Box 29.3 Preparations for angiography

- Informed consent
- Check for allergies to contrast/asthma
  - pre-intervention steroid administration
  - low iodine contrast
- Check for renal impairment
  - pre-hydration with i.v. fluids
  - monitor fluid balance and U&E closely
  - stop nephrotoxic drugs
  - limit contrast load and consider alternative imaging
  - consider *N*-acetylcysteine 1200 mg pre- and 1200 mg post-contrast if creatinine >120 mmol/L
- Check for diabetes
  - stop metformin the day before

intravascular contrast medium to highlight the arteries and veins. Modern computer software systems can also generate three-dimensional reconstructions of the vasculature. The quality of the reconstruction with the new powerful spiral CT scanners now approaches that of digital subtraction angiography and can be used even for assessing coronary vessels.

Magnetic resonance imaging (MRI)

By the use of different sequencing techniques, arteries and veins can be emphasised with or without the injection of contrast material. The use of MRI in cardiac imaging is relatively advanced, and by gating pictures to the electrocardiogram, real-time cine-loop images of the moving chambers and valves can be obtained. MR angiography (MRA) is a rapidly developing area. The addition of gadolinium contrast has significantly improved the quality of the images. Recently MRA has been increasingly used for imaging of aortic dissection and post surveillance of endovascular aneurysm repair.

Angiography

Despite the advances in non-invasive assessment described above, most surgeons still rely primarily upon angiography when procedures are planned. Careful patient preparation is necessary (Box 29.3).

Digital subtraction angiography (DSA)

Nowadays, virtually all angiography is performed using digital subtraction (Ch. 4), which allows fine detail in images of small vessels, such as those in the foot, to be obtained with relatively small amounts of contrast and less radiation exposure (Fig. 29.6).

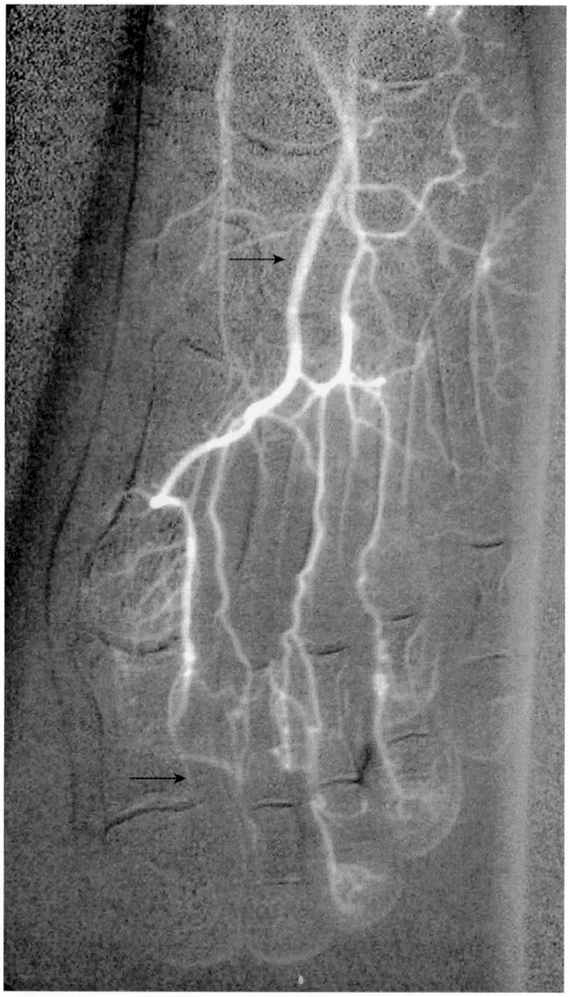

Fig. 29.6 Intra-arterial digital subtraction arteriogram showing filling of the plantar arch of the foot from the dorsalis pedis artery (arrow, upper). There is occlusion of the digital arteries to the great toe (arrow, lower) as a result of embolism from a proximal atheromatous plaque.

Route of contrast administration

Usually the contrast is injected directly into the artery to be examined – intra-arterial DSA (IA-DSA). This, of course, means that the arterial system has to be punctured, which has consequences: the potential for local wound complications; discomfort; and sometimes the need for the procedure to be done on an in-patient basis. Most often the common femoral artery is punctured in the groin. The brachial artery in the arm is also frequently used for coronary angiograms and when there is no femoral pulse. Some radiologists use the radial artery at the wrist to undertake IA-DSA as a day-case procedure. Contrast allergy, impaired renal function and administration of certain drugs (e.g. metformin) can all be relative contraindications for contrast use. In patients with renal impairment, administration of contrast can result in deterioration of their renal function or even renal failure.

Reasonable images may also be obtained when the contrast is injected peripherally into a vein – intravenous DSA (IV-DSA). The advantages of this approach for the patient are obvious. It also means that the procedure can be performed more quickly, less expensively and as an out-patient procedure. The disadvantages are that the images are not as clear, especially in the smaller peripheral arteries (as they are dependent upon a fast circulation time and a good cardiac output, which is often not the case in vascular patients), and more contrast is required. CT angiography and MRA are rapidly becoming credible non-invasive alternatives to DSA for diagnostic purposes. This allows IA-DSA to be used for therapeutic interventions.

TECHNIQUES

GENERAL CONSIDERATIONS

Vascular prostheses

Synthetic materials

Many of the techniques and prosthetic materials available and very much taken for granted in modern-day vascular surgical practice were not available as recently as 20 or 30 years ago. In particular, the development in the 1960s and 1970s of durable, non-thrombogenic, sterile, prosthetic materials for the construction of arterial bypasses was a major advance.

Prosthetic materials are used routinely in aorto-iliac surgery where the long-term patency of a relatively short, large-calibre, prosthetic replacement at a high-flow, high-pressure site is extremely good. The inner surface quickly becomes coated with protein, and at each end there may be some limited endothelial ingrowth. However, in humans, as opposed to animals, a neo-endothelium never comes to line the entire length of any prosthetic conduit. Externally reinforced grafts are coated with rings or a spiral of polypropylene. Many surgeons now use them routinely in order to overcome fears of kinking or external compression, a particular hazard where a graft crosses a joint. In an axillofemoral graft, compression may be from a waist band or because the patient sleeps on the side of the graft.

Biological materials obtained from cadavers (allografts or homografts) or animals (xenografts) and chemically treated have been used since the late 1940s, but problems of availability, concern about cross-infection and late structural degeneration led to their abandonment after the advent of synthetic alternatives. New methods of preserving and sterilising these materials may allow their use in the future.

Vein

Autologous vein (usually the long saphenous [LSV] from the thigh) undoubtedly provides the best long-term results in medium- to small-calibre arterial reconstruction; specifically, the results of lower limb bypass with vein are better than with prosthetic materials. The longer the graft, the more distal the distal anastomosis, and the poorer the run-off vessels, the greater the advantage. However, in a proportion of patients, the ipsilateral LSV is either unusable because of disease or has been extirpated by varicose vein operations or for coronary bypass surgery. In such circumstances, vein can be harvested from other sites – the contralateral LSV, the short saphenous system or the arm. Pieces of vein can be spliced together to obtain the desired length for the bypass. Another advantage of autologous material is resistance to infection. A potential disadvantage is the relatively small size of arm and leg veins, which makes them generally unsuitable for aorto-iliac reconstruction. However, in exceptional circumstances such as a grossly contaminated field, lengths of veins can be spliced together in ingenious ways to form short lengths of large-calibre conduit.

Use of blood and blood products

Vascular operations are frequently associated with greater blood loss than are general surgical procedures, additionally contributed to by full anticoagulation. For these reasons, there is a particular requirement for effective and sometimes extremely rapid blood replacement. Interruption of the circulation to relieve occlusion or carry out bypass usually involves a temporary period of ischaemia for substantial areas of the body. The combination of loss of blood volume, ischaemia and reperfusion predisposes to coagulopathy, which may require correction with blood products such as fresh frozen plasma (FFP), cryoprecipitate and platelets.

Blood transfusion has its own shortcomings and complications. There is increasing enthusiasm for autotransfusion, which can be achieved in several different ways:

- *Predonation*. If the need for surgery can be predicted several weeks in advance, the patient can attend the blood bank and predonate their blood for their own later use. Although this overcomes problems with infection and incompatibility, the blood transfused still has the properties of that from the bank.
- *Isovolaemic haemodilution*. Blood is taken from the patient immediately before operation and replaced with crystalloid; it may then be transfused back during the procedure. The advantage is that the retransfusion is of fresh whole blood.
- *Autotransfusion (cell saving)*. Blood shed during operation can be collected by suction, washed and re-infused.

Pre- and postoperative management

(see also Ch. 6)

Preoperative management

The history obtained from the patient with arterial disease is the most important information to guide the surgeon in management. Preoperative assessment (Box 29.4) should answer three essential questions:

- Is vascular disease the cause of the patient's symptoms?
- What are the physiological effects or potential risks of the lesion?
- What is the operative risk?

Patients who undergo vascular operations are usually older, have more cardiorespiratory and cerebrovascular comorbidity, are more likely to be diabetic, are on more medications, and suffer more postoperative morbidity and mortality than those who have general surgical procedures. Because of

Box 29.4 Preoperative management of the vascular patient

- Check indication and side of operation (if relevant)
- Consent, with explanation of risks and benefits
- Measure ABPI where relevant
- Routine bloods and cross-match
- Consider beta-blockers
- Continue aspirin until day of surgery
- Thromboembolic prophylaxis with LMWH
- Antibiotic prophylaxis according to local protocol
- Intravenous hydration whilst nil by mouth

ABPI, ankle: brachial pressure index; LMWH, low-molecular-weight heparin.

their widespread arterial disease and frequent lifelong heavy smoking, they are at especially high risk of cardiac, respiratory and cerebrovascular complications. Multisystem disease (e.g. ischaemic heart disease, hypertension, COPD, renal impairment, diabetes) is the rule rather than the exception. Information gathered from the history and examination together with the planned procedure guides the preoperative investigations. This allows the weighing of the benefit of an operation (relieving symptoms, prevention of mortality or morbidity in the future) against the risk of the procedure. The anaesthetist is closely involved in preoperative assessment and risk-factor management, the operation itself and in post-operative care.

Postoperative management

Postoperative management (Box 29.5) varies according to the operative procedure. Careful monitoring of blood pressure is important after a carotid endarterectomy. Judicious management of the fluid balance is important after abdominal aortic aneurysm repair, with careful monitoring of the hourly urine output. Distal limb perfusion needs to be assessed frequently for signs of graft blockage or distal embolisation (see Fig. 29.7, trash foot). Haematological parameters, electrolytes and indices of renal function need to be carefully monitored in all postoperative patients until normal diet has been resumed. Anticoagulants are not routinely employed, but all patients should be restarted on best medical therapy for atherosclerosis: anti-platelet therapy, usually aspirin, lipid-lowering therapy, and an ACE inhibitor in patients without pre-existing renal impairment.

Box 29.5 Postoperative management of the vascular patient

- Regular observations, particularly measurement of parameters assessing intravascular filling
- Observation of pulses distal to any reconstruction
- Neurological observations after CEA
- Wound or radiological puncture site observation
- Recommencement of anti-platelet treatment, prophylactic heparin or formal anticoagulation
- Objective measurement of ABPI if relevant

ABPI, ankle:brachial pressure index; CEA, carotid endarterectomy.

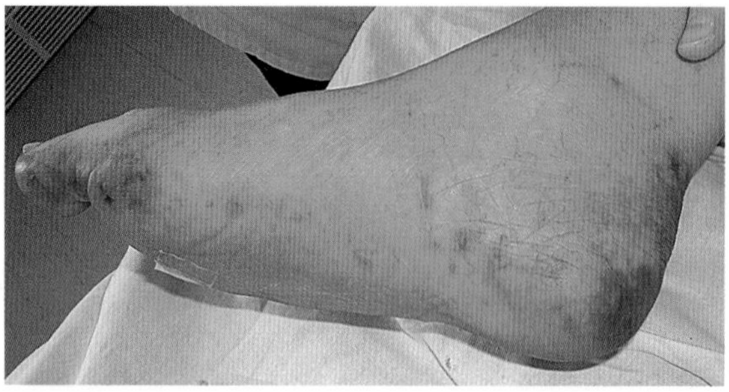

Fig. 29.7 Trash foot – note patchy discoloration caused by a shower of small emboli.

PERCUTANEOUS TRANSLUMINAL ANGIOPLASTY AND THROMBOLYSIS

Percutaneous transluminal angioplasty (PTA)

A guide wire is passed through the site of stenosis or occlusion via a percutaneous puncture of an accessible adjacent artery. A catheter-mounted balloon is then inserted over the guide wire and the balloon is inflated within the lesion to open the artery by disruption of the plaque. A small metal mesh tube (stent) may then be placed over the guide wire and deployed within the recanalised artery to reduce the risk of restenosis (Fig. 29.8).

Since PTA was first described, there have been major technical advances in the available equipment, and interventional radiologists are becoming increasingly adventurous in the scope of the procedures done. Despite these trends, there appears to be no reduction in the number of open arterial reconstructions being carried out, and PTA should be viewed as widening the scope of treatment rather than as a rival to surgery.

Indications and results

The TASC II document has categorised aorto-iliac and femoral lesions into four categories and suggested optimal treatment methods. TASC A and B lesions are best treated by PTA, whereas TASC D lesions would be best treated by surgery. Controversy exists about TASC C lesions that can be treated by either method after careful consideration and according to each centre's experience.

Aorto-iliac disease

The results of PTA are undoubtedly best in large, high-flow vessels, and it is often the treatment of choice in stenoses and occlusions of the aorto-iliac system. There is some evidence that, unless the lesion in question is a short stenosis, and the result of PTA alone is technically perfect, angioplasty should be followed by stent placement, although the initial cost is considerably increased.

Infra-inguinal disease

Except in the uncommon case of a short stenosis of the superficial femoral artery (Fig. 29.9), the results of infra-inguinal PTA (usually performed for claudication) are disappointing. Some interventional radiologists strongly disagree with that view and claim good long-term success even after recanalisation of long occlusions of arteries both above and below the knee.

Critical limb ischaemia

This is discussed in detail below.

Other sites

Although the bulk of PTA is performed for lower limb ischaemia, the technique has been used in the carotid, renal and mesenteric arteries. The long-term results of PTA and stenting in these areas remain to be defined. PTA is also used to dilate stenoses within bypass grafts (graft surveillance).

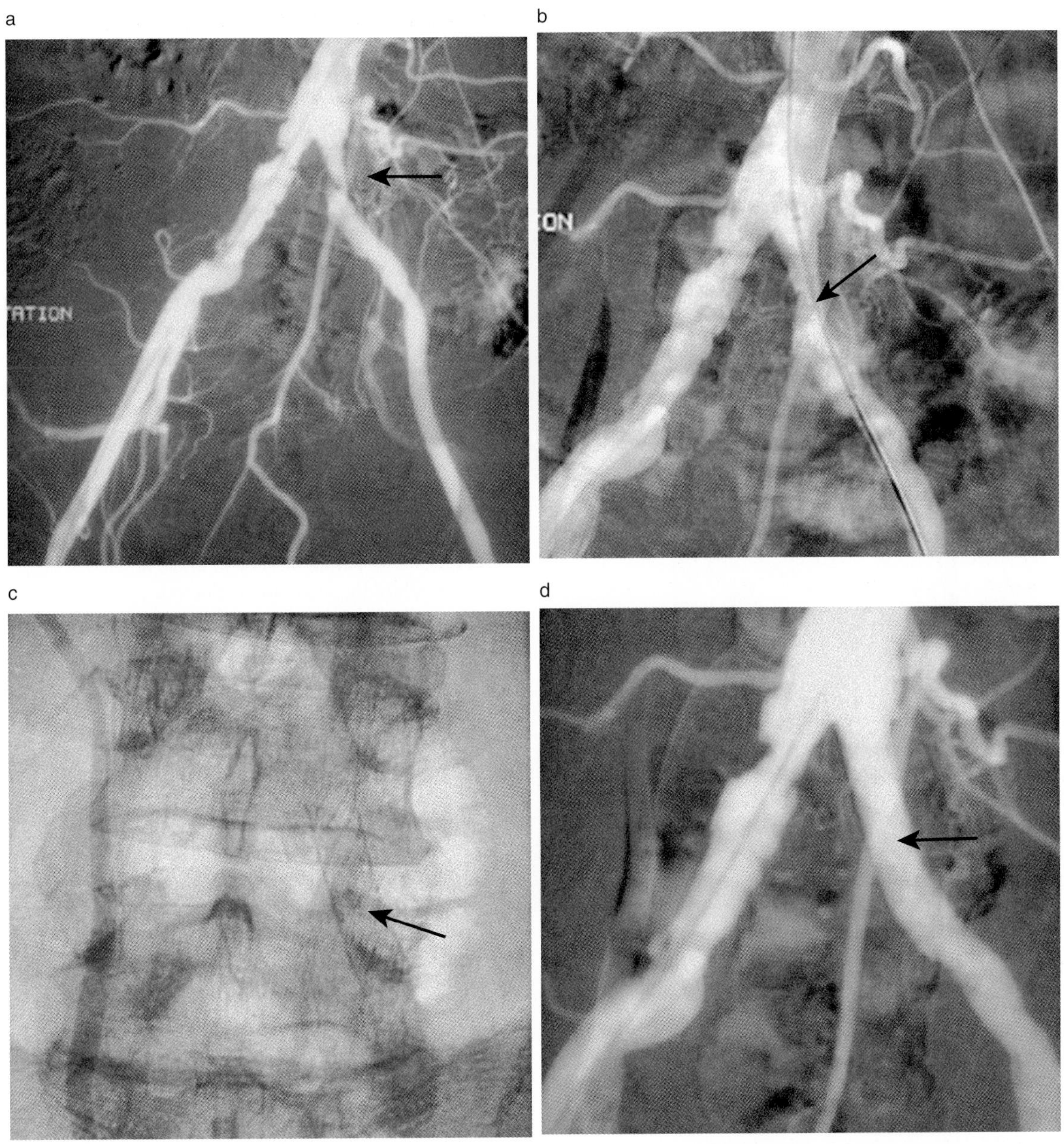

Fig. 29.8 Angiograms showing stages of percutaneous transluminal angioplasty. (a) There is a 90% stenosis of the left common iliac artery (arrow). (b) A guide wire (arrow) has been passed across the stenosis from a left common femoral arterial puncture, and the lesion has been stretched open by a 10 mm angioplasty balloon. (c) A metal stent has been positioned across the lesion (arrow) to prevent restenosis. (d) A final angiogram shows a widely patent left common iliac artery without residual stenosis.

Complications

Although percutaneous techniques are associated with less morbidity and mortality than open surgery, they are not without complications, and there is a significant early technical failure rate which depends on the clinical indications and the anatomical site. The main complications are related to the arterial puncture required to enter the arterial tree: haematoma, false aneurysm, occlusion and thrombosis. Although many of these can be treated non-operatively, a proportion require direct operative repair. Less commonly, angioplasty of a stenosed artery may lead to acute occlusion, worsening of ischaemia and the need for emergency surgical revascularisation or sometimes amputation.

Thrombolysis

Thrombolytic agents, such a streptokinase, urokinase and tissue plasminogen activator (TPA), are different from heparin and warfarin in that, rather than preventing clot formation, they actually lyse pre-formed thrombus. The technique involves infusing a drug into an artery in the hope that, after lysis, the diseased section that caused the thrombosis can be visualised and treated either by operation or PTA. The precise indications for thrombolysis are difficult to define.

Complications

Thrombolysis is not without morbidity and mortality, especially in the elderly. Most complications are the consequence

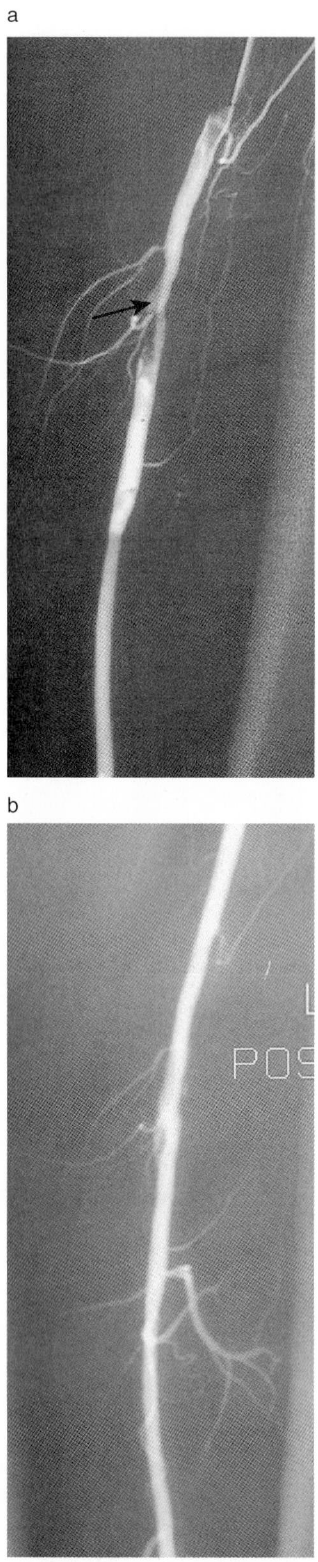

Fig. 29.9 Focal atheromatous plaque with attached thrombus in the right superficial femoral artery (arrow, [a]). This plaque had been the source of emboli to the toes and was treated successfully by angioplasty (b) and 6 months of anticoagulation with warfarin.

of haemorrhage. Therefore thrombolysis is contraindicated after recent surgery and in the presence of any other likely bleeding point such as a peptic ulcer or a recent haemorrhagic stroke. Dissolution of clot can lead to distal embolisation; particularly to be dreaded is embolus from the heart or carotid vessels to produce an ischaemic stroke.

OPEN SURGICAL TECHNIQUES

Endarterectomy

Before the advent of reliable prosthetic bypass materials, endarterectomy (open removal – coring out – of atheroma from inside a diseased artery) was the standard operation for occlusive arterial disease, especially that in large-calibre vessels. However, the technique poses a number of problems:

- The operation is technically demanding and maximally invasive.
- Unlike bypass surgery (see below), endarterectomy requires a very wide dissection of all, or almost all, of the length of the artery to be cleared.
- Arterial disease is generalised, and there are few instances where a diseased artery can be cleared to normal artery above and below the lesion: thus there is always a point of transition between the endarterectomised surface and the diseased intima of the adjacent vessel which, especially downstream, can form a ridge or a flap which is a focus for thrombosis, vessel occlusion and distal embolisation.

Closure of the vessel wall following endarterectomy often necessitates using a piece of vein or prosthetic material as a 'patch' in order to prevent narrowing of the lumen.

Endarterectomy is now much less frequently done except in certain specific sites, notably the carotid bifurcation and common femoral artery (Fig. 29.10).

Bypass

This is now the commonest procedure for occlusive arterial disease.

Technique

The operation proceeds as summarised in Clinical Box 29.1.

Most bypasses done in the UK are for critical lower limb ischaemia, when failure to revascularise the leg often results in amputation.

Bypass grafts are usually described in terms of their inflow, outflow and conduit (e.g. femoral to popliteal with reversed vein). Bypasses can generally be grouped into those that are anatomical – the conduit follows more or less the same course as the native vessel (e.g. femoropopliteal) – and those that are extra-anatomical, where a different path is used (e.g. axillofemoral).

Embolectomy

There has been a steady decline in the proportion of patients who develop acute ischaemia because of an embolus, as opposed to a thrombosis from chronic obliterative atherosclerosis. There are several reasons:

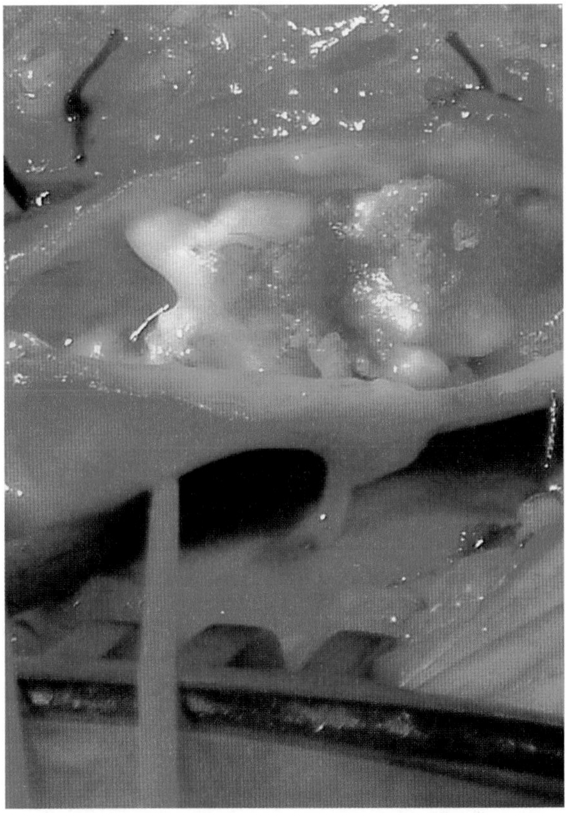

Fig. 29.10 Common femoral artery exposed and opened to reveal 'coral-like' plaque which is best treated by endarterectomy.

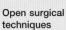

Clinical Box 29.1 **Bypass procedure**

- Dissect out and control arteries above and below the occlusion
- Make a tunnel through the tissues to allow passage of the bypass
- Give systemic heparin
- Clamp arteries
- Construct proximal and distal anastomoses
- Flush out native vessels and the graft to expel any air or clot
- Complete anastomoses
- Remove clamps
- Re-establish flow
- Assess adequacy of graft flow and distal perfusion

- a declining population of patients with atrial fibrillation and valve damage after rheumatic fever
- increased use of warfarin in the management of atrial fibrillation
- increased use of thrombolysis for myocardial infarction, which limits infarct size and the development of left ventricular mural thrombus.

Nevertheless, embolectomy is still frequently done – especially in the arm, where embolus has always been the commonest cause of acute ischaemia. Once the diagnosis of embolus has been reliably made on clinical assessment, perhaps supplemented by the use of angiography, the operation can be performed under local, regional or general anaesthesia.

Clinical Box 29.2 **Embolectomy procedure**

- Dissect out the relevant artery, usually the brachial in the arm or the common femoral in the leg, and control flow proximally and distally with tapes or plastic slings
- Give systemic heparin
- Open the artery
- Pass balloon catheters (Fogarty) into the artery with the balloon deflated and then remove with the balloon inflated to extract the clot to establish inflow first and then outflow
- Establish the adequacy of clot extraction clinically or by means of on-table angiography
- Close the arteriotomy (with a patch of vein if there is concern about the artery being narrowed at that point)
- Re-establish flow and consider further procedure if not adequate

Technique

The operation is summarised in Clinical Box 29.2.

Postoperatively, anticoagulation is continued. A search for a definite source of the embolus is usually made, although its origin may prove elusive. An echocardiogram and imaging of major vessels should be performed and coagulation disorders excluded. In the absence of a proven source, a judgement must be made as to the appropriateness and duration of anticoagulation.

Although most emboli lodge in the arm or leg, any arterial bed may be involved: e.g. the carotid artery, leading to stroke, or the superior mesenteric artery with bowel ischaemia (Ch. 24). Only a small minority of emboli are the result of infective endocarditis or of tumour. However, it is routine to send a portion of the extracted clot for bacteriological culture and histopathological examination.

Sympathectomy

Limb ischaemia

The sympathetic nervous system causes arteriolar constriction and in the past it was believed that by interrupting the sympathetic nerve supply to an ischaemic area, vasodilatation might improve the flow of blood. However, blood vessels in ischaemic tissues are already maximally dilated and, if sympathectomy does provide any benefit in severe distal ischaemia, it is likely that other mechanisms, such as alteration of pain perception, are responsible. With the increased use of arterial bypass for lower limb ischaemia, sympathectomy is used less and less.

Hyperhidrosis

The sympathetic nervous system also innervates sweat glands. Upper limb (cervical or thoracic) sympathectomy is most often used for severe axillary and palmar hyperhidrosis if medical treatment fails. The operation used to be performed through the root of the neck but is now done safely and expeditiously by thoracoscopy. Lumbar sympathectomy is also of value in patients with severe plantar hyperhidrosis. The effect on sweat gland function is usually permanent. Repeated injections of botulinum toxin is an alternative for axillary hyperhidrosis. Cervical sympathectomy is less successful at this site compared to the palms. Complications of sympthectomy include 'compensatory' increased sweating at other sites (trunk, thighs, face). Cervical sympathectomy carries a small risk of Horner's syndrome (drooping ipsilateral eyelids, constricted pupil and reduced facial sweating) and lumbar sympathectomy of sexual dysfunction.

Raynaud's phenomenon

Cervical sympathectomy has been recommended for Raynaud's phenomenon (RP), but the long-term results in the hand are poor. For an unexplained reason, however, lumbar sympathectomy may provide long-lasting relief in RP which affects the toes.

Amputation

Indications

Ideally, no patient with critical ischaemia should undergo major limb amputation for peripheral vascular disease without assessment by a vascular surgeon. Arterial reconstruction is by far the better option because of:

- mortality – 10–20% for amputation
- stump infection and ischaemia – both are common and, in up to 10%, lead to further amputation at a higher level; deep venous thrombosis and pulmonary embolus are also well-recognised complications
- failed rehabilitation – 2 years later, less than two-thirds of below-knee and less than one-third of above-knee, unilateral amputees are independently mobile
- financial cost – although a distal bypass operation for limb salvage may entail hospital expenditure in the region of £5000, a major limb amputation frequently costs 10 times as much once rehabilitation, artificial limbs and long-term care are considered.

It is a medical, humanitarian and economic disaster to do a reconstruction which fails early. However, in that 50–75% of patients with critical limb ischaemia are dead within 5 years (mostly from cardiac and cerebrovascular events), not all bypass procedures are required to work for a prolonged period. Reconstruction should be attempted if there is at least a 75% chance of the bypass remaining functional for 2 years. Sometimes, however, amputation is the only option in those with unreconstructable arterial disease and advancing tissue loss or with symptoms that cannot be controlled by medical means.

Level

Because rehabilitation is directly related to level of amputation, every effort should be made to preserve the knee if it is mobile and there is a prospect of a prosthesis. Although numerous investigations have been proposed, there is not a single test which reliably predicts at which level an amputation will heal.

Level remains, therefore, largely a matter of clinical judgement.

Perioperative pain

Preoperative

Many patients who need amputation for ischaemia have considerable preoperative pain. Adequate analgesia around the time of operation is vital for both humane reasons and because it hastens recovery and rehabilitation. The anaesthetist is usually closely involved in this aspect of care (Ch. 6).

Postoperative

Phantom pain, a continuation or worsening of the pain experienced in the limb before amputation, often accompanied by a distressing sensation that the limb is still present, is common. Various treatments have been advocated such as electrical stimulation, the anticonvulsant carbamazepine and the tricyclic antidepressant amitriptyline. There is some evidence that, if the patient is transferred to the operating room in a pain-free state, then the incidence of phantom pain is reduced. Epidural pain relief (Ch. 6) may achieve this end.

Rehabilitation

Although an amputation might be considered a technically straightforward procedure, there are important surgical principles which have to be observed if the chances of healing the amputation stump are to be maximised. In addition to the surgical team, the successful postoperative rehabilitation of an amputee depends upon the close cooperation of other disciplines – physiotherapists, occupational therapists and prosthetists.

MANAGEMENT OF ANEURYSMAL DISEASE

Abdominal aortic aneurysm (AAA)

Epidemiology and aetiology

This condition is present in 5% and responsible for the death of 1% of men over the age of 60. The principal cause of death is rupture, but distal embolism from thrombus in the aneurysm sac and, rarely, a thrombotic occlusion can also set the scene for death. The aetiology of aneurysmal disease is discussed above. The other complications of AAA are inflammation of the wall, leading to abdominal or back pain and compression of surrounding structures.

Pathological features

In keeping with the law of Laplace, an aortic aneurysm inevitably slowly expands, a process made more likely by hypertension and continued smoking. The rate of expansion is highly variable both between patients and for an individual patient over time. Thus the lifetime threat posed by a 5 cm AAA is considerably greater for someone aged 50 years than it is for someone over 75. Eventually rupture takes place through all the layers, with either the initial formation of a retroperitoneal haematoma or immediate free intraperitoneal bleeding sufficient to cause death. The risk of rupture is related to the size of the aneurysm: the normal aorta is 1.5–2.5 cm in diameter and is defined as aneurysmal when it is larger than 3 cm. The reported annual risk of rupture varies quite widely but is probably in the region of:

- 6 cm: 5–10%
- 7 cm: >20%.

Balancing the risks of surgery against those of rupture can be difficult in smaller aneurysms. The UK Small Aneurysm Trial found that for stable AAAs of 4–5.5 cm diameter, surveillance was safer than surgery, as the rupture risk was about 1% per annum. This does not apply to saccular or mycotic aneurysms, rapidly expanding or symptomatic aneurysms and perhaps equivalent-sized AAAs in small females. Such patients should all be treated surgically. Currently, elective repair is normally offered to suitable patients if their AAA is above 5.5 cm or the rate of growth is more than 1 cm per year.

Only a third of patients with rupture reach hospital, and of those that are operated upon, only half survive. Thus, the overall (community) mortality for rupture is as high as 80–90%, and possibly many other deaths occur from rupture of an undiagnosed, asymptomatic aneurysm.

Screening

The mortality for elective AAA repair in asymptomatic or mildly symptomatic disease is, in the best centres, less than 5% (endovascular repair lower than open repair). It thus makes clinical sense to detect and repair as many aneurysms as possible before rupture. Ultrasound-based screening of a defined population has been used to find asymptomatic aneurysms. Recent studies have shown that mass screening in men over the age of 65, and elective repair of asymptomatic aneurysms, can significantly reduce aneurysm-related mortality. The Department of Health has recently endorsed AAA screening and regional programmes will be established in the near future. Screening may be extended to first-degree relatives of known patients with AAA.

Clinical features

In thin patients, the aneurysm itself as well as its transmitted pulsation may be visible on inspection. On palpation there will be a pulsatile, expansile swelling in the midline of the abdomen, usually extending towards the left-hand side. However, it is important to appreciate that clinical examination alone, even when performed by an experienced vascular surgeon, may be unreliable for confirming the presence or absence of aneurysmal disease and for estimating the size of the aorta. This is one reason why so many AAAs go unrecognised until there are life-threatening complications such as rupture. Any suspicion of AAA should therefore prompt an ultrasound examination, and indeed a number of experts have advocated ultrasound-based population screening for AAA. Although it is frequently taught that AAA tenderness indicates actual or impending rupture, or the presence of an inflammatory component, this too is unreliable. Healthy persons will often feel pain if their aorta is palpated firmly. There may be a bruit on auscultation in association with origin stenoses of the branches of the abdominal aorta (coeliac axis, superior mesenteric, renal arteries). There is an association between AAA and aneurysms elsewhere, so the examiner should specifically exclude the presence of femoral and popliteal aneurysms. The surface marking of the aortic bifurcation is at the level of the umbilicus, so any pulsation felt below this level is likely to denote the presence of iliac aneurysmal disease.

Management

Although, as described above, most AAAs gradually increase in size, the unpredictable nature of this process means that vascular surgeons usually organise repeat ultrasound examination at 3- to 12-monthly intervals for those who do not require urgent management.

Indications for elective repair

The decision to operate involves weighing the known risk of leaving the AAA in place against that of operation. The first depends upon:

- size
- presence of symptoms
- age and physiological state.

Guidelines on size criteria for treatment of AAAs are given in Table 29.2. The risk of operation depends primarily upon cardiorespiratory status. Anaesthetists (Ch. 6) and cardiologists can help the surgeon assess this, and also life expectancy, more precisely. There is no advantage to be gained in repairing a small aneurysm at low risk of rupture in an elderly person with severe myocardial disease whose cardiac prognosis is poor.

Technique

Procedure for AAA repair is summarised in Clinical Box 29.3. Use of the high-dependency or intensive-care unit is routine (Ch. 10).

Operation for rupture proceeds in a similar manner except that systemic heparin is not given (Emergency Box 29.1).

Endovascular treatment of aneurysms

An alternative approach is to deploy an endoluminal stent in the aneurysm through a femoral approach (Fig. 29.11). Fixation of the stent relies on radial forces in the neck of the aneurysm just below the renal arteries and in the iliac vessels. Aneurysms with a suitable-length neck of 1.5 cm and fairly straight iliac arteries can be stented. The techniques of endovascular aneurysm repair (stenting) are still being developed. The technical success rate in experienced centres is more than 95%. The durability of endovascular aneurysm repair (EVAR) is still uncertain. Intermediate and long-term follow-up data have shown that the incidence of secondary interventions in patients with EVAR is around 10% per year. Endoleak, graft kinking, stenosis or thrombosis and device migration are causes for secondary interventions,

Table 29.2 Guidelines on size criteria for treatment of abdominal aortic aneurysms

Criteria	Treatment
Symptomatic aneurysms regardless of size	Urgent surgery
Asymptomatic aneurysms of diameter <5.5 cm	Surveillance if increasing by <1 cm/year Elective surgery if increasing by >1 cm/year
Asymptomatic aneurysms of diameter >5.5 cm	Elective surgery

Clinical Box 29.3 Procedure for repair of abdominal aortic aneurysm

- Open the abdomen through a long vertical midline or transverse incision
- Confirm the presence of an operable aneurysm and the absence of other disease which might affect prognosis, particularly colorectal cancer
- Dissect the neck of the aneurysm free by mobilising the fourth part of the duodenum to the right with care to avoid injury to the left renal vein
- Dissect the iliac arteries free
- Administer a bolus dose of i.v. heparin, usually 3000–5000 units, and, after a delay of 1–2 minutes, clamp the aorta and iliac vessels
- Open the aneurysm longitudinally, and deal with any back-bleeding from lumbar arteries or the inferior mesenteric artery by suture ligation
- Evacuate thrombus – most aneurysms are full of organised blood clot with only a small central lumen to allow blood flow
- Suture an appropriately sized graft end-to-end with non-absorbable sutures to the infrarenal neck of the aneurysm and then to the iliac bifurcation of individual iliacs
- Before the lower anastomosis is completed, thoroughly flush the arteries and the graft to expel any clot
- Restore flow to the legs, one side at a time to minimise the stress on the heart of the fall in blood pressure upon reperfusion; then evaluate haemostasis and lower limb perfusion
- Close the sac of the aneurysm and the posterior peritoneum over the graft to exclude it from the peritoneal cavity (inlay technique) and to separate the graft from the duodenum to minimise the risk of an aortoduodenal fistula
- Close the abdomen in the standard manner

Emergency Box 29.1

Management of suspected leaking abdominal aortic aneurysm

- Take brief history and examine to assess comorbidity and quality of life
- Establish i.v. access and colloid replacement to maintain systolic BP at 90–110 mmHg; monitor O_2 and saturation
- Arrange urgent blood tests and cross-match 8 units plus products
- Carry out ECG and rectal examination to exclude myocardial infarction or GI bleed (which may also lead to abdominal pain and collapse)
- Inform senior surgeon, anaesthetist, theatres and ICU
- Remain with patient and transfer directly to theatre
- Occasionally a CT scan is appropriate to determine open or endovascular treatment

emphasising the need for lifelong surveillance; however, these may decrease with use of new-generation grafts, better selection of patients and experience.

Popliteal aneurysm

One in 10 patients with AAA also have a popliteal artery aneurysm (PAA), and 50% of patients with PAA have an AAA.

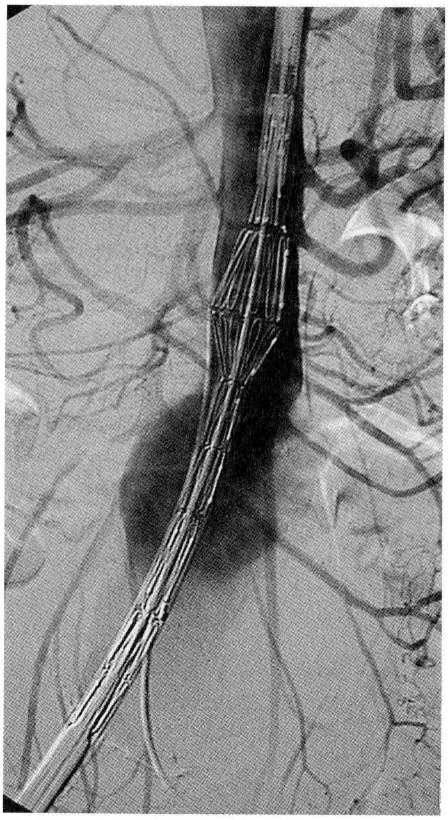

Fig. 29.11 Fluoroscopic image of an endovascular stent being deployed within an abdominal aortic aneurysm. (Courtesy of Mr D Baker, Royal Free Hospital, London.)

Pathological features

This type of aneurysm develops in the same way as others. The main complication is thrombosis with or without distal embolisation. Because the aneurysm itself is nearly always asymptomatic, presentation is usually as an emergency with the symptoms of acute limb ischaemia, unless an incidental diagnosis has been made on vascular examination.

Management

Emergency

Acute thrombosis of a PAA is associated with a high rate of limb loss, because usually the distal calf vessels thrombose simultaneously. Small thrombi from within the PAA may have embolised to obliterate the vessels of the calf and foot, which makes surgery technically difficult because there is no distal run-off for the surgeon to use for a bypass. Thrombosis in a PAA is an accepted indication for thrombolysis, which can be used to dissolve clot in the calf vessels either preoperatively by the radiologist through a femoral catheter or by the surgeon directly in the operating room. Despite these techniques, 50% of those who present with an acute thrombosis of a PAA lose their limb.

Elective

Many would operate when the diameter exceeds 2.5 cm or when a significant amount of thrombus has been seen on ultrasound. Symptomatic PAA with evidence of distal embolisation should also be prepared. About 20% of patients have bilateral disease, so the other limb should be carefully examined and if a PAA is found it should be repaired.

Technique

A reversed vein bypass is constructed from the superficial femoral artery above to the popliteal artery below the aneurysm. The PAA is tied off and thus excluded from the circulation. Endovascular stents can also be used if the anatomy is suitable.

Thoraco-abdominal aortic aneurysm (TAAA)

Epidemiology

The general view has been that 90% of all AAAs affect the infrarenal aorta. However, with increased awareness and better imaging techniques, particularly CT, it has become apparent that a greater proportion of aortic aneurysms than was previously thought (perhaps 15–20%) involve the abdominal aorta above the level of the renal arteries and/or the thoracic aorta (Fig. 29.12).

The risk of rupture appears to be the same as for infrarenal aneurysms. TAA may also lead to aortic dissection and compress surrounding structures such as the oesophagus to cause dysphagia or a main bronchus to produce lobar collapse and recurrent pneumonia. TAA may also cause severe chest and back pain, especially if it is large and there is erosion into the vertebral column.

Management

Repair is attempted in only a few centres in the UK, and the technique is highly specialised. The complexity, and thus the risks, are considerably higher than for infrarenal AAA repair.

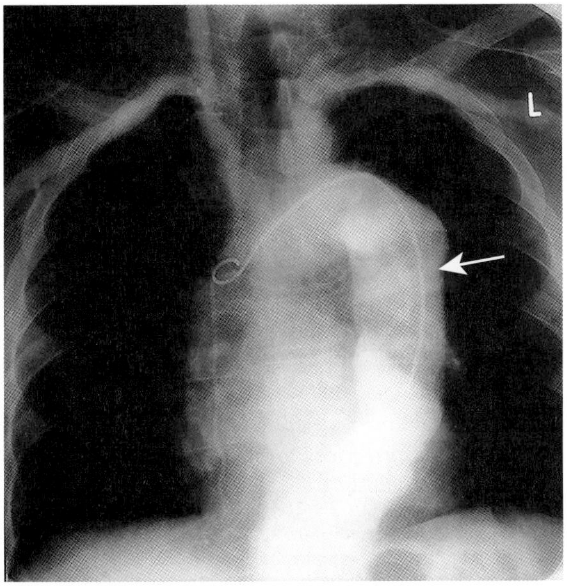

Fig. 29.12 Angiogram showing aneurysmal dilatation of the thoracic aorta. The guide wire is lying within the lumen (arrow). Angiography may underestimate the size of an aneurysm because it only demonstrates the lumen and not the large amount of thrombus that also usually lies within the aneurysm sac.

As a result, many surgeons will defer TAAA repair until the patient has severe symptoms or, in asymptomatic patients, the aneurysm has reached a size where the risk of rupture is thought to be particularly high. Endovascular repair (stenting) is an attractive alternative treatment for isolated thoracic aortic aneurysms. Hybrid repair which includes open debranching of visceral vessels and stenting of the aorta as well as the use of fenestrated/branched stents have increased the treatment options for TAAAs. Further developments in this field will probably change the way TAAAs are treated in the future.

False aneurysm

Aetiology

In civilian practice, most false aneurysms are the consequence of arterial puncture of the common femoral artery. After the procedure, the hole in the artery fails to close and blood enters the perivascular space to form a haematoma which liquefies to create a fluid cavity into which arterial blood still circulates and which is walled off from surrounding tissues by a fibrous capsule.

Management

If a false aneurysm is small then it may close spontaneously provided that the patient is not on anticoagulants. It is also possible to induce thrombosis by compression under ultrasound guidance. Most false aneurysms can be treated successfully with thrombin injection into the sac. However, if the aneurysm is very large, with a wide neck and continuing to expand, then surgical repair is necessary. This is usually a straightforward procedure – closure of the hole in the artery and obliteration of the sac.

Anastomotic false aneurysm

A false aneurysm can also develop at the site of an anastomosis between prosthetic material and native artery. In these circumstances, the surgeon should always consider the possibility of infection. Such anastomotic aneurysms may require operative repair to prevent rapid expansion and haemorrhage.

CHRONIC LOWER-LIMB ISCHAEMIA

Intermittent claudication

Intermittent claudication (IC) is the mildest manifestation of lower-limb ischaemia and affects approximately 5% of men over 60 years. In the majority it is the consequence of atherosclerotic narrowing or occlusion of the superficial femoral artery in the thigh.

Clinical features

Symptoms

Arterial insufficiency causes ischaemic muscle pain on walking which is quickly relieved by rest. To begin walking again causes re-arrest after the same distance has been travelled. This depends on whether the patient is walking on the flat or uphill but otherwise is quite constant under the same conditions. At rest, the blood requirement is met by the collateral circulation through the profunda femoris system which joins the popliteal artery below the blockage usually just above the knee. However, exercise produces a demand which cannot be met, and the calf muscles become ischaemic. Because the thigh muscles still have a normal blood supply, the pain is usually felt only in the calf. Cycling may be used as an alternative to walking because this activity depends primarily on the thigh rather than on the calf muscles. If stenosis is more proximal (aorto-iliac), then pain is felt in the whole leg and even the buttock if the blood flow to the internal iliac artery is compromised. A penile erection may also be impossible or difficult to sustain (Leriche syndrome) consequent upon an aorto-iliac obstruction.

Physical findings

On examination, the limb may be obviously ischaemic. Pulses are usually diminished or absent below the femoral (there is nearly always an associated bruit) but, if they are present, exercise causes their disappearance.

Diagnosis

There are many causes of pain in the leg, of which arterial disease is only one. Much of the time of a vascular service is spent excluding other disorders. Pain that radiates from the back, hip and knee joint, osteoarthritis and venous outflow obstruction (venous claudication, Ch. 30) may all be difficult to distinguish from true arterial claudication, especially if there is some coexistent but asymptomatic arterial disease.

Management

Arterial claudication is common, but progression to critical ischaemia is unlikely. Anxious patients should be reassured that amputation is unlikely. The risks for arterial surgery or amputation are less than 1–2% per year.

However, certain patients are at risk of disease progression, including those who:

- present with severe claudication of less than 50 m
- have low (less than 0.5) ABPI
- have multilevel or distal disease
- are diabetic
- continue to smoke.

Such patients need careful assessment, aggressive treatment of risk factors and the offer of reconstruction or endovascular therapy if and when critical limb ischaemia develops.

Medical therapy

For many years the standard treatment for the majority of patients has been to advise them to stop smoking and keep walking. All should be:

- reassured that the legs are not in imminent danger
- encouraged to stop smoking
- monitored and treated for hypertension
- started on anti-platelet therapy
- started on lipid-lowering therapy
- started on an ACE inhibitor if it is not contraindicated
- monitored and treated for additional risk factors such as diabetes
- told to exercise regularly to the point of pain in order to develop collateral circulation.

The majority accept the wisdom of this advice and attempt to alter lifestyle. However, a proportion will not comply and/or will not accept their level of disability, and in these intervention may have to be considered.

Percutaneous transluminal angioplasty

Experts disagree on the role of this procedure in claudication. There have been few direct comparisons between PTA and best medical therapy (BMT), but where patients have been randomly allocated to one or the other, PTA has not been shown to confer any additional long-term benefit. In the first 6 months, while BMT is taking effect, PTA of suitable lesions might provide better short-term symptomatic improvement.

In the longer term, however, there are clear advantages to BMT because not only does it lessen symptoms bilaterally but it also increases longevity by reducing the risk of death from ischaemic heart disease, stroke and bronchial carcinoma – by far the most frequent causes in this group. Furthermore, PTA costs £500–1000 per procedure and, although arguably safer than open operation, is associated with a 1–2% major morbidity rate. To some extent, comparisons between BMT and PTA are clinically inappropriate and the two procedures should be viewed as complementary and not competitive. The fundamental question is not in which patients should PTA be considered instead of BMT, but rather in which patients will PTA augment the results of BMT.

There is no doubt that the results of PTA are better in the aorto-iliac than in the femoropopliteal segment. If clinical examination (reduced femoral pulse and/or the presence of a bruit) suggests that aorto-iliac (inflow) disease is significantly contributing to symptoms, then angiography with a view to PTA should be considered. By contrast, if the femoral pulses are normal and the clinical diagnosis is one of femoropopliteal or infrapopliteal occlusion, routine investigation in greater detail is not indicated and is usually reserved for those with a threat to the limb or livelihood.

Operation

Contention also surrounds this option. As mentioned previously, the natural history is benign in terms of limb loss, and potential mortality or morbidity from intervention must be set against this.

Aorto-iliac (supra-inguinal) disease

There is a lower threshold for reconstruction in this arterial segment because:

- The ability to compensate for aorto-iliac occlusion by formation of collaterals is not as good as it is in infra-inguinal disease.
- The long-term result of aorto-iliac reconstruction is considerably better than in infra-inguinal bypass; more than 80% of aortobifemoral grafts for claudication are patent at 10 years.

- Bilateral claudication can be corrected by a single operation.
- Those affected by aorto-iliac disease are generally younger and more likely to have their livelihood threatened by their disability.

Infra-inguinal disease

By contrast, there is much less enthusiasm for infra-inguinal bypass because:

- Compensation by collateral development is often good.
- At 5 years, less than 70% of femoropopliteal grafts are still patent.
- Bilateral claudication is common, requires two operations and so doubles risk.
- Insertion of a bypass graft leads to involution of collateral pathways; if the graft blocks, the patient nearly always returns to a worse level of ischaemia than that present before operation.
- Rest pain may develop after a failed graft and force reoperation; the long-term results of such procedures are less impressive than those of primary reconstruction.

Recently, the BASII trial has questioned the approach of 'having a go first' with PTA and then proceeding to surgery as those patients with failed PTA seem to have worse results after surgery. It is imperative then that careful selection of patients for each treatment modality is essential.

There can be few experienced vascular surgeons who have not seen a patient die or lose a limb as a result of vascular surgery done for claudication. In the UK, most adopt an extremely conservative approach, and less than 10% of infra-inguinal grafts are for claudication.

CRITICAL LIMB ISCHAEMIA

Critical limb ischaemia (CLI) is defined as rest pain which requires strong continuous (opiate) analgesia for a period of 2 weeks or more, and/or tissue loss, in association with an ankle pressure of less than 50 mmHg or toe pressure less than 30 mmHg. The inference is that, without intervention, a patient with CLI will come to major amputation within weeks or months.

Clinical features

Symptoms

Rest pain is indicative of severe ischaemia, usually felt in the forefoot, and the pain is typically worst at night and disturbs sleep. The reasons for this are:

- Metabolic rate in the foot is increased under the warm bedclothes.
- Cardiac output and blood pressure fall during sleep.
- A beneficial effect of gravity on pedal blood pressure is lost.

For these reasons, relief at night is often sought by hanging the leg over the side of the bed or walking about on a cold floor.

Physical findings

In addition to findings of arterial insufficiency, there may be evidence of multilevel disease. Constant pain in the foot with single-level arterial disease is uncommon and should lead to a search for other causes.

Ischaemic tissue is extremely sensitive to injury: even minor wounds fail to heal and ulceration follows. Ulceration is usually on the tips of the toes (Fig. 29.13). Minor damage quickly leads to infection, and bacterial toxins destroy yet more tissue. Frank gangrene then ensues and can spread extremely rapidly, especially in diabetics.

Relatively limited arterial occlusion may sometimes be enough to cause CLI if the heart is inadequate – pump failure. For example, after myocardial infarction or another cardiac event, cardiac output and systolic blood pressure may fall to a point where even a small increase in peripheral vascular resistance cannot be overcome. Management is difficult because of the hazards of major procedures, and the outlook is poor.

Management

Medical

In contrast to a presentation with claudication, rest pain is a warning that tissue loss is imminent. In the great majority, CLI does not improve without surgical intervention, but medical measures have important roles:

- assessment and treatment of heart failure, intercurrent infection and anaemia
- control of diabetes

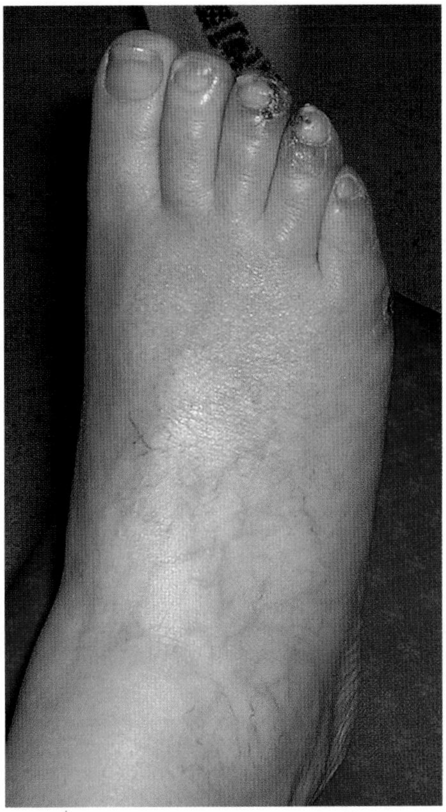

Fig. 29.13 Critically ischaemic foot. Note pallor on elevation and ulceration at the tips of the toes.

- antibiotic therapy of local infection (although the poor blood supply limits the tissue concentration that can be achieved)
- pain relief
- use of anticoagulants and occasionally prostacyclin-based drugs when tissue loss is minimal.

All of these measures can ensure that an optimum condition is achieved before surgical intervention is performed.

Balloon angioplasty

The majority view is that, in patients with early rest pain and/or minimal tissue loss (subcritical ischaemia), PTA may tip the balance just enough to salvage the limb when surgical reconstruction is not feasible. However, some believe that all patients with CLI should in the first instance be managed with PTA and that operation should be reserved for those who do not respond. This however has been challenged by the results of the BASIL trial that indicated a worse outcome for those patients treated with surgery following unsuccessful PTA.

Sympathectomy

This has little role to play in CLI, although those with early rest pain may achieve some relief.

Amputation

This is a last resort. Primary amputation can be the best option in the elderly frail patient with extensive tissue loss, but mortality is inevitably high.

Palliation

There are circumstances in which the patient and the family interests are best served by the provision of terminal care only.

Surgery

Bypass surgery and, to a far lesser extent, local endarterectomy are the mainstays of treatment, although the frequently present multisystem medical and vascular problems dictate a mortality for limb salvage surgery of up to 10%.

Aorto-iliac disease

In CLI, this is usually associated with infra-inguinal disease. As already implied, the results of PTA and stenting are optimal at this site, as are the long-term results of open arterial reconstruction. In younger, fitter patients who are considered unsuitable for PTA, the standard operation is aortobifemoral bypass graft. In those not fit for aortic surgery, an extra-anatomical bypass may be suitable. For example, if there is an iliac occlusion on one side and a relatively disease-free vessel on the other, a femorofemoral crossover graft (Fig. 29.14) is possible. An alternative is an axillobifemoral graft, where the inflow for the graft is taken from the axillary artery below the clavicle (Fig. 29.15).

Femorodistal bypass

This refers to an arterial reconstruction below the inguinal ligament in which common femoral or superficial femoral arteries are the site of proximal anastomosis and the popliteal or tibial vessels are the site of distal anastomosis. A popliteo-pedal bypass is a variant (Fig. 29.16).

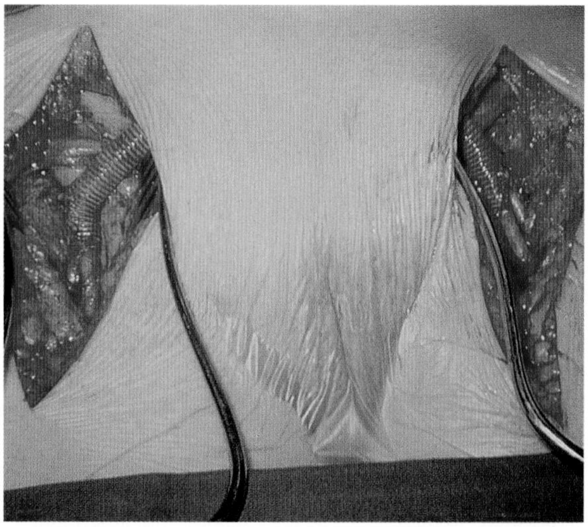

Fig. 29.14 An operative photograph showing a Dacron graft carrying blood from the left to the right common femoral artery below a right iliac occlusion.

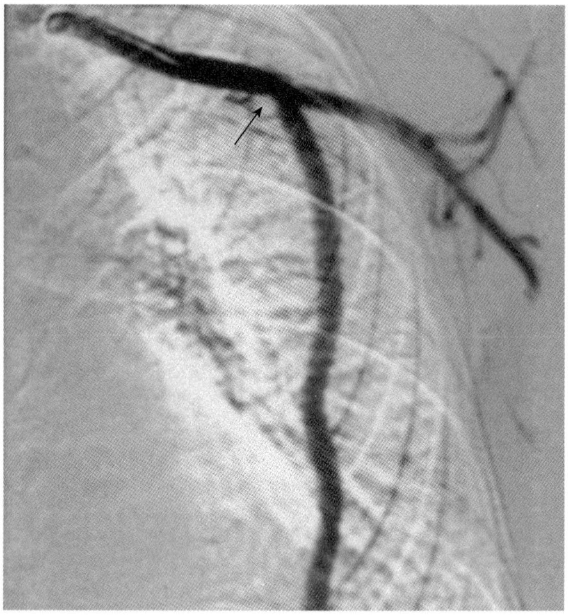

Fig. 29.15 Angiogram showing a graft using the left axillary artery as an inflow site (arrow) in order to revascularise both legs below an aorto-iliac occlusion. The patient was not considered fit enough to undergo aortic surgery.

Technical aspects of limb salvage surgery. Most femorodistal bypass grafts originate from the common femoral artery, but in certain patients, particularly diabetics, who have patent vessels to knee level and tibial vessel occlusion, there is no reason why the graft should not come from the popliteal. In general, the shorter the graft, the easier it is to construct and the better the patency.

The requirements for a successful distal bypass are:

- good inflow
- a reliable conduit
- good outflow.

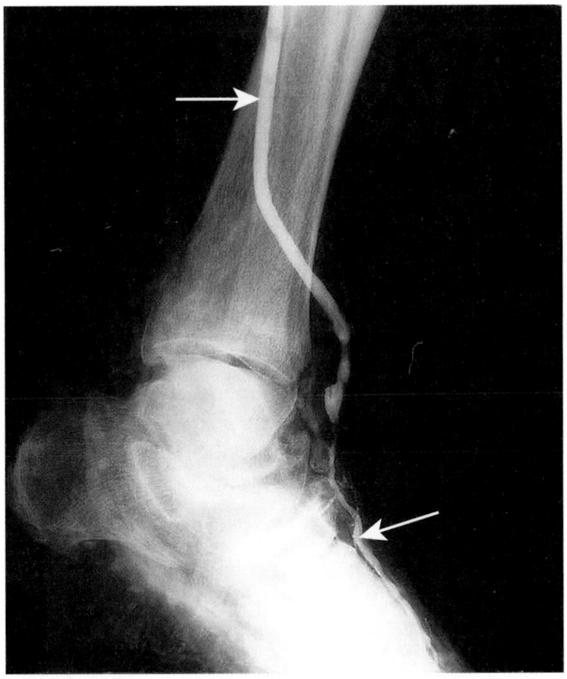

Fig. 29.16 An on-table angiogram to show flow of contrast from an in-situ femorodistal vein graft (upper arrow) into the dorsalis pedis artery (lower arrow) on the dorsum of the foot. The operation was carried out for critical limb ischaemia in a diabetic patient.

Inflow is usually provided by the ipsilateral iliac system, and any iliac disease must be corrected by PTA with or without placement of a stent.

Conduit. There is no doubt that autogenous vein provides the best long-term results, especially if the distal anastomosis is below the knee. The patency of long prosthetic bypasses (PTFE or Dacron) can be improved by using a vein interposition cuff at the distal anastomosis. Vein grafts may be placed in a reverse manner or in situ (non-reversed). In the first, the vein is reversed to remove any obstruction to flow that may occur from intact valves. In the second, the vein is not reversed and the valves are cut. Although no significant difference in patency between the two techniques has ever been demonstrated, from a technical point of view there are advantages to the in-situ technique when a long bypass to calf and foot vessels is to be constructed.

Outflow refers to the vessels into which the graft is to deliver blood. If the bypass is delivering blood to a dead end then thrombosis is inevitable.

Long-term patency. Femorodistal bypasses have a finite life expectancy which should be explained to the patient. Telephone contact should be available for those who feel that the graft may not be working. The chances of resurrecting a failed graft, particularly of vein, are often directly related to how quickly the problem can be tackled.

Most of those who have had a bypass are prescribed aspirin, because this both increases the rate of graft patency and reduces the risk of future coronary and cerebrovascular events. Anticoagulants are also sometimes used, although there is no definite evidence that these enhance patency, and anticoagulation in an elderly population is not without hazard.

Graft surveillance. It has been known for some time that certain grafts develop stenoses over time and that these predispose to occlusion. There is some evidence that, if such a graft can be identified and corrective measures applied before thrombosis occurs, the long-term patency may be significantly improved.

Stenosis most frequently takes place either at the distal anastomosis or within the body of a vein graft. The cause is neo-intimal hyperplasia – in simple terms, scarring where the intima has been damaged and which then impinges on the lumen to create a stenosis. Detection is best achieved by colour-flow duplex ultrasound; the concept of duplex-based vein graft surveillance is now well established. The patient returns for a scan every 3 or 6 months. If a tight stenosis is detected, a confirmatory angiogram is done and the lesion is corrected by either PTA or open operation. Most stenoses develop within the first 18 months and, to save cost and effort, most graft surveillance does not routinely go beyond this point. Late failure is more often the result of disease progression in the native arteries proximal or distal to the bypass.

Management of thrombosis in a graft

The options are:

- *surveillance* – if the leg is viable then it may be sensible to do nothing and wait for collaterals to develop; however, in that the majority of grafts are inserted for CLI, many (but not all) thromboses lead to redevelopment of a critical state
- *thrombolysis* – if successful, the underlying lesion which caused the graft to occlude can then be identified and corrected by either surgery or PTA
- *thrombectomy* – mechanical removal of thrombus, followed by an intraoperative angiogram to identify the underlying lesion and surgical correction
- *construction* of a new graft – some believe that in virtually all circumstances, the graft must be replaced by a new bypass in order to optimise long-term patency.

THE DIABETIC FOOT

Clinical features

Diabetics have a tendency to develop, often quite suddenly, severe ischaemia and infection in the feet which progresses to rapid tissue necrosis and amputation. The reasons for this are as follows.

- Vascular disease – which, in diabetes, develops earlier in life and tends to be more extensive and distal – makes intervention, by means of either angioplasty or surgery, more difficult and technically demanding. The clinical features are similar to those of non-diabetic vascular disease except that a palpable popliteal pulse is more frequently present, because of the more distal distribution of disease, particularly affecting the tibial vessels.

- Sensory neuropathy reduces or abolishes protective reactions to minor injury and to symptoms of infection or ischaemia.
- Autonomic neuropathy causes a lack of sweating and the development of dry, fissured skin which permits entry of bacteria.
- Motor neuropathy results in wasting and weakness of the small muscles, loss of the longitudinal and transverse arches of the foot, and development of abnormal pressure areas such as over the metatarsal heads (Fig. 29.17).

Management

Tissue loss is neuropathic or ischaemic, or more commonly a combination of both (neuro-ischaemic). The principles of management are best medical care for the diabetes, wide debridement of devitalised tissue, drainage of pus and, if ischaemia is present, revascularisation. Foot care is essential with involvement of podiatrist, early removal of calluses, moisturising of skin and protection of the foot from injury.

ARTERIAL DISORDERS OF THE UPPER LIMB

The arm is affected by ischaemia eight times less commonly than the leg because:

- atherosclerosis affects the leg more frequently
- the arterial supply of the leg in relation to muscle bulk is much poorer than that of the arm
- the ability of the arm to derive collateral supply appears superior.

Unlike the leg, the commonest cause of ischaemia is embolism. Ischaemia can progress rapidly, and loss of any part of the upper limb has a devastating functional result.

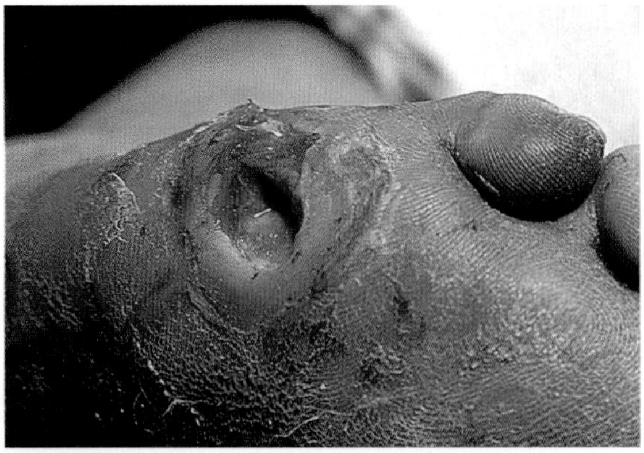

Fig. 29.17 Typical 'punched-out' ulcer over the head of the fifth metatarsal in a patient with diabetic peripheral vascular disease and neuropathy.

Thoracic outlet syndrome

Aetiology

Thoracic outlet syndrome (TOS) occurs when the lower trunk of the brachial plexus and/or the subclavian vessels are compressed as they pass over the first rib or a cervical rib or cervical band which runs from the transverse process of the seventh vertebra towards the first rib. The majority of patients are female and aged between 20 and 40 years.

Clinical features

Symptoms

The symptoms are predominantly neurological, typically pain, weakness, and/or paraesthesia over the ulnar aspect of the hand and forearm, often extremely vague and difficult to assess. Compression of the subclavian vein at the thoracic outlet may cause axillary vein thrombosis (Ch. 30). Only 5% present primarily with arterial ischaemic symptoms, most commonly claudication or Raynaud's phenomenon (below). Turbulent flow caused by a subclavian stenosis may progress to post-stenotic dilatation of the subclavian artery, which in turn may develop into an aneurysm; thrombus within this may cause a distal embolism.

Physical findings

A cervical rib can be palpable. On external rotation and hyperabduction of the shoulder, the radial pulse may be lost and the hand may go pale and numb (these signs are not specific because a proportion of normal people will also lose the radial pulse). Wasting of the small muscles of the hand is always pathological but can occur in a wide variety of conditions. Obvious digital ischaemia may be present after embolisation (Fig. 29.18) but also occurs in Raynaud's phenomenon where it is, however, always bilateral.

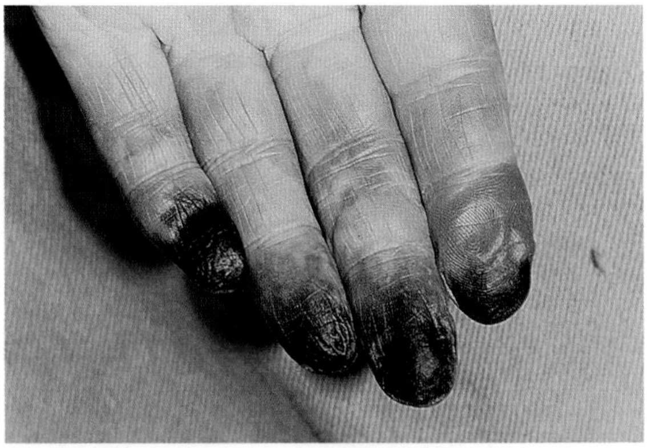

Fig. 29.18 Clinical photography showing extensive digital gangrene in a patient who had been treated medically for presumed Raynaud's phenomenon despite the fact that the symptoms had only ever affected one hand. More recently, gangrene had developed over only a few weeks. In fact, this patient had a cervical rib associated with a subclavian aneurysm containing thrombus which had been embolising down into the digital arteries. The rib was excised, the subclavian aneurysm replaced with a PTEE graft, and the tips of the affected fingers amputated.

Investigation

Plain radiography

A plain radiograph of the neck may show a cervical rib (Fig. 29.19) or a prominent transverse process which suggests but does not establish the presence of a fibrous band.

MRI

This is now the investigation of choice in that compression of the nerve roots and the artery can be demonstrated.

Angiography

A fixed stenosis in the neutral position, especially when it is associated with post-stenotic dilatation or aneurysm, is always pathological and remains the clearest indication for arterial surgery. Stenosis present only on abduction is present in 10% of normal individuals.

Duplex ultrasound

If present, a subclavian aneurysm together with any intraluminal thrombus can be identified, as can venous obstruction. Dynamic duplex with assessment of vessels with the arm in various positions can help diagnosis. As with angiography, 10% of normal population may show changes in blood flow in abduction and these should be interpreted with caution.

Venography

This investigation confirms venous obstruction and/or impingement; however, it is now rarely used.

Nerve conduction studies

These are useful in localising the problem to the thoracic outlet and should be considered before operation.

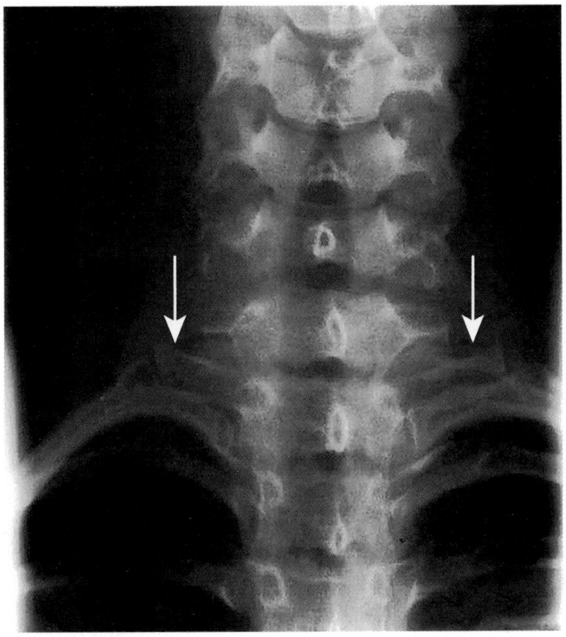

Fig. 29.19 Plain radiograph of the cervical spine showing the presence bilaterally of cervical ribs (arrows).

Management

Non-operative

In the absence of objective neurological damage or arterial ischaemia, treatment is symptomatic by physiotherapy in an attempt to improve posture and strengthen the muscles of the neck and shoulder girdle.

Surgery

Failure of conservative measures suggests the need for operative decompression. If a cervical rib or fibrous band is present, it can be excised via a supraclavicular approach. If not, many advocate excision of the first rib through a trans-axillary approach; a few suggest this even if a cervical rib is present. A subclavian aneurysm is excised and replaced by a graft.

When the symptoms are clear-cut and the diagnosis certain, the results of surgery are good. In other circumstances, when the surgeon and the neurologist are uncertain and operation is done as a diagnostic test or as a last resort, they are poor.

ACUTE ISCHAEMIA OF A LIMB

Aetiology

The great majority of cases of acute limb ischaemia are caused either by embolism or by thrombosis at a site of previous atherosclerotic narrowing. Differentiation is of clinical importance because the management is quite different (Table 29.3). However, even the experienced may be unable to distinguish between the two with confidence, and it is not uncommon for a patient with established peripheral vascular disease to have an embolus.

Embolism

Embolic material comes from:

- mural cardiac thrombus after a myocardial infarct
- left atrial appendix in atrial fibrillation
- vegetations from a heart valve in endocarditis or rheumatic disease

Table 29.3 Clinical features of acute embolism and thrombosis

Embolus	Thrombosis
Ischaemia is of sudden onset and very severe because of lack of preformed collaterals	Onset often insidious and less severe because of the pre-existence of collaterals
A potential source of embolus can usually be identified	No obvious source of embolus
Hospital records may indicate the presence of previous normal pulses	Previous records indicate long-standing peripheral pulse deficit
No history of arterial disease	History of arterial disease, e.g myocardial infarction, stroke, peripheral vascular disease
Normal pulses in contralateral limb	Absent or reduced pulses in contralateral limb

- thrombus from the aorta or other major vessel that is aneurysmal or atherosclerotic
- thrombus formed within a graft.

Embolic material tends to lodge at the site of major branches because of a match between it and the decreased vessel diameter.

Thrombosis

Surgical thrombectomy alone rarely succeeds, because of early rethrombosis; some form of arterial bypass or thrombolysis is usually necessary.

Clinical features

Symptoms

Symptoms are often described as the six Ps:

- pulseless
- pain
- pallor
- 'perishing' cold
- paralysis
- paraesthesia.

Physical findings

These reflect the symptoms. The presentation of an acutely ischaemic limb may not fulfil all the 'six Ps' criteria at the time of presentation. The limb is usually pale and pulseless, with painful toes/foot. Reduced sensation is not always easy to assess especially in patients with peripheral neuropathy such as diabetics. Deterioration of sensory neurologic function is an indication of progressive ischaemia. Proprioception and light sensation are first to be reduced or lost. Loss of pressure sensation, pain and temperature are late features of prolonged ischaemia. Loss of movement is a late feature. In embolic occlusion, events occur rapidly with early loss of motor and sensory function. In these circumstances the diagnosis of ischaemia, as well as the need to act quickly, is usually obvious. In those with thrombosis the presentation is often acute on chronic.

Management

Faced with the acutely ischaemic limb, the following questions must be addressed:

- Is the limb salvageable?
- Is the limb threatened?

The non-viable limb

Features that indicate the limb is no longer salvageable include:

- fixed staining of tissues
- lack of blanching on pressure
- anaesthesia with rigid muscles – rigor mortis.

Acute-on-chronic limb ischaemia may be the manifestation of another terminal illness such as cardiac failure or malignancy. To subject such a patient to amputation just before death from the underlying disease is not good practice.

In all circumstances, the decision must be whether it is appropriate to offer amputation or palliation. The wishes of the patient must be respected. If informed consent cannot be obtained, then the next of kin or other relatives should be involved.

The threatened limb

Features of an ischaemic limb that is likely, in the absence of revascularisation, to become non-viable include:

- loss of sensation
- loss of active movement
- pain on passive movement and when the calf muscles are squeezed.

When these features are present, there is a maximum of 6 hours in which to re-establish normal flow to avoid irreversible nerve and muscle injury.

If embolism is obvious, embolectomy is performed, but if the diagnosis lacks certainty, an angiogram avoids a blind procedure; alternatively, operative angiography achieves the same purpose. The surgical revascularisation required depends on the images obtained. In those whose limb is threatened but whose general condition precludes long and complicated arterial surgery, amputation may be the only option.

Management is summarised in Emergency Box 29.2.

The non-threatened limb

If sensation and movement are present and calf tenderness is absent, then the limb is not immediately threatened and it is safe to delay intervention. A period of medical optimisation and heparin therapy may lead to spontaneous improvement as a collateral circulation opens. Angiography and reconstruction can then be done on a semi-elective basis. An alternative is to start thrombolysis, but this requires 12–24 hours to complete. It is imperative that the limb is assessed frequently as changes may occur rapidly and valuable time may be lost if revascularisation becomes essential.

VASOSPASTIC DISORDERS (RAYNAUD'S PHENOMENON)

Understanding of this area has been hampered by the use of inconsistent terms. Here, standard European definitions are used:

- Raynaud's phenomenon (RP) is the general term which describes the clinical features of episodic digital vasospasm in the absence of an identifiable associated disorder

Emergency Box 29.2

Management of a limb threatened by acute ischaemia

- Make cardiorespiratory assessment of the patient
- Provide O_2 therapy and BP optimisation as necessary
- Provide analgesia
- Arrange blood tests (including clotting and cross-match), ECG and chest X-ray
- Keep nil by mouth and give i.v. fluids
- Start i.v. heparin – 5000 IU stat and 1000 IU/hour
- Arrange imaging – duplex ultrasound, arteriogram or on-table arteriogram depending on local availability
- Obtain consent
- Perform arterial reconstruction and consider fasciotomies

- Secondary Raynaud's syndrome (RS) is when the phenomenon occurs secondary to one of the conditions listed in Box 29.6.

Epidemiology and aetiology

Raynaud's phenomenon is 10 times more common in women than in men and may, in a mild form, affect up to 25% of the young female population. An episode in the fingers typically occurs in response to cold and emotion, but other predisposing factors such as the oral contraceptive pill, certain migraine drugs and tobacco have been identified. The toes and other extremities may be involved, and there is increasing evidence that RP may be a manifestation of a total body microvascular disorder.

Clinical features

There are three phases:

- pallor – because of digital artery spasm
- cyanosis – from the accumulation of deoxygenated blood
- redness (rubor) – reactive hyperaemia as blood flow returns.

Pain is unusual unless there are other complications, e.g. digital ulceration and gangrene.

Diagnosis

In the majority, the diagnosis of RP can be made on symptoms and physical findings; additional investigations are not required unless secondary RS is suspected. The proportion of patients who have an underlying disorder is uncertain; experts who run specialist clinics tend to collect the more intractable and severe examples, and, with adequate long-term follow-up, as many as 80% of all referred patients will eventually develop features of an underlying cause. Conversely, a GP who sees a small number of mildly affected patients may only occasionally identify one with a defined connective tissue disease (CTD) (Box 29.6). Only a minority have clear evidence of CTD on presentation. However, those with current tissue loss or scars from its previous occurrence must be assumed to have secondary RS, and a careful enquiry into the presence of isolated features of CTD should be made. Abnormal dilated nail-fold capillary loops, visible with an ophthalmoscope, are suggestive of, but not specific for, RS. Presentation for the first time in childhood or over the age of 30 increases the likelihood of RS. Eighty percent of those who present at over 60 years of age have an underlying disorder, although it is most often atherosclerosis. An asymmetrical distribution should also alert the vascular surgeon to the possibility of microembolisation from a proximal lesion (TOS), and a full vascular examination should be done in all.

Box 29.6 Conditions associated with Raynaud's syndrome

Connective tissue disorders
- Systemic sclerosis (90%)
- Systemic lupus erythematosus (30%)
- Mixed connective tissue disease (80%)
- Dermatomyositis/polymyositis (20%)
- Sjögren's syndrome (30%)

Macrovascular disease
- Thoracic outlet obstruction
- Atherosclerosis
- Buerger's disease
- Radiation arteritis

Occupational trauma
- Vibration white finger (VWF)
- Chemical exposure, e.g. nitrates, polyvinyl chloride
- Repeated exposure to extreme cold

Drugs
- Cytotoxic drugs
- Ergotamine
- Beta-blockers
- Ciclosporin

Miscellaneous
- Malignancy
- Reflex sympathetic dystrophy
- Arteriovenous fistula

Management

Medical

Most often, reassurance about the usually benign nature of the condition, advice to stop smoking and to avoid exposure to cold are sufficient; chemical handwarmers and electrically heated gloves are available. There is controversy over whether the oral contraceptive pill should be discontinued, but hormone replacement therapy appears to be safe. Numerous drugs have been used, the best of which appears to be the calcium channel blocker nifedipine, although side-effects are relatively common. Vasodilators may also be useful. In those with severe attacks, admission to hospital for a 5-day infusion of prostacyclin may provide great symptomatic relief in the winter months and, for unknown reasons, the beneficial effects may last up to 6 weeks.

Surgical

Secondary Raynaud's syndrome caused by macrovascular arterial disease is nearly always unilateral and may progress rapidly to tissue loss in the hand if the underlying lesion is not identified and treated expeditiously. In RS in the hand, sympathectomy is associated with poor long-term results, but the procedure appears to be more useful in the feet. In the variant CREST syndrome, digits affected by severe ulceration or calcium deposits may require amputation, although every attempt should be made to preserve as much tissue as possible.

CEREBROVASCULAR DISEASE

Carotid artery disease

Pathological features

Approximately 80% of all strokes are ischaemic rather than haemorrhagic; of these, as many as half are caused by atherosclerosis at the carotid artery bifurcation, which leads to either distal embolisation or thrombotic occlusion.

Clinical features

Symptoms

Micro-embolisation to the eye leads to ipsilateral transient loss of vision (amaurosis fugax), often described by the patient as a black curtain coming across the eyes, which usually lasts from a few seconds to a few minutes. A larger embolus may cause permanent blindness due to retinal infarct. Embolisation to the middle cerebral artery leads to hemispheric symptoms, usually a contralateral hemiparesis and, if the dominant hemisphere is affected, loss of speech. A cerebral event which does not cause brain infarction and therefore does not leave residual symptoms and signs is termed a transient ischaemic attack (TIA).

A completed stroke progresses to brain damage with a residuum of neurological features.

Physical findings

The neurological findings and their duration are consistent with the size of the area of brain affected.

Diagnosis and investigation

CT or MRI scanning should be performed urgently. Carotid artery stenosis may be visualised by angiography (see Fig. 29.1), but this technique may be associated with a 1–2% stroke rate and is not suitable therefore as a first-line investigation. Colour flow duplex scanning can give accurate information on the presence and degree of stenosis, and an increasing number of centres use this investigation as a basis for operation. A CT brain scan before operation is done to define the presence of pre-existing cerebral damage or to exclude other pathology.

Management

Early management

Immediate assessment in a specialist acute stroke unit should be arranged whenever possible. Urgent imaging is undertaken and thrombolysis with alteplase given (if appropriate) for ischaemic stroke within 3 hours of symptom onset. Aspirin is prescribed for ischaemic stroke and TIAs, while anticoagulation (heparin/warfarin) is used for acute venous stroke (cerebral venous sinus thrombosis). Nutritional support should be given, usually by tube feeding, if required. Antihypertensive treatment is used only if there is a hypertensive emergency (encephalopathy, nephropathy, cardiac failure or infarct, aortic dissection, or eclampsia) or with thrombolytic therapy (controlled to 185/110 or lower).

Carotid endarterectomy (CEA)

Indications. Two large randomised controlled trials have indicated that in cases of amaurosis fugax, TIA or stroke with good recovery plus an internal carotid artery stenosis of 70% or greater, the risk of future stroke is significantly reduced by CEA carried out as a supplement to best medical therapy, as compared with best medical therapy alone. Surgery should be performed within 2 weeks of developing symptoms whenever possible. Most stenoses less than 70% should be treated medically. The risks of surgery in patients with acute stroke and in those with completed stroke with poor recovery outweigh the benefits. There is also recent evidence from randomised trials that certain patients with high-grade asymptomatic stenoses may benefit from endarterectomy.

Technique. The major complication of CEA is a stroke. The benefits of the operation depend crucially upon a low perioperative stroke rate, which should be less than:

- 7.5% after a previous stroke
- 5% in amaurosis fugax or TIA
- 3% in those who are asymptomatic.

Balloon angioplasty

Trials are underway to compare CEA with angioplasty and stenting in both asymptomatic and symptomatic patients. Early data indicate that the immediate complication rate from endovascular treatment in symptomatic patients is higher than that associated with CEA. More recent results from centres using a cerebral protection device (umbrella-like system in the distal internal carotid artery to prevent debris embolising to the brain) and stents in addition to angioplasty are much improved. It is likely that both carotid stenting and CEA will have a place in future treatment of carotid disease.

Carotid body tumour

Pathological features

These rare lesions arise in the carotid body or less commonly in one of the adjacent nerves such as the vagus. They are paragangliomas, but it is not clear what proportion is malignant. Lymph node deposits may be found in up to 25%, but distant metastases are extremely rare and local recurrence is uncommon.

Clinical features

The usual presentation is a painless lump in the neck. It is frequently mistaken for a lymph node or a parotid lesion and may have been explored previously. The lump is not tender, is fleshy and, most importantly, can only be moved transversely in relation to the carotid sheath.

Diagnosis

A typical lump in the neck is investigated by either angiography, duplex scanning, CT or MRI. Angiography reveals a tumour blush and typical splaying of the internal and external carotid arteries into a wine glass shape (Fig. 29.20). Other imaging gives more detailed information on the feasibility of resection. Few carotid body tumours are part of the multiple endocrine neoplasia (MEN) syndromes. Those are more likely to secrete active substances. If there is adequate suspicion, then levels of circulating catecholamines and thorough investigations should be sought prior to any intervention.

Management

Carotid body tumours should be excised because they grow locally: the larger the tumour, the more difficult the operation becomes. Preoperative embolisation of tumours to reduce vascularity during operation has not been met with success and hence is rarely performed. Radiotherapy is reserved for symptomatic treatment of an inoperable lesion.

VISCERAL ISCHAEMIA

Acute mesenteric ischaemia

This condition is discussed in detail in Chapter 24.

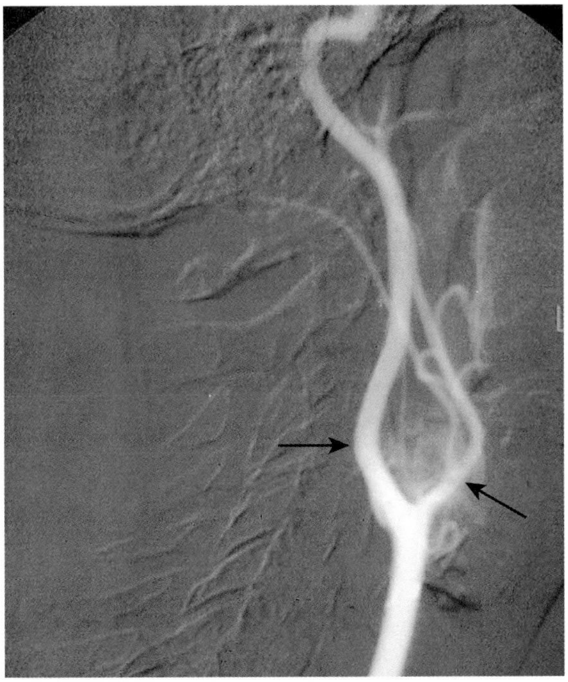

Fig. 29.20 Angiogram showing a 'blush' of contrast and splaying of the internal (left arrow) and external (right arrow) carotid arteries because of the presence of a carotid body tumour.

Chronic mesenteric ischaemia

The ability of the gastrointestinal circulation to develop collaterals ensures that the great majority of patients with arterial inflow obstruction are asymptomatic. It is generally believed that at least two of the three arteries which supply the gut (coeliac axis, superior and inferior mesenteric arteries) must be critically stenosed or occluded for symptoms to develop.

Clinical features

A typical complaint is of severe abdominal pain after eating – mesenteric angina. Fear of eating develops, so that mesenteric ischaemia is always associated with significant weight loss. This presentation mimics many other abdominal disorders, and frequently the patient has had numerous inconclusive investigations before the diagnosis is finally made.

Apart from weight loss, which is universal, there are rarely any physical findings. Occasionally an epigastric bruit is present, but this is often audible in those who are otherwise normal.

Diagnosis and management

Although, in these slim patients, an experienced ultrasonographer can often identify mesenteric disease on duplex scanning, the diagnosis can only be made with certainty on angiography.

Surgical revascularisation is the mainstay of treatment, although balloon angioplasty and stent placement is playing an increasing role. The commonest operation is to take a graft from the aorta to the superior mesenteric artery and the coeliac axis. This is a major surgical undertaking and is associated with significant risk, but the long-term results are good. The alternative is often a slow and painful death from progressive cachexia.

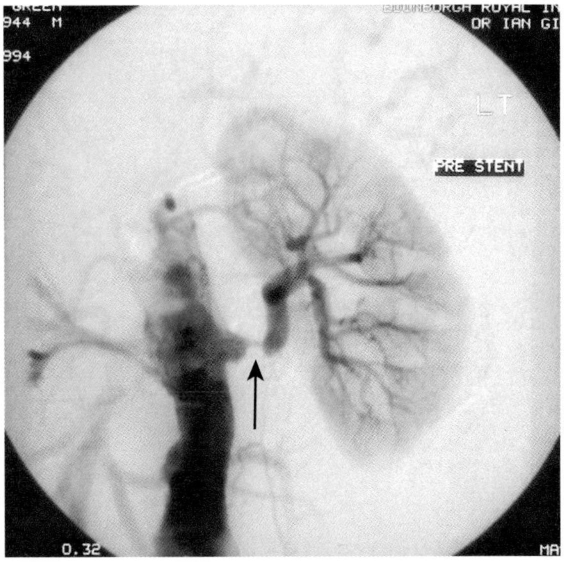

Fig. 29.21 Angiogram showing almost compete occlusion of the left renal artery from atherosclerosis (arrow). This was successfully treated by percutaneous placement of a stent.

RENAL ARTERY DISEASE

Renal artery stenosis

Pathophysiological and pathological features

In most patients, renal artery stenosis (RAS) is asymptomatic and merely an incidental finding at postmortem or on angiography done for another indication (Fig. 29.21). RAS leads to decreased renal perfusion and the release of renin from the juxtaglomerular apparatus. Renin converts angiotensinogen to angiotensin I, which is in turn converted to angiotensin II in the lung. Angiotensin II causes vasoconstriction and the release of aldosterone from the adrenal cortex. The renal excretion of sodium is reduced and blood pressure rises, which may in the short term return renal perfusion to normal. However, a progressive stenosis leads to worsening ischaemia, hypertension, loss of nephrons, atrophy and irreversible renal failure. The two main causes of RAS are atheroma (60%) and fibromuscular dysplasia (up to 40%). These two disease processes are quite different (Table 29.4). Less common causes include renal artery aneurysm thrombosis and embolism arteritis and trauma.

Clinical features

Renovascular hypertension affects a large number of people. For example, in the UK, approximately 10% of the adult population is hypertensive, and in these a renal cause is thought to be responsible for about 10%. Suggestive

Table 29.4 Comparison of renal artery atherosclerosis and fibromuscular dysplasia

Atherosclerosis	Fibromuscular dysplasia
60%	40%
Males aged 60 years and over	Females usually aged 40–60 years; may affect children
Stenosis at or within 1–2 cm of ostium	Affects distal two-thirds of renal artery ± segmental branches
30% have aortic occlusive or aneurysmal disease	Often multifocal
Part of generalised atherosclerotic disease	'String of beads' on angiogram
10–20% may occlude in 3 years	Occlusion uncommon
30% have bilateral disease	Unknown aetiology

features are onset before the third and after the fifth decade and the presence of peripheral vascular disease. The hypertension is typically of abrupt onset, severe or malignant in nature and difficult to control with standard medical therapy.

Renal failure caused by RAS is much less common but it should always be considered in the differential diagnosis of renal failure, particularly when there is other evidence of peripheral vascular disease. Deterioration of renal function after administration of an angiotensin-converting enzyme (ACE) inhibitor may be the trigger for clinical detection because these drugs prevent the adaptive responses described above. Discontinuation of the ACE inhibitor usually returns renal function to pre-treatment levels.

Diagnosis

Renovascular hypertension can be successfully corrected by surgical and/or radiological means and will reduce the long-term complications of hypertension (stroke and heart failure), the need to continue lifelong anti-hypertensive medication and the risk of renal failure. Therefore it is important to make a precise diagnosis, but this can be difficult. Clinically suspected RAS is usually confirmed by angiography. Although many other less invasive and expensive investigations have been advocated, none is sufficiently sensitive or specific to be a satisfactory screening test (Box 29.7). Occasionally the clinical significance of the diagnosis of RAS can only be confirmed by reduction in blood pressure and/or improvement in renal function after its correction.

Management

Medical

Drugs can control all but the most severe forms of hypertension and may limit hypertensive nephropathy in an unaffected contralateral kidney. However, medical treatment cannot arrest progression of stenosis, and information from non-randomised studies suggests that surgical correction is associated with an increased survival when compared with medical therapy. In particular, the risks of renal failure, stroke and myocardial infarction are reduced.

Surgical

Balloon angioplasty is now the first-line treatment of most cases of RAS, particularly that associated with fibromuscular dysplasia. Although restenosis is relatively common, the procedure can be repeated and is associated with less risk than open surgery. The long-term results of angioplasty are considerably better in non-ostial than in ostial lesions. Placement of a stent may offer better long-term patency in ostial disease. Open operation provides better long-term results than PTA but requires considerable surgical skill and is associated with a significantly greater morbidity and mortality. Operation is usually reserved for instances in which medical therapy and PTA have failed. The commonest operation is aortorenal bypass with long saphenous vein. Extra-anatomic renal revascularisation can also be achieved through hepatorenal and splenorenal bypasses. These procedures can be expected to provide long-term blood pressure control in 85–90% of patients with a mortality of less than 5% and a major morbidity of less than 10%. If there is a small non-functioning kidney, nephrectomy may be the only option. Acute thrombosis of a chronically stenosed renal artery may not lead to renal infarction, because of the development of collateral capsular supply, and surgical bypass or PTA with stenting can sometimes be successful.

Box 29.7 Investigations of patients with renal artery stenosis

Technetium (Tc)-labelled DTPA or MAG3 scanning
- Poor take-up of radioisotope on affected side
- Reveals RAS if greater than 60%, especially after administration of an ACE inhibitor which exacerbates renal hypoperfusion

Colour flow duplex ultrasound
- Directly measures flow velocities in the renal arteries
- Very operator-dependent
- Probably not reliable at present

Renin levels
- Can be measured in general circulation or in renal vein
- High levels suggest renovascular hypertension but low sensitivity and specificity

MRI
- Provides images of the renal arteries without exposure to ionising radiation
- At present there are still problems with expense, availability and software

DTPA, diethylenetriaminepentaacetic acid; MAG3, mercaptoacetyltriglycine.

Renal artery aneurysm

This is an uncommon disorder that may lead to renovascular hypertension and renal failure. Rupture also occurs, and repair should be considered if the lesion exceeds 2 cm in diameter.

VASCULAR TRAUMA

Mechanisms

The commonest non-iatrogenic cause of injury to blood vessels in the UK is road traffic accidents (usually blunt injuries). Penetrating injuries – e.g. knife and gunshot wounds

– are much less frequent. Iatrogenic injury to the brachial and common femoral arteries from angiography and angioplasty are by far the commonest examples. If the injury is caused by a sharp instrument such as a knife, the arterial or venous wound tends to be limited to the area of immediate injury and the remaining vessel is undamaged. In some, particularly high-velocity, missile wounds (Ch. 3) or in blunt trauma, the extent of the injury is often more extensive, in terms of both the vascular injury and associated injuries in other systems.

Clinical features

The two principal consequences of arterial injury are:

- Haemorrhage – external and obvious or internal and thus clinically unapparent until hypovolaemia develops. Blood loss tends to be greater if there is only partial rather than complete transection, because in partial transection the laceration is held open by the continuity of part of the wall, whereas in complete transection vasospasm and intimal retraction with thrombosis occur, which limits loss.
- Ischaemia – this is often severe because the injury is acute and the vasculature has previously been normal; there has not been any opportunity for collaterals to become established.

History and symptoms

An obvious story of injury is common, but sometimes, in the context of multiple trauma, this may not be apparent. Otherwise the symptoms are those of acute vascular interruption.

Physical findings

In young people, provided that the systolic blood pressure is above 100 mmHg, peripheral pulses should be readily palpable. Absent or diminished pulsation should immediately alert the clinician to the likelihood of vascular injury. In closed injury, an expanding haematoma may be palpable.

Doppler examination. An audible Doppler signal may be present from a collateral circulation even if the artery is transected proximally.

Investigation

Angiography should be considered in any instance where there is doubt about the diagnosis or where the site of injury is uncertain (Fig. 29.22).

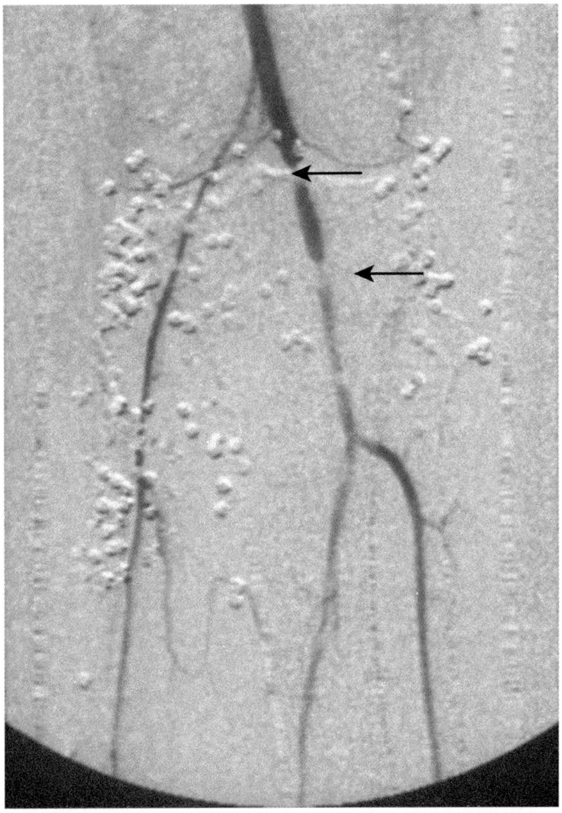

Fig. 29.22 This young man had a close-range shotgun wound of the knee. Although peripheral pulses were still present, the angiogram indicates severe multilevel injury to the popliteal artery (arrows). The vessel was reconstructed successfully with a vein graft, but unfortunately, because of extensive nerve injury, above-knee amputation was eventually required. Numerous shotgun pellets are also seen in the soft tissues.

Management

As in any acutely ill patient, management begins with resuscitation (Ch. 3). Immediate control of haemorrhage by direct pressure and then operation rapidly to restore normal flow are essential. The latter is achieved either by direct repair of the artery and accompanying large veins, if possible, or by means of a bypass graft. Because of the risk of infection, prosthetic materials should be avoided wherever possible.

All patients who sustain vascular trauma should receive appropriate antibiotics and, when indicated, tetanus prophylaxis (Chs 3 and 9). The use of thromboembolic prophylaxis has to be decided on an individual basis and must balance the risks of thrombosis against those of haemorrhage. The risk of reperfusion injury is greatest in vascular trauma, and fasciotomy is frequently indicated for prevention (Fig. 29.23).

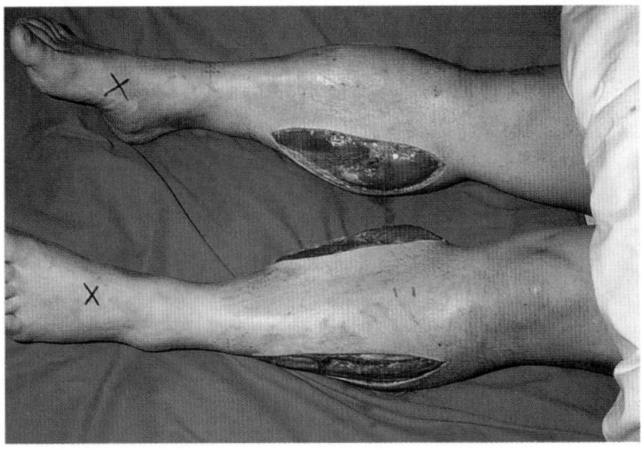

Fig. 29.23 Bilateral fasciotomies done following revascularisation of bilateral severe leg ischaemia. Note how the muscles are bulging through the skin incisions.

Traumatic arteriovenous fistula

If, as a result of trauma, there is damage to an adjacent artery and vein, a fistula between them may develop.

Clinical features

Symptoms include pain, swelling and sometimes other features of distal ischaemia. If the shunt is large, then, over some weeks and months, cardiac failure may develop.

There is often a thrill on palpation and, on auscultation, a machinery bruit throughout the cardiac cycle. Distal venous engorgement may develop.

Management

Surgical repair is indicated, but various endovascular techniques such as embolisation and covering the fistulous opening in the artery with a stent may also be used.

False aneurysm

As discussed above, arterial injury may lead to false or pseudo-aneurysm (Fig. 29.24). Treatment is by ultrasound-guided compression, thrombin, surgical repair, or, in certain circumstances, embolisation with a coil or placement of a stent. Large false aneurysms causing compression of local structures may require an open surgical approach. Recently combinations of stenting, coiling and thrombin injections can be used in experienced centres to deal with more complex pseudoaneurysms.

ARTERIOVENOUS MALFORMATION

These types of malformation are congenital but not hereditary abnormalities, almost invariably present at birth, although they may not present for medical attention until much later in life. A number of rare syndromes are recognised including the Klippel–Trènauny–Weber (port-wine stain, varicose veins, and bony and soft tissue hypertrophy involving an extremity), which has an identified genetic abnormality. Haemangiomas, by contrast, present a few days or weeks after birth and are much more likely to regress spontaneously. The more proximal an arteriovenous malformation (AVM) is in the circulation, the greater the transmitted flow. A proportion of malformations appear to be entirely venous. The terminology is often mixed when describing vascular malformations with the term AVM being wrongly used to describe even pure venous malformations.

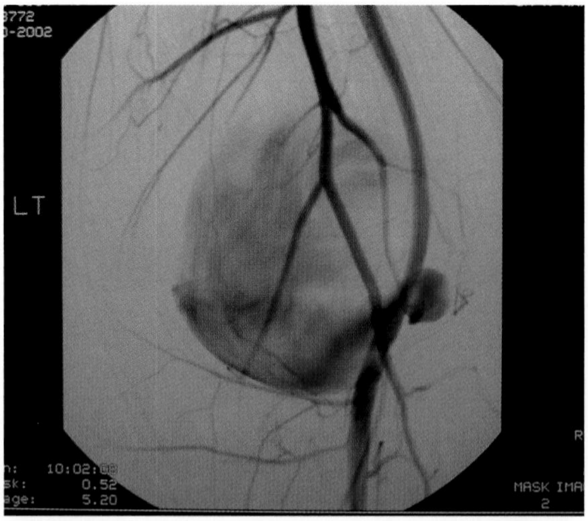

Fig. 29.24 Angiogram showing a large false aneurysm of the superficial femoral artery. The course of the native artery is seen to deviate as a result of the mass effect of the false aneurysm.

Clinical features

Symptoms

Patients present at almost any age; onset of symptoms may be related to the appearance of the menarche, to pregnancy or to an episode of minor trauma. There is swelling, discoloration and/or bleeding which is usually not life-threatening; pain, high-output cardiac failure, limb hypertrophy and ulceration are less common.

Physical findings

Lesions with an arterial component are usually pulsatile, a machinery-type murmur is heard on auscultation and, using a hand-held Doppler device, flow is easily detected in all phases of the cardiac cycle. Venous lesions engorge and empty with dependency and elevation, respectively.

Diagnosis

Appearance in later life requires distinction from malignant lesions such as sarcoma and metastatic deposits. Apart from biopsy to exclude malignancy in cases of doubt, the diagnosis is usually clinical.

Investigation

In venous lesions, phleboliths may be seen on plain radiographs. A chest X-ray allows assessment of cardiac size. Ultrasound, with or without venography, can be used to assess venous lesions. CT and particularly MRI (now the investigation of choice) give valuable information about deep extent when excision is contemplated. Angiography is invasive, should not be done for diagnostic purposes and is reserved for those lesions in which therapeutic embolisation is under consideration.

Management

AVMs may not require treatment except for counselling and reassurance for both the patient and, in children, the parents. When necessary, the principles are control of symptoms and prevention of complications with minimal intervention. Radiologists, cardiologists and vascular, orthopaedic, plastic and maxillofacial surgeons may all be involved in therapy.

Operation may occasionally be required to exclude malignancy. Complete excision provides good long-term control but is rarely feasible. The technique of dissection and ligation of feeding arteries is always associated with recurrence, compromises arterial access for interventional radiologists and should not be performed. Amputation is sometimes required as a last resort. Therapeutic embolisation, in which the lesion is filled from within with thrombogenic coils, gel or onyx is the mainstay of treatment but requires high skill and careful planning. This carries a risk of ischaemia in surrounding or distal vital tissues – inadvertent embolisation of neural tissues, fingers and toes is a particular concern. Venous lesions can be treated by direct injection of sclerosant and/or partial excision of prominent veins once the normality of the deep venous system (sometimes absent or hypoplastic) has been assured.

FUTURE DIRECTIONS

Many of the techniques described in this chapter have been developed only over the last 20–30 years. This rapid pace of technological advance continues, particularly that of minimally invasive and endovascular techniques – for example, the repair of abdominal aortic aneurysms by a stent – graft placed percutaneously through the femoral artery without the need for an abdominal incision. More complex aneurysms can now be treated with hybrid repairs combining open surgery and stenting or with fenestrated custom made stents. Laparoscopic intra-abdominal arterial surgery, although still in its infancy, shows promise for the future. Stenting of a carotid artery stenosis may become an alternative to carotid endarterectomy.

Equally impressive have been the advances in non-invasive imaging. High-quality, real-time, colour flow duplex ultrasound imaging has already revolutionised the imaging of arteries and veins. New ultrasound contrast media may allow certain vessels such as the renal and mesenteric arteries, previously inaccessible to ultrasound diagnosis, to be imaged with increasing ease and accuracy.

It is likely that there will also be major advances in the development of prosthetic grafts to match the long-term performance of autologous vein. In addition, there is much basic science work directed towards allowing human cadaver and animal arteries to be used as arterial conduits in humans. Research into gene tharapy and growth factors is rapidly growing and is likely to play an important role in prevention and/or treatment of vascular disease in the near future. With an ageing population and little evidence of a major decline in tobacco consumption or in the prevalence of diabetes, there is undoubtedly going to be a growing need for arterial surgery for many decades to come.

FURTHER READING

Beard JD, Gaines PA 2009 Vascular and endovascular surgery: a companion to specialist surgical practice, 4th edn. Elsevier Saunders, Philadelphia

Donnelly R, London NJM 2009 ABC of arterial and venous disease. 2nd edn. Wiley-Blackwell, Chichester

Hands L, Ray-Chaudhuri S, Sharp M, Murphy M 2007 Vascular surgery (Oxford specialist handbook in surgery). OUP, Oxford

Hallet JW, Mills JL, Earnshaw J, Reekers JA 2009 Comprehensive vascular and endovascular surgery, 2nd edn. Mosby Elsevier, Philadelphia

NICE clinical guidance 2008 Stroke: diagnosis and initial management of acute stroke and transient ischaemic attack (TIA). Available online. Accessed: 24 January 2011 from www.nice.org.uk

30 Venous and lymphatic disorders

VENOUS DISORDERS

The venous system is affected by conditions that cause clotting within it. This may in turn have consequences for the return of blood from the tissues and input from the arterial side. In addition, anatomical abnormalities (usually in the valves of the veins) may interfere with the fluid dynamics of the venous circulation and impair tissue nutrition, especially oxygenation, in the periphery.

Anatomical and physiological considerations (Fig. 30.1)

Superficial veins in the limbs and head and neck drain the skin. They contain valves which permit central flow but oppose reflux. The deep venous system comprises all channels within the investing (deep) fascia. In the limbs, these contain valves similar to those in the superficial veins. Communication between the superficial and the deep veins is provided by veins which perforate the investing fascia – reflux in these is also prevented by valves which only allow flow from superficial to deep. In the trunk the deep veins are without valves, so creating a central pool in which changes in pressure are uniformly distributed. Changes in central venous volume and pressure are one of the major methods by which cardiac output is maintained (see Ch. 17).

The detailed physiology of the veins of the lower limbs, whose function is much influenced by the upright posture of humans, is considered below.

Pathological features

Thrombosis

The fluidity of blood within veins is dependent on:

- free flow, although stagnation is probably only an accessory factor to other causes of thrombosis
- normal composition
- an intact endothelial surface. All vessels, but veins in particular, contain plasminogen activators which initiate the lysis of fibrin and so cause the dissolution of small accumulations of fibrin.

These three factors were first invoked as the underlying causes of venous thrombosis by the German pathologist Virchow (Box 30.1, Table 30.1).

Clotting of blood within a vein takes two clinicopathological forms (Fig. 30.2):

- *thrombophlebitis*, in which there is a strong element of endothelial trauma, either from a physical cause, or inflammation, or both
- *venous thrombosis*, which may have a local (usually trauma) or general precipitating cause, but acute inflammation is not initially present.

Although these are two distinct pathological entities, there may be an element of overlap in an individual case. The first is more common in superficial vessels and the second, in the deep system.

The pathological distinction between the two types is of clinical importance. In thrombophlebitis the clot is deposited on damaged endothelium and is therefore attached to the vein wall throughout its (damaged) length. Spread takes place proximally (downflow) but usually only to the point of the next venous confluence where flow, if sufficient, will prevent further propagation. In venous thrombosis the clot is loosely attached to the vein wall at the point of origin and extension proximally is as a free-floating mass (propagated thrombus) which may be of considerable extent and can easily become detached to pass proximally into the heart and lungs (pulmonary embolus) and can cause sudden death by obstruction of cardiac output. In both types of thrombosis

Box 30.1 Virchow's triad

Venous thrombosis occurs when there is:

- stasis
- increased viscosity of blood
- endothelial trauma

Table 30.1 Factors in the development of venous thrombosis (Virchow's triad)

Factor	Causes	Effects
Stasis	Obstruction Varicosity	Encourages aggregation of platelets and margination of leucocytes
Increased viscosity of blood	Increased platelets (thrombocytosis) Cell surface factors (malignancy) Surgery and trauma	Affects factors? Reduced fibrinolysis
Endothelial trauma	Direct injury	Provides point for adherence of platelets

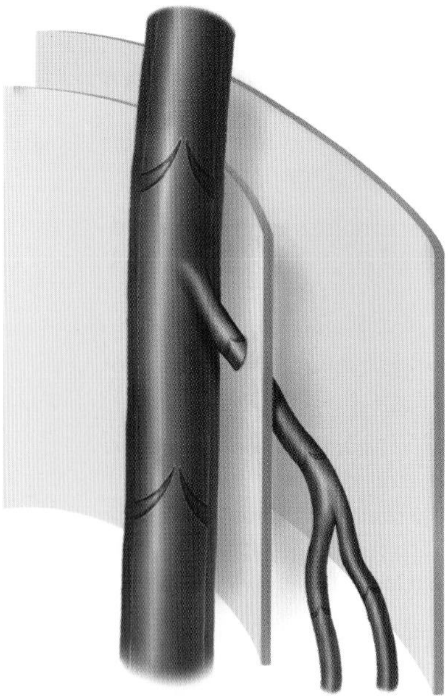

Fig. 30.1 The superficial and deep venous systems. The superficial vein passes through deep fascia to the deep venous system. A valve exists between the superficial and deep vein, permitting one-way passage of venous blood from superficial to deep systems.

(and in contrast to thrombosis in an artery – see Ch. 28) resolution takes place largely by fibrinolysis and the action of lysosomal enzymes secreted by leucocytes. The lumen is usually re-established (re-canalised) so that blood flow is restored. However, there may be a varying amount of damage to the wall of the vein (and its delicate valves), so that it undergoes some fibrous replacement with loss of elasticity. In consequence:

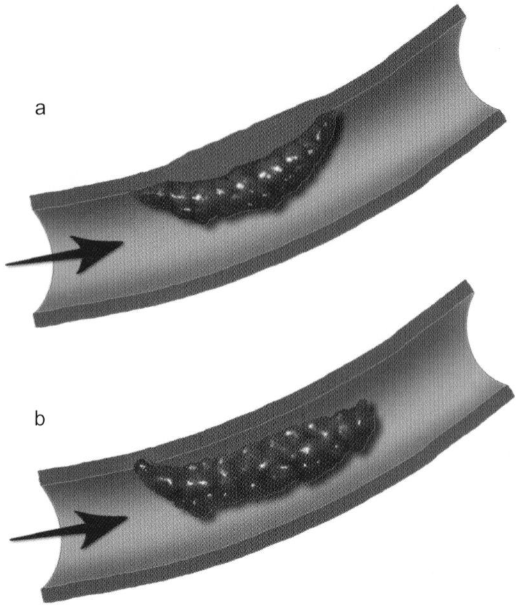

Fig. 30.2 Pathogenesis of venous clotting: (a) thrombophlebitis – blood clotting in vein secondary to inflammation of endothelium of the vein; (b) phlebothrombosis – blood clotting in vein due to stasis or factors other than inflammation.

- valves are destroyed or rendered incompetent
- the vein can become dilated, predisposing to stagnation.

The effect of this on venous function in the lower limb is considered below.

Recanalisation can be prevented if the vein is kept empty after the thrombotic episode – for example, by wearing firm support stockings. Permanent obliteration then occurs – a process which is used in the management of varicose veins (see 'Sclerotherapy', below).

VARICOSE VEINS

A vein is said to be varicosed when it becomes dilated and tortuous. Veins anywhere in the body can be affected but for practical purposes this common condition affects the lower limbs. The following section considers the lower limb only.

Anatomy

Venous drainage of the lower limb is by both the deep and superficial systems.

- Superficial veins lie in the subcutaneous tissue, i.e. external to the deep fascia.
- Deep veins are within the enveloping deep fascia and drain all structures within the fascial compartments, the most important of which are the muscles.

The two systems are connected by communicating veins, each of which contains a valve that permits flow only from the superficial to the deep system. There are upwards of 100 perforators in each leg, of which only a small number are of clinical importance. The two major ones are:

- the entry of the long saphenous vein into the common femoral vein at the saphenous opening in the groin – the sapheno-femoral junction;
- the junction of the short saphenous vein with the popliteal vein in the popliteal fossa – the short sapheno-popliteal junction.

Other communications are found along the line of the subsartorial canal (mid-thigh, medially – the so-called Hunterian perforator) and on the medial aspect of the leg – Cockett's perforators. Perforators also exist on the lateral aspect of the leg and thigh, but they are clinically less significant. A poorly recognised superficial-to-deep communication is via the perineal veins which drain from the superficial system in the thigh, via the vulva and peri-vaginal plexus, to both the internal iliac and ovarian veins.

The major deep veins follow the same paths as the arteries and below the knee are known as their venae comitantes. Above the knee, the veins join up to form a single companion trunk, the superficial femoral vein. This is then joined by the profunda vein just distal to the inguinal ligament to form the common femoral vein, into which the long saphenous vein drains before it (the CFV) becomes the external iliac vein at the level of the inguinal ligament. The valves in the deep system prevent reflux.

Venous physiology in the lower limb

The energy required to propel blood from the heart to the periphery is generated by left ventricular contraction. In the erect position, the return of blood to the right side of the heart from the lower limbs is assisted by:

- inspiration, which lowers intrathoracic pressure
- the muscle pumps of the thigh, calf and feet – of the two, this mechanism is by far the more important.

Contraction of the muscles in the relatively rigid compartments deep to the investing fascia causes intracompartmental pressure to rise. Furthermore, the veins and venous sinuses in the muscles are directly compressed by the muscular contraction. Blood is expelled and directed proximally by the one-way valves. The valves in the perforating veins prevent its escape into the superficial system. This sequence can be illustrated by measurement of venous pressure in a superficial vein on the dorsum of the foot. With the patient horizontal and at rest pressure is around 15 mmHg. On standing, but without muscle activity, blood continues to flow towards the heart but the pressure is increased to around 100 mmHg – an amount equivalent to the hydrostatic effect of a column of blood from the right atrium to the dorsum of the foot. Contraction of the muscles in the calf and foot (e.g. by rising on tiptoe) pumps blood towards the heart – the one-way valves prevent reflux into both the superficial system and distally. Relaxation of the muscles results in a transient fall in pressure to 40 mmHg, which then allows blood to flow in from the superficial veins via the perforators.

As seen in the cardiac pump, failure of the leg muscle pump, the valves, or the presence of obstruction, impairs the normal fall of superficial venous pressure on exercise and causes an accelerated return to resting pressure upon standing.

The common factor in the production of venous disease in the lower limbs is loss of valvular competence in the:

- superficial system – leading to cosmetic tortuosities (varicose veins) without disturbance of pump function
- communicating veins – resulting in deep-to-superficial incompetence (DTSI) with reflux of blood and high pressures in the superficial system on exercise. Pressures transferred to the superficial system by contracting calf muscles in the presence of DTSI can be significantly greater than the pressure generated in the standing individual with incompetent superficial veins alone – and may result in gross skin damage – see 'lipodermatosclerosis' below.
- deep valves – which raises the pressure in the deep system.

Epidemiology

Varicose veins are common. The prevalence is often stated as around 2% of the population, with a female: male ratio of 3:1. However, although varices are less common in the young, 30 to 50% of 35 to 75 year olds may have them.

The major complication of chronic venous hypertension is chronic inflammation and damage to the skin. This may eventually go on to ulceration and even malignancy – the eponymous 'Marjolin's ulcer', which is an aggressive, ulcerating, squamous cell carcinoma arising in an area of chronic ulceration.

Classification and aetiology

It is customary to classify varicosities into:

- primary – there is DTSI only (usually at either the sapheno-femoral or short sapheno-popliteal junction) where the varicosities appear without an obvious underlying cause
- secondary – where the varicosities occur because of some other cause: obstruction, or thrombo-inflammatory destruction of valves in both the communicating and deep veins.

Primary varicose veins

The exact mechanism by which valve failure occurs is still disputed. It was originally assumed that a valve or valves in a communication between the deep and superficial systems became incompetent from above downwards, followed by progressive proximal to distal destruction of the valves in the superficial system exposed to increased hydrostatic pressure. For example, in the long saphenous system, first sapheno-femoral valve incompetence, followed by dilation of the vein itself and thus valve failure throughout its length. Studies with Doppler ultrasound, however, have suggested that branches of the long saphenous vein (LSV) may become incompetent without or before incompetence at the sapheno-femoral junction. In addition, use of the saphenous vein for cardiac and arterial surgery (see Chs 18 and 29) suggests that its muscular wall makes it resistant to dilation when pressure is raised.

There is little doubt that there is a familial component but, this apart, there is no convincing hypothesis of cause. Contributing factors are:

- obesity
- multiple pregnancy – possibly through hormonal effects on the muscle of the vein wall – progesterone and oestrogen cause relaxation of smooth muscle.

Secondary varicose veins

These are less common than the primary type but are still frequent in some groups, such as women who have had multiple or complicated pregnancies. Causes are:

- deep or, less commonly, superficial venous thrombosis with recanalisation and consequent deep and/or deep-to-superficial valve destruction
- obstruction with venous hypertension – e.g. injury to a proximal vein, or obstruction by a tumour
- congenital or acquired arteriovenous fistulae, with increased pressure and flow being transmitted from the arterial side of the circulation.

Secondary varicose veins are associated with the syndrome of chronic venous insufficiency, which is considered below.

Secondary effects

Peri-venous tissue changes

Chronic venous hypertension causes characteristic changes in the skin and subcutaneous tissues of the lower limb. A rise in pressure at the venular end of the capillary loop to a value greater than the plasma oncotic pressure – normally 25 mmHg (about 34 cmH_2O) – causes:

- accumulation of interstitial oedema fluid which, at least initially, may be compensated for by increased removal by greater lymph flow
- impaired delivery of oxygen to cells, which predisposes the skin to break down from minor trauma – thus causing ulceration
- egress of plasma and red cells into the surrounding tissues.

Skin changes

The changes in the skin and subcutaneous tissues seen in chronic venous hypertension are described collectively in the term lipodermatosclerosis (LDS). It is characterised by:

- inflammation – caused by extrusion of plasma proteins, which are recognised as foreign by the macrophages and against which an immune (inflammatory) response is mounted. This is sometimes misdiagnosed as infection (bacterial cellulitis) and inappropriately treated with antibiotics. It should however be recognised that trauma to the skin can become secondarily infected. Thus the 'sterile inflammation' is complicated by bacterial inflammation (cellulitis). This has practical implications in that the sterile inflammation will not respond to antibiotics. Usually, however, non-infective inflammation responds to anti-inflammatory agents.
- pigmentation – secondary to the extrusion of red cells and their subsequent destruction by macrophages. Hemosiderin, the end-product of the breakdown of haemoglobin, is brown and causes the brown pigmentation characteristic of LDS.
- thickening of the subcutaneous tissues – oedema and patchy fibrosis.
- atrophy of the skin – often with depletion of normal pigment cells and white dermal patches – '*atrophie blanche*'.

Microscopic assessment of lipodermatosclerosis shows additional changes which stem from the venous hypertension and poor cellular nutrition:

- dilation and tortuosity but a decrease in the number of capillaries
- trapping of white cells within capillary loops
- peri-capillary deposition of a cuff of fibrin
- increased numbers of extravasated leucocytes.

All of these may play a role in the progression of the disorder. The dilated capillaries may be more permeable, so exacerbating the oedema. The fibrin cuff has been thought to reduce diffusion and so interfere with nutrition. However, this is currently regarded as unlikely and more probably a secondary phenomenon. Tissue oxygenation is certainly reduced. White cell activation associated with the release of cytokines, proteolytic enzymes and free radicals could result in further damage. Finally, tissue repair is inhibited by the physical presence of extravasated fibrinogen and by alpha-2-macroglobulin which binds growth factors, so making them unavailable (trap hypothesis).

A further, though uncommon, event is for squamous carcinoma to develop in a long-standing ulcer – Marjolin's ulcer, named after the French surgeon, Jean Nicolas Marjolin, who first described the condition in 1828.

Calf perforating veins – 'perforators'

Normally, during walking or running, the superficial veins in the lower limbs drain the skin into the deep veins via perforating veins (a.k.a. 'perforators') in both the calf and thigh – here we are not considering the sapheno-femoral and popliteal junctions as 'perforators'. The load on these perforators is increased in proportion to the incompetence in the superficial system – usually from either the sapheno-femoral or short sapheno-popliteal junctions. With increased load they dilate. The superficial incompetence may be of an order that causes the perforating vein/s to dilate beyond the point where their valves are competent. At this stage the significant pressures generated by the calf muscles during ambulation are transferred retrogradely through these now incompetent calf perforators to the skin where the changes of chronic venous hypertension can develop. After the superficial incompetence has been addressed surgically the load is removed and the perforators usually decrease in diameter to the point where they once again become incompetent. However, this may not occur and the patient can be left with chronic isolated calf-perforator incompetence and the consequences of the chronic venous hypertension. It is common for clinicians to miss this and, worse, if recognised, to feel that nothing can be done for these patients except for them to wear support stockings for life with the consequence that they may well develop chronic recurrent leg ulceration. This is unfortunate as this source of incompetence may be successfully addressed surgically, by either endovenous or open methods, thus providing the tormented patient with relief and even cure. Duplex Doppler scanning will confirm the diagnosis – see below.

The pathological and other features of ulceration are considered in more detail below.

Clinical features

History and symptoms

The symptoms of varicose veins may vary considerably. Because both varicose veins and leg symptoms are common, it is important to realise that they may neither be causal nor even related.

A family history is obtained in more than a third of patients and is often coupled with onset at a relatively young age. In secondary varices, there may be a history of deep-vein thrombosis (see below) although absence of this does not exclude such an event having taken place.

Patients with varicose veins may ascribe symptoms to them which, in fact, have other causes. Common symptoms which can be associated with varicose veins (some of which may have alternative causes) are listed in Table 30.2.

Discomfort. Aching is traditionally regarded by patients as a symptom they should have and may dominate their complaints – even though in fact they are more concerned about the unsightliness. Relief of discomfort on elevation or through the use of an elastic stocking is common although non-specific. Patients who have incompetent or obstructed deep veins may complain of discomfort of a bursting type on exercise. This will become more pronounced if a tourniquet is placed around the patient's thigh at a pressure higher than that in the superficial venous system (but, of course, lower than arterial pressure) – Perthe's test.

Pain may follow the development of a skin complication such as ulceration and will increase when complicated by cellulitis. Blood clot within a vein excites a non-bacterial inflammatory response – superficial thrombophlebitis – and is accompanied by acute pain along the line of the affected vein. Infection of a vein – e.g. where a cannula is present to administer intravenous fluids – may even cause thrombosis by initially damaging the wall of the vein.

Table 30.2 Symptoms of varicose veins and alternative explanations

Symptom	Alternative causes
Ugly appearance	Obesity Vascular disorders
Aching	Simple fatigue Musculoskeletal disorders in limb or trunk (sciatica, arthritis of hip or knee)
Pain on exercise	Arterial claudication Spinal claudication
Ankle swelling	Oedema of other cause – cardiac, renal, lymphoedema
Restless legs	Neurological disorder
Pigmentation and depigmentation	Skin disorders
Eczema	Skin disorders
Attacks of superficial phlebitis	Systemic causes – neoplasia – thromboangiitis obliterans
Ulceration	See Table 30.11
Bleeding into the subcutaneous tissues	Blood disorders with reduced clotting ability or increased bleeding tendency

Varices may bleed

- into the subcutaneous tissues. This is usually minor and causes only discomfort and bruising.
- externally, from the rupture of a varix. This is usually precipitated by minor trauma. If the patient remains upright there can be considerable blood loss because the haemorrhage is at high pressure. Deaths from such bleeding, which is in effect from the right side of the heart, have been recorded. However, they are rare – presumably because the patient has the insight to apply pressure and/or assumes the horizontal position (voluntarily or otherwise), thus reducing the pressure and allowing a thrombus to plug the leak.

'Venous eczema'. Early inflammation gives rise to itching This may lead the patient to scratch and further damage the skin – and this may become infected, causing bacterial cellulitis. Venous eczema may be seen in patches in relation to prominent varicosities and especially in the legs (i.e. below the knee where the venous pressure in the superficial system is higher than in the thigh).

Ulceration is usually painless, although episodes of inflammation caused by infection may change this.

Upon completion of taking a history from a patient it is important to have developed some idea of the severity of the symptoms and whether they are related to their varicose veins or are the consequence of another disorder.

Signs in the lower limbs

Variceal pattern. The initial examination is in the upright position with the groin and foot fully exposed. The pattern of varices (Figs 30.3 and 30.4) is usually easily recognised as being in the territory of either the long saphenous (most common, see Fig. 30.5) or the short saphenous vein (next most common), or both (unusual in primary varices). However, the patterns seen cannot on their own be used to make an anatomical diagnosis – because of the intercommunication between the two systems. Unusual variations in the distribution of varices suggest a possible pelvic obstruction; if associated with apparent enlargement of the limb and port wine stains of the skin, there is the possibility of an arteriovenous malformation or of the rare Klippel–Trènaunay–Weber syndrome – a complex developmental anomaly with multiple arteriovenous fistulae and overgrowth of the limb and which is associated with hypoplasia of the deep veins. The clinical manifestations of ovarian vein insufficiency are usually brought on by pregnancy, where the combination of raised progesterone levels (which causes smooth muscle cell relaxation) and the bulky uterus produce dilation in the vein and thus valvular insufficiency. Vulval and lower-limb varicosities can be impressive. The condition usually recedes after delivery but may persist and treated varicosities may recur. Patients with significant ovarian vein incompetence usually also have pelvic congestion syndrome – cyclical

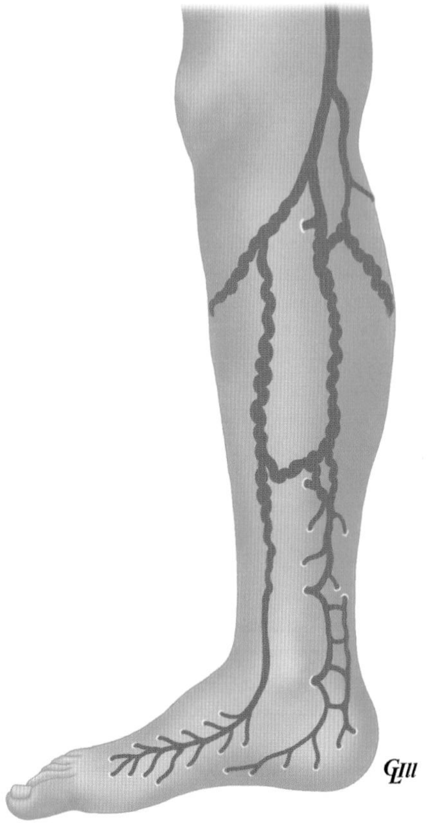

Fig. 30.3 Variceal pattern in long saphenous system in leg.

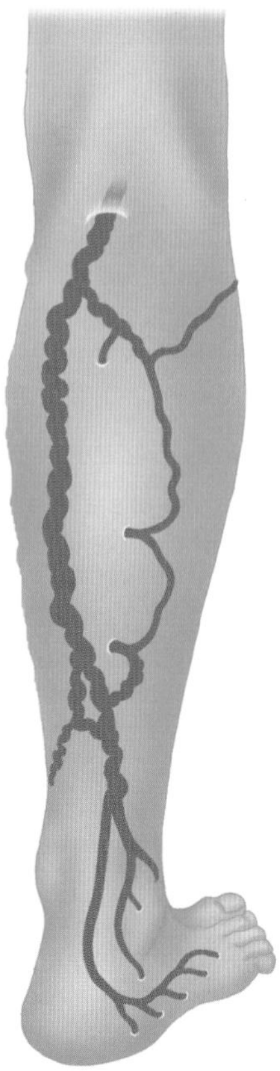

Fig. 30.4 Variceal pattern in short saphenous system in leg.

lower abdominal discomfort and menorrhagia. These symptoms may be debilitating to the extent that treatment of the underlying condition (ovarian vein incompetence) is considered – by endovenous embolisation.

With the patient supine and on raising the leg, varices either disappear completely or reduce significantly in size. An exception is when there is obstruction to venous outflow from the limb, causing secondary varices. The variceal pattern then includes the groin and adjacent abdominal wall.

Blow-outs. These are localised dilations and may be visible and palpable along either saphenous vein. They are sometimes associated with a palpable defect in the deep fascia and the presence of an incompetent perforating vein. A pronounced dilation is sometimes seen at the site of major incompetence between the deep and superficial systems: e.g. a saphena varix in the groin, which must be distinguished from a femoral hernia (Ch. 27); and a mass of tortuous vessels in the popliteal fossa. Blow-outs may also be seen in relation to incompetent medial calf perforators and should alert the clinician to their presence. Treating them (see later) may cure the patient of unpleasant manifestations of chronic venous hypertension including inflammatory sclerosis and lipodermatosclerosis (LDS).

Oedema associated with primary varices is usually relatively mild, pits readily and is typically seen at the site of the grip of an ankle sock. Gross oedema, except when associated with ulceration, is more likely to have a secondary cause: cardiac

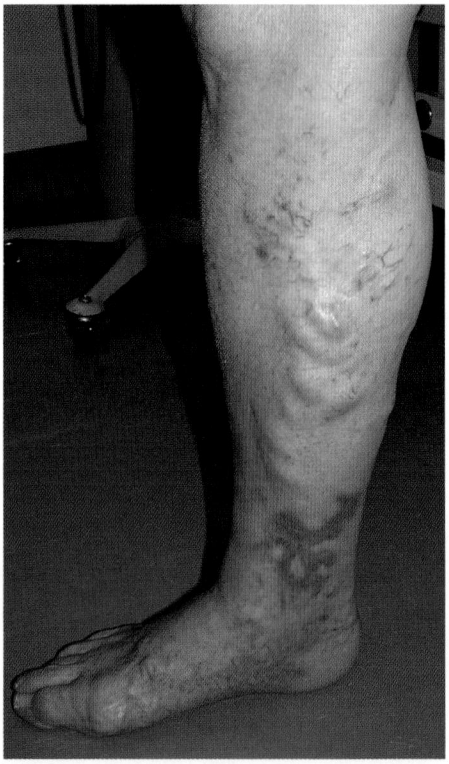

Fig. 30.5 Leg showing varicosities within the distribution of the long saphenous vein and skin changes above the medial malleolus. (Courtesy of Mr D Baker, Royal Free Hospital, London.)

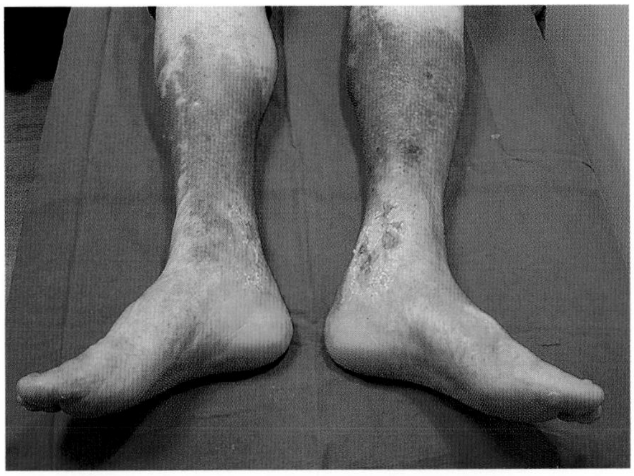

Fig. 30.6 Extensive bilateral lipodermatosclerosis and dark brown pigmentation (from the deposition of haemosiderin) with an area of ulceration as a result of long-standing deep venous incompetence.

disease, renal disease, or lymphoedema. Other causes of leg enlargement are lipoedema and primary cyclic oedema syndrome. In lipoedema there is a primary (usually familial) thickening of the subcutaneous tissues of the lower limbs, but sparing the feet – most frequently seen in women. The condition can be associated with a seemingly inexplicable, local tenderness. In primary cyclic oedema syndrome there is an idiopathic cyclic swelling of the legs, again, almost exclusively seen in females. As its name implies, the cause is unknown.

Skin and subcutaneous tissues. In mild varices, the skin is usually normal. However, where there has been long-standing superficial venous hypertension, whether caused by DTSI alone or associated with damage to the deep system, the characteristic changes of lipodermatosclerosis develop (see above and Fig. 30.6).

General examination

This may reveal underlying causes to explain symptoms and signs in patients who present with varices, particularly heart failure and musculoskeletal or pelvic disease in the elderly. Examination of the peripheral arterial system (skin temperature, nutritional changes and peripheral pulses) is essential to distinguish venous from arterial disorders, or to assess the relative contribution of each to a complication such as ulceration.

Clinical tests of valve function

Percussion of the column of blood in a vein with the patient standing – the 'tap test' – causes upward transmission of a palpable wave, especially when the vein is distended. In a varicose vein that has incompetent valves along its length, the wave is also transmitted downward. This procedure is most useful in the long saphenous system.

The Trendelenburg test (Fig. 30.7) is done by elevating the leg to 45° to empty the superficial veins by gravity and this may be assisted by stroking them from distal to proximal. A tourniquet is then lightly applied to the leg (the degree can only be learnt by practice but, in essence, it should be tight enough to prevent reflux of blood in the superficial system but sufficiently light not to impair arterial flow to the limb) just

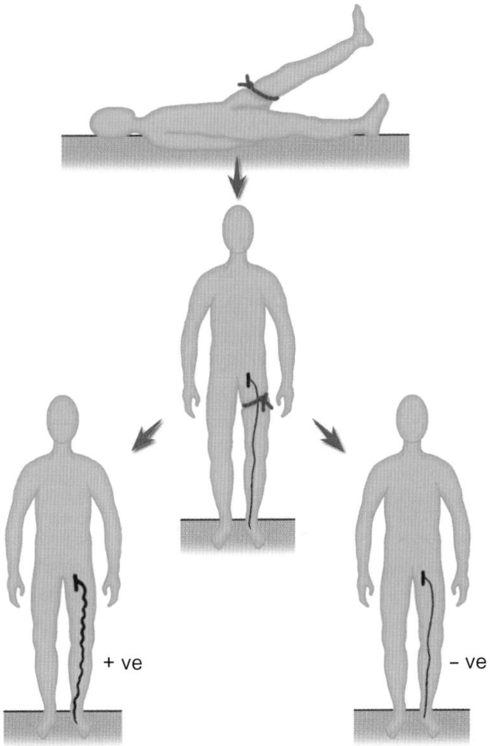

Fig. 30.7 The Trendelenburg test.

distal to the sapheno-femoral junction and the patient asked to stand. The tourniquet should be tight enough to prevent reflux of blood in the superficial system but sufficiently light not to impair arterial flow to the limb. If there is isolated sapheno-femoral valve incompetence the varicosities remain empty for at least 15–30 seconds and then gradually refill as blood continues to flow in from the arterial side of the circulation. The test is repeated with release of the tourniquet immediately on standing when, in the presence of significant venous insufficiency, reflux from the deep system will cause rapid filling of the varicose veins. Finally, if the veins fill at once even with the tourniquet in place, the sequence is repeated, moving the tourniquet down the limb until the lowest point of DTSI is found. If there is still rapid filling when the compression is below the level of the termination of the popliteal vein (just below the knee) then it is likely that there are incompetent perforating veins in the calf. However, localisation of these is not usually successful by this simple clinical procedure.

The Trendelenburg test may be done with finger pressure alone rather than a tourniquet, but experience is required; a precisely applied tourniquet is preferable.

Investigations

The investigations described below are for localisation of incompetent deep-to-superficial communications and for identification of valvular insufficiency in deep veins.

Continuous wave ultrasound

The Doppler directional probe (see Ch. 4) generates continuous waves which are reflected after striking their target. The reflected waves are then perceived by a sensor and transformed into a visual signal or sound. If the target is moving (as with the red cells in blood), on reflection, the frequency of the waves is altered – thus flow can be assessed. This principle is used to detect points of incompetence such as at the sapheno-femoral junction. With the probe just distal to this point, flow upwards in the saphenous vein is accelerated by compressing the calf or a prominent varix. Release of compression in the presence of competent valves causes a sharp cut-off of the signal. However, if there is incompetence, reflux occurs and generates a new signal. The test can be repeated at other sites of suspected DTSI such as the popliteal fossa (short sapheno-popliteal junction) and on the medial aspect of the leg where there are perforating veins. However, the accuracy of this investigation, except at the sapheno-femoral junction, is not very high and other investigations, such as duplex ultrasound Doppler scanning, provide more accurate information.

Duplex scanning

Duplex scanning is commonly used in the assessment of venous conditions and many surgeons use it routinely. It provides a combination of ultrasound imaging of the vessel and Doppler detection of the direction of flow (see Ch. 4). The underlying principles of assessment of flow are similar to those for the hand-held continuous-flow instrument. The advantages are:

- Valves at these junctions and in the deep veins can be seen.
- The anatomy, particularly at the sapheno-femoral and sapheno-popliteal junctions, can be clearly shown.
- Reflux is demonstrated by the reversal of the direction of flow, using the same principle as continuous-flow Doppler. Colour-coding the direction of flow improves the precision with which reflux can be detected.

Modern, easily-portable machines, enable surgeons to manage their patients in clinics and theatre more confidently.

Venous pressure and volume studies

The physiology of the venous muscular pump has been discussed in a previous section. Dynamic changes in volume of the leg are measured by various techniques, known collectively as plethysmography. They are not used in routine investigation but can be helpful when clarifying complex recurrence after surgery.

Radiological imaging

Since the advent of reliable duplex scanning, invasive, contrast-based radiological investigations are rarely indicated. They are still occasionally used in complicated cases where duplex investigation has been inconclusive.

Ascending venography is used to show the anatomy of the deep veins. Contrast medium is injected into a dorsal vein on the foot and, encouraged by the application of a tourniquet at the ankle, fills the deep system. It can be outlined in even more detail by application of a further venous tourniquet above the knee (Fig. 30.8). The technique can help to:

- identify sites of incompetent communicating veins (perforators) in the calf or thigh, although it does not necessarily reveal all of them
- demonstrate pathology in the deep veins caused by thrombosis – persistent occlusion or valvular incompetence. Its use is reserved for difficult problems associated with deep venous insufficiency.

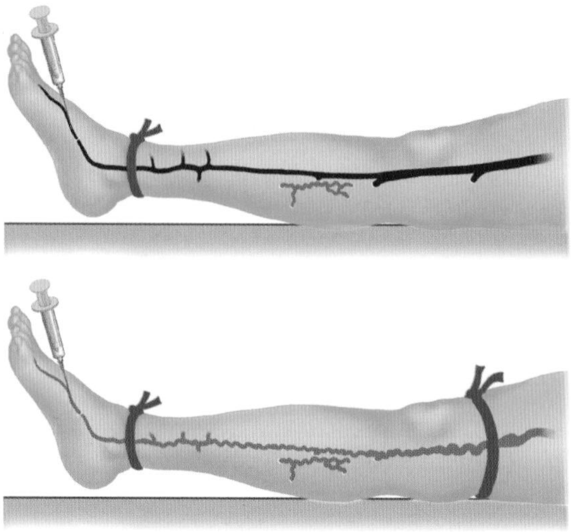

Fig. 30.8 Ascending venography. The deep venous system is outlined in more detail by applying a tourniquet above the knee.

Management of primary varices

By definition, these are varices in the superficial system with no evidence of disease in the deep venous system. Almost invariably they are associated with DTSI at one or more sites.

Once it is reasonably certain that the symptoms and signs in the leg are associated with the varices there are three management options: compression hose, sclerotherapy or surgery.

Compression hose

The indications are:

- mild symptoms
- those without skin changes
- the elderly – however, this group of patients may have difficulty pulling on these tight stockings, especially with arthritic hands
- those who refuse other forms of treatment
- most pregnant women.

The type of support and the choice are given in Table 30.3. It is important that any garments used should produce linear graduated compression, with the highest compression just above the malleoli and pressure decreasing towards the knee. Badly fitted support stockings or those which do not achieve graduated compression may produce more annoyance than relief and can, on occasion, cause damage to the skin. Poor choice of stockings increases the frequency of non-compliance. Patients should be instructed to apply compression hose before they rise in the morning and to remove them only before retiring.

Compression sclerotherapy

The principle of compression sclerotherapy is to produce sterile chemical inflammation in a vein with a sclerosant and

Table 30.3 Choice of support garment

Indication	Class	Pressure applied (at ankle, mmHg)[a]	Garment
Young patients; mild symptoms	I	14–17	Compression tights
Severe varices; early skin changes	II	18–24	Graduated compression: elastic stockings
Advanced skin changes; ulcer	III	25–35	Heavy-duty elastic stockings or initially elastic bandaging

[a]The compression pressure quoted is obtained by measuring the elastic tension at different sites on the stocking and deriving pressure from Laplace's equation: pressure = tension × radius. Methods for measuring the pressure under the stocking when it is in use are also available.

then keep it emptied by compression for a number of weeks – obliteration of the lumen follows. Commonly used sclerosant solutions are sodium tetradecyl sulphate 1% – 3% (Fibro-Vein™) and polidocanol (ScleroVein) – the latter is not licenced in the UK. Traditionally the method has been found suitable only for isolated varices without a large site of DTSI because, if this exists, recurrence rates are high. However, in recent years, ultrasound-guided injection of foam sclerosants has been demonstrated to increase the success rate. Nevertheless, many surgeons still find the recurrence rate of about 15% unacceptable. Furthermore, though small, with foam sclerotherapy there is the documented risk of embolisation to the brain via an occult patent foramen ovale, which can cause transient scotomata and even stroke. Trans-oesophageal echocardiography demonstrates that 25% of the population at large has an asymptomatic patent foramen ovale.

Further possible uses for sclerotherapy are:

- obliteration of isolated incompetent perforating veins, though recurrence is a problem
- vulval varices which persist after pregnancy – but these patients should first be investigated for underlying ongoing pelvic and / or ovarian vein incompetence as, if present, recurrence is likely
- treatment of telangiectasia (thread veins / spider veins / star-burst veins / etc.) by micro-injection sclerotherapy (MIST) – this is sought by patients for cosmetic reasons.

A common and frequently bothersome complication of injection sclerotherapy is skin-staining. The risk of this occurring is diminished by careful attention to adequate compression of the injected varices for up to 6 weeks, with intermittent inspection and aspiration of any liquefied intra-luminal haematoma. Potential complications are listed in Table 30.4. All are uncommon, but their possibility means that sclerotherapy should not be undertaken lightly and only after adequate training.

Surgery

The indications and contraindications for surgery are given in Table 30.5. The aim is to interrupt by ligation the major points of incompetence between the superficial and deep venous systems and, if appropriate, to remove the varices for both functional and cosmetic reasons. The two most common operations are sapheno-femoral and sapheno-popliteal ligation (Fig. 30.9) both of which can be done using day-care facilities. The procedure should be combined with removal of the saphenous trunk down to the knee by stripping, i.e. passing a flexible guide down the lumen of the vein, securing it to the divided vein and forcibly removing the vein subcutaneously. This not only improves the cosmetic result but also seems to be associated with fewer recurrences, probably because small incompetent perforating connections are avulsed – notably, in the thigh, the Hunterian perforator, which drains from the long saphenous vein (LSV) into the deep venous system, medially, at the mid-thigh level. Not infrequent causes of 'groin recurrence' are inadequate attention to removal of the anterior (or lateral) thigh vein (ATV) and the unrecognised presence of an accessory (or duplicated) long saphenous vein. In both instances neovascular tissue (numerous small venous channels which develop post-surgery) can reconnect the remaining vein (ATV or accessory LSV) to a patent sapheno-femoral junction. Some believe that the use of non-absorbable suture material like polypropylene (Prolene) to ligate the sapheno-femoral junction

Table 30.4 Complications of sclerotherapy

Cause	Reason	Outcome
Subcutaneous injection	Inexperience; failure to check reflux of blood into syringe	Pain, skin necrosis, ulceration
Intra-arterial injection	Failure to observe arterial pressure in syringe	Possible loss of limb from arterial thrombosis
Sclerosant entering deep veins	Inadequate compression	Deep-vein thrombosis
Escape of sclerosant into general circulation	Inadequate compression	Anaphylaxis, haemolysis

Table 30.5 Indications for surgery in primary varicose veins

History or physical finding	Indication	Contraindication
Pain	Definite if established as not due to another cause	Doubt as to cause
Phlebitis	Varicose veins the only cause	Other conditions not excluded
Bleeding	Episode of considerable bleeding to exterior	Minor bleeding: systemic blood disorder not excluded
Skin and subcutaneous changes, including eczema	To alleviate itch and prevent cellulitis and ulceration	Deep venous disease must be excluded
Ulceration	Adjunct to healing	Surgery not able to correct venous hypertension

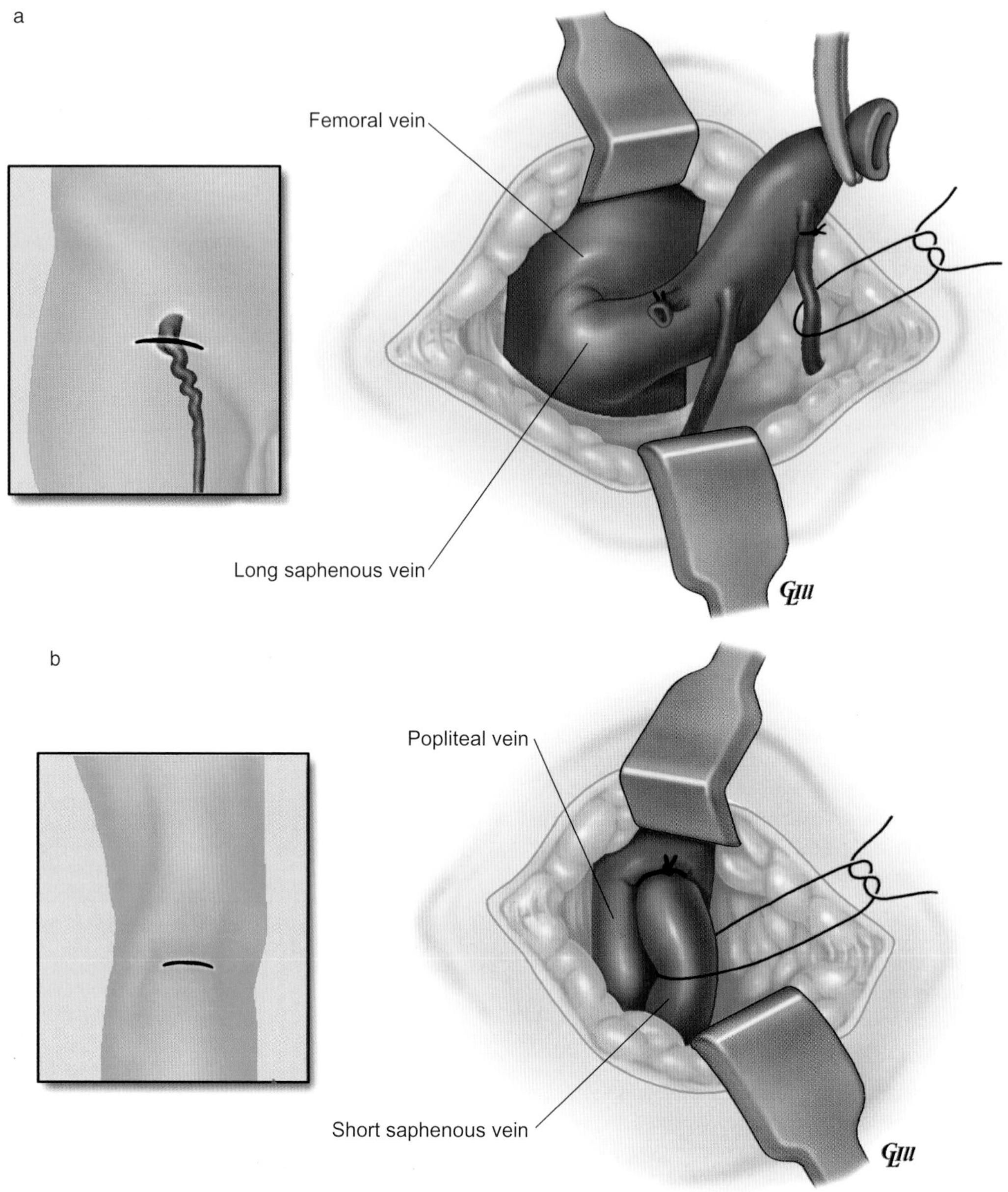

Fig. 30.9 Operations for (a) sapheno-femoral and (b) sapheno-popliteal ligation.

can help prevent this. Neovascular tissue in the groin post-surgery can be demonstrated with Duplex ultrasound but, in the absence of a remaining ATV or LSV, is almost invariably not associated with clinical recurrence.

If, in addition to sapheno-femoral or sapheno-popliteal incompetence, other incompetent sites have been identified, these too are ligated. Variceal channels are avulsed through small 'stab incisions' to give a pleasing cosmetic result – these incisions can be as small as 1 to 2 mm in length but sometimes need to be enlarged to accommodate larger varicosities. These incisions are sufficiently small to allow closure with Steri-Strips alone – no sutures are necessary.

The incidence of recurrence after surgery for primary varices is low when adequate clinical assessment supplemented, if necessary, by ancillary investigation, has been undertaken. The commonest causes of recurrence are:

- poor operative technique, including failure to adequately ligate the sapheno-femoral junction, and strip the long saphenous vein to the extent that the Hunterian (mid-thigh) perforator is not removed
- failure to recognise concomitant short saphenous incompetence
- failure to flush-ligate the short saphenous vein at its junction with popliteal vein
- failure to recognise incompetent perforators.

Recurrent primary varices require careful investigation, including, most importantly, Duplex ultrasound assessment.

It is imperative that patients are given realistic expectations of varicose vein surgery during the informed consent procedure. Problems after varicose vein surgery (Box 30.2) are among the commonest causes of medical negligence

Box 30.2 Complications of varicose vein surgery

- Bruising, which is inevitable
- Bleeding or haematoma
  - groin wound
  - avulsion sites
- Wound infection
- Neuropraxia
- DVT
- Recurrence
- Rarely, arterial or major nerve injury

claims but are largely avoidable with careful attention to detail during the history, investigation, consent, operative and postoperative periods.

Endoluminal venous obliteration A relatively new method of treatment of varices is currently available. It achieves obliteration of the long saphenous vein by thermal coagulation of the vein wall through means of either radiofrequency or LASER energy from a catheter placed within the lumen of the vein – 'endoluminal'. The catheter is inserted percutaneously under ultrasound guidance and the procedure can be carried out under local anaesthesia. Initially it was only the long saphenous vein that was treated but, increasingly, the short saphenous and perforator veins are being targeted. Postoperative pain and bruising may be reduced but results of long-term durability are not yet available. However, these techniques are increasingly being used and are becoming the standard treatment for varicose veins.

A concern about the method is that the catheter tip cannot be placed closer than 2 cm to the sapheno-femoral and sapheno-popliteal junctions – for fear of damage to the deep vein. This means that branches that drain into this untreated 2 cm length may be responsible for recurrence – typically the anterior thigh vein in the groin and popliteal area veins in the popliteal fossa. As time passes these questions will be answered.

What is seldom mentioned in the marketing of these minimally invasive techniques is that not infrequently the treated vein can develop an unpleasant thrombophlebitis which can last for several weeks and even months. The symptoms can usually be ameliorated with a non-steroidal anti-inflammatory agent. Where the vein is stripped, however, whilst the discomfort may be significant for the first few days, after a week or so, if the stripping has been done carefully and significant haematoma formation prevented (by the judicious use of compression bandaging during the stripping), the patient may be less symptomatic than if the vein had been endovenously treated and developed thrombophlebitis.

Ideally, the vein surgeon should have all the above methods available in her/his surgical armamentarium. A combination of patient preference, anatomical pathology and fitness for anaesthesia will then allow the most appropriate choice to be made.

VENOUS THROMBOSIS

Thrombosis may develop in superficial or deep veins anywhere in the body through any one or a combination of the three events which constitute Virchow's triad (see Table 30.1). This can occur in a wide range of circumstances.

SUPERFICIAL THROMBOPHLEBITIS

Aetiology

There are three main causes:

- stasis – e.g. varicose veins
- local trauma and inflammation – may be of any type but in surgical practice is frequently the result of i.v. therapy
- generalised hypercoagulability – e.g. malignancy and thromboangiitis obliterans.

Stasis is frequently a contributing factor to the other two.

Clinical features

An inflammatory response (thrombophlebitis) to the thrombus is produced in the vein wall and surrounding tissues – this is frequently associated with pain. There may be fever and, if the process is a pyogenic one, rigors, as bacteria are shed into the general circulation.

An obvious cause, such as an intravenous cannula and infusion, may be present. There is usually a red line along the skin over the vein – this is tender and firm to the touch.

Management

If there is a precipitating factor, this should be removed. Thereafter the condition is usually self-limiting and is treated symptomatically with non-steroidal anti-inflammatory agents. Spreading thrombophlebitis with systemic features may require blood culture and antibiotic therapy – and occasionally there is suppuration for which drainage is necessary. In recurrent attacks of migratory phlebitis, a search should be instituted for either arterial disease or an underlying malignancy – classically, carcinoma of the pancreas. Significant thrombophlebitis of a large superficial vein may lead to DVT as a consequence of the thrombus extending via a perforator into the deep system.

DEEP-VEIN THROMBOSIS (DVT)

Although thrombosis in the deep veins of the lower limb draws most attention (because of its frequency and potentially serious consequences) the process is not limited to this part of the circulation and can occur anywhere in the deep system. The causes are summarised in Table 30.6 and follow the pattern of Virchow's (Table 30.1).

Axillary–subclavian vein thrombosis

Aetiology

Only 2% of deep-vein thromboses occur in these vessels. The subclavian vein, along with the artery and nerves to the upper limb, pass through the so-called thoracic outlet which is bounded anteriorly by the subclavius muscle (attached to the inferior border of the clavicle) and first rib postero-inferiorly. This space can be narrowed by poor posture (e.g. carrying a heavy rucksack for prolonged periods), exercise (butterfly swimming and weight-lifting are good examples), trauma (fractured clavicle), etc. Narrowing of this already

Table 30.6 Major antecedents of deep-vein thrombosis

Factor	Circumstances
Immobilisation (venous stasis)	Bed rest during serious illness or injury Long-distance air travel Unconsciousness
Changes in clotting	Contraceptive pill – oestrogen containing Injury and operation Pregnancy/childbirth Malignant disease Hyperviscosity (e.g. polycythaemia) Antithrombin III, protein S and protein C deficiency Other thrombophilias
Effects on vein wall	Trauma – accidental or from cannulation Extrinsic compression – inflammation, tumour, bony abnormality

narrow space may lead to obstruction of venous return and precipitation of venous thrombosis. Further anatomical causes in the area are cervical ribs and hypertrophy of the scalenus anticus muscle. The condition is more frequent in men and is often associated with physical exercise which involves the shoulder girdle – the so-called Paget–Schrötter syndrome (effort thrombosis of upper extremity), which was described independently by Paget in 1875 and Schrötter in 1884. Forcible abduction of the shoulder may cause intimal damage which is a starting point for thrombosis. Thrombophilia is another underlying cause – from use of the contraceptive pill and congenital deficiencies (in antithrombin 3, protein C and protein S deficiencies and other blood clotting disorders which cause hypercoaguability). Finally, the common use of axillary / subclavian vein catheters for i.v. therapy may cause thrombosis from irritant solutions, local trauma or bacterial infection. It is said that DVT in the upper limb carries a 10% incidence of pulmonary embolus, but this is rarely life-threatening.

Clinical features

History

There may or may not be an obvious precipitating cause. The onset is fairly rapid (2–3 days) with the development of swelling of the upper limb, dragging pain and heaviness. Not infrequently the limb will take on a dusky-blue colour due to venous congestion.

Physical features

The limb is obviously swollen from the axilla to the fingers. The oedema initially pits readily but may become firm. Dilated (collateral) veins coursing over the shoulder girdle are seen, unless obscured by obesity or oedema.

Investigation

The diagnosis is usually obvious. However, subsequent investigation for an underlying cause may be required once the acute condition has subsided.

Management

The limb should be elevated to minimise the development of induration from prolonged oedema and to make the patient more comfortable. As the swelling subsides, elastic support is substituted for elevation. Anticoagulant therapy, initially with heparin and thereafter with oral agents, is continued until the limb has returned to normal. Thrombolytic therapy with tissue plasminogen activator (t-PA) is increasingly used but should be used with extreme caution because of the potentially devastating complication of haemorrhage, especially cerebral. On occasion, if there is an obvious local cause, surgical exploration or stenting is indicated. Provided an underlying cause is excluded, recurrence is unusual.

Lower-limb DVT

This is the condition that has attracted most attention because of its frequency and well-established relation to surgical procedures, particularly in the elderly. However, because of the factors outlined in Table 30.6, it is not confined to the surgical patient: those with serious illnesses that require or are traditionally associated with immobilisation, those with congestive heart failure and those with malignant disease are also at high risk. There is mounting evidence that the incidence of DVT amongst people travelling on long-haul flights may be higher than realised.

Anatomical considerations

The deep venous system of the lower limb has already been described – it comprises all the venous channels within the investing deep fascia. In clinical practice lower-limb thrombosis in the deep system commonly includes thrombus in the pelvic veins, in particular, the external iliac and common iliac veins, either in isolation or in continuity with thrombus which originates in the leg. For both diagnosis and management it is helpful to qualify a lower-limb DVT by referring to the particular segment or segments of vessel involved, e.g. a popliteal vein thrombus or an iliofemoral vein thrombus – the latter carries a higher risk of life-threatening pulmonary embolus.

Aetiology and epidemiology

All the factors given in Table 30.6 apply to DVT in the legs. Of particular importance in the postoperative patient are:

- immobility during the operation and postoperatively
- techniques of anaesthesia that promote muscular flaccidity and low rates of blood flow – prolonged general anaesthesia with paralysis and assisted ventilation
- posture of the patient on the table – continuous pressure on the calves of the supine patient or the position used for hip replacement
- application of partial or full limb casts
- venous obstruction in the pelvis during a surgical procedure
- increased tendency to clotting following surgical or other injury
- other thrombogenic changes in endothelial cell and leucocyte function after injury – this area is still under study.

Table 30.7 Percentage risk of postoperative deep-vein thrombosis without prophylaxis

Circumstance	Average risk (%)	Reported range (%)
General surgery		
– Abdominal	30	3–50
– Malignancy		40–70
Urology		10–50
– Open prostatectomy	40	
– Transurethral resection	10	
Vascular operations		
– Femoro-popliteal bypass	10	
– Aorto-iliac	5	
Traumatic operations in orthopaedics		
– Trauma	35	
– Hip fracture		40–60
– Tibial fracture		40–50
Elective orthopaedic procedures		
– Hip replacement	50	40–60
– Knee replacement	80	50–90
Immobilised patients with major medical illness (no surgery)	20	10–30

The incidence of DVT has been thoroughly studied in the postoperative patient and with which this account is chiefly concerned. Table 30.7 (compiled mainly from prospective studies which have employed highly sensitive detection techniques using radioisotope labelling of the thrombus) shows an average incidence of DVT of 30% in patients undergoing general surgical procedures. The incidence varies widely with age. Advancing age is associated with a rise, although this may partly reflect the type of surgery that is required, e.g. an incidence of more than 60% in hip replacement. The high figures do not necessarily reflect the need for therapy, in that small thrombi can undergo spontaneous lysis.

Risk factors for DVT in surgical patients

The risk of DVT associated with various surgical procedures has been indicated in Table 30.7. Additional factors for individual patients are shown in Table 30.8. In practice it is important to remember that the following increase risk:

- age – particularly over 40
- obesity
- operation for malignant disease
- a previous episode of DVT or pulmonary embolism
- consumption of the contraceptive pill within 30 days of a surgical procedure and for 2 weeks after. However, the increase in risk is relatively small.

Pathological considerations

Origin

Seventy-five percent of thromboses originate in the calf, particularly the soleal sinusoids, and in the valves of the calf veins; the remaining 25% are isolated to the proximal femoral or iliofemoral veins. Approximately 30% of thrombi in the calf spread in continuity to the popliteal and superficial femoral vein segments.

Table 30.8 NICE algorithm for VTE and bleeding assessment (Reproduced from NICE Quick Reference Guide Venous thromboembolism: reducing the risk, 2010)

Assessing risks of VTE and bleeding

Patients who are at risk of VTE

Medical patients	*Surgical patients and patients with trauma*
If mobility significantly reduced for ≥ 3 days **or** If expected to have ongoing reduced mobility relative to normal state plus any VTE risk factor	If total anaesthetic + surgical time > 90 minutes **or** If surgery involves pelvis or lower limb and total anaesthetic + surgical time > 60 minutes **or** If acute surgical admission with inflammatory **or** intra-abdominal condition **or** If expected to have significant reduction in mobility **or** If any VTE risk factor present

VTE risk factors[a]

- Active cancer or cancer treatment
- Age >60 years
- Critical care admission
- Dehydration
- Known thrombophilias
- Obesity (BMI > 30 kg/m^2)
- One or more significant medical comorbidities (for example: heart disease; metabolic, endocrine or respiratory pathologies; acute infectious diseases; inflammatory conditions)
- Personal history or first-degree relative with a history of VTE
- Use of HRT
- Use of oestrogen-containing contraceptive therapy
- Varicose veins with phlebitis

Patients who are at risk of bleeding

All patients who have any of the following.

- Active bleeding
- Acquired bleeding disorders (such as acute liver failure)
- Concurrent use of anticoagulants known to increase the risk of bleeding (such as warfarin with INR >2)
- Lumbar puncture/epidural/spinal anaesthesia within the previous 4 hours or expected within the next 12 hours
- Acute stroke
- Thrombocytopenia (platelets <75 × 10^9/L)
- Uncontrolled systolic hypertension (≥230/120 mmHg)
- Untreated inherited bleeding disorders (such as haemophilia or von Willebrand's disease)

[a]For women who are pregnant or have given birth within the previous 6 weeks: see page 23 of NICE Quick Reference Guide.

Natural history

As already indicated, many small calf vein thrombi undergo spontaneous lysis. When propagation occurs and occlusion of a main trunk such as the tibial or popliteal vein takes place, the thrombus is initially free-floating but after a relatively short time becomes adherent to the vessel wall and the process of organisation begins with either lysis or the replacement of fibrin by fibrous tissue, or a combination of the two. The subsequent events are described in the section on the postphlebitic limb.

The possibility of a portion of clot becoming separated and a pulmonary embolus occurring is at its greatest while the clot remains free-floating and continues to acquire thrombus.

Clinical features

Symptoms

Particularly in the postoperative patient, there are rarely any complaints while the thrombus is confined to the small veins. Extension into the main vessels may cause the patient to become symptomatic with calf pain and swelling.

Signs

Physical signs, particularly in the early stages, are also minimal and the accuracy of clinical diagnosis is no greater than 50% when compared with objective methods.

Calf tenderness. If possible, the knee should be flexed, the calf muscles relaxed and systematic bimanual palpation of each calf should take place up to the popliteal fossa. It is important to identify areas of tenderness, particularly in the soleal and gastrocnemius muscle masses. The consistency is compared in both limbs because the affected calf may feel more solid or less floppy than the normal one.

Oedema. Ankle oedema in a limb that has not been the site of surgery and was not swollen before the operation should arouse suspicion. Spread onto the dorsum of the foot almost always means that, if venous thrombosis is responsible, the popliteal segment is involved.

Distension of superficial veins. Unilateral distention may be present because blood has been diverted from the (blocked) deep system to the superficial but can also occur in association with hyperaemia or local infection.

Superficial thrombophlebitis. This can occur independently of DVT in the postoperative patient but may be associated with extension into the deep system. A tender cord-like thickening is usually easily palpable over the course of the normal or varicosed superficial vein. The overlying skin is erythematous and the site itself often very tender.

Limb discoloration. A diagnosis should have been made long before the limb has become so oedematous and engorged with venous blood as to produce what has long been known as *phlegmasia caerulea dolens* – inflamed blue painful (leg). Occasionally the obstruction to venous outflow is so severe as to impair arterial inflow. This, combined with arterial spasm induced by thrombophlebitis in the co-axial deep veins, may produce *phlegmasia alba dolens* – inflamed white painful (leg) (see 'white leg' later).

Pain on dorsiflexion of the ankle (Homans' sign). This much-quoted sign of pain in the calf on passive dorsiflexion of the ankle is, as its originator always maintained, unreliable in the diagnosis of DVT and potentially dangerous in its presence as it may precipitate embolisation.

Diagnosis

All postoperative patients should be regarded as at risk of DVT and pulmonary embolus. This implies that, whatever procedure has been undertaken, the legs should be examined at least daily and that minor, unexplained, fluctuations in temperature should arouse suspicion. It is also important to ensure that the method of prophylaxis in use is being adhered to. Screening in high-risk groups is appropriate.

Many of the mechanical problems which can mimic DVT, such as a ruptured popliteal cyst or a tear of the fibres of the gastrocnemius, are rarely relevant in the postoperative patient. However, the diagnosis can be confounded by local trauma within the limb itself, such as surgery to varicose veins or hip replacement. Objective methods are then required to exclude thrombosis. Oedema from fluid overload, or cardiac or renal failure, causes bilateral swelling. Haemorrhage into the limb may occur in a patient on anticoagulants, after an arterial puncture or direct arterial surgery, or even spontaneously after muscle strain. Superficial thrombophlebitis may be present in isolation but may coexist with DVT.

Investigation

The techniques used for the investigation of the peripheral veins have been described above.

Continuous-wave ultrasound

In the presence of obstruction to major (axial) veins there is no change in flow rate on calf compression. The technique cannot however detect thrombi confined to the calf vessels. It can be a useful first-line approach when used regularly by an experienced operator, usually a trained technician.

Duplex scanning

The vessel and the flow rate through it are both visible and, in skilled hands, the accuracy of diagnosis is greater than 90%.

^{125}I fibrinogen uptake tests

Fibrinogen labelled with iodine-125 is taken up by an actively growing thrombus and can be detected as a hot-spot by a scintillation counter. This test is of particular value in:

- the investigation of the effectiveness of new methods of prophylaxis or treatment
- the screening of patients who are at high risk following surgical procedures.

It is, however, not applicable in surgery that involves the limb below the inguinal ligament and is unhelpful in detecting thrombus above the mid-thigh and in the iliac segment. ^{125}I scanning is about 70–75% accurate but may take up to 5 days to establish a diagnosis if accretion to the thrombus is slow. It is now regarded as a research tool only, except in special circumstances.

Venography

Many of the above techniques were developed because of the invasive nature of venography. Until the development fairly recently of non-irritant radio-opaque materials, the contrast agent used could itself cause thrombosis and, if extravasation occurred, tissue necrosis. With the development of low-osmolality contrast material these risks have effectively disappeared. There are, however, other disadvantages:

- the discomfort associated with needle insertion and the bursting sensation on injection of the contrast medium

- the time and expense involved in any radiological technique.

Routine ascending phlebography is performed as described above. Because up to 50% of patients with DVT have involvement of both limbs, venography should be performed bilaterally. Thrombi show up as contrast-lucent filling defects (Fig. 30.10). The segment(s) involved can be defined and the upper limit outlined. It is difficult to recognise the age of a thrombus on venography but very fresh clot can be seen to float in the lumen. Although invasive, the method is more than 90% accurate and is the last court of appeal should the diagnosis remain in doubt after other investigations – a fresh clot can be difficult to see on ultrasound, but abnormality in flow can usually be detected using the Doppler component of Duplex Ultrasound.

Management

It is a prerequisite in most clinical situations that an accurate diagnosis reached before treatment is begun, particularly where that treatment may have undesirable side-effects. However, when there is a clinical likelihood of a DVT, treatment should not be withheld while awaiting confirmatory imaging. Heparin can usually be administered quite safely in most patients and then stopped if the duplex scan proves negative. Warfarin is not commenced until the diagnosis is proven.

Once the diagnosis is established treatment aims to:

- prevent extension
- reduce the chance of pulmonary embolisation
- limit the short- and long-term morbidity in the limb
- take measures to avoid late recurrence of thrombosis.

Anticoagulant therapy

Thrombus confined to the calf

Spontaneous lysis is common. Anticoagulation therapy can be avoided provided the patient is mobile. An appropriately measured and fitted below-knee support stocking and avoidance of sitting with the legs dependent are important supplementary measures.

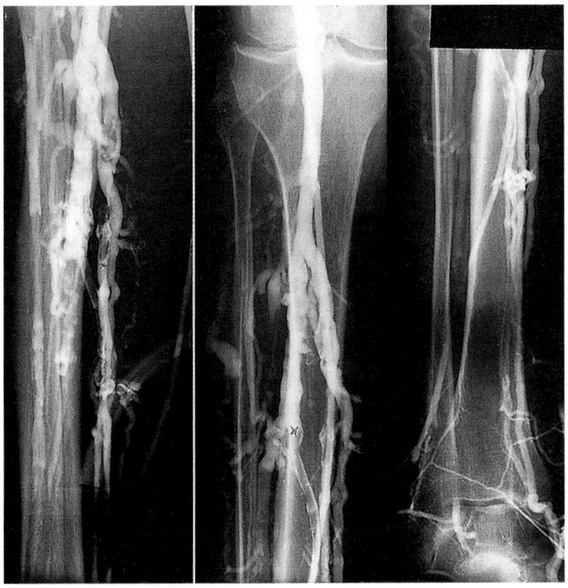

Fig. 30.10 Phlebogram of lower limb showing multiple thrombi in the tibial veins.

About 20% of thrombi which begin in the calf extend proximally. If a decision is made to withhold anticoagulants, it is important to continue monitoring the limb.

Thrombus in tibial, popliteal, superficial femoral and iliofemoral veins

Immediate anticoagulation is essential, provided there is not an absolute contraindication. Although heparin has been used for the treatment of DVT for more than 40 years, controversy still exists on the optimum dose and the duration of treatment.

Traditionally, heparin (unfractionated) is administered by continuous i.v. infusion at a rate of 20–25 units/kg per hour. The patient's own pretreatment activated partial thromboplastin time (APPT) should be at least doubled to ensure a therapeutic effect; comparison with a laboratory baseline normal is more likely to lead to inappropriate levels of anticoagulation. Plasma heparin levels should be maintained at more than 0.3 units/mL.

The duration of heparin therapy and the time when oral anticoagulation should be substituted remain debatable. Clinical experience suggests that in extensive DVT it is correct to continue heparin therapy for up to 10 days, introducing oral anticoagulation with warfarin between days 5 and 7. This gives time for the international normalised ratio (INR) (Box 30.3) to reach the therapeutic range of 2–3.

This traditional treatment plan is disadvantaged by the requirement for continuous intravenous infusion and constant blood monitoring during this phase. A more practical approach is to use low-molecular-weight heparin (LMWH) sometimes referred to as fractionated heparin (a reference to the method by which it is manufactured – i.e. whole heparin is separated in fractions and the active one is used). This is given as a once-daily subcutaneous injection and does not require constant blood monitoring – this allows its use in the community. A disadvantage of LMWH is that it is difficult to reverse and this can lead to problems when confronted with bleeding or the patient needs to undergo surgery within the next 24 hours. Extensive iliofemoral DVTs, however, still require longer in-patient treatment for elevation and investigation.

To reduce discomfort and potential morbidity the leg should be elevated during the early days of treatment and the patient should not be mobilised until the bulk of the swelling

Box 30.3 Calculation of the international normalised ratio (INR) for anticoagulant therapy with warfarin

Measurement – the time for fibrin clot to appear in citrated plasma after the addition of thromboplastin reagent and calcium – prothrombin time (PT)

Standardisation – all thromboplastin reagents are given an international sensitivity index (ISI) as recommended by the World Health Organization

Calculations

$$\text{Prothrombin ratio} = \frac{\text{patient PT}}{\text{control PT}}$$

$$\text{INR} = \text{prothrombin ratio} \times \text{ISI}$$

has subsided and the clot has fixed to the vessel wall and no longer has a free-floating apex. Before mobilisation the patient is fitted with high-compression support hose, full-length or below-knee, depending on the extent of the thrombosis.

Management of a suspected lower-limb DVT is summarised in Clinical Box 30.1.

Complications of anticoagulant therapy

Bleeding may occur:

- subcutaneously or into joint spaces
- intra-cerebral
- urinary tract or gut
- from wounds or puncture sites.

Early warning signs include the development of extensive areas of spontaneous bruising or ecchymoses in pressure areas which can only be detected by regular observation. Daily urine testing can reveal microscopic haematuria. In the postoperative patient bleeding from surgical wounds and raw areas may occur. Careful control of therapy is important but it must be said that the risk of bleeding does not correlate well with the tests used to monitor anticoagulation.

Heparin-induced thrombocytopenia is a well-recognised but uncommon complication which causes bleeding. When heparin is continued for more than 4 or 5 days, regular platelet counts should be done.

If there is bleeding, the initial action should be to stop the heparin (which has a relatively short half-life) and, if necessary, administer protamine sulphate by slow i.v. infusion (1 mg neutralises 100 units of heparin) and the dose is judged against the time since the infusion was stopped – heparin is rapidly excreted by the kidneys giving it a half-life of less than 6 hours. Thrombocytopenia is an indication to discontinue the drug and to substitute it with an oral anticoagulant.

Continuing management

The risk of recurrent thrombosis is greatest in the first 3 months after an acute episode. When extensive DVT has occurred, a minimum of 6 months of oral anticoagulant therapy is prescribed. The role of subcutaneous LMWH in the continuing management of established thrombosis is under assessment at present. It may well be that, when full anticoagulation is contraindicated, the antithrombotic effect of daily subcutaneous LMWH will be an acceptable substitute.

Anticoagulant therapy does not alter the effect of established thrombus in causing damage to the deep veins. To try to reduce the long-term local impact, patients should be discharged with instructions to wear graduated high-compression stockings – 25 to 36 mmHg. These should be worn continuously during oral anticoagulant therapy and duplex assessment of venous function is carried out at the end of this period before a decision to discontinue support is made – there is a case for continuing anticoagulation therapy until the recanalisation process is complete or shows no further progress.

Clinical Box 30.1 Management of a suspected lower-limb DVT

- Adopt a high index of clinical suspicion
- Administer LMWH or dabigatran at a therapeutic dose immediately
- Arrange duplex scan to confirm
- Elevate limb and fit compression stocking when mobilising
- Load with warfarin (while continuing LMWH) or continue dabigatran therapy
- Exclude thrombophilia or pelvic mass

LMWH, low-molecular-weight heparin.

Alternative methods

Thrombolysis

In DVT after operation, thrombolytic therapy has little place because of the risk of haemorrhage. Its use is more appropriate in spontaneous extensive iliofemoral thrombosis where the limb itself is threatened (see 'White leg/*phlegmasia alba dolens*') and where pulmonary embolus is a danger.

Surgery

Removal of the thrombus by surgery (usually by the use of a balloon catheter passed through a small incision or percutaneously) is now seldom used. The remaining indication is threat to life or limb and failure to respond to non-operative management.

Percutaneous methods

Recently, percutaneous (catheter-based) methods of clot dissolution and extraction have become available and are undergoing clinical evaluation. Initial results are encouraging.

Prophylaxis against deep-vein thrombosis (DVT) and pulmonary embolus (PE)

Increased emphasis has been placed on the prevention of DVT and PE in hospitalised patients. PE is one of the major causes of avoidable hospital death. DVT is a cause of significant morbidy – see above. The National Institute for Health and Clinical Excellence (NICE) has issued guidance on this important subject (see Further reading below). All patients admitted to hospital should be assessed at the time of admission for both the risk of venous thromboembolism (VTE) and the risk of bleeding. If appropriate, VTE prophylaxis is offered using one or more of the methods available (Table 30.9), but pharmacological prophylaxis should not be given if the risk of bleeding exceeds the risk of VTE. The assessment of risk for both VTE and bleeding is shown in Table 30.8. The assessment should be repeated at 24 hours after admission and whenever there is a significant change in the patient's condition.

The methods of prophylaxis available (Table 30.9) are of two types:

- mechanical: preservation of calf muscle flow and emptying of veins in the leg
- pharmacological: alterations in the dynamics of the clotting mechanism designed to discourage venous thrombosis but not lead to bleeding.

Mechanical

These techniques are less effective than pharmacological ones and are reserved for either low-risk patients or for specific surgical circumstances. Intermittent inflation of gaiters on the legs causes increased venous flow during (and sometimes after) operation. Low-compression graduated stockings should also be used.

Table 30.9 Prophylaxis of deep-vein thrombosis (especially postoperative)

Method	Efficacy	Disadvantages
Mechanical		
Physiotherapy by leg exercises	No proven effect	None
Early mobilisation	No proven effect although useful for other reasons	None
Graduated compression stockings	Probably minor influence	Must be good quality and individually fitted
Intermittent calf compression	Known reduction	Cumbersome
Pharmacological		
Oral anticoagulants	Known reduction, especially orthopaedics	Takes time to be effective Needs careful control Increased bleeding risk
Unfractionated heparin	Successful in general surgery Ineffective in orthopaedics Used in renal failure	8- to 12-hourly injections
Low-molecular-weight heparin	Known reduction	Risk of thrombocytopenia
Dabigatran etexilate	Proven in orthopaedics	Expense
Rivaroxaban	Proven in orthopaedics	Expense
Fondaparinux	Proven in orthopaedics	Injections Expense

Pharmacological

These techniques interfere in different ways with normal blood coagulation. Their relative merits must be balanced against the possibility of causing excessive or uncontrollable bleeding, their time course of action and their ease of administration.

Unfractionated heparin given subcutaneously at either 8- or 12-hour intervals is most effective when the dose is calculated for each individual and based on a known response in preoperative APPT, or heparin levels. Calcium heparin is said by some to be more effective than sodium heparin when each is administered at a dose of 5000 units. The use of unfractionated heparin reduces the incidence of DVT by up to 60% in general surgery and up to 50% in most orthopaedic procedures. Prophylactic low-dose heparin also lowers the frequency of both fatal and non-fatal pulmonary emboli. Unfractionated heparin has been largely replaced by low-molecular-weight heparins (see below) although it is still used in patients with renal failure.

Low-molecular-weight heparins (LMWHs) cause a more specific antithrombotic effect through their ability to inhibit factor Xa. Furthermore, in experimental models they produce less bleeding for an equivalent antithrombotic effect. A similar or greater reduction in the incidence of venous thrombosis has been demonstrated in general surgical patients using a single daily dose begun the day before operation. In orthopaedic surgery (particularly hip replacement) the same may also be true, although a higher dose is needed.

Warfarins given in appropriate dosage clearly reduce the risk of thrombosis but they also carry a higher potential for bleeding complications unless their administration is very carefully controlled. The agent must be started several days before operation to prolong the prothrombin time so that the INR is approximately two. A modification of this is to start the warfarin on the evening of surgery and to aim to bring the INR to a similar level by the fifth postoperative day.

Dabigatran etexilate is a direct thrombin inhibitor that can be taken orally and is used as VTE prophylaxis in othopaedic surgery.

Fondaparinux is a factor Va inhibitor given subcutaneously as an alternative to LMWH in orthopaedic surgery. Unlike LMWH there is no risk of heparin-induced thrombocytopenia.

Rivaroxaban is a factor Xa inhibitor that is given orally and is used in orthopaedic surgery.

VTE prophylaxis algorithms

As the complexity of decision making in VTE prophylaxis has become greater, NICE have designed algorithms for different clinical situations. Those for elective and non-elective orthopaedic surgery and for non-orthopaedic surgery are shown in Figures 30.11 and 30.12, respectively. Similar algorithms for other situations can be found in the guidance (see Further reading below).

Duration of prophylaxis

Pharmacological prophylaxis is normally continued for 7 days after operation or until the patient is fully mobile. In patients at high risk or with limited mobility, it may need to be prescribed for several weeks. Continuing self-administration at home of a single daily subcutaneous dose of LMWH or use of the oral rivaroxaban for 5 weeks postoperatively is recommended in high-risk patients, such as after hip replacement surgery.

Pulmonary embolism in DVT

The life-threatening complication of DVT is pulmonary embolism (PE). This is where the thrombus becomes detached, is carried proximally and lodges in the pulmonary artery or its branches, thus obstructing right heart output.

Aetiology

The great majority of pulmonary emboli occur after surgical procedures complicated by the development of DVT. However, DVT and consequent PE can occur in immobilisation for any cause. Other causative factors are shown in Table 30.9.

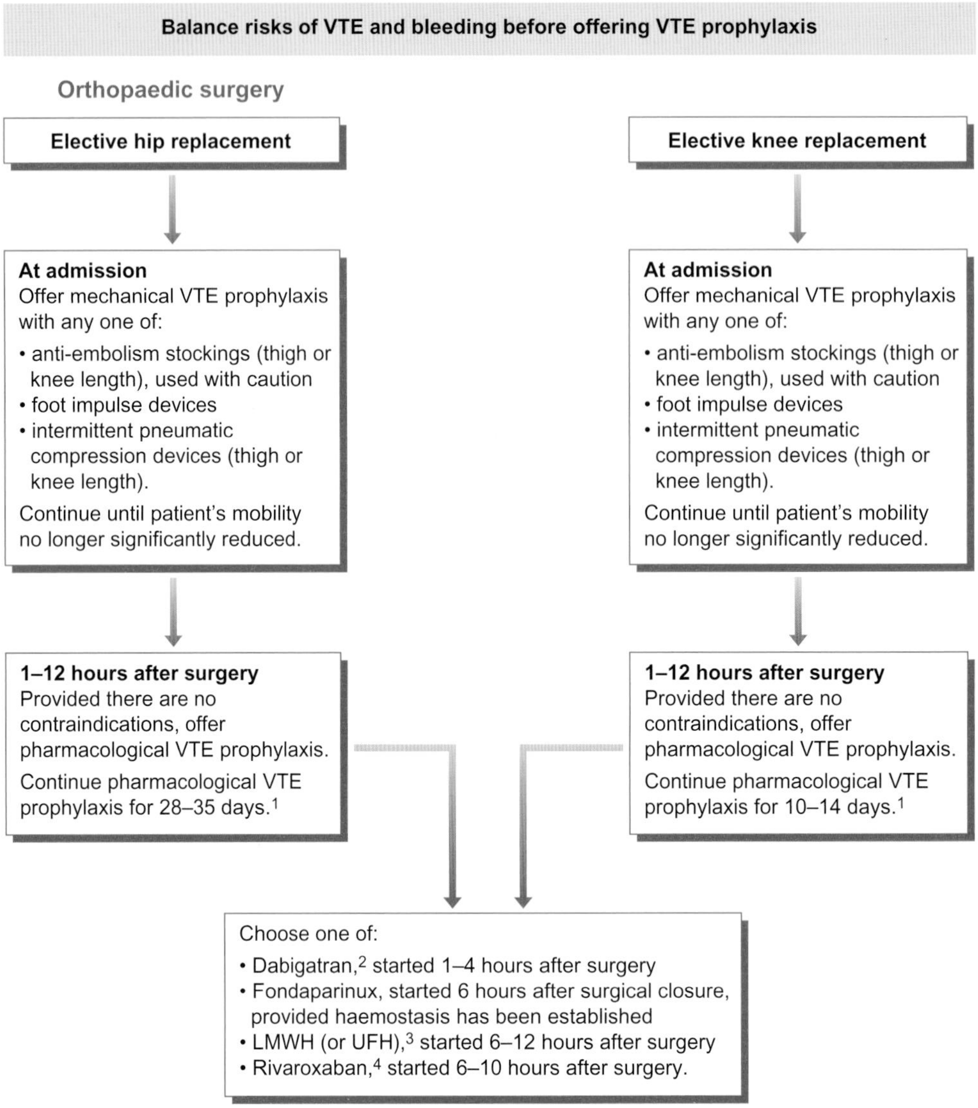
Balance risks of VTE and bleeding before offering VTE prophylaxis
Orthopaedic surgery
Elective hip replacement
Elective knee replacement
At admission
Offer mechanical VTE prophylaxis with any one of:
• anti-embolism stockings (thigh or knee length), used with caution
• foot impulse devices
• intermittent pneumatic compression devices (thigh or knee length).
Continue until patient's mobility no longer significantly reduced.
At admission
Offer mechanical VTE prophylaxis with any one of:
• anti-embolism stockings (thigh or knee length), used with caution
• foot impulse devices
• intermittent pneumatic compression devices (thigh or knee length).
Continue until patient's mobility no longer significantly reduced.
1–12 hours after surgery
Provided there are no contraindications, offer pharmacological VTE prophylaxis.
Continue pharmacological VTE prophylaxis for 28–35 days.[1]
1–12 hours after surgery
Provided there are no contraindications, offer pharmacological VTE prophylaxis.
Continue pharmacological VTE prophylaxis for 10–14 days.[1]
Choose one of:
• Dabigatran,[2] started 1–4 hours after surgery
• Fondaparinux, started 6 hours after surgical closure, provided haemostasis has been established
• LMWH (or UFH),[3] started 6–12 hours after surgery
• Rivaroxaban,[4] started 6–10 hours after surgery.

[1] According to the summary of product characteristics for the individual agent being used.
[2] In line with 'Dabigatran etexilate for the prevention of venous thromboembolism after hip or knee replacement surgery in adults' (NICE technology appraisal guidance 157); dabigatran etexilate, within its marketing authorisation, is recommended as an option for the primary prevention of venous thromboembolic events in adults who have undergone elective total hip replacement surgery or elective total knee replacement surgery.
[3] For patients with renal failure.
[4] In line with 'Rivaroxaban for the prevention of venous thromboembolism after total hip or total knee replacement in adults' (NICE technology appraisal guidance 170), rivaroxaban, within its marketing authorisation, is recommended as an option for the prevention of venous thromboembolism in adults having elective total hip replacement surgery or elective total knee replacement surgery.

Fig. 30.11 NICE algorithm for orthopaedic surgery VTE prophylaxis. (Reproduced from NICE Quick Reference Guide Venous thromboembolism: reducing the risk, 2010.)

Epidemiology

In England and Wales (population *c.* 55 million) there are approximately 20 000 deaths a year from pulmonary embolism. In the 1960s, prior to the use of heparin prophylaxis, 6 in every 1000 patients undergoing total hip replacement died as a result of PE. Currently, with the use of prophylactic measures as documented above, the fatal PE rate in hip surgery patients is 0.1%. In pelvic operations for malignancy this rises to 1% despite prophylaxis. The mortality of untreated symptomatic PE, however, remains at 30%. Following massive PE, of those who die, 50–70% do so in the first hour.

Physiological and pathological considerations

Embolism occurs when either the whole or the proximal propagated part of a free-floating clot detaches from the wall of a vein. The event may be spontaneous, or stripping of the

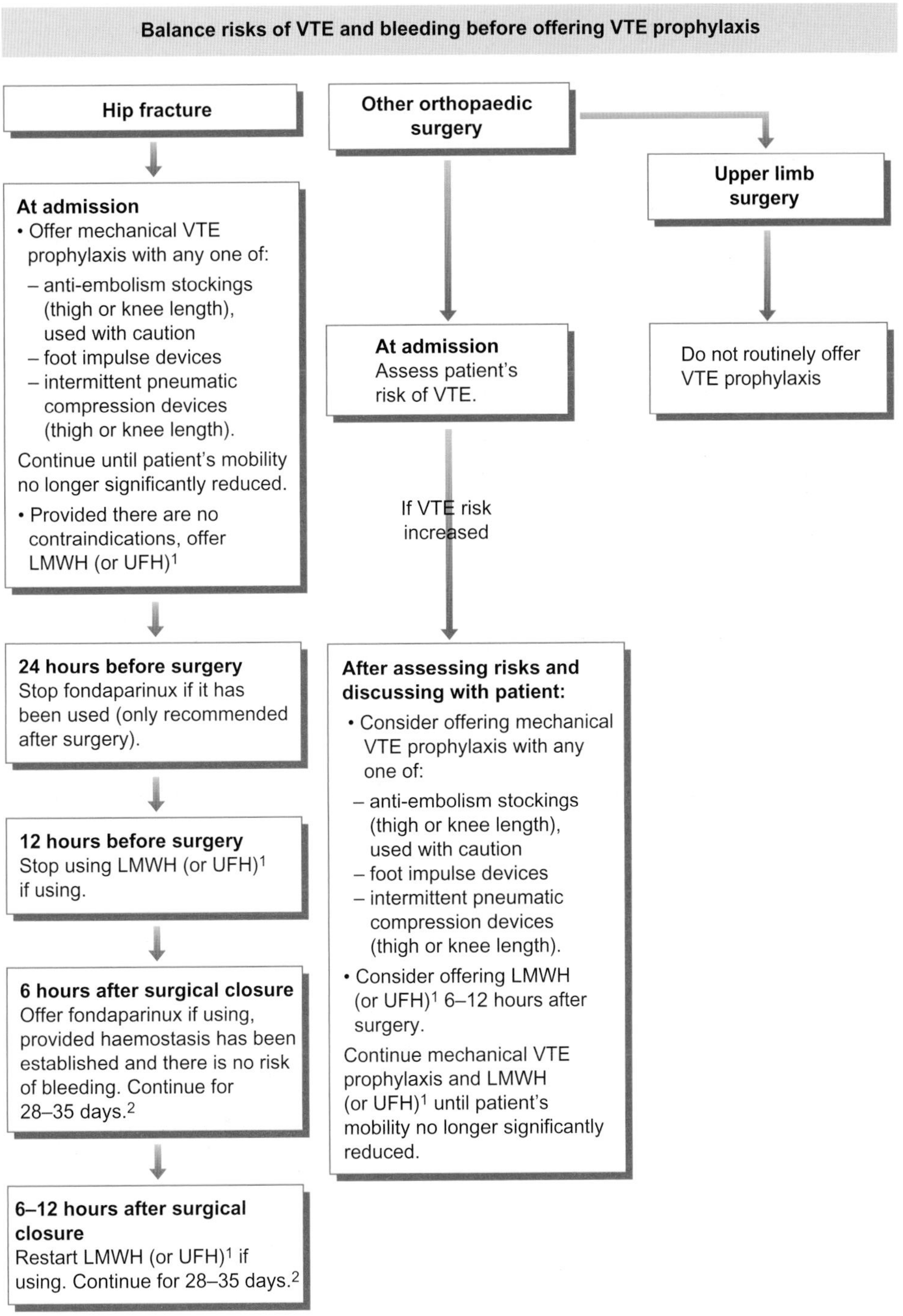
Balance risks of VTE and bleeding before offering VTE prophylaxis
Hip fracture
At admission
• Offer mechanical VTE prophylaxis with any one of:
– anti-embolism stockings (thigh or knee length), used with caution
– foot impulse devices
– intermittent pneumatic compression devices (thigh or knee length).
Continue until patient's mobility no longer significantly reduced.
• Provided there are no contraindications, offer LMWH (or UFH)[1]
24 hours before surgery
Stop fondaparinux if it has been used (only recommended after surgery).
12 hours before surgery
Stop using LMWH (or UFH)[1] if using.
6 hours after surgical closure
Offer fondaparinux if using, provided haemostasis has been established and there is no risk of bleeding. Continue for 28–35 days.[2]
6–12 hours after surgical closure
Restart LMWH (or UFH)[1] if using. Continue for 28–35 days.[2]
Other orthopaedic surgery
At admission
Assess patient's risk of VTE.
If VTE risk increased
After assessing risks and discussing with patient:
• Consider offering mechanical VTE prophylaxis with any one of:
– anti-embolism stockings (thigh or knee length), used with caution
– foot impulse devices
– intermittent pneumatic compression devices (thigh or knee length).
• Consider offering LMWH (or UFH)[1] 6–12 hours after surgery.
Continue mechanical VTE prophylaxis and LMWH (or UFH)[1] until patient's mobility no longer significantly reduced.
Upper limb surgery
Do not routinely offer VTE prophylaxis

[1] For patient's with renal failure.
[2] According to the summary of product characteristics for the individual agent being used.

Fig. 30.11, continued

attachment may occur as a result of an acute rise in venous pressure such as occurs during a Valsalva manoeuvre on defecation. The clot is swept proximally into the pulmonary artery and, if sufficiently large to be arrested in the main stem or across the bifurcation of the vessel, reduces cardiac output so much that death results instantly or within a very short time. Lodgement in branches produces a volume of lung tissue that is initially ventilated but underperfused – the so-called 'ventillation-perfusion mismatch' that can be detected on certain special investigations. There is arteriolar spasm in the involved segment so reducing inflow and causing infarction. If the block to the pulmonary circulation

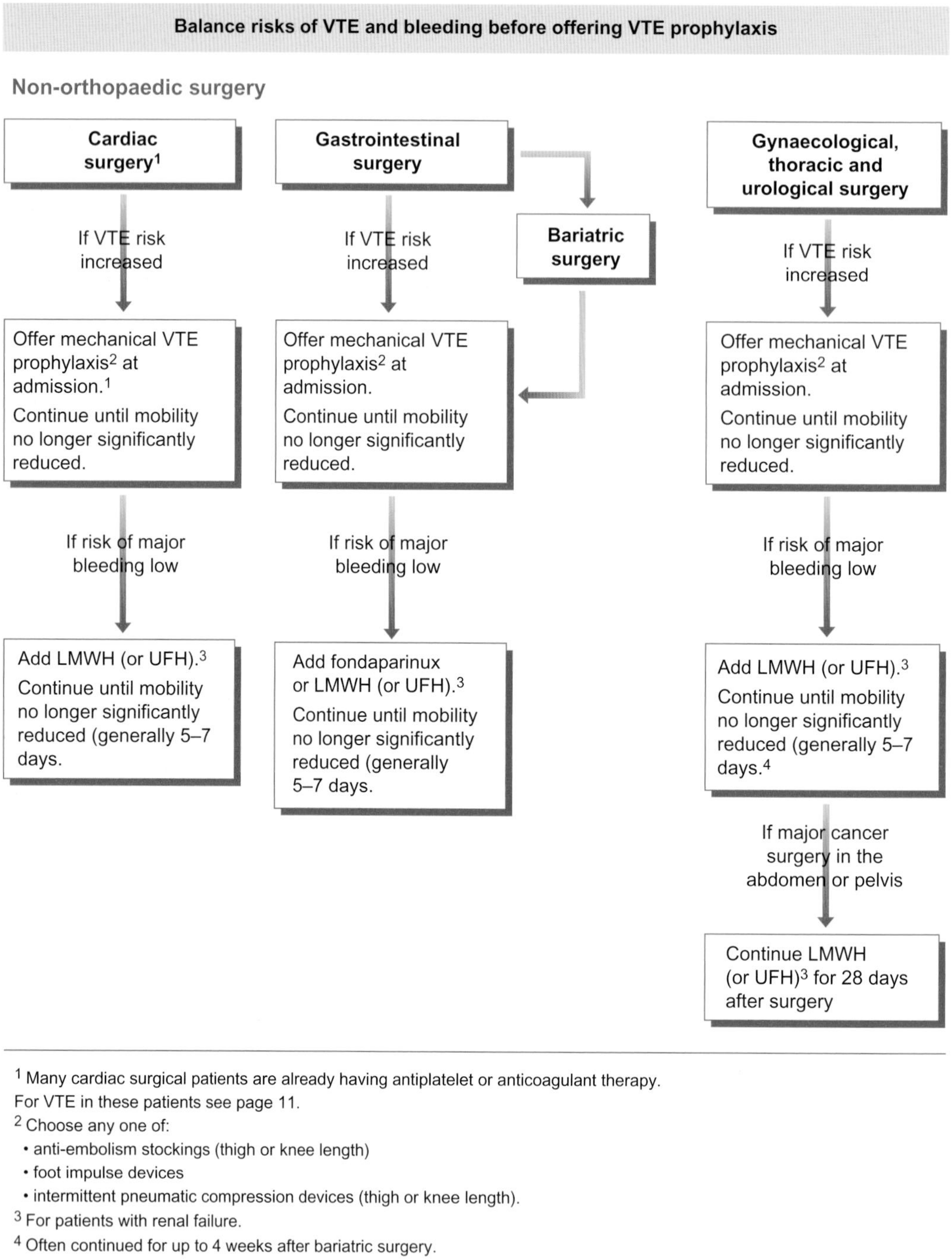
Balance risks of VTE and bleeding before offering VTE prophylaxis
Non-orthopaedic surgery
Cardiac surgery1
Gastrointestinal surgery
Bariatric surgery
Gynaecological, thoracic and urological surgery
If VTE risk increased
If VTE risk increased
If VTE risk increased
Offer mechanical VTE prophylaxis2 at admission.1
Continue until mobility no longer significantly reduced.
Offer mechanical VTE prophylaxis2 at admission.
Continue until mobility no longer significantly reduced.
Offer mechanical VTE prophylaxis2 at admission.
Continue until mobility no longer significantly reduced.
If risk of major bleeding low
If risk of major bleeding low
If risk of major bleeding low
Add LMWH (or UFH).3
Continue until mobility no longer significantly reduced (generally 5–7 days.
Add fondaparinux or LMWH (or UFH).3
Continue until mobility no longer significantly reduced (generally 5–7 days.
Add LMWH (or UFH).3
Continue until mobility no longer significantly reduced (generally 5–7 days.4
If major cancer surgery in the abdomen or pelvis
Continue LMWH (or UFH)3 for 28 days after surgery
1 Many cardiac surgical patients are already having antiplatelet or anticoagulant therapy.
For VTE in these patients see page 11.
2 Choose any one of:
• anti-embolism stockings (thigh or knee length)
• foot impulse devices
• intermittent pneumatic compression devices (thigh or knee length).
3 For patients with renal failure.
4 Often continued for up to 4 weeks after bariatric surgery.

Fig. 30.12 NICE algorithm for non-orthopaedic surgery VTE prophylaxis (Reproduced from NICE Quick Reference Guide Venous thromboembolism: reducing the risk, 2010)

is large, pressure in the right heart rises. Subsequently the segment becomes consolidated as a consequence of haemorrhagic infarction. If the patient survives, the clot can lyse (50% within 2 weeks) and the circulation will be restored. Alternatively, or even when there has been initial but incomplete lysis, organisation and fibrosis take place with a pulmonary scar detectable up to a year later on perfusion studies. Repeated emboli may, by this mechanism, cause the development of pulmonary artery hypertension and right heart failure.

Clinical features

Symptoms

Symptoms may be sudden in onset and without warning. However, in retrospect, a swollen ankle or leg may have been

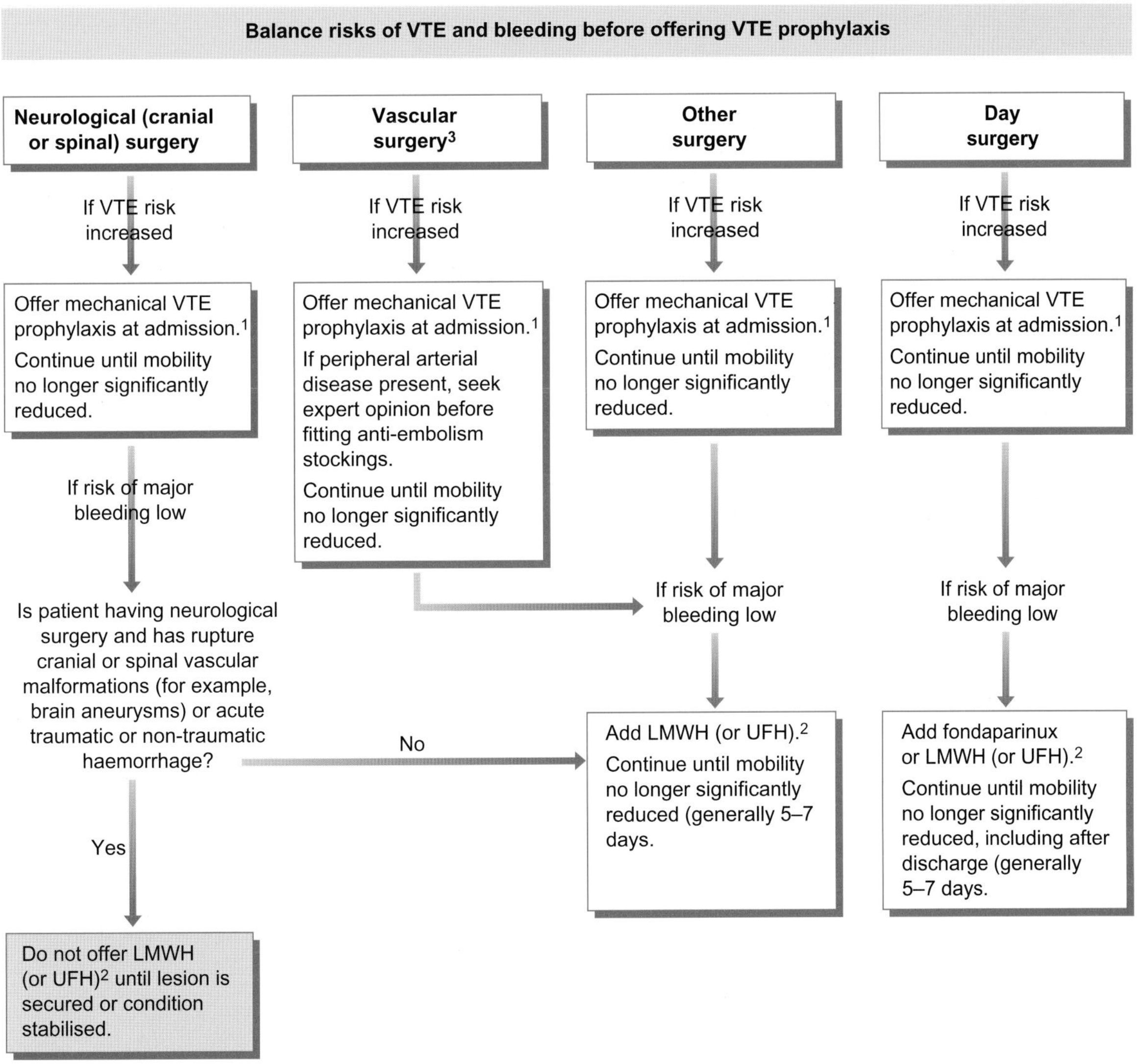
Balance risks of VTE and bleeding before offering VTE prophylaxis
Neurological (cranial or spinal) surgery
Vascular surgery3
Other surgery
Day surgery
If VTE risk increased
If VTE risk increased
If VTE risk increased
If VTE risk increased
Offer mechanical VTE prophylaxis at admission.1 Continue until mobility no longer significantly reduced.
Offer mechanical VTE prophylaxis at admission.1 If peripheral arterial disease present, seek expert opinion before fitting anti-embolism stockings. Continue until mobility no longer significantly reduced.
Offer mechanical VTE prophylaxis at admission.1 Continue until mobility no longer significantly reduced.
Offer mechanical VTE prophylaxis at admission.1 Continue until mobility no longer significantly reduced.
If risk of major bleeding low
If risk of major bleeding low
If risk of major bleeding low
Is patient having neurological surgery and has rupture cranial or spinal vascular malformations (for example, brain aneurysms) or acute traumatic or non-traumatic haemorrhage?
No
Yes
Add LMWH (or UFH).2 Continue until mobility no longer significantly reduced (generally 5–7 days.
Add fondaparinux or LMWH (or UFH).2 Continue until mobility no longer significantly reduced, including after discharge (generally 5–7 days.
Do not offer LMWH (or UFH)2 until lesion is secured or condition stabilised.

[1] Choose any one of:
- Anti-embolism stockings (thigh or knee length)
- Foot impulse devices
- Intermittent pneumatic compression devices (thigh or knee length).

[2] For patients with renal failure.

Fig. 30.12, continued

present, and it is a source of chagrin to notice this for the first time while trying to save the life of a patient with acute circulatory collapse. Small emboli may not cause any symptoms. Those that involve up to half of the pulmonary circulation give rise to symptoms confined to the lung. Greater involvement causes additional cardiac and systemic effects. Pre-existing pulmonary disease increases the effects of a given amount of obstruction.

- **Chest pain**. Infarction of the lung causes well-localised pleuritic pain over the affected segment, worse on inspiration or coughing. A large embolus may be associated with crushing substernal rather than pleuritic pain and rapidly followed by cardiac arrest.
- **Dyspnoea** may be present but is not a striking feature except in very large emboli.
- **Haemoptysis** may follow within minutes or hours in those that survive but is usually confined to blood streaking of the sputum.
- **Transient or prolonged loss of consciousness** implies a large embolus with circulatory effects.

Signs

Circulatory. With a large embolus there is:

- arterial hypotension, usually with a pale, vasoconstricted skin, although sometimes with cyanosis
- raised jugular venous pressure

- tachycardia and, in large emboli, gallop rhythm
- dysrhythmias.

Respiratory. Examination of the chest may show:

- pleural friction rub with associated crackles (*syn.* crepitations)
- later, signs of consolidation will appear.

General. There may be evidence of DVT in the lower limbs, but detachment of the whole or the greater part of the clot from a relatively proximal vein may mean that the limb is normal.

Investigation

Plasma D-dimer

This is the first investigation, a negative test effectively ruling out a pulmonary embolus (sensitivity 99%). However, false positives are common after surgery and further confirmatory investigation is necessary.

Chest X-ray

In small emboli there may be no abnormality on chest X-ray. If infarction has occurred, a wedge of consolidation with its apex centrally located may be present or there may be evidence of areas of reduced vascularity – loss of vascular markings.

Pulmonary radioisotope ventilation/perfusion (V/Q) scans

Technetium-99m-labelled albumin given intravenously may demonstrate areas of underperfusion of the lung. A normal ventilation/perfusion (V/Q) scan excludes a significant PE. Other causes of underperfusion (such as previous PE) may confuse the clinical picture but in an abnormal scan there is an approximately 75% chance that a recent embolus is present. Specificity is greatly enhanced if ventilation is simultaneously assessed by the inhalation of xenon-133: there is a mismatch between perfusion (decreased) and ventilation (initially maintained).

Multislice CT scan

This is the investigation of choice because it is generally readily available and is non-invasive. Multislice scanners reliably detect even small emboli (sensitivity 83%, specificity 96%).

Electrocardiography

In a small to moderate-sized PE, the ECG is frequently normal. A large embolus, which produces dilation of the right heart, causes tall and peaked P waves in lead II, right axis deviation, right bundle branch block and T-wave inversion in precordial leads. Large emboli can produce changes which are difficult to distinguish from inferior myocardial infarction.

Blood gas analysis

Reduction in pO_2 occurs if cardiac output is profoundly depressed and/or a large volume of lung is underperfused. Dyspnoea increases the elimination of carbon dioxide and the pCO_2 is therefore also reduced. This situation is uncommon except in collapse/consolidation of the lung (see Ch. 16) and, given the clinical circumstances, provides confirmatory evidence of PE.

Investigation of possible DVT

Provided the patient is in a stable circulatory state the usual investigations are undertaken.

Diagnosis

It is important to be aware that the finding of a normal ECG, chest X-ray and negative duplex scan (excluding DVT) does not exclude a diagnosis of PE. If there is any clinical suspicion the patient should be anticoagulated pending diagnostic confirmation with CT angiography or V/Q scan.

Other events may present a clinical picture very similar to that of a large embolus:

- myocardial infarction – usually with the features of left rather than right ventricular failure
- massive fluid overload – generalised features are present in addition to right heart failure
- severe sepsis
- haemorrhage – the jugular venous pressure is low
- tension pneumothorax
- cardiac tamponade
- aortic dissection.

Management

Resuscitation

When cardiac arrest is thought to have occurred, the standard techniques need to be instituted in an attempt to establish adequate cardiac output and also to reach a diagnosis which is used to guide further treatment. A loading dose of 10 000 units of heparin should be given intravenously.

Continuing treatment

Resuscitation successful. An adequate cardiac output to sustain systemic perfusion is achieved. A continuous heparin infusion is begun at 25 units/kg per hour. Assuming progress is maintained, a similar regimen to that described for the management of venous thrombosis is followed and the patient is subsequently changed to oral anticoagulation for a minimum of 6 months.

Resuscitation unsuccessful. Hypotension and an inadequate cardiac output persist. The options are:

- establish cardiopulmonary bypass and remove the clot at open operation
- right heart catheterisation and regional administration of a thrombolytic agent such as streptokinase or alteplase
- pulmonary artery catheterisation and suction removal of the clot – a method which can be combined with thrombolysis.

In the past, dramatic, occasionally successful, transthoracic embolectomies without cardiopulmonary bypass were described. However, without the availability of bypass, patients who survive to reach operation would also get to the preferable alternatives of thrombolysis or direct suction. Streptokinase thrombolysis has been shown to be beneficial in a randomised controlled trial with a significant survival advantage. This therapy should be adopted more widely.

Emergency Box 30.1

Management of a suspected pulmonary embolism

- Assess arterial blood gases (on air)
- Measure plasma D-dimer
- Arrange portable chest X-ray and ECG (to help exclude other pathologies)
- Start oxygen
- Administer therapeutic i.v. heparin or subcut. LMWH
- Arrange multislice (or spiral) CT or V/Q scan to confirm diagnosis
- Consider streptokinase thrombolysis
- Arrange venous duplex or MRI (venous phase) scan as indicated to assess lower-limb and pelvic veins
- Prescribe long-term anticoagulation
- Consider use of IVC filter

LMWH, low-molecular-weight heparin.

Management of a suspected PE is summarised in Emergency Box 30.1.

Recurrent pulmonary emboli

If treatment of the DVT is rigorous, survival after PE may not be followed by recurrence. However, further episodes of circulatory collapse, dyspnoea and chest pain are not infrequent. Extension of underperfusion or infarction in the lung can be confirmed by further isotope scanning or pulmonary angiography.

Management involves:

- making sure that anticoagulation with heparin has been achieved and is at a therapeutic level
- consideration of interruption of the venous pathway above the most proximal level of thrombosis.

The methods available for interruption are:

- surgical plication either by sutures or clips – now rarely used
- percutaneous insertion of a filter into the vena cava below the renal veins. These filters can usually be removed (percutaneously) a few weeks later when the patient has been stabilised.

Opinions vary about the need for such intervention if anticoagulation is adequate, but they probably do have a small place. Indications for IVC filtration include:

- recurrent PE despite adequate anticoagulation
- PE with contraindication to anticoagulation
- free-floating thrombus in a proximal vein (contentious).

White leg

Extensive venous thrombosis in the lower extremity can produce a clinical syndrome known as 'white leg' – historically known as *phlegmasia alba dolens* – inflamed white painful (leg); so-named because it was originally thought that the condition had an inflammatory element.

Aetiology

Rapid thrombosis along the whole length of the deep venous system and into the iliac segment so obstructs drainage that arterial input is reduced. Furthermore, thrombophlebitis in the coaxial deep veins induces arterial spasm. The condition used to be common in the puerperium but is now more often seen in those with generalised hypercoagulability, e.g. in malignancy, sometimes occult.

Clinical features

Symptoms

Pain and swelling in the whole limb are the dominant features. Systemic disturbance is often quite considerable.

Signs

The affected limb is:

- grossly swollen up to the inguinal ligament, and oedema may spread onto the abdominal wall
- cool and white because of reduced arterial input
- often without arterial pulsation at the ankle from swelling, which makes it difficult to feel, but also because arterial pressure in the limb is reduced
- characterised by dusky cyanosis at the tips of the toes.

The last suggests that necrosis is about to supervene, but in fact this is limited to the skin (see below).

Management

The initial treatment is that of any DVT, with anticoagulants and limb elevation. Thrombolysis or clot extraction is reserved for those who do not improve in the first 24–36 hours or in whom there is extension of the distal cyanosis. Even then, it is doubtful if the results are improved over those of standard therapy, in that what appears to be a limb that requires major amputation (so-called venous gangrene) turns out, on continued non-intervention, to have only very limited loss of tissue in the skin and subcutaneous layers of the toes.

Once the acute episode is over, investigation of venous function follows the lines already outlined.

POSTPHLEBITIC LIMB – CHRONIC VENOUS INSUFFICIENCY/CALF PUMP FAILURE SYNDROME

Postphlebitic limb – chronic venous insufficiency/calf pump failure syndrome

These and other terms are used to describe a limb in which there is damage to the deep veins, their valves and the valves in the communicating veins with the production of:

- raised static pressure in the deep veins
- transmission of this hypertension to the superficial system
- exacerbation of hypertension by the activity of the muscle pump which, in the presence of incompetent valves in the communicating (DTSI) veins, allows deep-to-superficial reflux.

Aetiology and pathological features

The most common cause is a previous DVT. It should be noted, however, that although destruction of deep veins is the rule, a number of patients with only DTSI can develop symptoms and signs which are clinically indistinguishable from those of chronic deep venous insufficiency. Furthermore, there may also be a group of patients who have deep venous incompetence without an underlying acquired cause.

Pathological features are of venous hypertension (described earlier) in the superficial tissues. Damage to the deep valves is usually secondary to a DVT with recanalisation; however, rarely, there may be congenital absence of valves in the deep system.

Clinical features

History

There may be a history of DVT, although its absence does not mean that an asymptomatic DVT did not occur in the past. Over some years, the patient will have noticed the development of increased aching on exertion, ankle and calf oedema, venous eczema and ulceration. A bursting feeling on walking is relatively common. Otherwise the symptoms are the same as for other causes of venous hypertension (see above).

Signs

The findings are of venous insufficiency as already described. Oedema is often quite marked and, although predominantly venous and compressible may, with time, develop a lymphoedematous component, which is firm and non-pitting.

Investigation

From the foregoing definition it is clear that it is essential to establish whether there is deep-vein involvement or the condition of the limb reflects only severe DTSI. The methods of achieving this have already been outlined. Both deep and superficial incompetence may coexist. Great care should be taken in excluding any obstructive component in the deep veins before giving consideration to treating superficial venous incompetence.

Management

The potential for limb morbidity in patients with advanced changes of venous hypertension is often poorly recognised by clinicians.

Prophylaxis

Adequate prophylaxis and treatment of DVT and the subsequent use of effective well-tailored high-compression garments can be expected to dramatically reduce the development of the chronic changes of deep venous insufficiency.

Treatment

Deep-to-superficial incompetence only. If clinical and other tests show that this is the cause, improvement up to complete cure can be produced by standard treatment with surgical ligation of points of incompetence, such as the sapheno-femoral and sapheno-popliteal junctions, and obliteration of varices. Long-term use of support hose is a valuable supplement.

Deep-vein incompetence with deep-to-superficial incompetent communications but without ulceration. A full-length high-compression support stocking is the least radical and most acceptable method of treatment, possibly coupled with sclerotherapy for clearly incompetent perforating veins. A below-knee stocking may suffice in milder cases: the compression should be graduated, with a value of 36 mmHg at the ankle; ankle, calf and leg-length measurements should only be taken after oedema has been reduced to ensure an accurate fit. Techniques of venous bypass for obstruction and for valve reconstruction have been developed, but follow-up is still short and they remain to be proven in the long term.

LEG ULCERATION

Epidemiology

Eighty to eighty-five percent of leg ulcers are of venous origin, although, particularly in the elderly, an arterial element may be co-causative. Ten percent are entirely the consequence of arterial disease. It is probable that approximately 1% of the population have, or have had, a leg ulcer and that at any one time 30–40% of ulcers are active. Approximately 70% of those with active ulcers are over 70 years of age and there is a prevalence of 2% in the over-80s. Females exceed males by a factor of three, perhaps reflecting the risks of pregnancy and childbirth.

Some years ago it was estimated that management of leg ulceration caused by venous disease costs the NHS in the UK at least £55 million a year.

Aetiology

Oedema from venous hypertension and raised pressure at the venular end of the capillary loop, skin and subcutaneous hypoxia, and an episode of minor trauma are the usual antecedents of ulceration. They are most likely to occur when there is damage to the valves of the deep veins, but long-standing superficial hypertension caused by DTSI alone is also a well-recognised cause. Once an ulcer is established, healing of the poorly nourished skin is difficult, and granulation tissue and a fibrous base develops. Chronic recurrent inflammation causes scarring (fibrosis), which in turn impairs arterial input – this is a further impediment to healing. Secondary infections by skin flora such as staphylococci are common and may cause painful spreading cellulitis.

Other causes of leg ulceration may have to be taken into consideration; these are given in Table 30.10. Venous hypertension is however by far the commonest cause.

Clinical features

Venous ulcers occur most commonly just above the medial malleolus. They are usually oval in shape, flat and without a raised edge, look relatively healthy and have a granulating base usually covered with a thin layer of fibrin. Weeping eczematous change may be seen in the surrounding skin which often arises from the use of inappropriate local applications. The tissues are indurated and there may be scarring in the adjacent paper-thin skin where healing has occurred in the past. Concomitant infection, with either surrounding erythema or extensive cellulitis, may be present.

A venous ulcer (Fig. 30.13) is recognised easily when it is situated in the typical position close to the medial malleolus, surrounded by pigmentation and oedema. However, venous ulcers also occur on the lateral side of the leg and on the foot, principally the dorsal surface. The circumferential size

Table 30.10 Causes of ulceration of the leg

Underlying cause	Mechanism
Venous disease	Superficial venous hypertension – hypoxia, oedema, trauma
Arterial disease	Reduced inflow – hypoxia
Trauma	Skin loss, infection, persistent pressure in prolonged bed rest
Rheumatoid arthritis (often with an added arterial or venous component)	Autoimmune inflammation in subcutaneous tissues (vasculitis)
Pyoderma gangrenosum	
Systemic sclerosis	Inflammation of skin and subcutaneous tissues – cause unknown
Malignant disease	Squamous-cell carcinoma (usually de novo but occasionally associated with long-standing varicose veins and ulceration) Malignant melanoma Basal cell carcinoma
Diabetes mellitus	Neuropathy; possibly an arterial component with skin infarction Lesions more frequent at pressure points – ball of foot and heel
Blood disorders	Microvascular thrombosis in sickle cell disease and spherocytosis

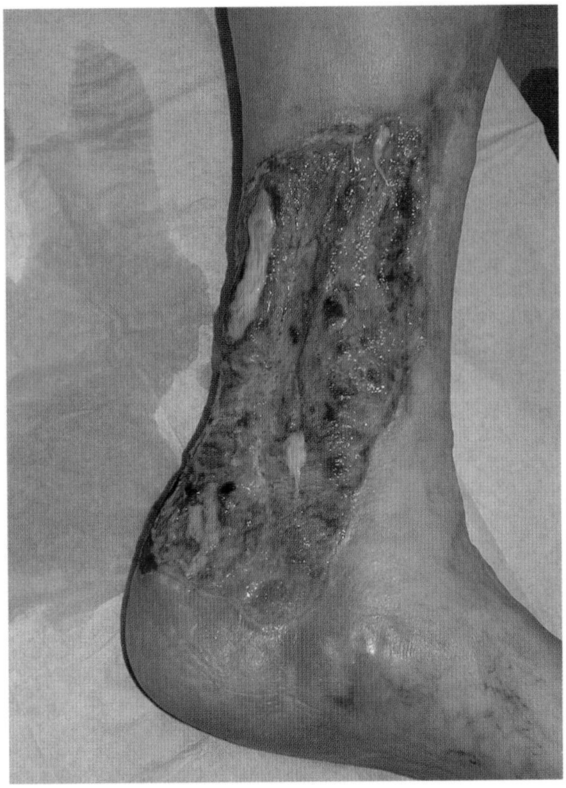

Fig. 30.13 Untreated venous ulcer overlying the medial malleolus. Note the covering of slough and lack of granulation tissue. (Courtesy of Mr D Baker, Royal Free Hospital, London.)

Table 30.11 Distinctive characteristics of venous and arterial ulcers

	Venous	Arterial
History	Previous deep-vein thrombosis; varicose veins	Intermittent claudication; ischaemic heart disease; hypertension; diabetes
Pain	Occurs only in severe oedema, secondary bacterial infection, thrombosis, varicose veins	Nearly always present; worse at night; relieved by dependency
Site	Usually near medial malleolus but do occur on lateral side of leg	Common on toes, heel, foot and lateral aspect
Size/development	Variable but increases slowly if untreated	Variable but increases rapidly
Oedema	Common and worse at end of day	Uncommon unless the leg is dependent and patient immobile
Skin appearance	Pigmentation and atrophy; white patches; induration of subcutaneous tissues	Shiny, thin, atrophic nails
Skin temperature	Usually warm	Cool
Skin colour	Normal or slight cyanosis accentuated by dependency and improved by elevation	Pallor made worse by elevation and slow to recover; cyanotic on dependency
Appearance of ulcer	Shallow flat margin; looks healthy; no deep invasion	Often involves deep fascia; tendon may be exposed
Foot pulses	Present, although can be difficult to feel because of oedema	Reduced or absent

of the lesion does not indicate its cause, and venous ulcers may be multiple.

Diagnosis

An exact diagnosis must precede management. Apart from the obvious distinctions that have to be made from the conditions shown in Table 30.10, a venous ulcer must be differentiated from an ischaemic one because the treatment is so different. The features that permit this are shown in Table 30.11. Awareness of the association of ulceration with diabetes mellitus is well understood, but the association with rheumatoid arthritis, systemic sclerosis (scleroderma) and other generalised diseases is less well recognised. The more elderly the patient, the more likely there are to be multiple aetiological factors.

It is rare in hospital practice to see an ulcer which has not been 'treated' for some considerable period of time elsewhere, often without adequate determination of the cause – particularly the nature of the venous component which may be easily treated.

Management

Most venous ulcers which are correctly diagnosed and treated respond readily to conventional treatment, but even relatively small lesions can take up to 3 months to heal. More chronic lesions – the result of inappropriate or inadequate initial assessment and treatment – require a more precise and rigorous regimen:

Step 1 is to establish if there is correctable superficial venous hypertension which is the consequence of DTSI only. If this is so, surgery as described above is indicated, although it is highly desirable to heal the ulcer first, using the methods described below.

Step 2. If there are multiple points of incompetence or, what almost always pathophysiologically amounts to the same thing, deep venous damage, the starting point is non-operative management. The majority of venous leg ulcers fall into this category. The essential component is to apply effective compression to the limb and sustain it until the ulcer has healed. Most venous ulcers heal if the patient is confined to bed with the foot elevated to at least the level of the heart so that venous hypertension is abolished, the microenvironment improved and healing promoted. However, bed rest is a costly and therefore usually inappropriate method. Adequate local compression in a patient who is otherwise mobile is an effective alternative. It can be achieved by:

- *bandaging* – usually multilayer and dependent on the skill of the nurse or doctor who applies it. Four-layer bandaging (Charing Cross method) has been used successfully for many years – it aims to produce a pressure of up to 40 mmHg at the ankle and 16 mmHg in the upper calf. This method does require a certain degree of skill that may not be readily acquired. Short-stretch bandaging is an equally effective method that is increasingly used these days. Here, a bandage that is designed so that it cannot be overstretched and thus produce too high a compression force is used. Venous ulceration is a condition of the elderly, often with coexisting arterial disease, and it is therefore vital to check the ABPI (see Ch. 29). Compression therapy is contraindicated if the ABPI is less than 0.8
- *fitted elastic hosiery* with known compression – more expensive but does not require great expertise to apply; inappropriate if ulcers are very wet.

Step 3, which runs concurrently with steps 1 and 2, is local management of the lesion. The ulcer should be kept clean with regular saline cleanses: at least daily, and more frequently if there is substantial exudate (exacerbated by not elevating the limb and/or poor compliance regarding the wearing of support hose). The inappropriate use of topical agents, including impregnated bandages, should be avoided. Dressings are kept simple, and pharmacologically active substances applied only for specific and logical reasons – which means hardly ever. If the underlying causes are treated, then bland dressings are all that is required (see also Ch. 3). Saline-gauze dressings are effective at cleansing ulcers but do need to be changed regularly, i.e. before they dry out, otherwise removal is painful and any delicate, rejuvenating epithelial layer will be removed. Antibiotics are not appropriate; all leg ulcers are contaminated with bacteria and most will yield a positive culture which frequently shows multiple organisms, a so-called 'Garden of Eden' bacteriological culture. Systemic therapy is indicated only if there is spreading cellulitis; topical applications are ineffective in controlling contamination unless the causes of the ulcer are dealt with.

Surgical measures in ulceration

Occasionally, before non-operative treatment is begun, severely contaminated long-standing ulcers with infected granulation tissue at the base may benefit from surgical debridement (Ch. 3). Once measures have been undertaken to reverse the pathophysiological processes, if the surface area of the ulcer is relatively large, consideration may be given to skin-grafting to decrease the patient's hospital stay or number of clinic visits. Either split-skin or pinch grafts (Ch. 39) are used.

Surgery to varicosities

Once an ulcer is healed, surgical attention may need to turn to whether or not the venous hypertension can be corrected to prevent recurrence. The circumstance in which this may be possible has already been indicated – correctable deep-to-superficial valvular incompetence, without incompetence in the valves of the deep veins. Full support of the limb will need to be continued indefinitely in all cases where there is deep vein insufficiency, and where DTSI has not been surgically corrected.

LYMPHATIC DISORDERS

Anatomical and physiological considerations

The lymphatic system comprises a network of capillaries and vessels lined by endothelial cells. The capillaries allow the absorption of protein-rich interstitial fluid across their walls and the vessels possess valves to prevent lymph reflux. Lymphatic vessels run alongside the venous system but drain directly to lymph nodes where the lymph fluid is filtered through lymphoid tissue. This permits phagocytosis of cellular and bacterial debris. In addition, lymph nodes provide a setting for immunological response to foreign antigens. The efferent lymphatic vessels eventually drain into the central venous system.

Pathological conditions

These include lymphadenopathy (node enlargement), lymphangitis and lymphoedema.

Lymphadenopathy may occur as the result of local infection or tissue injury, or as a feature of malignancy – either metastatic tumour (e.g. breast cancer, malignant melanoma) or lymphoma. Node enlargement may be detected on examination or imaging such as ultrasound, CT or MR scanning (see Ch. 4). Open biopsy or fine-needle aspiration cytology of an enlarged node should provide a pathological diagnosis when required and allows appropriate treatment, e.g. radiotherapy or cytotoxic chemotherapy for lymphoma. Excision of local and regional nodes with a primary cancer (e.g. breast, colon, stomach) is described as a radical operation, gives prognostic information by staging the tumour and may also improve local control and survival for some cancers (see Ch. 13).

Acute lymphangitis, or inflammation of the lymphatic vessels, occurs typically with streptococcal infections, when tender red lines may be seen and palpated in the dermis. There is associated regional lymphadenopathy – e.g. groin or axilla. Penicillin therapy combined with rest and elevation is usually effective.

LYMPHOEDEMA

Oedema is an excess of fluid between tissue cells. Lymphoedema is the swelling which results from the accumulation of interstitial fluid as a consequence of failure of the lymphatic system to drain it.

Classification and aetiology

The condition is classed as either primary (disorder of the lymphatic system itself) or secondary (some other condition outside the lymphatic system which interferes with drainage).

Primary lymphoedema

The subject is not well understood The following factors are probably of importance:

- Very few patients are born with a hypoplastic lymphatic system, usually in the lower limb (*congenital hereditary lymphoedema*).
- Obliteration of lymphatic channels by fibrosis of unknown cause may develop at or after puberty.
- Obstruction of a group of lymph nodes (e.g. in the pelvis) may also occur for the same reason.
- Hyperplastic tortuous lymph channels can sometimes be shown at lymphangiography (see below), suggesting another type of congenital disease (often associated with capillary naevi); the defect may be in the valves of the lymphatics.

Primary lymphoedema is six times more common in women than men. Cases of primary lymphoedema may be referred to as 'Lymphoedema Congenita', 'Lymphoedema Praecox', and 'Lymphoedema Tarda'. These terms are more descriptive than diagnostic, reflecting the stages in life when they manifest themselves clinically.

Secondary lymphoedema

In Western countries the causes are:

- surgical removal of a group of lymph nodes – either in the axilla (mastectomy for breast cancer) or the groin (usually for malignant melanoma, less commonly for other malignancies)
- radiotherapy for malignancy – usually both factors (surgical removal and radiotherapy) are involved – it is not common for surgical excision alone to cause lymphoedema
- malignant invasion of lymphatics and nodes
- chronic venous disease, which may, particularly if recurrent infections occur, cause secondary lymphoedema in addition to the hydrostatic oedema that is present because of raised venous pressure. The lymphoedema of chronic venous disease is caused by constrictive fibrosis of the lymph channels induced by chronic inflammation.

In developing and tropical countries intra-lymphatic infection is the commonest cause:

- *Filariasis* caused by the worm *Wuchereria bancrofti* induces fibrosis in the lymphatics. The incubation period after the initial mosquito bite may be up to 18 months, and the condition should therefore be borne in mind in those who have returned from tropical to temperate climates.
- Silica particles enter through the skin of those walking barefoot on silica-rich soils; lymphatic drainage is interfered with, and secondary infection of cuts further damages the partially obstructed lymphatics and nodes.

Functional classification

An alternative approach combines developmental lymphatic abnormalities with an acquired element (probably repeated infection). The lymphoedema that follows is either:

- obliterative – from progressive intimal thickening
- obstructive – from developmental abnormalities in proximal nodes and possible fibrotic replacement
- valvular – from the presence of incompetence.

Pathophysiological and pathological features

The interstitial space contains not only water and electrolytes but also proteins (mostly albumin), other large molecules, cellular debris and sometimes bacteria. Most of the water and electrolytes are reabsorbed at the venular end of the capillary loop. The rest enter the lymphatics and pass to the nodes and thence to the thoracic duct. In consequence, if lymph flow is obstructed, there is an increase in their concentration in the interstitial space. This stagnant fluid may:

- be invaded by granulations and become organised into fibrous tissue
- provide an ideal culture medium for pathogenic bacteria and so cause recurrent episodes of cellulitis which further aggravates interstitial fibrosis and destruction of lymph channels.

Clinical features

Although either primary or secondary lymphoedema may occur in any part of the body drained by lymphatics, the common clinical presentation is in the limbs – chiefly the lower – and the description that follows relates mainly to this. However, many of the principles apply elsewhere.

Primary lymphoedema

Symptoms

There is often a family history, particularly on the female side, though this may be confused with one of venous disease. The most typical presentation is a teenage girl with the insidious and apparently spontaneous onset of unilateral swelling of the dorsum of the foot and the ankle. At first the swelling is most obvious in warmer weather and tends to disappear with a night's rest, but once it has been present for some time it fails to resolve completely. Pain is usually absent, but discomfort is associated with heaviness as the swelling increases. Oedema gradually becomes more marked and frequently ascends into the calf and from the dorsum of the foot forward to the toes. Onset in older patients is often similar and may occur at a more proximal level in the limb, for example the thigh, without foot and calf swelling. The skin remains healthy for many years and, in contrast to venous disease, complaints of pigmentation and ulceration are rare unless they develop because of recurrent cellulitis.

Signs

In half the patients, at initial presentation, the oedema is unilateral but, if bilateral, one limb frequently shows more advanced changes. The early oedema principally accumulates on the dorsum of the foot and initially pits on pressure. The pitting oedema and involvement of the dorsum of the foot distinguishes lymphoedema from lipoedema (or lipodystrophy), which is a non-pitting condition of the subcutaneous fat of the lower limbs where the foot is spared. Even at a late stage there is frequently an element of removable fluid even though fibrosis may also have taken place. With more extensive oedema, this is uniformly distributed from the calf down into the toes. The skin is nearly always intact but may show visible and palpable thickening.

Dilation of dermal lymphatics and subsequent fibrosis gives rise to fine dermal papillae (especially over the toes) known as papillomatosis.

Secondary lymphoedema

Symptoms

There may be a history suggestive of the underlying cause, and the onset of oedema may be closely related to this. Rapidity of onset may more closely mimic an acute venous thrombosis, with which secondary lymphoedema may occasionally coexist. Episodes of infection are more common in secondary disease.

Signs

The clinical appearances are similar to those of primary lymphoedema. When chronic venous disease is the cause, the features of venous hypertension will usually be apparent.

Investigation

The diagnosis is not usually in doubt, but distinction of primary from secondary lymphoedema – and, in both, detection of a cause – may require further investigation.

Distinction between lymphoedema and venous disease

Ultrasonography excludes disease of the deep and superficial veins.

Distinction between obliterative and obstructive disease

A bolus injection of technetium-labelled rhenium/sulphur colloid (lymphoscintigraphy) into the web space of the foot produces slow clearance from the tissues and minimal uptake of isotope in the draining lymph nodes in obliterative disease. A CT scan may also indicate a lack or absence of nodes draining the area involved.

Cause of obstruction

When, on clinical grounds, the cause is thought to be obstructive and the condition is intractable to conservative management, lymphangiography is indicated. This combination of circumstances is uncommon – less than 10% of patients.

Management

Non-operative

Management consists of:

- reduction of oedema – elevation, distal-proximal massage (MLD – manual lymphatic drainage), mechanical compression devices (Lymphopress®)
- continuous support with compression garments such as elastic stockings
- prophylaxis against infection – control of fungal infection, good skin hygiene and prevention of inadvertent skin trauma – scratching and wearing of shoes.

Ongoing encouragement and support is often required, as patients consider that non-operative management implies that 'nothing can be done for me'. The authors have found referring patients to the Lymphoedema Support Network website useful in their long-term management (www.lymphoedema.org). There is also a section on the condition lipoedema which, as discussed, is distinct from lymphoedema.

Surgical

There is no current treatment that will reliably restore function to the lymphatic system.

Anastomotic and bridging procedures include:

- improvement of lymphatic drainage in obstructive lymphoedema – microvascular anastomosis between lymphatics and veins
- provision of lymphatic bridges by anastomosis of an isolated loop of ileum without its mucosa to a lymph node just distal to an obstruction.

Debulking operations are:

- removal of the skin and thickened subcutaneous tissue with free split-skin grafting of the raw area
- removal of much of the involved tissue with a dermal flap buried beneath the deep fascia which it is hoped will provide new lymphatic pathways for drainage
- liposuction.

Symptomatic relief and cosmetic improvement may come from any of the above procedures. Selection is difficult and the operations are technically challenging and usually

Bacterial cellulitis as a complication of lymphoedema

Emergency Box 30.2

Differential diagnosis of an acutely swollen limb

- Venous – DVT is the most likely diagnosis
- Arterial – seen following successful revascularisation of an ischaemic limb (reperfusion oedema). If tense, consider reperfusion injury causing compartment syndrome
- Oedema – usually less acute, and bilateral. Most often associated with congestive cardiac failure or renal failure
- Lymphoedema – chronic, but acute exacerbation when secondarily infected
- Infection – severe cellulitis or necrotising fasciitis
- Factitious – suspected if there is a sharp cut-off, possibly resulting from the use of a tourniquet to produce distal swelling

complicated by significant blood loss. Liposuction is the least invasive.

Differential diagnosis of an acutely swollen limb is summarised in Emergency Box 30.2.

BACTERIAL CELLULITIS AS A COMPLICATION OF LYMPHOEDEMA

The condition is both a complication of lymphoedema and a cause of secondary forms. It is common and frequently misdiagnosed.

Aetiology

Organisms, usually beta-haemolytic streptococci though occasionally a synergistic combination, gain entry either through an apparently inconsequential injury or an insect bite. More commonly, there is a history of chronic fungal infection in the web spaces of digits.

Pathological features

The condition is usually a self-limiting subcutaneous cellulitis but necrosis of skin and fascia can occur.

Clinical features

Symptoms

The onset is usually with an acute influenza-like illness, with shivering and occasional rigors. Later, progressive swelling and erythema develop and spread with varying degrees of rapidity. If a limb is involved it is acutely painful.

Signs

The area involved is red, hot and tender. Swelling is increased. The regional lymph nodes, if they are present, are also tender.

Management

Early recognition and prompt antibiotic treatment in association with methods designed to reduce the oedema rapidly and enhance lymphatic drainage may reduce the immediate complication of skin necrosis and reduce the likelihood of further obliteration of lymphatics. A simple but effective initial antibiotic combination is high-dose penicillin 1.2 g 4-hourly, intravenously if severe, together with 500 mg of flucloxacillin 4- or 6-hourly. The initial site of entry should be dealt with concomitantly, e.g. fungal infection in the web space.

Once the acute phase has subsided, the patient may be mobilised and oedema reduced by a high-compression support hose. Six weeks of oral erythromycin is recommended for prophylaxis.

FURTHER READING

See Chapter 29.

Bergan JJ 2007 The vein book. Elsevier Academic Press, Amsterdam

Browse NI, Burnand KG, Irvine AT et al 1999 Diseases of the veins. Arnold, London

Dieter RS, Dieter RA 2010 Venous and lymphatic diseases. McGraw-Hill Medical, New York

National Institute for Health and Clinical Excellence, January 2010: Venous thromboembolism: reducing the risk. Available online. Accessed 24 January 2011 from http://guidance.nice.org.uk/CG92/QuickRefGuide/pdf/English

SECTION 3
SURGICAL SPECIALTIES

31 Neurosurgery

Neurosurgeons treat structural and functional lesions of the brain, spinal cord and peripheral nerves. The spectrum of disorders managed by neurosurgeons is broadening as our understanding of neuroanatomy and neurophysiology develops. The pathology encountered often demands a medical as well as surgical approach to treatment. The common disorders treated are shown in Box 31.1.

BASIC CLINICAL PRINCIPLES

Neurosurgery has benefited significantly from major technical advances over recent years. Modern imaging techniques provide assistance in diagnosis and treatment. However, neurosurgical patients often present in extremis, unable to co-operate with examination or provide a history, with imminently life threatening conditions. Therefore the neurosurgeon relies on basic clinical skills, and an understanding of the signs that can be elicited in order to make precise, quick decisions, that can make the difference between life and death. This combination of the modern medical science and traditional clinical techniques produces an exciting and challenging specialty.

History and examination

Clinical findings remain central to diagnosis in neurosurgery. A comprehensive history and neurological examination provide powerful diagnostic tools with which the neurosurgeon can identify the type of pathology and its location. The majority of conditions can be diagnosed based on this approach and the decision to operate or not to operate invariably depends on the clinical findings. A neurological history must identify salient features vital to establishing a diagnosis. The examination should include initial assessment of consciousness and higher cognitive function, then cranial nerves, upper limbs and lower limbs, trunk and sphincters.

Management of the unconscious patient

It is paramount that any professional looking after neurosurgical patients has an understanding of how to manage the unconscious patient. A patient in coma requires measures to save life and prevent deterioration before a precise diagnosis is made and definitive treatment undertaken. Whatever the cause of coma, management is along the lines given in Clinical Box 31.1. Once these objectives have been achieved, a diagnosis is made as soon as possible.

Assessment of the level of consciousness

The Glasgow Coma Scale (see Box 31.2) is now universally used. It consists of three components which deteriorate as coma deepens:

- Stimulus to produce eye opening
- Patient's verbal response
- Best motor response.

The score for each component is recorded and the total for the patient obtained. A fully conscious patient scores 15 points while one who is completely unresponsive scores 3. Coma is considered to be 8 points or less. Changes can be easily noted on a chart, and the scale is simple enough to be reproduced accurately by all grades of nurses and doctors.

Investigations

Computed tomography (CT)

CT has revolutionised diagnostic neurology since its introduction in the mid-1970s (see Ch. 4). It allows imaging of brain, skull bones, soft tissues and spine and has become the first line of investigation for many conditions treated by neurosurgeons. Latest technology allows 3D reconstruction of the bony skeleton and non-invasive cerebral angiography (CTA).

Box 31.1 Disorders treated by neurosurgeons

- Congenital abnormalities
- Trauma
- Tumours of the brain and spinal cord
- Cerebral haemorrhage
- Hydrocephalus
- Spinal degenerative disease
- Peripheral nerve entrapment
- Infections of the brain and spinal cord and their coverings
- Pain
- Movement disorders

Clinical Box 31.1 Management of the unconscious patient

- **A**irway: establish and maintain a clear airway
- **B**reathing: ensure adequate oxygenation, if necessary intubation and ventilation
- **C**irculation: make sure the patient is fully resuscitated and has a normal blood pressure and good urine output, allowing adequate cerebral perfusion
- **D**isability: exclude metabolic causes of coma, especially hypo- or hyperglycaemia. Calculate the Glasgow Coma Score. Assess pupils and perform a neurological examination tailored to the unconcious patient.

Box 31.2 The Glasgow Coma Scale

Event	Score
Eye opening occurs	
Spontaneously	4
In response to speech	3
On pain stimulation	2
Does not occur	1
Verbal response	
Alert and orientated	5
Confused	4
Inappropriate	3
Incomprehensible	2
Does not take place	1
Best motor response	
Commands are obeyed	6
Localises to pain	5
Withdraws to pain	4
Abnormal flexion to pain	3
Extension to pain	2
No response to pain	1

Magnetic resonance imaging (MRI)

The principles behind this technique are outlined in Chapter 4. In recent years the use of MRI has moved on from a purely diagnostic tool to one that has augmented our understanding of normal and abnormal brain function. Unlike CT, soft tissues can be imaged and it has now become the gold standard for imaging of the brain and spinal cord.

Angiography

Contrast medium is injected into the cerebral or spinal arteries to see and delineate aneurysms and arteriovenous anomalies. The blood supply of a tumour can also be visualised. Although diagnostic invasive angiography is declining in use whilst that of CT and MR angiography increases, therapeutic angiography to treat cerebral aneurysms and arteriovenous malformations (AVMs) is being used more frequently.

Computerised combination of CT, MR and angiography images allows the surgeon to be guided by 3D virtual images of a lesion and surrounding structures whilst operating. In some centres intraoperative MR scanning can allow the surgeon to gauge the extent of tumour resection during the procedure.

Lumbar puncture (LP)

Withdrawal of cerebrospinal fluid (CSF) by tapping the subarachnoid space in the lumbar region, LP is used to diagnose subarachnoid haemorrhage (uniform blood staining and xanthochromia) if CT scanning is non-diagnostic and meningitis (pus cells and bacteria). LP must only be performed after imaging to rule out a space-occupying lesion or decreased CSF volume around the brainstem.

Electrophysiology

The electroencephalogram (EEG) may be useful in the investigation of epilepsy. Nerve conduction studies are important in the diagnosis of peripheral nerve lesions.

TRAUMA

Head injury is a leading cause of death and disability in the UK and places a huge demand on individuals and society: 300 per 100 000 population are admitted to hospital every year and 9 per 100 000 die (25 per 100 000 in the USA). Although some injuries are immediately catastrophic and fatal, appropriate management of the remainder of cases can result in reducing disability and preventing death.

Pathophysiology

Traumatic brain injury (TBI) can be categorised as diffuse or focal, or primary and secondary, a description of the timing of cellular damage.

- Diffuse axonal injury results from shearing forces from the initial insult. The consequence of this ranges from mild concussion to death depending on the severity.
- Focal damage refers to the presence of cortical contusions, lacerations and intracranial haematomas (extradural, subdural and intraparenchymal). Contusions can occur on the same side as the impact or on the opposite side (contra-coup injury). If left untreated a rise in intracranial pressure, resulting from the focal lesion, may result in tentorial or tonsillar herniation (coning) and death from brainstem compression.
- Primary brain injury occurs immediately on impact. Movement of the brain within the skull results in tearing of neurons and blood vessels. The severity of injury is dependent on the force of impact but the mechanism is the same.
- Secondary brain injury results from ongoing cellular insult caused by hypoxia, cerebral ischaemia, swelling, infarction and infection and is potentially avoidable.

Secondary brain damage causes a rise in intracranial pressure (ICP). This rise compromises cerebral blood flow (CBF), which is directly influenced by cerebral perfusion pressure (CPP) using the following equation:

CPP = MAP (mean arterial pressure) − ICP

Intracranial pressure is normally kept constant by autoregulation. However, physiological control is disrupted in traumatic brain injury and autoregulation is lost. As a result the intracranial pressure increases. Therefore treatment is aimed at preventing secondary brain damage.

Causes of raised pressure

- *Expanding intracranial haematoma.*
- *Swelling.* Primary and secondary damage cause brain swelling either by hyperaemia or an increase in extracellular fluid. Because the brain is enclosed in a rigid box, the increase in brain volume raises intracranial pressure (Monro–Kellie doctrine). Cerebral perfusion pressure falls, which leads to ischaemia, causing further brain swelling.
- *Infection.* The usual cause is a skull fracture with tearing of the meninges and a leak of CSF through an open wound or into an air sinus or the middle ear. Infection can take the form of meningitis or abscess.
- *Epilepsy.* The brain uses glucose and oxygen abundantly when a fit is taking place, and ischaemia develops rapidly if fits are not controlled.

Management

Management of head injury patients can be considered in three parts:

1. **Resuscitation.** Initial resuscitation according to Advanced Trauma Life Support (ATLS) principles (ABCD). Head injury patients commonly have multiple injuries and a compromised airway can kill a patient much more quickly than an expanding intracranial haematoma. Attention to ABCD should also allow adequate ventilation, preventing cerebral hypoxia, and circulatory support, preventing cerebral ischaemia, by maintaining cerebral perfusion pressure (Emergency Box 31.1).
2. **Assessment of head injury.** This includes:
   - information regarding mechanism of injury
   - examining the head for lacerations and signs of skull and base of skull fracture (Emergency Box 31.2)
   - assessment of the Glasgow Coma Score (GCS)
   - pupillary response (dilated, non-reactive, pupil suggests expanding intracranial mass on ipsilateral side)
   - unilateral weakness (contralateral to a space-occupying lesion) and cranial nerve palsies allow localisation of a possible intracranial bleed
   - CT scanning is essential to identify injuries that may require neurosurgical intervention. NICE provide clear and useful guidelines regarding which patients should be scanned and when.
3. **Escalation of care.** Imaging and clinical findings allow early identification of patients likely to suffer secondary brain damage and those who require urgent surgical intervention or intensive care (Boxes 31.3 and 31.4).

Based on this assessment patients can be broadly divided into two groups:

1. *Mild head injury.* Defined as a GCS of 13–15 in the first 48 hours after injury. Those at risk of developing secondary complications, especially haematomas, must be identified early and managed appropriately:
   (i) Should the patient be admitted (Box 31.3)?
   (ii) Is neurosurgical intervention required (Box 31.4)?
   (iii) Supportive care:
   - oxygenate
   - adequate hydration

Emergency Box 31.1

Management of patients with severe head injury

- Immediately intubate and ventilate. (Fears of intubating a patient with an unstable spine and of masking physical signs by using sedatives/paralysing agents are not valid. All necks should be immobilised until cleared clinically and radiologically)
- Correct hypovolaemia by intravenous resuscitation
- Assess head and other injuries, including use of X-ray/CT scanning
- Treat other life-threatening injuries – abdominal, chest
- Refer/discuss with neurological centre

Emergency Box 31.2

Signs of skull base fractures

- CSF rhinorrhoea (glucose present in nasal discharge suggests CSF)
- CSF otorrhoea
- Bleeding from the ear
- Bilateral periorbital bruising (racoon eyes)
- Mastoid bruising (Battle sign)

Box 31.3 Indications for admission

- Focal neurological signs
- Skull fracture
- Depressed level of consciousness
- CSF leak, depressed fracture, penetrating wound

Box 31.4 Indications for neurosurgical referral

- Deterioration
- Drowsiness in a patient with a skull fracture – a significant clot is present in 1 out of 4 patients with this combination, and referral should be made before further deterioration takes place
- Depressed fracture/CSF leak
- Penetrating wound
- Failure to improve after 12–24 hours

- regular neuro-observation
- control seizures if present
- analgesia
- early referral if indicated.

Most patients in this group will be well enough to be discharged after 48 hours. Patients and relatives must be provided with information about signs of deterioration and of post-concussion syndrome (headaches, dizziness and loss of concentration that can persist for a number of weeks).

2. *Moderate* (GCS 9–12 in the first 48 hours) and *severe* (GCS 3–8 in the first 48 hours) *head injury.* Treatment is aimed at preventing secondary brain damage. This involves a combination of medical and surgical approaches to maintain cerebral perfusion pressure and control intracranial pressure. Patients should be admitted to a neurosurgical intensive care unit and managed with these objectives in mind. Figure 31.1 is an example of a protocol used to manage major head injury.

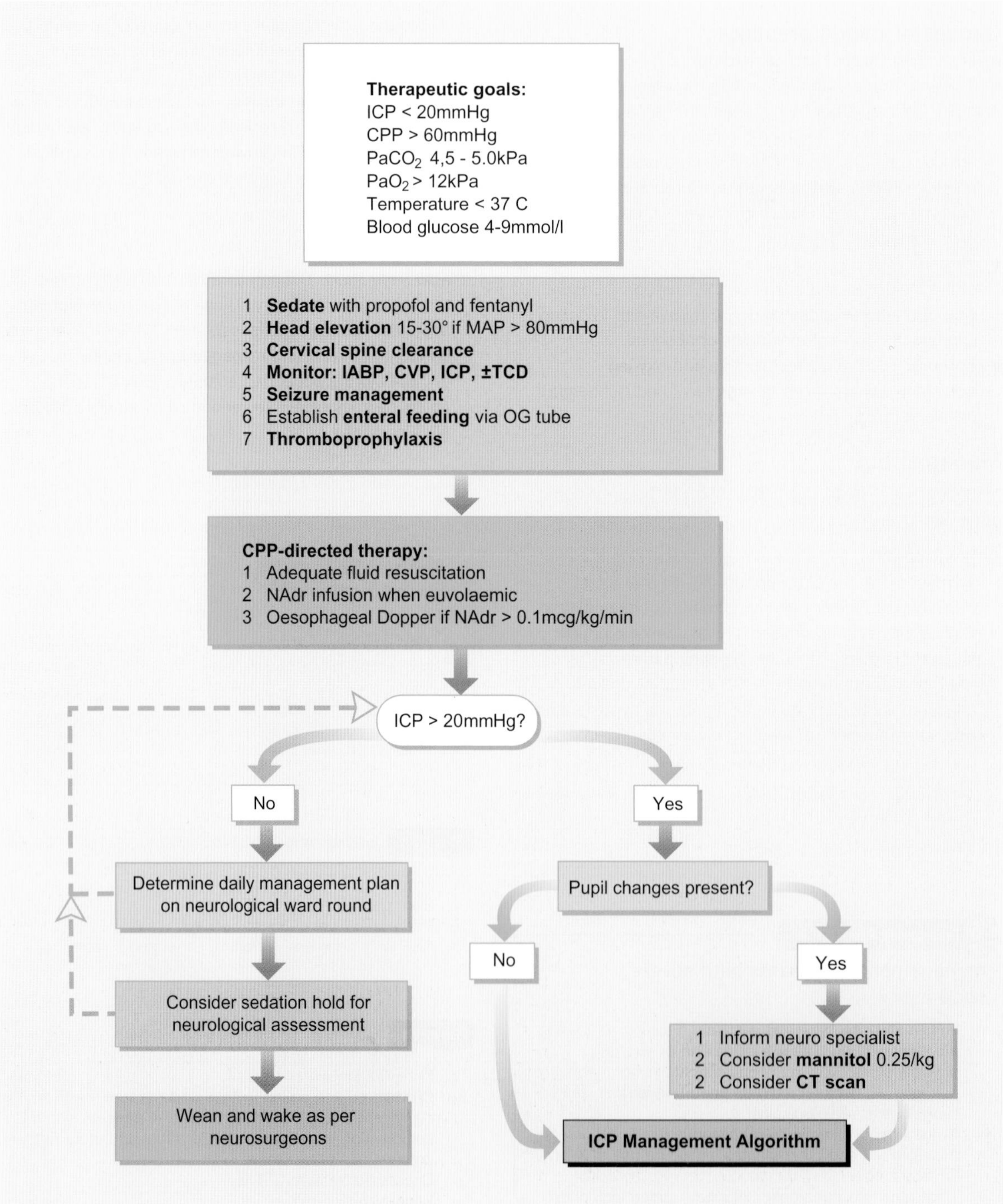

Therapeutic goals:
ICP < 20mmHg
CPP > 60mmHg
$PaCO_2$ 4,5 - 5.0kPa
PaO_2 > 12kPa
Temperature < 37 C
Blood glucose 4-9mmol/l
1 Sedate with propofol and fentanyl
2 Head elevation 15-30° if MAP > 80mmHg
3 Cervical spine clearance
4 Monitor: IABP, CVP, ICP, ±TCD
5 Seizure management
6 Establish enteral feeding via OG tube
7 Thromboprophylaxis
CPP-directed therapy:
1 Adequate fluid resuscitation
2 NAdr infusion when euvolaemic
3 Oesophageal Dopper if NAdr > 0.1mcg/kg/min
ICP > 20mmHg?
No
Yes
Determine daily management plan on neurological ward round
Consider sedation hold for neurological assessment
Wean and wake as per neurosurgeons
Pupil changes present?
No
Yes
1 Inform neuro specialist
2 Consider mannitol 0.25/kg
2 Consider CT scan
ICP Management Algorithm

Fig. 31.1 Protocol used to manage major head injury. (Produced by Oxford Neuro Intensive Care Unit, C Kearns and H Madder. Reproduced with permission.)

Surgical intervention is part of this approach and the procedure adopted depends on the intracranial pathology present:

- *Extradural haematoma* (Fig. 31.2a) requires emergency craniotomy to remove the clot. Cerebral compression from an extradural haematoma (usually haemorrhage from the middle meningeal artery) leads to raised intracranial pressure. Further compression leads to bilaterally fixed and dilated pupils, and the terminal stage of compression – coning (downward displacement of the brainstem into the foramen magnum) – is associated with hypertension, bradycardia, respiratory failure (Cushing's response) and finally cardiac arrest. Intervention at the stage of deteriorating conscious state can lead to a rapid full recovery, but this is rare after coning has taken place.
- *Acute subdural or intracerebral haematoma* (Fig. 31.2b): emergency craniotomy to remove the clot and prevent cerebral compression.
- *Decompressive craniectomy:* following craniotomy the bone flap is left out to allow space for the brain to swell. The potential benefit of this is as yet unknown in the treatment of closed head injury but is currently the subject of an international multi-centred randomised controlled trial.
- *Elevation of depressed skull fracture* to prevent intracranial haemorrhage, mass effect, CSF leak.
- *Repair of basal skull fractures* causing CSF leak.

a

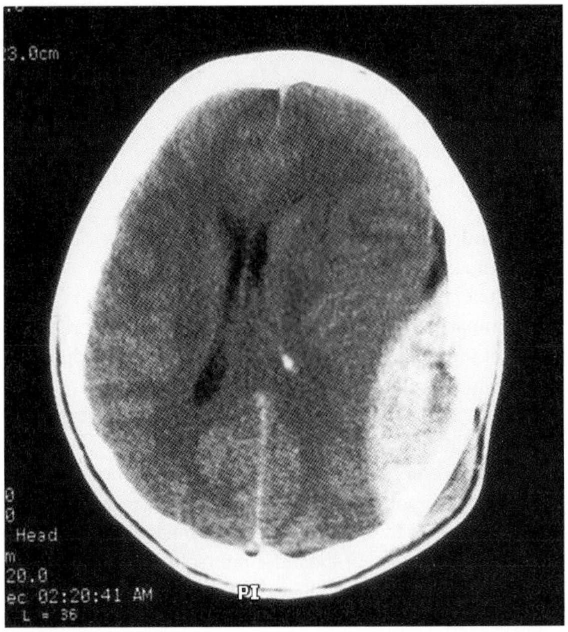

b

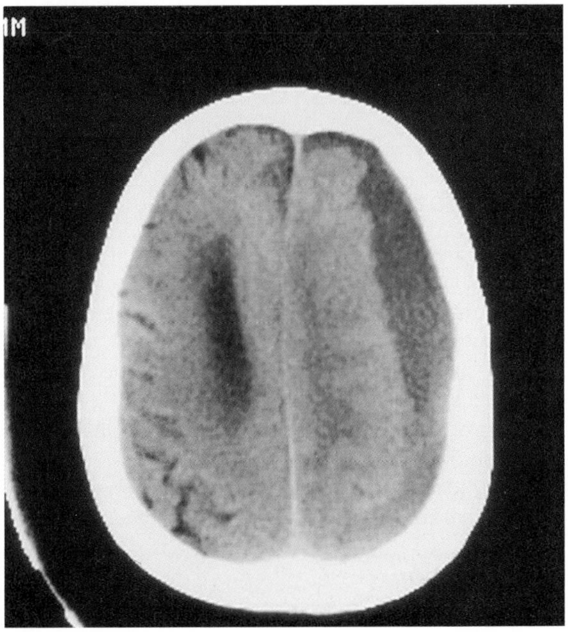

Fig. 31.2 CT scans: (a) left extradural haematoma obliterating the ventricle and shifting the midline to the right; (b) left chronic subdural haematoma.

Outcome after head injury

The best prognostic indicator for outcome is the patient's best GCS score after resuscitation. Table 31.1 shows the outcome for those in coma on admission to hospital. The consequences of even mild head injury can be very significant with patients suffering from poor memory, personality changes, physical disability, epilepsy and depression either alone or in combination. Families may be wrecked by the difficulties of caring for these people. Intensive rehabilitation with physiotherapy, speech therapy, occupational therapy and psychological help started soon after injury may reduce the difficulties and improve outcome.

Subdural haematoma

Subdural collections can be acute or chronic. Although trauma is clearly a significant factor in the aetiology of acute subdurals, it may only play a minor role in the aetiology of chronic subdurals. Chronic subdurals are far more common than acute subdurals and commonly occur in the over 50s.

Pathogenesis

Chronic subdural haemorrhage (SDH) is common in conditions of cerebral atrophy, notably old age and alcoholism. Minor trauma leads to a small amount of insignificant bleeding in the subdural space. As this blood breaks down over weeks or months, fluid is drawn into the subdural space by the hyperosmolar breakdown products, and a membrane forms. The collection gradually enlarges and compresses the

Table 31.1 Outcome in head injury patients with coma on admission

Status	Percentage of patients
Complete recovery	30%
Some disablement but able to look after themselves	20%
Severe disablement: vegetative state or unable to care for themselves	10%
Death	40%

brain, mimicking a tumour. Subdural haemorrhage in infants should always raise suspicion of non-accidental injury.

Diagnosis

CT or MR scan.

Treatment

Burr hole or mini-craniotomy drainage to let the fluid out of the subdural space, which is then washed through with warmed saline.

TUMOURS OF THE BRAIN AND MENINGES

Approximately 6 people per 100 000 are diagnosed with a primary brain tumour every year. Secondary tumours are more common but these are rarely treated by neurosurgeons unless the patient presents with a brain tumour in the absence of known/detectable cancer elsewhere. Occasionally solitary metastatic tumours are excised. Although brain tumours account for only 2% of all primary tumours in the UK, they are responsible for 7% of life years lost before the age of 70 and cause about 3500 deaths every year.

Pathology

Supratentorial tumours account for 80–85% while infratentorial tumours account for 15–20% (Table 31.2). The World Health Organisation (WHO) classifies adult primary brain tumours according to the lineage of differentiation and their histological grade.

- **Neuroepithelial origin.** Diffusely infiltrative gliomas are most common, and these are divided into:
  - Astrocytomas show features of astrocytic differentiation.
  - Oligodendrogliomas, the cells of which resemble oligodendrocytes. (Both types are assigned WHO grades II to IV according to the presence or absence of aggressive histological features.)
  - Ependymomas show features of ependymal differentiation. They are commonly intraventricular and can, rarely, spread through the CSF.
  - A variety of other, less common, intrinsic brain tumours including primitive neuroectodermal tumours (PNET) of various types, pineal parenchymal tumours and ganglion cell (neuronal) tumours.

Table 31.2 Tumours of the central nervous system

Tumour	Origin
Glioma	Supporting tissues
Meningiomas	Covering layers
Neuromas	Nervous tissues
Pituitary	Endocrine cells of anterior pituitary
Developmental	Abnormal islands of cells at points of closure of neural tube. Persistent primitive cells

- **Meningeal origin:**
  - Meningiomas usually arise from the arachnoid granulations and are mostly benign (WHO grade I). A minority are of higher grade and may show malignant behaviour. Benign lesions can cause significant distortion of normal intracranial structures and may, therefore, become life threatening. Surgical resection is often curative. They can be highly vascular and therefore enhance avidly on CT scan with contrast, showing clear attachment to the meninges.
- **Nerve sheath cell origin:**
  - Schwannoma: histological features of Schwann cells, commonly arising from the VIIIth cranial nerve.
  - Neurofibroma: histological features of Schwannn cells, perineural-like cells and fibroblasts
- **Blood vessel origin:**
  - Haemangioblastomas: highly vascular tumours of uncertain histogenesis which usually arise in the posterior fossa or spinal cord. They are the commonest presenting manifestation of Von Hippel–Lindau disease.
- **Tumours of the sellar region:**
  - Pituitary tumours can be functioning or non-functioning and can present with hormonal imbalance or visual disturbance due to compression of the optic chiasm, which passes over the top of the pituitary gland.
  - Craniopharyngiomas often present with pituitary dysfunction.
- Medulloblastoma, germ cell tumours including germinoma and choroid plexus tumours are all usually associated with children, but are sometimes also seen in adults. All except the latter are high-grade lesions. The typical position of these tumours may be different in adults than in children.

The degree of malignancy of a brain tumour is reflected in the cellular grading, which considers features such as:

- cellularity
- mitoses
- pleomorphism
- necrosis.

Clinical features

Brain tumours can present as follows:

1. Raised intracranial pressure (ICP). Examination of the fundi may reveal papilloedema. If the raised pressure is left untreated it will lead to coma and death.
2. Fits – patients presenting with seizures of late onset should be investigated.
3. Neurological deficit influenced by the site of the tumour.
4. Rarely tumours are picked up incidentally when patients are scanned for another reason such as trauma.

Investigation

Imaging is required to confirm the presence of a space-occupying lesion. Tissue is required to make a histopathological diagnosis. Investigation of intracranial masses is not limited to the brain and thorough investigation is paramount to rule out a primary lesion elsewhere in the body and to rule out the possibility of intracranial abscess.

Management

The aim of surgery in the management of intracranial tumours is twofold:

- To make a tissue diagnosis
- To reduce the mass effect.

Some patients may require urgent craniotomy to debulk the tumour if they present with a poor GCS due to mass effect. If the tumour is causing hydrocephalus then a shunt or extraventricular drain may be indicated. Following discussion with a neurosurgeon, patients should be started on the following drugs prior to surgery:

- Steroids to reduce oedema if present
- Anticonvulsants if the patient has fitted.

In some benign tumours such as meningiomas it is possible to achieve complete excision. For highly malignant tumours the aim is to remove as much as possible without damaging normal brain tissue.

Surgery forms part of the multidisciplinary approach to the management of brain tumours. Malignant gliomas can be treated with a combination of surgery, radiotherapy and chemotherapy. These are only suitable in patients who are well enough to tolerate the treatment. The use of temozolomide in patients with high-grade, aggressive astrocytomas has seen an increase in survival in recent years. The prognosis is still poor, however. Life expectancy without any treatment is less than 8 months, increasing to 12–14 months in patients fit enough to tolerate surgery, radiotherapy and chemotherapy.

Some tumours can be treated using the gamma knife, a form of stereotactic radiosurgery. This can be used in the treatment of some meningiomas, neuromas and pituitary adenomas.

Gene therapy is another modality that may provide an alternative treatment option. Currently it is experimental and results so far have been disappointing. Advances in molecular analysis of astrocytomas has allowed identification of growth signalling pathways which may provide a mechanism for more targeted therapy in the future.

Paediatric tumours

Brain tumours are the most common solid tumours in children and the second most common form of cancer, with an incidence of approximately 2–5 cases per 100 000. The intracranial distribution is different compared with adults, 40% occurring above the tentorium and 60% below. The principles of classification are identical to those used for adult tumours. In children, medulloblastomas and cerebellar astrocytomas predominate. Paediatric astrocytomas, such as pilocytic astrocytoma, are distinct in their histological features and behaviour. They are usually well circumscribed and of low grade and are often successfully treated by surgery alone. Again, the approach to treatment of paediatric tumours is multidisciplinary with combinations of surgery, chemotherapy and radiotherapy being employed.

CEREBRAL HAEMORRHAGE

Cerebral haemorrhage makes up a large part of neurosurgical practice. The emphasis has shifted away from surgical intervention for some forms of neurovascular disease such as aneurysms; however, decompressive craniectomies are becoming increasingly common in the management of patients who have devastating rises in intracranial pressure. Surgery is also required to manage some of the complications of haemorrhage such as hydrocephalus.

Intracranial haemorrhage

This is defined as spontaneous bleeding within the cranial cavity. Sites of haemorrhage are:

- Within the brain substance (intracerebral haemorrhage)
- In the subarachnoid space (subarachnoid haemorrhage)
- In the subdural space (subdural haemorrhage).

Intracerebral haemorrhage

This accounts for 10–20% of all strokes and is associated with the highest mortality and morbidity. The haemorrhage is most often deep within the cerebral substance and is usually associated with hypertension. It can also be caused by an arteriovenous malformation, aneurysm, amyloid angiopathy or, rarely, bleeding into a tumour.

Clinical features

The most common site in adults is within the basal ganglia and thalamic region. Presentation is often with sudden-onset headache, neurological deficit and possibly coma.

Surgical intervention

Recent studies now suggest that surgical decompression by craniectomy may have a role in a limited number of selected patients. Few debate that patient selection is key to successful outcome with decompression. If the patient has a dominant hemisphere haemorrhage and poor neurological state (e.g. fixed dilated pupils, extending to pain), then decompression will provide little benefit. If the patient is alert with a gradually deteriorating deficit and conscious state, decompression may help. Timing is crucial and clots should be removed early to prevent deterioration due to swelling.

Subarachnoid haemorrhage (SAH)

Epidemiology

Incidence: 10–15 per 100 000 population per year.

Bleeding into the subarachnoid space can be:

- traumatic (most common)
- spontaneous, due to:
  - aneurysmal rupture – 75–80%
  - arteriovenous malformation (AVM) – 5%
  - unknown – 15–20%.

Clinical features

- Severe, sudden-onset headache and neck stiffness are characteristic; this may be preceded by a headache for 2–3 days (sentinel headache)

- Loss of consciousness, seizure, coma
- Neurological deficit
- Meningism.

Prognosis

Thirty per cent of those who survive the initial episode die within the next 6 weeks from one of the following:

- failure to recover from the initial haemorrhage
- re-bleeding
- cerebral ischaemia which is the result of arterial vasospasm 3–10 days after the haemorrhage.

Ischaemia may be mild and without clinical effects. If severe it can be associated with hemiplegia and persistent coma.

Management

- Resuscitation: A, B, C, D.
- Establish diagnosis by:
  - CT scan – 91–98% sensitive.
  - Lumbar puncture if CT is negative: positive if the CSF is uniformly bloodstained and there is xanthochromia (the appearance of the CSF when bilirubin is present). Spectroscopy is required to detect bilirubin and oxyhaemaglobin.
  - CT or MR angiography (non-invasive) or cerebral angiography (invasive) to identify cause of haemorrhage.

Treatment

Considered in two parts:

1. **Securing the aneurysm.** Traditionally this was done by placing a small metal clip across its neck by open craniotomy. Alternatively, the aneurysm may be filled with platinum coils by endovascular techniques. The ISAT trial (Molyneux et al. 2002) has suggested that the mortality and morbidity following endovascular coiling of an aneurysm is significantly less than that for surgical clipping. Coiling has now become the treatment of choice for most aneurysms in most centres, although some aneurysms are better treated by open clipping.
2. **Managing the complications:**
   (i) Cerebral ischaemia secondary to vasospasm by the following:
   - Nimodipine (calcium channel blocker)
   - Haemodilution
   - Hypervolaemia
   - Hypertension.

   (ii) Hydrocephalus, requiring:
   - Extraventricular drain
   - Ventriculoperitoneal shunt.

An AVM, if superficial and in a suitable position, can be surgically excised. However, if deep or in an area of vital function, it can be treated by embolisation or stereotactically focused radiotherapy.

CONGENITAL ANOMALIES

With better intrauterine diagnosis, congenital anomalies of the central nervous system can be detected early in pregnancy. If remediable, the need for early post-delivery or even pre-delivery treatment can be anticipated and arranged.

Spinal dysraphism

A group of conditions where the neural tube fails to close, a process that normally takes place during the first 25 days of fetal development.

Epidemiology

Approximately 2/1000 live births, 2–3/100 if found in a sibling. It is commonly associated with other abnormalities such as hydrocephalus.

Conditions vary from asymptomatic spina bifida occulta to open myelomenigoceles:

- Spina bifida occulta – a bony defect where the spinal process is absent, usually with no clinical significance. However, if a tuft of hair, sinus, dimple or mark on the skin overlying the defect is present, it may be associated with underlying defects.
- Meningocele – a CSF-filled cavity formed by outpouching of the posterior wall of the neural tube through the space formed by the bony defect.
- Myelomeningocele – the CSF space has parts of the spinal cord or roots within it. The skin covering the defect may break down, allowing cord and roots to become externalized, and CSF to leak. As a consequence, meningitis often occurs and can be life threatening.

Presentation

- Skin defects over the lumbar spine
- Neurological deficit, including weakness in the legs, diminished pain response and bladder dysfunction
- Identification of associated pathology, including Chiari malformation, lipomas, cord tethering and sinuses.

Investigations

- Ultrasound
- MRI.

Management

Spina bifida occulta may not require any treatment. A meningocele associated with a CSF leak should be excised immediately. In the absence of a leak, excision can be delayed or may not be necessary at all.

Surgical intervention in myelomeningocele aims at replacing the neural tissue into the spinal canal. Surgical closure can be life-saving in preventing meningitis but may not improve neurological deficit, including paraplegia and loss of sphincter control. Some associated conditions may require surgical correction at an early age.

Encephaloceles

In this condition fusion of the neural tube fails at the cranial end. Meninges and brain herniate through the defects in the skull, most commonly in the occipital region and frontonasal areas. They are surgically corrected with great care as they often contain vascular structures.

Craniosynostosis

Premature fusion of one or more cranial sutures causes excessive compensatory growth perpendicular to the fused suture.

- Sagittal synostosis – the sagittal suture is fused and the head becomes elongated (scaphocephaly)
- Coronal synostosis – bilateral (one of the defects seen in Apert's and Crouzon's syndromes) or unilateral, causing superior and lateral elongation (brachiocephaly)
- Oxycephaly – multiple sutures
- Pansynostosis – all sutures.

Clinical manifestation

- Craniofacial deformity
- Exophthalmos
- Raised intracranial pressure.

Treatment

Surgery aims to reconstruct the cranial and facial skeleton, partly for cosmetic reasons but primarily to reduce raised intracranial pressure. Complex craniofacial deformities require a multidisciplinary team approach, which can be found in only a few centres throughout the world. Brain growth is the main stimulus for the growth and shaping of the skull and therefore any corrective surgery should be performed within the first 2 years while the brain is still growing.

Chiari malformation

Downward displacement of the posterior fossa structures causes an anatomical malformation at the medullary spinal junction. The reason for this is unknown.

- Type I – the cerebellar tonsils lie below the level of the foramen magnum. This is associated with syringomyelia (cyst or cavity within the spinal cord) and hydromyelia (excess CSF within the central canal of the spinal cord) in 50% of cases and hydrocephalus in 10%.
- Type II – structures including the medulla, cerebellar vermis and 4th ventricle herniate through the foramen magnum. The lower cranial nerves and upper cervical roots are displaced.
- Type III – a cervico-occipital myelomeningocele is present and parts of the posterior fossa structures lie within it.
- Type IV – severe anatomical deformity rarely compatible with life.

Clinical presentation

This is influenced by the severity of herniation and varies with age. Infants may present with lower cranial nerve lesions and respiratory difficulties that may become life threatening. Ataxia, motor and sensory deficits may be more predominant features in childhood. Only patients with mild forms of Type I or Type II will present in adulthood and commonly suffer from headaches, exacerbated by rises in intracranial pressure from straining or coughing.

Investigations

MRI of the brain and spine to look for an abnormality of the medullary spinal junction and disorders commonly associated with Chiari malformation such as syringomyelia, hydrocephalus and spina bifida.

Treatment

Surgical treatment is aimed at managing hydrocephalus if present with ventriculo-peritoneal shunts, or at decompressing the foramen magnum to allow more space for the contents of the posterior fossa. This may involve removing the arch of the atlas and the posterior rim of the foramen magnum and opening the dura.

HYDROCEPHALUS

Definition: enlargement of the normal CSF spaces.

Physiology

CSF is made by ultrafiltration through the choroid plexus, mostly in the lateral ventricles. It passes via the foramen of Munro to the third ventricle and through the aqueduct to the fourth ventricle. It then leaves the ventricular system and passes into the subarachnoid space through the foramina of Luschka and Majendie and is reabsorbed into the bloodstream through the arachnoid granulations over the surface of the hemispheres (Fig. 31.3).

Types and causes

Communicating

In this type, CSF can reach the subarachnoid space but is not absorbed. Causes are anything that interferes with reabsorption by action on the arachnoid granulations, e.g.:

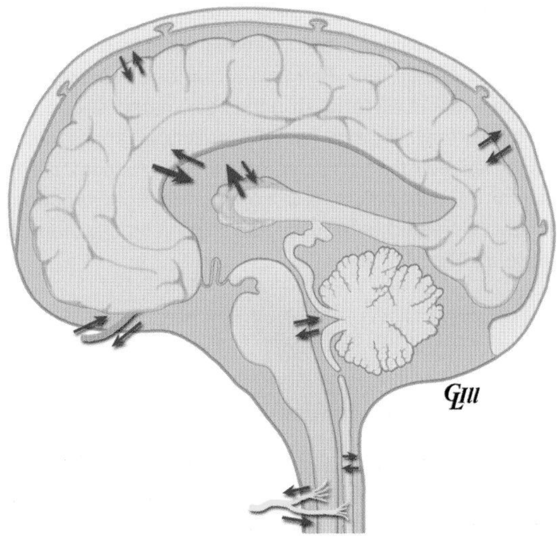

Fig. 31.3 The circulation of the CSF.

- subarachnoid haemorrhage
- head injury
- meningitis.

Non-communicating

Blockage prevents CSF reaching the subarachnoid space. Causes are:

- intraventricular haemorrhage
- congenital anomalies (Dandy–Walker cyst, aqueductal stenosis)
- intracranial masses.

Overproduction of CSF

This is a rare condition that results from a papilloma of the choroid plexus.

Clinical features

Presentation depends on the age of the patient and the cause.

In infants, features are:
- failure to thrive
- enlarging head
- tense fontanelle
- failure of upgaze (setting sun sign).

In adults, features are:
- typical features of raised intracranial pressure
- associated clinical signs of the cause – coma after head injury, subarachnoid haemorrhage or meningitis.

In the elderly, a normal-pressure hydrocephalus may occur in old age, which presents with:
- confusion
- ataxia
- incontinence.

Diagnosis and management

A CT or MRI scan will show the enlarged ventricles and may reveal a cause. In communicating hydrocephalus, lumbar puncture can be attempted safely, allowing pressure measurement and therapeutic drainage of CSF.

Temporary drainage can be achieved by intermittent ventricular tap in infants or by continuous ventricular drainage into an external system. Permanent drainage is achieved by inserting a shunt. This is an antibiotic-treated silicon tube with a one-way valve of varying pressure ranges, which passes between the ventricles and the peritoneum, pleural space or the right atrium. Non-communicating hydrocephalus may be treated by endoscopic third ventriculostomy to bypass an obstruction.

SPINAL DEGENERATIVE DISEASE

Degeneration of the vertebra and intervertebral discs results in pain and neurological deficit. The lumbar, cervical and thoracic regions are affected in descending order of frequency.

LUMBAR DEGENERATIVE DISEASE

Acute disc prolapse

This occurs when the nucleus pulposus of the intervertebral disc herniates through the surrounding annulus fibrosis causing compression of the nerve roots (when the protrusion is lateral) or compression of the cauda equina (when the protrusion is central). This causes acute back pain radiating down the leg, which is made worse by coughing or straining. The distribution of pain and neurological deficit are dependent on the level of disc prolapse:

- compression of the S1 root – pain down the back of the leg to the sole of the foot
- compression of the L5 root – pain down the outside of the leg to the big toe and weakness of extensor hallucis longus
- compression of the L4 root – pain on the inner aspect of the leg, weakness of ankle dorsiflexion and diminished ankle reflex.

Initial management

Non-operative

Bed rest with adequate analgesia and muscle relaxants. Failure to improve or the development of a foot drop are indications for imaging by MRI, with a view to surgery.

Surgery

If conservative management has failed, then surgery is indicated. This involves removing the prolapsed disc by open operation. Minimally invasive techniques have led to a reduction in postoperative recovery time and hospital stay, with some patients going home on the day of surgery.

Compression of the cauda equina

Occasionally, a large central disc prolapse, usually at L5/S1, compresses the cauda equina and causing a combination of symptoms that must never be ignored (Emergency Box 31.3). This condition is a surgical emergency and decompression must take place urgently to prevent permanent sphincter disturbance.

Lumbar canal stenosis

With increasing age and wear and tear on the spine, there is a general narrowing of the spinal canal by bony overgrowth and ligamentous hypertrophy. This gradually interferes with the blood supply to the cauda equina, leading to spinal claudication. This can be differentiated from arterial claudication by the presence of weakness and the relief the patient

Emergency Box 31.3

Cauda equina syndrome

- Back pain
- Saddle paraesthesia
- Bilateral sciatica
- Urinary retention

experiences with rest. Spinal claudication is only relieved by sitting or lying down, whereas arterial claudication can be relieved by just standing still.

Clinical features

- Numbness and weakness of the legs on walking, sometimes less than 100 m, relieved by rest.
- There are usually few clinical signs unless the patient is walked beyond the distance where symptoms develop.

Investigation and management

CT or MRI scanning will show a narrow spinal canal. Surgical treatment is by decompressive laminectomy.

CERVICAL DEGENERATIVE DISEASE

Acute disc prolapse or spondylosis due to chronic bony distortion can result in narrowing of the canal and consequent damage to the cervical spinal cord (myelopathy) or roots (radiculopathy), due to direct pressure or vascular change. The two can coexist, with radiculopathy at the level of the lesion and myelopathy below it.

Myelopathy

Clinical features

Compression causes a lower motor neuron lesion at that level and an upper motor neuron lesion below:

- Lower motor neuron lesion:
  - weakness
  - hypotonia
  - reduced or absent reflexes
  - fasciculations
- Upper motor neuron lesion:
  - hypertonicity
  - brisk reflexes
  - clonus
  - extensor plantar response.

Radiculopathy

Clinical features

An acute lateral disc prolapse or chronic osteophyte development can compress a nerve root in the lateral part of the spinal canal or the exit foramen, producing the following signs:

- pain (dermatomal)
- paraesthesia (nerve root distribution)
- sensory level
- weakness
- absent reflexes.

Investigation and management

If imaging is required, MR scanning, or rarely (nowadays) myelography, is used.

When there are cord signs, early surgical decompression is indicated. In stenosis of the canal, surgical decompression is performed. This can be by an anterior cervical discectomy and fusion (ACDF) or a posterior approach in order to perform a laminectomy. The aim of surgery is to prevent progression, although reversals of the neurological deficit can occur. Surgery for radiculopathy involves an anterior approach to remove the disc and osteophyte.

THORACIC DEGENERATIVE DISEASE

Thoracic degenerative disease is uncommon, probably because the thoracic spine is less mobile. Thoracic disc prolapses do occur and usually cause a chronic myelopathy. The treatment is surgical removal.

SPINAL TUMOURS

Spinal tumours other than metastases are far less common than those in the brain. The anatomical site and the histological appearances are the two main methods of classification (Table 31.3).

Anatomical site

Extradural

These tumours can cause:

- back pain, which is usually non-specific but may be radicular
- myelopathy.

Intradural extramedullary

These tumours can cause:

- root pain
- myelopathy in late cases.

Intradural intramedullary

- Slow onset of central cord syndrome – clinical characteristics of lower motor neuron signs in the arms and upper motor neuron signs in the legs.

Investigation

Detection by MRI.

Management

The management is outlined in Table 31.3.

Table 31.3 Tumours of the spinal cord

Site	Nature	Management
Extradural	Usually metastatic	Radiotherapy Surgery to prevent paralysis
Intradural extramedullary	Meningioma Neurofibroma	Surgical removal
Intradural intramedullary	Astrocytomas, ependymomas Cysts	Surgical decompression Radiotherapy

PERIPHERAL NERVE LESIONS

The common disorders are structural, e.g. trauma and entrapment.

Trauma

Injury may be by traction (e.g. a tear to the root of the brachial plexus when the arm is distracted in relation to the body) or by division in a penetrating wound.

Entrapment

Nerves that pass through bony or fibrous tunnels are affected (e.g. the median nerve in the carpal tunnel at the wrist and the ulnar nerve at the elbow).

Clinical features

Loss of function (of lower motor neuron type) and anaesthesia follow trauma. Entrapment causes pain and tingling in the distribution of the nerve, with muscle wasting if there is motor innervation.

Investigation and management

Further investigation is not required in obvious traumatic division, but a traction injury may require neurophysiological studies to confirm whether or not the injury is complete and therefore unlikely to recover. In entrapment, the symptoms and signs are often imprecise, and nerve conduction studies are required for confirmation.

Repair of traumatic division can be primary in a clean wound but is better delayed if there is contamination. Entrapments are treated by surgical decompression.

INFECTIONS

Intracranial

Intracranial infection can occur in the form of meningitis or abscess. Intracranial abscesses occur in 2–3 per million population. Although relatively uncommon due the advent of antibiotics, they are serious and life threatening. They can be classified according to anatomical location (subdural or extradural).

Pathophysiology

In 45% of patients spread occurs directly from the sinuses, infected dental caries or chronic otitis media/mastoiditis. Trauma accounts for a further 10% as fracture of the skull base provides a route for infection; 25% result from haematogenous spread from a distant focus. The source is unknown in 15% of cases.

The organism varies according to the source:

- Direct invasion form the sinuses or middle ear – *Streptococcus milleri*, *Bacteroides fragilis*, *Streptococcus pneumoniae*, *E. coli*.
- Haematogenous – *Staphylococcus aureus*, *S. milleri*, *S. pneumoniae*.
- In immunocompromised patients – *Candida*, *Aspergillus*, *Nocardia, Toxoplasma*, *Listeria.*
- Trauma – *S. aureus.*

Clinical presentation

Patients with intracranial abscesses present in a similar way to any others with a space-occupying lesion:

- headache
- vomiting
- reduced GCS
- focal neurological signs such as hemiparesis or dysphasia
- seizures due to parenchymal irritation.

Certain features raise suspicion of an abscess:

- signs of systemic infection: temperature, raised inflammatory markers
- signs of the source of infection: bacterial endocarditis, sinusitis, mastoiditis,
- immunocompromised patients.

Investigations

- CT or MRI with contrast
- X-rays to view sinuses and mastoids

Management

- Urgent abscess drainage
- Treatment of infective source
- Antibiotic therapy.

Meningitis

A diffuse infection of the meninges is actually far more common but shares the aetiological pattern for abscess. Features are:

- fever
- headache
- neck rigidity
- decline in level of consciousness
- fits.

Management

Antibiotics form the mainstay of therapy.

Spinal infection

Classification:

- intradural
- extradural.

Organism. *Staphylococcus* in 90% of cases.

Source: as for intracranial abscesses, this can be by direct spread from osteomyelitis of the vertebral column or haematogenous.

Clinical presentation. Spinal compression with rapidly progressing neurological deficit:

- Weakness
- Sensory level
- Urinary retention

- Signs of systemic infection
- Localised pain.

Immunocompromised and diabetic patients are at increased risk of developing abscesses.

Investigations

- Plain X-rays
- MRI.

Management

Urgent decompression of the spinal cord by laminectomy and drainage of the abscess. A long course of antibiotics for at least 6 weeks of intravenous therapy followed by oral.

Pain and movement disorders

Functional neurosurgical techniques target very specific intracranial pathways in an attempt to treat movement disorders, pain, epilepsy and psychological disorders. Originally, surgery aimed to create a permanent lesion in the targeted pathways. Now deep brain stimulation (DBS) by electrodes placed intracranially via burr holes allows reversible targeted therapy. The technique of stereotaxy, where patients are scanned with a frame fixed to their head, is used to locate specific lesions with remarkable accuracy. The range of conditions treated by this technique is broadening as our understanding of neuroanatomy and neurophysiology develops. Stereotaxy also allows us to perform biopsies and deliver radiotherapy with a degree of accuracy unobtainable previously. Another technique used increasingly to treat intractable pain involves implanting devices for delivery of analgesics directly to the CSF or epidural space.

REFERENCES

National Institute for Health and Clinical Excellence 2007 Head injury. NICE Clinical Guideline 56. Available online. Accessed 25 January 2011 from: www.nice.org.uk/nicemedia/pdf/CG56NICE Guideline.pdf

Molyneux A, Kerr R, Stratton I, et al 2002 International Subarachnoid Aneurysm Trial (ISAT). Lancet 2002 360 (9342): 1267–1274

FURTHER READING

Greenberg M S 2010 Handbook of neurosurgery, 7th edn. Thieme, New York (*Detailed and comprehensive, essential for the neurosurgical trainee, a good reference book for the student*)

Liebenberg W A, Johnson R D 2010 Neurosurgery for basic surgical trainees, 2nd edn. Hippocrates Books (*Useful practical guide for student or foundation doctor*)

Lindsay K W, Bone I, Fuller G 2010 Neurology and neurosurgery illustrated, 5th edn. Churchill Livingstone, Edinburgh. (*A good comprehensive text for student or foundation doctor*)

32 Surgery of the endocrine glands

PRINCIPLES IN ENDOCRINE SURGERY

Although surgeons have operated on the endocrine glands for more than a century, in the last 20–30 years, endocrine surgery has become a subspecialty. The reasons, apart from the technical demands, are that the biochemical and genetic understanding of the place of endocrinology has greatly increased. Many diseases require a multidisciplinary approach involving surgeon, endocrinologist, radiologist, pathologist, oncologist and geneticist. Nearly all endocrine disorders that have to be considered for surgical management fall into the following classes:

- neoplasia – either benign or malignant and, if the latter, either primary or secondary
- autoimmune
- genetic – and of varying inheritance.

In addition, disorders may or may not be associated with endocrine dysfunction, which is usually due to hypersecretion either of the hormone normally produced or of one or more of its analogues. Finally, hormones may be produced by tissues (usually neoplastic) which are not normally associated with an endocrine function (e.g. bronchial cancer, Ch. 16) to cause paraneoplastic syndromes.

Before individual organs and their disorders are considered, some principles that underlie all surgery on the endocrine glands are outlined.

Diagnosis

A precise diagnosis is essential and has the following characteristics:

- The exact nature of the disorder:
  - neoplastic: whether benign or malignant (primary or secondary)
  - autoimmune: the process involved
  - genetic: the mode of inheritance and the influence of this on counselling of both the patient and relatives.
- A clear biochemical confirmation of endocrine dysfunction.
- Exclusion of a paraendocrine syndrome.

Localisation of a tumour

A determination of the organ or organs involved; if an organ is paired (e.g. the adrenal), whether one or both are responsible. Accurate anatomical localisation is always of help, although in some special circumstances it can be omitted. Localising techniques are of three kinds:

- conventional imaging, including arteriography
- selective uptake of labelled precursors
- sampling of effluent blood from areas in the vicinity of the endocrine gland thought to be affected.

All of these techniques may also identify harmless, non-functioning adenomas which have been called (inelegantly) incidentalomas. The finding of such a lesion does not always confirm the clinical diagnosis of endocrine dysfunction. In addition, the presence of a tumour which has potential serious consequences must not be confused with one that is incidental.

Rendering the patient into a safe physiological state

Even if the ultimate treatment is surgical, it is often necessary, by preoperative medical management, to correct any deleterious effects of hormonal dysfunction (for example hypertension, hypoglycaemia, hypokalaemia). An urgent operation for endocrine dysfunction is rarely required.

Choice of management

Surgical treatment may not be the only option, and before it is undertaken other methods of management must be considered. Particularly in asymptomatic disorders (e.g. hypercalcaemia thought to be caused by a parathyroid adenoma or hyperplasia), the risks of operation must be balanced against those of progression of the disorder.

THYROID

Embryology

The thyroid gland is derived from an epithelial proliferation in the floor of the pharynx at a point that is later indicated by the foramen caecum at the junction of the anterior two-thirds and the posterior third of the tongue in the midline. The gland migrates downwards in front of the foregut to come to lie anterior to the trachea but, during this movement, remains attached to the floor of the mouth by a narrow canal – the thyroglossal duct – which ultimately disappears. Its persistence results in:

- thyroglossal sinus
- thyroglossal cyst (Fig. 32.1).

Surgical anatomy

The important features are:

- investment by a thick fibrous sheath (pretracheal fascia) which sends septa into the substance of the gland and also binds it to the larynx so that a normal gland rises on swallowing

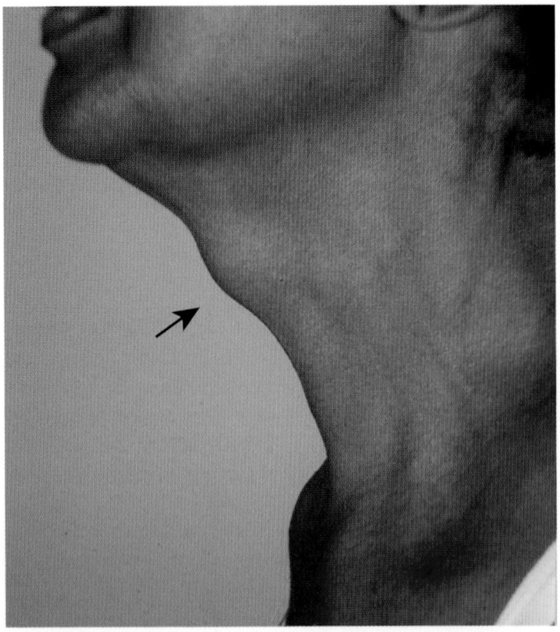

Fig. 32.1 Thyroglossal cyst overlying the hyoid bone.

- a rich blood supply from the paired superior and inferior thyroid arteries (Fig. 32.2) – increase in blood flow occurs in disease such as hyperthyroidism and may make surgical treatment more difficult
- lymphatic drainage to the middle and lower deep jugular, pretracheal and mediastinal nodes – the first two groups are initially involved in some malignant disorders
- proximity of the recurrent laryngeal nerve to the inferior thyroid artery, between whose branches it usually passes, although this is variable (Fig. 32.2) – injury, with paralysis of the vocal cord on the same side, may occur during operation
- application of the superior pole of the gland to the anterolateral aspect of the larynx, across which passes the external branch of the superior laryngeal nerve to supply the cricopharyngeus – damage to the nerve interferes with reaching a high note in speech and singing
- the close, though variable, relationship of the parathyroid glands to the posterior aspect of the thyroid – extensive dissection and/or inadvertent removal during surgical operations on the thyroid – may cause temporary or permanent hypoparathyroidism
- pyramidal lobe – a vertical tongue of thyroid tissue of variable size which arises from the isthmus and extends towards the hyoid bone; it is a remnant of the embryological descent of the gland
- aberrant thyroid tissue – found anywhere along embryological descent of the gland but always in the midline; common sites include the back of the tongue (lingual thyroid) and the anterior mediastinum (retrosternal extension).

Operations on the gland threaten adjacent vital structures, and these and the effects of injury are summarised in Table 32.5.

Histological features

The thyroid is composed of follicles (acini) which are roughly spherical with a diameter of 3 mm. Each is lined with epithelial cells which secrete the thyroid hormones that are stored in the colloid of the follicle. The cells are usually cuboidal but become columnar in response to the secretion of pituitary thyroid-stimulating hormone (TSH). A second group of cells – C cells – between the follicles, manufacture and secrete calcitonin.

Physiological features

The gland produces two types of hormones:

- those that regulate metabolic rate – thyroxine and its analogues
- calcitonin, which is concerned with calcium homeostasis.

Thyroxine and its analogues

Iodine is trapped by follicular cells and bound to tyrosine residues on the glycoprotein thyroglobulin. The iodine-containing residues – mono-iodotyrosine (MIT) and di-iodotyrosine (DIT) – are cleaved and coupled to yield tri-iodotyrosine (T_3) and thyroxine (T_4). Both the iodination reac-

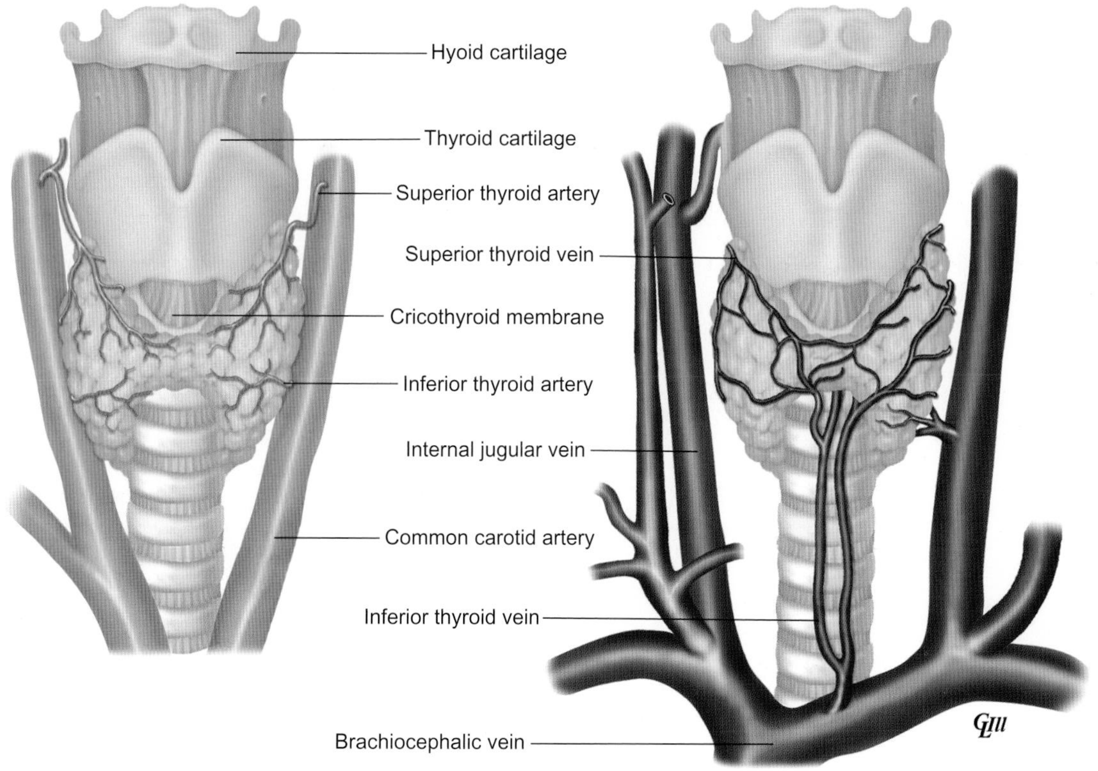

Fig. 32.2 Blood supply of the thyroid.

tion and the cleavage of MIT and DIT are catalysed by the enzyme thyroid peroxidase, which is membrane-bound and located at the apex of the follicular cell. T_3 and T_4 are bound in the circulation to thyroxine-binding globulin, thyroxine-binding pre-albumin and albumin. T_3 is believed to be the biologically active hormone formed predominantly from the peripheral de-iodination of circulating T_4.

The hypothalamic–thyroid axis regulates the production of T_3 and T_4. Thyrotrophin-releasing hormone (TRH) from the hypothalamus promotes the release of thyroid-stimulating hormone (TSH) from the anterior pituitary. TSH binds to its receptor on the follicular cell and stimulates synthesis and release of T_3 and T_4, whose presence in the blood decreases TRH and TSH output.

Thyroid hormones have wide-ranging metabolic and physiological effects, demonstrated by the variety of syndromes observed in both excess production (thyrotoxicosis) and deficiency (myxoedema).

Calcitonin

The hormone has actions that could decrease the concentration of calcium in the serum by inhibiting osteoclast-directed absorption of bone and by increased renal excretion of calcium. However, lack or excess of calcitonin has no overall effect on serum calcium (see page 540).

General pathological features

As described above, the thyroid is a target organ. It is influenced by:

- dietary intake of iodine – inadequate intake may cause hypertrophy (which may be followed by involution) because the gland seeks to extract as much of the element as possible so as to synthesise its hormones
- pituitary TSH
- other hormones – particularly oestrogens
- immune globulins which target the thyroid TSH receptor and may be important in causing thyrotoxicosis
- goitrogens – substances which block the normal pathways of synthesis of thyroid hormones.

In consequence, the gland undergoes cyclical hypertrophy and involution according to the internal environment to which it is exposed. Some pathological changes can follow. Repeated stimulation may result in areas of fibrosis – the gland becomes nodular, although only one nodule may be palpable. Most multinodular goitres are the consequence of this mechanism. Stimulation may be associated with clinical hyperactivity – thyrotoxicosis.

Evaluation of thyroid disease

The commonest symptom in thyroid disorder is goitre – an enlargement of the gland. Steps in the clinical assessment of a patient with goitre are given in Clinical Box 32.1.

Clinical features

History

Apart from presentation with a goitre, there may be other symptoms in the neck or of a change in thyroid hormonal status.

Clinical Box 32.1 Steps in the clinical assessment of a patient with a goitre

	History	Examination
Is there endocrine dysfunction?	Hypothyroid	Hypothyroid
	Hyperthyroid Euthyroid	Hyperthyroid Euthyroid
Is there suspicion of malignancy?	Rapid growth	Solitary hard mass
	Hoarseness Positive family history Exposure to ionising radiation	Lymphadenopathy
Is there compression of local structures?	Dysphagia	Tracheal deviation
	Dyspnoea	Stridor Retrosternal dullness

Associated neck symptoms are:

- dysphagia – compression of the oesophagus
- dyspnoea – compression or displacement of the trachea
- hoarse voice – infiltration of the recurrent laryngeal nerve, usually by carcinoma
- other lumps – usually lymph nodes.

Functional state may be:

- *euthyroid* – a normal level of thyroid function
- *hyperthyroid (thyrotoxic)* – increased levels of circulating thyroid hormones
- *hypothyroid* – decreased levels of circulating hormones.

An individual with a goitre may be in any of these three states.

Symptoms related to thyroid hyperactivity are:

- subjective – nervousness, irritability, behavioural change
- weight loss – in spite of a good appetite
- diarrhoea
- muscle weakness
- tremor
- intolerance of a hot environment, preference for cold
- loss of libido and, in addition, in women, oligomenorrhoea
- eye complaints (Table 32.1)

Symptoms of hypothyroidism are:

- slowness, tiredness and malaise
- weight gain, despite poor appetite
- intolerance of a cold environment, preference for warmth
- constipation
- depression, psychosis and (rarely) coma
- change in appearance – puffy eyes, dry skin and coarse hair
- poor libido and, in women, menorrhagia or oligomenorrhoea.

Table 32.1 Eye features in hyperthyroidism

Symptoms	Signs
Poor sight for both near and distant objects	Ophthalmoplegia
Double vision	
Grittiness in the eye	Conjunctival oedema (chemosis)
Exophthalmos – protrusion of the globes	Exophthalmos
	Lid retraction
	Lid lag

Features associated with cause are:

- place of long-term residence – an area of endemic goitre?
- family history – genetic causes
- drugs – antithyroid agents, iodide-containing medicines (asthma) and para-aminosalicylic acid (tuberculosis)
- age – puberty or the menopause
- pregnancy.

Physical findings

If a neck swelling is present and the thyroid is suspected as the cause, the matter can nearly always be decided by asking the patient to swallow: all thyroid swellings move upwards unless the neck is diffusely infiltrated with cancer.

Clinical features of thyrotoxicosis are:

- anxiety
- excessive purposeless movements
- diffuse fine tremor – best elicited in the outstretched fingers
- signs of recent weight loss – loose skin, little subcutaneous fat
- warm and often moist peripheries with vasodilatation
- sinus tachycardia and systolic hypertension
- atrial fibrillation and cardiac failure, especially in the older patient
- eye signs (Table 32.1)
- pretibial myxoedema – infiltration of the shin present only in those with eye signs
- proximal myopathy – particularly in the upper limbs.

Signs of hypothyroidism are:

- hypersomnolence
- slow relaxing tendon reflexes
- nerve entrapments – carpal tunnel syndrome
- cool, dry and thickened skin
- peripheral and periorbital oedema
- hoarse voice
- bradycardia
- cardiomegaly.

Examination of the thyroid. In addition to determining the usual features of consistency and contour, this should include:

- solitary or multiple nodules (Fig. 32.3)
- mobility of the gland on swallowing

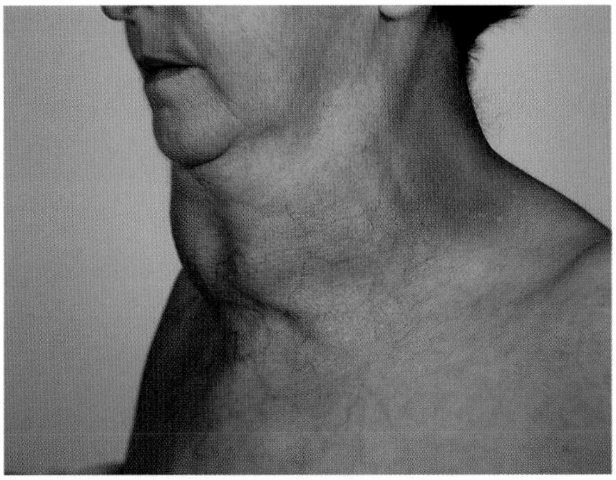

Fig. 32.3 Large, diffuse, nodular goitre.

- presence of cervical lymphadenopathy
- whether or not it is possible to get below any enlargement
- movement on protrusion of the tongue – characteristic of thyroglossal cyst
- palpation for a thrill and auscultation for a bruit – both features of an increased blood supply
- detection of tracheal deviation.

Diagnosis

After the history and clinical examination are complete, the clinical metabolic status (hyperthyroid, hypothyroid or euthyroid) and the nature of the goitre (diffuse, nodular or solitary nodule) will have been determined. This information allows the clinician to place the patient into a diagnostic category. However, some pitfalls of clinical assessment are as follows:

- Mild degrees of hyper- and hypothyroidism may not be clinically evident and may only be detected by tests of thyroid function.
- When a single nodule is thought to be present, there are often several others which are impalpable.

Some common diagnostic categories of goitre are described below.

Euthyroid – smooth enlargement. This is a diffuse, smooth, often firm goitre – it is most commonly an endemic condition, the result of the thyroid attempting to extract more iodine from the blood in circumstances when there is iodine deficiency; this may be an early phase which progresses to multinodular goitre. Thyroid enlargement in pregnancy is a similar condition.

Euthyroid – multinodular goitre. The majority of patients present with this. The most common cause is endemic (iodine deficiency in the diet) or sporadic goitre (isolated occurrences affecting few people), but these features may be seen in long-standing goitres that are the consequence of cell hyperplasia, including autoimmune thyroiditis.

Euthyroid – single palpable nodule (clinical solitary nodule). In this case, the rest of the gland may be truly normal; alternatively there may be other impalpable nodules.

Hyperthyroid – diffuse goitre. The whole gland is enlarged and soft and its surface is smooth – typical of Graves' disease. Other features such as eye signs may be present.

Hyperthyroid – gland multinodular. This is the so-called secondary thyrotoxicosis seen commonly in the older patient who usually gives a history of long-standing goitre.

Hypothyroid – varying goitre, either smooth or multinodular. The typical clinical signs of Hashimoto's thyroiditis are seen.

Investigation

There are three general methods:

- tests of thyroid function
- imaging
- biopsy.

Thyroid function

Most laboratories measure blood levels of free thyroxine, free tri-iodothyronine (T_3) and TSH. Many authorities recommend measurement of TSH as the initial investigation of patients with suspected hypo-or hyperthyroidism. If the outcome is abnormal, then output hormones are measured.

Thyroid function tests may be unreliable in three circumstances:

- severe acute or chronic illness – total and free T_3 and T_4 tend to be low and basal TSH normal or low (sick euthyroid syndrome); values return to normal when the underlying illness has resolved
- pregnancy and in those taking oral contraceptives – levels of thyroid hormones are often greatly increased but do not cause clinical problems
- intake of drugs that affect thyroid hormone protein binding – these include antithyroid drugs, lithium and amiodarone.

Imaging

Techniques available are:

- X-ray of neck, thoracic inlet and chest
- ultrasound
- CT or MRI
- isotope scans – ^{123}I and ^{99m}Tc pertechnetate.

These are used in three circumstances:

- hyperthyroidism – when the cause is thought to be a solitary nodule
- thyroid cancer
- ectopic thyroid.

Hyperthyroidism. ^{99m}Tc scan is the investigation of choice for patients assumed to be hyperthyroid. It is relatively cheap and exposes the patient to a lower dose of radiation than an iodine isotope scan. This imaging can reliably distinguish between the common causes of thyrotoxicosis.

Thyroid cancer. In primary tumour, ultrasound establishes whether the lesion is solid or cystic, and an isotope scan whether it is hot or cold (functioning or non-functioning).

However, neither investigation can reliably determine if a lesion is benign or malignant.

When there is metastatic disease after the thyroid primary has been removed (usually by total thyroidectomy), total body radionuclide scanning is very sensitive for the detection of deposits of differentiated thyroid cancer. Both CT and MRI are also useful in assessing the extent of undifferentiated cancer.

In postoperative follow-up, iodine scanning is valuable to detect recurrent disease.

Ectopic thyroid tissue. Abnormal locations include the midline of the upper neck and the anterior mediastinum. A correct diagnosis must be made because of the risk of excising what is the only functional thyroid tissue. Scanning with ^{123}I is the best technique because it is more specific for thyroid tissues than is ^{99m}Tc and avoids confusion with salivary glands which also take up technetium. The radiation dose for ^{123}I is much less than for ^{131}I, and it is therefore safely used in the young.

Biopsy

There are two methods of biopsy:

- fine-needle aspiration cytology (FNAC)
- core biopsy with a drill or wide-bore needle.

In both, a nodule is targeted either by palpation or with the help of ultrasound.

FNAC is a reliable method of providing a tissue diagnosis but is dependent on an experienced cytopathologist. There is a strict classification for FNAC results (Table 32.2). The technique is useful in suspected malignancy, particularly a solitary nodule in which ultrasound imaging and isotope scanning lack specificity for the prediction of a histological diagnosis. Although FNAC has a low incidence of false-positive results, the false-negative rate may be as high as 20%, and clinicians must be aware that a negative report does not exclude cancer. Liquid aspirates of cystic lesions are examined for malignant cells, although these are rarely found.

Core biopsy using a Tru-Cut or other wide-bore needle, is done under local anaesthesia and provides tissue that can be examined histologically. The risk of haemorrhage precludes its routine use other than in a hard, fixed mass such as a widely infiltrating carcinoma or lymphoma.

Table 32.2 Classification of thyroid FNAC

Classification	Cytology report
Thy 1	Acellular – no diagnosis can be made
Thy 2	Benign
Thy 3	Follicular neoplasm *Or* Some suspicious features of papillary cancer
Thy 4	Very suspicious for malignancy
Thy 5	Definite malignancy

NON-TOXIC GOITRE

A simple hyperplastic goitre is caused by stimulation of the thyroid from a raised circulation level of TSH, which is, in turn, the outcome of low levels of circulating thyroid hormones. The end stage of such hyperplasia is a multinodular goitre.

Epidemiology and aetiology

The underlying factor is an absolute or relative deficiency in dietary iodine. Causes are:

- in endemic areas from iodine lack in the soil (geographically on high ground where, on a geological time scale, rain has washed out soluble elements such as iodine)
- change in physiological demand
- blockage of normal uptake or processing of iodine within the gland – usually goitrogens in the diet or in medications
- enzyme malfunction in the gland.

Endemic iodine deficiency causes the gland to enlarge and produce a goitre as it attempts to extract sufficient iodine from the diet where this is deficient.

Physiological variations such as puberty and pregnancy may alter demand for thyroid hormones and cause temporary enlargement of the gland. In pregnancy, increased renal iodine excretion, raised TRH concentration and direct stimulation of the thyroid by β-hCG (human chorionic gonadotrophin) all induce hyperplasia.

Goitrogens are chemicals which interfere with thyroid hormone synthesis. They are found in foods such as cabbage and cassava, and goitres are common in areas where these are consumed in large quantities.

Enzyme malfunction is manifest clinically when, for example, peroxidase, responsible for organification of trapped iodine, is deficient. Syndromes of this type (e.g. Pendred's syndrome, a combination of goitre and congenital deafness) are genetic.

Hyperplastic goitres can occur in childhood in endemic areas, but those of physiological cause appear between 15 and 30 years. Goitres from goitrogens may be seen at any age. In almost all instances, females outnumber males by nearly 5:1.

Clinical features

History

The patient is euthyroid and complains of a painless, gradually progressive swelling in the neck. In later stages there may be discomfort or pain. Tracheal or oesophageal compression may develop with dyspnoea or dysphagia, particularly if there is retrosternal extension.

Physical findings

During the hyperplastic phase, the thyroid is often better seen than felt, its surface is smooth and the consistency soft. Later, nodules develop and the gland often becomes large – sometimes enormous – and firm. Occasionally only one nodule is palpable, although there are microscopic changes throughout the gland. Such a single clinical nodule is often referred to as dominant. The trachea may be displaced, and there may, in advanced enlargement, be signs of obstruction of the superior vena cava with distended veins coursing over the neck and chest. Regional lymphadenopathy or a hoarse voice suggests malignant change.

Investigation

The most important consideration is to establish whether or not there is a carcinoma. It used to be taught that multinodular goitres are almost never malignant, but recent studies indicate that the histological incidence of malignant change may be as high as 16%. However, in that the potential of such microscopic lesions to invade the thyroid capsule is not known, their clinical significance is questionable.

Thyroid function tests

Confirmation of the clinical status should be obtained. Most patients are euthyroid, but some are hypothyroid. An older patient with a goitre and features of cardiac disease such as arrhythmia or heart failure may be thyrotoxic without any other clinical features of overactivity.

Imaging

Plain X-ray of the chest and thoracic inlet (Fig. 32.4) may show:

- tracheal compression and deviation
- retrosternal extension
- glandular calcification.

Ultrasound is the best way to demonstrate multiple nodules. High resolution can distinguish cysts from solid lesions.

Isotope scans show irregular uptake. Cold nodules may be areas of cystic degeneration, fibrosis or malignancy. The main indications for the use of an isotope scan are:

- possible retrosternal extension
- recurrent multinodular goitre in which the quantity of thyroid tissue is uncertain.

Biopsy

Fine-needle aspiration cytology of the clinically dominant nodule should be done.

Management

Euthyroid goitre

This may well resolve spontaneously and requires reassurance only. Surgical intervention is necessary only if resolution does not occur and the goitre is cosmetically unacceptable, becomes nodular or produces compressive symptoms.

Hypothyroid goitre

Thyroxine treatment is necessary to restore and maintain the euthyroid state. It provides an extraneous source of hormone and so suppresses the cellular hyperactivity that causes the goitre.

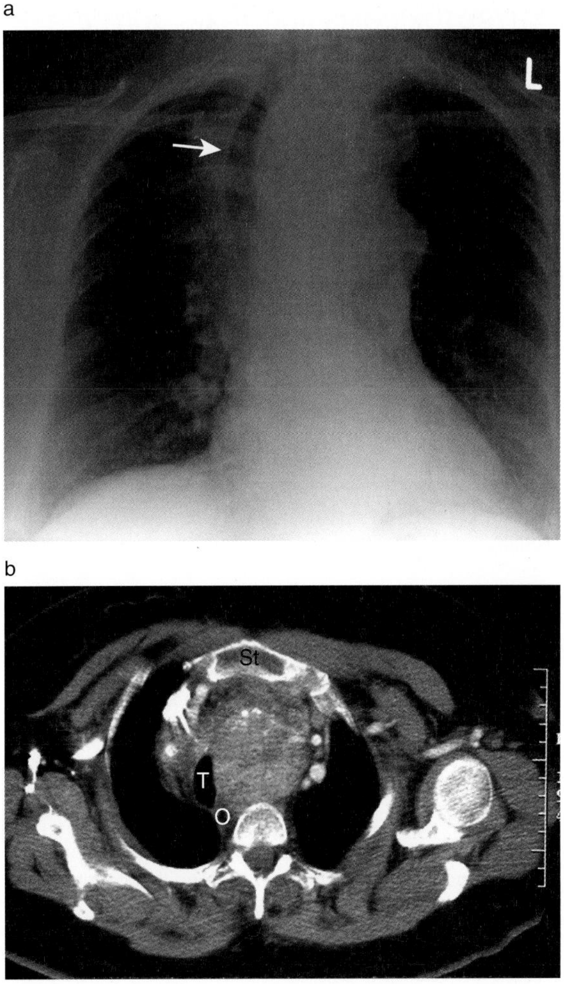

Fig. 32.4 (a) Chest X-ray showing mediastinal mass with displacement of the trachea to the right (arrow). (b) CT scan of same patient, demonstrating calcified goitre behind the sternum (St) displacing trachea (T) and oesophagus (O) to the right.

Multinodular goitre

Once nodules are associated with significant enlargement of the gland, return to normality with thyroid replacement is unlikely to succeed. Provided there is no suggestion of malignancy, it is acceptable to leave the gland alone and follow its progress by repeated clinical examination. Surgical excision is done if there is:

- suspicion of malignancy that has not been allayed by the investigations described above
- cosmetic problems
- pressure symptoms from tracheal or oesophageal compression.

In extensive disease, a total excision may be necessary but must be done only by experienced surgeons because of the risk of damage to the parathyroids and recurrent laryngeal nerves.

THYROTOXICOSIS AND TOXIC GOITRE

Thyrotoxicosis or hyperthyroidism is the clinical syndrome which results from the peripheral actions of raised levels of circulating thyroid hormones.

Clinical classification

Thyrotoxicosis is a relatively common problem affecting nearly 2% of females and 0.15% of males. It has several distinctive causes whose manifestations and treatment are different. Ninety-five per cent of instances are the result of the three most common causes:

- diffuse toxic goitre – Graves' disease
- multinodular toxic goitre
- solitary toxic adenoma.

Rarely, manifestations of the disease are the consequence of self-administration of thyroxine (thyrotoxicosis factitia).

Graves' disease

This is the commonest cause of thyrotoxicosis and can occur at any age, although the peak incidence is between 20 and 40 years. Women are affected five times more often than males.

Aetiology

It is caused by an autoimmune process characterised by the presence of a spectrum of abnormal autoantibodies, whose actions are directed against the thyroid TSH receptor (thyroid receptor antibodies, TRABs). Why they are produced is unclear but there is evidence that genetic factors are concerned. The eyes may be involved (Graves' ophthalmopathy) because of a cross-reaction between antibodies to eye muscles and thyroid antigens. There is a group of patients who have all the ocular features of Graves' disease but who are euthyroid – ophthalmic Graves' disease.

Clinical features

The natural history of Graves' disease is one of intermittent remission and relapse. Forty per cent of patients have a single episode only.

The symptoms of thyrotoxicosis are summarised above. There may be a history of autoimmune disease. Eye involvement may produce double vision.

The thyroid is often uniformly enlarged, firm, smooth and moves on swallowing. There may be a bruit. When there are eye problems chemosis and periorbital oedema may be seen. The specific eye signs are summarised in Table 32.1.

Investigation

Thyroid function tests. These confirm thyrotoxicosis with an elevated T_4 and T_3 and reduced TSH.

Thyroid autoantibodies. Anti-thyroglobulin and anti-microsomal antibodies are present when the cause is autoimmune.

Table 32.3 Comparison of multinodular toxic goitre and Graves' disease

Feature	Multinodular toxic goitre	Graves' disease
Onset	Over 50	Puberty to early 20s
Symptoms related to nervous system	Uncommon	Common
Cardiac involvement	Common	Uncommon
Thyroid enlargement	Usually slight and irregular	Can be considerable – diffuse, smooth and soft
Tracheal displacement	Not uncommon	Rare

Multinodular toxic goitre (Plummer's syndrome)

This is sometimes referred to as secondary toxic goitre in that a goitre has been present for several years before the development of toxic features. The disease is more common in women and usually presents after the age of 50. Eye disease is unusual but cardiac arrhythmias and heart failure are common presenting features. The goitre is nodular and may be large, sometimes displacing the trachea. Features which distinguish multinodular toxic goitre from Graves' disease are summarised in Table 32.3.

Toxic solitary adenoma/nodule

Aetiology

This is a solitary autonomous adenoma. The cause of toxicity is not known but it is clear that long-acting thyroid stimulators (LATS) are not involved. The condition is responsible for nearly 5% of all hyperthyroidism. A single nodule in the gland becomes overactive and produces high levels of thyroxine, causing suppression of all surrounding thyroid tissue. This property permits diagnosis of a solitary toxic nodule on an isotope scan because the nodule takes up isotope but the surrounding gland does not. Eye disease is unusual in thyrotoxicosis caused by a solitary nodule.

Management of thyrotoxicosis

General principles

It is important to distinguish between the three types of thyrotoxic disease, as their specific treatments differ. However, a common principle is to make all patients euthyroid before surgery is contemplated.

In addition, other secondary problems should be brought under control, although suppression of thyrotoxicosis may lead to their spontaneous resolution:

- eye complications (Table 32.4)
- cardiac complications – managed by medical means.

Antithyroid agents. Carbimazole and related drugs block thyroid peroxidase and therefore inhibit thyroxine synthesis.

Table 32.4 Management of eye complications in Graves' disease

Problem	Treatment
Exposed cornea with drying	Methylcellulose eye drops for lubrication
Failure of lid closure in marked exophthalmos	Tarsorrhaphy
Inflammation	Systemic steroids
Deterioration in sight from compressive optic atrophy	Surgical decompression of both orbits
Severe diplopia	Corrective surgery to eye muscles

They are the agents of choice in the UK for the initial management of the thyrotoxic state. The dose is 10–40 mg daily, and the major side effect is agranulocytosis. However, the long half-life of T_4 means that the therapeutic response is slow – up to 8 weeks may be required to reduce the metabolic and other effects of excess levels. Thyroxine is added to the above therapies in some instances to enable a larger dose of antithyroid drug to be given to suppress the gland as much as possible without producing hypothyroidism (block and replace regimen).

Beta-adrenergic blocking agents are effective in reducing the effects of T_4 on the sympathetic system, which is the way in which thyrotoxicosis is manifest both physiologically and clinically. Propranolol is most commonly used. It may be administered parenterally in a severely toxic patient.

Management of specific causes of thyrotoxicosis

Graves' disease

Non-operative

The nature of the disease and the possibility that only one episode will occur makes non-operative management the first-line approach. Antithyroid agents are continued for 6–18 months. One-third of those treated become permanently euthyroid. The majority of those who relapse do so in the first 2 years after treatment is stopped.

Radioactive iodine (I^{131}) may be used to ablate the thyroid gland permanently and is widely used an alternative to thyroidectomy. Contraindications include current or planned pregnancy and possibly also severe ophthalmopathy. There is a lifelong risk of developing hypothyroidism and long-term follow-up is necessary with replacement therapy as required.

Operation

Thyroidectomy is not usually required but is indicated for:

- patients unwilling to undergo prolonged drug treatment
- relapse after drug therapy
- intractable side effects of therapy
- failure of compliance
- large goitre after effective drug treatment.

Total thyroidectomy is the standard operation.

Specific complications of thyroidectomy for Graves' disease are:

Box 32.1 Causes of a clinical solitary nodule

- Dominant nodule of multinodular goitre
- Cyst
- Localised Hashimoto's disease
- Non-functioning adenoma
- Functioning adenoma
- Primary malignant tumour
- Metastatic deposit

- recurrence of hyperthyroidism (3%) if a less-than-total thyroidectomy is undertaken – managed by antithyroid agents and therapeutic radioiodine
- hypothyroidism (10% of patients within 1 year of operation) – it is particularly likely if microsomal antibodies were present before the operation, because they continue to destroy the thyroid remnant; the proportion rises with time.

Treatment of eye problems

Eye disease may improve or regress completely when the patient has reached a euthyroid state, but not always. The management is given in Table 32.4.

Multinodular toxic goitre

Non-operative

Antithyroid drugs very uncommonly induce remission.

Radioactive iodine is the definitive treatment for those with:

- small goitres
- absence of pressure symptoms
- disorders which preclude surgery – usually severe heart disease
- refusal of an operation.

Operation

Thyroidectomy. In large goitres, pressure symptoms may persist after medical treatment for thyrotoxicosis unless the bulk of the thyroid tissue is removed. In such instances, a total thyroidectomy is the preferred treatment provided that the risk is low for the individual patient.

Solitary toxic nodule

Radioactive iodine ablation is probably the best option. The remainder of the thyroid does not concentrate the ^{131}I because it has been suppressed secondary to the undetectable level of TSH. An alternative strategy is to surgically excise the nodule together with the lobe in which it is contained.

CLINICAL SOLITARY THYROID NODULE

Aetiology and pathological features

Between 1% and 3% of the population have an isolated thyroid nodule, and the proper approach to its presence must be understood. The causes are summarised in Box 32.1. The chance of malignancy being present is about 10%. Risk factors include:

- previous neck irradiation
- family history of thyroid carcinoma.

Clinical features

The history and physical findings are the same as in multinodular goitre, but only a single nodule is found in an otherwise apparently normal gland.

Investigation

Thyroid function tests

These are done to exclude toxicity, but in the majority the state is euthyroid.

Imaging

Ultrasound determines whether the nodule is truly solitary or multiple – a dominant nodule in a multinodular goitre is the commonest cause of a clinical solitary nodule. In experienced hands ultrasound can also identify lymphadenopathy.

FNAC

This is the preferred method of diagnosis and often makes a preoperative diagnosis available. However, as indicated above, in certain circumstances it may be unreliable.

Management

If a definite diagnosis of malignancy has not been achieved preoperatively, the operation is a total thyroid lobectomy. The resected tissue is examined histologically, and, if the result is malignant, a completion total thyroidectomy is done.

MANAGEMENT OF PATIENTS WHO ARE TO UNDERGO THYROID OPERATIONS

Preoperative management

Investigations specific to operations on the thyroid (and the parathyroids) are:

- direct laryngoscopy to assess vocal cord function
- measurement of baseline plasma calcium concentration
- white cell count in patients who have received antithyroid agents
- thyroid function tests to ensure that patients are euthyroid at the time of surgery.

Informed consent of possible complications should cover bleeding, nerve injury, transient hypocalcaemia and long-term hypoparathyroidism.

Medication. Antithyroid agents and beta-adrenergic blockers are continued up to the day of operation. It is now almost unknown for a patient to be operated upon without having been rendered euthyroid and without the other toxicity effects, such as cardiac arrhythmias, having been treated.

Operation

Dissection must be precise, and structures at risk of injury should be formally identified (Table 32.5). Because of the serious nature of bleeding into the neck, haemostasis must be rigorous.

Table 32.5 Important structures which must be safeguarded at thyroidectomy

Structure	Result of injury
Recurrent laryngeal nerve	Paresis or paralysis of vocal cord: • unilateral – hoarseness • bilateral – stridor; change in voice; risk of aspiration
Parathyroid glands	Hypocalcaemia – severity depends on amount of tissue that remains
External laryngeal nerve	Paresis or paralysis of cricothyroid muscle – inability to achieve high-pitched notes

Emergency Box 32.1

Postoperative (thyroid or parathyroid surgery) upper airway obstruction

Symptoms: distress, dyspnoea
Signs: stridor, hypoxia, altered consciousness

Action:

- High-flow oxygen
- Sit patient upright
- Call for help:
  - anaesthetist
  - ICU staff
  - surgical consultant
- If evidence of wound haemorrhage (swelling, bruising), immediately remove skin sutures and deep sutures to strap muscles to evacuate haematoma
- If evidence of recurrent laryngeal nerve injury (bovine cough, exertional stridor), resuscitate and wait for anaesthetist

Complications

Bleeding

Bleeding into the neck causes dyspnoea and stridor (respiratory obstruction) usually within 24 hours of operation. This is an emergency and may require the wound to be opened without return to the operating room (Emergency Box 32.1). Alternatively, reintubation and formal drainage may be necessary.

Hypocalcaemia

The condition is unusual if only one lobe has been operated upon. After a total thyroidectomy the calcium level is routinely measured on the day after the operation and, if it is low, administration of oral calcium carbonate may be indicated. The first clinical features are paraesthesia around the mouth and in the digits; later there is muscle spasm and finally tetany. The two typical clinical signs are:

- Trousseau's – occlusion of the circulation to the hand causes small muscle spasm
- Chvostek–Weiss – tapping the branches of the facial nerve in front of the ear induces spasm of the facial muscles.

Although not life-threatening, the condition is disturbing and is managed according to the protocol set out in Emergency Box 32.2.

Management of patients who are to undergo thyroid operations
Thyroiditis

Emergency Box 32.2

Postoperative (thyroid or parathyroid surgery) hypocalcaemia

Symptoms: paraesthesiae of extremities (fingers, toes, lips)
Signs: Trousseau and Chvostek–Weiss
Investigation: Plasma calcium (uncuffed) corrected to albumin of 40 g/L

Action:

Plasma calcium (mmol/L)[a]	Symptomatic	Asymptomatic
>2.15	Milk	Nil
2.00–2.15	Calcium carbonate 2.5G t.d.s.	Calcium carbonate 2.5G o.d.
1.90–2.00	Calcium carbonate 2.5G t.d.s. 1-Alfacalcidol 1 μg o.d.	Calcium carbonate 2.5G t.d.s.
1.80–1.90	Calcium carbonate 2.5G t.d.s. 1-Alfacalcidol 1 μg b.d.	Calcium carbonate 2.5G t.d.s. 1-Alfacalcidol 1 μg b.d.
< 1.80	Tetany – 10–30 m i.v. calcium gluconate over 10–15 min	L Calcium carbonate 2.5G t.d.s. 1-Alfacalcidol 1 μg t.d.s.

[a]Corrected to albumin of 40 g/L.

Nerve injury

The nerves at risk are the recurrent and superior laryngeal. Identification of injury to the recurrent laryngeal nerve at the time of surgery is followed by immediate repair. If recurrent nerve injury is diagnosed after operation (more commonly the case) the patient should be promptly referred to a specialist ear, nose and throat (ENT) surgeon. Invasive treatment is withheld for about 9 months as nerves that have been stretched or bruised can recover, and patients are prescribed speech therapy. If severe disability persists beyond this time, techniques such as injection of polytetrafluoroethylene (PTFE) into the vocal cord and surgical lateral fixation may be considered. The superior laryngeal nerve supplies sensation to the larynx and hypopharynx as well as motor innervation to the cricothyroid muscle. A superior laryngeal nerve palsy changes the pitch of the voice and causes an inability to make explosive sounds. A bilateral palsy presents as a tiring and hoarse voice. When diagnosed, specialist ENT referral is made.

Thyrotoxic storm (syn. *crisis)*

Adequate preoperative treatment to restore a euthyroid state has now almost abolished this major complication, which had a mortality of 10%. The cause is the release of large amounts of thyroxine into the circulation. Ancillary factors which may be involved in the thyrotoxic subject are:

- stress or infection
- operations, other than those on the thyroid
- therapeutic doses of radioactive iodine with consequent cell destruction.

Historically the condition was most common in the early postoperative period after manipulation and resection of the thyroid. Its clinical features include restlessness, confusion, tachycardia and hyperpyrexia. In severe cases, the patient may become hypotensive and may suffer cardiac arrest.

Prevention is to ensure the euthyroid state before operation, which, if there are urgent indications, can be done within a week by the use of a combination of carbimazole, iodine and, most importantly, a beta-adrenergic blocking agent.

Treatment is urgent and is with full doses of propranolol, potassium iodide and antithyroid drugs; propylthiouracil is preferred.

THYROIDITIS

Hashimoto's thyroiditis

This is an autoimmune disease of unknown cause. The thyroid is diffusely infiltrated by lymphoid and plasma cells with the formation of germinal centres and destruction of thyroid follicles.

Clinical features

History

In the early stages of the disorder, there may be thyrotoxicosis, but with progression, symptoms of hypothyroidism are typical. A goitre may occasionally be the presenting feature and produce pressure symptoms.

Physical findings

A diffuse goitre is characteristic and is firm with an irregular (bosselated) surface. Less commonly, the disease is focal and there is a solitary nodule.

Investigation and management

Titres of autoantibodies directed against thyroglobulin and thyroid microsomes are markedly elevated. The biochemical pattern of hypothyroidism (raised TSH and low T_4) is present. There is no need for isotope scanning. In focal thyroiditis, FNAC is used to confirm the diagnosis.

Management is by lifelong thyroxine replacement. Most goitres shrink to a minimal size, but those that persist rarely require thyroidectomy.

De Quervain's thyroiditis

This is an uncommon condition caused by viral infection. There is an acute inflammatory reaction in the gland, with histiocytes, multinucleate giant cells and granuloma formation.

Clinical features

The history is of an acute pain in the neck, accompanied by malaise and pyrexia. A tender enlarged thyroid will be seen.

Investigation and management

The ESR is raised and, in the early stages, there may be an elevated T_4 and a low TSH consistent with hyperthyroidism. Thyroid antibodies are absent.

The condition is self-limiting, and analgesics and NSAIDs are all that is required.

Reidel's thyroiditis

This is an exceptionally rare condition of unknown cause. There is dense fibrosis, not confined to the gland but extending into the surrounding soft tissues of the neck. It may occur in isolation or with other analogous disorders such as periaortitis (retroperitoneal fibrosis), sclerosing cholangitis and mediastinal fibrosis.

Clinical features

A rapidly increasing goitre is noticed by the patient, often with features of tracheal or oesophageal compression. A hard, woody goitre which is palpable will be found on examination.

Investigation and management

Diagnostic criteria do not exist. The priority is to exclude malignant disease. FNAC demonstrates scanty fibroblasts, but open biopsy may be required for diagnostic certainty.

Decompression of neck structures may be required, and tracheostomy is occasionally necessary.

CANCER OF THE THYROID

This condition is relatively uncommon, causing less than 0.5% of all deaths from malignant disease, but, perhaps because of interesting biological features, has attracted considerable clinical and research interest.

Aetiology

The cause of most thyroid cancers is not known. However, certain predisposing factors are:

- genetic – a quarter of patients with medullary carcinoma of the thyroid have a familial condition which may be associated with neoplasms in other endocrine organs MEN II
- radiation – either from external-beam radiotherapy given for malignant conditions of the head and neck, or from the environment (^{131}I), where exposure occurs because of high natural levels or from nuclear explosions (Hiroshima and Nagasaki) or accidents (Chernobyl).

Pathological classification

There are five types of thyroid cancers:

- papillary
- follicular
- medullary
- lymphoma
- anaplastic.

The first two are usually grouped together as differentiated carcinoma. The pathological features and behaviour are so different that they are considered in relation to each type of growth.

Modes of presentation

Incidental finding

Occult thyroid tumours may be encountered either within a resection specimen or at the time of surgery for benign disease.

Primary tumour

The patient notices a painless lump in the neck, and examination reveals a solitary thyroid nodule. Physical signs of local invasion are:

- hoarseness – typical of invasion of the recurrent laryngeal nerve
- stridor
- fixation of the lump.

Metastatic disease

An enlarged lymph node in the neck may first call attention to the disease, as may distant spread to lung, bone or brain.

Differentiated cancer

Papillary carcinoma

Pathological features

Papillary carcinoma accounts for two-thirds of all thyroid malignancies and is generally a slow-growing tumour with a good prognosis. Many tumours are found only at postmortem examination (13–28%). Histologically, finger-like tumour papillae are present, and the growth is often multifocal. Psammoma bodies are typical. The tumour invades lymphatics, and over 50% of patients have cervical lymph node involvement at presentation.

Investigation

Euthyroidism is the rule. The diagnostic investigation is FNAC. Ultrasound shows a solid lesion and may reveal enlarged lymph nodes.

Follicular carcinoma

Pathological features

Follicular carcinoma is a well-encapsulated solitary tumour which accounts for 20% of all thyroid malignancies and has a favourable prognosis. There is a uniform follicular structure, and the diagnosis of cancer as distinct from a follicular adenoma is dependent on the presence of extracapsular or vascular invasion. The tumour spreads by the bloodstream, whereas cervical node involvement is found in only 5%.

Investigation

Euthyroidism is always the case. FNAC is unreliable in distinguishing between follicular adenoma and carcinoma. Aspiration cytology that yields follicular cells (Thy 3) should be followed by removal of the involved lobe and histological examination for the features of cancer.

Management of differentiated carcinoma

Primary tumour

The minimal procedure is total thyroid lobectomy with resection of the isthmus. Thereafter, clinical opinion (rather than prospective studies) supports either thyroxine suppression of TSH production or destruction of all thyroid tissue by total thyroidectomy followed by ^{131}I therapeutic ablation. The thinking underlying the use of thyroid ablation is as follows:

- Papillary tumours are multifocal.
- Follow-up by repeated measurements of thyroglobulin and ^{131}I diagnostic scanning is more sensitive.

- The incidence of local recurrence is reduced.
- Survival is improved and local recurrence rates reduced.

However, total thyroid lobectomy with thyroid suppression is adequate treatment for small (<10 mm) solitary incidental tumours and avoids the greater morbidity of total thyroidectomy. Adverse prognostic indicators that influence surgeons to undertake total ablation are:

- age over 50 years
- tumour diameter greater than 10 mm
- presence of local invasion or distant metastases
- pronounced vascular invasion in follicular carcinoma.

Metastases

Cervical lymph nodes. Involvement of these by tumour is not an indicator of survival. Involved nodes are best resected because this reduces the incidence of local recurrence.

Distant metastases. The majority of differentiated tumours are functional, i.e. they concentrate iodine. This property not only facilitates their detection by a radioisotope scan but also their treatment with ^{131}I. However, metastases are only detected once the whole thyroid has been ablated. For the less-differentiated tumours that do not concentrate iodine, external-beam radiotherapy is used.

Follow-up

Total-body iodine scanning

In addition to regular clinical examination, patients who have undergone total thyroid ablation have a total-body radioiodine scan which necessitates stopping replacement therapy with levothyroxine for 6 weeks.

Thyroglobulin

Most differentiated tumours produce this protein; it is therefore a useful postoperative tumour marker.

Most clinicians measure the thyroglobulin on an annual basis and resort to total body scanning when a rise is detected.

Medullary carcinoma

Aetiology and pathological features

These tumours account for 5–10% of thyroid malignancies and are derived from C cells, which means that they produce calcitonin that can be detected in the blood. Three-quarters occur sporadically, but there is a genetic basis for the other quarter. Such familial medullary carcinoma:

- is inherited in an autosomal dominant manner with an age-related penetrance
- frequently has a pre-invasive phase – C-cell hyperplasia – which is diffusely distributed throughout the gland
- is often multifocal
- can be associated with other endocrine disorders such as phaeochromocytoma and parathyroid hyperplasia (see 'MEN II' syndrome, below).

Screening of relatives

Relatives of those with familial medullary carcinoma must be screened at the time of diagnosis. Historically, this has relied on biochemical tests of the blood and urine (plasma calcium concentration and 24-hour urinary excretion of metanephrines); but negative results do not exclude involvement, because the disorder may only become apparent in relatives several years after screening. The development of genetic tests for the presence of the specific mutations associated with MEN syndromes has removed the requirement for repeated screening when an individual is shown to be unaffected and has led to prophylactic thyroidectomy in those whose genetic test is positive.

Clinical features

History

For those with a family history, the diagnosis may be established by screening at a stage when symptoms are absent. Otherwise, the history is of a lump in the neck or of distant metastases. Rarely there is diarrhoea because of high plasma concentrations of calcitonin.

Physical findings

These vary with the stage of the disease:

- thyroid nodule or nodules
- mass in the neck either from lymph node metastases or advanced local disease
- features of distant metastases
- marfanoid phenotype (see MEN II).

Investigation

Familial tumours

Screen-detected individuals should undergo a 'prophylactic thyroidectomy'. The specific mutation dictates at what age the patient should undergo surgery, but for most, surgery is undertaken before school-age.

Sporadic tumours

Blood examination. Plasma calcitonin is elevated.

FNAC is done on a thyroid mass or lymph node enlargement.

Imaging. CT cross-sectional imaging is useful to detect both the primary tumour and secondary deposits.

Management

Total thyroidectomy with lymph node dissection and thyroid replacement therapy comprise the initial treatment. In the postoperative period, patients are monitored by measurements of plasma calcitonin. Surgical resection is preferred for local recurrence. The prognosis is determined by the stage of the disease but is less favourable than differentiated thyroid cancer.

Anaplastic carcinoma

These are aggressive tumours and are believed to arise from previously unrecognised differentiated tumours. They are more common in areas where endemic goitre is prevalent, but the incidence is decreasing. Usually the presentation is at or above 60 years.

Clinical features

Typically patients present with a rapidly enlarging goitre and hoarseness. A long-standing goitre may have been present which has recently increased in size and perhaps caused pressure symptoms.

The physical finding is of a hard woody mass with fixation to surrounding structures. Clinically the condition can be confused with lymphoma.

Investigation and management

FNAC or, if this is equivocal, core biopsy will confirm the diagnosis. Lung metastases are frequently found on a chest X-ray.

Surgery is avoided to prevent fungation through the operation wound, and the patient is usually treated by external-beam radiotherapy. These tumours do not respond to radioiodine.

Anaplastic carcinoma has a uniformly poor prognosis, and few patients survive beyond 12 months.

LYMPHOMA

This is a rare growth (2% of thyroid malignancies) typically affecting elderly females. Long-standing Hashimoto's thyroiditis is the only known risk factor. The condition is part of the non-Hodgkin's B-cell lymphoma group.

The presentation is similar to that of anaplastic carcinoma.

Investigation and management

The diagnosis is either made by cytology using flow cytometry or from a core biopsy. The tumour can be staged by a CT and PET scans.

Treatment is undertaken by haemato-oncologists and involves chemotherapy and sometimes radiotherapy. Surgery has no role in the management of thyroid lymphoma. The prognosis is much better than that for anaplastic carcinoma, and to make the distinction is therefore important.

PARATHYROID

Embryology

The superior parathyroid glands (IV) are derived from the fourth pharyngeal pouch, whereas the inferior glands (III) are from the more cephalad third pharyngeal pouch. The explanation for this apparent paradox is that of the common origin of the inferior glands and the thymus. From the fifth week of gestation, the thymus gland (also derived from the third pouch) descends into the superior mediastinum, dragging the inferior parathyroids with it. In consequence, some surgeons refer to the inferior parathyroids as 'parathymic'.

Anatomy

Because of their complicated embryological derivation, the precise location of individual glands is variable, although it tends to be symmetrical. The superior glands are usually found adjacent to the thyroid, typically within a 1 cm radius, above the junction of the inferior thyroid artery and the recurrent laryngeal nerve. The inferior glands are usually located in a condensation of fascia between the lower pole of the thyroid and the thymus (the thyro-thymic ligament). However, they may lie in the superior mediastinum or within the carotid sheath. The typical parathyroid gland is only 1 mm × 3 mm × 5 mm and weighs approximately 30 mg; the total weight of parathyroid tissue is thus about 120 mg. The blood supply for both pairs of glands is usually from the inferior thyroid artery. Fewer than 5% of individuals have five or more glands, with the supernumerary ones usually located within the thymus.

The cellular structure of the parathyroid gland is:

- abundant chief cells which manufacture and secrete parathyroid hormone
- sparse oxophil cells whose function is poorly understood.

Physiology of the control of the level of serum calcium

On the cell surface of every parathyroid cell is a calcium-sensing receptor. The concentration of plasma calcium is tightly controlled between 2.2 and 2.6 mmol/L. A reduction in serum calcium stimulates the secretion of parathyroid hormone (PTH) and vice versa.

Parathyroid hormone

The main product of the parathyroid glands has three principal actions:

- stimulation of the activity of osteoclasts in bone and thus mobilisation of calcium from bone into the bloodstream
- enhancement of the absorption of calcium from the gut into the bloodstream, an action facilitated by vitamin D
- increase of the reabsorption of calcium by the renal tubules, thereby reducing urinary calcium excretion.

All of these tend to increase serum calcium concentration, which then has negative feedback on the secretion of PTH.

Vitamin D

Vitamin D_3 is produced in the skin from the action of ultraviolet light upon 7-dehydrocholesterol; it is also ingested in the diet. This inactive form undergoes a two-stage hydroxylation process in the liver and kidney (Fig. 32.5) to produce the active vitamin D: 1,25-dihydroxycholecalciferol. The second hydroxylation is stimulated by PTH. Active vitamin D_3 enhances intestinal calcium absorption by PTH and facilitates bone mineralisation.

Calcitonin

Calcitonin is secreted by the parafollicular or C cells of the thyroid. Its actions are the direct opposite of those of PTH and, in particular, it decreases osteoclastic activity. However, its biological importance in calcium homeostasis is uncertain. Serum calcium concentration is normal both in patients who have undergone total thyroidectomy (and who therefore have negligible serum levels of calcitonin) and in those with medullary thyroid carcinoma (high levels of calcitonin).

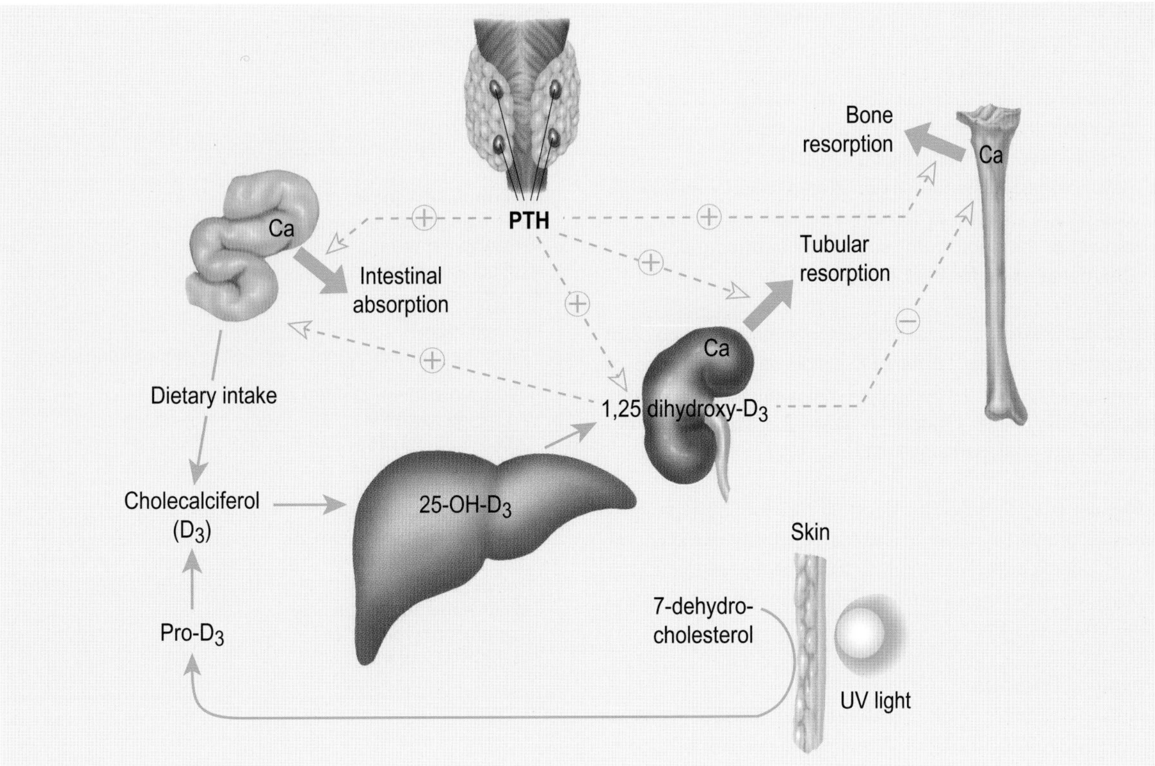

Fig. 32.5 Metabolism of vitamin D.

HYPERPARATHYROIDISM

In this condition, there is overactivity of one or more parathyroid glands with secretion of excessive amounts of PTH. Three subtypes are recognised, as follows.

- *Primary hyperparathyroidism.* Without any demonstrable stimulation, the parathyroid gland(s) secrete inappropriately raised amounts of PTH. Serum calcium concentration is raised and negative feedback is abolished, so the level of PTH is inappropriately high for the level of calcium. The cause is most commonly adenomatous change in one parathyroid, but less frequently there may be hyperplasia of all four or a carcinoma of one.
- *Secondary hyperparathyroidism.* This occurs in chronic kidney disease (failure of tubular reabsorption); intestinal malabsorption and vitamin D deficiency. There is a reduction in the plasma concentration of calcium, which causes hyperplasia of all four glands. Increased production of PTH is therefore appropriate and, if the cause of hypocalcaemia can be corrected, in most instances the parathyroids return to normal.
- *Tertiary hyperparathyroidism.* For patients with chronic kidney disease induced secondary hyperparathyroidism, the situation becomes chronic owing to dialysis. If a patient were then to receive a renal transplant, the implanted kidney retains the ability to activate vitamin D, which, in the presence of continuing parathyroid overactivity, leads to hypercalcaemia.

Primary hyperparathyroidism

Epidemiology

Primary hyperparathyroidism is the commonest subtype to present to the surgeon. The availability of the multichannel autoanalyser, which provides serum calcium concentrations on blood samples sent for other tests, has resulted in an increasing recognition of this disorder. It can occur at any age but its peak incidence is over 60 years. Women are more commonly affected. It has been reported to occur in 1 in 1000 patients in hospital, but community prevalence is much less.

Aetiology and pathological features

The cause remains obscure.

Eighty per cent of patients have a solitary adenoma. The adenomatous gland is enlarged, and the chief cells are hypertrophied and numerous. The other glands are suppressed, small, their chief cells few, and their stroma contains an abundant amount of fat. In 5% of patients, adenomas are multiple. The remainder (15–20%) have multiple-gland hyperplasia. Patients with hyperplasia may suffer from the multiple endocrine neoplasia (MEN) syndrome.

Clinical features

History

The symptoms are those of complications of the disorder, often summarised as 'stones, bones, abdominal groans and psychic moans' but more formally listed as:

- urinary tract stones – mainly renal colic (Ch. 32)
- bone decalcification, which may cause bone pain or a pathological fracture
- abdominal pain – often of obscure cause but occasionally consequent on the presence of a peptic ulcer or recurrent pancreatitis (Ch. 21)
- psychological disturbances of altered mood – mainly depression which may remain unrecognised by the patient or the doctor until successful treatment alters the mental state for the better.

Acute disturbances. Occasionally a rise of serum calcium concentration above 3.5 mmol/L produces a syndrome of vomiting, dehydration, renal failure and coma. The event may be potentially lethal. Emergency Box 32.3 summarises the management of hypercalcaemia.

Minimally symptomatic. Increasingly (up to 80%) patients are without overt symptoms and the possibility of the condition is signalled by an abnormal result on the autoanalyser profile. Most patients admit to fatigue, poor memory and bone and joint pains.

Physical findings

Examination rarely reveals any abnormality. It is most unusual to find a lump in the neck. Features of the complications outlined above may be present.

Investigation

Diagnostic criteria are as follows:

- Unequivocal hypercalcaemia – blood is taken without applying a tourniquet to the arm, because this may raise serum calcium concentration by provoking regional acidosis. At least three measurements are made on different occasions; since most calcium in serum is bound to albumin, results are adjusted to a standard albumin concentration of 40 g/L.
- Simultaneous finding of detectable or raised levels of PTH in the blood – excluding other causes of hypercalcaemia (see Table 32.6).
- Increased urinary excretion of calcium.
- Bone mineral density scan – severe osteopaenia is an indication for parathyroidectomy.

Localisation of abnormal parathyroid(s)

This used not to be necessary for a patient undergoing parathyroid exploration for the first time, because an experienced surgeon can identify no less than 95% of glands during neck exploration. The increased success of preoperative imaging has led to the development of a scan-directed 'targeted parathyroidectomy' via a unilateral approach to the neck. However, if the first operation fails to discover and remove the abnormal gland(s), successful localisation is mandatory before a repeat operation. There are two reasons:

- There is a greater chance that the disorder is in a gland (or glands) at an unusual site.
- Re-exploration of the neck carries a sixfold greater risk to the recurrent laryngeal nerves, and successful lateralisation of the parathyroid reduces this.

Emergency Box 32.3

Hypercalcaemia

Symptoms

Nausea, vomiting, thirst, weakness, malaise, confusional state

Differential diagnosis (Table 32.6)

- Primary hyperparathyroidism
- Multiple myeloma
- Bony secondaries
- Sarcoidosis

Investigation

Plasma calcium corrected to albumin of 40 g/L (uncuffed)

Action (only once calcium result known)

Mild hypercalcaemia (2.65–2.95 mmol/L)	Rehydrate: oral fluids 2–3 L/24 h
Moderate hypercalcaemia (3.00–3.50 mmol/L)	Intravenous saline 3–4 L/24 h
Severe hypercalcaemia (>3.50 mmol/L) or failure of fall in calcium despite rehydration	Bisphosphonate therapy: single i.v. infusion given slowly; plasma calcium begins to fall within 48 h
Definitive therapy for primary hyperparathyroidism is parathyroidectomy	

Table 32.6 Other causes of hypercalcaemia to be excluded in the diagnosis of primary hyperparathyroidism

Cause	Method of exclusion
Secondary carcinoma of bone (common sites: breast, bronchus, thyroid, kidney and prostate)	History Typical bone X-rays Bone scan
Multiple myeloma	Typical bone X-rays Plasma electrophoresis Bence–Jones proteinuria
Vitamin D intoxication	History of intake
Sarcoidosis	
Thyrotoxicosis	
Rare tumours (usually carcinoma of bronchus) which secrete PTH-related peptide	
Familial hypercalcaemic hypocalciuria – diminished renal calcium excretion	Family history Low renal calcium output

Methods of localisation are:

- *Non-invasive*
  - neck ultrasound; about 70% reliability
  - CT and MRI; more reliable for ectopic mediastinal tumours
  - isotope scanning; sestamibi-only scanning correctly lateralises glands with up to 90% success (Fig. 32.6).
- *Invasive*
  - selective venous sampling from veins draining the neck structures directs the surgeon to the area in which the abnormality lies (regionalisation).

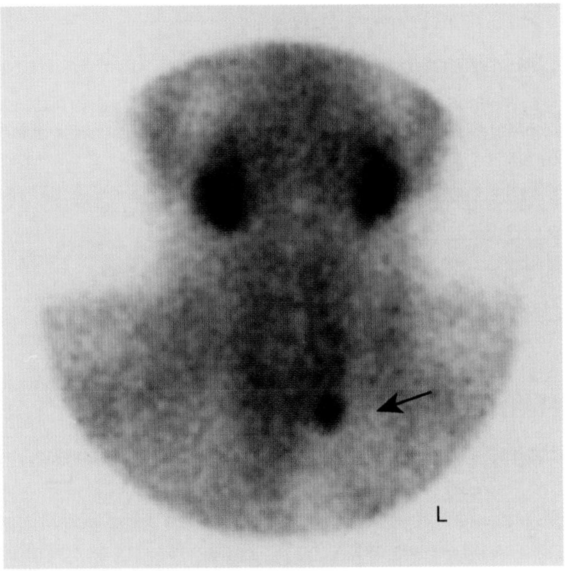

Fig. 32.6 Sestamibi-only isotope scan localises an adenoma of the left inferior parathyroid gland (arrow). Sestamibi is a synthetic molecule that passively crosses cell membranes. Its distribution after intravenous injection reflects blood supply.

Management

Hypercalcaemia

Severe hypercalcaemia (above 3.5 mmol/L) requires rehydration and the administration of bisphosphonates, which inhibit osteoclastic bone resorption. Calcium concentrations are measured at least daily and often need to be followed more frequently. Moderate hypercalcaemia (3.0–3.5 mmol/L) is usually controlled by intravenous rehydration.

Surgical

Surgical removal offers the only cure for primary hyperparathyroidism and should be offered to all symptomatic patients and those asymptomatic patients whose calcium concentration exceeds 2.75 mmol/L. The high success rate and low morbidity of exploration of the neck have led towards a more liberal surgical policy for minimally symptomatic patients with a plasma calcium between 2.60 and 2.75 mmol/L.

The preoperative preparation is as for thyroidectomy. Some surgeons use frozen section and others intra-operative (quick) PTH assay.

Operation

The approach and exposure are the same as for thyroidectomy. If an adenoma is found, it is removed. The surgical treatment of multi-gland hyperplasia is more difficult. The conventional management is subtotal parathyroidectomy (removal of three and a half glands), leaving half a gland in the neck. However, there is a chance of recurrence, and neck re-exploration is then more difficult and treacherous. Some surgeons now autograft the remaining half gland into the forearm. The graft survival rate is high (more than 90%) and further surgery in the neck is avoided. A third option is to cryopreserve some parathyroid tissue and delay its transplantation until hypocalcaemia is documented; however, graft survival is much lower. The fourth option is to excise all parathyroid tissue and place the patient on lifelong calcium and vitamin D supplements.

Postoperative care

Serum calcium concentration is measured the day after surgery. After a successful procedure, the calcium level often falls below normal before it rises to the normal range. If the calcium level does not fall, or returns to its original level after a transient decrease, the surgeon has failed to remove the disordered tissue.

The patient is questioned for early signs of hypocalcaemia such as paraesthesiae of the hands and lips. Trousseau's and Chvostek's signs may be elicited. It may be necessary to give oral calcium and vitamin D until the suppressed parathyroids recover.

Complications

Persistent or recurrent hypercalcaemia is the consequence of failure to remove an adenoma or enough hyperplastic tissue. Re-exploration must be carried out, but only by an experienced surgeon because the complication rate is much higher than for a first operation.

Hypoparathyroidism. Transient hypocalcaemia is common even after successful removal of a diseased gland but recovery occurs within a week. Permanent hypocalcaemia follows removal of too much parathyroid tissue. If cryopreserved tissue is available, some of it is implanted as already described; otherwise, the patient is treated with calcium and vitamin D for life.

PARATHYROID CARCINOMA

This condition is very rare. Usually there is invasion of local tissues and recurrence after excision. Metastases are uncommon. Death is often caused by hypercalcaemia.

Clinical features

There may be symptoms of metastatic disease in addition to the progressive effects of hyperparathyroidism.

Physical findings are of a mass in the neck which may be palpable; this should alert the surgeon to the possibility of carcinoma.

Investigation and management

The plasma calcium concentration is typically very high and is accompanied by a high level of PTH. CT of the neck demonstrates the local anatomy, and a chest X-ray should be taken to look for secondary spread.

The surgical strategy is en-bloc resection of the tumour. Adjuvant oncotherapy should be considered, and bisphosphonates may be required to control the hypercalcaemia.

ADRENALS

Embryology

The glands are derived from two components: the cortex and the medulla. The cortex is formed during the fifth week of life from proliferation of mesodermal cells. This is then invaded by ectodermal cells which have migrated from the neural crest (ectoderm) to form the adrenal medulla; these cells either differentiate into chromaffin cells containing granules of catecholamines (phaeochromocytes) or non-chromaffin sympathetic ganglion cells.

Neural crest cells are widely dispersed throughout the embryo but are usually replaced by lymphatic tissue shortly after birth. Ectopic nests of cells have been described in diverse sites including the urinary bladder, gonads and gastrointestinal tract. Persistence of these cells may give rise to extra-adrenal medullary neoplasms.

Anatomy

The adrenal glands are paired and similarly placed, bilaterally, above the kidneys; however, they are far from symmetrical. Each normal gland weighs approximately 5 g and is 5 cm long, 3 cm wide and approximately 1 cm thick. The right gland is pyramidal while the left is semilunar. The blood supply arises from three arteries: branches from the aorta, renal and phrenic arteries.

Physiology

The cortex secretes steroid hormones from three distinct zones. The outer zona glomerulosa secretes the mineralocorticoid aldosterone whose major actions are in the control of renal sodium and potassium excretion in conjunction with renin and angiotensin. The middle zona fasciculata secretes the glucocorticoid cortisol whose many physiological effects include hepatic gluconeogenesis, protein catabolism, some mineralocorticoid effects and regulation of the response to inflammation. Secretion of cortisol is regulated by adrenocorticotrophic hormone (ACTH) from the anterior pituitary. The inner zona reticularis secretes adrenal androgens and accounts for 15–20% of total androgen activity in males. The cells of the adrenal medulla are part of the amine precursor uptake and decarboxylation (APUD) system and secrete catecholamines noradrenaline (norepinephrine) and adrenaline (epinephrine).

Pathological features

The variety of disorders which arise from adrenal hyperplasia and tumours are summarised in Box 32.2.

Box 32.2 Adrenal syndromes associated with hyperplasia or tumour

Cortex

Benign
- Hyperplasia
- Adenoma

Malignant
- Carcinoma
- Metastases

Medulla

Benign
- Phaeochromocytoma
- Ganglioneuroma

Malignant
- Ganglioneuroblastoma
- Neuroblastoma
- Metastases

THE ADRENAL CORTEX

Classification of disorders

Hyperplasia or neoplasia of the adrenal cortex produces characteristic syndromes which are dependent on the zone of origin:

- zona glomerulosa – primary hyperaldosteronism
- zona fasciculata – Cushing's syndrome
- zona reticularis – virilism.

These entities can occur on their own or there may be a mixed picture which is suggestive of an adrenal carcinoma.

Primary hyperaldosteronism

Epidemiology and pathological features

This condition is relatively rare, occurring in less than 2% of patients with hypertension. It presents most commonly between the ages of 20 and 50 years and is more common in men. There are two subtypes:

- idiopathic hyperaldosteronism – bilateral adrenal hyperplasia
- Conn's syndrome – a single, usually small, canary-yellow tumour of the adrenal cortex, which is nearly always benign (98%).

Idiopathic hyperaldosteronism is three times less common than Conn's syndrome as a cause of primary hyperaldosteronism. It is important to distinguish between a single tumour, which is best treated surgically, and bilateral adrenal hyperplasia, which can be managed medically.

Inappropriate autonomous oversecretion of aldosterone leads to sodium retention and potassium loss, causing hypertension and muscle weakness. High levels of aldosterone suppress the renin–angiotensin–aldosterone axis and, in consequence, the plasma renin concentration is low.

Clinical features

Symptoms are either vague or absent. Patients may complain of lethargy, muscle weakness and thirst. Clinical examination is normal, but there is hypertension.

Investigation

There are two stages of investigation: initially to confirm the diagnosis and then to localise a tumour if one is thought to be present.

Initial

- Confirm primary hyperaldosteronism.
- Differentiate between Conn's syndrome and adrenal hyperplasia.

Localisation

CT scan may show a small (1 cm) tumour (Fig. 32.7), but it must be remembered that there is a significant incidence of adrenal incidentalomas.

Scanning with radiolabelled cholesterol can distinguish a solitary functional adrenal tumour from bilateral increased uptake. The gold standard test is bilateral adrenal venous sampling to measure aldosterone concentrations. However,

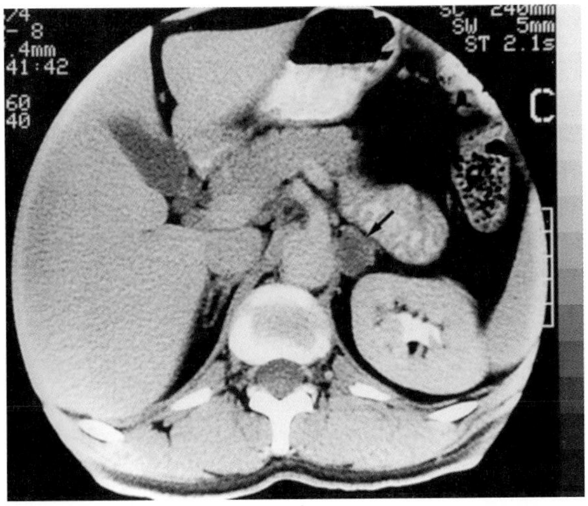

Fig. 32.7 Abdominal CT scan demonstrating a left adrenal tumour (arrow) in a patient with Conn's syndrome. Note the typical appearance of the normal right adrenal with its very dark medulla. (Courtesy of Dr A L Hine, Central Middlesex Hospital, London.)

this technique is difficult to undertake and carries a risk of infarction to one or both adrenals.

Management

Non-operative

If a tumour has been diagnosed, it is essential that serum potassium concentration be returned to normal before surgical treatment is considered; this can be achieved by the use of spironolactone, which blocks aldosterone receptors and reduces aldosterone secretion; 200–400 mg/day is used for 3–6 weeks before operation. Hyperplasia is not an indication for exploration and bilateral adrenalectomy because this renders the patient permanently dependent on steroids and restores the blood pressure to normal in only one-third of all patients. Spironolactone in doses of 200–400 mg/day controls the hypokalaemia, but other agents may be necessary to reduce blood pressure.

Operative

Adenomas are treated by unilateral adrenalectomy. This can be achieved laparoscopically. There is a high cure rate and virtually no morbidity or mortality. The hypokalaemia of primary aldosteronism is almost universally cured, but hypertension persists in 30% of patients and may recur in a further 20%, with, therefore, a long-term cure of hypertension of only 50%.

Cushing's syndrome

This condition is characterised by glucocorticoid excess. The underlying causes are shown in Box 32.3.

Epidemiology

Cushing's syndrome affects patients between 20 and 40 years old and has a predilection for women; however, ectopic ACTH secretion has an equal sex incidence which reflects the chief cause, which is bronchogenic carcinoma. Adrenocortical carcinoma as a cause is very rare.

Box 32.3 Causes of Cushing's syndrome

ACTH-dependent

- Ectopic ACTH secretion – 15%
- Cushing's 'disease' – 65%

ACTH-independent

- Adrenocortical adenoma – 10%
- Adrenocortical carcinoma – 10%
- Iatrogenic steroid therapy – variable but should never be forgotten

ACTH, adrenocorticotrophic hormone.

Pathophysiology

Primary ACTH-secreting tumours of the pituitary are described later in this chapter. Ectopic ACTH production stimulates both adrenal glands to produce excess cortisol. Adrenocortical adenomas and carcinomas secrete excess levels of cortisol with suppression of ACTH, and each accounts for about 10% of patients with Cushing's syndrome.

Clinical features

History

The effects of excess cortisol on the body are wide-ranging and produce characteristic clinical features. Typical symptoms are:

- facial and truncal obesity
- menstrual irregularity
- hirsutism
- muscle weakness
- osteoporosis.

Clinical findings

The typical physical signs are (Fig. 32.8):

- moon face
- buffalo hump
- central obesity ('lemon-on-sticks' appearance)
- muscle wasting and weakness
- striae
- hirsutism
- ecchymoses
- hypertension.

Adrenal carcinomas tend to be large, and a mass may be palpated. Patients with ectopic ACTH production are usually pigmented and may have clinical signs of a primary bronchial neoplasm.

Investigation

Biochemical and endocrinological

The following are used to confirm the presence of the disorder:

- The 24-hour urinary free cortisol is elevated, and a low-dose dexamethasone suppression test depresses the hypothalamic–pituitary axis in normals but not in Cushing's syndrome.
- ACTH-dependent and -independent disorders are distinguished by the methods given in Table 32.7.

Table 32.7 Methods to distinguish between ACTH-dependent and ACTH-independent disorders

Test	Cushing's disease	Adrenal tumour	Ectopic ACTH
Plasma ACTH	Normal to elevated	Undetectable	Elevated ++
High-dose dexamethasone suppression test	Suppression	No suppression	No suppression

ACTH, adrenocorticotrophic hormone.

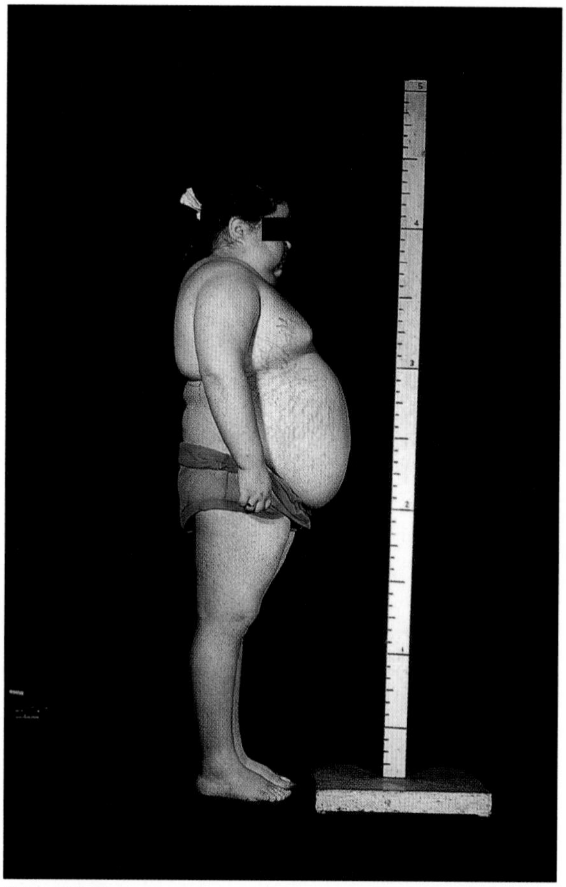

Fig. 32.8 Cushingoid ('lemon-on-sticks') appearance of a female adolescent. (By courtesy of Professor S R Bloom, Hammersmith Hospital, London.)

Localisation of a tumour

Methods used are CT and selective venous sampling.

Management

Medical

If an operation is indicated, steroid cover with hydrocortisone must be given both preoperatively and perioperatively and reduced to a maintenance dose of 20–30 mg/day of hydrocortisone usually within 10 days after operation. Patients with ectopic ACTH secretion are best treated by resecting the primary source, but all too often this is either not technically feasible or the patients have advanced metastatic disease and a poor prognosis. In such circumstances, drugs which block steroid synthesis, such as metyrapone and aminoglutethimide, are used.

Surgical

Adenomas are treated by unilateral adrenalectomy. Adrenal carcinomas are usually advanced, and metastases are common. Despite their poor prognosis (less than 50% survival at 2 years), surgery is the treatment of choice in an attempt to reduce the bulk of the tumour and palliate the symptoms of steroid excess. This can be aided in part by the use of mitotane (o,p′-DDD), a mitochondrial poison, which, in the majority of patients, reduces the secretion of both cortisol and adrenal androgens.

Virilising tumours

Overproduction of sex steroid hormones can lead to either virilisation (excess androgen) or feminisation (excess oestrogen). The cause is usually a congenital enzyme defect or an adrenal tumour.

Congenital adrenal hyperplasia

Pathophysiology

The underlying cause in 90% is an enzyme deficiency – absence of 21-hydroxylase, an enzyme essential for cortisol synthesis. The consequent reduction in plasma cortisol levels leads to an excess of ACTH, which in turn results in an increase of intermediate metabolites that become channelled into testosterone production.

Clinical features

The usual presentation is at birth with pseudo-hermaphrodite external genitalia in female children and precocious sexual maturation in affected males.

Investigation

The diagnosis is confirmed by finding high concentrations of the steroid precursors in blood and urine. The karyotype must be checked in affected females.

Management

Medical. Cortisol deficiency is corrected so as to suppress the ACTH secretion. Hydrocortisone 25 mg/m^2 is given daily in two or three divided doses.

Surgical. On occasions, surgical correction of the abnormal genitalia may be necessary.

Adrenocortical adenoma and carcinoma

Acquired syndromes of sex steroid excess are rare and usually secondary to an underlying adrenocortical tumour. Androgen-secreting tumours are much more common than are the feminising tumours.

Investigation and management

The diagnosis is made by a combination of CT and radionuclide scanning (iodocholesterol is the most favoured viewing agent).

When there is a benign tumour of the adrenal, surgical removal is curative. By contrast, adrenal carcinoma carries a poor prognosis.

THE ADRENAL MEDULLA

Tumours are the only conditions of surgical importance and are derived either from chromaffin cells (phaeochromocytoma) or non-chromaffin cells (neuroblastoma, ganglioneuroma and ganglioneuroblastoma).

Phaeochromocytoma

This is a catecholamine-secreting tumour of chromaffin cells in the adrenal medulla or in the paraganglionic tissues adjacent to the sympathetic chain at any level.

It is a rare tumour with an incidence of 1 per million and which therefore accounts for less than 1% of cases of hypertension.

Pathological features

It has been called the '10% tumour' because 10% are bilateral, 10% are malignant and 10% are extra-adrenal. Extra-adrenal tumours are more likely to be malignant and can be found anywhere from the pelvis to the base of the skull. The most common extra-adrenal site is the organ of Zuckerkandl, which lies at the aortic bifurcation, but instances in the urinary bladder, the mediastinum and the neck have all been described.

Malignancy is usually characterised by the presence of established metastases in liver, lymph nodes, bones and lungs.

Phaeochromocytoma occurs in half of patients with MEN II and is also associated with other uncommon disorders such as von Hippel–Lindau disease (phaeochromocytoma, angioma, renal carcinoma), neurofibromatosis and tuberous sclerosis.

Clinical features

History

The typical symptoms are secondary to the effects of excessive α-adrenoreceptor stimulation. Sweating is very common in phaeochromocytoma and occurs in almost 90% of patients. Attacks are usually spontaneous, but sometimes they are precipitated by exercise, overeating, defecation or sexual intercourse. Patients describe them as consisting of:

- paroxysmal headache
- palpitations
- profuse perspiration
- sometimes precordial pain
- a fearful feeling of impending death (angor animi).

These rarely last more than 15 minutes but tend to become more frequent over time.

Death from cardiovascular episodes and myocardial infarction has occurred during an attack. It must be remembered that invasive investigative procedures may precipitate an acute episode – an important consideration in efforts to localise the tumour.

Physical findings

Hypertension is the most common finding: over 50% of patients have persistent and sustained hypertension, but in the other 50% it is intermittent. Examination is otherwise normal but an abdominal tumour is occasionally found.

Investigation

Blood examination

The circulating plasma volume may be reduced by a combination of intense vasoconstriction and hypertension. A secondary rise in haematocrit is then evident.

Cardiac

There may be evidence of left ventricular hypertrophy on the ECG.

Hormonal

Twenty-four-hour measurement of the urinary metabolites of adrenaline and noradrenaline – nor- and metanephrines – is an effective screening test and is rarely normal in patients with symptomatic disease. If urinary metanephrines are high then plasma catecholamines are measured. Once an endocrine diagnosis has been made, abdominal CT will localise the tumour and whole-body radioisotope scan (MIBG, see Fig. 32.9) might be indicated for multiple tumours when metastases are suspected.

Management

Medical

Phaeochromocytomas are potentially lethal, and the major advance in their management has been the preoperative use of α- and β-adrenergic-blocking agents which have reduced operative mortality to 1%. Alpha-receptor blockade is mandatory before removal of the tumour and, when cardiac function is compromised, must be introduced gradually; phenoxybenzamine, a non-selective α-blocker, is the agent of choice. Phenoxybenzamine decreases the vasoconstriction, so that mild to severe postural hypotension develops,

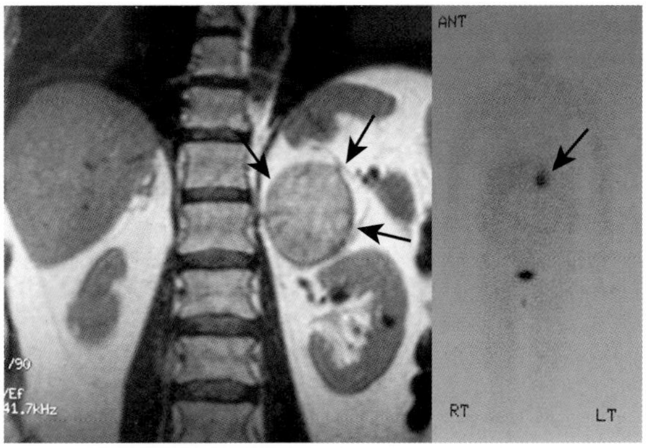

Fig. 32.9 (a) Sagittal MRI scan demonstrating a large left adrenal phaeochromocytoma (arrowed). (b) Corresponding whole-body localisation (MIBG) scan.

and the blood volume may need to be restored by increased oral fluid intake. The subjective symptoms are relieved, and the patient may appear to be drowsy as though sedated. Tachycardia may increase so that β-blockade becomes necessary but only after α-blockade is well established and the circulating blood volume has been restored.

Surgical

After the above preparation and precise localisation of the tumour, exploration and removal constitute the treatment of choice.

Neuroblastoma

Neuroblastoma is the third most common malignancy of childhood (after leukaemia and cerebral malignancy) and, in the UK, affects approximately 1 in 10 000 children alive at birth.

Pathological features

Neuroblastomas arise from the most primitive cells of the adrenal medulla. Local invasion of surrounding structures is frequent. Blood-borne metastases are common, particularly to the skull and orbit from left-sided primaries (Hutchinson type) and liver from right-sided primaries (Pepper type).

Clinical features

The child typically presents with malaise and weight loss. An abdominal mass will be felt. Hypertension is not usually a feature.

Investigation and management

Urinary levels of metanephrines are usually elevated.

Referral to a specialised centre is essential to ensure the highest rate of survival. A triad of chemotherapy, radiotherapy and debulking surgery occasionally produces excellent results. The overall prognosis, however, is poor although dependent upon how advanced the disease is at the time of diagnosis.

ACUTE ADRENAL INSUFFICIENCY

This is essentially a medical condition, but surgeons may encounter adrenal insufficiency as a post-traumatic (including postoperative) complication. It may be either acute or chronic, and the common causes are shown in Box 32.4.

Clinical features

In acute adrenal failure, patients present with hypotension, vomiting, abdominal pain and mental confusion. There is typically a history of recent surgery or associated sepsis, coagulation defect or cancer. Hypotension and circulatory collapse inevitably develop.

Investigation and management

The classical picture of hyponatraemia and hyperkalaemia may take several days to become apparent and can be confused by concomitant intravenous fluid regimens. A low plasma cortisol is diagnostic but the fundamental necessity is to be aware of the diagnosis.

Box 32.4 Causes of adrenal insufficiency

Acute
- Primary – Addison's disease
- Secondary – adrenal apoplexy in the newborn
- Sepsis – especially meningococcal (Waterhouse–Friderichsen syndrome)
- Bilateral adrenalectomy
- Postoperative haemorrhage

Chronic
- Idiopathic atrophy
- Adrenal destruction
  - tuberculosis
  - histoplasmosis
  - metastatic disease
  - lymphoma
  - amyloidosis
  - haemochromatosis
- Hypothalamic–pituitary axis disease
  - tumour
  - irradiation
  - infarction

Management is by urgent steroid replacement with the cooperation of an endocrinologist.

GASTROENTEROPANCREATIC TUMOURS

These are slow-growing tumours and tend to cause symptoms by their secreted peptides rather than by any bulk effect, although pressure and other mechanical events may occur in the late stages. With the exception of insulinoma, most gastroenteropancreatic tumours are malignant. However, despite extensive hepatic and other metastases, which are often present at the time of the original diagnosis, many patients may survive for years.

Insulinoma

Epidemiology

Insulinomas constitute about 70% of all pancreatic endocrine tumours and occur in approximately 1 in 1 million of the population. Although they are rare in children, in infants there may be an associated entity of nesidioblastosis – a very rare condition of beta cell hyperplasia which is diffuse throughout the pancreas and causes symptomatic hyperinsulinaemia and usually necessitates either a distal subtotal or a total pancreatectomy.

Pathological and pathophysiological features

The tumour arises from the beta islet cells, and 70–90% are benign, usually small (less than 2 cm in diameter) and equally distributed throughout the pancreas. Less than 10% are multiple, and about 10% are associated with MEN I. They intermittently secrete insulin, with consequent hypoglycaemic attacks.

Clinical features

History

Pre-coma – light-headedness, disorientation and sometimes disturbances of mood such as bad temper and rage – may go on to frank unconsciousness usually with spontaneous recovery, although brain damage may occasionally occur. Many patients have previously been investigated for mental illness, epilepsy or suspected drug abuse before the diagnosis is finally established.

Physical findings

Clinical signs are usually absent, although patients tend to be obese because they eat to avoid hypoglycaemia. The diagnosis is suspected when three criteria are met (Whipple's triad):

- Attacks are precipitated by fasting.
- Hypoglycaemia (less than 2.0 mmol/L) is documented at the time of an attack.
- Symptoms are relieved by the administration of glucose.

Investigation

Biochemical and endocrine

Patients are fasted and the plasma glucose is monitored. When the plasma glucose falls to 2.0 mmol/L or less, further samples are taken for insulin, C-peptide and sulphonylurea. C-peptide is cleaved from the pro-insulin molecule and should therefore be elevated in the presence of a raised endogenous insulin, which is not the case if self-injection of insulin is taking place. Patients may need to be rescued from a fast with intravenous 50% dextrose.

Sulphonylurea assay will not be detectable unless the patient is in a self-induced hypoglycaemic attack.

Localisation

Once hypoglycaemia in the presence of hyperinsulinaemia has been verified, attempts are made to localise the tumour. This can be achieved with a combination of CT scans, visceral angiography, portal venous sampling and intraoperative ultrasound scanning.

Management

Medical

Before surgical exploration is contemplated, diazoxide, which inhibits the release of insulin, is administered to return the blood sugar concentration to normal. In the perioperative period, patients receive an intravenous infusion of 10% dextrose and potassium 40 mEq/L.

Surgical

The only curative treatment for insulinoma is removal. Tumours can usually be enucleated, but for large ones (10%) it may be necessary to resect part of the pancreas.

Glucagonoma

This is a very rare malignant tumour with an estimated annual incidence of 1 in 20 million. It is an alpha-cell tumour of the pancreas which secretes glucagon. Most glucagonomas are solitary and, in the majority, liver and lung metastases have already occurred at the time of presentation.

Clinical features

There is a characteristic syndrome of migratory necrolytic erythema, diabetes mellitus and weight loss. The rash is so typical that a pancreatic endocrine tumour may be diagnosed from this alone. Its cause is uncertain but it may be consequent upon a deficiency of zinc in the skin.

Investigation

Confirmation of the diagnosis is achieved by demonstrating an elevated plasma level of glucagon in the absence of other causes of hyperglucagonaemia (e.g. renal or hepatic failure). Most tumours are large and readily detected on CT.

Management

Medical

Before attempted removal by operation, patients may require nasogastric or parenteral feeding. Zinc deficiency is corrected. Octreotide, a somatostatin analogue, often improves the rash but does not confer any survival benefit.

Surgical

Surgical resection for cure is the treatment of choice but is open to only a minority of patients. For those with extensive and metastatic disease, debulking of the tumour and selective hepatic artery embolisation of liver secondaries achieve reasonable palliation.

Gastrinoma

Epidemiology

This is the second commonest islet cell tumour, although it frequently occurs in extrapancreatic sites, particularly the duodenum. Approximately one-third of patients with gastrinomas have the MEN I syndrome.

Pathophysiology

Thirty per cent of gastrinomas are malignant, and over 70% of these present with metastases. Their secretion of gastrin stimulates an excess production of gastric acid and leads to the development of the Zollinger–Ellison syndrome – severe peptic ulceration, often multiple, with a progressive and complicated course and sometimes found in the distal rather than the proximal duodenum.

Clinical features

Symptoms

Patients typically complain of epigastric pain secondary to peptic ulceration. Other symptoms include:

- diarrhoea
- weight loss
- dysphagia secondary to oesophagitis.

Physical findings

Physical examination is usually normal. Clinicians are alerted to the diagnosis by the atypical nature and severity of peptic ulcers seen on upper-intestinal endoscopy and which are refractory to conventional anti-ulcer medication.

Investigation

Biochemical and hormonal

In the absence of anti-ulcer medication, the biochemical criteria for a diagnosis of gastrinoma are:

- elevated fasting levels of serum gastrin
- increased gastric acid secretion.

Gastrin in the serum can also be elevated in achlorhydria, pernicious anaemia, atrophic gastritis, renal failure and hyperparathyroidism. In doubtful instances, the level of gastrin rises in response to provocation with secretin.

Imaging

The role of preoperative imaging for localisation is controversial, and many tumours are not found until the patient is explored.

Management

Treatment is directed at both the tumour and the complications it produces.

Medical

Historically, the management of a gastrinoma syndrome was by total gastrectomy, which removed the target organ rather than the tumour, so preventing the complication of peptic ulcer. The advent of proton-pump inhibitors has provided a very effective means of palliating the symptoms/complications of excess gastric acid and rendered gastric surgery virtually obsolete.

Surgical

A well-localised tumour should be removed to endeavour to achieve a cure. However, half of those who undergo resection develop recurrence; nevertheless, the tumours are usually slow-growing, and up to 30% of patients will survive many years on long-term omeprazole, even in the presence of a large tumour load.

VIPoma

The estimated annual incidence of VIPoma is 1 in 10 million. These islet cell tumours are always malignant and oversecrete vasointestinal peptide (VIP). They produce the Verner–Morrison syndrome of watery diarrhoea, hypokalaemic acidosis and achlorhydria.

Clinical features

In addition to the increased stool volume, patients may complain of lethargy and flushing.

Clinical examination is typically normal, although occasionally an abdominal mass and hepatomegaly are found.

Investigation

The diagnosis is made by detecting an elevated concentration of VIP in the serum in patients with hypokalaemic alkalosis. A combination of CT (Fig. 32.10), ultrasound and visceral angiography localises the tumour.

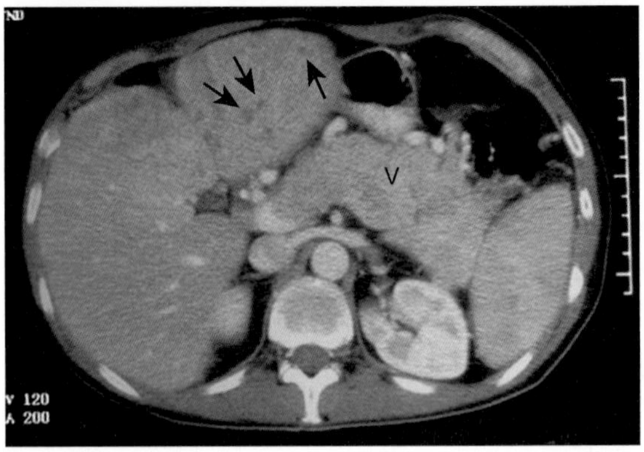

Fig. 32.10 CT scan of abdomen demonstrating a large VIPoma in the pancreatic tail (V) and multiple liver metastases (some arrowed).

Management

Medical

The electrolyte disturbances are corrected with intravenous fluids. Octreotide dramatically improves the secretory diarrhoea by inhibiting the release of VIP. In the presence of extensive metastases, the mainstay of treatment is cytotoxic chemotherapy rather than surgery.

Surgical

Resection of tumours is reserved for patients without metastases (approximately 50%).

Neuroendocrine tumours (NET)

Pathophysiology

Neuroendocrine tumours arise from the enterochromaffin (Kulchitsky) cells located throughout the body but principally within the intestinal submucosa (85%) and the main bronchi (10%). These cells are part of the APUD system and used to be termed carcinoid tumours. These tumours secrete vasoactive substances (serotonin, bradykinin, prostaglandin, substance P), which are rapidly metabolised by the liver. A characteristic desmoplastic reaction is often found in the mesentery with fibrosis and contraction, and this may compound bowel obstruction or cause mesenteric angina. They range in differentiation from well to poorly differentiated, and there is a spectrum of behaviour from benign to malignant.

Clinical features

Neuroendocrine tumours may present in a number of ways:

- incidental finding at laparotomy
- local physical complications – bowel obstruction, perforation, haemorrhage
- features of metastatic disease
- carcinoid syndrome (see below).

Clinical examination is often normal.

Investigation

In the absence of secondary disease, these tumours may be difficult to localise. They are predominantly submucosal and are not seen on contrast examination of the gastrointestinal tract. Visceral angiography may detect the tumour from the corkscrew appearance of the mesenteric vessels produced by the desmoplastic reaction. The tumour expresses somatostatin receptors on its cell surface. Radiolabelled agents which bind to these receptors (e.g. octreotide) can be used to make a diagnosis by scintigraphic scanning. Chromogranin A and B are serum markers of neuroendocrine tumours.

Management

Gastrointestinal NETs are classified according to their embryological site of origin.

Foregut

Gastric NETs are often (60%) associated with hypergastrinaemia, occasionally as part of the Zollinger–Ellison syndrome. In these instances the clinical course is typically indolent and the tumours can be adequately resected and progress kept under observation with the endoscope. The sporadic tumours (not associated with hypergastrinaemia) display a more aggressive tendency and necessitate surgical resection. Duodenal NETs are rare and usually adequately managed by local resection.

Midgut

Small-bowel NETs present in a non-specific way, usually with abdominal pain. Two-thirds of patients develop metastases and one-third the carcinoid syndrome. Tumours are sometimes multiple and associated with other malignancies, in particular adenocarcinoma of the small intestine.

Appendicular NETs are found in approximately 1:200 appendices, usually incidental findings during surgery for appendicitis. They most commonly occur at the tip of the appendix (90%), and appendicectomy is curative. If a tumour is at the base or larger than 2 cm in diameter, a right hemicolectomy is recommended.

Hindgut

Colorectal NETs have a predilection for the right colon and typically present with abdominal pain and haemorrhage. Treatment consists of regional hemicolectomy with removal of lymph node metastases.

Metastatic disease

Even in the presence of metastases, resection of the primary is recommended to avoid bowel complications. In selected patients, it may be feasible to resect a hepatic metastasis.

Prognosis

The prognosis of patients with a NET is relatively good. The most important factors are the site and stage of the primary disease. Favourable sites are the appendix and the bronchus, where 5-year survival rates of over 94% can be achieved in small tumours. Liver metastases reduce 5-year survival to about 30%.

Carcinoid syndrome

Pathophysiology

Carcinoid syndrome occurs when vasoactive substances (mainly 5-hydroxytryptamine – serotonin) are secreted and reach the systemic circulation in sufficient concentration to have a pharmacological effect. There are two circumstances:

- Large amounts of serotonin produced from a gut tumour saturate hepatic metabolic pathways.
- Hepatic or other metastases secrete directly into the systemic circulation.

In more than 90%, the underlying cause is a primary tumour of midgut origin.

Clinical features

The characteristic symptoms of the syndrome are:

- cutaneous flushing
- diarrhoea
- valvular disease on the right side of the heart – tricuspid and pulmonary valve stenosis
- bronchospasm.

In addition to hepatomegaly, the patient may be flushed, and a heart murmur may be heard. Bowel sounds are often hyperactive.

Investigation

The syndrome is diagnosed by detecting elevated levels of 24-hour urinary 5-hydroxy-indoleacetic acid (5-HIAA), the breakdown product of serotonin. Chromogranin A and B will be elevated. CT and ultrasound demonstrate the presence of hepatic metastases.

Management

The liver is usually diffusely involved, and fewer than 5% of affected patients have liver tumours amenable to surgical excision. The mainstay of treatment is octreotide, which suppresses hormone release. In addition, hepatic metastases may be embolised at selective hepatic angiography, and this procedure can be repeated. Any patient undergoing operation must have preoperative preparation with octreotide in order to avoid a carcinoid crisis, a potentially fatal event caused by a surge in the release of secretory products at the time of operation.

PITUITARY

Embryology

The pituitary gland develops from two distinct elements:

- an ectodermal outpocketing of the stomodeum known as Rathke's pouch produces the anterior lobe
- a downward extension of the diencephalon forms the posterior lobe.

Anatomy and physiology

The normal pituitary is bean-shaped with a concave upper surface bearing the pituitary stalk of the posterior lobe, which is attached to the hypothalamus. The gland lies in the pituitary fossa and is surrounded by a capsule which is continuous with the dura mater and is perforated on its upper surface for the pituitary stalk.

The pituitary gland produces many hormones, whose secretion is regulated by the adjacent hypothalamus.

TUMOURS OF THE ANTERIOR PITUITARY

Epidemiology and pathological features

Tumours of the pituitary account for approximately 10% of intracranial neoplasms. Carcinoma of the pituitary is very rare. In general, pituitary tumours are benign, epithelial neoplasms three-quarters of which secrete inappropriate amounts of pituitary hormones. Most secrete only one hormone. Those that produce either prolactin, growth hormone or ACTH account for 90–95% of secreting tumours. Rarely, these form part of the multiple endocrine neoplasia type I (MEN I) syndrome.

Clinical features

History

The mode of presentation depends upon:

- local pressure effects
- the endocrine consequences of hypersecretion of a specific hormone.

Non-secreting tumours cause symptoms of raised intracranial pressure and visual field defects because of the proximity of the optic chiasm.

Physical findings

In addition to the features of the individual endocrine syndrome, there may be visual-field defects, signs of raised intracranial pressure and other cranial-nerve lesions.

Investigation

Lateral skull X-rays may show enlargement of the pituitary fossa or erosion of its floor. MRI reveals in great detail the surrounding soft-tissue structures such as the pituitary stalk and optic chiasm. To show small tumours, it is possible to enhance the pictures using gadolinium-DTPA (diethylene-triamine-penta-acetic acid). The sensitivity of detection of tumours with MRI is over 90%, compared with about 50% with CT (Fig. 32.11), and, if available, it is the investigation of choice. When doubt exists after MRI, angiography and selective venous sampling of the petrosal sinuses may localise a tumour.

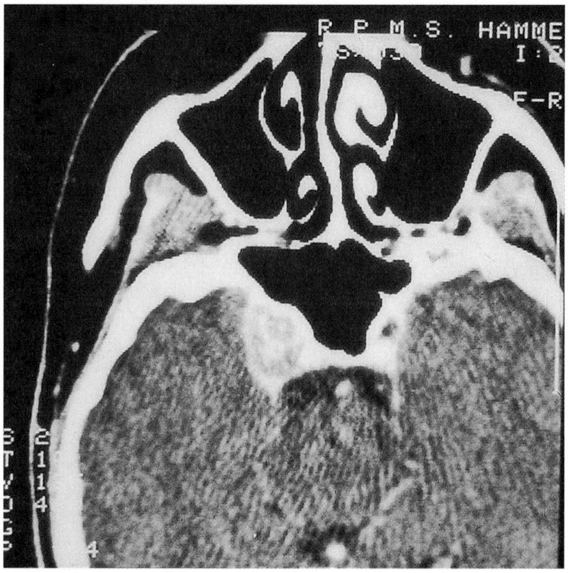

Fig. 32.11 CT image of a pituitary tumour adjacent to the right sphenoidal sinus. (By courtesy of Professor S R Bloom, Hammersmith Hospital, London.)

Prolactinoma

Pathological features

Prolactin-secreting tumours of diameter less than 1 cm (microprolactinomas) may be present in up to 10% of post-mortems; most are clinically without significance. Tumours larger than 1 cm (macroprolactinomas) have specific effects in women and in men.

Pathophysiology and clinical features

In women

- The onset of menstruation is delayed
- The menstrual periods may range from amenorrhoea to oligomenorrhoea, although they are occasionally normal
- Sterility is present even if the periods are normal
- Galactorrhoea can vary from large quantities of milk production to a minor discharge
- Reduction in libido is common.

In men

- Galactorrhoea
- Decreased libido with associated impotence
- Change in secondary sexual characteristics such as reduced growth of facial and body hair and small soft testicles associated with apathy and weight gain.

Management

Medical

Bromocriptine, an agent derived from ergot, is a dopamine agonist and inhibits the release of prolactin. In the majority of patients, it returns the prolactin concentration to normal. Menstruation is quite rapidly restored and galactorrhoea is reduced. The drug is not always well tolerated, because of side effects, including nausea and vomiting, which can sometimes be limited by careful adjustment of the dose or by taking tablets intra-vaginally. If intolerance is severe, other ergot derivatives may be tried.

Surgical

Long-term treatment with bromocriptine for microprolactinomas is popular because their prolactin secretion is very modest. Some expert centres do, however, consider microsurgery (endoscopic transsphenoidal hypophysectomy) which has the advantage that it can potentially cure the patient. For most macroprolactinomas, surgery is not curative and, when attempted, causes hypopituitarism. Bromocriptine often induces tumour shrinkage. Radiotherapy may be added in an attempt to induce a cure.

SYNDROMES OF GROWTH HORMONE EXCESS

Gigantism

Growth hormone-secreting pituitary adenomas are manifest as gigantism in the prepubertal population before fusion of the bony epiphyses arrests growth. Affected individuals can reach an abnormal height, although what is truly abnormal must be judged against the standards of the local population. However, this end-point is rarely seen nowadays because of early recognition and prompt surgical excision of the tumour.

Acromegaly

Growth hormone excess after fusion of the epiphyses is a more insidious disorder often not diagnosed until many years after its onset. It is a rare condition with a prevalence of only 40 cases per million.

Clinical features

The main appearances are of overgrowth of the hands and feet and coarse facial features (Fig. 32.12). In addition, there are physiological disturbances:

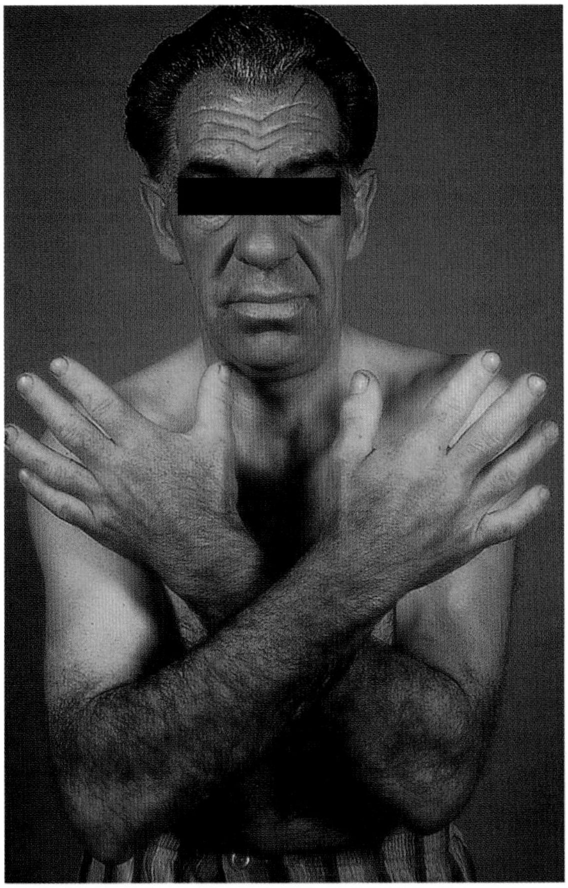

Fig. 32.12 Acromegaly. Note coarse facial features resulting from increased growth of connective tissue and cartilage, together with the typical broadening and enlargement of the fingers. (Courtesy of Professor S R Bloom, Hammersmith Hospital, London.)

- glucose intolerance – diabetes mellitus
- osteoporosis
- hypertension.

Investigation

The diagnosis is confirmed by finding elevated (or normal) plasma growth hormone levels which are not suppressed by a glucose tolerance test and by identifying a tumour as described above. Raised insulin-like growth factor 1 (IGF-1) levels are usually found. Visual fields should be checked because the pituitary tumour may press on the optic nerves.

Management

General

It is important to make a distinction between cure and control. Cure is achieved when growth hormone levels are undetectable on random blood samples or in response to a glucose tolerance test; control is obtained when levels of growth hormone are significantly reduced. Most centres attempt to control rather than eradicate the excess of growth hormone. The treatment of acromegaly in part depends on the expertise of the local centre.

Operation or radiotherapy

Transsphenoidal operation or the use of radiotherapy often shrinks rather than completely removes the tumour and both are equally effective. The disadvantages of radiotherapy are that it takes several years for the growth hormone level to fall to an acceptable value but continued decline may eventually result in hypopituitarism.

Medical

Octreotide (a somatostatin analogue) administered as an adjunct to surgery or radiotherapy is effective in further reducing growth hormone levels. Dopamine agonists (e.g. bromocriptine) and the growth hormone antagonist can also be used.

CUSHING'S DISEASE

Aetiology

Cushing's disease is pituitary-dependent bilateral adrenocorticohyperplasia secondary to ACTH secretion by a pituitary adenoma. The majority of affected patients are female, and they present with cushingoid features. The clinical description and diagnostic tests are detailed above. The differential diagnoses are adrenocortical adenoma/carcinoma, ectopic ACTH secretion and steroid therapy.

Management

Surgical

Transsphenoidal removal of the pituitary is considered the first-line treatment and gives an 80% chance of cure. For the remaining 20% of patients, it may be necessary to irradiate the pituitary. Used in isolation, radiotherapy can cure approximately 50% of adults but has a remarkable 80% success rate in children. Bilateral adrenalectomy remains an option, particularly in patients not cured by either surgery or radiotherapy, but it is considered a salvage technique in the presence of failure of other treatments.

Medical

There is little role for long-term drug treatment unless there has been a failure of radiotherapy or surgery. Metyrapone, which blocks steroid synthesis by the adrenal gland, is used preoperatively.

COMPLICATIONS OF MANAGEMENT OF PITUITARY DISORDERS

Nelson's syndrome

This is a combination of skin hyperpigmentation and a rapidly expanding pituitary tumour which may arise as a consequence of adrenalectomy for Cushing's disease. The lessening of feedback inhibition by cortisol results in markedly elevated levels of ACTH, associated with a transformation of a microadenoma into a fast-growing and aggressive pituitary tumour. Pigmentation occurs as a direct effect of the high concentration of plasma ACTH, whose molecular structure closely resembles melanocyte-stimulating hormone (MSH). This hyperpigmentation is also observed in ectopic ACTH syndrome. To prevent Nelson's syndrome after bilateral adrenalectomy, the pituitary must be irradiated.

Diabetes insipidus

This results from a deficiency of vasopressin (antidiuretic hormone, ADH) which is normally secreted from the posterior lobe. The commonest cause is as a complication of operations on the pituitary. There is polyuria and compensatory polydipsia. Dehydration (pure water lack) may result. The diagnosis is confirmed by a high plasma osmolality in the presence of a low urine osmolality. Treatment is with synthetic vasopressin (DDAVP) administered as a nasal spray.

Mixed tumours of the pituitary

It is sometimes possible to demonstrate production of more than one hormone by the cells of a pituitary tumour. Adenomas that produce both growth hormone and prolactin may cause acromegaly and mild features of hyperprolactinaemia. When surgical tumour samples are maintained in cell culture, it may be possible to demonstrate the secretion of multiple hormones in vitro which are not paralleled by multiple endocrine manifestations in vivo.

Thyrotrophic adenomas (TSH-producing adenomas)

These tumours are rare, very aggressive and account for approximately 1% of pituitary neoplasms. They present with mild thyrotoxicosis and are best treated by radical surgery.

Gonadotrophin-producing tumours

These tumours are exceptionally rare and large, often with compression of the pituitary stalk. Patients therefore present with the unusual combination of panhypopituitarism with retained libido and potency because of the effects of luteinising hormone on testosterone secretion. Treatment is by transsphenoidal hypophysectomy.

Craniopharyngioma

It is believed that this tumour arises from nests of misplaced tissue of the hypophyseal recess (Rathke's pouch). Although most are suprasellar, some develop within the pituitary fossa. They account for approximately 3% of all pituitary tumours and have been reported at birth. Increase in tumour size is slow, and presentation is with headaches, visual defects and failure of normal growth. Local pressure on the surrounding hypothalamic tissue by the tumour produces an intense gliosis, making total excision by the neurosurgeon not only difficult but also extremely dangerous.

Null-cell adenomas

So-called functionless tumours of the pituitary were in the past thought to be quite common. Many such adenomas are now shown by immunocytochemistry or tissue culture techniques to secrete a variety of hormones, although these are produced at an insufficient level to cause endocrine syndromes. Their major presentation is with severe headaches associated with destruction of the pituitary, consequent hypopituitarism and associated severe visual defects. Small tumours are often found incidentally at postmortem.

Carcinoma of the pituitary and secondary deposits

Carcinoma of the pituitary is exceptionally rare and, when it occurs, rarely metastasises outside the brain. Secondary deposits in the pituitary are quite common. They are blood-borne and associated with carcinomatosis, particularly from primary growths in the bronchus or breast. It is rare for these tumours to produce specific clinical entities.

MULTIPLE ENDOCRINE NEOPLASIA

During embryonic life, the cells destined to form the endocrine organs arise from a single group in the neuro-ectoderm of the fetus. These cells, despite their widespread location in the body, have common histochemical features summarised by the acronym APUD (amine precursor uptake and decarboxylation). When such a tumour arises from one endocrine gland, it is likely that it is associated with tumour in other endocrine organs. The distribution of these tumours is not haphazard; certain associations are more common. Multiple endocrine neoplasia types I and II (MEN I, MEN II) are such autosomal dominant familial cancer syndromes.

MEN I

This is the more common type and involves the MEN I tumour suppressor gene on chromosome 11. The syndrome comprises neoplasia or hyperplasia of the parathyroids, the pancreatic islet cells, the pituitary and the thyroid, and rarely adrenal cortical tumours, carcinoids and lipomas. The pattern of neoplasia most commonly present is shown in Table 32.8. Not all tumours are present in any one patient. The likelihood of a particular tumour being found in a patient with MEN I, and the effects of these disorders, are also shown in Table 32.8.

Table 32.8 The pattern of neoplasia in MEN I

Gland(s)	Abnormality	Frequency	Effect
Parathyroids	Hyperplasia	90%	Hyperparathyroidism
Pancreatic islets	Multiple adenomas	60–80%	Zollinger–Ellison syndrome or insulinoma or glucagonoma or VIPoma
Pituitary chromophobes	Adenoma	50–70%	Prolactinoma or acromegaly
Thyroid	Adenoma	20%	Non-functional

Management

Parathyroid hyperplasia

There is a very high recurrence rate following subtotal parathyroidectomy, and some surgeons advocate total parathyroidectomy and lifelong maintenance with calcium and vitamin D supplementation.

Pancreatic islet cell hyperplasia

Pancreatic adenomas tend to be multiple and recur after partial pancreatectomy. Insulinomas are treated by either distal pancreatectomy or enucleation of tumours that are in the pancreatic head. Gastrinomas frequently present at a late stage and are successfully managed medically.

Pituitary adenomas

These can be treated medically (see above) or by excision if medical treatment is unsuccessful.

Thyroid adenoma

The main consideration is to exclude malignancy and for this reason the adenoma is best excised.

MEN II

This is an inherited cancer syndrome characterised by medullary thyroid cancer (MTC) and its precursor C-cell hyperplasia. There are three distinct subtypes:

- familial – MTC is the sole feature
- MEN IIa – MTC, phaeochromocytoma and parathyroid hyperplasia
- MEN IIB – as with MEN IIA (although parathyroid involvement is rare) but with the additional developmental abnormalities of marfanoid features, mucosal neuromas and intestinal ganglioneuromas.

Genetics

The MEN II gene has been identified as the *ret* proto-oncogene on chromosome 10, which encodes the transcellular tyrosine kinase receptor. Mutations of the *ret* proto-oncogene have also been identified in patients with Hirschsprung's disease.

Management

Thyroid medullary carcinomas

See above for a discussion.

Adrenal tumours

These must be removed. Recurrence is likely and patients must be carefully followed up.

Parathyroid hyperplasia

The disease is usually mild, and surgical resection is limited to the enlarged gland(s).

Screening relatives

See 'Thyroid medullary carcinomas' (above).

FURTHER READING

Clark O H, Duh Q-Y Kebebew E (eds) 2005 Textbook of endocrine surgery, 2nd edn. Elsevier Saunders, Philadelphia

Lennard TW 2009 Endocrine surgery: a companion to specialist surgical practice, 4th edn. Elsevier Saunders, Edinburgh

33 Urology

Urology deals with diseases and disorders of the male genitourinary and female urinary tracts. Urologists have been responsible for the introduction of many new techniques. These include the development and widespread use of endoscopes, lithotripsy, prosthetic stents, laparoscopic surgery including robotic surgery, and high intensity focused ultrasound (HIFU).

KIDNEYS AND URETERS

Symptoms arising from the kidney and ureter

Systemic

Fever

Acute pyelonephritis is usually associated with a high fever (40°C). In infants and children there may not be any associated urinary symptoms. Chronic pyelonephritis is not associated with fever. Swinging pyrexia is often a feature of renal carcinoma.

General malaise and weight loss

These are often seen – as in diseases of other systems – with cancer or chronic infection. They may also be features of chronic kidney disease.

Pain

Pain may be perceived at the surface directly over the area of involvement: local renal pain is felt in the flank and costovertebral angle. It is typically a dull, constant ache and related to distension of the renal capsule. However, many renal diseases progress slowly and may not be associated with such pain until some secondary event occurs to cause acute capsular distension. Examples are cancer, tuberculosis, polycystic disease, staghorn calculi and hydronephrosis secondary to congenital pelviureteric junction obstruction (Fig. 33.1).

Pain may also be experienced at the surface further away from the site of origin. Such pain is often called 'referred', but it is being felt at the surface representation of the segment in which it originates. Thus the severe pain of ureteric colic

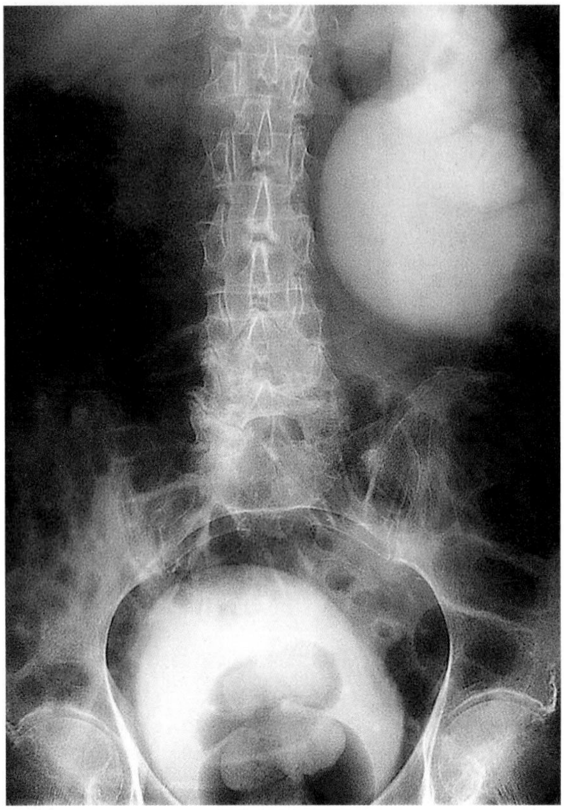

Fig. 33.1 An intravenous urogram of a congenital obstruction of the left pelviureteric junction.

Clinical Box 33.1 Haematuria diagnosis and investigation

- Haematuria may be painful or painless
- Painful haematuria is usually associated with an infection but may result from stones, carcinoma in situ of the bladder, self-induced foreign bodies or urethral trauma
- Painless haematuria is a sinister sign and most likely due to renal or bladder cancer. Other conditions are shown in Box 33.1
- A cystoscopy investigation and ultrasound scan are mandatory

Box 33.1 Common causes of haematuria

Systemic
- Anticoagulants
- Sickle cell disease
- Bacterial endocarditis (emboli)
- Henoch–Schönlein purpura
- Cyclophosphamide

Nephrological
- Mesangial IgA disease
- Glomerulonephritis
- Renal infarcts
- Urinary infection
- Tuberculosis
- Polycystic disease

Urological
- Carcinoma of kidney
- Urothelial tumours
- Stones
- Schistosomiasis
- Benign prostatic

which occurs in waves and is often associated with vomiting may be felt in the testicle (T11 to T12). A stone in the lower ureter may cause pain referred to the scrotal wall (L1) and the bladder.

Oliguria and anuria

A reduced or absent urine output may be caused by underperfusion of the kidney as a result of shock from blood, water and electrolyte loss or in sepsis. Bilateral ureteric obstruction or injury to a solitary kidney are other causes.

Anaemia and its symptoms

These are invariable in chronic kidney disease but also occur as a result of renal tumours, chronic infection and blood loss.

Local

Haematuria

Haematuria always requires full investigation (Clinical Box 33.1). The additional presence of proteinuria and abnormal red-cell morphology on microscopy are more suggestive of a renal cause. Common causes of haematuria are shown in Box 33.1.

Clinical examination of the upper urinary tract

Tongue

Because water and electrolyte disturbance are common in urological disease, the tongue should be examined for dryness and at the same time the breath smelt for the characteristic fishy smell of uraemia.

Abdominal inspection

In children, inspection is the most reliable method of identifying a renal mass, which may be seen in the upper abdomen or inferred from fullness or oedema in this area, the latter implying perinephric infection.

Palpation

The patient should lie supine on a firm surface. The kidney is lifted by one hand placed in the costovertebral angle. On deep inspiration, the kidney moves downwards. When it is at its lowest, the other (anterior) hand is pressed firmly backwards beneath the costal margin in an effort to trap the kidney below that point. The anterior hand can then palpate the size, shape and consistency of the kidney as it slips back into its normal position. The left kidney should be examined from the left side. The right kidney lies lower than the left and it is sometimes possible to feel the lower pole even if it is normal. The left cannot usually be felt unless it is enlarged or displaced.

Enlargement of the kidney suggests polycystic disease, a renal cyst, tumour or hydronephrosis.

Percussion

Renal masses are frequently soft and difficult to feel. They can often be more easily outlined by percussion.

Auscultation

A bruit may be heard over the upper abdomen. Possible causes are renal artery stenosis, aneurysm of the renal artery and an arteriovenous fistula.

Investigation

A combination of haematological, biochemical, bacteriological, radiological, isotopic and endoscopic examination is needed to achieve an accurate, rapid, cost-effective determination of the probable diagnosis and requirements for treatment.

Examination of the urine

Technique

A timed urine collection may be required for assessment of renal function (see 'Creatinine clearance', below), proteinuria or the excretion of substances associated with stone formation.

It is best to examine a freshly voided specimen taken midway through the act of micturition. Many of the details in the collection of this midstream (MSU) sample are shrouded in rituals which are mostly a waste of time and money. Specimens collected from women who have not undergone any special preparation and who void into disposable plastic cups show a 95% concordance with a catheter specimen. In addition, genital cleaning makes little difference to the bacterial count. The most important factor is rapid transport of specimens to the laboratory.

Urine is usually collected into a clean polystyrene cup and then transferred without spillage to a sterile universal container. In younger children, a plastic bag is attached around the urethral meatus. In girls, catheterisation with a fine catheter is appropriate, although, in either sex, suprapubic needle aspiration is easy to perform, particularly if hydration is adequate and the bladder full. The suprapubic area is cleansed; local anaesthetic is injected to raise an intradermal wheal 1–2 cm above the pubic symphysis. A 10 mL syringe with a 22 gauge needle is inserted perpendicularly through the abdominal wall into the bladder, maintaining gentle suction with the syringe so that the urine is aspirated as soon as the bladder is entered.

Colour and appearance

Overtly bloody urine is usually unmistakable. However, red urine can result from:

- betacyanin excretion after beetroot ingestion
- myoglobinuria, the result of muscle trauma
- haemoglobinuria after haemolysis.

Chemical tests

Chemically impregnated reagent strips permit the simultaneous rapid performance of a number of tests, including the presence of blood, protein, ketones, glucose, nitrites and leucocyte esterase. These tests can be useful for screening and show excellent correlation with more-extensive laboratory examination. Positive tests for nitrites and leucocytes has a high predictive value for urinary infection and treatment should be started immediately before culture results are available.

Microscopy

Examination of the centrifuged urinary sediment allows identification of red blood cells (which always requires further investigation), white blood cells, bacteria and casts. Cytological examination for malignant cells is also possible.

The presence of more than five white blood cells per high-powered field is abnormal (pyuria) and, if associated with bacteria, indicates a urinary infection. Sterile pyuria – white blood cells but without bacteria – occurs in:

- tuberculosis of the urinary tract
- urinary stones
- recovery from urinary infection.

Culture

Culture enables the organism present to be identified and a prediction made of which antibiotics may be effective in treatment.

Serum creatinine concentration and creatinine clearance

Creatinine in serum is the end-product of the metabolism of creatine in skeletal muscle, which takes place at a fairly steady rate. The molecule is filtered through the glomerulus and its clearance is approximately equal to the glomerular filtration rate (GFR). The serum creatinine concentration remains within the normal range until approximately 50% of renal function has been lost.

Kidney function used to be estimated by measuring creatinine clearance, which required a 24-hour urine collection in addition to serum creatinine estimation. This has been replaced by a calculated estimate of glomerular filtration (eGFR) – see Box 33.2.

Serum urea concentration

The amount of urea in the blood is also related to the GFR. However, it is more influenced by factors external to the kidney, e.g.:

- dietary protein intake
- endogenous sources of nitrogen in the gut such as a gastrointestinal haemorrhage
- rate of urine production, which is the outcome of a number of factors including the state of hydration.

Approximately two-thirds of renal function must be lost before a significant rise in the serum urea concentration takes place. The measurement is less specific as an index of renal function than is creatinine clearance.

Box 33.2 Factors used for calculating estimated glomerular filtration rate (eGFR)

- Serum creatinine
- Age
- Sex
- Race

Serum calcium concentration

The level of serum calcium should be routinely measured in patients with renal stones to identify hyperparathyroidism and alterations in vitamin D metabolism in those with chronic kidney disease. Calcium concentration may also be elevated in patients with renal-cell carcinoma either as part of a paraneoplastic syndrome caused by the secretion of parathyroid hormone-like substance or from bone destruction by secondary deposits.

Serum alkaline phosphatase

The concentration may be elevated as part of a paraneoplastic syndrome in renal-cell carcinoma or from bone deposits in patients with genitourinary or other cancer.

Imaging

Abdominal plain X-ray

A plain abdominal radiograph is frequently called a KUB (kidneys, ureters, bladder) and is the preliminary exposure taken in any radiological study of the urinary tract. It is always the first film to be examined before reporting on any contrast study and can avert pitfalls (Fig. 33.2) and yield a great deal of information (Fig. 33.3).

X-ray contrast studies

Some water-soluble preparations that contain iodine can be administered by several routes, including directly into blood vessels. All procedures which use intravascular contrast media carry a small but definite (≈5%) risk of an adverse reaction. Most are minor and include nausea, vomiting,

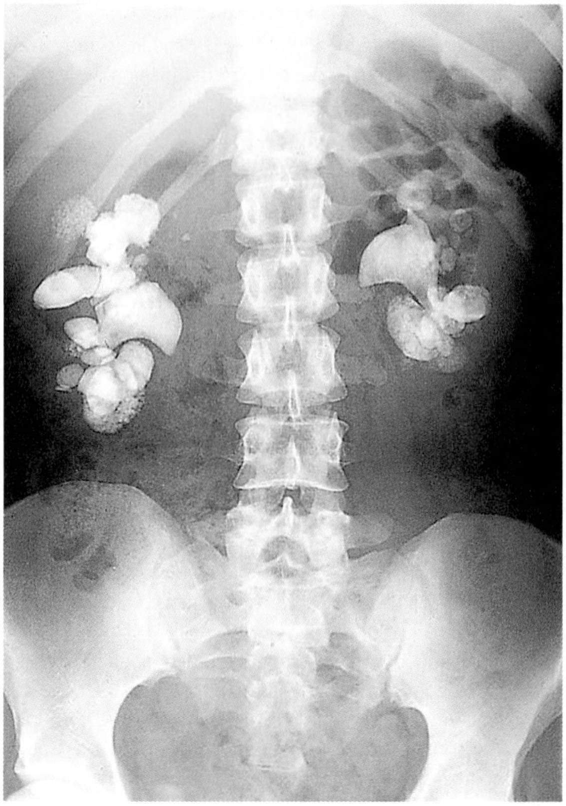

Fig. 33.2 Plain film of the abdomen. Bilateral renal calculi, which could be mistaken for an intravenous urogram, are shown.

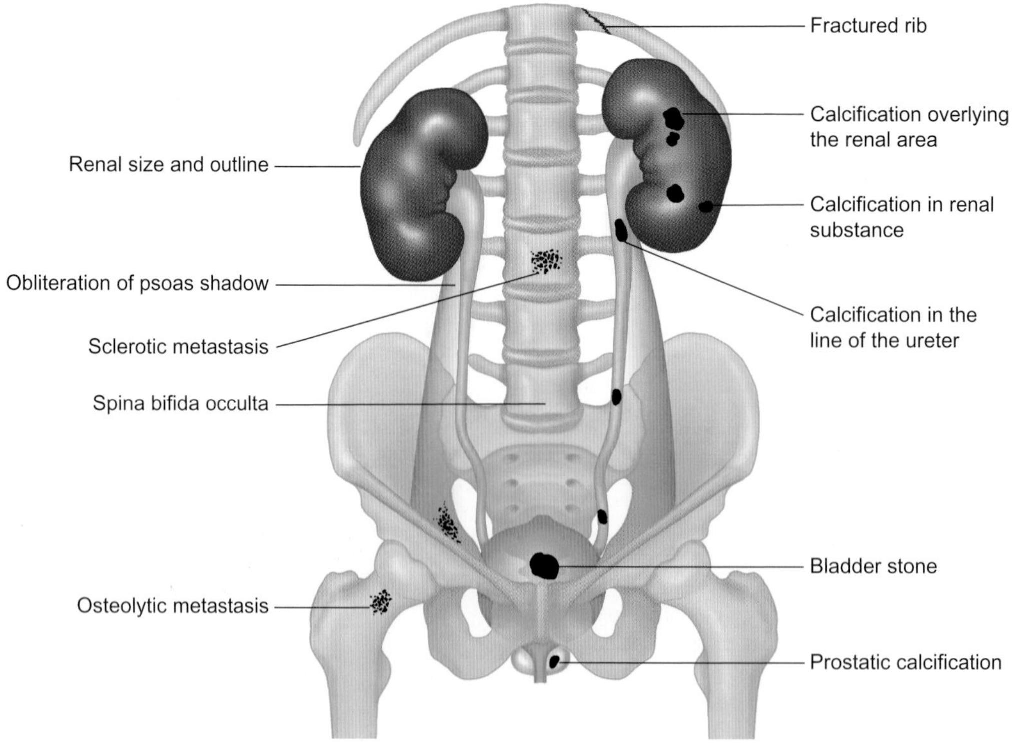

Fig. 33.3 A guide to the interpretation of a plain abdominal X-ray.

itching, rash or flushing. Cardiopulmonary adverse reactions can occur but are rare (1:40 000), although they may be life-threatening or fatal. The contraindications to the use of intravascular contrast to image the urinary tract are shown in Box 33.3.

Patients with relative allergic contraindications can be given corticosteroids. However, there is little evidence to indicate conclusively that their prophylactic use is efficacious.

Intravenous urogram (IVU)

IVU was the most frequently used contrast investigation, but has largely been replaced by a combination of ultrasound and CT scanning. Many of the items shown in Figure 33.4 may also be elicited or confirmed by urography and additional information also obtained (Fig. 33.5).

Those with chronic kidney disease are unable to excrete the usual dose of contrast media at a concentration sufficient to provide an image, and a larger than usual dose is required. It is usual to restrict fluids before an IVU so as to concentrate the urine, but this should not be done in diabetics.

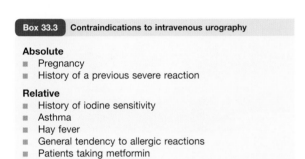

Box 33.3 Contraindications to intravenous urography

Absolute
- Pregnancy
- History of a previous severe reaction

Relative
- History of iodine sensitivity
- Asthma
- Hay fever
- General tendency to allergic reactions
- Patients taking metformin

Retrograde ureterography

A cystoscopy and the placement of a catheter in the ureter are required. Radio-opaque contrast medium is then introduced directly into the renal pelvis or ureter.

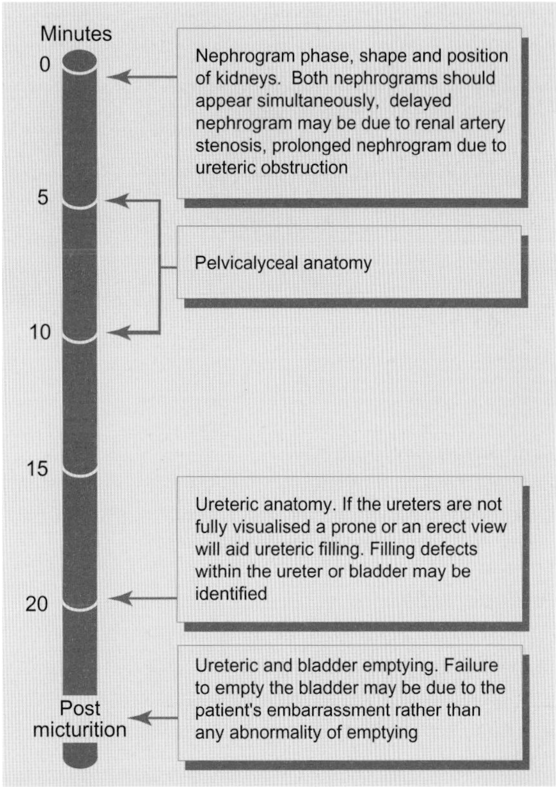

Fig. 33.5 Additional information from an IVU.

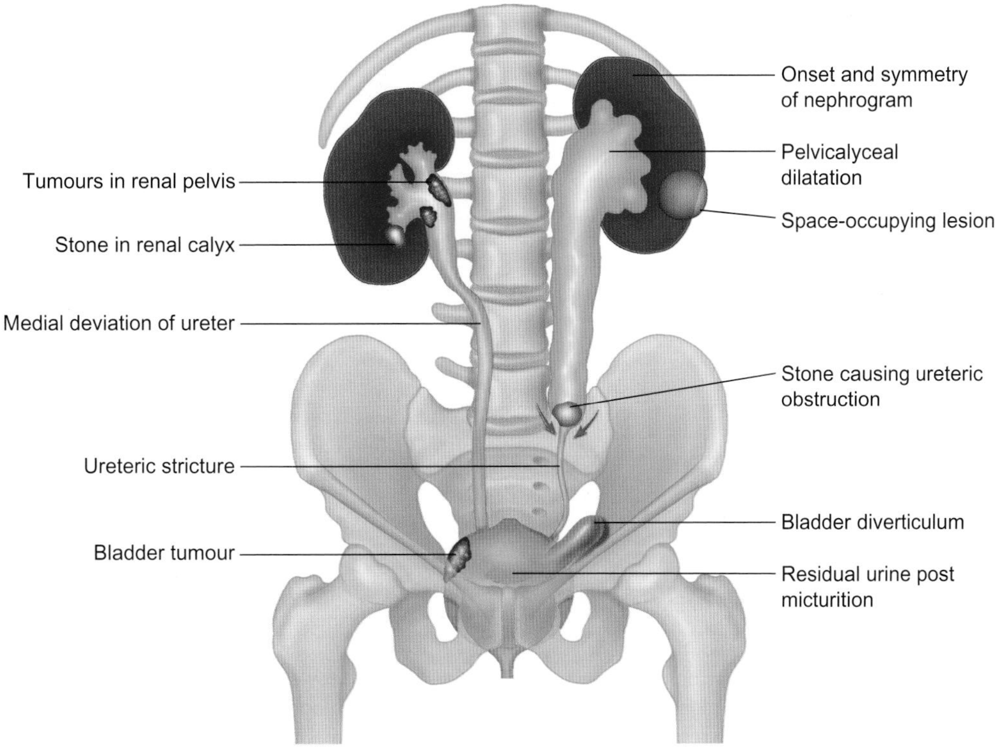

Fig. 33.4 A guide to the interpretation of an intravenous urogram (IVU).

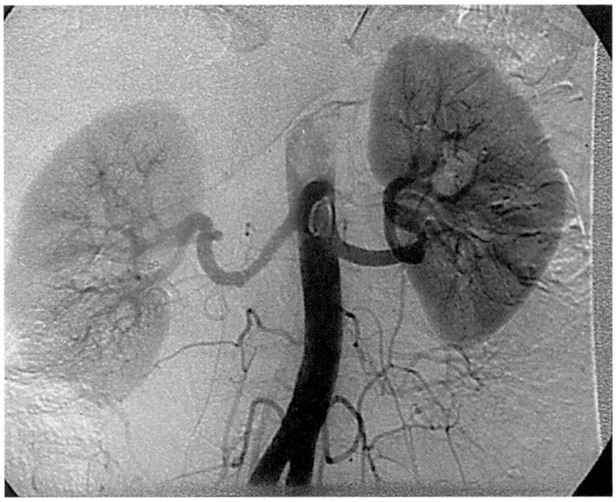

Fig. 33.6 A normal renal arteriogram showing single arteries to both kidneys.

Antegrade pyelography

Contrast medium is introduced either through a nephrostomy tube (nephrostogram) or by direct injection into the renal pelvis via a percutaneous needle puncture.

Arteriography

Arteriography (Fig. 33.6) is most frequently done to evaluate:

- possible causes of renovascular hypertension
- anatomical suitability of potential live related kidney donors
- vascular anatomy before surgery.

It is being superseded by magnetic resonance angiography.

Arteriographic techniques can also be used for therapy. Arteriovenous fistulae and bleeding vascular renal tumours can be embolised and renal artery stenoses dilated.

Micturating cystourethrography

This is done to determine the presence of vesicoureteric reflux. Contrast medium is introduced into the bladder via a urethral catheter which is then removed. Dynamic X-ray studies are made during voiding, and contrast may be seen to reflux up the ureter(s) (Fig. 33.7). The urethra is also delineated and an assessment of residual urine can be made.

Computed tomography

The principal uses of CT are:

- diagnosis and staging of tumours (Fig. 33.8)
- delineation and diagnosis of retroperitoneal masses
- identification and classification of renal trauma
- identification of urinary tract stones.

Ultrasonography

Ultrasound is used in the upper urinary tract to:

- determine the size of the kidneys and the presence of pelvicalyceal dilatation, which may be due to obstruction in patients with chronic kidney disease
- distinguish between solid and cystic renal masses
- identify non-opaque renal stones.

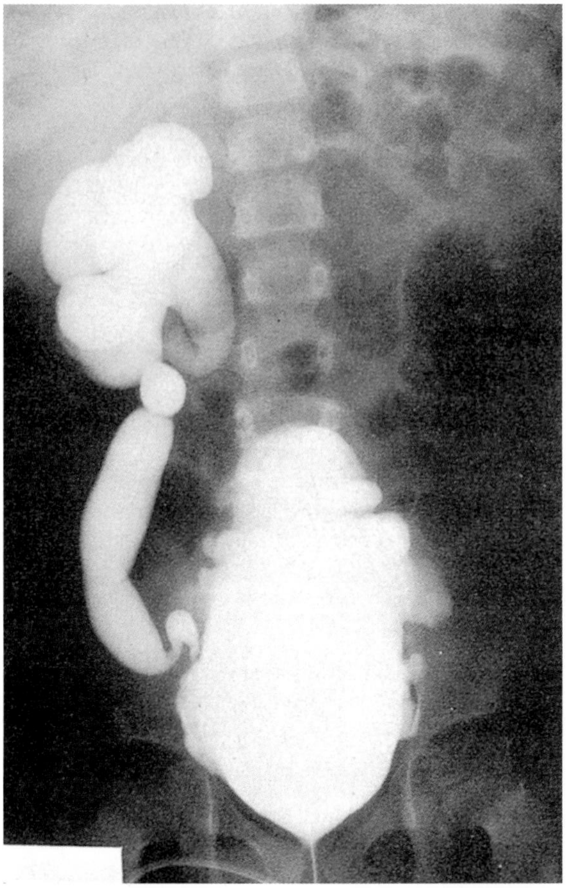

Fig. 33.7 A micturating cystogram which shows reflux and renal scarring.

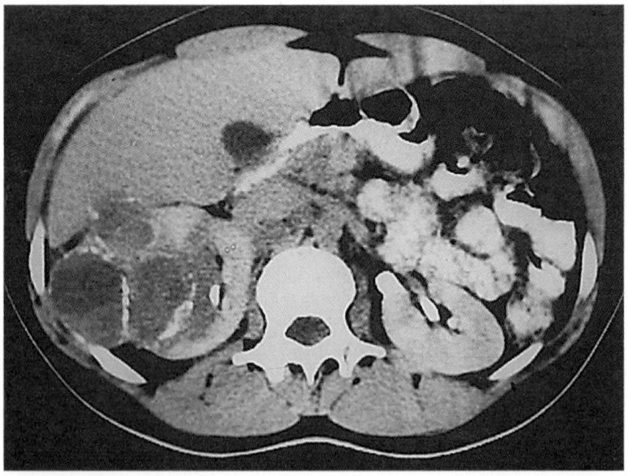

Fig. 33.8 A CT image showing a right renal tumour with extension into the vena cava.

Ultrasonography cannot provide detailed visualisation of the calyces and pelvis, nor does it outline an undilated ureter or provide functional information about the upper urinary tract.

Magnetic resonance imaging

The main advantages of MRI and contraindications to its use are given in Box 33.4. Now new contrast medium such as gadolinium are beginning to improve the imaging ability of

MRI, particularly in the interpretation of prostate architecture. The ability to visualise tumours of the prostate is also enhanced by the latest 3-G magnetic coils.

Radioisotope studies

There are two types of radioisotope study:

- dynamic, in which the function of the kidney is examined over a period of time
- static, which involve imaging of a radiopharmaceutical taken up and retained by the renal tubules.

Dynamic studies. Diethylenetriamine pentaacetic acid (DTPA) is actively secreted by the renal tubules. It is labelled with technetium-99m and administered intravenously. There is a progressive accumulation of the isotope followed by excretion which is recorded over each kidney by a gamma camera (Fig. 33.9) to give quantitative data on excretory function. The information can be used to demonstrate the degree of obstruction in a kidney. Progressive uptake of isotope may also occur in a dilated but unobstructed system, but this can be distinguished from obstruction by the rapid clearance of the isotope after the intravenous injection of furosemide (frusemide; Fig. 33.10). Technetium-99m mercaptoacetyltriglycine (MAG3) is rapidly cleared by tubular secretion and is not retained in the parenchyma of normal kidneys. Due to a much smaller volume of distribution and faster clearance, MAG3 is replacing DTPA in diuretic renography.

Static studies. Dimercaptosuccinic acid (DMSA) is taken up by tubular cells in proportion to their function. The same technique is used as for DTPA scanning: labelling with ^{99m}Tc, intravenous injection and counting with a gamma camera. The relative function of each kidney can then be determined. The investigation is of value in identifying ectopic kidneys, renal scarring and pseudo-tumours in which normally functioning renal tissue is abnormally placed within the substance of the kidney.

Box 33.4 Magnetic resonance imaging

Advantages
- It does not involve the use of ionising radiation
- It permits multiplanar imaging
- It is non-invasive
- It allows greater tissue contrast than do other modalities, particularly for bladder and prostate

Contraindications
Patients who should not undergo MRI include:
- those with cardiac pacemakers
- those with ferromagnetic metallic foreign bodies, including ones that have been placed surgically

DISORDERS OF THE KIDNEY

CONGENITAL ANATOMICAL ABNORMALITIES

The developing kidney is lobulated and becomes kidney-shaped at around 34 weeks of intrauterine life. Persistence of such lobulation into adult life is not of significance. Renal agenesis (the absence of a kidney, ureter and half the trigone of the bladder) has an incidence of 1 : 450 and is important in the context of trauma. A solitary kidney undergoes compensatory hypertrophy. Renal aplasia is associated with a small number of nephrons and undeveloped pelvis and ureter. A hypoplastic kidney is a miniature adult organ commonly associated with the development of hypertension and infection for either of which nephrectomy may be indicated. An ectopic kidney may cause confusion by presenting as an abdominal or, more usually, a pelvic swelling.

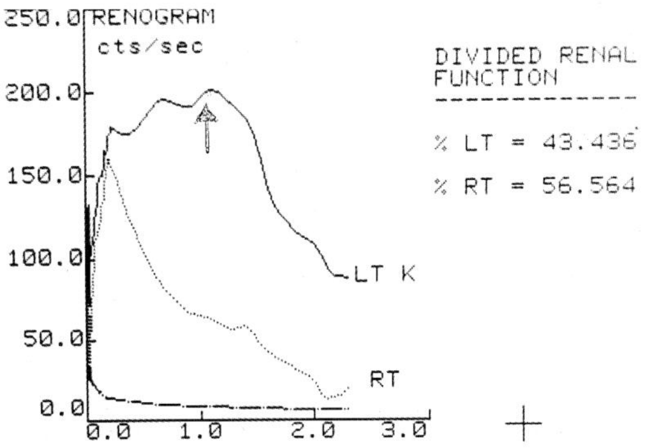

Fig. 33.10 A DTPA renogram following furosemide (frusemide; arrow) showing clearance of the isotope, which refutes a diagnosis of obstruction.

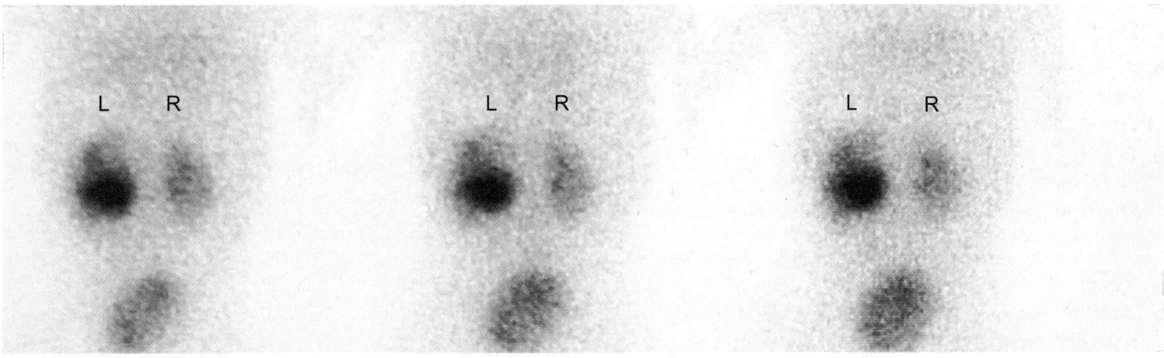

Fig. 33.9 A DTPA renogram which is suggestive of an obstructed left kidney.

Renal cysts

True cysts occur in three circumstances:

- a solitary cyst
- multicystic kidney
- polycystic kidney.

Solitary cysts

The aetiology is unknown. Symptoms are usually absent and the cyst is found during investigation of the urinary tract for other reasons. Very occasionally there may be pain or obstruction of urine drainage, and only then is treatment required by percutaneous aspiration under ultrasound guidance.

Multicystic kidney

Multiple cysts may be found in either dysplastic or otherwise normal organs. In a poorly functioning dysplastic kidney, a nephrectomy is indicated if pain, infection or hypertension is a feature. Multiple cysts in an adult kidney with normal function do not usually warrant treatment. However, if there is pain, aspiration under ultrasound guidance is done.

Polycystic kidney disease

There are two types: infantile and adult.

Autosomal recessive polycystic renal disease

Infantile disease is inherited as an autosomal recessive and presents within the first 9 months of life with gross abdominal distension because of renal masses. The child is pale, has easily palpable kidneys and renal failure. Most infantile polycystic disease has a hopeless prognosis and, without dialysis or transplantation (see Ch. 13), death takes place before the age of 18 months.

Autosomal dominant polycystic renal disease

This is 10 times more common than autorecessive disease. Its relatively common occurrence makes it important, especially as 10% of patients who require renal replacement therapy have this condition.

Aetiology and pathological features. A single gene defect linked to the alpha-haemoglobin gene on the short arm of chromosome 16 is inherited as an autosomal dominant. The precise mechanism of cyst formation is unknown. They are present in infancy and, with advancing age, enlarge to cause progressive loss of intervening renal tissue and the development of renal failure. The following can be associated:

- berry aneurysms of the cerebral vessels
- polycythaemia
- cysts in other organs – liver, thyroid, breast and pancreas
- hypertension.

Clinical features. The common presenting age is between 25 and 50 years. Symptoms include:

- loin pain from increase in size of the kidneys
- acute loin pain with haematuria because of haemorrhage into the cysts
- hypertension and its associated sequelae.

General examination commonly reveals hypertension. There may be features of chronic kidney disease. The kidneys are large and irregular (Fig. 33.11). Occasionally there is hepatomegaly from cystic involvement of that organ.

Diagnosis. A definitive diagnosis can be made by ultrasound, which shows the pelvis of each kidney elongated and attenuated by the smooth surface of adjacent cysts. Ultrasonography confirms the presence of multiple cysts in the kidneys and other organs. This investigation should be used to screen children who are the offspring of parents known to have the condition.

Management

In the majority, the disease is progressive and ultimately necessitates renal replacement by dialysis and/or transplantation (Ch. 13). Failure to control hypertension accelerates the loss of kidney function.

URINARY INFECTION

Urinary tract infection is the most common bacterial infection in humans of all ages. The incidence and sequelae of urinary infections, their diagnosis and treatment all vary with age. By the time adolescence is reached, 1–2% of boys and 5% of girls will have had a urinary infection.

Infection in children

Aetiology and pathological features

Organisms that ascend from the urethral meatus are usually Gram-negative faecal flora. *E. coli* and *Proteus* spp. are the commonest. Vesicoureteric reflux or other anatomical abnormalities may be associated. If infection ascends to the growing kidneys (up to the age of 5 years) and is repeated, renal damage occurs with progressive scarring (the outcome of healing of a cortical abscess) and the development of chronic kidney disease and hypertension. Infection is one of the few preventable forms of chronic kidney disease.

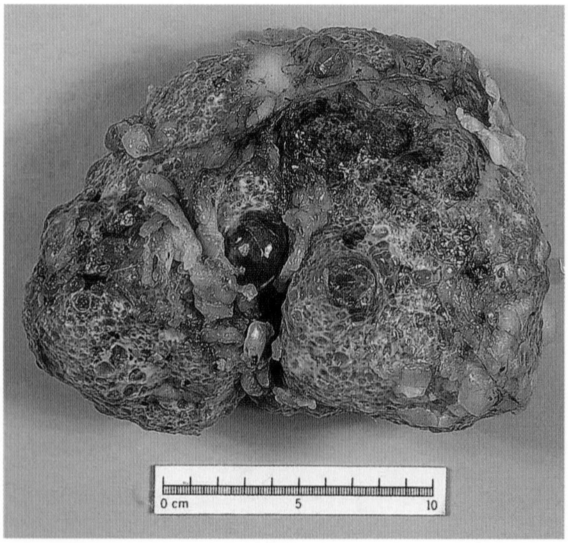

Fig. 33.11 A polycystic kidney.

Clinical features

The younger the child, the less specific the symptoms (see Box 33.5). Older children may complain of:

- loin pain
- increased frequency
- burning on micturition
- haematuria
- enuresis.

Specific signs are absent, but there may be some tenderness in one or both renal angles.

Investigation

Bacterial culture

Urine should be obtained for dipstick testing (see above) and for culture and antibiotic sensitivities before antibiotic therapy is begun.

Imaging

Any child with an infection must be thoroughly investigated to find out if there is an anatomical abnormality.

Ultrasound identifies congenital abnormalities, dilatation of the renal pelvis and ureter, urinary stones and renal scarring.

Micturating cystourethrography is done, after the urine has been made sterile, to identify and quantitate vesicoureteral reflux, scarring and the adequacy of bladder emptying (see Fig. 33.7).

DMSA renography is the best way of identifying renal scarring.

Management

Infants and children with a normal ultrasound and micturating cystogram

A single course of an appropriate broad-spectrum antibiotic (amoxicillin, trimethoprim, and cephalosporins are among the most effective) should be given for 5–7 days. Thereafter, follow up for a year with monthly urine specimens for bacterial analysis. Because of the risk of renal scarring in infants, prophylactic low-dose antibiotics are given until the age of 2 years. In older children, prophylaxis is limited to 6 months. Clinical recurrence requires further antibiotic therapy and full investigation.

Children with vesicoureteric reflux and/or renal scarring

The treatment of the acute episode is as above. Thereafter, prophylaxis up to the age of 5 years is essential. Ultrasound examination of the kidneys is done at yearly intervals. A direct cystogram is done up to the age of 2 years if the reflux has not resolved. An indirect cystogram using MAG3 renography is performed annually up to the age of 5 years. The reflux resolves spontaneously in 80% and, in consequence, there has been a move away from its surgical correction. Indications for surgery are not clearly defined but include:

- recurrent infection in the presence of antibiotic prophylaxis
- persistent loin pain or fever
- poor compliance with prophylaxis
- progressive scarring.

Box 33.5 Non-specific symptoms associated with urinary tract infection in children

- Vomiting and diarrhoea
- Jaundice
- Weight loss
- High fever
- Unexplained screaming attacks

Acute pyelonephritis

Aetiology

Aerobic Gram-negative bacteria which ascend from the urethra and genital tract are the principal cause; haematogenous infection is infrequent. Once infection is established in the bladder, its ascent to the kidney is the consequence of:

- microbial virulence
- presence of vesicoureteric reflux
- quality of ureteric peristalsis.

Clinical features

Symptoms are:

- high fever, sweating and often vomiting
- dull ache in the loin
- increased frequency
- dysuria
- haematuria.

The only specific sign is loin tenderness.

Investigation

Urine

This is turbid and contains protein and blood. Organisms, red cells, white blood cells and debris may be seen on direct microscopy. Culture is essential.

Blood

Apart from routine investigations, a blood culture may identify the pathogen responsible.

Imaging

Plain X-ray of the abdomen may show renal enlargement or obliteration of the renal outline by perirenal oedema or the presence of a radio-opaque stone.

Ultrasonography may identify a radiolucent stone but, more importantly, may show dilatation of the renal pelvis which suggests an obstruction that needs urgent relief (Fig. 33.12).

Management

There is no need to wait for the results of bacterial culture and sensitivity tests. Antibiotic therapy should begin at once. The majority of infections are caused by organisms that are sensitive to trimethoprim, amoxicillin, cephalosporins or quinolones. The urine is re-cultured a week after treatment is complete to ensure that the infection has been eradicated.

Once the acute episode has settled, any correctable precipitating cause is dealt with.

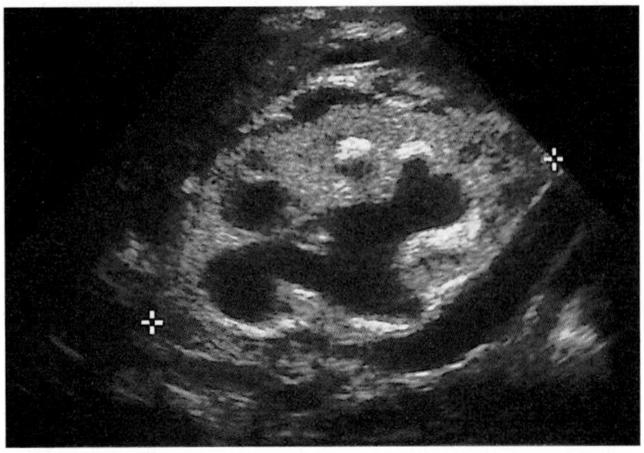

Fig. 33.12 Ultrasound examination showing dilatation of the renal pelvis, a result of ureteric obstruction.

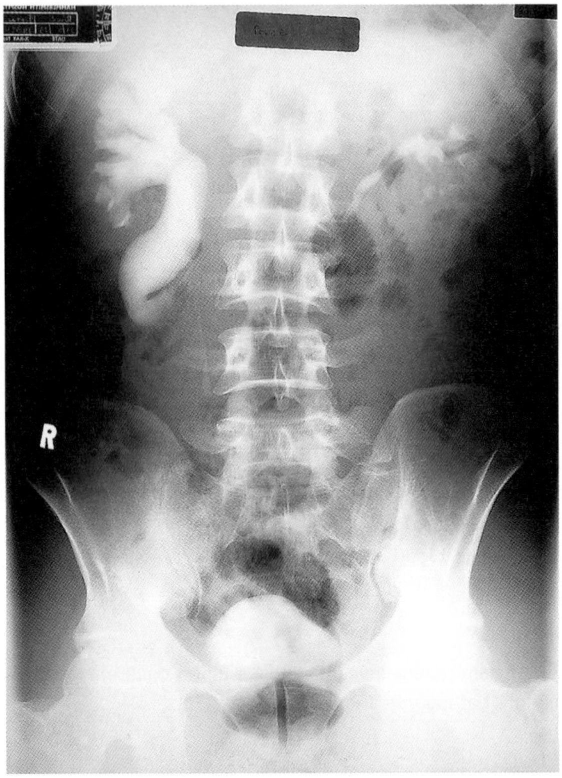

Fig. 33.13 An IVU showing reflux nephropathy. The right kidney is shrunken and scarred with calyceal clubbing.

Reflux nephropathy

This is largely a radiological diagnosis based on the finding of shrunken kidneys with an irregular outline because of cortical scarring – the end result of cortical abscesses. The calyces are clubbed (Fig. 33.13).

Clinical features

The symptoms are those of:

- urinary tract infection
- chronic kidney disease
- hypertension.

There are no specific signs. Most patients are hypertensive, while some are normotensive due to the development of a salt (Na^+)-losing nephropathy.

Management

Existing infection must be eradicated and recurrence prevented by long-term continuous antimicrobial prophylaxis. If hypertension is associated with unilateral disease, a nephrectomy may be indicated.

Renal abscess

Aetiology and pathological features

There are two causes:

- Haematogenous spread – usually of *Staphylococcus aureus* – from a distant site. The condition is common in drug abusers and diabetics. Abscesses are usually multiple and in the cortex.
- Acute pyelonephritis, often with obstruction, causes medullary abscesses which are more common.

Clinical features

Symptoms

There may be a history of recurrent urinary tract infection or parenteral administration of therapeutic (insulin) or other non-therapeutic substances. The patient is often acutely ill with high fever and loin pain.

Signs

In cortical abscess, signs are of:

- flank tenderness
- palpable mass
- erythema of the skin of the loin
- clear urine.

In medullary abscess, signs are of:

- flank tenderness
- obvious pyuria.

Investigation

This is as for acute pyelonephritis. Ultrasonography can identify a renal abscess, but it is difficult to distinguish this from a cystic-necrotic renal carcinoma. However, percutaneous needle aspiration, under ultrasound guidance, confirms the presence of pus.

Management

Management is with systemic antibiotic therapy. Percutaneous drainage of any collections seen on ultrasound is carried out. In medullary abscess, there is subsequent correction of any precipitating factor.

Perinephric abscess

Aetiology and pathological features

The majority of perinephric abscesses result from rupture of a cortical abscess into the perinephric tissue. They therefore lie between the renal capsule and perirenal fascia. A large collection may point posterolaterally over the iliac crest (Fig.

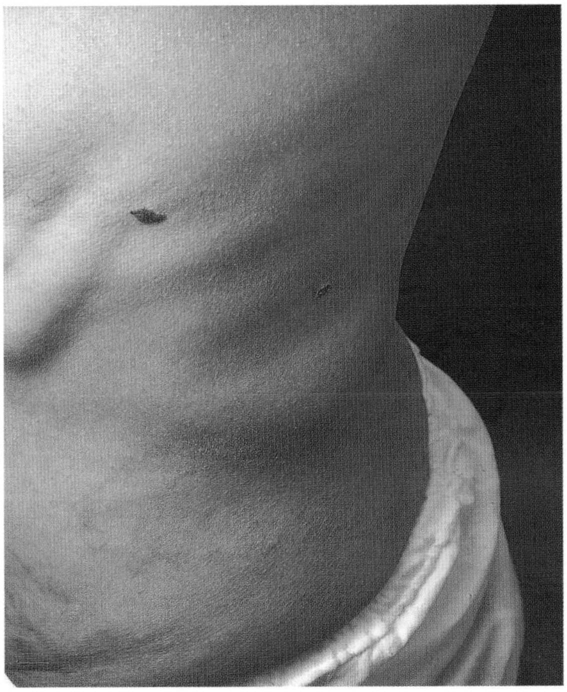

Fig. 33.14 A perinephric abscess pointing posteriorly over the iliac crest.

33.14). The organisms are the same as those found in renal abscesses. There may be an underlying infected hydronephrosis (pyonephrosis).

Clinical features

The onset tends to be slower than in renal abscess. The patient has a fever and complains of loin pain.

Signs are of:

- tenderness over the affected kidney
- large mass
- pleural effusion on chest examination.

Investigation

Blood

There will be a marked leucocytosis.

Imaging

Plain X-ray of the abdomen shows a soft-tissue mass in the flank with obliteration of the renal and psoas shadows. A stone in the renal pelvis may be seen. Because of spasm of the lumbar muscles, there is often a scoliosis with the concavity towards the affected kidney. Gas – produced by coliform or other organisms – may be seen in the renal collecting system or around the kidney.

Ultrasonography may demonstrate a hydronephrosis as well as delineating the extent of the abscess.

CT scan may also outline the mass (Fig. 33.15).

Management

Percutaneous drainage under ultrasound guidance may be adequate, but an open operation is sometimes required.

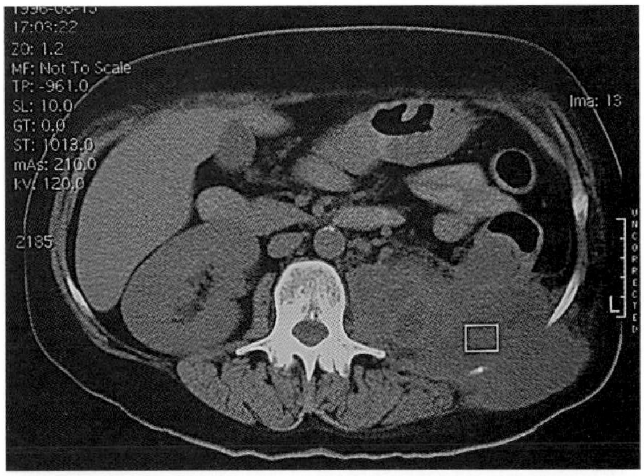

Fig. 33.15 A CT scan of a patient with a perinephric abscess and pyonephrosis.

Nephrectomy is often needed because of underlying kidney disease.

Complications

Ureteric stenosis because of periureteric fibrosis is a common sequel. If the kidney has not been removed, the patency of the ureter should be assessed after 1 month.

Renal tuberculosis

Epidemiology

The condition is on the increase in the UK. There are three known reasons:

- influx of migrants from developing countries where the disease is endemic
- tuberculosis in patients with the acquired immune deficiency syndrome (AIDS)
- tuberculosis in drug users.

However, in addition, renal tuberculosis is reappearing in those that do not meet the above criteria.

Aetiology and pathological features

The organism reaches the genitourinary tract by haematogenous spread from a focus in the lung, which is often asymptomatic. The kidney is usually the primary site, and other organs become involved by shedding of bacteria into the urine. The progress of the disease is slow; in a patient who is otherwise in good condition, it may take many years to destroy the kidney. Involvement of the renal pelvis and ureter may lead to stricture and hydronephrosis. Infection of the bladder wall causes progressive fibrosis and ultimately a shrunken bladder.

Clinical features

The slow evolution of the disease means that, in a patient with an involved kidney, years may elapse before symptoms occur, although occasionally there may be a dull ache in the flank and haematuria. Spread to the bladder may cause increased frequency and pain on moderate bladder distension and at micturition. Rarely, the first presentation is when the patient discovers a painless epididymal swelling.

There are no specific signs.

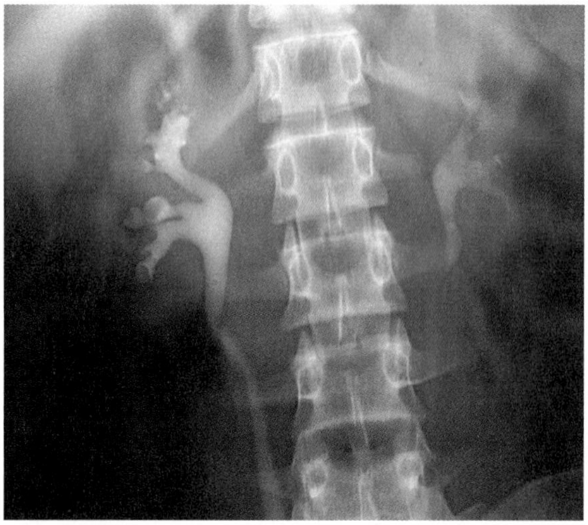

Fig. 33.16 A tuberculous abscess cavity in the upper pole of the right kidney in a patient who presented with an epididymal swelling.

Investigation

Urine

The finding of persistent pyuria without pyogenic organisms on ordinary culture is an indication to collect a first morning specimen on at least three separate occasions for culture for tubercle bacilli. Although a negative result does not exclude the disease, a positive one – which is obtained in a high percentage of samples – is confirmatory. If there is strong presumptive evidence for the presence of tuberculosis, but a negative result, cultures should be repeated, because not only is it necessary to be certain that genitourinary tuberculosis is present, but also the antimicrobial sensitivity must be determined before treatment is begun.

Imaging

Chest X-ray may show evidence of tuberculosis.

IVU may demonstrate calcification in the kidney, an abscess cavity or dilated calyces (Fig. 33.16). Absence of function is a consequence of complete destruction – autonephrectomy.

Management

Management is by chemotherapy. Treatment does not usually need to exceed 9 months and consists of a combination of rifampicin, isoniazid and pyrazinamide. During this treatment, repeated examination by ultrasound is required to make sure that a ureteric stricture does not develop as the tuberculous lesions heal (Fig. 33.17).

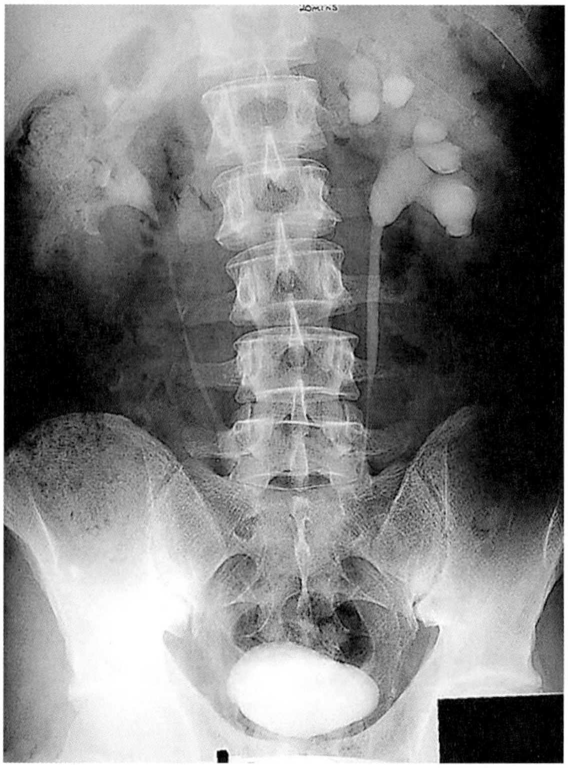

Fig. 33.17 An IVU which demonstrates a left ureteric stricture after treatment for renal tuberculosis.

RENAL TRAUMA

Injury to the kidney is not uncommon, but it rarely results in an urgent life-threatening problem.

Aetiology and pathological features

Closed trauma follows road traffic accidents and sporting injuries and may be accompanied by fracture of the 11th and 12th ribs and injuries to the liver and spleen.

Box 33.6 Classification of renal injuries

- Minor renal trauma (85% of cases) – renal contusion, subcapsular haematoma, superficial cortical laceration. These injuries rarely require surgical exploration
- Major renal trauma (15% of cases) – deep corticomedullary lacerations which may extend into the collecting system. Extravasation of urine into the perirenal space may occur along with large retroperitoneal and perinephric haematomas
- Vascular injury (1% of blunt trauma) – there may be total avulsion of the artery or vein or partial avulsion of the segmental branches of these vessels

Penetrating injuries by knives, bullets and a diagnostic biopsy may, in the first two instances, be associated with other abdominal and thoracic damage. A classification of renal injuries is given in Box 33.6.

Clinical features

No symptoms may be attributable to the kidney, especially in multiple trauma. An otherwise well patient may complain of loin pain and haematuria.

Signs of renal trauma are:

- haematuria
- bruising over the ribs posteriorly
- evidence of penetrating injury
- tenderness and guarding in the loin
- hypotension
- expanding mass
- localised bruit in arteriovenous fistula.

Renal trauma
Renal tumours

Investigation

Imaging

Plain X-ray may show fractures of the 10th, 11th or 12th ribs.

CT scan with contrast is now the investigation of choice. It will accurately assess:

- absence of function on the affected side but a normal contralateral kidney
- absence of function and no contralateral kidney
- the extent of injury
- lacerations
- extravasation
- surrounding haemorrhage
- vessel injury
- non-renal injuries.

CT angiography has largely replaced invasive, but therapeutic angiography may be required in the following circumstances:

- non-function on CT
- persistent severe haematuria which might require embolisation
- presence or development of a bruit
- late development of hypertension in a patient who has recovered from an injury.

Management

Some factors influencing management are given in Clinical Box 33.2.

Any patient with a renal injury should be at rest in bed and have the usual observations. All urine passed is examined for blood.

Penetrating injury

Depending on the type of injury (e.g. gunshot or knife) and the findings on CT scanning, surgical exploration may be required for non-renal damage. Other injuries take priority and the kidney is explored only if there is evidence on preoperative evaluation or at operation of major damage. Nephrectomy may be inevitable.

Closed injury

Treatment is initially non-operative with careful continued assessment. Prophylactic antibiotics are administered. Unless one of the more severe injuries listed in Box 33.6 is present, most injuries resolve, although a relatively prolonged period of stay in hospital may be required. The incidence of later surgical intervention to manage complications is also increased but, in contrast to early exploration, nephrectomy is less commonly needed.

Persistent haematuria or arteriovenous fistula

Selective arterial embolisation of the site is the management of choice.

Clinical Box 33.2 Factors influencing management of renal trauma

- Only 2% of patients with blunt renal injuries, but up to 55% with penetrating injuries, will require exploration
- Nearly all patients with renal gunshot wounds have associated intra-abdominal injuries, compared with 12% with stab wounds posterior to the anterior axillary line
- Urine dipstick testing should be obtained early
- Radiographic imaging should not delay urgent surgery
- CT scanning provides optimal definition of the injury and is the investigation of choice. It also detects other abdominal injuries
- Ureteric and renal pelvic injuries are usually the result of a penetrating injury

RENAL TUMOURS

Tumours of the kidney account for approximately 2% of all malignancies. Benign solid tumours are extremely rare.

There are four types of malignant tumour, apart from the very rare fibro- and liposarcomas:

- nephroblastoma (Wilms' tumour)
- adenocarcinoma
- transitional cell carcinoma of the renal pelvis
- squamous carcinoma of the renal pelvis.

Nephroblastoma

This is also known as a Wilms' tumour. This is the commonest genitourinary neoplasm in infants and second only to brain tumours as a cause of death in this age group. Sex distribution is equal, there is a peak incidence at 2 years and the tumour is bilateral in 5%.

Pathological features

It is an undifferentiated embryonic tumour which contains primitive glomeruli and tubules as well as irregular areas of collagen, cartilage, bone and adipose tissue. Spread is by direct infiltration of the kidney and surrounding structures, by lymphatics and by the bloodstream to the liver, lungs, long bones and brain.

Clinical features

There is often failure to thrive, and a thin, ill infant or child presents with a visible abdominal mass. One-third have haematuria.

Investigation

Imaging

Ultrasonography demonstrates a solid renal mass. CT or MR scanning is required for staging.

Management

In all patients, a radical nephrectomy (a procedure in which, through an abdominal approach, the kidney, perirenal soft tissue and adjacent lymph nodes are removed as a block and the renal vessels divided as close to their origin as possible) is done. The renal vessels are ligated early in the operation to reduce the risk of escape of malignant cells during manipulation.

Additional treatment with radiotherapy and/or chemotherapy depends on the stage of the disease.

Table 33.1 Paraneoplastic syndromes in renal cell carcinoma

Event	Cause
Raised ESR	Changes in plasma proteins
Anaemia	Depressed erythropoiesis and haemolysis
Polycythaemia	Erythropoietin secretion
Hypercalcaemia	Tumour secretion of parathormone-like substance
Raised alkaline phosphatase concentration	Secretion from the tumour
Pyrexia	Circulating pyrogens
Hypertension	Secretion of renin
Amyloid deposition	Unknown
Peripheral neuropathy and myopathy	Unknown

Table 33.2 T component of TNM staging of carcinoma of the kidney

Stage	Findings
T1a	Tumour <4 cm
T1b	4–7 cm limited to kidney
T2	Tumour >7 cm limited to kidney
T3	Tumour extends into major veins or invades adrenal or perinephric tissue but not beyond Gerota's fascia
T4	Tumour invades beyond Gerota's fascia

Prognosis

For localised tumours, there is a 5-year survival of over 90%, but this falls in the presence of anaplastic histology, lymph node metastases and/or metastases to solid organs.

Adenocarcinoma

Epidemiology and pathological features

The peak incidence is in the fifth generation, and the condition is commoner in men. The tumour arises from the renal tubules, is usually well-encapsulated and contains areas of haemorrhage and necrosis. On histological examination, it consists of columnar or cuboidal cells with clear cytoplasm and dark nuclei. Spread is by local infiltration and chiefly by the blood to distant organs. Direct growth may take place into the renal vein and vena cava. Paraneoplastic syndromes may occur (Table 33.1).

Staging

TNM staging is used, based on the preoperative investigations, operative findings and the histological examination of the excised tissues. T stages are shown in Table 33.2 and N and M stages in Table 33.3.

Clinical features

Twenty percent of tumours are detected on ultrasound examination during the course of investigations for non-specific symptoms or for features that suggest a paraneoplastic syndrome.

Table 33.3 N and M components of TNM staging of carcinoma of the kidney

Stage	Findings
NX	Regional lymph nodes cannot be assessed
N0	No regional lymph node metastases
N1	Metastases in a single lymph node <2.0 cm in diameter
N2	Metastases in single lymph node 2–5 cm in greatest diameter or multiple lymph nodes, none >5 cm in greatest diameter
N3	Metastases in lymph node >5 cm in greatest diameter
M0	No distant metastases
M1	Distant metastases

Symptoms

Specific symptoms are not common, but there are some which are semi-specific:

- aching loin pain
- episodes of acute pain – caused by haemorrhage into the tumour and sometimes of sufficient severity for the patient to present as an emergency
- haematuria (60%)
- symptoms of paraneoplastic syndromes (Table 33.1)
- pathological fracture.

Signs

A loin mass is the only finding unless there is clinical evidence of distant metastases. By the time that the triad of loin pain, loin mass and haematuria is present, the tumour is usually advanced.

Investigation

Urine

Haematuria should be sought. Significant proteinuria may indicate involvement of the renal vein.

Blood

Analysis should be done for any of the paraneoplastic syndromes. Hypercalcaemia or a raised alkaline phosphatase does not necessarily imply metastatic disease.

Imaging

Chest X-ray may show typical 'cannonball' metastases.

IVU demonstrates a space-occupying lesion best seen in the nephrogram phase and also calyceal distortion.

Ultrasonography can distinguish between a cyst and a solid tumour and is an effective way of identifying involvement of the renal vein and the vena cava.

CT scan is the most precise way of staging the tumour (Tables 33.2 and 33.3; Fig. 33.8).

Renal angiography is less commonly used but is essential in bilateral tumours or a tumour in a solitary kidney.

Management

Surgery

Radical nephrectomy is the primary treatment in the absence of metastatic disease. There is increasing utilisation of laparoscopy both for removal of the whole kidney and more limited resections of small peripheral tumours. Large tumours and those with tumour tissue invading the renal vein or inferior vena cava are not suitable for a laparoscopic approach.

Non-operative treatment

In symptomatic patients who are unsuitable for surgical treatment, embolisation of the renal artery is effective in controlling pain and haematuria.

Radiotherapy to the primary tumour is ineffective but may help in reducing the pain of a bony metastasis. Endocrine therapy and chemotherapy are both ineffective. Newer treatments for patients with metastatic disease include sunitinib (a tyrosine kinase inhibitir), bevacizumab (a vascular endothelial growth factor inhibitor) and sorafenib (another tyrosine kinase inhibitor), which are showing improved effectiveness compared with previous treatment regimens.

Prognosis

Seventy percent of those with T1 tumours survive for 5 years, and prolonged survival has been reported after removal of secondary deposits. However, there may be long intervals between the presentation of the primary and of metastases. Very rarely, secondary deposits may regress after removal of the primary. Nevertheless, very few patients who present with evidence of metastatic disease survive for more than 2 years.

Carcinoma of the renal pelvis

Carcinoma of the renal pelvis accounts for 10% of all renal tumours, and may be bilateral in up to 25% of cases.

Aetiology and pathological features

Ninety percent are derived from the transitional epithelium (urothelium) and are likely to be associated with similar tumours elsewhere in the urinary tract. However, urothelial tumours of the bladder are 60 times more common than those of the renal pelvis. The remaining 10% in the renal pelvis are squamous carcinomas – a consequence of metaplastic change – and are almost invariably associated with stones. The aetiological factors for transitional cell cancer are similar to those for the same lesion in the bladder.

Clinical features

These are loin pain and haematuria.

Investigation

Cytology

Malignant urothelial cells may be present in the urine.

Imaging

An IVU may show a filling defect in the calyces or renal pelvis (Fig. 33.18), which must be distinguished from a non-opaque renal calculus by ultrasound. CT scanning with and without intravenous contrast is required to provide further information about the primary tumour and to exclude metastatic disease.

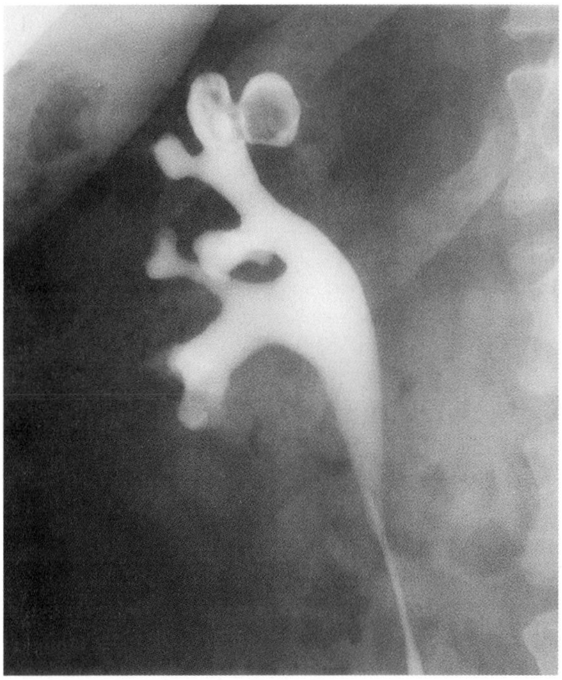

Fig. 33.18 An IVU showing multiple transitional-cell carcinomas of the right renal pelvis.

Management

Management is by removal of the kidney and ureter together with a cuff of bladder mucosa around the ureteric orifice. The reason for such radical surgery is the possibility of the occurrence of a further tumour; in the bladder it is simple to diagnose by cystoscopy, but the ureteric stump cannot be so easily examined.

More conservative management has been attempted by endoscopic resection through a percutaneous nephrostomy tube, direct instrumentation of the ureter or instillation of chemotherapeutic agents directly into the renal pelvis.

Prognosis

In localised transitional-cell tumours of the renal pelvis the outlook is good, but squamous-cell carcinoma of the renal pelvis has a poor prognosis.

STONE DISEASE

Epidemiology

The incidence and site of occurrence of urinary stones vary in different parts of the world and in different parts of the UK. Renal stones are more common in affluent communities whereas bladder stones remain the common site in developing countries. In the UK, the incidence of upper urinary tract stones varies from 15 per 100 000 in the north of England (Burnley) to 47 per 100 000 in the south-east (Canterbury). There are similar differences in the type of stone between countries: uric acid stones make up only 5% of the total in the UK, but this rises to 40% in Israel.

Aetiology

In the majority of instances aetiology is unknown.

Metabolic disorders

Conditions that alter the composition of the urine, chiefly (but not exclusively) to increase its calcium content, are shown in Box 33.7.

Other causes

The commonest of these is infection with the urea-splitting organism *Proteus*. The result is the production of ammonia, an alkaline urine and triple phosphate stones (staghorn calculi) (see Fig. 33.2), which are a mixture of calcium, magnesium and ammonium phosphate. Other factors are dehydration and immobilisation.

Characteristics of stones

These are given in Table 33.4.

Clinical features

Symptoms

These depend on the size and position of the stone and the presence or absence of infection. The patient may be asymptomatic or give a history of occasional haematuria or dysuria. In cystine stone, there may be a family history, and in all stones there may have been previous episodes. A stone lodged at the neck of a calyx or at the pelviureteric junction causes renal colic, in which there are waves of increasing pain in the loin often superimposed on a background of continuous nagging pain at the same site. Radiation downwards into the groin or scrotum is not common, in contrast to the symptoms of a stone in the ureter. The pain from a stone in the renal pelvis is continuous in the loin and often aggravated by movement.

Physical findings

Tenderness may be found in the loin and is increased in severity if there is infection or obstruction when pyrexia is common.

Differential diagnosis

Pain in stone disease is notorious for causing diagnostic confusion with other acute abdominal conditions, some of which require urgent surgical management (Box 33.8).

There are two reasons for making as precise a diagnosis as possible: first, to undertake relief of pain when one of the alternative conditions is present and may mask the clinical features and compound the misdiagnosis; second, many substance abusers have learned the symptoms of renal colic in order to obtain analgesics or narcotics.

Investigation

Any patient who has formed a renal stone stands a greater than 20% chance of producing another. It is important to identify metabolic or structural abnormalities because appropriate management may reduce the risk of recurrence.

Urine

- Culture and sensitivity, measurement of pH and screening for cystine.
- Two 24-hour collections with the patient on a normal diet for measurement of calcium, uric acid, oxalate and citrate concentrations.

Blood

Concentrations of the following are measured:

- urea
- creatinine

Box 33.7 Metabolic causes of urinary tract stones

Hypercalcaemia and hypercalciuria
- Hyperparathyroidism
- Idiopathic hypercalciuria
- Hypervitaminosis D
- Disseminated malignant disease
- Myeloma
- Prolonged immobilisation
- Sarcoidosis
- Milk alkali syndrome
- Cushing's disease
- Hyperthyroidism

Increase in other substances
- Cystinuria (tubular transport defect for cystine, lysine, ornithine and arginine)
- Xanthinuria
- Primary hyperoxaluria
- Secondary hyperoxaluria (ileostomy)
- Hyperuricuria (gout; chemotherapy for leukaemia)
- Indinavir therapy

Box 33.8 Conditions which may mimic ureteric colic

- Appendicitis
- Cholecystitis
- Diverticulitis
- Pyelonephritis
- Leaking aortic aneurysm

Table 33.4 Characteristics of stones

Stone	Incidence	Colour	Appearance	Radio-opacity
Calcium oxalate (mulberry stone)	80%	Pale yellow-brown	Sharp projections	Opaque
Triple phosphate[a] (magnesium ammonium phosphate – struvite stone often causing a staghorn calculus)	10%	Chalky white	Soft	Opaque
Uric acid	5%	Light brown	Facetted	Lucent
Cystine[b]	2%	Yellow-brown	Smooth	Moderately opaque
Xanthine	Rare	Yellow-brown		Lucent

[a]Often associated with infection with urea-splitting organisms, e.g. *Proteus*.
[b]Often a family history and/or episodes of repeated stone formation.

- electrolytes
- total protein
- calcium
- alkaline phosphatase
- uric acid
- phosphate.

In a patient with a stone causing complete obstruction, the bladder urine may be sterile. Urine should then be obtained by the insertion of a percutaneous nephrostomy, which is almost certainly required for relief of obstruction.

Imaging

A patient who presents with acute symptoms and signs and a suspected stone must have an urgent imaging. The use of CT with its ability to identify non-opaque stones is the investigation of choice.

The diagnosis can be firmly established, the size of the stone determined, together with the degree of obstruction, the likelihood of the stone passing spontaneously, and the need for hospital admission.

Non-operative management

Asymptomatic stone

A small, asymptomatic, non-obstructing stone in an elderly, unfit patient can be left alone.

Acute episode

The pain of renal colic is severe and is treated with intravenous diclofenac and if necessary narcotic analgesics, and antispasmodics such as hyoscine. Stones less than 0.5 cm in diameter will usually pass spontaneously, and, if they are opaque, their progress can be assessed by repeated plain abdominal X-ray.

Oxalate stones

The commonest abnormality detected is idiopathic hypercalciuria. A low-calcium diet and a high fluid intake to dilute urine calcium concentration is often recommended. However, it is usually unsuccessful in that tap water in many areas contains significant amounts of calcium and a reduction in dietary calcium intake leads to an increased intestinal absorption of oxalate.

Attempts to reduce urine calcium excretion with bendrofluazide have only been shown to reduce calcium stone formation after prolonged periods of therapy. Sodium cellulose phosphate decreases calcium excretion but is often unacceptable because of the foul diarrhoea it may cause.

Cystine stones

Cystinuria is an inherited defect of amino acid transport involving cystine, ornithine, lysine and arginine. Cystine is relatively insoluble, particularly in acid urine, and this can lead to stone formation. Because its excretion is relatively constant, the stones can be both dissolved and prevented by maintaining a high fluid intake throughout the 24 hours and alkalinising the urine. The latter can be achieved with either sodium bicarbonate or potassium citrate, or a combination of both. If this fails, treatment with penicillamine, which produces a more soluble cystine–penicillamine complex, is sometimes successful. However, it may be associated with the development of skin rashes and the nephrotic syndrome.

Uric acid stones

Uric acid is less soluble in acid urine and, as a result, patients with chronic diarrhoea or an ileostomy are more likely to produce uric acid stones. They can be dissolved or prevented by increasing the fluid intake and alkalinisation of the urine. In addition, allopurinol (100 mg three times a day) should be given to those with an elevated serum level.

Triple phosphate stones

The prevention of recurrent phosphate stones associated with infection is dependent on three factors:

- complete removal of the initial stone(s)
- correction of any anatomical abnormalities of urine drainage
- maintenance of sterile urine.

The last can be achieved with long-term low-dose antibiotic therapy. If this proves difficult, treatment with a urease inhibitor (acetohydroxamic acid) should be considered.

Surgical management

Indications for intervention

Urgent percutaneous nephrostomy drainage is required when:

- fever does not resolve after 24 hours of appropriate antibiotic therapy in a patient with an obstructed kidney
- severe pain persists in spite of the medical management outlined above.

The nephrostomy track can be used at a later stage for endoscopic stone destruction or removal. An indwelling stent can be inserted to establish drainage down the ureter before treatment by lithotripsy (see below).

Intervention in persistent stone

Major advances have been made in the management of stones over the past decade by techniques other than open operation.

Destruction of the stone in situ can be done with:

- extracorporeal transcutaneous techniques (extracorporeal shock wave lithotripsy, ESWL)
- direct application of shock waves or laser to the stone by a probe inserted endoscopically or percutaneously.

Removal can be achieved either endoscopically or percutaneously.

DISORDERS OF THE URETER

CONGENITAL ANATOMICAL ABNORMALITIES

Ureteric duplication

Incomplete duplication is much more common than complete ureteric duplication and occurs in approximately 1% of individuals. Complete duplication is present in about 1 in every 500–600 individuals. The extent of incomplete ureteral duplication may vary from a bifid renal pelvis (which could be considered as a normal variant) to two separate ureters joining with each other at some point during their course. A complete duplication results in two separate ureters with two separate ureteric openings in the bladder. The orifice of the upper-segment ureter always enters the bladder more medial and caudal to the lower-segment orifice. The ureter from the lower part of the kidney is more likely to be associated with vesicoureteric reflux, as the orifice of this ureter is more lateral and cephalic. As the orifice of the ureter from the upper pole is more caudal, it can be located in an ectopic position which may open at the level of the bladder neck, urethra, vestibule or vagina and may result in either obstruction or incontinence.

Clinical features

Duplication of the ureters is commonly asymptomatic. Vesicoureteral reflux into the lower moiety can result in infection, haematuria or flank pain.

Management

Asymptomatic duplications do not require any treatment. If one of the moieties of the kidney is non-functioning, a heminephroureterectomy is the procedure of choice. In cases of complete duplication, vesicoureteral reflux is managed in the usual way. An ectopic ureter can either be re-implanted or a heminephroureterectomy can be performed, depending on the function of that portion of the kidney.

Congenital obstruction at the pelviureteric junction

The pelviureteric junction (PUJ) is the most common site of obstruction in the upper urinary tract.

Aetiology

In the congenital type, intrinsic abnormalities of the PUJ are the most common cause of obstruction. They result from an aperistaltic segment at the level of the PUJ, resulting in a functional obstruction to the passage of urine. In some cases, valve-like processes and polyps have been found.

Extrinsic abnormalities are seen in about one-third of patients with PUJ obstruction. Aberrant vessels may cause obstruction, especially when they cross in front of the PUJ or when the ureter appears to be trapped between two such vessels. PUJ obstruction occurs in approximately 1:1500 births. It is more common in males and is bilateral in 5% of cases. Obstruction is acquired as a result of stricture formation following surgery for stones, trauma or tuberculosis.

Clinical features

Symptoms

The typical clinical presentation has changed since the advent of widespread antenatal sonographic screening. A significant number of babies with antenatal hydronephrosis are subsequently found to have a PUJ obstruction.

Symptoms in infants and children are:

- abdominal mass
- urinary tract infection
- haematuria
- failure to thrive.

Symptoms in adults are:

- intermittent loin pain sometimes associated with alcohol consumption
- urinary infection
- haematuria following mild trauma
- symptoms of stones.

Signs

In infants and children, the sole sign is abdominal mass.

In adults, signs are:

- loin tenderness
- rarely, abdominal mass
- an incidental finding during the course of investigation for another condition.

Investigation

To diagnose PUJ obstruction, both anatomical and functional studies of the kidney are required. Anatomical information of the kidney can be obtained by ultrasound examination. Ultrasound examination reveals dilatation of the pelvicalyceal system and also demonstrates the state of the renal cortex.

Intravenous urography with diuretic enhancement of urine flow

IVU gives an indication of the anatomical as well as the functional state of the kidney (Fig. 33.5). IVU can also be combined with diuretic enhancement of urine flow by giving 40 mg furosemide (frusemide) intravenously. Following contrast and furosemide (frusemide) injection, if there is no increase of dilatation of the pelvicalyceal system and there is good washout of contrast, this indicates a non-obstructed system.

Nuclear isotope scan

A prolonged excretory third phase occurs when there is pelvicalyceal dilatation. If furosemide (frusemide) is given, the counts may rise (obstructed) or fall (non-obstructed).

Management

Broad options of management include:

- observation
- surgical reconstruction
- percutaneous balloon dilatation
- retrograde balloon dilatation
- percutaneous incision (endopyelotomy)
- laparoscopic surgery.

Most PUJ obstructions are now discovered antenatally and hence are asymptomatic. Management is decided on the basis of anatomical and functional information provided by different scans. After birth, the kidneys are observed by repeated scanning with ultrasound and/or isotope renography.

Indications for surgery

These are:

- deterioration of renal function
- worsening of renal dilatation
- thinning of renal cortex
- the presence of symptoms, pain, haematuria or infection.

For primary PUJ obstruction, if operative intervention is required, surgical reconstruction is the method of choice. The percutaneous or retrograde dilatation/incision techniques are usually reserved for secondary PUJ obstruction. The most common surgical technique is the Anderson–Hynes pyeloplasty which disconnects the pelvis from the ureter, reduces the size of the pelvis but requires re-anastomosis of the ureter to the pelvis. A Culp pyeloplasty is useful for those with a small extrarenal pelvis. Re-anastomosis of the ureter is not required (Fig. 33.19). Laparoscopic surgery is being increasingly utilised.

DISORDERS THAT MAY BE EITHER CONGENITAL OR ACQUIRED

Disorders that may be either congenital or acquired

Megaureter

Aetiology

The underlying cause of the congenital variety is the same as that of PUJ obstruction, but the muscular imbalance in megaureter is at the ureterovesical junction. The ureter proximal to this becomes dilated and hypertrophied. The condition may be bilateral, and a secondary hydronephrosis may develop with the formation of stones.

Secondary megaureter may be caused by schistosomiasis or bladder outflow obstruction.

Pathophysiology

Classification on the basis of reflux and the presence of obstruction to flow is shown in Box 33.9 and is used to guide management. Very rarely, reflux and obstruction may coexist. A combination of ultrasound scanning, micturating cystograms and renography permits appropriate categorisation.

Clinical features

Symptoms of megaureter are:

- incidental finding during investigation for another condition
- loin pain
- urinary infection.

Box 33.9 Pathophysiological classification of megaureter

Congenital
- Non-refluxing or refluxing
- Non-obstructed or obstructed

Secondary
- Non-refluxing or refluxing
- Non-obstructed or obstructed

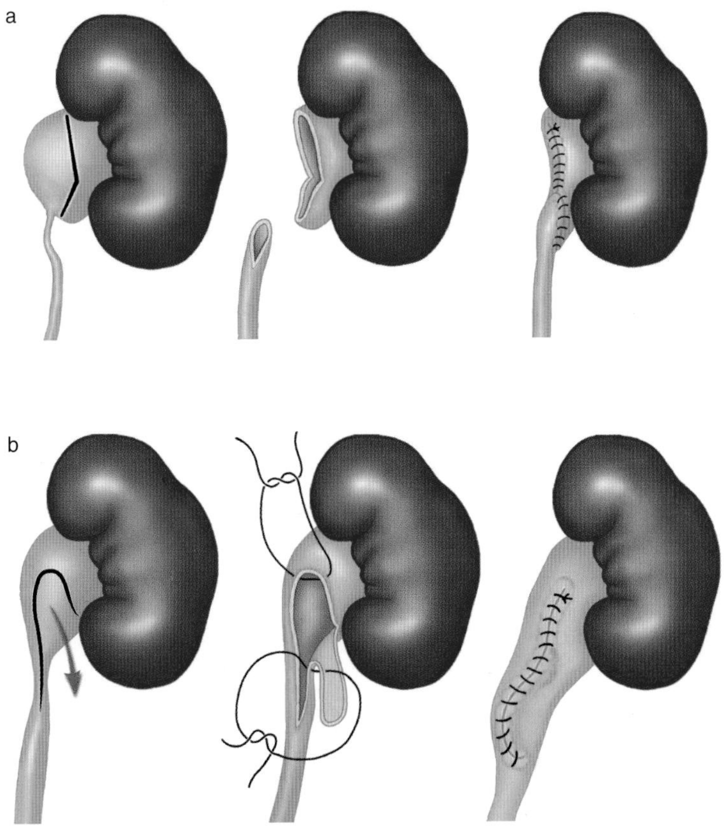

Fig. 33.19 Pyeloplasty operations: (a) Anderson–Hynes; (b) Culp.

Management

Non-obstructed, non-refluxing megaureters do not require treatment.

Congenitally obstructed megaureters should be re-implanted after the narrowing at the distal end has been removed. Those with reflux are treated along the lines of management of vesicoureteric reflux. A secondarily obstructed megaureter requires treatment of its cause.

Vesicoureteric reflux

Aetiology and pathological features

Primary reflux is the result of a defective valvular mechanism at the ureterovesical junction; when compared with a normal ureter, the intramural course is short and more horizontally directed. The condition is bilateral in 50%, and 90% of affected patients are female. There is a familial incidence. As the ureterovesical junction matures, reflux may cease spontaneously.

Secondary reflux may occur because of bladder outlet or urethral obstruction or in neurogenic bladders.

Inflammatory conditions of the bladder wall (schistosomiasis, tuberculosis) can hold the ureteric orifice open.

Clinical features

In primary reflux, the onset is in the first decade. Symptoms may include fever, lethargy, anorexia, nausea and vomiting. There is often mild haematuria, but the main symptoms are those of recurrent urinary infections. Older children may complain of pain in the loin or on micturition. In secondary disease, the onset is later, and again symptoms of infection predominate.

There are no specific signs.

Investigation

Ultrasound is often normal but may show ureteric dilatation or renal scarring.

Micturating cystogram. Cystoureteric reflux is best demonstrated at the time of micturition (Fig. 33.7).

Isotope scanning. A DMSA scan can be used to identify current renal damage.

Management

The majority of patients can be satisfactorily managed by antibiotic therapy. Long-term therapy to suppress infection is necessary up to the age of 6 years. The incidence of renal scarring after this age is very low. Surgical re-implantation of the ureter is indicated when medical management fails to suppress the development of new urinary infections or there is non-compliance with antibiotic treatment. The injection of inert, non-absorbable substances around the ureteric orifice to prevent reflux offers a non-surgical option to treat this condition.

Ureterocele

Ureterocele is a cystic dilatation of the terminal portion of the ureter and may occur in either a normally placed ureter or rarely in an ectopic one. This usually involves the upper-segment ureter of a duplex system. They may become very large and occupy most of the available space in the bladder. A stone impacted in the lower end of the ureter is one cause.

Clinical features

Some patients are asymptomatic. When symptoms do occur, they are usually secondary to complications, such as:

- obstruction of the bladder outlet
- infection
- loin pain.

Signs are minimal. An ectopic ureterocele in a female may present as a vaginal tumour at birth or in childhood. Occasionally they may present at the urethral meatus.

Diagnosis

The diagnosis is made on an ultrasound which shows a rounded swelling in the bladder associated with a dilatation of the ureter – hydroureter.

Management

Asymptomatic ureteroceles do not need treatment. If the ureter is dilated or there is a stone, the ureterocele can be transected endoscopically. The cut is made on the inferior surface because this makes reflux less likely. Ectopic ureteroceles require a heminephroureterectomy.

ACQUIRED CONDITIONS

Ureteric injuries

Aetiology

Open injuries occur from gunshot or stabbing. A closed avulsion of the ureter from the renal pelvis may follow rapid deceleration. However, surgical injuries during abdominal or pelvic operations are the commonest cause. The ureter is at particular risk if it is displaced from its usual anatomical position by the condition under treatment. Operations most frequently associated with ureteric injuries are listed in Box 33.10.

Pathological features

One or both ureters may be ligated. The kidney stops secreting once the intraureteric pressure has risen to the filtration

Box 33.10 Operations most frequently associated with ureteric injuries

Gynaecological
- Hysterectomy
- Ovarian cystectomy
- Repair of vesicovaginal fistula
- Anterior colporrhaphy

General surgery
- Sigmoid colectomy
- Abdominoperineal resection of the rectum
- Repair of aortic aneurysm

Urology
- Excision of bladder diverticula
- Ureterolithotomy
- Ureteroscopy

pressure. In consequence, dilatation of the renal pelvis is mild and, if the condition goes untreated, atrophy of the kidney takes place. Less commonly the lumen is incompletely obstructed by inclusion in a stitch, in which case the kidney continues to secrete and hydronephrosis develops often with accompanying infection. Alternatively, the ureter is divided or suffers a crushing injury. The latter may be ischaemic. Urine then leaks to the exterior or into the retroperitoneal tissues and, less commonly, the peritoneal cavity.

Clinical features

The injury may be recognised at the time of surgery. If not, bilateral ligation will be recognised very soon. Leak usually presents around the fifth postoperative day but may be delayed for 10–14 days if it results from ureteric ischaemia. The features are:

- bilateral ligation – immediate postoperative anuria
- unilateral ligation – either absence of clinical features or, if there is proximal infection, fever and persistent loin pain
- division – urine appears from the drain, the wound or the vagina
- retroperitoneal leakage of sterile urine leads to abdominal distension secondary to ileus and intraperitoneal leakage to signs of free fluid in the peritoneal cavity
- retro- or intraperitoneal leakage of infected urine is associated with the features of peritonitis and generalised sepsis.

Investigation

In the early stages of complete obstruction, an IVU shows a nephrographic effect – contrast medium outlines the whole kidney, but little change in radiodensity is seen in the renal pelvis or ureter. In incomplete obstruction or transsection, there is some delay in excretion, and ureteric dilatation on the side of the injury down to the site of damage is usually seen. If, however, this is not identified, retrograde ureterography may help.

Management

Prevention

A CT scan should be done before any operation in which the ureters are at risk, particularly if there is the possibility of ureteric displacement.

Treatment

The insertion of a ureteric stent may allow a small fistula to close. In critically ill patients, a temporary percutaneous nephrostomy is the procedure of choice to allow drainage of the obstructed and usually infected kidney. In all other instances, surgical repair is necessary, and complicated procedures may be required.

If the injury is recognised at the time of surgery, ligatures should be removed, the crushed area resected, the cut ends should be spatulated and a primary anastomosis performed over a ureteric stent (Fig. 33.20b). Other techniques include:

- re-implantation of the damaged ureter into the bladder (Fig. 33.20d)
- anastomosis of one ureter to the other (Fig. 33.20a)

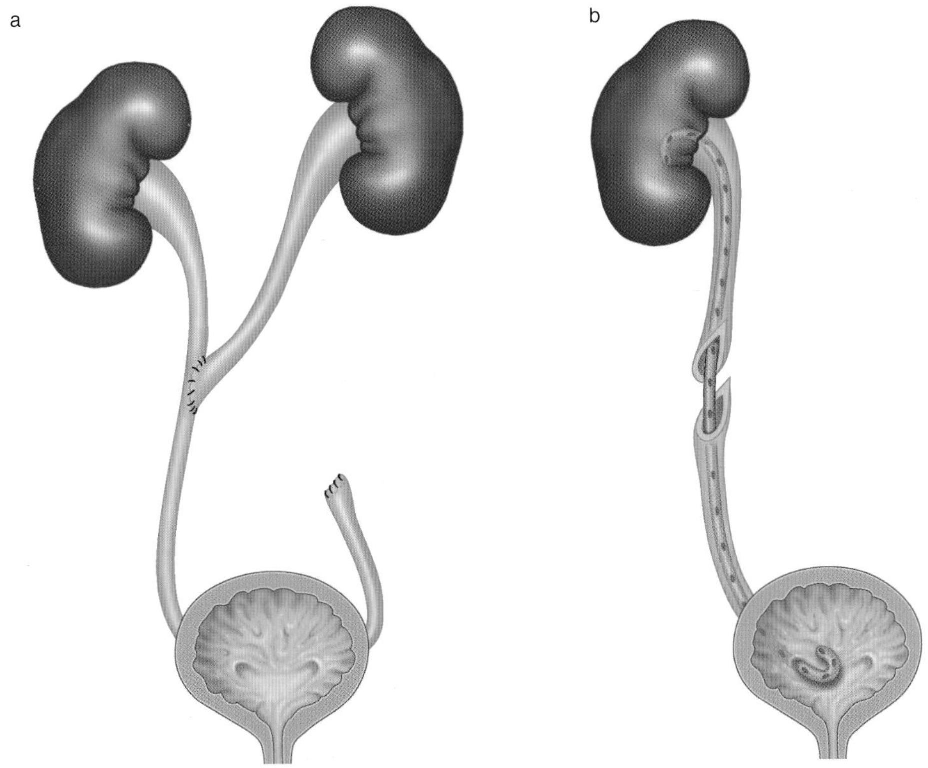

Fig. 33.20 Techniques which may be used for repair of an injured ureter.

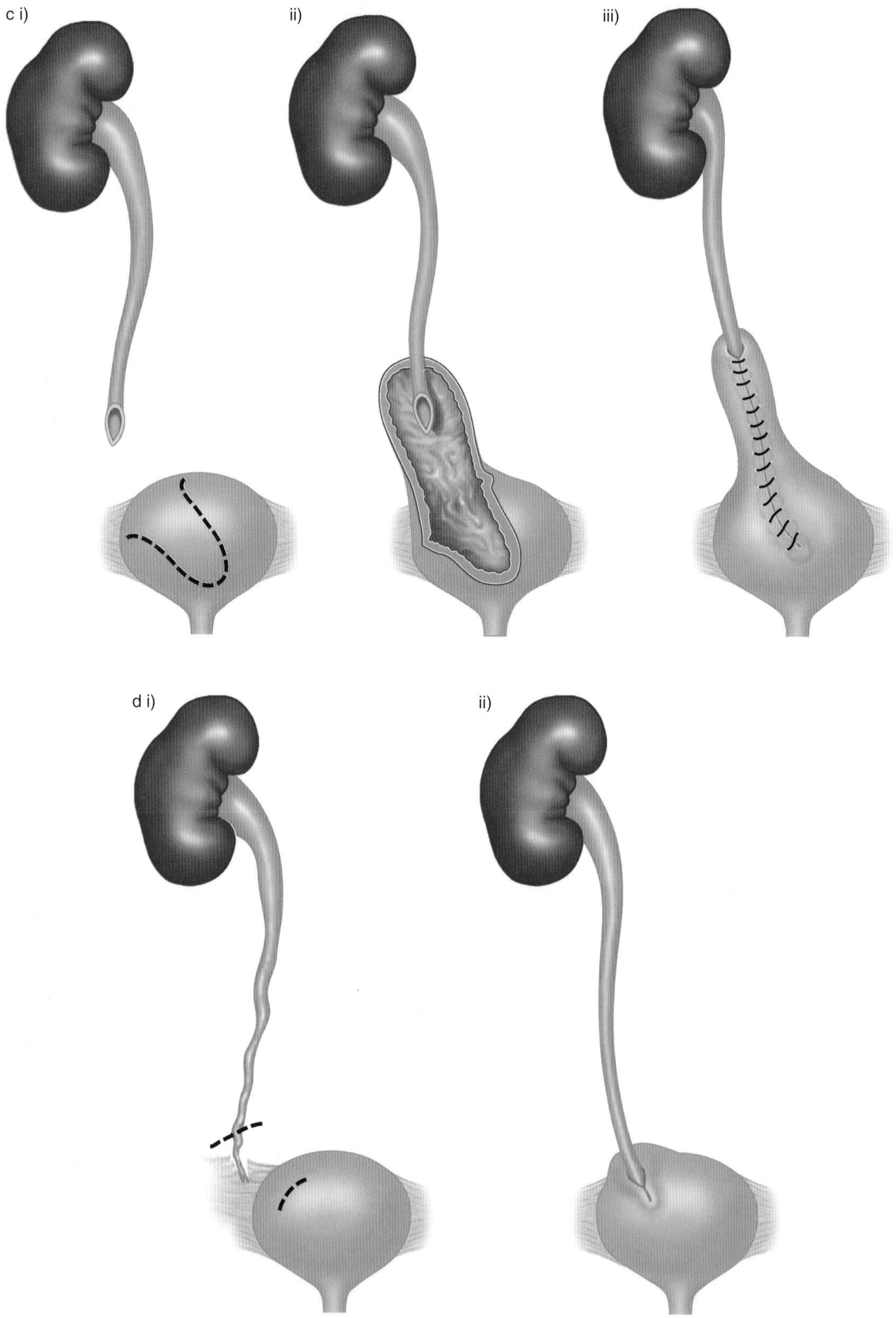

Fig. 33.20, continued

- replacement of the ureter by small intestine
- use of the bladder flap (Boari) to replace the damaged segment (Fig. 33.20c).

Retroperitoneal fibrosis

Aetiology

There are two forms: idiopathic and secondary. In the first, as its name implies, the cause is not known. Secondary retroperitoneal fibrosis may follow:

- treatment with methysergide
- extravasation of urine
- retroperitoneal sepsis
- aortic or iliac aneurysms
- radiotherapy
- most commonly, retroperitoneal spread of malignant disease – cervix, ovary, testis, prostate and lymphomas.

Pathological features

In the primary idiopathic form, one or both ureters become encased in and obstructed by a retroperitoneal plaque of fibrous tissue between the pelviureteric junction and the pelvic brim, although involvement may be more extensive.

Clinical features

Symptoms are non-specific but include backache, low-grade fever and malaise, as well as those of hypertension, renal failure or anuria.

The physical findings are also non-specific and related to the renal failure or hypertension.

Investigation

ESR is invariably raised.

Ultrasound may show upper urinary tract dilatation.

CT scanning shows upper urinary tract dilatation, with medial deviation of one or both ureters, and is useful to define the extent of the retroperitoneal mass.

Bilateral retrograde ureterography often results in complete anuria from ureteric oedema and should be avoided.

Management

Treatment is surgical. A definitive diagnosis of possible underlying causes can only be made by histological examination of tissue from the retroperitoneum, and ureterolysis can be done at the same time. To prevent recurrence of obstruction, both ureters are either wrapped in omentum or brought laterally and intraperitoneally to distance them from the fibrotic mass. Idiopathic retroperitoneal fibrosis does respond to treatment with steroids, but long-term therapy is required. A histological diagnosis to exclude retroperitoneal malignancy is not made unless therapy is preceded by surgical exploration.

Ureteric stone

Aetiology and site of lodgement

These stones originate in the kidney and migrate downwards. Arrest is likely at the three sites of relative narrowing: the pelviureteric junction, the pelvic brim where the ureter crosses the iliac vessels, and the intravesical termination.

Clinical features

Ureteric stones almost always cause renal colic, and they account for one of the most frequent urological presentations in the Accident and Emergency Department.

Symptoms

The patient is in severe pain which is intermittent and radiates from the loin to the groin and sometimes into the testicle, scrotum or labia. Vomiting frequently occurs and the patient is unable to find any comfortable position or to lie still. The urine is often bloodstained.

Signs

Fever suggests the presence of a pyonephrosis. The abdomen is tender with slight guarding. An impacted stone may be complicated by paralytic ileus which produces a silent distended abdomen.

Investigation

Urine

Examination of the urine is carried out for red blood cells and bacterial culture.

Imaging

A plain abdominal X-ray may show a calcified opacity lying in the course of the ureter. A CT scan should always be done urgently to confirm the diagnosis and to assess the degree of obstruction and the likelihood of the stone passing spontaneously; 90% of stones less than 0.5 cm in diameter will do so (Fig. 33.21).

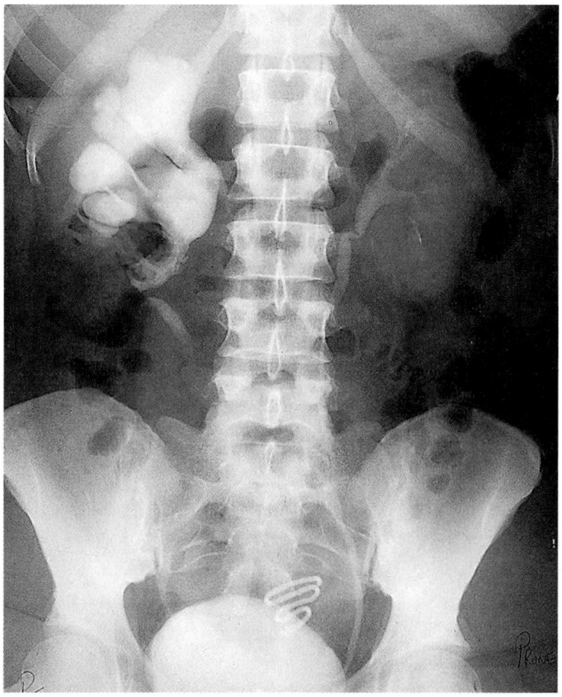

Fig. 33.21 An intravenous urogram showing clubbed calyces secondary to ureteric obstruction.

Management

Most patients are admitted to hospital for relief of pain, although the majority require only one parenteral injection of opiate. Antispasmodics and non-steroidal anti-inflammatory agents are effective thereafter.

Indications for intervention

These are:

- evidence of infection
- recurrent or persistent pain
- failure of the stone to progress downwards
- deterioration of renal function determined by isotope scanning.

Methods of intervention

In an emergency, intervention is by either percutaneous nephrostomy or the passage of a ureteric stent to bypass the obstruction (Fig. 33.22).

Definitive treatment is by:

- extraction – snaring small stones in the lower 5 cm of ureter in a basket passed up the ureter; or very rarely by open ureterolithotomy
- extracorporeal destruction by shock wave lithotripsy
- in-situ destruction with lithotripsy or laser via a ureteroscope.

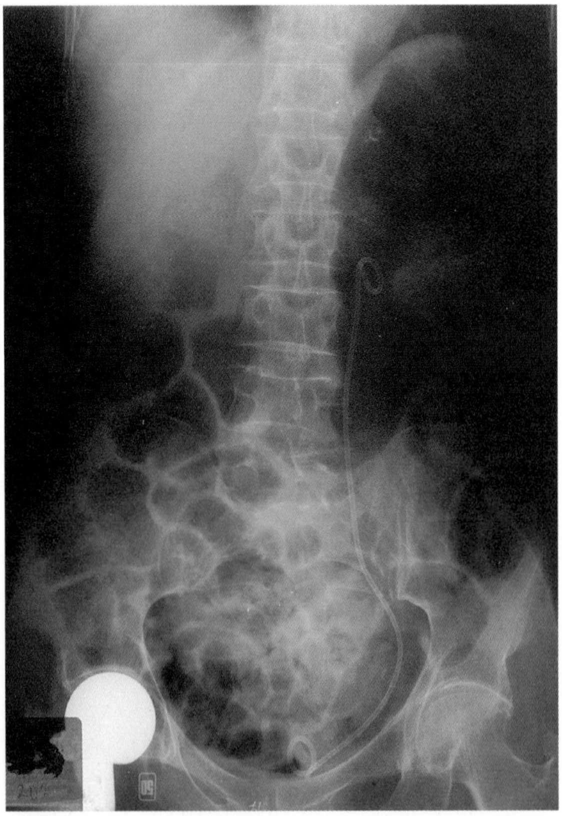

Fig. 33.22 Double pigtail catheter providing drainage of the renal pelvis and stenting of the left ureter.

URINARY DIVERSION

Decompression or drainage of the urinary tract is frequently employed in urological practice. It is now usually done under radiological control rather than at open operation.

Nephrostomy and pyelostomy

In nephrostomy, a drainage tube is passed through the kidney substance into its pelvis; in pyelostomy the pelvis is intubated directly. Either procedure is most frequently employed to decompress and drain a kidney obstructed at the pelviureteric outflow. Decompression may also be needed after operations such as reconstruction of the pelviureteric junction. An external drainage bag can be avoided if it is possible to intubate an obstruction or suture line by placing a ureteric stent across it so that one end lies in the renal pelvis and the other in the bladder (Fig. 33.22). The technique is frequently used before lithotripsy, to prevent fragments of stone causing ureteric obstruction.

Other forms of urinary diversion

Surgical diversion of urine to the exterior is required if the bladder is removed or is so congenitally deformed (exstrophy) or diseased that adequate function is impossible. Diversion is most frequently achieved by using an isolated segment of ileum into which the ureters are implanted. The segment acts as a conduit to bring the urine to the abdominal wall (Fig. 33.23). Intestine can also be used to make a new

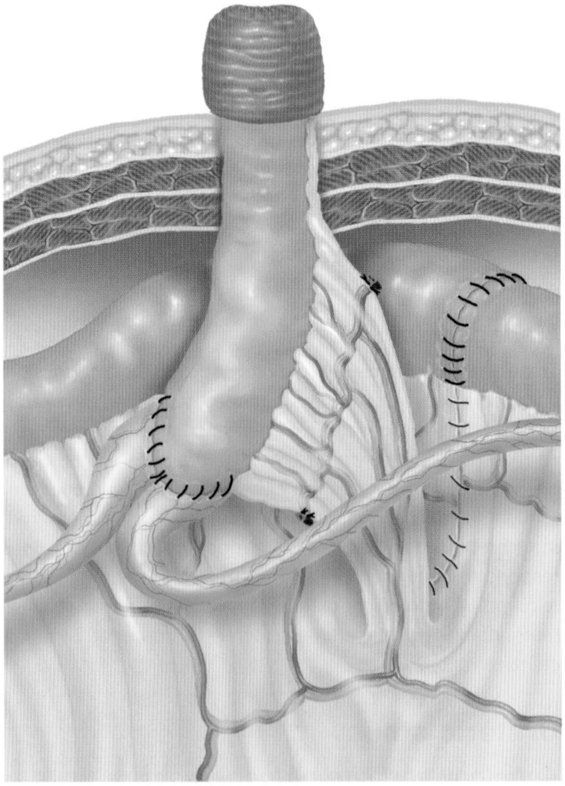

Fig. 33.23 An ileal conduit.

bladder with a continent external opening on the abdominal wall which the patient catheterises intermittently (cf. continent ileostomy). Rarely, the ureters may be implanted into the intact sigmoid colon. However, that technique often leads to ascending urinary infection and chronic pyelonephritis; and, because of reabsorption of urinary constituents from the intestine, hyperchloraemic acidosis develops. Yet a further complication is the development of adenocarcinoma at the site of ureteric implantation. This procedure has now been superseded by the creation of a pouch in the sigmoid colon (Mainz II). This has a much lower incidence of complications.

THE LOWER URINARY TRACT

Symptoms in the lower genitourinary tract

Bladder pain

This may be sharp or dull and is located in the midline of the lower abdomen. Rapid overdistension of a previously normal bladder causes severe pain, but if the distension is gradual over weeks or months, pain is absent.

Prostatic pain

This is a dull ache which may be felt in the lower abdomen, the rectum, perineum and anterior thighs.

Urethral pain

This is usually felt at the tip of the penis and ranges from a mere tickling discomfort to severe and sharp pain exacerbated by passing urine.

Scrotal pain

Pain may be referred to the scrotum as in renal colic. Similarly, pain arising from the scrotal contents may be referred to the groin or abdomen. Most scrotal pain is the result of stretching of the tunica albuginea; if this happens acutely, pain is severe, but slow distension, as in a tumour, causes a dragging sensation or a dull ache.

Disorders of micturition

Increased frequency may occur during the day and the night (nocturia) and may be a response to an excess fluid intake or failure of the kidneys to concentrate the urine, as occurs in diabetes insipidus, hypercalcaemia, chronic kidney disease and diseases which produce a high solute load such as diabetes mellitus.

Urological causes of increased frequency are:

- urinary infection
- incomplete bladder emptying
- detrusor irritability
- small bladder volume
- bladder cancer.

Dysuria. The term describes a burning sensation during the passage of urine. It may occur throughout micturition or just at its end (terminal dysuria). Infection with inflammation of the urethra is the commonest cause.

Strangury is a repeated desire to pass urine but with little to show for it other than pain related to the urethra or the penile tip. Infection is likely.

Intermittency. The urine stream is interrupted during micturition. The symptom is associated with bladder stones, ureteroceles and benign prostatic obstruction.

Hesitancy is the need to wait before the urine stream begins. Prostatic obstruction to urine flow and stricture are causes.

Incomplete emptying is, as the phrase implies, a feeling that the bladder is not emptied at the end of micturition. Prostatic disease and detrusor dysfunction are possible causes.

Terminal dribbling is a progressive reduction in the rate of urine flow at the end of the urine stream and is associated with prostatic obstruction.

Post-micturition dribbling is leakage after the patient believes that micturition is complete and is associated with detrusor irritability, urethral diverticula or the failure to empty the urethra manually after micturition.

Incontinence is of five types (Box 33.11).

Abnormal urine stream. The stream may be:

- slow – prostatic obstruction or detrusor insufficiency
- forked – often associated with a urethral stricture.

Examination

A distended bladder is visible and palpable in most patients examined in the supine position. Dullness to percussion in the midline of the abdomen above the pubic symphysis nearly always means bladder distension in a male.

Box 33.11 Types of incontinence

- True – a fistula between the urinary tract and the exterior
- Giggle – in young girls, provoked by bouts of unrestrained mirth
- Stress – leakage during a transient increase in abdominal pressure such as caused by coughing or laughing
- Urge – a desire to pass urine of such severity that the patient is unable to reach the toilet; it may be associated with urinary infection, bladder stones, detrusor instability or bladder cancer
- Dribbling or overflow – there is a continual loss of urine from a chronically distended bladder

The external genitalia are often not examined, because of embarrassment. The foreskin, glans penis and urethral meatus must be examined for meatal stenosis, phimosis, anatomical abnormalities such as hypospadias, penile tumours and warts. The scrotal contents are examined with the patient both supine and standing to aid identification of a varicocele.

Rectal examination

In the UK, it is traditional to examine the male in the left lateral position. The purpose is to identify abnormalities within the anal canal and rectum and to determine the size, contour and consistency of the prostate. A similar position is used in the female but is usually preceded by a vaginal examination with the patient supine and the knees flexed. In the latter, oestrogenisation of the perineum, urethral prolapse, urethral diverticula and gynaecological abnormalities of the vagina, cervix, uterus and its adnexa can be detected.

Investigation

General

Bacteriological and biochemical investigation for the upper urinary tract are also relevant to the lower tract.

Imaging

Urethrography

Water-soluble contrast medium is introduced into the urethra via a catheter to outline urethral strictures, urethral diverticula and urethral injuries.

Ultrasonography

Transabdominal, transurethral and transrectal routes are available (Fig. 33.24). The techniques provide precise information on:

- residual urine
- bladder tumours
- prostatic size
- nature of prostatic enlargement – benign or possibly malignant
- staging prostatic cancer.

Transrectal ultrasound (TRUS) guidance also improves the accuracy with which a prostatic biopsy is obtained when confirmation of malignant disease is required.

CT and MRI are the most accurate way of assessing the depth of invasion of bladder and prostate cancer.

Bladder function

Urinary flow rate

The patient voids into a device which records the rate of accumulation of the expelled urine (flow meter). The total voided, which should be greater than 150 mL, and the peak and mean flows are recorded (Fig. 33.25). A peak flow of less than 15 mL/s may indicate bladder outflow obstruction or detrusor failure.

Urodynamics

The investigations are more invasive to the extent that urethral catheterisation with a filling catheter and a pressure transducer is required. A further pressure transducer is placed in the rectum to measure intra-abdominal pressure. Subtraction of pressures recorded by the two catheters is done automatically and gives a true intravesical pressure which is measured both during bladder filling and on micturition (Fig. 33.26). After micturition, residual volume is measured by emptying the bladder through the filling catheter.

Endoscopy

A flexible cystoscope passed under local anaesthetic, or a small rigid cystoscope using sedation or general anaesthesia, is used. The whole of the urethra and bladder can be examined and ureteric catheters passed.

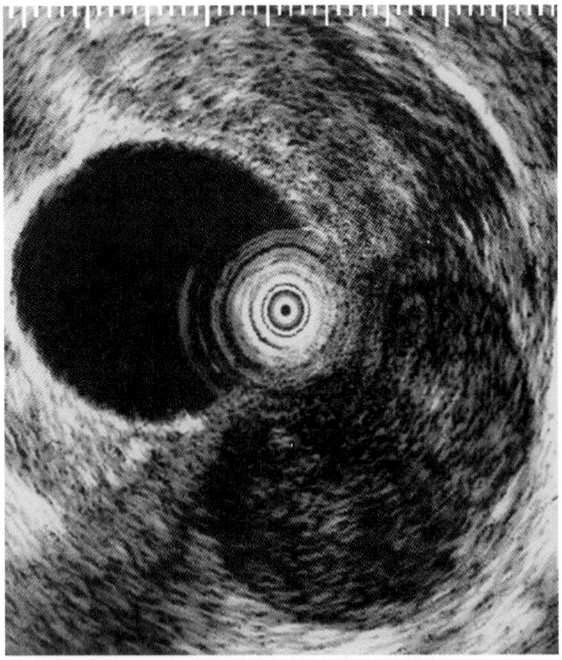

Fig. 33.24 Transrectal ultrasound scan showing benign enlargement of the prostate.

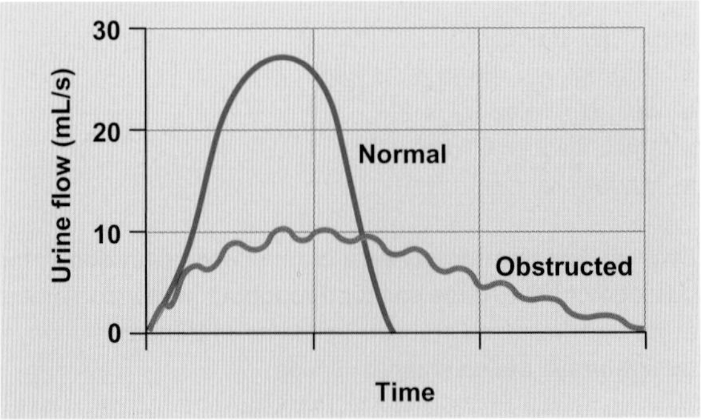

Fig. 33.25 Measurement of urinary flow rate using a flow meter.

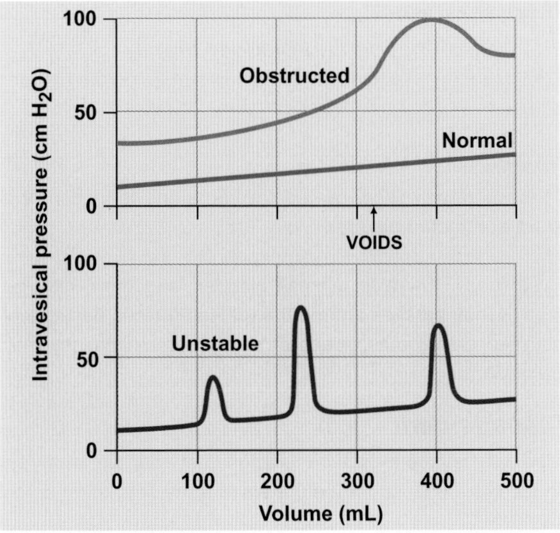

Fig. 33.26 Urodynamic pressure studies showing obstructed and unstable responses.

DISORDERS AND DISEASE OF THE BLADDER

CONGENITAL ABNORMALITIES

Urachus

Failure of the urachus to close results in a urachal fistula with leakage of urine from the umbilicus at birth. Persistence of the mid-part of the urachus produces an urachal cyst palpable in the midline below the umbilicus, which may undergo malignant change.

Exstrophy of the bladder (ectopia vesicae)

Epidemiology and aetiology

The incidence is approximately 1:50 000 live births, with 50% being male and 50% female. The cause is unknown. The bladder does not infold, so that its mucosa is exposed as a flat plate on the surface of the abdomen.

Pathological findings

There is failure of development of the anterior wall of the urogenital sinus and of the lower abdominal wall. The abnormality is associated with:

- wide separation of the symphysis pubis
- epispadias – failure of dorsal closure of the urethra
- inguinal hernia
- imperforate anus.

A secondary problem is the development of adenocarcinoma if the exposed bladder mucosa remains untreated.

Management

The bladder and penis are reconstructed in stages after a pelvic osteotomy to allow approximation of the symphysis pubis. The insertion of an artificial sphincter is usually necessary to maintain continence. Urinary diversion and excision of the deformed bladder may be required. Continence can be achieved in 80% of cases.

INFECTIONS OF THE LOWER URINARY TRACT

Acute cystitis

In men, this is invariably bacterial and often associated with other bladder abnormalities such as outflow obstruction, foreign bodies, stones and tumours. In women, it is most commonly bacterial but may also be allergic or chemical. The agent responsible can easily ascend the short female urethra.

Clinical features

Frequency, dysuria, lower abdominal pain, strangury, haematuria and pyrexia all occur to a varying degree.

Mild suprapubic tenderness may be present, and the urethral meatus may be inflamed. Apart from these, specific signs are absent unless there is evidence of underlying disease.

Investigation

Urine

It is essential to send a urine specimen for culture and sensitivity before antibiotic therapy is begun. In females, a high vaginal swab should be sent for analysis to exclude *Candida, Trichomonas* and other vaginal pathogens, because such infections may precipitate an attack of cystitis.

Imaging

Patients who present with haematuria must have both an ultrasound and a cystoscopy, which are also indicated when the MSU shows no bacterial growth. Carcinoma in situ of the bladder may present with cystitis-like symptoms.

Management

An episode requires a high fluid intake and antibiotic administration (e.g. amoxicillin), which may need to be modified once the results of urine culture and bacterial sensitivities are available. Seven days after the course of antibiotics, a further MSU and high vaginal swab should be obtained to ensure that bacteria have been eradicated. In women, it is essential to identify those who have developed *Candida*, because this needs to be treated to stop the development of a vicious cycle of cystitis → antibiotic administration → persistent *Candida* infection → further symptoms.

Chronic cystitis

The cause is usually inadequate treatment and investigation of an acute attack. Postmenopausal women are prone to recurrent episodes of cystitis and can benefit from topical or systemic oestrogen replacement therapy. Ten percent of patients who receive pelvic irradiation suffer from haemorrhagic cystitis without bacterial infection. Most cases subside spontaneously during the 12–18 months after completion of therapy, although it may lead to bladder fibrosis with a small contracted bladder.

Interstitial cystitis

This occurs most frequently in women who have irritative voiding symptoms and negative urine cultures. Many develop severe bladder pain, frequency, urgency and incontinence.

Tuberculosis of the bladder

In those who present with intractable symptoms that resemble cystitis and have a sterile pyuria, repeated examinations of early morning urine should be carried out to identify the tubercle bacillus.

Management

The treatment of contracted bladder is considered below.

Schistosomiasis (bilharzia)

Epidemiology and aetiology

The blood fluke *Schistosoma haematobium* is endemic in the Middle East and the Nile valley and other rivers and lakes of eastern and southern Africa. Human infestation is acquired by contact with infected water. Adult worms produce ova in the pelvic and vesical veins. The ova migrate through the bladder wall into the urine, which is passed into the irrigation ditches, where miracidia penetrate the water snail. These develop into cercaria which can pass through human skin and are carried to the pelvic venous plexuses where they develop into the adult fluke (Fig. 33.27).

Pathological features

The eggs in the bladder wall cause an inflammatory reaction which goes on to fibrosis, calcification and secondary infection. Stone formation and squamous carcinoma are secondary consequences. The ureters may be involved directly or may become secondarily dilated because of the small, thick-walled and fibrotic bladder.

Clinical features

Symptoms

In acute presentations, pyrexia, itching, dysuria, frequency and haematuria are seen. In those who are in a chronic state, frequency, haematuria and episodes of infection resistant to treatment are usual.

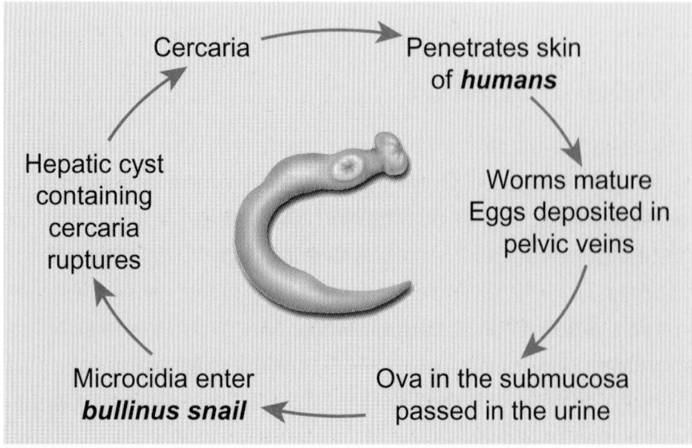

Fig. 33.27 Life cycle of *Schistosoma haematobium*.

Investigation

Urine examination and bladder biopsy

Eggs can be identified in either the urine or on bladder biopsy.

Imaging

Ultrasound may show dilated ureters, stone formation or a small contracted bladder.

Cystoscopy. There is a small bladder, and there may be small sandy patches around the ureteric orifices because of calcified granulomas. Areas of squamous malignancy may be obvious.

Management

Medical treatment is with praziquantel. Surgery may be required to reconstruct the ureters and the small contracted bladder.

BLADDER TRAUMA

Because of its anatomy, the bladder may rupture into either the peritoneal cavity or the extraperitoneal plane. The differences in cause between the two forms of rupture are summarised in Box 33.12.

Intraperitoneal rupture

Clinical features

Symptoms

Usually there is a history of injury. Patients with a very full bladder have often consumed large quantities of alcohol, and a clear history may be difficult to obtain. There is usually also severe lower abdominal pain – modified by the patient's clinical state – and anuria.

Signs

These are as follows:

- If the urine is sterile, increasing abdominal distension and discomfort
- If the urine is infected, features of peritonitis
- Attempted micturition results in the passage of a few millilitres of bloodstained urine
- Urethral catheterisation is easy, but urine is not forthcoming, although there may be a little blood.

Box 33.12 Causes of bladder rupture

Intraperitoneal
- Blunt abdominal trauma with a full bladder
- Penetrating injury (rare)
- Gross overdistension at endoscopy
- During endoscopic surgery on the bladder vault

Extraperitoneal
- Fracture of the pelvis
- Resection of prostate
- Difficult lower abdominal surgery
- During repair of a direct hernia with bladder in the medial aspect of the sac

Management

The abdomen is explored, the bladder laceration repaired and the bladder drained.

Extraperitoneal rupture

Trauma is the only cause – a fracture of the pelvis, or during transurethral resection of the prostate or bladder tumours.

Clinical features

There is a history of injury, either accidental or surgical. Symptoms are:

- lower abdominal pain, although this may be masked by the effects of pelvic fracture
- inability to micturate or, at most, a few drops of bloodstained urine.

Urine and blood extravasated into the perivesical space cause the following:

- tender suprapubic thickening
- palpable mass (occasionally).

Management

Extravasation of urine after transurethral resection of the prostate or of a bladder tumour usually responds to a period of urethral catheterisation. For severe injuries which are a consequence of pelvic fracture, suprapubic drainage of the bladder and drainage of the retropubic space are required.

BLADDER TUMOURS

The bladder, like the rest of the urinary tract, is lined with transitional-cell epithelium and, because it acts as a store for urine and any carcinogens that may be present, it is the commonest site for the development of malignant urinary tract tumours. Benign tumours of the urothelium are exceedingly rare, as are benign tumours of the bladder muscle. Rhabdomyosarcomas of the latter occur in childhood. However, the great majority of bladder tumours arise from the urothelium, 95% of which are transitional-cell lesions. Carcinoma in situ (CIS) refers to flat areas of epithelium composed of cells with anaplastic features and disorderly pattern of growth without extension into the bladder lumen. They are multicentric and commonly occur in association with obvious transitional-cell tumours. Squamous-cell tumours occur in schistosomiasis, and adenocarcinomas are the consequence of untreated bladder exstrophy or an urachal remnant.

Epidemiology

For urothelial cancer there is a 5:1 male predominance, although the incidence in females is increasing and may be related to cigarette smoking. The highest incidence of bladder cancer is in the sixth and seventh decades.

Aetiology

Chronic irritation and carcinogenic chemicals are associated with the development of the disease.

Chronic irritation may be caused by:

- schistosomiasis
- exstrophy with persistent infection and physical trauma.

Carcinogens include:

- tobacco smoke
- products of the chemical industry – aniline dyes, printing, rubber processing, pesticides.

Because of the known association with the above industries, there are now regular surveillance programmes which use cytological examination of the urine. If a worker in an industry that is known to have a high risk develops bladder cancer, both the victim and dependents may be entitled to compensation.

Clinical features

Symptoms

The great majority of patients present with painless haematuria. A small proportion have urinary infections. A few tumours are found coincidentally in patients who undergo a cystoscopy for other reasons. Advanced cases have lower abdominal pain, severe dysuria, strangury and incontinence of bloodstained urine. Similar irritative findings are found in patients with carcinoma in situ and must be distinguished from bacterial cystitis.

Signs

Unless the disease is advanced, abnormalities are usually absent. A careful bimanual examination may reveal a mass in the bladder wall, but if the diagnosis is established by other means (usually endoscopically) then bimanual examination is better done under anaesthesia to stage the lesion.

Investigation

Urothelial tumours are often multicentric. Any patient who presents with symptoms suggestive of a urothelial tumour requires full investigation of the urinary tract, which includes:

- urine microscopy and culture for evidence of haematuria and infection
- cytological examination of the urine – most likely to be positive in those with carcinoma in situ or well-differentiated tumours
- assessment of renal function
- IVU used to be used to search for other tumours in the renal pelvis, ureter or bladder (Fig. 33.28), although small tumours were difficult to detect
- Ultrasound and CT scanning give additional information about the primary tumour stage and show other synchronous lesions or metastatic disease and are now used instead of IVU.
- endoscopic examination of the urethra and bladder; endoscopy identifies the number, position and macroscopic type of urethral or bladder tumours and obtains a biopsy for histological examination of both the tumours and apparently normal mucosa
- bimanual examination (rectum and abdomen in the male; vagina and abdomen in the female) to assess spread of tumour beyond the bladder wall
- chest X-ray and bone scan to seek distant metastases.

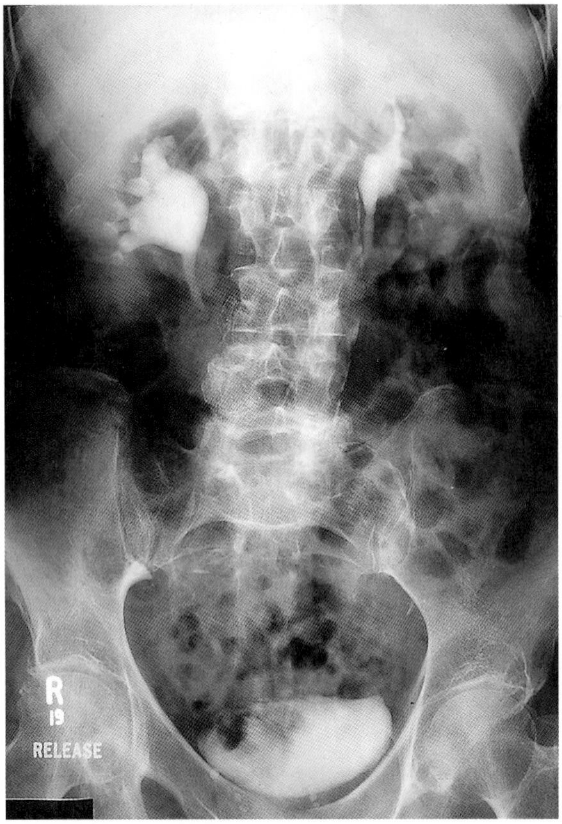

Fig. 33.28 Intravenous urogram showing a large filling defect in the right side of the bladder as a result of a tumour.

Table 33.5 Local staging of superficial bladder cancer from histological examination of the resected specimen

Stage	Histological findings
pT(CIS)	Carcinoma in situ
pTa	Papillary carcinoma with basement membrane intact
pT1	Tumour has penetrated the basement membrane

Table 33.6 Local staging of bladder cancer that is no longer superficial

Stage	Findings
T2	Superficial muscle is involved
T2a	Through superficial muscle
T2b	Into deep muscle
T3a	Through deep bladder muscle into fat (microscopic)
T3b	Extending beyond muscle into fat (macroscopic) but bladder still mobile
T4a	Adjacent structures involved
T4b	Fixed to pelvic wall

Table 33.7 Nodal staging in bladder cancer

Stage	Findings
N0	No nodes involved
N1	Single regional node <2 cm
N2	Multiple regional nodes <5 cm
N3	At least one node >5 cm

In tumours which show histological evidence of invasion into bladder muscle, a CT or MRI scan is essential to determine the stage of the disease (see below) and the need for more radical treatment.

Histological grading

The grades used are:

- carcinoma in situ – this is a high-grade lesion
- well differentiated – Grade 1 (G1)
- moderately differentiated – Grade 2 (G2)
- undifferentiated – Grade 3 (G3).

Most tumours contain a mixture of cell types. Grade is assigned on the worst pattern of differentiation.

Tumour staging

The TNM classification is used.

Tumour category is best assessed by histological examination of the resected specimen (pT category). The depth of penetration into or through the bladder wall is used as the criterion for the T component. A tumour is nominally regarded as superficial (pTa) if it has penetrated no further than the basement membrane (Table 33.5). Tumours that have transgressed the bladder wall to a greater degree are pT2–pT4, and their classification is based on a combination of histological and bimanual examination (Table 33.6).

Node category. The lymphatic spread is to nodes on the surface of the bladder, the internal iliac and para-aortic nodes and then more distally. The classification is shown in Table 33.7.

Management

Treatment depends on the site, size and histological grading of the tumour. At the initial endoscopic examination, the tumour is resected as far as possible, with deeper areas of resection being sent separately for histological examination to assess spread into the bladder muscle. Random biopsies of apparently normal bladder mucosa should also be obtained, as these may show changes of dysplasia or carcinoma in situ and provide useful prognostic information on the likelihood of recurrence. The treatment of superficial cancer (pTiS–pT1B) is summarised in Table 33.8. pT2 to pT4 tumours, unless they have advanced nodal involvement or distant metastases (N3 or M1), are managed by radical resection, radical radiotherapy or systemic chemotherapy, or a combination of these modalities. Radical cystoprostatectomy is usually followed by urinary diversion. The simplest form of urinary diversion is the ileal conduit (see above). However, orthotopic neobladder reconstructions have been developed, such as the Studer pouch to allow voiding through the urethra with no need for a stoma or external appliance. With T2 disease there is a 5% improved survival rate with the addition of chemotherapy. External

Table 33.8 Management of superficial bladder cancer

Stage	Treatment
pT(CIS)	Endoscopic removal of local areas and intravesical BCG
pTa	Transurethral resection (TUR)
pT1	TUR For recurrence – repeated resection and intravesical BCG, or mitomycin
pT1 with poorly differentiated tumour (G3)	BCG and TUR
pT2	Radical surgery or radiotherapy

Table 33.9 Survival in bladder cancer

Stage	Grade	5-year survival (%)
pTiS		75
pT1A	1	95
pT1B	1	72
pT1	3	39
pT2		45
pT3		39
pT4		5

beam radiotherapy to the bladder is usually reserved for those patients that are not fit enough for surgery.

Surveillance

Once a diagnosis of urothelial carcinoma has been made, regular lifelong follow-up is required; 50% of patients will develop further tumours (unless they presented with a single pTa, G1 tumour).

Prognosis

Five-year survivals are summarised in Table 33.9; 95% of those with pT1A tumours survive 5 years.

BLADDER DIVERTICULA

A diverticulum is a protrusion of mucosa through the bladder muscle (Fig. 33.29).

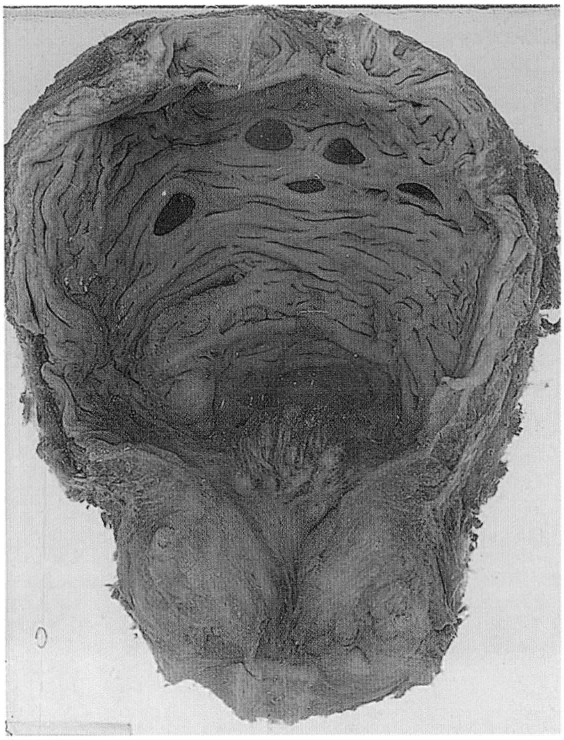

Fig. 33.29 Bladder showing the openings of multiple diverticula.

Aetiology and pathological features

The majority are acquired and associated with bladder outflow obstruction.

Diverticula are often multiple, not surrounded by muscle fibres and therefore unable to empty when the detrusor contracts. Stagnation of urine in a diverticulum or the urinary tract leads to infection, stone formation and squamous metaplasia with the possibility of tumour. A tumour in a diverticulum has a worse prognosis than one in the intact bladder because invasion into surrounding tissues occurs earlier.

Clinical features

Uncomplicated single or multiple diverticula are usually asymptomatic and found coincidentally during the course of investigation of a patient with bladder outflow obstruction. Complications lead to haematuria, dysuria and frequency.

There are no signs which are specific to the condition but infection may cause local tenderness.

Investigation and management

Diverticula are frequently seen on ultrasound, intravenous urography and at cystoscopy.

Bladder outflow obstruction should be relieved. If diverticula do not cause problems thereafter, treatment is not required. Persistent infection is an indication for removal.

BLADDER FISTULAE

A fistula is an epithelium-lined track between one hollow viscus and another or between a viscus and the exterior. Bladder fistulae are classified in Table 33.10.

Vesicovaginal fistula

Aetiology and pathological features

The commonest cause of vesicovaginal fistula in developing countries is prolonged obstructed labour and ischaemic necrosis, by the descending fetal head, of the anterior vaginal wall and bladder. In developed countries, they occur as a result of gynaecological surgery, pelvic malignancy and irradiation damage to the vagina and bladder following treatment for cervical cancer.

Clinical features

There is a constant leak of urine through the vagina.

There may be features of the underlying cause apparent. Examination of the vagina shows urine trickling down from the vault, and the fistula may be thickened and palpable.

Table 33.10 Classification of bladder fistulae

Type	Origin	Condition
Bladder to exterior	Congenital	Extrophy of bladder Urachal fistula
Bladder to vagina	Acquired	Injury (prolonged obstructed labour) Hysterectomy Cancer Radiotherapy
Bladder to colon	Acquired	Diverticular disease Cancer Radiotherapy
Bladder to small intestine	Acquired	Crohn's disease Radiotherapy
Bladder to rectum	Acquired	Post-prostatectomy Carcinoma of rectum Radiotherapy for prostatic cancer Laser therapy to the prostate
Bladder to uterus	Acquired	Malignancy of either organ Caesarean section Radiotherapy

Investigation

CT and MRI scanning

These imaging techniques are used to assess pelvic and urinary tract disease following previous treatment for pelvic malignancy.

Dye test

If there is doubt about the source of leakage, a swab is placed into the vagina and methylene blue inserted into the bladder via a urethral catheter. Blue staining of the swab in the vagina confirms the presence of vesicovaginal fistula. A swab soaked in clear urine suggests a ureterovaginal fistula. Patients with a vesicovaginal fistula often have multiple fistulae. The dye test should be repeated without the swab and the vagina examined directly using a Sim's speculum.

Management

Very few fistulae close spontaneously, however prolonged is bladder drainage.

Fistulae caused by irradiation or malignancy

Urinary diversion via an ileal or sigmoid conduit is most appropriate because the tissues are unsuitable for repair and life expectancy is short. In women with a long life expectancy, a continent urine diversion or Mainz II pouch may be appropriate.

Obstetric and post-traumatic fistulae

Repair should not be attempted within 3 months of confinement, to allow control of infection and revascularisation of the ischaemic tissues. For postoperative fistulae, an immediate repair is done.

Fistulae from bladder to gut (enteric fistulae)

These are usually between the large bowel and the bladder.

Clinical features

The patient complains of:

- recurrent urinary infections
- bubbles in the urine (pneumaturia)
- faecal material in the urine (uncommon).

Signs are non-specific but include those of cystitis.

Investigation and management

The diagnosis is not usually in much doubt, but a barium enema often identifies the site and extent of underlying disease. This is usually diverticular disease or, more rarely, carcinoma of the large bowel.

Management is by resection of the abnormal bowel and closure of the bladder.

NEUROPATHIC BLADDER

This term is used to describe bladder dysfunction of neural origin. The neurophysiology of bladder function is incompletely understood, and clinical classifications are therefore the most useful in therapy and widely used. Three types are recognised:

- acute atonic bladder
- chronic atonic bladder
- hyperreflexic bladder.

Aetiology

The causes may be divided into congenital and acquired. The latter are further divisible into trauma, cord compression, primary central nervous system disease, and spinal cord disease secondary to that elsewhere.

Pathological features

Whatever the type of neuropathy, the secondary effects are:

- urinary stasis with dilatation of the upper urinary tract
- recurrent ascending infection
- progressive loss of renal function
- secondary stone formation.

Clinical features

Symptoms

These range from painless retention of urine to uncontrolled incontinence, frequency, urgency and poor urine stream. In long-standing neuropathy, there may be systemic symptoms of chronic kidney disease.

Signs

There is commonly evidence of other neurological involvement from the underlying cause. A full neurological examination is essential. Depending on the clinical nature of the neuropathy, the bladder may be distended with a trickle of overflow or empty with urine constantly emerging from the urethral meatus.

Investigation

Urine

Because of the likelihood of infection, bacterial culture is carried out repeatedly.

Renal function

Standard techniques are used.

Ultrasonography

Upper urinary tract dilatation and bladder emptying can be assessed.

Urinary flow studies

These are an essential part of the diagnosis and management of the neuropathic bladder. The patient with a full bladder voids into a machine which measures both the volume voided and the maximum flow (Q_{max} in mL/s). The pattern of voiding can also be observed. Voided volumes of <150 mL may lead to erroneous results. A patient who has a normal bladder outlet and normally functioning detrusor will void with a flow rate of >15 mL/s.

Pressure flow studies

Bladder and intra-abdominal pressure (usually rectal) are measured simultaneously. The abdominal pressure is automatically subtracted from the bladder pressure to give detrusor pressure. The bladder is filled at a standard rate and the detrusor pressure measured. Rises in pressure during filling are recorded, as is the detrusor pressure at maximal urine flow. After completion of voiding, the residual urine can be measured. Bladder emptying can be recorded using a video system.

Management of clinical types of neuropathy

The general aims of treatment are to restore continence and preserve renal function.

Acute atony

This condition typically occurs after spinal cord injury in the stage of spinal shock (see Ch. 31) and may last up to 3 months. The internal involuntary sphincter remains closed and the detrusor inactive so that the bladder is distended and empties by overflow. However, this situation should not be allowed to occur, because it results in delay of return of function to the bladder spinal reflex centres (sacral 2, 3 and 4). Intermittent urethral catheterisation performed by either the patient or the carer four to five times a day, best carried out in a specialised centre, prevents distension. The eventual result is an automatic bladder which empties involuntarily every 2 or 3 hours or a bladder from which the urine can be expelled by manual compression.

Chronic atony

The cause is either a peripheral neuropathy or long-standing outflow obstruction. The former is usually irreversible, and either intermittent self-catheterisation or urinary diversion should be considered. It may be possible to correct the latter without producing incontinence (see 'Prostatic hyperplasia'). Urodynamic studies are essential in assessing residual detrusor function and the likelihood of the bladder being able to empty once the obstruction is relieved.

Hyperreflexia

Uninhibited high-pressure detrusor contractions are found on urodynamic studies but are not diagnostic of systemic neuropathy. Other features which may be found are:

- detrusor sphincter incoordination
- high voiding pressure
- significant residual volume
- poor and intermittent flow rate.

The bladder assumes a fir tree appearance on IVU or cystography (Fig. 33.30).

Management includes:

- bladder conditioning – the patient is asked to delay voiding for longer and longer periods
- anticholinergics – these are usually used in combination with bladder conditioning and are effective in mild to moderate cases
- clam cystoplasty – an opened segment of small bowel is sutured into the opened bladder. This decreases the bladder pressure and increases the bladder volume. The reduction in bladder pressure results in poor bladder emptying, and intermittent self-catheterisation is usually necessary
- urine diversion if indicated.

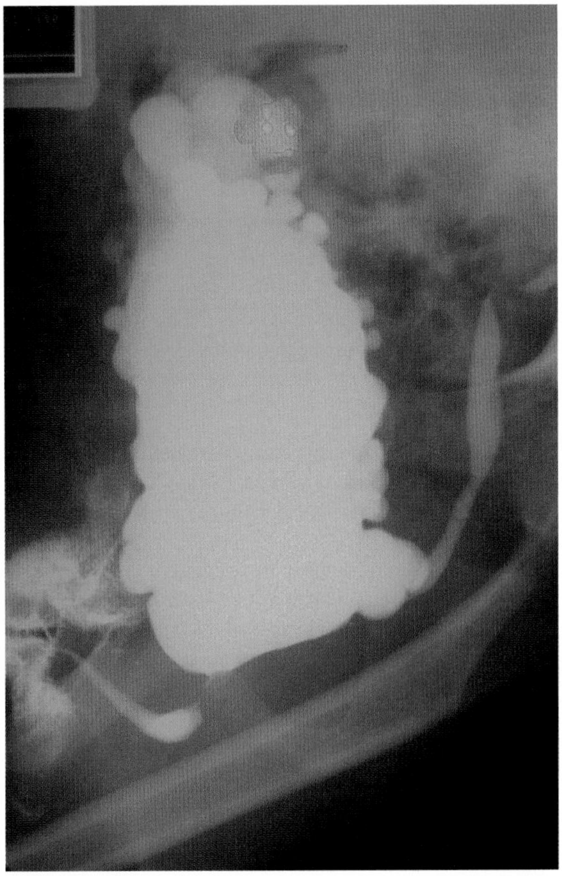

Fig. 33.30 Fir tree appearance of a neuropathic bladder.

INCONTINENCE

Incontinence is the involuntary passage of urine from the urethra and occurs as a result of either sphincter weakness or bladder instability.

The most common cause of stress incontinence in women is descent of the bladder neck so that any sudden increase in abdominal pressure acts only on the bladder and not the sphincter mechanism. In men it results from a prostatectomy.

Clinical features

Symptoms

Stress incontinence results in involuntary loss of urine whenever intra-abdominal pressure is raised – by coughing, sneezing or exercise. Symptoms of detrusor instability include frequency, urgency, urge incontinence, nocturia and bed-wetting. Not all of these symptoms may be present.

Signs

Patients with detrusor instability may have evidence of a neuropathy. Stress incontinence may be demonstrable when the patient coughs or strains.

Investigation

Urine examination

Bacterial culture is essential. Cytology should be obtained because the clinical features of detrusor instability can be mimicked by carcinoma in situ of the bladder. The two conditions can coexist.

Urodynamic studies

Patients with symptoms of detrusor instability may have normal urodynamic findings.

Management

Stress incontinence

Conservative treatment includes:

- weight loss
- pelvic floor exercises
- pelvic floor stimulation
- local or systemic oestrogen therapy
- ephedrine 15–30 mg t.d.s. (at least 3 months' treatment is usually required).

In men pelvic floor exercises and ephedrine are worth a trial. Failure to respond requires surgical therapy with the insertion of an artificial sphincter or injection of inert substances into the sphincter area.

In women who have failed to respond to a conservative regimen, surgical treatment aims to elevate the bladder neck by a retropubic approach (colposuspension) or a transvaginal approach inserting an inert sling to support the urethra.

Detrusor instability

Whether or not detrusor instability has been identified by urodynamic studies, the majority of patients respond to bladder training. After a full explanation of the condition, the patient is asked not to pass urine for increasingly lengthy periods. An accurate fluid chart of input and output and of the timing of micturition is also kept. In the few patients who fail to respond, anticholinergic agents are of value (e.g. oxybutynin hydrochloride or tolterodine), but they must not be used in patients with a history of glaucoma.

THE PROSTATE

The gland is subject to hormonal influences throughout life. In utero, it is stimulated by maternal oestrogen, and an alteration in the androgen–oestrogen balance may be responsible for the enlargement of the prostate which occurs in later life. During the active sexual period, androgenic stimulation predominates. Testosterone produced by the testes, adrenals and the peripheral conversion of other steroids is converted in the prostate by the enzyme 5α-reductase to dihydrotestosterone, the most active androgen within the prostate.

Clinical assessment

Rectal examination allows direct assessment of the size, shape, consistency and other features of the gland by digital palpation through the anterior wall of the rectum.

The normal gland has the following characteristics:

- It is soft to firm
- It has a well-defined median sulcus
- It is not tender.

Abnormalities are as follows:

- Increased size causes the prostate to bulge backwards into the rectum so that the finger inserted through the anus passes a posterior overhang. The median sulcus becomes less obvious.
- Changes in consistency are either diffuse or localised. A very hard and irregular gland is characteristic of prostatic cancer but can occur in other conditions.
- Tenderness is present in inflammation.

It is notoriously difficult to judge accurately absolute prostatic size.

Diseases of the prostate

The prostate is subject to three major disorders:

- infections
- benign prostatic hyperplasia (BPH)
- carcinoma of the prostate.

INFECTIONS

There are three clinical entities:

- acute bacterial prostatitis
- chronic bacterial prostatitis
- chronic pelvic pain syndrome.

Acute bacterial prostatitis

Aetiology

This condition is more common in patients with diabetes mellitus. *E. coli*, *Staphylococcus aureus* and *Neisseria gonorrhoeae* are the common organisms. *Chlamydia* may also be found. The route by which these organisms reach the prostate is unknown, but some instances may be by retrograde spread from the urethra.

Clinical features

There is general malaise with fever, rigors, dysuria and frequency. Pain is felt in the perineum, the rectum, and the suprapubic and sacral areas. Rectal examination reveals an acutely tender but soft prostate.

Investigation and management

Bacterial culture of urine should be performed and, if possible, fluid obtained from the urethra after gentle prostatic massage.

Management is with bed rest and appropriate antibiotic therapy. If *Chlamydia* is identified, tetracycline or erythromycin are the agents of choice. The patient's partner will also need to be treated.

Chronic bacterial prostatitis

Aetiology

This condition may arise as a result of a blood-borne infection or failure adequately to treat an episode of acute prostatitis. The prostate becomes the site of chronic inflammation with fibrous tissue formation.

Clinical features

There are symptoms of generalised ill health, frequency, dysuria, haematuria, haemospermia and perineal discomfort.

Rectal examination reveals a tender, hard and sometimes slightly irregular prostate. The prostate may also be normal.

Investigation and management

Culture of expressed prostatic secretion usually does not result in a growth of bacteria, but white blood cells are present.

The condition is difficult to eradicate. Long-term antibiotic therapy with a quinolone antibiotic, trimethoprim or tetracycline may be of value with alpha-adrenergic blocking agents to relax the smooth muscle of the prostate.

CHRONIC PELVIC PAIN SYNDROME

These patients do not have prostatic infection but suffer from chronic pelvic pain and require symptomatic relief.

BENIGN PROSTATIC HYPERPLASIA

This condition is present in almost all men over the age of 40. Benign prostatic hypertrophy (BPH) occurs in 75% of men in the eighth decade, and 20% of men over the age of 40 will require treatment during their lifetime for bladder outflow obstruction.

Aetiology and pathological features

The cause of BPH is unknown, but the condition is generally regarded as a consequence of fluctuating levels of both androgen and oestrogen (and consequently the ratio between them) at different times of life. The effect is to produce hyperplasia of the glandular cells of the central zone with associated myoepithelial and fibrous tissue development. The cells involved vary in their proportionate contribution in any one patient. Perhaps because of this, the condition is variably referred to as benign prostatic hyperplasia and benign prostatic hypertrophy, but both are subsumed under the shorthand BPH. The hyperplastic central zone cells displace the peripheral zone so that a pseudo-capsule is formed. Hyperplasia also variably compresses the urethral lumen, but this has little relationship to the overall size – glands of less than 40 g can cause as much trouble as those in excess of 100 g. The only relevance of the size of the prostate is that it may affect the type of treatment given.

Clinical features

The patient may present in one of three ways:

- prostatic obstruction
- acute retention of urine
- chronic retention of urine.

Prostatic obstruction

This may present with lower urinary tract symptoms (LUTS), which include:

- hesitancy
- poor stream
- intermittancy
- terminal dribbling
- increased frequency during the day or at night
- nocturia
- urinary tract infection.

The last two symptoms are due to incomplete bladder emptying. In addition, patients with bladder outflow obstruction frequently have detrusor instability and may therefore complain of urgency, urge incontinence and post-micturition dribbling. Not all patients with LUTS have benign prostatic hypertrophy. Not all patients with benign prostatic hypertrophy have outflow obstruction. The inter-relationship of these phenomena – LUTS, benign prostatic hypertrophy and bladder outflow obstruction – is best illustrated by a Venn diagram (Fig. 33.31).

Acute retention of urine

Forty percent of patients who present in this way do not have a preceding history of prostatic outflow obstruction. The episode may be precipitated by anticholinergic drugs, diuretics (including alcohol), prolonged voluntary suppression of micturition, and surgery for conditions outwith the urinary tract.

Symptoms are a sudden inability to pass urine and, after a very short period, acute severe suprapubic pain because of distension of what is usually a previously normal bladder.

Signs. The patient is in severe pain and frequently unable to stay still. The bladder is palpable and tender in the midline above the pubis and below the umbilicus. Rectal examination shows an enlarged prostate, but the gland is pushed down by the overfull bladder so that the size may be exaggerated.

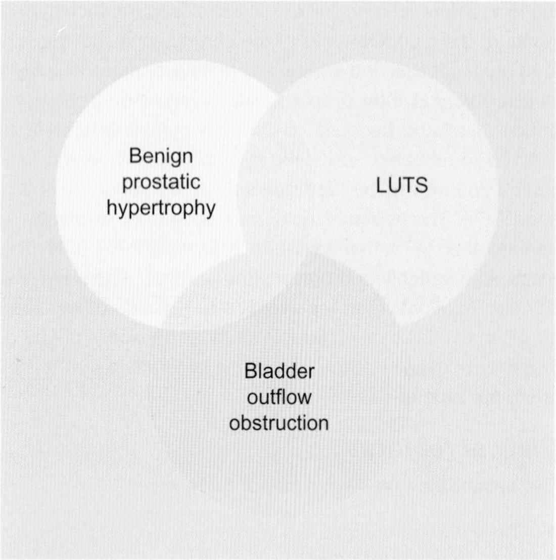

Fig 33.31 The inter-relationship between benign prostatic hypertrophy (BPH), lower urinary tract symptoms (LUTS) and bladder outflow obstruction (BOO).

Chronic retention

Symptoms. Chronic retention is painless. The patient may be ill from the metabolic effects of back pressure on the kidneys. There is characteristically the passage at frequent intervals of small quantities of urine and of rising on a number of occasions at night.

Signs. The patient's clothes and underwear may be wet and smell of urine. Apart from the systemic features of chronic kidney disease, there is a visible suprapubic swelling, dull to percussion. A search is made for any neurological abnormality because a painless bladder enlargement from such a cause may be confused with BPH and chronic retention.

Rectal examination shows the same general features as those of acute retention.

Investigation

Lower urinary tract symptoms (LUTS)

Urine is taken for culture. Renal function tests in the form of U&Es are sent. Only in the presence of urinary blood or abnormal renal function should upper-tract ultrasound be performed. In the absence of these patients perform a micturition flow test. Ninety percent of people with a flow rate of less than 12 mL/s have a degree of bladder outflow obstruction characterised by a peak maximum detrusor pressure in excess of 50 mmHg. Bladder ultrasound residual post micturition is performed and transrectal ultrasound of the prostate to assess the size of the gland and look for the possibility of a middle lobe.

Management of prostatic obstruction

Not all men require treatment in the absence of marked outflow obstruction demonstrated by very poor flow and high post-micturition residuals or upper-tract dilatation. In the absence of bothersome lower urinary tract symptoms a period of watchful waiting to see whether patients have become more symptomatic or quiescently obstructed can be justified. Medical treatment includes alpha-androgenergic blocking agents and these are subdivided into selective and non-selective alpha blockers. These drugs have an effect on all prostates of all sizes, but are particularly useful in the smaller glands where outflow obstruction is largely due to failure of relaxation of the bladder neck rather than benign prostatic hypertrophy characterised by the condition of bladder neck dyssynergia. 5α-Reductase inhibitors are deemed from large trials to be largely ineffective in men with smaller glands under the size of 40 g. In men with larger glands in excess of 40 g, the reduction in volume over a 3–6-month period on the drug is between 20 and 30%. 5α-Reductase inhibitors can improve lower urinary tract symptoms and also reduce the risk of presenting with acute urinary retention by as much as 10%.

Minimally invasive surgical treatments

Thermotherapy

This can be delivered either using microwaves or radiofrequency and temporary prostatic stents may be suitable for patients who are not fit for surgery, who are in retention and do not want to have an indwelling catheter.

Surgical treatment

The treatment of choice for prostates with an estimated weight of less than 100 g is transurethral surgical treatment of the prostate with TURP. Traditionally, this is performed using an endoscope and radio-frequency diathermy loop. Prostatic chips are resected – this is called transurethral resection of the prostate (TURP). However, over the last few decades other transurethral surgical methods have been developed. These include transurethral incision of the prostate where the bladder neck is incised, usually at the 5 or 7 o'clock position from the ureteric orifice to the verumontanum. This is a good alternative where the prostate is not enlarged and the bladder neck is the cause of obstruction.

Transurethral laser therapy of the prostate is the commonest althernative surgical method using green light laser, either to desiccate and destroy the prostatic tissue, or the holmium laser to enucleate the adenoma. Transurethral vaporisation of the prostate is radio-frequency diathermy using a corrugated diathermy ball to desiccate tissue rather than dissect tissue.

For large glands in excess of 100 g an open Milan's retropubic prostatectomy may be the best treatment. This is usually performed through a lower midline or Pfannenstiel incision. The prostatic capsule is left intact, incised and opened and the obstructing adenoma is enucleated.

The advantages of transurethral prostatectomy are:

- absence of wound infection
- significant reduction in pain
- less frequent urinary infection
- postoperative incontinence reduced
- lower incidence of general complications such as chest infection, deep-vein thrombosis and pulmonary embolus
- hospital stay and early mortality are reduced.

Disadvantages include:

- a long period of training is required to learn the technique
- a high incidence of reoperation for recurrent disease
- possible increased incidence of later postoperative mortality.

Complications are:

- bleeding – primary, reactionary or secondary haemorrhage
- absorption of irrigation fluid into the systemic circulation which can cause hyponatraemia with epileptiform fits and cardiovascular collapse (the TUR syndrome)
- failure to void
- urinary infection
- epididymo-orchitis
- incontinence
- erectile dysfunction.

Retrograde ejaculation is an invariable sequel of prostatectomy about which patients must be warned.

Prognosis. Only 70% of patients are completely satisfied with the result of a prostatectomy. The main reasons for this are that either the operation was performed for detrusor instability rather than bladder outflow obstruction or, where both conditions existed, detrusor instability did not resolve after prostatectomy.

Acute retention of urine

The patient is in severe pain, and catheterisation is required (Emergency Box 33.1). It is best achieved by the suprapubic route, though the majority of patients still receive a urethral catheter. The advantages of a suprapubic catheter include:

- lack of damage to the urethra
- urethral stricture from an indwelling catheter does not occur
- false passages are avoided
- ease of introduction in a patient with a large prostate
- trial of voiding is simple
- the operative field is left clear for a subsequent TUR.

Emergency Box 33.1

Acute retention of urine

- This is a urological emergency. The aim of treatment is to relieve pain. If a urethral catheter is to be used, it should be the smallest, softest self-retaining catheter, e.g. 12 Fr Foley
- If retention is due to blood clot then a large (22 Fr) three-way catheter, to allow irrigation, should be used. The volume of urine drained (<700 mL) is a good predictor of the likelihood of spontaneous voiding when the catheter is removed
- A short course of an alpha-adrenergic blocker, e.g. alfuzosin, may aid initiation of voiding
- Insertion of a catheter by the suprapubic route has significant advantages (see main text)
- If it is not possible to insert a catheter, do not persevere. Call for more senior help
- Only those trained in their use should utilise a catheter introducer
- A rectal examination with the bladder distended will give misleading information as to the prostate size
- Acute urinary retention will significantly increase the level of serum prostate-specific antigen, misleadingly suggesting a diagnosis of carcinoma of the prostate

Suprapubic catheters should be inserted under ultrasound guidance to avoid the risk of bowel or vascular injury at the time of insertion.

Because 40% of patients with acute retention have no previous history of outflow obstruction, it is reasonable to allow them to attempt to void after clamping the suprapubic catheter. Those who are able to void usually had a residual urine of less than 700 mL when initially catheterised and avoid a prostatectomy in the short term. Patients who revert back into retention require a prostatectomy.

Chronic retention

The treatment is by prostatectomy. The only indication for preoperative catheter drainage is in patients with impaired renal function secondary to back pressure on the kidneys. Catheterisation eventually leads to the development of a urinary infection, which increases the morbidity and mortality of a subsequent operation and is difficult to eradicate in a large floppy bladder. If a catheter is required, attempts should be made to decompress the bladder slowly, as this reduces but does not completely do away with the development of severe bleeding from distended submucosal veins. The renal concentrating mechanism is usually impaired, and bladder catheterisation may result in diuresis leading to dehydration, hypotension and further impairment of renal function. Close monitoring of the patient's weight, blood pressure, pulse, fluid input and urine output is required. Once renal function has improved and stabilised, definitive surgery can be undertaken.

CARCINOMA OF THE PROSTATE

Epidemiology

This tumour is rapidly becoming the most common malignancy to affect men. The disease is one of ageing, rarely discovered under the age of 50 and with a peak incidence in the 70s. Examination of serial sections of the prostate of men who have died from other causes has demonstrated that 29% of those aged between 50 and 60, 49% of men in the age group 70–79 and 67% of those aged 80–89 had unsuspected prostate cancer. Not all are clinically apparent and, even when identified, they do not express the same malignant potential. At one extreme are those tumours which are found only at death, while at the other there are rapidly progressive tumours with invasive and metastatic potential. In between there are tumours with intermediate degrees of aggression and long periods of local growth only. However, current techniques are unable to identify which are which. In consequence, there is much confusion and controversy about whether or not to screen for the condition. To do so would lead to a significant over-treatment of the many men discovered. The same dilemma exists about treatment: diagnosis does not necessarily imply progression or a need to treat.

Aetiology

Prostate cancer appears to have multi-factorial causal factors. There is a genetic relationship to males within a family who have had the disease and also a relationship to the female line in a family who have had breast cancer. There are genetic studies showing predisposition to the disease with certain genetic phenotypes including *BRCA1&2*. There is also increasing evidence in relation to diet in that it is a disease of the developed countries. In populations that have a predominately vegetarian diet the incidence is low; when these individuals adopt a Western diet the incidence increases to that in developed countries.

Pathological features

Tumours are usually adenocarcinoma, arising in the periphery of the gland in 70% of cases. The tumour spreads along neuronal pathways, via the lymphatic and via the blood principally to bone. Tumours may locally invade into the periprostatic tissue, and spread by lymphatics to the iliac and para-aortic nodes, obdurator nodes and pre-sacral nodes.

Clinical features

The commonest presentation of prostatic cancer is now due to screening with PSA rather than presenting with symptoms. However, clinical features may include the following.

Symptoms

These include:

- bladder outflow obstruction (see above)
- metastatic disease – bone pain, leg swelling from lymphatic obstruction
- renal failure from bilateral ureteric obstruction.

Signs

These include:

- a nodule in a palpably benign gland
- hard irregular prostate on rectal examination, sometimes with perirectal and periprostatic thickening
- ankle and leg oedema
- other signs of metastases.

The disease may only be discovered at an incidental rectal examination or on histological examination of prostatic tissue removed during a prostatectomy for clinically benign disease.

Investigation

Histological diagnosis is required in the vast majority of cases and this is performed using usually transrectal ultrasound guided biopsy and to a lesser extent transperineal biopsy. For rare central tumours transurethal resection of the prostate may be required.

Other investigations include:

- routine evaluation of renal function
- serum alkaline phosphatase concentration – elevated in patients with bone metastases.

Serum prostate-specific antigen (PSA) concentration

PSA is a protein secreted by prostatic cells and may be elevated in benign prostatic hypertrophy, inflammatory change of the prostate and least commonly in malignant prostatic disease. Twenty percent of men with prostate cancer have a normal PSA. Further understanding and usage of PSA has shown clinical value in the serum free to serum total PSA ratio, with a percentage below 24% indicating a higher risk of cancer and a value above 24% showing a lower risk of cancer. There is a small group of patients who have non-PSA expressing tumours. They are often poorly differentiated.

PCA3 is a new genetic marker which is measured from secreted prostatic cells in urine. The specimen is produced after the first void following vigorous prostatic massage. Shed prostatic cells are spun down and a risk index is given. An index above 35 is indicative of a high risk of cancer and a PCA3 below 35 indicates low risk. This test is becoming more widely used.

Gleason grade

Histopathological grade is classified using the Gleason system. The histopathologist scores two separate areas of cancer with a grade from 1 to 5, with 1 being benign and 5 being highly malignant. However, most pathologists have dispensed with the 1 annotation. Most prostate cancers are between 2 and 4, with few poorly differentiated Gleason 5 cancers. A joint Gleason score is described by giving the predominant grade first and the less predominant second. Thus, Gleason 4+3 will have a more predominant 4 pattern as opposed to a 3+4 where the moderate 3 grade is more predominant. The Gleason score, the sum of the two grades, has a high relationship to the risk of metastasis, margin positive status and disease recurrence.

There is also the further histological pre-cancerous classification of prostatic intraduct neoplasia (PIN). The original classification of PIN was from grade 1 to 3, with 3 being the most likely to be related to the risk of developing adenocarcinoma. However, more recent studies have shown that PIN grades 1 and 2 are rarely associated with progression to adenocarcinoma. However, PIN grade 3 has a significant chance of conversion to cancer over a 5–10-year period. Patients with this finding need careful follow-up with regular PSA and digital rectal examinations.

Ultrasonography

Abdominal ultrasound may identify unilateral or bilateral hydronephrosis because of ureteric involvement. Transrectal ultrasound is used both as an aid to diagnosis and for staging prostate cancer, but unfortunately it is not particularly accurate in either. It is unable to detect microscopic spread beyond the prostate.

MRI scanning

Further staging investigations include MRI scan of the prostate, which is used to look at the state of capsular penetration or seminal vesicle involvement. This is largely reserved for patients with higher presenting PSA levels of over 15, higher Gleason scores of 7 or above, or palpable digital rectal findings suggestive of either locally advanced disease. MRI is not indicated for moderate to well-differentiated tumours with low presenting PSA of less than 10, unless as part of an active surveillance protocol.

Bone scanning

Radioisotope bone scan can detect areas of increased bone activity irrespective of their cause (Fig. 33.32). Confirmatory X-rays need to be taken of areas of increased isotope uptake. Bone metastases from carcinoma of the prostate are sclerotic (osteoblastic). Bone scintigraphy is required in all patients who present with a PSA of greater than 15 or who present with poorly differentiated disease (Gleason 7 or above). There is no indication for bone scan in well to moderately differentiated disease with a PSA of less than 10. The chances of a positive scan are extremely low.

Staging

Staging is by the TNM classification, given in Table 33.11.

Management

The management of prostate cancer can largely be divided by patient stage into those with organ-confined disease and those that present with metastatic disease.

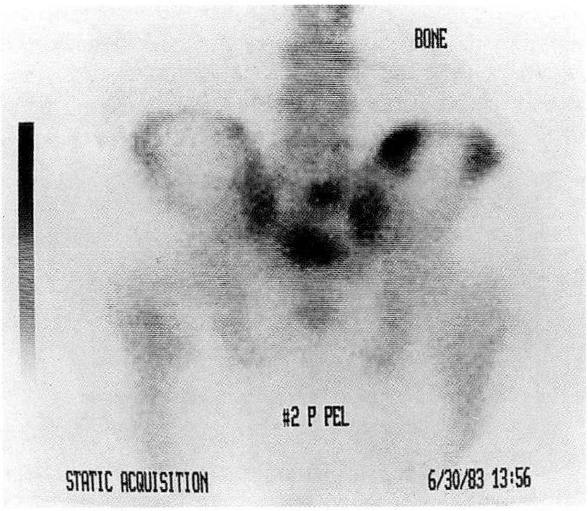

Fig. 33.32 A bone scan showing multiple hot spots caused by metastatic carcinoma of the prostate.

Table 33.11 Staging of prostate cancer

Stage	Findings
T1a	An incidental finding of tumour with low biological potential for aggressive behaviour in a prostate removed for clinically benign disease
T1b	An incidental finding of a tumour with potentially biological aggressive behaviour found in a prostate removed for clinically benign disease (high-grade or diffuse)
T1c	Tumour identified because of an elevated serum prostate-specific antigen
T2a	Tumour involving half a lobe or less
T2b	More than half a lobe but not both
T2c	Both lobes
T3	Tumour extends through capsule and may involve seminal vesicle
T4	Tumour fixed invasive of adjacent structures other than seminal vesicle

Management of organ-confined prostate cancer

The widespread use of PSA testing over several decades, the patient outcome data after radical prostatectomy and histological specimen analysis has led to an improved understanding about the variable natural history of prostate cancer. Whilst it remains one of the commonest cancers in men, the number of men who die from the disease is relatively small in relation to its overall incidence. Recent studies have questioned the validity of PSA screening and its value in reducing prostate cancer mortality and have emphasised the considerable potential cost to the patient. It has become clearer from a number of studies that active surveillance has a clear rationale, based on the fact that patients with moderate to well differentiated disease of small volume, i.e. involving a small percentage of any one core or cores involved, together with a low presenting PSA are very unlikely to develop progressive disease, particularly in men over the age of 65. Based on recent studies, active surveillance is a very good option for these men. The role of active surveillance becomes less clear in younger men. More long-term follow-up needs to be established to relate the actual risk of progression over time in such individuals. There is a trend to treat with curative intent in men under the age of 60 – that is by radical prostatectomy. That said, however, there still may be a role for closely monitoring patients who have small volume tumours of low grade, histological Gleason score, low PSA and low PSA ratio scores. The term 'watchful waiting' is used when men present with the disease over the age of 70 and are considered unlikely to benefit from primary treatment either in the form of surgery, radiotherapy or other modalities. Such patients should be monitored and treatment can be instituted if the disease progresses usually in the form of hormone manipulation and possibly external beam radiotherapy.

Primary treatment modalities for prostate cancer

- no treatment, with assessment of progress
- endocrine therapy
- radiotherapy
  - conformal external beam
  - external beam proton therapy
  - seed implant brachytherapy
- surgery
  - open – perineal or retropubic
  - laparoscopic ± robotic assisted
  - cyroablation
- HIFU (high-intensity focused ultrasound)
- Chemotherapy.

No treatment

Men with asymptomatic low-stage, low-grade disease and those with significant comorbidity can be offered follow-up with regular observation. Those who show signs of disease progression can then be treated with one of the therapies outlined below.

Early treatment by hormone therapy provides a slight survival advantage and reduction in morbidity from disease progression in men who have asymptomatic advanced localised or metastatic prostate cancer.

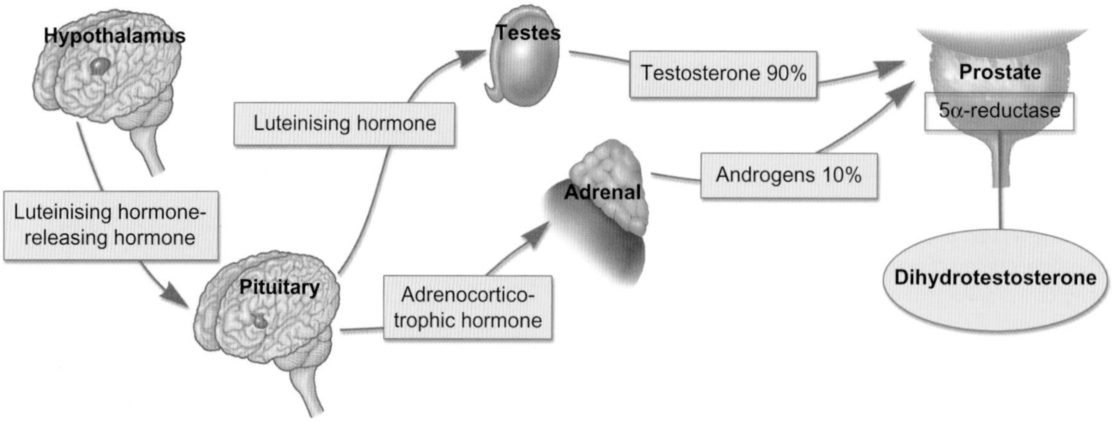

Fig. 33.33 Hormonal control of the prostate.

Endocrine therapy

Most of the cells of the prostate are dependent for their multiplication on the male hormone testosterone. Ninety percent of circulating testosterone is produced by the testes under the influence of luteinising hormone (LH), which is in turn controlled by the hypothalamic secretion of luteinising hormone-releasing hormone (LHRH; Fig. 33.33). The remaining 10% of testosterone is produced by the adrenals and by peripheral conversion of other steroids. Eighty percent of patients with symptomatic prostate cancer respond subjectively and 60% respond objectively to androgen suppression or ablation. The mean duration of response is 2 years. Once the tumour is no longer hormone-responsive, the mean survival is 6 months.

Androgen suppression. This is only used in men with locally advanced or metastatic disease. LHRH analogues initially stimulate the pituitary, but after approximately 7 days the pituitary receptors become blocked and downregulation occurs. Serum testosterone falls to castrate levels. These substances are long-acting and are administered subcutaneously every 1 or 3 months. Because of the initial stimulation of the pituitary, an anti-androgen should be given for 10–14 days before the analogue is given to prevent disease progression.

Androgen ablation is by bilateral subcapsular orchidectomy, which can be done under local anaesthesia on an out-patient and removes the testosterone-producing part of the testicle. There is no difference in response between orchidectomy and LHRH analogue therapy, and the choice of treatment should lie with the patient.

Radiotherapy

Radiotherapy is effective in controlling the pain of bony metastases. It is also used for the treatment of the primary if it is thought that the tumour is confined to the prostate. There have been no useful randomised controlled trials to assess its benefit compared with radical surgery. More recently, brachytherapy, in which radioactive seeds are placed throughout the prostate with the aid of a template and ultrasound guidance, has been used. Long-term results are awaited.

Surgical treatment

Transurethral resection is used in patients who present with symptoms of outflow obstruction or acute retention.

Radical prostatectomy is one of the most controversial aspects of the treatment of carcinoma of the prostate. Its use for disease that is believed to be localised to the prostate is widespread in the USA and Europe and is increasing in the UK. Some concerns include:

- The purpose of the operation is to remove the whole of the prostate with its confined cancer; this is not always accurately assessed before surgery.
- A high proportion of prostatic cancers have low malignant potential, and radical prostatectomy is over-treatment.
- There is a hospital mortality of 1%.
- Morbidity is considerable and includes incontinence, erectile dysfunction and anastomotic strictures.

Against this, it is probably indicated in men with poorly differentiated tumours which are thought to be localised to the prostate and who would otherwise have a 10-year life expectancy. A radical prostatectomy correctly performed will eradicate the disease if it is confined to the prostate.

HIFU and cryoablation

These are newer alternative less invasive techniques for the treatment of localised prostate cancer. Long-term results are awaited.

Chemotherapy

When patients with metastatic disease fail to respond to endocrine therapy, chemotherapy should be considered. Twenty percent will respond to treatment with docetaxel and a number of other agents are also used including mitoxantrone and epirubicin.

Prognosis

In men with prostate cancer confined within the capsule who undergo radical prostatectomy, approximately 55% survive 10 years, whereas only 25% of those who have metastatic disease at presentation can be expected to survive 5 years with current therapy.

THE MALE URETHRA

CONGENITAL ABNORMALITIES

These are:

- urethral valves
- hypospadias
- epispadias.

Urethral valves

Pathological features

Folds of urothelium develop in the posterior urethra in utero to form a valve-like obstruction to the passage of urine. Gross dilatation of the prostatic urethra (Fig. 33.34), distension of the bladder and ureters and hydronephrosis result. Severe renal impairment follows. With increasing use of antenatal ultrasound, many boys with urethral valves are diagnosed in utero by antenatal screening.

Clinical features

The bladder may be palpable, and the infant constantly dribbles urine. The development of a urinary infection may draw attention to the problem before end-stage renal failure develops.

Management

When diagnosed in utero, a stent can be inserted to drain the baby's bladder into the amniotic cavity, so preserving renal function. Endoscopic division of the valves is required, sometimes with urinary diversion to improve renal function.

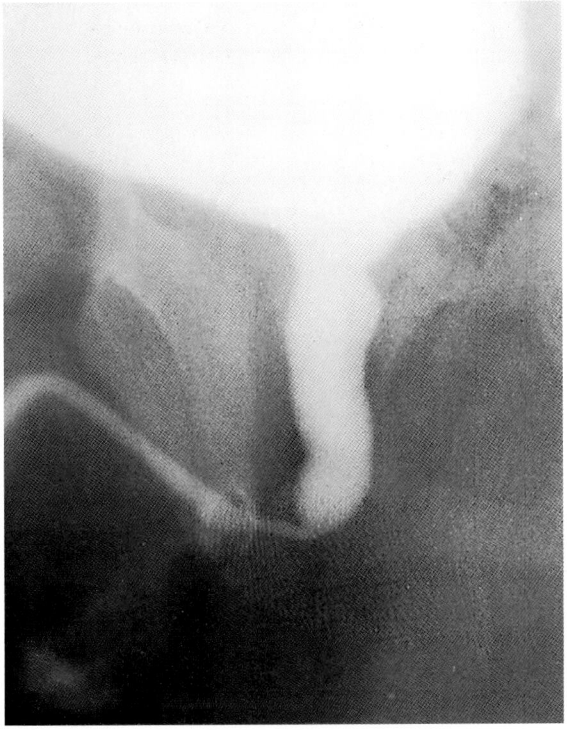

Fig. 33.34 Urethral valves causing bladder distension and dilatation of the prostatic urethra.

Hypospadias

Aetiology

The two genital folds on the ventral aspect of the phallus fail to fuse and form the anterior urethra of the male. The meatus is therefore displaced posteriorly for a variable distance. Hypospadias is classified according to where the opening lies (Fig. 33.35). Other genital abnormalities, such as failure of testicular descent, are often present, and there may be a family history.

Clinical features

Apart from the abnormal opening of the urethra, the foreskin is hooded and the penis is bent (chordee) ventrally because of secondary fibrosis in the area of the absent urethra.

Management

Surgical repair, usually utilising the foreskin, is carried out at around the age of 3 years before the child goes to school and has to face his 'normal' contemporaries.

Epispadias

This is extremely rare. The urethra opens on the dorsum of the penis, and there may be exstrophy of the bladder. No clear embryological mechanism has been formulated. Complex repair is required.

URETHRAL INJURY

Aetiology

The male urethra is more frequently injured than that of the female. The most common cause is instrumentation of the urethra by a catheter or cystoscope. Up to 30% of pelvic

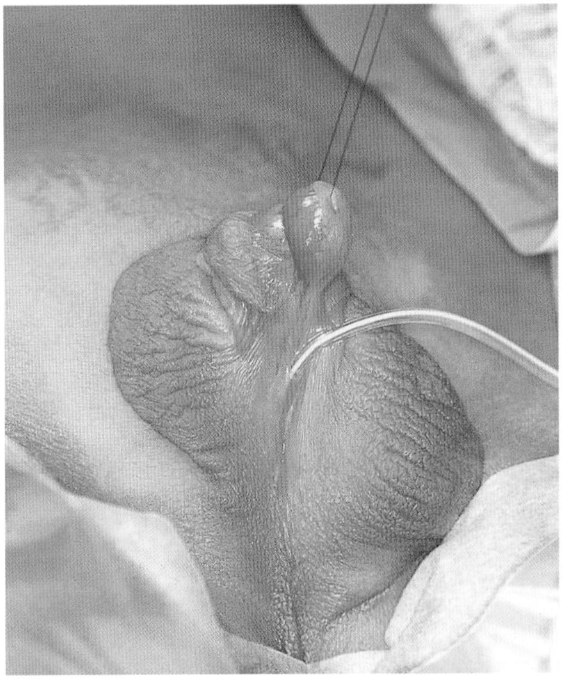

Fig. 33.35 An example of a penile hypospadias.

fractures are associated with urethral damage, and 10% of urethral trauma, beyond the pelvic floor, is caused by a fall-astride injury.

Clinical features

History

A urethral injury should always be suspected in a patient who has been injured and who presents with any of the following:

- blood at the urethral meatus
- haematuria
- anuria.

Signs

Physical examination may reveal a palpable bladder. Lower abdominal tenderness is always present in a patient with a pelvic fracture and does not necessarily imply bladder or urethral damage. In fall-astride injuries there may be bruising and swelling in the perineum. In rupture of the membranous urethra, the prostatic area is said to be boggy and the prostate high-riding. However, anyone who has attempted to perform a rectal examination in a man with a fractured pelvis realises how difficult this physical sign is to elicit.

Investigation

It is unwise to make repeated attempts to pass a urethral catheter. If the diagnosis is in doubt, urethrography using water-soluble contrast media is done.

Management

The urethral injury takes low priority in the overall management of patients subjected to severe multiple trauma.

Anterior urethral injuries

If the rupture is complete, the perineal haematoma is evacuated and a primary repair done. If incomplete, either a well-lubricated soft, small urethral catheter should be passed by an experienced urologist and left in situ for 10 days or a suprapubic catheter inserted.

Posterior urethral injuries

Either a suprapubic catheter should be inserted or a urethral catheter should be railroaded into the bladder (Fig. 33.36). This allows alignment of the divided ends, and if a stricture develops, subsequent management may be easier.

Complications

These are as follows:

- urethral stricture
- incontinence
- erectile dysfunction (neurogenic and vascular).

Urethral stricture

Aetiology

Strictures may be congenital, traumatic or inflammatory (Box 33.13).

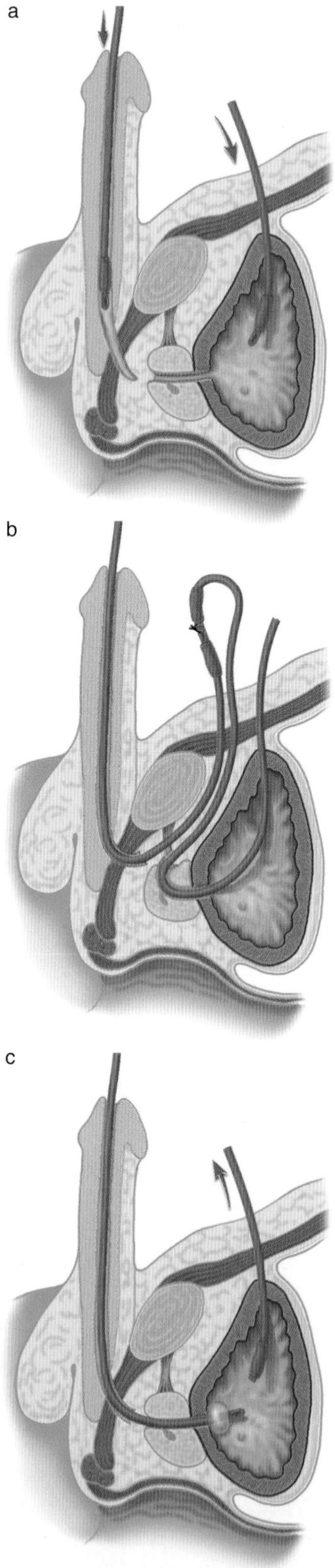

Fig. 33.36 A technique for railroading a urethral catheter in a patient with a ruptured urethra.

Box 33.13 Causes of urethral stricture

Congenital
- Meatal stenosis

Traumatic
- Urethral catheterisation
- Cystoscopy
- Transurethral resection
- After rupture of urethra

Inflammatory
- Gonorrhoea
- Non-specific urethritis
- Long-term urethral catheter

Clinical features

There may be a history related to the underlying cause. The patient complains of difficult and incomplete micturition with a poor stream. There is a thin, divergent urine stream with terminal dribbling. The bladder may be palpable.

Investigation and management

Urine flow rate is reduced and prolonged with intermittent peaks signifying temporarily improved flow due to abdominal strain. Urethrography demonstrates the site, length and number of strictures.

Urethral dilatation used to be the only treatment but invariably had to be continued indefinitely to prevent recurrence. Today the treatment of choice is direct endoscopic incision or a urethroplasty.

PENIS

Phimosis

Definition and aetiology

This is inability to retract the foreskin.

Congenital

It is not usually possible to retract the foreskin without the application of undue force until the age of 2–3 years, because the inner surface of the foreskin adheres to the glans. No active measures are required for uncomplicated, unretractile foreskin even when the foreskin is reported as ballooning when the child passes urine.

Acquired

This is the result of:

- recurrent infections (balanitis) of which diabetes mellitus is an associate
- underlying tumour of the glans penis.

Clinical features

The preputial orifice is white and scarred and indurated, presenting symptoms including secondary intractability of the foreskin, irritation at or bleeding from the preputial orifice, dysuria and occasionally acute urinary retention.

Management

Treatment is by circumcision. The operation should not be carried out until infection is under control.

Paraphimosis

Aetiology and pathological features

The foreskin contains fibrous tissue because of previous attacks of inflammation usually as a result of forceful retraction of the prepuce. It normally cannot be retracted, but if this occurs either by manipulation or during sexual intercourse, the fibrous band encircles the penis in the subcoronal area to cause congestion of the glans.

Clinical features

There may be a suggestive history. Pain in the glans is usually moderate to severe, and there may be difficulty on micturition.

It is not possible to reduce the retracted foreskin. The glans is oedematous. A tight band may be palpable in the subcoronal area.

Management

An injection of hyaluronidase with lidocaine (lignocaine) into the constricted area, followed by gentle pressure and traction, will usually result in reduction. Failure necessitates incision of the constricting band. Patients should subsequently be circumcised if it is a recurrent problem.

Circumcision

Indications

Indications are:

- religious ritual circumcision – Muslims, Arabs and Jews
- phimosis
- paraphimosis
- recurrent balanitis
- preputial injuries.

Complications

The operation should not be undertaken lightly. There is an anaesthetic mortality. In addition there may be:

- primary or secondary haemorrhage
- secondary infection
- meatal ulceration and stenosis because of the absence of protection by the foreskin
- injury to the glans
- over-radical excision with scarring.

Peyronie's disease

Aetiology and pathological features

The cause of this condition is unknown. There is fibrous thickening in the corpora cavernosae which results in bending or angulation of the penis when erect. Circumferential fibrosis may result in distal flaccidity during an erection.

Clinical features

The penis is angulated during erection, which may make intercourse impossible or painful (Fig. 33.37). The degree of

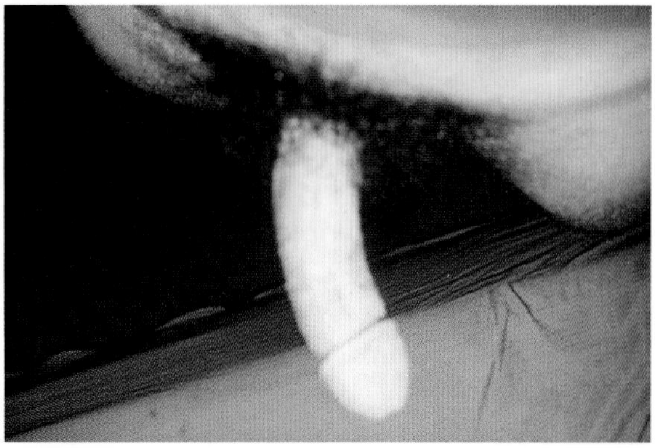

Fig. 33.37 Peyronie's disease with penile bending.

Box 33.14 Causes of priapism

- Idiopathic (80%)
- Intracavernosal injections of vasoactive drugs for the treatment of erectile dysfunction
- Sickle cell anaemia
- Leukaemia
- Malignancy

angulation can be assessed by inducing an artificial erection with an injection of intracavernosal prostaglandin E1.

Management

The penis can be straightened but made shorter by excising a wedge from the corpora opposite to the maximum angulation. Resuturing the excised edges straightens the penis.

Priapism

This is a persistent and painful erection of the penis.

Aetiology and pathological features

The great majority (80%) have no underlying cause. Those known are summarised in Box 33.14, and some relate to episodes of blood sludging. If detumescence does not take place within 8 hours, venous and arterial thrombosis ensues with fibrosis in the corpora and permanent erectile failure.

Management

Because of the risk of irreversible damage to the erectile apparatus, this is a urological emergency. Aspiration of the thick viscid blood from the corpora may be sufficient. If that fails, a shunt is created between the corpora cavernosa and the glans penis, the corpora cavernosa and the corpora spongiosa, or the corpora cavernosa and the saphenous vein.

Carcinoma of the penis

Aetiology

The occurrence of the disease mainly in the uncircumcised and elderly suggests that poor standards of subpreputial hygiene allow the accumulation of carcinogens, but there is no direct evidence for this. The tumour is a squamous carcinoma. It is now rare in developed countries.

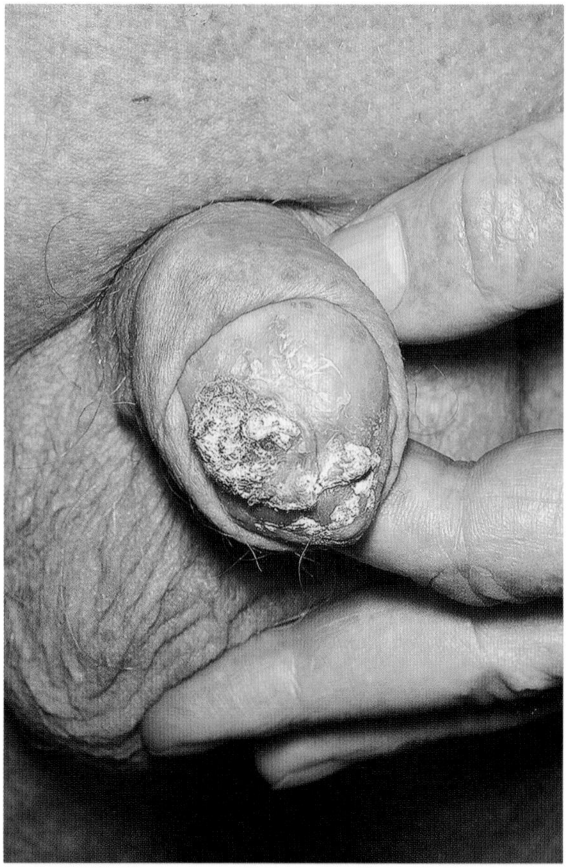

Fig. 33.38 An early carcinoma of the penis involving only the glans.

Clinical features

There is an offensive bloody discharge issuing from beneath a non-retractile foreskin. Inguinal lymphadenopathy is invariably present as a result of either infection or secondary spread. An early carcinoma is shown in Figure 33.38.

Management

This depends on the extent of the disease. Treatment options include:

- partial amputation
- radical amputation with block dissection of inguinal lymph nodes
- radiotherapy
- chemotherapy.

TESTIS, EPIDIDYMIS AND CORD

Undescended testis

Epidemiology

Both testes are undescended in 30% of premature infants: at term this has fallen to 3%; and at one year 1%. Spontaneous descent after 1 year is exceedingly rare.

Aetiology

The cause is failure of migration along the normal line of descent. In an ectopic testis the testicle deviates away from the line and may lie in front of the penis in the superficial inguinal pouch, in the perineum or in the thigh. The cause is not known.

Clinical features

An empty scrotal sac or hemiscrotum at 1 year indicates that the testicle is:

- proximal to the external inguinal ring (undescended)
- truly absent
- retractile – the cremaster muscle reflexly pulls the organ up towards the inguinal canal
- ectopic.

A retractile testis can usually be coaxed into the scrotal sac, or will enter spontaneously if the child is asked to crouch. An ectopic testicle may be palpable in the areas described above but cannot be brought into the scrotum. An incompletely descended testis may be palpable at the external ring or in the neck of the scrotum. A testicle in the inguinal canal is impalpable.

Complications

Complications are:

- infertility – inevitable in bilateral and common in unilateral undescent, and frequent in those who have had undescent treated
- torsion
- trauma
- inguinal hernia
- malignant disease.

Investigation

If the testicle is not palpable, ultrasonography, CT and laparoscopy are useful investigations to determine whether the testicle is truly absent and, if not, where it is situated.

Management

The aim is to bring the testicle with its blood supply into the scrotum as early as possible, usually between 1 and 2 years. Boys who present with a well-developed undescended testis before puberty should undergo an orchidopexy, an operation to bring the testicle and its blood supply into the scrotum. However, if the testis is poorly developed, an orchidectomy is advised. Beyond puberty, orchidectomy should be done. A testicular prosthesis can be placed in the scrotum.

Torsion

Aetiology and pathological features

Torsion is a recognised complication of testicular maldescent. The episode occurs any time between birth and early adolescence but is uncommon thereafter. A horizontally lying testicle with a long mesorchium and cord within the vaginal sac, so that the testis hangs like the clapper of a bell, is most prone to torsion. This anatomical arrangement is usually bilateral, so that both testes are at risk. The twist deprives the organ of its blood supply; if untwisting does not take place within 6 hours, ischaemia is irreversible, gangrene develops and the testis either suppurates or atrophies.

Clinical features

There may be a history of previous episodes of testicular pain. The pain may be initially felt in the iliac fossa or over the cord and is often associated with vomiting.

The testicle is extremely tender, swollen and drawn up in the scrotum. The unaffected testicle may have a horizontal lie.

Other conditions which must be considered are:

- torsion of an appendix of the testis
- acute epididymo-orchitis
- idiopathic scrotal oedema.

Investigation

Urinalysis will reveal a sterile, acellular urine.

Ultrasonography will demonstrate the absence of blood supply to the affected testicle.

Management

Treatment of testicular torsion is, for the reasons given above, a surgical emergency.

Non-operative

It may be possible to de-rotate the testis. Standing at the foot of the bed, the testis is rotated towards the thigh and may have to be rotated through two or three turns. If this manoeuvre is successful, the testicle and that on the other side should be surgically fixed on the next operating list.

Surgical

Failure of non-operative reduction requires immediate operation. The testis is de-rotated and fixed. The unaffected testis is dealt with at the same operation. A gangrenous testis is removed.

Orchitis and epididymo-orchitis

Aetiology and pathological features

Primary orchitis is rare except in association with mumps. The testis is often secondarily infected from epididymitis which originates by retrograde spread from the prostate and seminal vesicle; a blood-borne infection is the alternative source. A surgical procedure on the lower urinary tract, such as a TUR, may also be a precipitating factor. The organisms are *Neisseria gonorrhoeae*, *Escherichia coli* and *Chlamydia*. Chronic infection or a discharging sinus may be the consequence of tuberculosis.

Clinical features

There may be a preceding history of an operation or of dysuria, frequency and haematuria. Pain in the scrotum is acute, and the patient is conscious of swelling. Fever and rigors are not uncommon.

The epididymis is acutely tender and enlarged, although it may be difficult to distinguish it from the equally tender testis. Overlying redness and oedema may be present.

Investigation

Blood count. Leucocytosis is present.

Blood culture. A positive culture is useful to direct antibiotic treatment, although this should be started on an empirical basis before the result is available.

Urinalysis. This will reveal a pyuria, and the organism may be revealed by culture.

Aspiration of the epididymis. Chlamydia is best grown from this source.

Ultrasonography. Increased blood flow may be demonstrated.

Management

In a young man the commonest infecting organism is *Chlamydia*. Bed rest, scrotal elevation and tetracycline or erythromycin are appropriate. Other antibiotics may be needed according to the bacteriological analysis. The partner should also be investigated and treated.

SCROTAL SWELLINGS

A non-inflammatory swelling of the scrotal contents may be a:

- testicular tumour
- epididymal cyst (spermatocele)
- varicocele
- hydrocele
- hernia.

Clinical examination

The following points enable distinctions to be made:

- If it is possible to get above the swelling and palpate a normal cord, the swelling is not a hernia.
- If there is a cough impulse in the groin or, with the patient lying flat, the scrotal mass disappears or is reducible, the swelling is a hernia.
- The testicle lies anteriorly and the epididymis posteriorly, gentle palpation establishes where the swelling lies and therefore its origin.
- Hydroceles transilluminate.
- Varicoceles are more apparent with the patient standing and feel like a bag of worms.

Hydrocele

Aetiology

These may be congenital or acquired. Congenital hydroceles follow failure of obliteration of the processus vaginalis. Peritoneal fluid can then enter the scrotum. The great majority of acquired hydroceles are of unknown origin, but 10% are associated with tumour or infection of the testicle.

Clinical features

An infant presents with a large scrotal sac, and the hydrocele is easily demonstrated by transillumination.

In adult life, there is a firm painless transilluminable swelling which it is possible to get above.

Management

The majority of congenital hydroceles resolve spontaneously by the age of 3, but persistence beyond this time requires operative treatment by division and ligation of the processus. In acquired hydrocele, an ultrasound scan will identify any underlying cause. If the hydrocele is symptomatic, surgical excision of the outer wall of the hydrocele is required.

Epididymal cysts and spermatoceles

These may be single or multiple and are usually related to the head of the epididymis. They lie posterior or superior to the testicle and may transilluminate.

Management

Asymptomatic cysts do not require treatment. If they cause discomfort, simple aspiration is often satisfactory: spermatoceles yield a turbid milky fluid and epididymal cysts a fluid the colour of lemon barley water. Should recurrence occur after aspiration, surgical excision is required.

Varicocele

Aetiology and pathological features

The venous valve at the junction of the left spermatic vein with the renal vein is incompetent or becomes so. It is most uncommon for the same to take place on the right. Very occasionally, a tumour in the kidney with extension along the renal vein may be present. Varicocele is a common finding in men presenting with subfertility but is equally common in men requesting vasectomy for contraception. The veins of the pampiniform plexus become enlarged and tortuous.

Clinical features

There is a dragging sensation in the scrotum which is worse in hot weather and on prolonged standing. Subfertility may be mentioned.

Physical examination reveals the 'bag of worms', which becomes more obvious if the patient stands. A cough impulse is present in the same position. The left testicle may be smaller than the right.

Management

Treatment is required for those with symptoms and for those with subfertility. The procedure of choice is embolisation of the testicular vein under radiological control.

Testicular tumours

Benign, interstitial cell and Leydig cell tumours of the testis are exceedingly rare. Malignant tumours are uncommon (1–2% of all neoplasms in males) but do occur in young adults with an otherwise long expectation of life. In the age range 20–35 years, testes tumours are the most common malignancy excluding leukaemia. The psychological effects of a diagnosis of malignancy are, in consequence, considerable.

Aetiology and epidemiology

Maldescended testes – particularly those retained within the abdomen – have a 40% greater chance of malignant change than does a normal testis. Otherwise the cause is unknown. The overall incidence is 2–3 per 100 000 of the population per year. They are rare before puberty. Teratomas (see below), which account for 60% of germ cell tumours, have a peak incidence at 20–30 years. Seminomas (see below), which account for the remaining 35%, have a peak incidence at 30–40 years. Lymphomas, which are often bilateral, occur in the 60–70-year age range.

Pathological features

Classification of germ cell tumours is as follows:

- seminoma
- teratoma (Fig. 33.39)
- mixed – these consist of both seminomatous and teratomatous elements but should be treated as teratomas.

The further subdivision of teratomas is shown in Box 33.15.

Clinical features

Symptoms

Ten percent of patients give a history of previous orchidopexy, and in 5% the tumour is bilateral. There is often a recent history of trauma, although this is not a cause but merely draws the patient's attention to the presence of a lump. The most frequent complaint is of a painless swelling which causes a dragging sensation in the scrotum. In one-third, the swelling is painful. Patients with a choriocarcinoma may develop gynaecomastia. Others present with symptoms from secondary deposits such as backache, haemoptysis or neurological complaints.

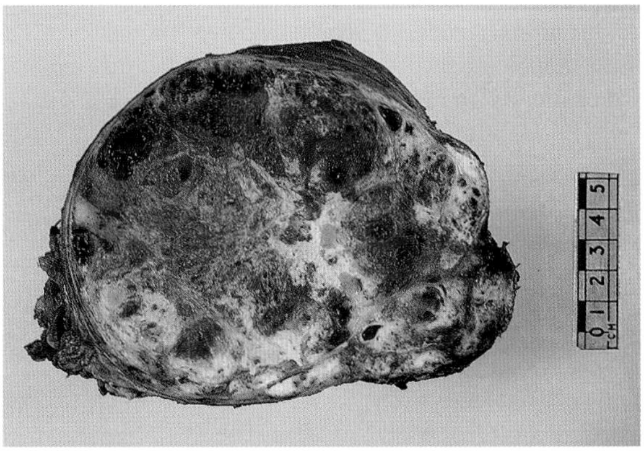

Fig. 33.39 A malignant teratoma showing cystic degeneration and haemorrhage.

Box 33.15 Teratomatous tumours of the testis

- Differentiated (TD) – teratoma differentiated
- Intermediate (MTI) – malignant teratoma intermediate
- Undifferentiated (embryonal) carcinoma (MTU) – malignant teratoma undifferentiated
- Trophoblastic (chorionic) carcinoma (MTT) – malignant teratoma trophoblastic

Signs

These include:

- a hard lump in the body of the testis
- diffuse testicular enlargement
- absence of tenderness on gently squeezing the testicle
- hydrocele.

Investigation

Tumour markers

Testicular teratomas secrete alpha-fetoprotein (AFP) and beta-human chorionic gonadotrophin (β-hCG). Both teratomas and seminomas may secrete lactic dehydrogenase, and seminomas may secrete placental alkaline phosphatase. These should be measured preoperatively and at regular intervals postoperatively. They are good indicators of the likelihood of complete excision of the tumour or, alternatively, the presence of residual disease which requires further treatment.

Imaging

Ultrasound. If it is not possible to determine the nature of the mass in the testicle clinically, ultrasound is particularly helpful. The normal testis has a homogeneous appearance. Malignant tumours are inhomogeneous, may be cystic and are often associated with speckled calcification.

CT scan of the chest and abdomen is done to identify pulmonary deposits and lymphadenopathy. Regular repeated examination is required postoperatively.

Staging

The stage of an individual tumour and its pathological type have considerable influence on management (see below). The Royal Marsden Hospital Staging System is summarised in Table 33.12.

Management

Patients with testicular tumours should be dealt with in specialist centres. There is no doubt that the earlier the diagnosis, the better the results. Improvements in therapy mean that the majority of testicular tumours should be regarded as curable.

Surgery

Orchidectomy is done through a groin incision – operations through the scrotum have a high incidence of tumour implantation. In order to reduce the risk of disseminating malignant cells by manipulation of the testis, the cord is mobilised and occluded before the testis is delivered from the scrotum. In men with a small or atrophic contralateral testis, or a history of subfertility, a biopsy from the contralateral testis should be taken. Up to 5% of men will have carcinoma in situ involving the other testis.

Supplementary management

The management options of seminoma and teratoma are given in Table 33.13. If chemotherapy is to be used, the patient should be advised to store semen prior to the chemotherapy. Patients with testicular tumours are often subfertile, and chemotherapy may result in irreversible germ cell damage.

Prognosis

Seminoma. For a tumour localised to the testis, over 95% of patients should survive 5 years. For those who present with metastatic disease, the 5-year survival is approximately 75%.

Non-seminomatous germ cell tumours. For those with a tumour confined to the testis and low tumour markers, 90% survive 5 years. If the tumour markers are grossly elevated and metastases are confined only to the lungs, 80% survive 5 years, but if there are visceral metastases and grossly elevated tumour markers, the 5-year survival falls to 45%.

ANDROLOGY

Infertility

Ten percent of couples have difficulty in conception. In approximately one-third, the problem lies with the male and in a further one-third there are contributory factors from both. Unless the male is found to be azoospermic (a complete absence of sperm), investigations of both partners should proceed simultaneously. The purpose of investigation is to give the couple a prognosis on the likelihood of conception. Couples who have been trying for more than 5 years with regular unprotected intercourse are unlikely to conceive without assisted conception.

Table 33.12 Royal Marsden Hospital Staging System

Stage	Details
I	Tumour confined to testis
IM	Rising concentrations of serum markers with no other evidence of metastasis
II	Abdominal node metastasis
A	≤2 cm in diameter
B	2–5 cm in diameter
C	>5 cm in diameter
III	Supradiaphragmatic nodal metastasis
ABC	Node stage as defined in stage II
M	Mediastinal
N	Supraclavicular, cervical or axillary
O	No abdominal node metastasis
IV	Extralymphatic metastasis
Lung	
L1	≤3 metastases
L2	≥3 metastases, all ≤2 cm in diameter
L3	≥3 metastases, one or more of which are ≤2 cm in diameter
H+, Br+, Bo+	Liver, brain or bone metastases

Clinical features

History

Relevant questions include:

- age of both partners
- length of time trying to conceive
- previous children of both
- frequency of intercourse
- whether intercourse is taking place in the vagina.

A previous medical history of orchitis, venereal disease, inguinal or scrotal surgery, testicular injury or fallopian tube injury or disease should be sought. The occupation of both may be of significance, as may their general health and social habits (drug and alcohol intake).

Physical examination

In the male, testicular and epididymal size should be assessed, the presence of a vas on both sides confirmed and gynaecomastia excluded.

In the female, further examination is the province of a gynaecologist and is not further considered here.

Investigation

Semen analysis

This is the most useful investigation. The patient should abstain from intercourse for at least 4 days, and the specimen should be produced by masturbation into a sterile container and examined within 1 hour of production. The measurements provided by the laboratory and their normal values are shown in Table 33.14.

Table 33.14 Semen analysis

Measurement	Normal value
Volume	2–6 mL
Sperm concentration	More than 50 million/mL
Sperm motility	More than 60%
Abnormal sperms	Not more than 30%
White blood cells	None
Mixed agglutination reaction (MAR)	Negative

Table 33.13 Supplementary management of seminoma and teratoma after orchidectomy

Stage	Seminoma	Teratoma
I	Pelvic and para-aortic irradiation for relapse	Surveillance Platinum-based chemotherapy for relapse
IIa & b	Irradiation	Platinum-based chemotherapy Radical retroperitoneal lymphadenectomy for residual disease
IIc	Platinum-based combination chemotherapy	Platinum-based chemotherapy Radical retroperitoneal lymphadenectomy for residual disease

If white blood cells are found, a further semen specimen should be cultured for bacteria. The mixed agglutination reaction (MAR) test screens for antisperm antibodies and should be negative.

Endocrine analysis

Measurements of testosterone and prolactin are only required if a patient complains of lack of libido. In those with small testes, the FSH concentration in the blood should be measured. If it is elevated and the patient has azoospermia, no further action is required as no treatment is available.

Management

In patients with oligospermia, it may be possible to separate out the most actively motile sperm and use these for artificial insemination. Azoospermia and a normal FSH suggest a diagnosis of testicular obstruction, which may be amenable to surgical correction.

Treatment of varicocele may improve both the sperm count and motility but not necessarily conception. Infected semen is an indication for treatment with antibiotics as for prostatitis. In the presence of antisperm antibodies, there is some evidence that treatment with prednisolone improves pregnancy rates, but using high-dose steroids has significant risks and side-effects. It is now possible to directly aspirate sperm from the epididymis or extract viable sperm from a testicular biopsy. These sperm can be directly implanted into an ovum. These techniques are used in cases of severe oligospermia and azoospermia.

Impotence

A better term is erectile dysfunction. The definition is the inability to achieve and maintain an erection for completion of satisfactory intercourse. Approximately 80% of men have a predominantly organic cause, but the fact that they cannot make love introduces an additional psychological element.

Aetiology

Organic

Organic factors are:

- generalised atherosclerosis
- diabetes mellitus
- multiple sclerosis
- pelvic fracture with urethral injury
- arterial disease at the aortic bifurcation
- endocrine dysfunction
- anti-hypertensive therapy
- corporeal venous dysfunction
- other drugs.

Psychogenic

The psychodynamics are poorly understood and probably multifactorial.

Clinical features

Organic

The findings are those of the underlying cause.

Psychogenic

In this form, the following are more likely to be present:

- age less than 50
- non-smoker – smokers may have vascular disease
- absence of neurological or endocrine disorder
- no anti-hypertensive therapy
- nocturnal and early morning erections
- erections with different partners
- erection is present up to the time of attempted penetration.

Investigation

These are required only in the following situations:

- The patient presents with lack of libido, when measurements of serum testosterone and prolactin concentrations are required.
- Young patients with impotence as a result of pelvic trauma, to ensure that there is not a correctable arterial problem.
- Failure to respond to an artificial erection test with vasoactive drugs – corporeal venous incompetence may be present and requires specialist investigation.

Management

Those with obvious psychogenic causes may benefit from psychosexual counselling. Correctable organic disease should be treated.

Therapies are as outlined below:

- Sildenafil, vardenafil and tadalafil are type 5 phosphodiesterase inhibitors which prevent the breakdown of cyclic GMP, a second messenger for smooth muscle relaxation. They improve erectile ability sufficiently to allow intercourse to take place in approximately 60% of men with organic disease.
- Intraurethral prostaglandin E1. A small pellet of prostaglandin is inserted into the anterior urethra in men with organic erectile dysfunction – 66% achieve an erection satisfactory for intercourse.
- Intracavernosal prostaglandin E1. The patient administers an injection of prostaglandin E1 directly into the corpora cavernosa – 80% of men with organic erectile dysfunction achieve an erection.
- Vacuum erection devices. These consist of a plastic cylinder placed around the penis. By creating a vacuum within the cylinder, the penis becomes erect. The erection is maintained by placing a rubber constriction device around the base of the penis prior to removal of the cylinder.
- Penile prostheses. These are of two types: a semi-malleable and an inflatable. They are inserted at operation into both corpora cavernosa. They should only be used when other treatments have failed.

Complications

Complications are:

- phosphodiesterase inhibitors – facial flushing, headache, visual disturbances

- intraurethral prostaglandins – penile pain and discomfort
- intracavernosal prostaglandin – penile discomfort, penile fibrosis, prolonged erection
- penile prostheses – pain, infection, extrusion
- vacuum devices – penile oedema and bruising.

FURTHER READING

Mundy AR, Fitzpatrick J, Neal DE, George NJ 2010 The scientific basis of urology, 3rd edn. Informa Healthcare, London

Reynard J, Brewster S, Briers S 2009 Oxford handbook of urology, 2nd edn. OUP, Oxford

Tanagho EA, McAninch JW 2008 Smith's general urology, 17th edn. McGraw-Hill Medical, New York

34 Principles of orthopaedics

Orthopaedics is concerned with the surgical treatment of bone and joint conditions. The word is derived from the Greek for 'straight child', and the symbol that has been adopted by most orthopaedic associations is the twisted sapling (symbolising the bent child) lashed to a straight supporting stick.

Orthopaedic terms. A number of terms with particular definitions are used in orthopaedic practice, and these are summarised in Box 34.1.

SPECIAL FEATURES OF ORTHOPAEDIC HISTORY AND EXAMINATION

History

Pain

This is usually the presenting symptom. Onset and duration are important. Was it sudden or was it slow over a few months? Is the pain constant or exacerbated by standing? The site is obviously important. There are some characteristic patterns: hip pain is classically felt in the groin but may also be apparent in the knee, particularly in children; if there is a nerve root trapped in the spine, pain may radiate down the arm or leg. Factors that may bring about relief include rest, load reduction with a walking stick, or drugs. Exacerbation from causes other than weight-bearing include particular movements such as a twist of the knee with a meniscal tear or lifting in low back pain. Night pain is an important symptom: it is common with arthritic joints when muscular tone relaxes. When sleep is lost, this may be an indication for joint replacement. Pain at night is also classical in benign osteoid osteoma (although a rare tumour).

Weakness

Patient may have weakness secondary to pain or due to tendon tears as in rotator cuff tears of the shoulder. Weakness due to neurologic damage will usually be associated with sensory disturbances unless it is a pure motor nerve damage (e.g. posterior interosseous nerve damage). Even the so-called pure motor nerves carry proproceptive sensations to the joints they cross.

Stiffness and loss of function

Stiffness and pain are hallmarks of arthritis but are also a feature of contractures around any joint (typical example will be a frozen shoulder).

Feeling of instability

This occurs with altered joint stabilisers as seen with cruciate ligament injuries of the knee, labral tears of the shoulder or fractures.

Trauma

Is there a history of injury? Mechanism of injury is important as it gives a clue to the degree of damage and in fractures the directions of displacements that allow one to reverse the mechanism to reduce fractures (e.g. Colles' fractures).

Secondary osteoarthritis may follow:

- direct disruption of a joint
- malunion which places undue loads on a joint.

Box 34.1 Orthopaedic terms

Proximal[a] Closer to the trunk
Distal[a] Further away from the trunk
Varus[b] Deformity or angulation towards the midline
Valgus[b] Deformity or angulation away from the midline
Genu Knee
Recurvatum Abnormal hyperextension of the knee joint
Cubitus Elbow
Coxa Hip
Pes Foot
Cavus[c] Abnormally arched
Planus[c] Flat
Alta[d] High
Baja[d] (pronounced Ba-ha) Low
Scoliosis[e] Abnormal lateral curvature
Lordosis[e] Posterior curvature – normal in cervical and lumbar regions
Kyphosis[e] Anterior curvature – normal in thoracic region
Crepitus Grating or grinding sound or sensation from an abnormal joint (usually degenerative) when moved
Ankylosis Joint fusion secondary to a pathological process (usually inflammatory) – usually fibrous
Arthrodesis Joint fusion brought about by operation – always bony
Osteoporosis Normal bone mineral content but reduction in bone mass or matrix
Osteosclerosis Increased bone mineral content
Osteomalacia Reduced bone mineral content
Polydactyly Duplication of digits
Macrodactyly Enlarged digits
Syndactyly Fused digits
Camptodactyly Deformed digits

[a]Example: at the distal end of the arm is the hand and at the proximal end is the shoulder.
[b]The description is applied to the distal part.
[c]Terms applied to the foot.
[d]Terms describing the position of the patella.
[e]Terms used to describe the shape of the spine; may be combined.

Need to use an 'aid'

The need for a walking stick or special cutlery may give an indication of the severity of the problem or of the use of past conservative management by the patient or doctors.

Occupation

Certain occupations which involve continued or repetitive movements can cause tenosynovitis (tendon inflammation) for example in typists, chicken pluckers or keyboard operators. Osteoarthritis of the spine is seen in miners and farm workers. Osteonecrosis of the femoral heads occurs in deep-sea divers and is termed 'caisson's disease'.

Dominant hand

The dominant hand may be affected more commonly, as in carpal tunnel syndrome.

Past medical history

This includes:

- similar problem on the contralateral side
- recent infections – urethritis, gastroenteritis or a streptococcal sore throat, all of which predispose to reactive arthritis
- pregnancy – which often precipitates low back pain or carpal tunnel syndrome
- diabetes – which is often associated with frozen shoulder.

Table 34.1 Phases of normal gait

Phase	Movement
Heel strike	The heel makes contact with the ground
Stance	Weight is being transferred from the heel to the toes
Toe-off	A final push is given to the foot as it leaves the ground
Swing-through	The leg is brought forward with the knee lightly flexed to allow the foot to clear the ground

Family history

Dupuytren's contracture, gout, rheumatoid arthritis and bone dysplasias may all run in families.

Medication

Current and past medication should be identified. The use of steroids predisposes to osteonecrosis of the femoral head. Patients on steroids often have problems with wound healing. Dupuytren's contracture is observed in association with phenytoin.

Examination

General assessment

Two classes of information result:

- specific indications of the cause of the problem
- suitability and fitness for surgery to correct the condition.

Joints

The examination of any joint has four components:

- look
- feel
- measure (not always applicable)
- move

... and special tests pertinent to the joint examined.

Look at:

- gait – assessment is made when the patient walks into the clinic or takes a few steps on the ward; normal gait has four phases (Table 34.1) which flow smoothly one into the other but there are many abnormalities (Box 34.2)
- skin – for scars and colour
- shape of the joint in general, the presence of swelling and lumps, and the position of the limb.

Feel for:

- temperature
- crepitus
- abnormal movement
- swelling – is it fluctuant and therefore fluid, or soft tissue or bone?

Measure the length of the limb to determine inequality in the two sides by using the distance between fixed bony points. Is it possible to determine if the whole limb or only a part of it is short? Muscle wasting can be documented by measuring and comparing girths.

Move. Joint movement may be painful, and care should be taken not to cause pain. First, the patient is asked to move the joint in question actively. This gives the examiner an indication of the degree of pain and disability within an affected joint. Next the limb is passively moved. Often there is no significant difference between the active and passive ranges. Local weakness due to muscular or neurological dysfunction may result in limited active movement but a full range of passive movement; in the shoulder, rotator cuff lesions may limit active abduction, but passive abduction is often unaffected.

The range of movement is recorded in the notes to allow for later comparisons (see Table 34.2).

Box 34.2 Abnormal gaits

Antalgic Painful and with a short stance phase; seen in any condition of the lower leg where the pain is exacerbated by weight-bearing, e.g. osteoarthritis of the hip

Stiff leg A fused hip or knee joint causes abnormal swing-through when the pelvis has to be rotated to bring the leg through

Trendelenburg With proximal muscle weakness the pelvis on the opposite side sags during the stance phase – seen in developmental dysplasia of the hip, poliomyelitis and in osteoarthritis of the hip

Short leg During the stance phase, the short leg results in the pelvis and shoulder on the affected side sagging down

Shuffling Seen in Parkinson's disease, it has a short swing-through and no real heel strike or toe-off

Stamping The swing-through phase is abnormal with a broad base and high stepping – often caused by peripheral neuropathy with tabes dorsalis

Ataxic Broad-based with unsteadiness on turning – cerebellar disease, multiple sclerosis or head injury

Foot drop During swing-through, the foot scuffs on the ground – an L5 root lesion, common peroneal nerve palsy or old poliomyelitis

Scissor Occurs in children with cerebral palsy with adductor spasm, so the swing-through of one leg is blocked by the other

Investigation

Imaging

Plain X-ray can allow differentiation between a disorder in bone and one in soft tissue and will nearly always confirm its nature. Old trauma may be evident. If arthritis is present, the type may be apparent (Table 34.3). Calcification within the joint suggests chondrocalcinosis (Fig. 34.1).

Arthrography. Injection of a radio-opaque contrast medium into a joint delineates its anatomical boundaries and shows abnormal communications such as those that occur in rotator cuff tears of the shoulder. Intra-articular structures may become apparent, e.g. loose bodies or the menisci in the knee. Arthrography is widely used in countries where MRI is unavailable. It can be combined with CT or MRI to give further information.

Computed tomography (CT). In orthopaedics, this technique is used for imaging bony pathology, fractures, the spine and bone tumours.

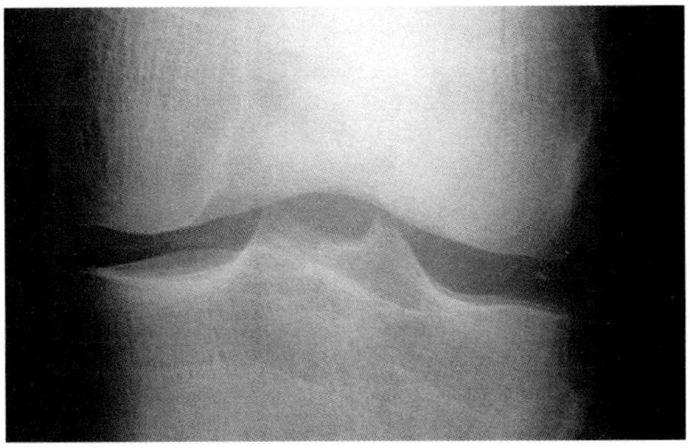

Fig. 34.1 Radiological calcification in a meniscus in the knee joint.

Table 34.3 Radiological appearances in arthritis

Feature	Osteoarthritis	Rheumatoid arthritis
Loss of joint space	Yes	Yes
Sclerosis	Yes	No
Osteophytes	Yes	No
Subchondral cysts	Yes	No
Erosions	No	Yes
Osteoporosis	No	Yes

Table 34.2 Normal degrees of large joint movement

Joint	Flexion	Extension	Abduction	Adduction	External rotation	Internal rotation
Shoulder	180	50	180	30	80	100
Elbow	150	5	–	–	–	–
Wrist	Dorsi- 90	Palmar 90	Ulnar 30	Radial 15	Supination 90	Pronation 90
Hip	150	0	45	30	80	45
Knee	140	10				
Ankle	Dorsi- 15	Plantar 70	Eversion 10	Inversion 25		

Magnetic resonance imaging (MRI). This is now the standard investigation for many musculoskeletal problems. This technique (Ch. 4) provides excellent images in both coronal and sagittal planes, and with appropriate computer software, three-dimensional reconstruction is possible. MRI of the brain and spinal cord now provides unparalleled detail (Fig. 34.2). MRI scans are also useful in the staging of bone tumours: intraosseous as well as extracompartmental spread can be identified and local oedema defined.

Isotope scanning (see Ch. 4) is frequently used in orthopaedics. Technetium-99m diphosphonate is concentrated in areas of increased osteoblastic activity usually associated with increased blood supply. These areas occur in such conditions as arthritis, fractures or bone secondaries. Scans also reveal zones of relative underactivity when the blood supply is reduced in osteonecrosis. Radiolabelled white blood cells are used to localise infection within a painful joint replacement or a nidus of osteomyelitis (see below).

Ultrasound is used extensively in the assessment of dislocation or investigation of possible infection in the hips of babies and children. It is also in adults to identify soft-tissue problems such as rotator cuff tendonitis (shoulder) or trochanteric bursitis (hip).

Blood investigations

ESR and C-reactive protein (CRP) are non-specific markers of inflammation which can be used to follow the course of an orthopaedic disease and its treatment. They are raised in such conditions as osteomyelitis, active rheumatoid arthritis, malignant disease and infected joint replacement.

Rheumatoid factor is an IgM autoantibody present in the serum of patients with a number of conditions, including rheumatoid arthritis (80%), Sjögren's syndrome (90%) and systemic lupus erythematosus (50%). Cyclic citrullinated peptide antibody (CCP test) is a newer test for rheumatoid arthritis, being useful particularly in early disease and rheumatoid factor negative patients.

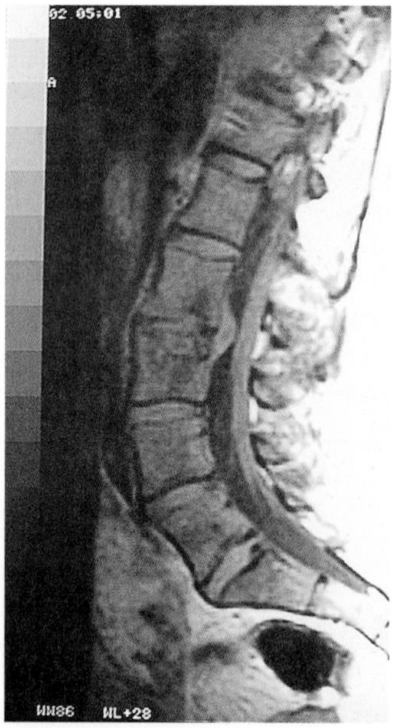

Fig. 34.2 MRI of a disc abscess in the spine at L2/3.

Uric acid. Raised levels in the serum predispose to gout but are not always raised in acute attack.

Antistreptolysin (ASO) titres are increased in recent streptococcal infection, which may be helpful in confirming an occult infection in a joint replacement.

Protein electrophoresis for a specific monoclonal antibody is diagnostic of myeloma.

Alkaline phosphatase is raised in Paget's disease, secondary malignancy in bone and osteomalacia.

Synovial fluid examination

Joint aspiration is an out-patient procedure which must be performed with aseptic technique and may reveal:

- the presence of crystals in both gout and pseudogout (seen using a polarising light microscope) organisms and a very high white cell count (50×10^9/L) in septic arthritis and lower levels in any inflammatory arthritis ($1–3 \times 10^9$/L).

Arthroscopy

Endoscopic principles are considered in Chapter 4. The interior of the knee joint was first examined in 1918, using a cystoscope. The techniques were refined over subsequent years until 1957 when the first purpose-built instrument was introduced. An arthroscope is a rigid instrument with an outer sheath and an inner lens system.

Almost any joint can be arthroscoped, although some require specialised instrumentation. The commonest ones are the knee (most frequent), shoulder, elbow, wrist, hip and ankle. Arthroscopy of the phalangeal joints has been described, as well as that of the facet joints of the lumbar spine.

The technique consists of the introduction of the sheath into the joint by a small puncture wound (portal) followed by distension with saline. The lens system can be slid down within the sheath and the joint inspected. Procedures can be performed with instruments introduced through other portals. A large variety are available. They range from simple hooked probes to scissors, grasping forceps, knives, specialised meniscal sutures and powered tools to shave or cut. Lasers can also be used to trim intra-articular structures such as meniscal tags or to shrink the capsule in unstable shoulder or ankle joints.

ARTHRITIS

Osteoarthritis

Epidemiology and aetiology

Osteoarthritis (OA) is the most frequent type of arthritis and is more common in women than in men. The incidence increases with age, and by 80 years, 80–90% of hips show radiographic evidence of osteoarthritis. The condition is usually primary but can be secondary to other conditions (Box 34.3). Primary OA is of unknown cause, although repeated minor trauma and a genetic predisposition are probable factors. It affects the main weight-bearing joints – the spine, hips and knees – although it rarely occurs in the ankle. The distal interphalangeal joints of the hand and, in the thumb, the carpometacarpal joints can also be sites of the disorder. Secondary osteoarthritis can affect any joint.

Clinical features

History

Joint pain and stiffness are usual and tend to be progressive over time but they may be variable from day to day. Pain initially occurs on weight-bearing, then at rest and subsequently wakes the patient at night. As well as pain during movement, joint crepitus may be felt and heard by the patient.

Deformity of the affected joint from local swelling and destruction may be noted and, on weight-bearing, these may increase.

Physical findings

- *Look* for:
  - local swelling
  - deformity – weight-bearing may make this worse
  - scars or sinuses that suggests a secondary cause.
- *Feel* to detect if:
  - the swelling is bone, soft tissue or fluid
  - crepitus is present.
- *Move* the joint to test:
  - active and then passive range of movement
  - stability of ligaments.

Investigation

Few investigations are required. Plain X-rays are needed to assess the extent of the disease, but the radiological appearances (Table 34.3) may not correlate well with clinical symptoms.

Box 34.3 Causes of osteoarthritis

Primary (or idiopathic)
- Unknown

Secondary
- Abnormal joint contour
- Trauma (dislocation in particular)
- Developmental dysplasia of the hip
- Slipped upper-femoral epiphysis
- Osteonecrosis
- Kienbock's disease of the lunate
- Panner's disease of the capitellum
- Scheuermann's disease of the vertebral end plates
- Perthe's disease of the hip
- Osgood–Schlatter's disease of the tibial tuberosity
- Sever's disease of the calcaneum
- Kohler's disease of the navicular
- Freiberg's disease of the metatarsal heads
- Drugs
  - Systemic steroids and cytotoxics
  - Intra-articular steroids
- Local radiotherapy
- Sickle cell disease
- Alcoholism
- Neoplasia – leukaemia and lymphoma
- Occupational – caisson's disease
- Cartilage destruction
  - Infection
  - Recurrent haemarthrosis – haemophilia
  - Gout and pseudogout
  - Rheumatoid arthritis

Metabolic and endocrine disorders
- Alkaptonuria
- Wilson's disease
- Acromegaly

Neuropathic disorders
- Diabetes mellitus
- Tabes dorsalis

Rheumatoid arthritis

Epidemiology and aetiology

This is a systemic inflammatory disease which affects 3% of the female and 1% of the male UK population. Small joints in the hands and wrists, elbows, shoulders, cervical spine and feet are particularly involved, but any joints may be affected except the lumbar spine and the distal interphalangeal joints. The cause remains unknown, although various organisms and an exaggerated immune response to them have frequently been invoked.

Clinical features

History

There is usually a long history of systemic illness with multiple joint involvement and extra-articular problems including weight loss, low-grade fever, subcutaneous nodules, arteritis and tendon sheath involvement.

Joint symptoms are pain, morning stiffness and progressive deformity with loss of function.

Physical findings

- *Look:*
  - at the hands, which have the characteristic deformity of ulnar deviation of the fingers and subluxation at the metacarpophalangeal joints
  - for rheumatoid nodules on the subcutaneous border of the ulna.
- *Feel* for:
  - subcutaneous nodules
  - local warmth in the affected joint
  - soft-tissue swelling around joints and tendon sheaths
  - joint crepitus.
- *Move* to detect:
  - active rather than the passive range of movement
  - abnormal joint mobility secondary to subluxation.

Investigation

The diagnosis of rheumatoid arthritis has usually been made by the time the patient is seen in the orthopaedic clinic.

Imaging

Plain X-ray may help to confirm the diagnosis (Table 34.2). However, there may be radiological features of superimposed (secondary) osteoarthritis. MRI scanning is best for investigation of early disease.

Blood examination

Anaemia is common and is either a leucoerythroblastic type or reflects iron deficiency (secondary to chronic gastrointestinal bleeding after NSAID ingestion).

ESR is usually raised.

Rheumatoid factor is detectable in 80% of cases. CCP test is usually positive (see above).

Management

Rheumatoid arthritis is predominantly managed by medical means. Patients are referred to the orthopaedic clinic or to one conducted jointly with rheumatologists when correction of deformity and restoration of function may be beneficial.

Other arthritides

Systemic lupus erythematosus (SLE)

This systemic inflammatory condition mainly affects young women. Ninety percent of patients develop joint symptoms that include polyarthritis of the hands.

Polymyalgia rheumatica

This affects the elderly and is more common in women. It presents with aching and morning stiffness in the shoulders and pelvis. Locally, there is muscle tenderness and a reduced range of active movement but normal passive movement. There may be associated temporal arteritis. The ESR is markedly raised (>100). Management is with steroid therapy.

Gout

Arthropathy with urate crystal deposition affects mostly men at the metacarpophalangeal joint of the big toe, although the knee is also a common additional site. Acute attacks may occur spontaneously or be precipitated by local trauma. Gout may also be secondary to myeloproliferative disorders with increased purine production or renal disease with reduced urate excretion. Urate crystals may also be deposited as tophi in soft tissues: the Achilles tendon, around joints, in bursae and on the pinna of the ear. The diagnosis is made by demonstrating the presence of urate crystals within the joint or soft tissues. Management includes treatment of the acute attack with NSAIDs and long-term prophylaxis with allopurinol to reduce uric acid production after the acute attack has settled.

MANAGEMENT OF ARTHRITIS

Arthritis is rarely reversible, and treatment is directed at symptomatic relief and the preservation or restoration of function.

Non-operative

Conservative management

Conservative measures are tried initially in patients with osteoarthritis. Pain relief with simple analgesics, NSAIDs or cyclo-oxygenase 2 (COX-2) selective inhibitors will be helpful. For patients with early rheumatoid arthritis, treatment with disease modifying anti-rheumatic drugs (DMARDs) provides good results. The medical treatment of rheumatoid and other forms of arthritis is beyond the scope of this chapter.

Intra-articular steroid injection

The role of this is controversial and it is not used in young people. An intra-articular injection often provides pain relief, because the inflammatory reaction within the joint is reduced, but repeated steroid injections may increase joint degeneration by the inhibition of the normal processes of repair. In general, two or three injections should be the maximum at any one point.

Weight reduction

Weight loss is encouraged. Not only is the load transmitted through the damaged joint reduced but also obesity is associated with an increase in the complications of operation should this ultimately be required.

Aids to daily living (ADL)

These should be considered; they include walking sticks and crutches. The rheumatoid patient with limited hand function may require special large-handled cutlery and easy-open containers for medication.

Operative

When conservative measures have failed, surgical options need to be considered.

Arthroscopy

A joint that is swollen and inflamed may benefit from an arthroscopic washout which removes inflammatory mediators and fragments of cartilage, although there is no evidence of benefit for this procedure in patients with uncomplicated osteoarthritis.

Synovectomy

The role of synovectomy has reduced as more effective medical treatments for rheumatoid arthritis have become available. Surgical excision of the synovium or tendon sheath in rheumatoid arthritis can occasionally be beneficial. In the past it was done as an open procedure with consequent considerable joint morbidity, but this has been replaced by arthroscopic synovectomy with special powered instruments.

Joint surgery

Long-term or permanent relief of the symptoms of arthritis requires surgery on the bones of the affected joint. A variety of options are available (Table 34.4) and the choice depends on a number of factors, including:

- age
- patient expectation
- occupation
- the joint affected.

In the younger patient with osteoarthritis, prosthetic replacement (Table 34.5) is avoided, if possible, because of the limited lifespan of the prosthesis. The results of further replacements after initial failure (revision surgery) are not as good as those of the primary procedure, and with

Table 34.4 Surgical options for an arthritic joint

Procedure	Effects	Example
Arthrodesis	Stiff but pain-free joint	Fusion of the lumbar spine, ankle or wrist
Excision	Removal of one aspect of the joint may relieve pain; shortening of the limb beyond the resection	Keller's operation on the big toe for hallux valgus
Osteotomy	Alteration of the line of load transmission to an unaffected part of the joint – now an infrequently performed procedure	High tibial osteotomy for unicompartmental osteoarthritis of the knee
Prosthetic replacement	Excision of diseased joint surfaces and replacement of surfaces with metal and high-density polyethylene	Hip, knee and shoulder and other joints

Table 34.5 Types of joint replacement

Type	Nature	Comments	Examples
Constrained	Simple hinge	Loosening because of inevitable rotational movement	Elbow, wrist
Semi-constrained	Simple hinge, but some rotation possible	Still subject to loosening	Elbow, wrist
Unconstrained	Two independent parts so that stability depends on sound anchorage in bone and the soft tissues	Most common type in use; highly satisfactory	Hip, knee, ankle, shoulder, elbow

In the knee, the replacement can be unicompartmental if one side only is affected; more usually, all three compartments are replaced.

each subsequent attempt the surgery becomes more challenging.

Almost any joint in the arm or leg can be replaced. Usually the replacement consists of a metal component bearing on a high-density polyethylene surface. The prosthesis may be cemented into place with methyl-methacrylate bone cement or be uncemented, with the surface textured to encourage bone ingrowth. New surfaces include the use of hydroxyapatite (HA), which is the basic mineral of bone. With HA chemically bonded to the surface of the prosthesis, the patient's bone can directly bind the implant.

The first successful replacement was the hip joint developed by Charnley in the 1960s although previous attempts had been made to replace the hip as far back as the 1930s. The modern hip joint can be expected to last for 15–20 years but this depends upon:

- surgical experience
- state of the recipient bone
- prosthesis design
- stresses placed upon the implant
- the materials used at the bearing surfaces – recent research has supported hard-on-hard articulation with ceramic-on-ceramic or metal-on-metal.

Approximately 50 000 hips and 40 000 knees are implanted each year in the UK.

Complications of joint replacement surgery include:

- general complications of any major operation
- specific complications of the procedure, including intraoperative fractures, postoperative dislocations and fractures, infection of the implant and loosening.

Loosening may be secondary to infection or an aseptic mechanical process. If the prosthesis is mechanically loose, it can be removed and replaced, but when infection is present, the safest option is to remove all the foreign material, identify the infective agent and treat this vigorously. At a second procedure, it may then be possible to insert another prosthesis.

Joint replacement surgery in rheumatoid arthritis carries particular risks. The immune response is altered, and infection rates are higher. At operation, the bones are often osteoporotic with an increased risk of intraoperative fractures. When multiple joints are involved, the surgeon may be embarking on an extended programme of replacement.

INFECTIONS

Acute osteomyelitis

Before the introduction of antibiotics, acute osteomyelitis was a common infection with a 50% mortality. In the Western world the condition has now become much less common – although the reason for this is not entirely clear – and fatalities are rare.

Aetiology

Haematogenous

Organisms transported by the bloodstream from a distant site lodge in the capillaries of bone (usually, but not always, the metaphysis of a long bone) and set up a focus. Their origin is usually not clear but occasionally there may be a distant infected focus, such as a boil. Localisation of the infection may be determined by a minor injury to the bone, although this is not well established in pathological terms. Individuals of any age may be infected but the condition is more common in children.

Exogenous

Direct inoculation of bone from the outside takes place as a result of some surgical procedure or after an open fracture.

Pathological features

Organisms

In haematogenous osteomyelitis, the agent is most commonly *Staphylococcus aureus* (85%), now often penicillin-resistant. *Streptococcus pyogenes* and *Pseudomonas aeruginosa* are other pus-producing organisms sometimes involved. Occasionally, *Salmonella typhimurium* is found either with or without an intestinal infection and is more common in patients with sickle cell disease. *E. coli* may infect the bones of neonates.

Infection from without can be with any organism and is often mixed.

Pathological course

In haematogenous osteomyelitis, a short period of intense inflammation is speedily followed by pus formation within the medulla. Because bone is not expandable, pressure rises rapidly with two effects:

- pus is forced through the Haversian canals to reach the periosteum, so forming a subperiosteal abscess
- blood vessels in the Haversian canals thrombose, and the bone dies; stripping of periosteum contributes to this infarction.

Eventually, if treatment does not take place, pus breaks through the periosteum, tracks up to the skin surface and discharges to produce an infected sinus. There is dead bone in its depths which gradually separates to form a sequestrum.

Exogenous infection does not usually pursue such an acute course, and damage to bone is less. However, it is often persistent and chronic.

Clinical features

History

There is often a history of minor trauma. The patient, usually a child, is unwell with a high pyrexia and – if old enough to voice this – a complaint of severe localised bone pain. The affected limb is held still (pseudoparalysis).

Physical findings

- *Look:*
  - redness and oedema may be seen over the affected metaphysis
  - the limb is held still.
- *Feel:*
  - warmth at the affected site
  - focal bony tenderness – an important sign
  - fluctuant swelling overlying the bone
- *Move:*
  - pain on movement.

Investigation

Imaging

Plain X-ray is initially normal. Changes occur after 10–14 days, when the periosteum is lifted and there is local rarefaction. Later, dead bone and sequestra show up as sclerosis.

Ultrasound may identify a subperiosteal abscess.

Radioisotope bone scan shows increased activity after a few days but well before anything is seen on X-ray.

MRI is extremely sensitive in identifying intraosseous oedema and pus.

Blood examination

White cell count, ESR and CRP are raised.

Blood culture (before the administration of antibiotics) is positive in half of those with haematogenous osteomyelitis.

Management

Non-operative

High-dose intravenous antibiotics are begun immediately after a blood culture has been taken. The affected limb is elevated and splinted because this helps to relieve pain. Antibiotic therapy is continued until the ESR has returned to normal, which may take 6 weeks or longer.

Surgical

If the patient fails to respond by speedy return of temperature to normal and relief of pain, or if there is a fluctuant abscess on presentation, then the site is explored. The periosteum is incised and the underlying bone drilled to drain and decompress the medullary cavity.

Complications

Complications are:

- acute septic arthritis secondary to direct spread from adjacent bone
- pathological fracture through bone that is rarefied because of infection
- growth impairment from epiphyseal involvement
- chronicity because of dead bone
- chronic osteomyelitis.

Chronic osteomyelitis

This condition occurs because of inadequate treatment of acute osteomyelitis, or it may complicate the management of an open fracture or the surgical treatment of a closed one. It is now rare in the UK.

Clinical features

History

There has usually been an episode of acute haematogenous osteomyelitis often followed by a discharging sinus. Evidence of infection is dormant for months or years with an occasional flare-up in which there is local pain and swelling with discharge of pus.

Physical findings

There are often scars from old sinuses, one or more of which may still be open with a purulent discharge.

Investigation

Imaging

Plain X-ray shows grossly abnormal bone with areas of rarefaction and sclerosis. A sequestrum appears as a separate piece of dense bone lying within a cavity.

Isotope bone scan may show increased activity although, if there is a sequestrum, reduced uptake is present in relation to it.

CT may give useful information on the exact size and position of a sequestrum.

Examination of the blood

This is usually unhelpful, but the ESR may be raised. Blood culture is negative except during a flare-up.

Management

Non-operative

Antibiotics are insufficient by themselves as they are unable to penetrate the dense soft-tissue fibrosis and the relatively ischaemic bone. The occasional flare-up can be managed with dry dressings until the sinus stops discharging.

Surgical

The aim of surgery is to remove all dead bone and infected material. A chain of antibiotic impregnated beads can then be implanted in the cavity to give a very high but localised concentration of antibiotic.

Complications

Complications are:

- pathological fracture
- amyloidosis
- squamous cell carcinoma in the sinus tract.

Septic arthritis

Any joint may be affected but the common site is the knee and hip.

Aetiology

Causes are:

- haematogenous spread from a distant focus of infection
- secondary to acute osteomyelitis
- direct inoculation after trauma or surgery – the incidence after arthroscopy is less than 0.2%.

Pathological features

Organisms

- *Staphylococcus aureus*
- *Streptococcus pyogenes*
- *Neisseria gonorrhoeae.*

Course

The hyaline cartilage is destroyed by a combination of ischaemia and toxic enzymes released by white blood cells and bacteria. As with osteomyelitis, unchecked development of pus eventually ruptures the joint capsule, and discharge occurs through the skin. Such a damaged joint heals with either a fibrous or a bony ankylosis.

Clinical features

History

The patient complains of increasingly severe pain in the joint and is unwell with a high swinging pyrexia.

Physical findings

- *Look* for:
  - a red and swollen joint
  - immobility because of pain
  - rarely evidence of a local wound.
- *Feel* for:
  - local warmth
  - local tenderness.
- *Move:*
  - marked pain on movement.

Investigation

Imaging

Plain X-ray is normal in the early stages. After 2–3 weeks, there is local rarefaction of the adjacent bone and loss of joint space. Still later, the necrosis of cartilage reduces the joint space still further. Finally, bony ankylosis can be seen.

Blood examination

The white cell count, ESR and CRP are raised and blood culture may be positive.

Joint aspiration

This should always be done (before commencing antibiotics) and is both diagnostic and therapeutic. The aspirate is sent for culture. At the same time, the toxic content of the effusion can be reduced by washing out the joint cavity. The reduction of intra-articular pressure provides relief from pain.

Management

Medical

High-dose intravenous antibiotics are begun (flucloxacillin up to 8 g 6-hourly or clindamycin up to 1.2 g 6-hourly if allergic to penicillin), adjusted on the results of culture and continued until the ESR has returned to normal, which may take 6 weeks. The joint is rested.

Surgical

Pus within a joint must be washed out as a matter of some urgency. This may be performed via an arthrotomy; however, some joints such as the knee, ankle, shoulder and elbow can easily be washed out through the arthroscope. This is simply because of the larger bore of the instrument, a more efficient form of aspiration.

Complications

Complications are:

- dislocation – in particular, the hip in children
- joint stiffness
- secondary osteoarthritis.

Table 34.6 Bone tumours

Cell of origin	Benign	Intermediate	Malignant
Osteoblast	Osteoid osteoma	Osteoblastoma	Osteosarcoma
Osteoclast		Giant-cell tumour (osteoclastoma)	
Chondroblast	Chondroma Osteochondroma		Chondrosarcoma
Fibroblast	Non-ossifying fibroma (unicameral bone cyst)		Fibrosarcoma
Vascular	Haemangioma	Aneurysmal bone cyst	Haemangiosarcoma
Marrow		Plasmacytoma	Ewing's sarcoma Lymphoma Myeloma Leukaemia

BONE TUMOURS

These are either primary or secondary. Primary tumours may be either benign or malignant, but some are in an intermediate group which, although showing locally invasive features, do not metastasise. A detailed classification is given in Table 34.6.

Clinical features

History

When the tumour is secondary, there may be symptoms from the primary malignancy, although sometimes the first presentation is with bone pain or a pathological fracture. Pain is common and is localised at the site of the tumour. It is usually constant with no relieving factors and often worse at night. A lump may be noticed.

Physical findings

A thorough general examination is required. Most bone tumours are secondary deposits, and so the common sites of a possible primary (breast, lung, prostate, thyroid and kidney) must be examined (Table 34.7):

- *Look* for a lump.
- *Feel* for:
  - a lump
  - local bony tenderness
  - crepitus under the fingers when there is a history of possible pathological fracture.
- *Move* – possible abnormal movement in the presence of a pathological fracture.

Table 34.7 Common sites of primary in secondary bone tumour

Site	Incidence (%)
Breast	35
Prostate	30
Bronchus	10
Kidney	5
Thyroid	2

Investigation

Imaging

Plain X-ray is always needed. Benign tumours have a sharp margin and the cortex is intact. By contrast, malignant growths are expansive with indistinct margins and destruction of the cortex. In osteosarcoma, new bone formation is seen – so-called 'sun-ray spicules'.

Isotope scan differentiates secondary deposits – which produce multiple areas of increased activity – from a primary tumour in which there is usually a solitary active area.

MRI is also useful for the assessment of local spread within the bone and adjacent soft tissues.

CT is required to assess the local spread of malignant tumours and so to aid in the planning of surgery. The lungs are scanned for evidence of metastases.

Biopsy is essential for a histological diagnosis for all suspicious lesions.

Benign tumours

These occur in young adults. They may be found in any bone; however, chondromas favour metacarpals, metatarsals and the phalanges.

Clinical features

History

Benign tumours are often without symptoms unless a pathological fracture occurs. Constant local pain often worse at night may be the presenting feature. In osteoid osteoma, relief is obtained from aspirin but not opioid analgesics. Local pressure symptoms is typical of osteochondromas.

Physical findings

- *Look* for any evidence of a fracture – chiefly deformity.
- *Feel* for:
  - a hard lump
  - localised bony tenderness
  - crepitus.
- *Test* for unusual movement – indicative of a pathological fracture.

Management

If there are symptoms, curettage and bone grafting may be required. A pathological fracture through the tumour can lead to spontaneous cure.

Locally aggressive tumours

These tumours are not truly malignant, and metastatic spread is very rare. There is, however, local destruction, and there may be local recurrence after surgery.

Aneurysmal bone cysts

These are blood-filled cavities that usually occur in the spine and at the ends of long bones. On plain X-ray, the cyst is seen as an expansive lesion with thinning of the cortex. The management is curettage and bone grafting, which is usually curative. Radiotherapy may be required for recurrent lesions. Embolisation may represent optimal treatment for inaccessible lesions.

Giant-cell tumour (osteoclastoma)

This occurs at the end of long bones in adults between the ages of 20 and 40 – the knee is a common site. There is local pain and possibly a pathological fracture. The X-ray appearance is that of a multiloculated lesion; the tumour extends up to the joint surface. Metastases are rare but can occur especially after local recurrence.

Curettage with bone grafting is often followed by recurrence. The cavity should be filled with bone cement which sets by an exothermic reaction that is cytotoxic to residual tumour cells. Local recurrence necessitates wide excision and then either bone grafting or a prosthesis.

Malignant tumours

These are rare – only 125 new osteosarcomas and 60 new chondrosarcomas a year in the UK. They spread via the bloodstream to the lungs and other sites.

Osteosarcoma

This tumour occurs mainly in the young between the ages of 10 and 30 years. There is a second peak in the elderly in association with Paget's disease of bone.

The tumour occurs in the metaphyseal region of long bones, the knee being the most common site. Its management used to be by amputation, but now, with more effective chemotherapeutic agents and consequently a better prognosis, surgical resection is less radical. Excision of the affected bone and replacement with a custom-made or modular prosthesis now form the standard approach. Radiotherapy is usually reserved for inaccessible sites or for recurrence. With radical surgery and chemotherapy, there is a 90% survival at 1 year and over 50% at 3 years. Survival for more than 3 years means a probable cure.

Chondrosarcoma

This occurs in an older age group than that of osteosarcoma: between 30 and 70 years. Tumours commonly involve the flat bones: scapula, ribs and pelvis. They vary widely in their degree of differentiation, from high-grade anaplastic to low-grade with only slow growth. Their management is by wide local excision with bone grafting or reconstruction with a custom-made prosthesis. Radiotherapy is ineffective. The 5-year survival ranges from 20% to 80%, depending on size, location and histological grade.

Fibrosarcoma

This is a rare growth in the age range of 40–60 years and occurs at any site. Management is surgical, with wide excision or amputation. The outlook is poor, with a 5-year survival rate of about 30%.

Ewing's sarcoma

This is a highly malignant tumour that affects children and adolescents of 5–20 years. Males are slightly more frequently affected. The common site is the diaphyseal region of long bones. The clinical features, in addition to local pain and a lump, may include general ill health and fever. The lump may be red and warm. Ewing's sarcoma is often initially misdiagnosed as acute osteomyelitis. On the plain X-ray, a characteristic 'onion peel' appearance is typically seen. Management is by chemotherapy followed by surgical excision and radiotherapy. The outlook has been poor. However, with radical and aggressive treatment, survival rates are now approaching 50% or more at 5 years.

Plasmacytoma

This condition is rare and consists of a mass of plasma cells in bone or soft tissue which may prove to be a focal manifestation of multiple myeloma. Isolated lesions may be excised followed by a course of radiotherapy.

Secondary tumours

Secondary bone tumours are common: about 30% of patients who die of a malignancy have bone secondaries. Common sources of the primary growth are given in Table 34.7.

The patients are often over 60, because of the nature of the primary. Any bone may be affected, but the skull, vertebrae, ribs and pelvis are common sites. On plain X-ray, most secondary tumours are osteolytic but bone deposits from carcinoma of the prostate and about 10% of breast cancers are osteosclerotic. Treatment which is appropriate for the primary – such as hormone manipulation in breast and prostate cancer and chemotherapy – may alleviate the symptoms of secondary deposits. The pain may respond to anti-inflammatory drugs and local radiotherapy. Pathological fractures do not unite spontaneously and should therefore be internally fixed, by which quality of life is improved and nursing made easier, although life expectancy remains unchanged. Prophylactic internal fixation should be considered when there is:

- rapid increase in local pain
- destruction of 50% or more of shaft diameter in a long bone
- a femoral lesion greater than 3 cm in diameter.

SHOULDER

The shoulder is the most mobile of all joints and, with the elbow, has the prime function of manoeuvring the hand to the best position required for function, particularly to the mouth.

General clinical features

History

Pain is felt over the deltoid insertion in impingement syndromes (see below); at the front in arthritis; and at the top in acromioclavicular disorders. Radiation down the arm is common. Pain around the shoulder may also be the result of reference from other sites such as the heart, lung, diaphragm or cervical spine.

Stiffness is a common symptom in shoulder disease, and loss of function such as inability to brush the hair can be socially embarrassing.

Trauma frequently figures in the history and may cause fractures, dislocations or soft-tissue injury to the joint capsule, particularly the rotator cuff.

Mechanical derangement may be a presenting symptom, as in recurrent dislocation.

Physical findings

- *Look* for:
  - muscle wasting of the deltoid, biceps, supraspinatus and infraspinatus
  - scars – indications of previous injury or surgery
  - the contour of the shoulder – in dislocation, the normal rounded appearance is lost and the shoulder looks squared off because of the prominence of the acromion
  - winging of the scapula because of weakness of the serratus anterior muscle.
- *Feel* for the belly of biceps during resisted elbow flexion – rupture of the long head of biceps tendon results in an abnormal contour of the muscle.
- *Move:*
  - through the active and passive ranges (see Table 34.2)
  - note any painful arcs of movement during elevation of the arm – pain during mid-elevation is caused by subacromial impingement, but pain at full elevation is from an acromioclavicular disorder.

Investigation

Imaging

Plain X-ray is required, both an anteroposterior and an axillary view. This can show degenerative arthritis, loose bodies and abnormal calcification – usually in tendons. In recurrent dislocation, a defect (Hill–Sachs lesion) may be seen on the posterosuperior humeral head and is caused by repeated impingement of the rim of the glenoid on the humerus.

Ultrasound scanning is commonly used as the first investigation after plain X-rays.

Arthrograms were commonly performed and are still used where MRI is unavailable. Rotator cuff tears are demonstrated by leakage of contrast medium into the subacromial bursa. Alternatively the rotator cuff can be assessed by ultrasound scan.

CT and MRI are of increasing value. A tear may be visualised, loose bodies seen and bicipital tendonitis can be diagnosed.

Arthroscopy

The procedure is both a diagnostic tool and of therapeutic value. It is possible to repair tears in the labrum of the glenoid, to stabilise the shoulder in recurrent dislocation, to decompress the subacromial space, to repair rotator cuff, or SLAP (Superior Labrum from Anterior to Posterior at the point where the biceps tendon inserts on the labrum) lesions, synovectomy or release contractures and remove loose bodies.

ACROMIOCLAVICULAR DISORDERS

Acromioclavicular osteoarthritis

Aetiology

This condition is often secondary to trauma.

Clinical features

History

Pain is the usual feature often felt on the top of the shoulder in relation to the joint and aggravated by lifting the arm above the head or across the body.

Physical findings

- *Look* for:
  - prominence of the acromioclavicular joint
  - muscle wasting, in particular in the supraspinatus.
- *Feel* for:
  - localised tenderness at the joint
  - crepitus on movement.
- *Test movement* – pain is found when passive movement above shoulder level is attempted.

Management

Surgical excision of the outer end of the clavicle provides relief.

Rheumatoid arthritis

The shoulder and acromioclavicular joint are often affected by rheumatoid arthritis. In addition to pain, there is often prominent swelling.

Management

Non-operative

Medical management of the disease is important and provides pain relief.

Surgical

Excision of the outer end of the clavicle is performed.

SUBACROMIAL DISORDERS

The subacromial bursa, the rotator cuff and the tendon of biceps lie between the acromion and the head of the humerus. Any one of these structures may become trapped between the two bones and cause pain.

Impingement

This often affects the rotator cuff tendons of subscapularis and supraspinatus.

Clinical features

A painful arc occurs on abduction of the humerus. On examination, the arc is confirmed and can be precisely defined. There is tenderness in the anterior cuff and signs of impingement are present. The most commonly used is the Hawkins sign where a forceful internal rotation on a forward flexed shoulder at 90° produces subacromial pain.

Management

Non-operative

Analgesics such as NSAIDs may help the local swelling to settle. Local steroid injection into the subacromial space is also helpful.

Surgical

If symptoms fail to improve with conservative measures then surgery is advisable. The subacromial space is decompressed by excising the undersurface of the acromion as a wedge.

Rotator cuff tears

There are two causes:

- acute injury as a result of trauma and seen with dislocations of the shoulder in the elderly
- more commonly, chronic lesions from degeneration within the cuff.

Pathological features

There is a spectrum of disorders that are interconnected and which range from superficial abrasions of the rotator cuff from impingement through incomplete (partial-thickness) tears to complete full-thickness ones. However, there is not inevitable progression from one to another. Other factors such as ischaemic degeneration within the cuff coupled with trauma may determine the extent of tear.

Clinical features

History

There may be a history of significant shoulder injury, but more usually there is chronic shoulder pain felt over the deltoid muscle, especially at one point of abduction. Adduction may also be difficult.

Physical findings

- *Look* for muscle wasting – especially in the supraspinatus.
- *Feel* for localised tenderness along the lateral border of the acromion.
- *Test for shoulder movement* – active movement, particularly abduction, is reduced but there is a full range of passive movement.

Management

Non-operative

Partial tears of the cuff heal and the symptoms settle after resting the shoulder. Once acute symptoms have settled, a graduated programme of rehabilitation is begun. Tears in the elderly should be managed conservatively; surgical repair in this age group is difficult, and severe stiffness after surgery is likely.

Surgical

When symptoms fail to settle, then it is likely that the tear is complete. In the young, it should be repaired. The rotator cuff is exposed and repaired with interrupted sutures, which is now achieved by arthroscopic surgery, reducing morbidity. Very large tears may require grafts of fascia lata to close the defect.

Acute calcific tendonitis

Deposition of calcium hydroxyapatite within the tendon of supraspinatus may occur for unknown reasons. There is a local inflammatory reaction.

Clinical features

History

The inflammation that takes place causes pain that is dull initially but over a few hours becomes increasingly severe. There is considerable muscle spasm, and a septic arthritis may be suspected, but the joint itself is not inflamed.

Physical findings

- *Look* for:
  - a pale, sweaty patient in severe pain
  - the arm held still by the side.
- *Feel* for diffuse tenderness of the whole shoulder region.
- *Test for movement* which will be resisted because of pain.

Management

Non-operative

Rest, anti-inflammatory drugs and local anaesthetic injections may help.

Surgical

Incising the tendon releases the calcific deposit. It squeezes out under pressure like toothpaste from a tube, and pain relief is immediate.

Adhesive capsulitis (frozen shoulder)

This condition is characterised by increasing pain and relative immobility of the joint. It fundamentally is a contracture of the shoulder capsule. The aetiology is unknown, but there may be a history of minor trauma, and the disorder may also complicate other illnesses such as a myocardial infarct or pneumonia. Recent research has highlighted an association between adhesive capsulitis, insulin-dependent diabetes and Dupuytren's contracture.

Clinical features

Pain and stiffness are the only complaints. Joint movement is limited, and attempts to increase the range of passive movement cause pain. Over a period of about a year, the symptoms may gradually improve, and within 2 years the shoulder may have returned to normal but sometimes the stiffness can be protracted.

Management

Non-operative

The mainstay of treatment is that resolution eventually takes place. Cautious physiotherapy is helpful, and steroid injections into the shoulder joint may also help during the painful phase.

Surgical

When recovery is slow and stiffness persists, a manipulation under anaesthesia is often beneficial.

GLENOHUMERAL DISORDERS

Osteoarthritis

This condition is uncommon and usually secondary to trauma. Pain is felt at the front of the joint and may radiate through to the posterior aspect. Conservative measures such as anti-inflammatory agents and steroid injections into the joint help in the early stages. Persistent disability requires:

- arthroscopy – the joint is washed out and any loose bodies are removed, which gives some relief for most patients
- arthroplasty – replacement with a prosthesis; many designs are available but most consist of a metal humeral head and a high-density polyethylene glenoid
- arthrodesis – fusion of the shoulder is rarely done except as a salvage procedure after failed joint replacement.

Rheumatoid arthritis

The shoulder is commonly affected by this disease. Management is usually non-operative by treating the underlying condition and using intra-articular steroid injections. Surgical options are the same as for osteoarthritis.

Avascular necrosis of the humeral head

This is much less common than the same condition in the femoral head. The causes and mechanisms are the same. Management is by treating any underlying cause and by the use of anti-inflammatory agents and physiotherapy. Surgical core decompression is indicated in early disease to arrest progress. In the late stages, when there has been collapse of the humeral head and secondary osteoarthritis has developed, an arthroplasty may be required.

ELBOW

The elbow joint is a hinge that works in consort with the shoulder in positioning the hand.

General clinical features

History

- **Stiffness** is noticed early by patients because of difficulty in getting the hand to the mouth.
- **Pain** is common and often aggravated by movement.
- **Locking** is an occasional feature, particularly in degenerative disease.
- **Past trauma** to the joint is not uncommon.

Physical findings

- *Look* at:
  - the shape of the joint – compare with the other side
  - contour for swellings – a bursa, rheumatoid nodule or effusion
  - carrying angle of the arm in extension – normal is 8–10° of valgus.
- *Feel* for:
  - crepitus
  - bony landmarks – two epicondyles and the olecranon: do they form an equilateral triangle with the elbow flexed (Fig. 34.3)?
  - effusion – best felt between the lateral epicondyle and the olecranon; the normal hollow is filled out by a soft swelling
  - radial head during pronation and supination – does it dislocate as the forearm moves?
- *Test* for:
  - ulnar nerve function in the hand
  - movements – ask the patient to demonstrate the active range of movement; measure the passive range of movement (see Table 34.2).

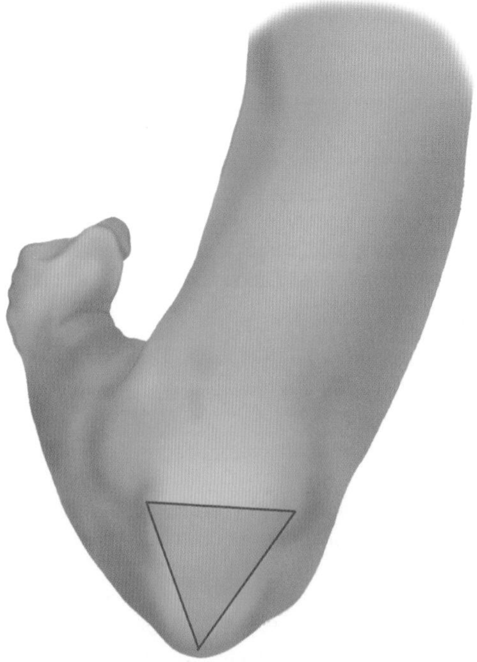

Fig. 34.3 Equilateral triangle formed at the elbow by two epicondyles and the olecranon.

Investigation

Imaging

Plain X-ray is usually the only investigation required and can show old injuries, the presence of arthritis, loose bodies and subluxation of the radial head.

Nerve function

If an ulnar nerve lesion is suspected, electromyography is required.

Osteoarthritis

Clinical features

The condition is almost always secondary to trauma. Pain and stiffness are the common symptoms. Locking can sometimes occur.

Management

Non-operative

The usual initial – and often the only – treatment required consists of analgesia, local strapping and physiotherapy.

Surgical

The indications for surgery are:

- symptomatic loose bodies which can be removed arthroscopically
- ulnar neuritis – usually the consequence of a valgus deformity; this is treated by transposition of the nerve in front of the medial epicondyle.

Fusion is indicated when there is failure of conservative treatment, with severe pain. The joint is fixed in a position of function that allows the hand to reach the mouth – about 100° of flexion.

Total elbow replacement is possible, and the long-term results are less satisfactory in the joint with degenerative disease as compared with rheumatoid arthritis.

Rheumatoid arthritis

The elbow is often involved in rheumatoid arthritis, and clinical features are of pain, swelling and stiffness.

Management

Non-operative

Most patients can be managed by control of the systemic disease and local measures including splints.

Operative

If conservative measures are not sufficient, then there are a number of surgical options.

- **Synovectomy** can produce good relief of pain and is usually done through the arthroscope.
- **Excision of the radial head** can reduce symptoms if this structure is particularly involved.
- **Fusion and replacement** can both be considered.

HAND AND WRIST

Loss of hand function is very disabling in that nearly all daily activities require the hands to a greater or lesser extent. The wrist, in conjunction with the elbow and shoulder, positions the hand in space while the fingers and thumb hold and manipulate.

General clinical features

History

Pain is often felt in the wrist but less commonly in the hand. Pain which originates in the hand may be felt across the wrist joint or be localised to a styloid process. In the fingers, it is usually related to pathological change in a joint. Pain at night which affects the hand and is associated with numbness is characteristic of compression of nerves in the carpal tunnel.

Stiffness in the wrist may not cause significant problems, but in the fingers it is an early complaint because it is so disabling.

Swelling in the hand or fingers is noticed early. Rings may become tight and so draw attention to the fingers.

Paraesthesia is usually in the distribution of a peripheral nerve.

Weakness is a common symptom in median or ulnar nerve lesions. Patients often complain of difficulty in fine finger movements such as in knitting or writing.

Physical findings

- *Look* for:
  - the position of the hand at rest – are the fingers in fixed flexion because of fascial contractures in the palm (Dupuytren's contracture)?
  - finger deviation with ulnar drift as seen in the rheumatoid hand
  - muscle function in the hand – the thenar eminence may be atrophied in median nerve compression, and the hypothenar eminence and interossei in ulnar nerve compression
  - the pattern of any swelling at the joints of the fingers; Heberden's nodes are seen at the distal interphalangeal joints in osteoarthritis.
- *Feel:*
  - the palmar aponeurosis – thickened areas may indicate aponeurotic fibrosis
  - the skin – warmth and dryness are present if there is a peripheral nerve lesion.
- *Test:*
  - sensation to light touch and pinprick and establish the distribution of any loss found
  - for crepitus at the wrist on movement
  - ulnar and median nerves for Tinel's sign; this is often positive in fascial compression at the wrist or other causes of nerve excitability
  - active and passive ranges of movement (see Table 34.2).

Investigation

Imaging

Plain X-ray is often needed and can confirm if a lump arises from bone. Arthritic change and its underlying cause can be demonstrated (see Table 34.3). Old trauma may be evident. Unusual conditions such as Kienbock's disease (osteochondrosis of the lunate – often post-traumatic) or Madelung's deformity (subluxation of the distal radioulnar joint, see below) can be confirmed.

Electromyography (EMG)

If a peripheral nerve lesion is suspected, EMG is essential. It confirms the diagnosis and site of the lesion and may help to avoid unnecessary surgery.

Arthritis at the wrist

At the wrist, osteoarthritis is often secondary to trauma. Rheumatoid arthritis also affects the wrist.

Clinical features

The symptoms are pain, stiffness and swelling. The swelling is often accompanied by deformity from a previous fracture. Crepitus may be felt.

Management

Non-operative

Measures such as a removable wrist splint can relieve symptoms, as do mild analgesics.

Surgical

The indications for surgery are pain and incapacity which have failed to respond to non-operative measures, such as in the young adult with post-traumatic arthritis. Of the options available (see Table 34.4), fusion is the procedure of choice. The joint is removed and a bone graft inserted. A plate is normally required for stabilisation until the bone unites.

Wrist joint replacement is technically feasible but remains controversial.

Arthritis of the hand

The distribution in the hand follows a pattern characteristic of the cause.

Clinical features

Stiffness and deformity of the fingers are common symptoms. In rheumatoid arthritis, the hand deforms in a characteristic way. Progressive destruction of the metacarpophalangeal joints causes the fingers to drift to the ulnar side, and later there is subluxation at these joints. In addition, inflammatory tenosynovitis may lead to tendon rupture with one or more dropped (semi-immobile and flexed) fingers.

Management

Because arthritis, in particular rheumatoid, is a continuing process, management varies with the stage of the disease. A series of procedures may be required as deformities develop and progress.

Non-operative

Physiotherapy to conserve and improve hand function is essential. The occupational therapist can provide crucial aids to assist in the activities of daily living: modified cutlery with curved or flattened handles, special fasteners for clothes, and other devices may all preserve independence. Hand splints are often used. They rarely prevent deformity but do allow rheumatoid joints to be rested during an acute exacerbation of the disease.

Surgical

Various operative procedures are appropriate at different stages of the disease, but the potential problems of undertaking surgery should always be carefully discussed. Many badly deformed hands are still able to function usefully. Ruptured tendons should be repaired and, in rheumatoid arthritis, early synovectomy may delay destruction. In later stages, or in osteoarthritis, damaged joints may be replaced by Silastic implants. These correct deformities and relieve pain but rarely increase grip strength and some residual stiffness persists.

Dupuytren's contracture

This is a condition of the hand in which there is thickening and contraction of the palmar aponeurosis, which may be due to a local change in collagen metabolism.

Aetiology and pathological features

The precise cause is not known, but there are nevertheless a number of well-recognised associated factors, including:

- a family history
- male sex
- regular high consumption of alcohol
- insulin-dependent diabetes mellitus
- adhesive capsulitis
- phenytoin therapy
- trauma.

Contracture is bilateral in 45%; similar lesions in the plantar aponeurosis (Lederhosen's disease) occur in 5%; and the penile fascia (Peyronie's disease) is affected in 3%.

Clinical features

The condition usually develops at the base of the ring and little fingers. As the lesion progresses, the fingers gradually develop fixed flexion deformities, and the thumb web may also be involved.

Management

Non-operative

Although many measures have been tried, none is effective. The condition may be self-limiting but is usually progressive.

Surgical

Five operations may be considered, and these are outlined in Table 34.8. The choice depends on the extent of the disease, the degree of disability and whether or not previous operations have been done.

Table 34.8 Operations for Dupuytren's contracture of the palmar fascia

Procedure	Technique	Outcome
Percutaneous fasciotomy	Simple division of fibrous bands through percutaneous stab wounds	Recurrence rates high and damage may occur to nerves and blood vessels
Selective fasciectomy	Thickened areas are excised	Most common operation; successful in limited disease
Complete fasciectomy	Whole aponeurosis excised even if not obviously involved	Potentially curative but high incidence of skin necrosis
Complete fasciectomy and skin graft	Aponeurosis excised together with the skin of the palm followed by split-skin grafting	Curative but requires high skills
Amputation	Removal of a single digit (usually little finger), severely contracted into the palm and interfering with hand function	Can be procedure of choice in special circumstances

Nerve entrapment syndromes

These commonly affect the hand. Usually it is compression of the median nerve that gives rise to symptoms, but ulnar nerve entrapment at the elbow or occasionally the wrist can also occur.

Aetiology

Median nerve compression in the carpal tunnel is usually without an identifiable cause, but any abnormal structure within the tunnel can produce the condition. Examples are:

- wrist fracture – early from local haematoma and oedema or late because of a malunion and bony encroachment
- ganglion within the carpal tunnel
- tenosynovitis from rheumatoid arthritis or repetitive strain injury
- changes in the interstitial space – obesity, diabetes mellitus, hypothyroidism, pregnancy, acromegaly and amyloidosis.

Ulnar nerve compression is usually at the elbow adjacent to the medial epicondyle of the humerus. There may not be an obvious cause, but a fracture which causes a valgus deformity of the elbow may attenuate the nerve. Compression at the wrist in the ulnar canal between the pisiform and the hook of the hamate is less common.

Clinical features

History

In **median nerve compression** – the characteristic carpal tunnel syndrome – there is often pain in the distribution of the median nerve, and this is frequently worse at night. Loss of grip and clumsiness in handling objects are other complaints.

In **ulnar nerve compression** at the elbow there may be a past history of trauma in the region of the joint. Weakness and clumsiness of the hand are the chief complaints.

Physical findings

Median nerve. Wasting of the thenar eminence and the first dorsal interosseous is seen. There is loss of sensation in the median nerve territory of lateral three and a half fingers.

Ulnar nerve. If the compression is at the elbow, evidence of elbow deformity may be apparent with an abnormal carrying angle. An elbow lesion also causes weakness of the ulnar half of flexor digitorum profundus, but flexor carpi ulnaris is weak only when the lesion is above the elbow. Wasting of the hypothenar and interosseous muscles is present (most noticeable in the first web space). The hand may appear flattened with the ring and metacarpophalangeal joints hyperextended because of lumbrical paralysis. Attempts to grip a sheet of paper between the thumb and index finger cause the trick movement of flexion of the distal phalanx of the thumb to compensate for the weak interossei (Froment's sign – Fig. 34.4).

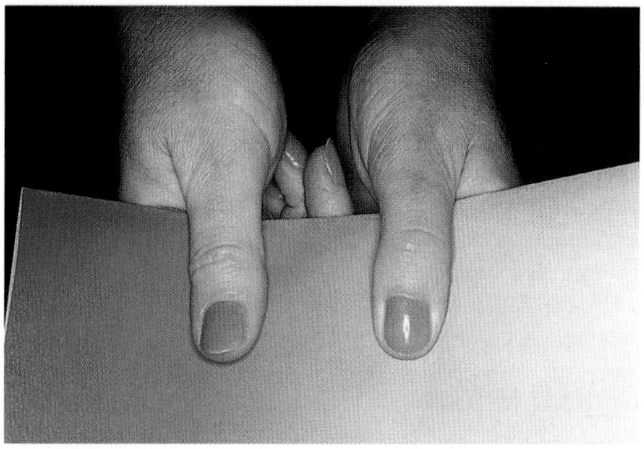

Fig. 34.4 Froment's sign, positive in the patient's left thumb.

Management

Non-operative

Underlying causes at the wrist are treated. In pregnancy, the symptoms often resolve rapidly after delivery. Injections of steroid into the carpal tunnel may help in mild cases but should not be repeated more than twice or irreversible fibrosis may take place in the median nerve. Non-operative treatment of ulnar nerve problems usually fails.

Surgical

Median nerve. Decompression of the median nerve by dividing the carpal ligament is a highly effective and simple procedure that can be carried out under local or general anaesthesia. Relief of symptoms is often immediate and any thenar wasting recovers with time.

Ulnar nerve. For lesions with their cause at the elbow, the nerve is released in situ (releasing the nerve as it pierces the flexor carpi ulnaris distally and proximally the medial intermuscular septum) or rarely transposed to lie in front of the medial epicondyle after dividing the medial intermuscular septum which, if left intact, can chafe the nerve and cause persistent problems. At the wrist, the ulnar canal is explored and decompressed. Recovery is slow compared with the median nerve but symptoms do generally improve.

Ganglion

Ganglions are tense cysts containing viscous, jelly-like material. They often occur on the dorsum of the wrist and are associated with joints or tendon sheaths. They are commonly found around the wrist and ankle but also occur in the hand and in the foot.

Aetiology and pathological features

Many explanations have been advanced but none has been conclusively established. It is possible that they are derived from small extra-articular fragments of synovium and at times a communication with the underlying joint or tendon sheath can be demonstrated and this would certainly explain both their inspissated contents and their tendency to recur if incompletely removed.

Clinical features

Symptoms are cosmetic only unless previous inadequate surgery has caused secondary problems.

Signs are of a tense, fluctuant usually globular swelling deep to skin and incompletely mobile on the deep aspect because of attachment to a neighbouring joint or tendon sheath.

Management

Non-operative

An asymptomatic lesion which does not cause cosmetic embarrassment is best left alone. Traditional treatment has also included subcutaneous rupture – the family bible was often used as the weapon. More modern therapy consists of aspiration followed by steroid injection, but 15% or more recur.

Surgical

Excision of the ganglion is effective provided the technique is meticulous and undertaken in a bloodless field.

Trigger finger

The cause is unknown. There is localised thickening of a flexor tendon pulleys with associated narrowing of the sheath. The thickened part is then unable to pass smoothly under the entrance to the synovial sheath at the base of the finger.

Clinical features

The patient recognises that the affected finger catches in flexion and straightens suddenly with assistance and a snap. The features can usually be produced to order.

Management

Surgical treatment is the only option. The sheath is incised to allow the tendon to move freely.

de Quervain's syndrome

Tenosynovitis of the tendon sheaths of extensor pollicis brevis and abductor pollicis longus may be the result of local trauma, but usually no cause is found. It is most frequent in middle-aged women.

Clinical features

The symptoms are pain and weakness of the thumb.

The sheath is palpably thickened and tender. Adducting and flexing the thumb and wrist (Finkelstein's test) are painful.

Management

Non-operative

Injection of steroid into the tendon sheath is often effective, but it is important that only the sheath (and not the tendon) is injected because the tendon may otherwise be weakened and rupture.

Surgical

The tendon sheath is slit, so freeing up movement. The procedure is curative and that of choice if the condition is chronic.

Kienbock's disease

This condition is avascular necrosis of the lunate. In most instances the cause is unknown, but it may occasionally follow dislocation of the bone.

The patient – a young adult – complains of local ache and stiffness at the wrist. There are no clinical findings except slight tenderness over the dorsum of the wrist.

Investigation and management

Plain X-ray shows sclerosis of the lunate. As the condition progresses, there is fragmentation, and secondary osteoarthritis develops in the wrist joint.

In the early stages a splint may help. Attempts have been made to revascularise the bone with part of the pronator quadratus muscle, but these have met with limited success. Other surgical options include:

- removal of the bone and insertion of a Silastic prosthesis
- shortening of the radius to decompress the lunate
- fusion if osteoarthritis is present.

Madelung's deformity

This is a growth disorder of the distal radial epiphysis. It becomes apparent after the age of 10 years and is more common in girls.

The patient complains of a prominent lump alongside the ulnar styloid with stiffness at the wrist. Examination of the mother's wrist often reveals the same deformity. There is some limitation of the range of movement.

Investigation and management

Plain X-ray shows the distal radius to be shortened slightly and curved, with the lunate tending to sublux between the radius and ulna. The ulna is of normal length and therefore appears more prominent.

Operations should be avoided if possible. Excision of a segment of distal ulna leaves a weak wrist. In gross deformity, elongation of the abnormal radius may improve the appearance and function of the wrist but is technically challenging.

HIP

General clinical features and examination

History

Pain originating from the hip tends to be felt in the groin or thigh. It may be referred to the knee, particularly in children. Pain is worse at the end of the day and on weight-bearing. Nocturnal pain may cause much loss of sleep.

Past trauma. In chronic disorders there may be a past history of trauma, e.g. fracture of the pelvis and dislocation or fracture-dislocation of the femur.

Limp and gait. Limp may be noticed by others or by the patient, and there may be increasing difficulty in walking. Causes may be:

- pain as the patient tries to protect the joint
- short leg
- muscle weakness.

For abnormal gaits associated with hip disorders, see Box 34.2.

Physical findings

- *Look* at:
  - skin for scars
  - the position of the hip – in established osteoarthritis the hip is in fixed flexion, internal rotation and adduction
  - gait; this can be protective (antalgic), Trendelenburg (abnormal abductor mechanism which included the hip joint fulcrum), short- or stiff-legged.
- *Feel:*
  - for crepitus on movement
  - to measure leg length – from the anterior superior iliac spine to the medial malleolus.
- *Move:*
  - to establish active range of movement
  - to measure the passive range of movement.

The normal range is shown in Table 34.2.

It is important to ensure that movement is taking place at the hip alone and not the pelvis as well. Fully flexing the other hip to abolish the normal lumbar lordosis demonstrates a fixed flexion deformity as the affected leg rises up off the examination couch. On flexion, a hand under the lumbar spine can feel when the pelvis starts to tilt (Thomas hip flexion test). During abduction and adduction, a forearm across the pelvis prevents pelvic tilt.

Investigation

Imaging

- **Plain X-ray** is usually sufficient to confirm a clinical diagnosis.
- **Isotope scan.** In lytic lesions, there is increased uptake; avascular necrosis appears as a relatively dense area.
- **CT and MRI** can help to determine the site or extent of bony and other damage in more detail.

Blood examination

In osteoarthritis, the ESR is normal and rheumatoid factor is absent. The reverse is usually true in rheumatoid arthritis.

Osteoarthritis

This condition is extremely common. Its treatment to relieve pain and restore mobility has been revolutionised by the development of prosthetic hip joints.

Epidemiology and aetiology

The factors that can contribute to the development of the condition have been discussed above. By far the most common is wear and tear on the joint in a population with an increased life expectancy – by the age of 80 years, 80–90% of hips show radiographic evidence of the condition. Women are more commonly affected than men (3:1). The condition can be unilateral or bilateral. More than 10% of unilateral instances become bilateral over 5–8 years.

Management

Decisions on management depend on:

- the wishes of the patient
- age – although with modern techniques of surgery and anaesthesia, chronological age is rarely a bar to operation
- general physical condition
- degree of disability and its interaction with lifestyle.

Non-operative

Those with only minor symptoms can be managed by losing weight, physiotherapy, foam heel wedges, a walking stick and NSAIDs. Loss of 1 kg of body weight reduces the forces acting across the hip by roughly 3 kgf.

Surgical

Surgery for osteoarthritis of the hip is now essentially joint replacement, although in the past there were other options (see Table 34.4). An osteotomy can provide short-term relief of pain, but a subsequent joint replacement may be difficult because of the altered anatomy. Excision is reserved for the infected hip replacement. The modern total hip replacement was introduced in 1961 and can be expected to last for at least 15–20 years. However, this depends on a number of factors, as described above.

The chief causes of failure are:

- infection, which should be less than 1%
- loosening without infection and recrudescence of pain.

Infection means that the prosthesis must be removed, although it may be possible to insert a replacement after the organism has been eliminated. Loosening without infection is treated by a revision procedure. A variety of surgical approaches to the hip are used, as shown in Table 34.9. Typical pre- and postoperative management is given in Clinical Box 34.1.

Rheumatoid arthritis (RA)

This is a systemic condition which is initially managed medically. The hip and knee are involved but, in particular, it affects the upper limbs and the feet. There are a number of problems encountered with hip joint replacement in the patient with RA. When, as is often the case, multiple joints are involved, rehabilitation may be difficult. Bone quality is often poor, so that intraoperative fractures occur. Infection rates are higher than for replacement in OA.

Nevertheless, hip replacement for RA has a definite place provided that the joint is the principal site of the problem and there is a good chance of restoring mobility.

Table 34.9 Surgical approaches to the hip joint

Approach	Advantages	Disadvantages
Anterior/anterolateral	Reduced risk of dislocation Sciatic nerve not at risk	Increased muscle dissection Femoral nerve at risk
Posterior	Faster and easier approach Muscle-splitting approach, so preserving muscle power Femoral nerve not at risk Improved access to femoral canal and acetabulum, especially in revision hip surgery	Increased risk of dislocation Sciatic nerve at risk Increased risk of infection?

Clinical Box 34.1 Total hip replacement – pre- and postoperative management

Preoperative
- Obtain adequate and up-to-date radiological images
- Exclude intercurrent infection
  - Midstream urine sample
  - Skin infection and venous ulcers
- MRSA swabs to groin and axilla to determine carrier status
- Anaesthetic assessment
- Group and save

Postoperative
- Abduction pillow for 24 hours, to minimise risks of dislocation
- Early mobilisation
- Low molecular weight heparin, dabigatran etexilate, fondaparinux sodium, or rivaroxaban continued for 4–5 weeks to reduce risks of venous thrombosis (unfractionated heparin in patients with renal failure)
- Crutches or sticks to reduce risk of falling
- In-patient stay for 4–7 days
- Raised toilet seat for 6 weeks
- Avoid low chairs for 6 weeks

Osteonecrosis of the femoral head

In this condition, the femoral head becomes ischaemic and infarcts. As a result, there is structural weakness and collapse of the bone.

Aetiology

The underlying process is not fully understood. The following have been postulated:

- arterial insufficiency following a fracture or dislocation
- venous occlusion – a feature of Perthe's disease
- raised intraosseous pressure – possibly the cause in sickle cell disease, alcoholism, systemic steroids and decompression from high atmospheric pressure with the formation of gas bubbles (the bends in deep-sea divers).

Management

Non-operative

Treatment of any correctable underlying cause is instituted. Anti-inflammatory drugs are symptomatically helpful.

Surgical

Surgery is often required to provide pain relief:

- core decompression – drilling a core of bone out of the femoral head and neck is thought to be effective by reducing the intraosseous pressure and improving venous drainage but is less helpful in later stages III or IV
- arthroplasty is reserved for the late stages when there is collapse and secondary osteoarthritis.

Tuberculosis

Aetiology and pathological manifestations

The disease is now less common, although the incidence has recently increased in the poor and groups with immunosuppression from such causes as AIDS. The route of infection is haematogenous and the pathological features are the same as for tuberculosis in other organs – tissue destruction, abscess formation and fibrosis. Untreated, the joint progresses to fibrous ankylosis.

Clinical features

As well as systemic symptoms of malaise and fever, local ones include a mild ache and limp.

Initially, there is little to be found – only the features of an irritable hip. Later, there is marked muscle wasting, joint stiffness, pain and shortening. This chronic picture is in contrast to the acute, severe pattern of septic arthritis.

Investigation and management

X-ray changes are of osteoporosis and, later, joint destruction.

As in septic arthritis, pus is drained, the organism is cultured to establish sensitivity to chemotherapy and appropriate anti-tuberculosis therapy begun. With these measures, damage can be limited. A hip that heals with ankylosis may require a raised shoe when walking is resumed. A painful joint may need to be arthrodesed. Arthroplasty is considered with caution because reactivation of the infection can occur.

KNEE

General clinical features

History

Age. Young adults commonly suffer injury in sport; their first presentation is often to general practitioners and casualty departments. In older individuals, the joint is more frequently affected by osteoarthritis, although injury may be a precipitating factor. In an acute event, the patient may be able to pinpoint the exact moment of injury.

Pain. Generalised or localised pain is a frequent symptom. The location is important because it may indicate the diagnosis. Generalised pain over the whole knee is a feature of arthritis and acute injury. In meniscal tears, pain is localised to the joint line, including posteriorly in the popliteal fossa. Collateral ligament sprains cause pain above or below the joint line. Anterior pain is a symptom of disorders of the patella such as chondromalacia. Such anterior pain is frequently worse when the knee is loaded in flexion – characteristically when going up or down stairs. Deficiency of the anterior cruciate ligament is often associated with a sensation of giving way; the pain is diffuse.

Mechanism in injuries. Commonly, there is a twisting injury, often with an associated tearing or popping sensation from the joint which is accompanied by pain. The patient may well fall to the ground and if playing a sport then has to stop.

Swelling may be immediate (within an hour) and implies an acute haemarthrosis (the usual causes are given in Table 34.10). Swelling delay for several hours suggests a meniscal injury. Arthritic knees are chronically swollen from either an effusion or thickened synovium.

Locking and giving way occur when the knee is unstable. Locking may fix the knee, usually in flexion, or it may unlock with a pop or a click and indicates a bucket handle tear of the meniscus. The arthritic knee may also give way because of instability and may lock because of loose bodies trapped within.

Table 34.10 Causes of acute haemarthrosis of the knee

Lesion[a]	Percentage
Anterior cruciate ligament rupture	39
Peripheral meniscal tear	26
Collateral ligament injury	13
Capsular tear	9
Osteochondral fracture	7
Posterior cruciate ligament rupture	6

[a]Seventy percent have more than one lesion, 29% have only one lesion, and in 1% no cause is found.

Physical findings

- *Look* for:
  - swelling – by assessing contour
  - wasting of the quadriceps
  - position at rest – is the joint in fixed flexion or is there a varus or valgus deformity?
  - scars – previous arthroscopy portals can be missed unless examination is meticulous
  - abnormal skin colour.
- *Feel* for:
  - swelling – if present, is it bone, boggy synovial thickening or fluid?
  - the presence of an effusion (see below)
  - altered temperature
  - the joint line – medially, laterally and in the popliteal fossa
  - local tenderness, which suggests a meniscal tear
  - tenderness over the femoral condyles when the knee is flexed; they may be tender when damaged, as occurs in arthritis
  - the patella – is it very mobile; when pushed laterally, does the patient flinch (such positive apprehension is seen with recurrent dislocation of the patella); is there tenderness on the retropatellar surface?
  - loose bodies which may shoot from under the fingers
  - crepitus when the joint is moved.

Effusion is diagnosed by two methods. The first, cross-fluctuation, is the more sensitive of the two. The second, patellar tap, confirms a large effusion but may not be elicited with a small collection.

Cross-fluctuation. The suprapatellar pouch is emptied by placing one hand proximal to the patella, so pushing any fluid down into the main cavity of the joint. The hand stays in position and the medial and lateral sides are examined. In the normal knee, a soft hollow is seen, but this is absent with a large effusion. With a stroking motion of the other hand to the medial and lateral sides, fluid can be pushed across the joint. In the presence of an effusion, a soft swelling appears on the opposite side of the knee to the hand.

Patellar tap. The suprapatellar pouch is emptied as before and kept empty by leaving the hand above the patella. The other hand gently presses the patella down onto the underlying femoral condyles. There is a distinct feeling of the patella sinking down and coming to a sudden stop when it hits the condyles with a 'tap'.

Collateral ligament stability is assessed with the knee in 20° of flexion. A varus strain is applied to test the lateral collateral ligament; a valgus strain for the medial collateral.

Cruciate ligaments. The integrity of the anterior cruciate is assessed by performing the Lachman test (Fig. 34.5), and the posterior cruciate by looking for 'posterior sag' (Fig. 34.6).

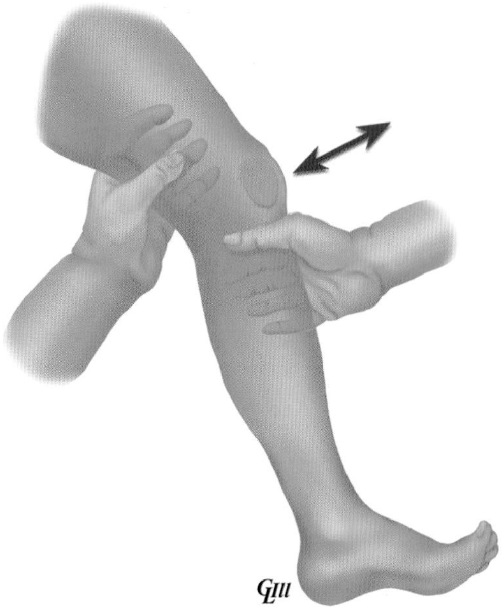

Fig. 34.5 Lachman's test for integrity of the anterior cruciate.

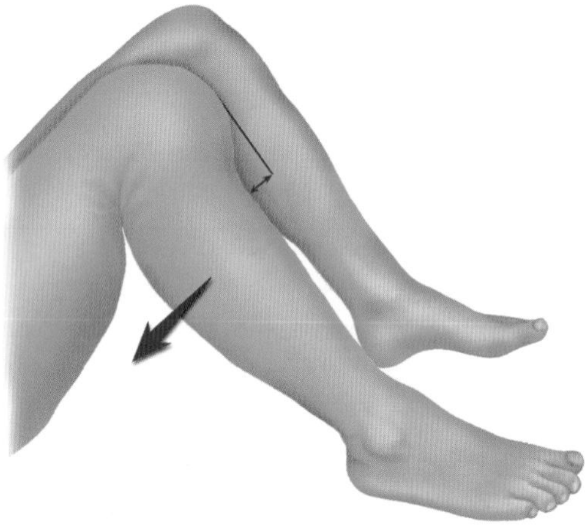

Fig. 34.6 Posterior sag in a lesion of the posterior cruciate.

Quadriceps wasting. The circumference of the leg is measured on both sides at a fixed distance (usually 10 cm) above the upper border of the patella.

Movement. The patient is asked to walk. On bearing weight, does the knee go into a valgus or varus deformity? There may be an antalgic, short leg or stiff leg gait (see Box 34.2).

The range of active movement is then assessed and compared with the passive range. Is it possible to get the knee to full extension, or is there a block? Finally, in a normal knee, the patella tracks evenly on the trochlear surface of the femur. Maltracking occurs when it is seen to sublux or dislocate laterally as the knee moves.

Investigation

Imaging

Plain X-ray reveals any arthritis. Loose bodies may be seen, often in the intercondylar notch. On the lateral film, the length of the patella should be about equal to the distance from the inferior pole of the patella to the tibial tuberosity. If it is less than this, then the patella is riding high (patella alta) which predisposes to dislocation.

Skyline views show the patellofemoral joint and are taken with the knee flexed. The patella should be horizontal and centrally positioned within its trochlear groove.

Tunnel views are taken with the knee flexed to 45° and provide a view of the intercondylar notch. They are useful if loose bodies are suspected. If an avulsion of the anterior cruciate is possible, then a small flake of bone torn off the tibial plateau may be seen.

Weight-bearing films accentuate any loss of joint space and also show up varus/valgus deformities.

Arthrography can show meniscal and capsular tears. With the advent of MRI and diagnostic arthroscopy, its use is declining.

CT is not often used in the knee but can show arthritis, loose bodies and patella malalignment.

MRI can demonstrate meniscal and cruciate injuries. It is non-invasive and in most centres has replaced arthrography.

Radioisotope scan shows increased activity in degenerative conditions which may be localised to one compartment.

Meniscal injuries

A meniscus trapped between the joint surfaces may tear. There are five main types of tear (Fig. 34.7). The distribution is:

- medial meniscus 70%
- lateral meniscus 25%
- both 5%.

The frequent involvement of the medial meniscus is because it is firmly adherent to the medial capsule and therefore less mobile than the lateral one.

Clinical features

History

There has usually been a painful twisting injury, often during sport. There may be an associated 'pop', 'crack' or tearing sensation within the joint and swelling quickly appears. Subsequently there is persistent swelling and a feeling of something catching. Occasionally the knee locks for some hours as the torn meniscus becomes lodged between the joint.

Physical findings

- *Look* for:
  - effusion
  - wasted quadriceps by comparison with the other side.
- *Feel* for:
  - effusion
  - tenderness at the joint line.

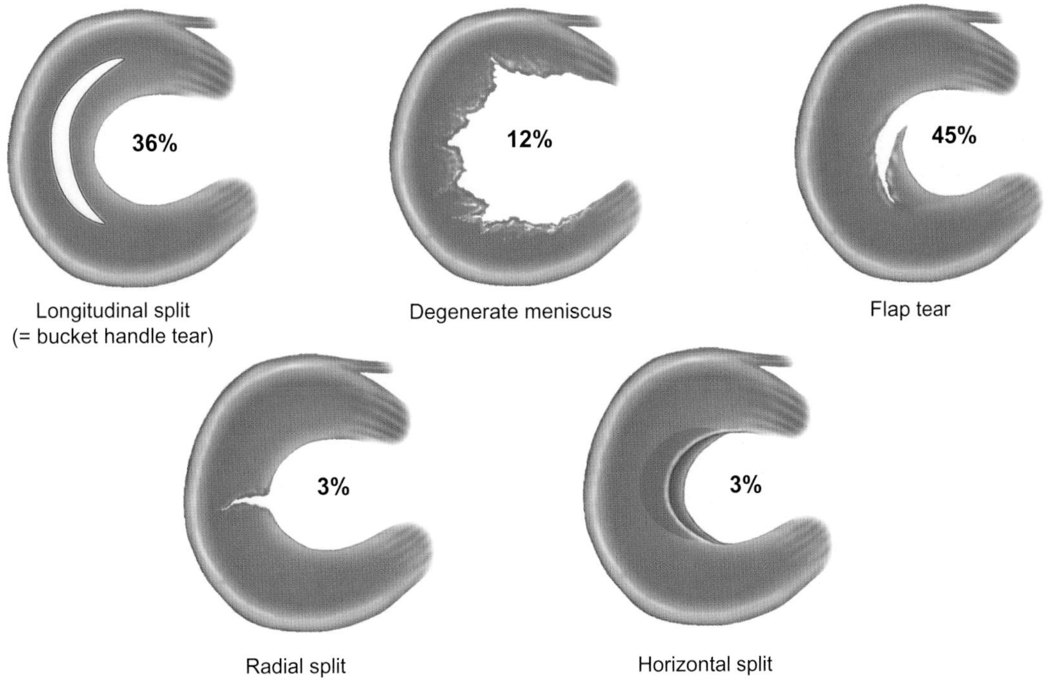

Fig. 34.7 Types of meniscal tear in the knee.

- *Test movement* for:
  - springy feel in a locked knee
  - McMurray's test – with the knee at 90° of flexion, the tibia is rotated on the femur to try to trap the meniscal tear between the two bones; internal rotation of the tibia catches a lateral meniscus and external rotation the medial; in either event pain is felt at the joint line.

Management

Non-operative

When there is doubt about the diagnosis, then it is reasonable to treat the symptoms with a review in 2–3 weeks. In those with improvement, a graduated programme of knee rehabilitation is continued. When symptoms and signs persist, surgery should be considered.

Surgical

When the clinical features are typical, then the management is surgical. Arthroscopy (see below) is both diagnostic and therapeutic – the tear can be seen and then either excised or repaired depending on the type of tear. Repairable tears are acute in the red zone (more vascular) of the meniscus near the periphery. After operation, it is vital that formal rehabilitation is undertaken to avoid further injury to the joint. This starts immediately with quadriceps exercises, and once the portals have healed, swimming, cycling and weight training of the muscles can begin. Only when all these activities are managed with ease is return to exercise which involves weight-bearing on the knee surface allowed (such as jogging, low-impact aerobics and, finally, contact or high-impact sporting activities).

Anterior cruciate ligament (ACL) injuries

Mechanism and pathological features

These injuries are sustained after a twisting and valgus strain is applied to the knee. Typically they are seen in the footballer who twists on the knee during a tackle on an opposing player. In women, the most common cause of ACL rupture is skiing. The medial collateral ligament and medial meniscus are often damaged at the same time. Hyperextension on its own can also produce an isolated ACL rupture. Occasionally, any of these mechanisms may avulse a fragment of bone at the insertion of the ACL onto the tibial plateau.

Clinical features

Physical examination demonstrates only about 70% of ruptures of the ACL. The diagnosis is confirmed by MRI.

Management

Non-operative

The knee with a ruptured ACL can often be managed without resort to surgery. Intensive rehabilitation is used to strengthen the hamstring and quadricep muscles and improve proprioception at the knee. Swimming, cycling and weight training followed by gentle jogging can then be attempted. Change in lifestyle with withdrawal from some sports or other activities may be necessary. A brace can help to stabilise the knee. A large variety are available but all rely on firm strapping above and below the knee with metal or carbon fibre supports for tennis or skiing.

Surgical

With effective non-operative management, surgery may often be avoided. If it is, urgent operation has no advantage over delayed repair. The only unequivocal indication for early repair is when a fragment of bone has been avulsed from the tibial plateau, in which case the fragment should be reattached with a screw.

Delayed reconstruction may be required if the torn ACL continues to cause instability (giving way). Various methods to stabilise the knee have been used in the past, including an extra-articular reconstruction or use of synthetic intra-articular grafts however the current favoured surgical technique is an intra-articular reconstruction using either patellar tendon or hamstring tendons harvested from the patient's knee.

Posterior cruciate ligament (PCL) injuries

Rupture of the posterior cruciate is much less common than that of the ACL and is often not recognised. The tibia is forced posteriorly on the femoral condyles – as in a head-on car crash when the lower leg hits the dashboard.

Clinical features

The functional instability after PCL rupture may be minimal, with the symptoms of pain, stiffness and an effusion only developing after degenerative changes in the knee have occurred.

In an acute injury there is a tense haemarthrosis with perhaps soft-tissue abrasions on the front of the tibia.

Investigation and management

Plain X-ray shows an effusion and sometimes a piece of bone that has been avulsed off the back of the tibia (PCL insertion).

A change in lifestyle, including the form of sporting activity, may allow the patient to lead a near-normal life.

An avulsed fragment should be exposed through the popliteal fossa and reattached. In a rupture with chronic problems, the indications for surgical treatment are the same as for repair of the ACL, and the methods are also similar.

Recurrent dislocation of the patella

The patella is a mobile sesamoid within the quadriceps tendon and is in a vulnerable position in front of the knee. True dislocation must be differentiated from maltracking in which there is painful subluxation.

Clinical features

History

Full dislocation. The patella always dislocates laterally, and there is usually a history of direct trauma to the medial side, often during sport. The patient sees and feels the bone displaced, and the knee is locked in 30–40° of flexion. Anterior pain and rapid swelling develop.

Subluxation. The patella is felt to 'pop' out of place, often during a turning movement. Pain is momentary and sharp over the front of the knee, which may feel unstable or give way. Minor swelling is noted over 24 hours.

Physical findings in acute dislocation

- *Look* for:
  - the patella on the lateral side of the knee
  - knee locked in flexion
  - effusion.
- *Feel* for:
  - position of the bone to the lateral side
  - tenderness on the medial side of the patella after reduction
  - effusion.
- *Test* for reducibility by applying firm pressure on the lateral side and simultaneously extending the knee; the bone may reduce with a 'snap'.

Investigation

Plain X-ray shows the displacement. After reduction, patella alta (see below) may be seen. Skyline views are helpful and may reveal an osteochondral fracture that occurs as the patella dislocates over the lateral femoral condyle.

In subluxation, X-rays may be normal or show patella alta (high riding patella).

Arthritis

Arthritis of the knee is very common, and the usual form is osteoarthritis. Rheumatoid arthritis also occurs but less frequently. As in the hip, the management of this painful, disabling condition has been transformed by the development of prosthetic replacement.

Clinical features

History

Pain is the main complaint. Initially this is felt only after walking but later also at rest. Accompanying stiffness and swelling, initially intermittent but eventually permanent, occur. It is also common for the joint to lock because of loose bodies and painfully give way.

Physical findings

- *Look* for:
  - varus or valgus deformity with the patient standing
  - swelling.
- *Feel* for:
  - effusion
  - tenderness at the joint lines and over the femoral condyles
  - crepitus.
- *Test* for:
  - movement – fixed flexion deformity is common
  - collateral ligament laxity when there is varus or valgus deformity.

Management

Non-operative

Weight loss, analgesics, physiotherapy, a walking stick and foam heel wedges all help in those with mild symptoms.

Surgical

There are several surgical options. The choice depends on:

- wishes of the patient
- age
- degree of disability.

Arthroscopy is a useful first step and allows the surgeon to assess the extent of the disorder. Debris in the joint is washed out and can provide pain relief for a year or more. Loose bodies can be removed and degenerative meniscal tears trimmed. In rheumatoid arthritis, an arthroscopic synovectomy is symptomatically useful in that synovial hypertrophy contributes to the inflammatory process.

Osteotomy. Often the medial compartment of the knee is affected by the arthritis but the lateral side is relatively spared. An osteotomy can be performed to realign the knee, and forces are transferred to the relatively healthy side. This procedure is of use in the younger patient and may provide 8–10 years of pain relief. Once the lateral side starts to wear, a knee replacement can be done.

Total knee replacement. Knee replacements with a hinge were inserted in the early 1950s, and later in that decade metal discs were interposed but with poor results. However, it was not until the early 1970s, with the development of dedicated instrumentation and unconstrained (no hinge) prostheses, that the results improved. 'Unconstrained' means that stability relies on the surrounding tissue tension to hold the two parts in correct alignment. A large variety of knee replacements are now available. These fall into three main groups as shown in Table 34.5.

Arthrodesis. This operation has largely been superseded by joint replacement. It can be a salvage procedure after joint replacement has failed. The knee is fused in a functional position of about 5–10° of flexion, which allows the limb to be swung through during the relevant phase of the gait cycle.

ANKLE AND FOOT

ANKLE

General clinical features

History

Pain from the ankle joint is often felt as a band across its front. When there is a problem at the malleolus, the symptoms may be to one side or the other. Pain from the subtalar joint tends to be felt below the ankle and may radiate forward into the foot.

Instability is a sensation of unusual movement, usually from side to side, and is common because of the frequent exposure of the ankle to twisting strains.

Swelling around the ankle may be the consequence of local disease such as arthritis or of more general problems – cardiac or renal. In chronic instability, it is often localised at one or other malleolus.

Trauma is often an important factor. In addition to predisposing to chronic instability, it can also cause secondary osteoarthritis – the result of joint surface irregularity or of avascular necrosis in a fragment of a fractured talus.

Physical findings

- *Look* for:
  - swelling
  - scars.
- *Feel* for:
  - localised tenderness in the malleoli
  - crepitus (gently) in the area as a whole
  - swelling – boggy synovial thickening, pitting oedema or an effusion within the joint
  - local warmth.
- *Move* the ankle for:
  - walking – the gait (see Box 34.2) may attempt to avoid pain or there may be foot drop, which causes the toes to contact the ground when normally the heel should strike first; this gait is seen after injury to the sciatic nerve at the buttock, or the common peroneal nerve at the knee
  - active and passive range – the ankle joint is capable of both plantarflexion and dorsiflexion from a neutral position; inversion and eversion occur at the subtalar joint; the test is done by holding the lower leg with one hand and grasping the heel with the other so that the subtalar joint can then be moved separately
  - excessive movement – laxity of the collateral ligaments is detected on inversion and eversion; drawing the foot forwards and backwards on the lower leg may reveal subluxation.

Investigation

Imaging

- **Plain X-ray** may show arthritis or evidence of old trauma. When the history is one of instability, there may be localised arthritic changes at the malleolus with perhaps a loose body at the tip of the malleolus from an old avulsion fracture. Avascular necrosis of the talus results in sclerosis and collapse of the bone. If the history and examination suggest that the site of the problem is in the subtalar joint, it may be necessary to request plain films of this joint.
- **Stress X-ray** is done by applying a valgus or varus strain to the joint while films are taken – when this is painful, general anaesthesia may be required. If there is significant instability, the talus may be shown to tilt within the mortice of the ankle joint.
- **Isotope bone scan** may show an increase in activity in the ankle or subtalar joint or at a malleolus. In avascular necrosis of the talus, there is an area of reduced uptake.
- **CT or MRI** confirm the presence of arthritis and are also helpful when avascular necrosis is suspected, as its extent can be clearly seen.

Chronic instability

This condition is better prevented than cured. The cause is an inversion or eversion injury that tears the collateral ligament which is put under stress.

Clinical features

There is usually a history of the relevant injury. There is tenderness over the ligament just distal to the malleolus. Evidence of bruising is only present in the early stages.

Investigation and management

Stress X-ray will demonstrate talar tilt, although this investigation may be difficult in the acute phase because of pain.

In a patient with an acute injury in whom a diagnosis of a collateral tear has been made, the traditional treatment has been 3 weeks in a below-knee plaster cast to allow the ligament to heal. More recently, early intensive physiotherapy with proprioceptive training on a 'wobble board' (a board balanced on a ball) has been advocated, and the results are possibly better.

In spite of adequate treatment, chronic instability may become established and is treated:

- *non-operatively* – which may be sufficient if the patient alters lifestyle, changes to a different sport or wears boots that support the ankle
- *surgically* – a number of operations have been described; as well as reconstituting the affected ligament, further support is provided by using a local structure such as the tendon of peroneus brevis. The joint capsule may be shrunk with a thermal technique.

Arthritis

As a weight-bearing joint, the ankle is prone to osteoarthritis but much less commonly than the hip or the knee. The reason is unclear but may be in part because the ankle is essentially a hinge joint whereas at the hip and knee there is also rotation and therefore extra shear forces on the cartilage. Nevertheless, post-traumatic secondary osteoarthritis of the ankle is common in young adults involved in athletics.

Involvement by rheumatoid arthritis is to a similar extent as the hip and knee.

Management

Non-operative

This is the most common method: a walking stick, firm boots to limit movement at the joint and anti-inflammatory drugs.

Surgical

Operation is less satisfactory in the ankle than in the hip or knee; the options are fusion, providing a stiff painless joint, or arthroplasty.

Prosthetic replacements are available but the long-term results are not as good as in the hip or knee.

FOOT

Painful feet are common. The hazard of attempts at surgical management of an individual lesion is that it may merely transfer the problem from one part of the foot to another and so never achieve a cure.

Clinical features

History

Pain is the usual presentation, most commonly localised to one point, but it may radiate, be worse on weight-bearing and be relieved by rest. There is often difficulty in finding shoes that can be worn without pain.

Physical findings

The appearance of the foot can be the presenting feature.

- *Look* for:
  - shape, including any callosities and their site
  - the shoes and in what areas they show signs of wear – an indication of how load is being transferred
  - evidence of vascular insufficiency – the presence of peripheral vascular disease may contraindicate surgery on the foot.
- *Feel* for:
  - local tenderness
  - pulses in the foot (dorsalis pedis and posterior tibial).
- *Move:*
  - the midtarsal joint by holding the heel with one hand and the forefoot with the other
  - the toes – are any deformities correctable?

Investigation

Imaging

Plain X-ray of the foot may be required so as to plan an operation. The presence of radiological evidence of arthritis may influence what procedure, if any, is performed.

Films taken during weight-bearing may be useful.

Other investigations

Pedobarography produces a pressure profile of the foot. However, the device is not widely available. It can confirm the areas of high pressure and can be used to assess the effect of surgical procedures.

Most other investigations are usually not helpful. A very painful, red and swollen first metatarsophalangeal joint may raise the suspicion of gout.

Hallux valgus

This is a progressive valgus deformity of the big toe. Once the toe starts to angulate, progression is inevitable because the pull of the tendons increases the deformity.

Aetiology

A number of factors can be identified in the development of hallux valgus:

- family history
- sex – more common in females
- age – tends to occur in the middle-aged; with the passage of time the foot tends to splay, so making any deforming forces worse
- metatarsus primus varus – if the first metatarsal is in varus, there is a greater tendency for the big toe to go into valgus because of the pull of the extensor tendon

- shoes – modern shoes tend to be very tight at the toes, so forcing the big toe into valgus; hallux valgus rarely occurs in the unshod.

Clinical features

History

There is cosmetic deformity and discomfort over the prominent bunion at the metatarsophalangeal joint. Inflammation occurs as this rubs on the shoes. Crossing of the first toe under or over the second and third increases discomfort.

Physical findings

- Look for the deformity and the bunion.
- Feel for localised tenderness.
- Test for movement, which is often reduced, and to find out if the valgus deformity is reducible.

Management

Non-operative

In the elderly with poor peripheral blood flow, conservative management is best. Surgical shoes can be made to fit the foot, as opposed to the normal practice of squashing the deformed toe and foot into the shoe. Regular chiropody is important to care for the skin and nails.

Surgical

Over 40 operations have been described for hallux valgus. A simple bunionectomy is usually not enough because the deformity will recur. When there is osteoarthritis at the joint, surgery is either an excisional arthroplasty (Keller's) or joint replacement with a Silastic or ceramic implant. These relieve the pain and correct the deformity, but the joint is often stiffer than normal and, after a Keller's procedure, the big toe is short. In the younger age group, surgery is directed at correcting the underlying deformity – the varus displacement of the first metatarsal. Various operations have been described to lateralise the head of the first metatarsal and therefore correct the deformity.

Hallux rigidus

This condition of a stiff, painful big toe is caused by degenerative arthritis at the first metatarsophalangeal joint. During walking, the big toe is unable to extend as the foot rolls forwards to toe-off (see Table 34.1). This is painful.

Management

Non-operative

A rocker-bottom sole on the shoe allows the foot to roll forward more easily during walking. This is often cosmetically unacceptable and so is of use only in those unable to undergo an operation.

Surgical

A dorsal cheilectomy is performed. This operation involves excision of the dorsal osteophytes and so allows a greater range of extension. Arthrodesis of the metatarsophalangeal joint provides good pain relief although the big toe will rest in a somewhat extended position. Other methods such as excisional arthroplasty may be useful in the frail or elderly population.

Metatarsalgia

In this condition, the distal foot is painful. The source of the pain is high pressure on the metatarsal heads as the patient walks. It is often associated with claw toes (see below), and as a result, instead of the toes sharing in weight-bearing, all the weight is taken on the metatarsal heads. It can also occur when the foot has a high longitudinal arch (pes cavus) for either unknown reasons or in neuromuscular conditions such as cerebral palsy, spina bifida or Friedreich's ataxia.

Morton's metatarsalgia (neuroma) is a specific condition in which there is an interdigital neuroma between the metatarsal heads. This is then irritated by the adjacent bones, so resulting in pain and sensory disturbance at the corresponding cleft.

Management

Non-operative

A padded metatarsal bar fitted into the shoes to offload the metatarsal heads helps to spread the load across the foot. Surgical shoes may also be required to accommodate the foot comfortably.

Surgical

An oblique osteotomy of the metatarsal necks allows the heads of the metatarsals to ride up. It is important to divide the second, third and fourth metatarsals because operating on one alone is not sufficient. In Morton's metatarsalgia, the affected space is explored and the neuroma excised. After operation, sensation is absent in the cleft.

Claw toes

Toes hyperextended at the metatarsophalangeal joints and flexed at the interphalangeal joints are clawed and do not touch the ground. As a result, they rub on the shoes and callosities develop over the proximal interphalangeal joints. There is also a tendency to develop an associated metatarsalgia. The cause is usually unknown, but claw toes are seen in neuromuscular disorders such as spina bifida.

Management

Non-operative

Local measures such as felt pads and attention to footwear may be sufficient.

Surgical

Fusion of the proximal interphalangeal joint allows the toe to straighten. This is usually done by excising the joint and then using a small wire to hold the toe straight for 6 weeks until the bone ends unite. A single, grossly deformed toe should be amputated.

Plantar fasciitis

This is a painful condition of the heel caused by a localised area of inflammation of the plantar fascia at its origin from the os calcis. It is sometimes precipitated by local trauma or excessive weight-bearing.

Clinical features

A relevant history of focal trauma may be obtained. Otherwise, the only complaint is of well-localised pain in the heel on weight-bearing.

There is tenderness over the most prominent point of the calcaneus in the sole of the foot.

Investigation and management

Plain X-ray may show a spur on the plantar aspect of the os calcis.

Non-operative management with use of a cushioned heel wedge, night splints or local steroid injection is usually successful. Surgery to release the plantar fascia is occasionally required.

Achilles tendonitis

This is a similar condition to plantar fasciitis in which there is an area of local inflammation at the insertion of the Achilles tendon. It may be precipitated by local trauma or a new pair of shoes that rub on the heel. Treatment consists of a heel wedge to reduce the tension in the tendon and a local steroid injection to the tendon sheath. Surgery is occasionally required to incise the inflamed tendon sheath.

Freiberg's disease

This condition is of an unknown cause in which there is fragmentation and collapse of the second metatarsal head. It occurs in young adults, and there may be a history of local trauma. The enlarged metatarsal head produces local pressure symptoms and metatarsalgia. Treatment is conservative with felt pads to relieve pressure. Surgery is occasionally done to reduce the size of the metatarsal head.

Gout

This is a medical condition which does not usually concern the orthopaedic surgeon, but patients may present initially to the A&E department or the orthopaedic clinic. The metatarsophalangeal joint is red, hot, swollen and extremely painful. There may be a precipitating history of minor trauma to the big toe, dietary excess, recent surgery or the use of drugs such as a thiazide diuretic. In the acute stage, the treatment is with NSAIDs. Prophylaxis with allopurinol may prevent recurrent attacks and should be undertaken if these are frequent.

PAEDIATRIC ORTHOPAEDICS

HIP

Problems with the hip are common. Patients present with a limp and pain which may be felt in the knee alone, and any child with knee pain must have his or her hip examined. Whereas trauma and infection can occur at any age, other conditions tend to occur within particular age brackets (Table 34.11).

Table 34.11 Age ranges for paediatric hip conditions

Age	Condition
0–5 years	Congenital dislocation of the hip
5–10 years	Perthe's disease
10–15 years	Slipped upper-femoral epiphysis

Developmental dysplasia of the hip

The hip is unstable at birth either because of ligamentous laxity or because of dislocation out of an undeveloped (dysplastic) acetabular socket.

Epidemiology

The incidence is 15/1000 at birth but falls to 1.5/1000 at 6 weeks. The left side is affected in 60%, the right in 20% and the condition is bilateral in 20%.

Aetiology

Genetic

There may be a family history:

- affected sibling – 6% chance
- affected mother – 12% chance
- affected sibling and mother – 35% chance.

Sex

It is more common in girls than in boys in a ratio of 9:1. This is probably because the girl fetus is more sensitive to the maternal hormone relaxin secreted during pregnancy.

Perinatal

Associated factors are:

- first birth
- an extended breech presentation
- coexistent talipes (see below)
- any other congenital anomaly
- oligohydramnios.

Postnatal

Wrapping the infant in extension and adduction can cause hip dislocation.

Clinical features

History

Often the condition is diagnosed at birth, as part of the routine postnatal check (clicky hips). Occasionally, the parents may notice asymmetry of the skin creases. In older children there is a history of abnormal gait (see Box 34.2).

Physical findings

- *Look:*
  - at the skin creases – there may be asymmetry of the gluteal creases but not if the condition is bilateral
  - for limited abduction in flexion
  - at the gait of an older child – it is a characteristic Trendelenburg gait.
- *Feel and move* – the head may dislocate and relocate when Ortolani's or Barlow's tests are performed (Box 34.4); they must be done gently and not repeated,

because avascular necrosis of the femoral head may result.

Investigation

Plain X-ray. Up to 15 signs can be identified on a plain X-ray of the pelvis. The common ones are shown in Figure 34.8. The ossification centre of the femoral head does not appear until the age of 5 months. For the acetabulum to develop normally, the femoral head must be within it. If not, it remains shallow with a large acetabular angle.

Ultrasound. In experienced hands, as well as being diagnostic, it is a useful screening technique. Under the age of 5 months, it is the investigation of choice to diagnose a dislocated hip.

Arthrography is required only for planning surgical correction in the older child.

Management

The final result depends to a great extent on the age at which the diagnosis is made and treatment begun. If this is at birth, the developed hip is normal. The aim of treatment is to achieve a complete and stable reduction. Patients who are missed at birth may present late – up to the age of 3 or 4 years – and in these circumstances the outlook for good function is poor and treatment difficult.

Birth to 6 months

A splint is used to hold the hip joint in approximately 60° of abduction and 90° of flexion. A variety is available, but the most common type used is the Pavlik harness. The splint is worn all the time until the acetabulum is seen to be developing normally.

Box 34.4 Special tests for developmental dysplasia of the hip

Barlow's test
With the hips adducted and flexed to 90°, gentle pressure is applied along the femoral shaft to dislocate the head posteriorly

Ortolani's test
The femoral head is dislocated as for Barlow's test. The hips are then abducted and the head is felt to relocate with a 'clunk'

Six months to walking

At this age, the hip is dislocated. Gentle traction is applied over a few weeks with progressive abduction (an adductor tenotomy may be required). The hip is then assessed under a general anaesthetic. If it is stable, a plaster of Paris hip spica is applied. If unstable or still dislocated, then an arthrogram is done which may show an inverted, thickened and folded acetabular labrum (limbus). This requires surgical removal to permit reduction.

The older child

An open operation is required to remove the limbus (contracted acetabular labrum and capsule) which is in the way of reduction of the femoral head into its socket. At a later stage, femoral osteotomy may also be required. Over 7 years of age, there is a case for non-operative management and, when secondary osteoarthritis develops in adult life, a total hip replacement.

Perthe's disease

There is, in this condition, a variable degree of osteonecrosis of the femoral head.

Aetiology and pathological features

The cause is essentially unknown. An effusion forms, perhaps as a result of minor trauma or a viral infection. Pressure within the joint rises and impairs venous return from the femoral head, which then undergoes avascular necrosis. The incidence is 1:9000, and the condition occurs four times more frequently in boys than in girls. It is bilateral in 10%.

The degree of collapse of the femoral head and the subsequent secondary arthritis is such that, by the age of 45, nearly half require a hip replacement, and by 65, secondary osteoarthritis is evident in 86%.

Clinical features

The age of onset is between 5 and 10 years with a limp and a complaint of a dull ache. There are few signs, but abduction in flexion is reduced.

Investigation

Imaging

Plain X-ray. An effusion may be seen. As the condition progresses, the femoral head becomes increasingly sclerotic

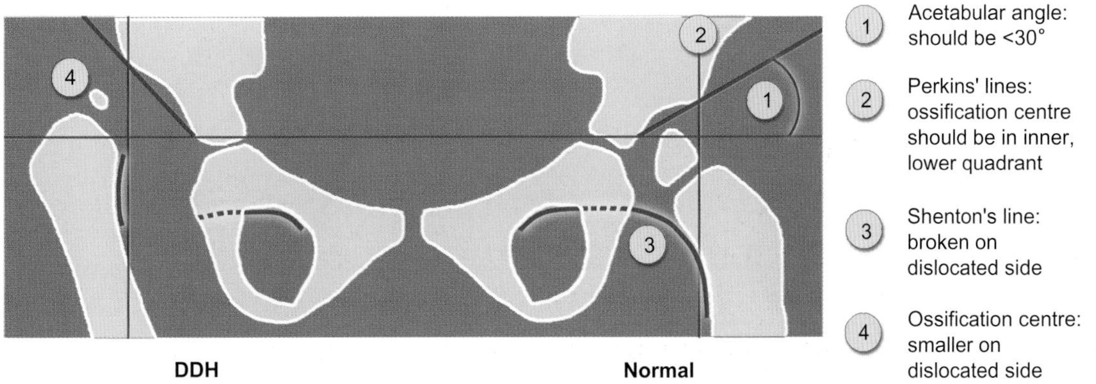
4
2
1
3
DDH
Normal
1 Acetabular angle: should be <30°
2 Perkins' lines: ossification centre should be in inner, lower quadrant
3 Shenton's line: broken on dislocated side
4 Ossification centre: smaller on dislocated side

Fig. 34.8 Common radiological features of the dislocated hip.

and fragmented. Collapse of the head is associated with lateral subluxation.

Bone scan is rarely required but, if undertaken, shows an area of reduced uptake that corresponds to the femoral head.

Blood examination

Standard tests are normal.

Management

Non-operative

Weight-bearing should be avoided while there is pain. The child should rest the hip whilst it is painful. A conservative approach can be employed if the progression of the disease is slow with limited involvement of the femoral head.

Surgical

If the femoral head subluxes laterally on X-ray, surgery is aimed at containing it within the acetabulum. This can be achieved by wide abduction of the hip in a hip spica, or a femoral osteotomy to bring the head back into the acetabulum.

Slipped upper-femoral epiphysis

The upper-femoral epiphysis can sometimes slip on the adjacent cartilaginous growth plate (physis). The epiphysis then slides off posteriorly.

Epidemiology

The incidence varies with race. In Caucasians it is 2 in 100 000, but in Afro-Caribbeans it is 7 in 100 000. Boys are affected twice as often as girls. The age of onset is between 10 and 15 years and is younger in girls (12 years) than in boys (14 years). The condition is slightly more common on the left side and is bilateral at presentation in 10%. If one side slips, there is a 25% chance that the other side will follow.

Aetiology

Trauma

There may be an acute slip after injury to the hip.

Hormonal

A relative deficiency of sex hormones which play a part in the ossification of cartilage is thought to be a factor in the development of a chronic slip. As growth progresses, the cartilaginous plate is then unable to resist the increasing load placed upon it.

Clinical features

History

In 70%, the history is of chronic pain and a limp. In 30%, there is an acute slip with a correspondingly short history.

Physical findings

- *Look:*
  - the child is often fat and sexually underdeveloped
  - the hip is held in extension, external rotation and adduction.
- *Measure* – the leg is short by 1–2 cm.
- *Move:*
  - abduction in flexion is reduced – there may be fixed external rotation
  - possibly a Trendelenburg gait (see Box 34.2).

Investigation

On an anteroposterior X-ray, the presence of a mild slip may be missed: look at Trethowan's line (Fig. 34.9). On a lateral film, however, the slip is easily seen. The amount is usually expressed as the percentage of the head uncovered on the lateral film.

Management

There is no place for conservative management. When there is a mild slip of up to 30%, the epiphysis should be pinned where it is without attempting reduction, because forcible manipulation may precipitate avascular necrosis. Greater

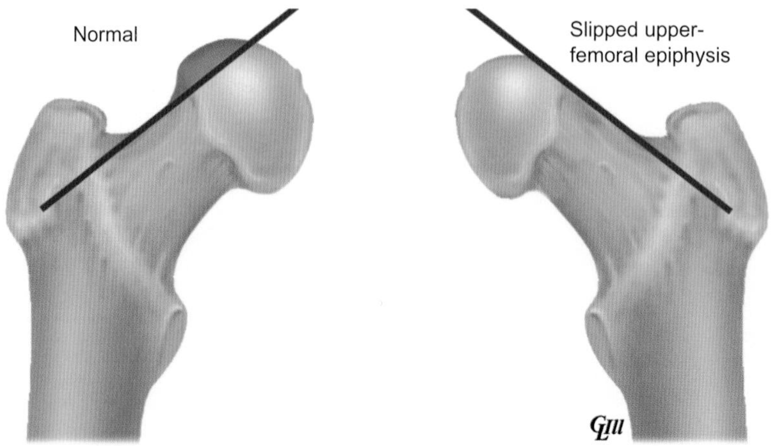

Fig. 34.9 Trethowan's line in slipped femoral epiphysis compared with normal.

than 30% displacement is managed by either of the following:

- open reduction and pinning – there is a 14% risk of avascular necrosis of the femoral head
- pinning without reduction and later femoral osteotomy to bring the epiphysis back into the correct position.

Late secondary osteoarthritis frequently occurs when there has been a slip of 50% or more.

It is generally accepted that if there is unreliable parental care or follow-up, consideration should be given to pinning the contralateral hip prophylactically.

TALIPES

This term is applied to a congenital deformity of the foot. A more detailed classification follows below.

Epidemiology and aetiology

The incidence is 2 in 1000 of live births in the UK. It is twice as common in boys as in girls and is bilateral in one-third.

In most instances, the condition is present at birth, and it used to be thought that the intrauterine position might be causative. However, deformities from this cause rapidly recover after birth. Other causes are neuromuscular, e.g. spina bifida, polio and arthrogryposis – the last is a joint malformation of unknown but possible neurogenic cause.

Types

The disorder is classified by the direction in which the heel points and the deviation of the forefoot. A foot that points down is said to be in equinus and one that points up in calcaneus. The forefoot may be in either varus or valgus.

The types in order of frequency are then:

- equinovarus – most common
- calcaneovalgus – second most common; may be associated with congenital dislocation of the hip
- equinovalgus – rare
- calcaneovarus – rare.

Clinical features

The deformity is usually noticed at routine postnatal examination or by the parents within a few days or weeks of birth.

Physical findings are of uncorrectable deformity in one of the directions described above.

Management

Non-operative

The initial treatment is to gently stretch and manipulate the foot into the correct position. A number of methods have been described to do this. The Ponsetti technique of serial casting is started in the first week after birth and can result in a very good outcome in experienced hands. The technique is time-consuming and requires close attention to detail. With this technique, an achilles tenotomy may be required after 4 to 6 weeks of casting and this can performed in the clinic. After the deformity has been corrected, the baby will need to continue to wear special shoes (Dennis Brown boots) for 3 to 4 years.

Surgical

If non-operative methods are unsuccessful or if there is a relapse in the older child then surgery will need to be considered. The tight soft tissue posteriorly and medially will need to be released and in the older child bony surgery may also be required.

MINOR LEG DEFORMITIES

Knock-knees, bow-legs and an in-toeing gait are all common and a source of much parental anxiety.

Knock-knee and bow-leg

In babies and toddlers, there is physiological bowing that corrects at 2–3 years of age. Later, at 4 or 5, there may be knock-knee of unknown cause. All but 2% of these correct spontaneously.

In a few children there is an underlying cause. Rickets is rare in the UK (but not unknown in some dark-skinned ethnic groups accustomed to more sunlight than they get in Britain). However, worldwide it is a common cause. Osteochondrosis deformans is a rare epiphyseal dysplasia which is associated with knock-knee.

In-toeing

This is the consequence of torsional deformity of either the tibia or the femur. Children then have a tendency to trip over their own feet. Treatment is not required until at least 6 or 7 years because almost all will correct spontaneously. If correction is required, then the affected long bone is derotated by an osteotomy.

35 Principles of management of fractures, spinal injuries and peripheral nerve

Surgeons tend to forget that they are not masters but only servants. They can assist the natural powers within all living flesh but cannot replace them.

John Hunter

FRACTURES

A fracture is a break in the continuity of a bone, ranging from an incomplete hairline crack to a complete break with many fragments. The majority of fractures are the result of force applied to the bone. If the bone is weakened by a disease process it may appear to break spontaneously, although this is usually as a result of a minor, and often overlooked, injury (pathological fracture, see below). Fracture is also defined as a soft-tissue injury with a broken bone inside it, to emphasise the importance of the soft tissue envelope.

Classification

The shape of the fragments that result from a fracture are the outcome of the magnitude and direction of the damaging forces applied. Careful study of these forces allows them to be reversed at the time of reduction and also indicates the extent of associated soft-tissue damage. In consequence, it is necessary to have some idea of the mechanisms producing specific fracture types (Fig. 35.1).

Direct (localised) force applied to a bone often produces a *transverse* fracture at the point of impact with associated soft-tissue injury. Higher levels of direct energy or a crushing force produce a *comminuted* (multi-fragmentary) fracture, often with significant soft-tissue injury. Indirect forces, applied to the bone away from the fracture site, produce fragments which demonstrate the direction of force and may produce soft-tissue injuries distant to the fracture. A compression force usually produces a *short oblique* fracture while a twisting force produces a *spiral* or *long oblique* fracture. Bending forces frequently produce a fracture with a triangular ***'butterfly'*** fragment on the side of compression.

Specific types of fracture

Greenstick fractures

The bones of children are more yielding because they contain more connective tissue matrix and less mineral than those of adults. The resulting greenstick fracture is an incomplete break with buckling of the bone.

Crush fractures

Direct compression of cancellous bones may cause its trabeculae to collapse so that there is a crush fracture. Common sites include the os calcis and the vertebral bodies.

Open fractures

A closed (synonym: simple) fracture is not in contact with the exterior. By contrast, in an open (synonym: compound) fracture, there is a communication between the site of fracture and the surface of the body. Most often this is through a wound of the skin and subcutaneous tissues but it can also take place through a mucous membrane, such as in the perineum or skull. Open fractures are classified as shown in Table 35.1.

Pathological fractures

In a pathological fracture, the bone is weakened by disease. Often, it gives way after a trivial application of force such as might be encountered in normal activity. Any fracture occurring in such circumstances should prompt a search for a cause of the bone weakness. Common underlying causes are given in Table 35.2.

Fracture healing

Nearly all fractures can and will heal without surgical intervention. However, the surgeon harnesses the ability of the body for repair, and this requires a thorough knowledge of the mechanisms and course of fracture union. As with healing of a soft-tissue wound (Ch. 2), different stages in healing can be identified, but these form a continuum and blend into one another to varying degrees. They are summarised in Figure 35.2.

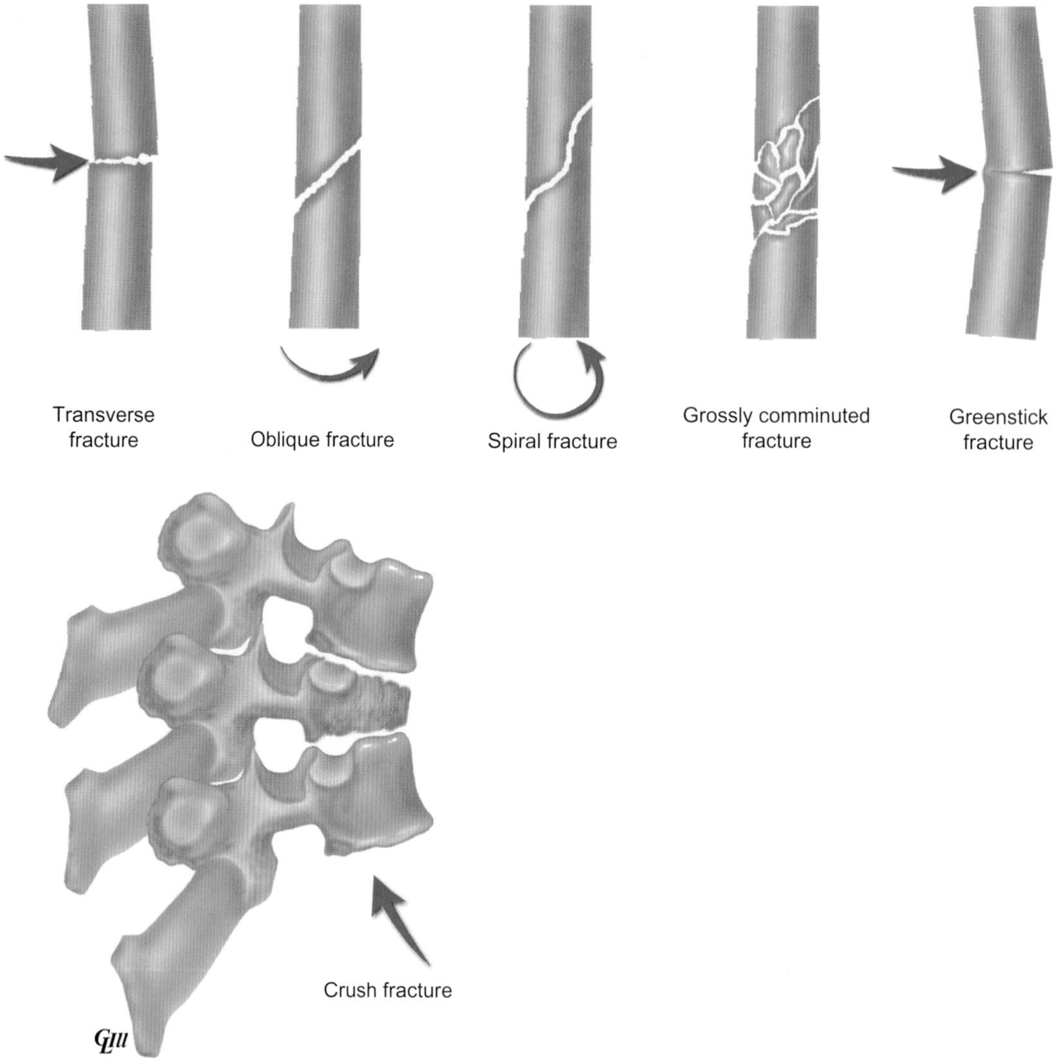

Fig. 35.1 Types of fracture and fragments produced.

Table 35.1 Classification of open (compound) fractures[a]

Type	Surface	Associations	Risk of wound infection
I	≤1 cm	Low velocity Minimal soft-tissue damage	0–2%
II	>1 cm	Low velocity Minimal soft-tissue damage	0–10%
III	Any size	High velocity or severe soft-tissue injury. Gross contamination as in military or agricultural injuries	>10%

Type III injuries are further subdivided into:
- IIIA – adequate cover of exposed bone still possible
- IIIB – wide periosteal stripping with possible devascularisation of bone
- IIIC – vascular (usually arterial) or nerve injury which requires repair.

[a]After Gustilo & Anderson.

Haematoma formation

A fracture tears blood vessels in the surrounding soft tissue, periosteum and medulla. A haematoma forms around and between the ends of the bone. Osteocytes in the fractured ends are deprived of nutrition, and local cell death occurs. If a fragment of bone becomes completely detached from its blood supply, it undergoes avascular necrosis.

Cellular proliferation and organisation (inflammatory phase)

The next stage is similar to that in healing soft tissues (see Ch. 2) – an acute inflammatory reaction with vasodilatation, plasma exudation and inward migration of acute inflammatory cells. The haematoma is replaced by granulation tissue with slender capillary loops in a loose connective tissue.

Table 35.2 Causes of pathological fracture

Class	Example
Congenital	Osteogenesis imperfecta
Infection	Chronic osteomyelitis
Metabolic	Osteoporosis Osteomalacia Hyperparathyroidism
Benign neoplasms	Bone cyst Enchondroma
Malignant neoplasms	Metastatic carcinoma (common are breast, kidney, prostate, thyroid, lung) Primary bone tumours (rare)
Other	Paget's disease of bone

Box 35.1 Assessment of union of a fracture

Clinical
- Absence of movement at the fracture site
- Little or no tenderness on direct pressure over the fracture site
- Little or no pain when the fracture site is stressed manually or by bearing weight through the limb

Radiological*
- Continuous callus seen spanning both sides of the fracture in 2 views

*Radiological evidence usually occurs a few weeks after clinical evidence.

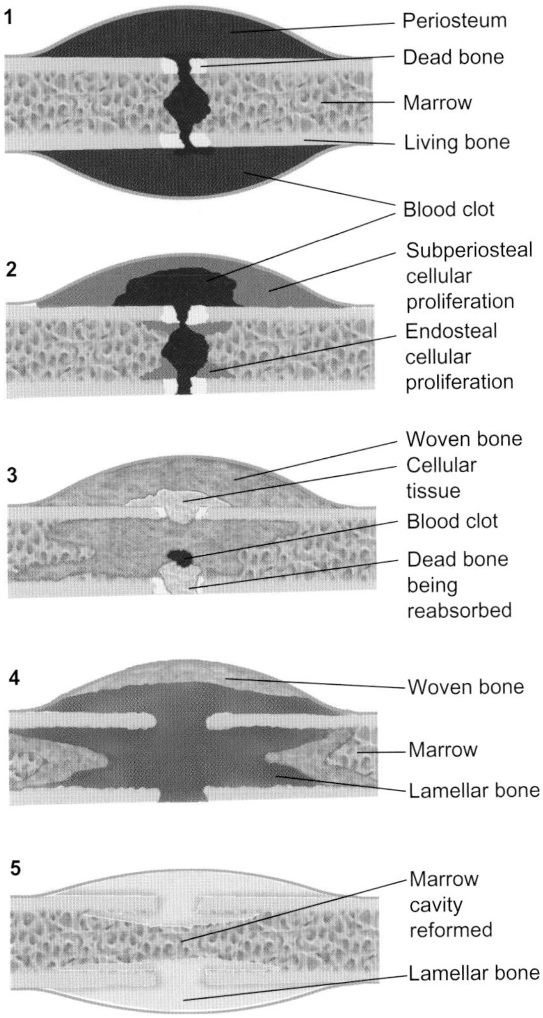

Fig. 35.2 Stages of fracture healing.

Formation of callus

Specialised cells invade the granulation tissue, including mesenchymal cells, fibroblasts and osteogenic precursor cells. These cells are derived from both local damaged tissue and the systemic circulation. The cells are stimulated to produce a randomly organised mass of fibrous tissue and cartilage, called *soft callus*, which provides an enveloping scaffold across the fracture, under the neighbouring periosteum and inside the medullary cavity. This callus is at first weak and flexible so that stressing the fracture at this stage is associated with some movement and pain. Soft callus is progressively replaced, from about 2 weeks onwards in a child and 3 weeks onwards in an adult long bone, by immature (or *woven*) bone, forming *hard callus*. With the progressive increase in hard callus, and thus mineral content, the callus becomes visible on radiographs and becomes increasingly stiff.

Union

Once both surfaces of a fracture are connected by callus strong enough to hold the bone rigidly, *union* is said to have occurred. The practical assessment of union is summarised in Box 35.1. When the fracture is regarded as having united, external immobilisation should be discarded and the limb rehabilitated. As a rough guide, external splintage needs to be maintained for 4–8 weeks for fractures in cancellous bones and 6–12 weeks for fractures in long bones in adults. Fractures in children heal in approximately half these times.

Consolidation and remodelling

In the months that follow, the immature woven bone is reorganised and replaced with mature, or *lamellar*, bone in a process called *consolidation*. This new bone is indistinguishable histologically from uninjured bone, with the bone laid down along lines of stress. Radiologically, the fracture line will be obliterated with clear bony trabeculae crossing it. The bone has returned to its original strength and the fracture is said to be consolidated. For several years later, the fusiform mass of healing bone is gradually removed and the bone's shape is further refined along its whole length in response to the normal stresses across it. This process, called *remodelling*, is most remarkable in children (Fig. 35.3).

Bony healing with callus formation does not always occur if a surgeon intervenes. The amount of callus produced is in direct response to the mobility of the fracture. Treatment options which give relative stability (see 'Immobilisation', below) will produce less callus than fractures left to heal naturally. The extreme of this occurs if the fracture is reduced and held rigidly with internal fixation; there is no movement and no gap for callus to fill. Instead, the bone heals by direct cortical healing, a process which resembles remodelling. The lack of callus formation can make radiological confirmation of union difficult.

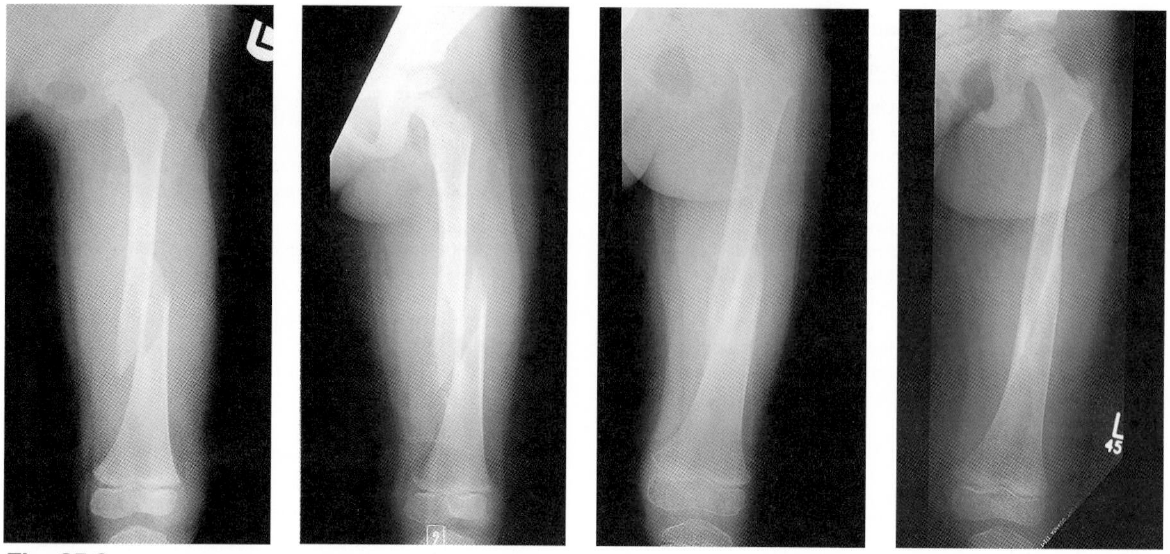

Fig. 35.3 Consolidation/remodelling of fracture site (left to right).

Clinical features

History

The history may throw light on the circumstances that led to the injury and the underlying causes. The following are of significance:

- An injury may have been caused by a simple mechanical fall but may be due to a fall secondary to a medical condition, such as cardiac or neurological problems.
- Fracture after trivial injury or stresses within the normal range of physical exertion may indicate a pathological fracture, requiring careful investigation.
- The way the injury was sustained should lead to a search for other skeletal injuries from the same cause; a fracture of the os calcis after a fall from a height may be accompanied by vertebral or hip injuries, and a knee injury in a front seat passenger in a head-on collision may be associated with a posterior dislocation of the hip.
- Time since injury should be ascertained as accurately as possible because of its association with complications such as infection in an open fracture or with ischaemia distal to a vascular injury.

Unless there is a neurological condition, a limb with a fracture is acutely painful and held as immobile as possible. However, there are circumstances in which a history cannot be obtained, such as unconsciousness or the overriding importance of other injuries; then the history of the injury obtained from others may be of importance.

Examination

- **Swelling** caused by haematoma formation and oedema is usually evident.
- **Deformity** is seen in displaced fractures and is described anatomically as displacement of the distal fragment with respect to the proximal, e.g. anterior or posterior. Varus and valgus are terms also used, but in descriptions of fractures these are best avoided.
- **Abnormal mobility** may be present but should be sought with gentleness.
- **Crepitus** is the grating sensation elicited on palpation as the broken ends of bone grind against each other with movement; it must not be deliberately elicited, as it causes intense pain.
- **Skin integrity** must always be assessed: abrasions or mild ischaemia may lead to later breakdown and infection of the fracture.
- **Vascular perfusion and neurological function** distal to the injury must be evaluated in all limb fractures. The presence of arterial pulses must be elicited and recorded. Sensation may be reduced in a glove and stocking manner in vascular insufficiency. Injury to peripheral nerves produces specific neurological deficiencies which must be tested for.
- **Pelvic fractures** may be associated with bladder and urethral injuries and disruption of the muscles of the pelvic floor. Examination for such accompanying injuries is essential.

Radiological investigation

If a fracture is suspected, radiographs in two planes at right angles to each other (usually anteroposterior and lateral views) are initially taken and should include the whole length of the fractured bone including the joint above and below. Only in this way can the full extent of the injury and the associated bone injuries be detected (Fig. 35.4).

In some circumstances, additional oblique or tangential views may be required. Computed tomography (CT) and magnetic resonance imaging (MRI) are valuable in the investigation of certain intra-articular fractures and specific fractures, such as of the pelvis and spine. Radioisotope bone scanning detects increased vascularity, which begins with the inflammatory phase of healing, and is useful in the diagnosis of fractures that are not immediately obvious on plain X-ray because of lack of displacement (e.g. fracture of the scaphoid).

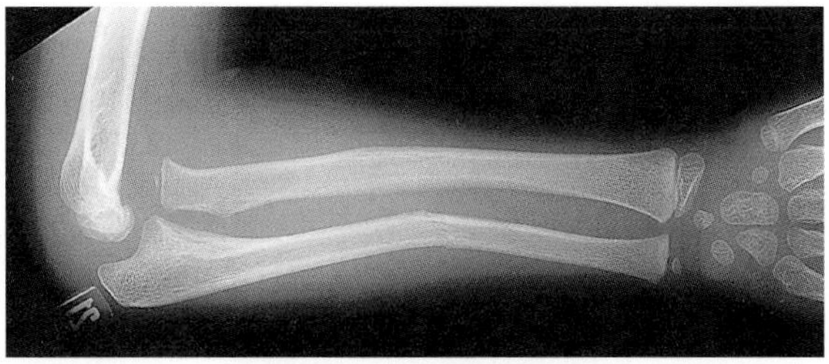

Fig. 35.4 Radiographic examination of a fracture. The X–ray is of a fracture of the ulna accompanied by anterior dislocation of the radial head at the elbow joint (Monteggia fracture–dislocation). The dislocation would not have been detected without an X-ray that included the elbow joint.

Box 35.2 Principles of fracture management: FRIAR

- First aid and management of the whole patient – always
- Reduction – if necessary
- Immobilisation – if necessary
- Active movement of injured limb – as much as possible
- Rehabilitation – always

Principles of management

The management of a patient with a fracture can be summarised by the mnemonic FRIAR (Box 35.2).

First aid and management of the whole patient

Patients who have suffered violence sufficient to fracture part of their skeleton often have injuries to other systems, some which may be life-threatening. In the management of such multiply injured patients, priority should be given to the ABCs – Airway maintenance, Breathing and Circulation. The matter is considered in more detail in Chapter 3. Pain relief is also important and is discussed in Chapter 6.

Reduction

Reduction is the manipulation of the fractured bone to restore normal anatomy. In diaphyseal fractures it is to restore length, alignment and rotation and in intra-articular fractures to restore normal anatomy and perfect congruence of joint. Some fractures do not require reduction either because deformity is not present or because its nature is immaterial to the final functional result (e.g. many displaced clavicle fractures heal without functional deficit).

Closed reduction

This is the preferred initial method. It can be carried out under general anaesthesia, regional anaesthesia or, in some instances, after injection of anaesthetic into the fracture haematoma. Reduction is achieved by:

- longitudinal traction which disimpacts any interlocked fragments
- reversal of the forces that caused deformity.

Reduction must be confirmed by radiography.

Mechanical traction

This method may be used to gradually reduce fractures, such as of the spine or of the femur. The weight pulling on the fracture gradually overcomes the tension in the surrounding muscles and straightens the bone.

Open reduction

Open reduction by operation is necessary when:

- closed reduction fails
- very accurate reduction is required, e.g. a fracture which involves a joint surface
- the fracture has caused a vascular or (sometimes) a nerve injury.

The injured limb is opened surgically and the fracture manipulated under direct vision. It is then usually stabilised by internal fixation (see below).

Immobilisation

A fracture is held in reduction to:

- relieve pain
- prevent redisplacement of the fragments
- avoid shearing movements at the fracture site which damage the delicate capillaries in callus and consequently interfere with the process of union.

Immobilisation is not always necessary, e.g. in fractures of the ribs or metatarsals. In some other injuries, relatively rigid immobilisation is essential if union is to occur, e.g. the shaft of the ulna.

The methods of immobilisation are summarised in Box 35.3.

Box 35.3 Methods of immobilisation of fractures

- External splints
  - casts made of plaster of Paris or synthetic resins
  - specially designed splints
- Continuous traction
  - applied to the distal fragment by skeletal pin or adhesive tape applied to the skin
- Internal fixation
  - screws, plates and pins inserted at open operation
- External fixation
  - a rigid bridging device held in place by bone pins either side of the fracture

External splints

Casts made from plaster of Paris (POP) or synthetic resins are, in most circumstances, the standard method. POP is commercially available as bandages coated with hemihydrated calcium sulphate which reacts with water to form a solid cast. Newer synthetic-resin materials are available which are stronger and lighter, but they are more expensive and harder to apply.

When applying an external cast, a layer of cellulose padding is placed deep to the cast to prevent the plaster from sticking to the hairs and skin and to allow for expansion from swelling at the fracture site. Initial immobilisation should not be by completely encircling the limb; continued swelling within a rigid cast can lead to ischaemia distal to the fracture site – compartment syndrome (see below). In consequence, casts used on a newly injured limb are applied either as a slab on one aspect only held in place by a crepe bandage or as a cylinder which is then immediately split longitudinally.

Immobilisation of the adjacent joints above and below is usually necessary to stabilise a fracture managed in a cast but increases the risk of disuse muscle atrophy and joint stiffness. Any form of immobilisation inevitably causes some muscle atrophy and joint stiffness. The splint must be discarded as soon as union of the fracture is deemed to have occurred. In some long bone fractures, a hinge may be inserted in the splint (functional bracing) as union progresses.

Continuous traction

This method is used when it is difficult to hold the bone reduced with an external splint because the fracture site is surrounded by soft tissue and/or because of absence of bony points above and below which can be used to gain purchase. Typical examples are fractures of the shaft of the femur and of the lower humerus. Traction of up to 2 kg may be applied with longitudinal adhesive strapping applied to the skin (skin traction) but a careful watch must be kept for skin damage, especially in the elderly and in patients on steroids. If more force is required, traction may be exerted through a pin inserted into the bone distal to the fracture site (skeletal traction). The pin site must be kept clean to prevent infection tracking down to the bone.

Continuous traction confines the patient to bed and thus increases the risk of pressure sores, chest infection, disuse osteoporosis and other problems. It is therefore usually only used as a temporary measure until formal, usually surgical, immobilisation can be performed.

Internal fixation

Internal fixation by open operation is used to secure reduction, to ensure it is maintained and to allow earlier mobility of the patient (Fig. 35.5). The advantages of earlier return of function, shorter hospital stay and quicker resumption of work or of pre-injury style of life have to be weighed against the risks of neurovascular damage, infection and of delaying healing by devascularisation of the bone. Unless the surgical team is experienced, closed means are preferable for simple fractures. Internal fixation is strongly indicated in patients with:

- multiple injuries
- pathological fractures
- associated neurovascular injury
- fractures where accurate reduction is required (e.g. those involving joints)
- the need to avoid a long period of immobilisation in bed, e.g. an elderly patient with a fracture of the femur.

External fixation

This is mainly used in the management of open or infected fractures (see 'Open fractures', below). Pins are inserted through the skin into the fragments of bone and fixed rigidly to an external device such as a metal bar (Fig. 35.6). The skin overlying the fracture site can be dressed or grafted without disturbing the fracture.

Observation

In the early stages after reduction and immobilisation, careful and repeated observation is required to detect insufficient distal blood supply or a neurological injury. A tightly applied circular dressing which becomes soaked with blood and then dries may similarly impair the circulation (see also 'Compartment syndrome'). Suggestive features include:

- persistent or increasing pain
- paraesthesia or tingling in digits
- sluggish capillary return
- cyanosis distal to the fracture (late finding)
- absent pulses (late).

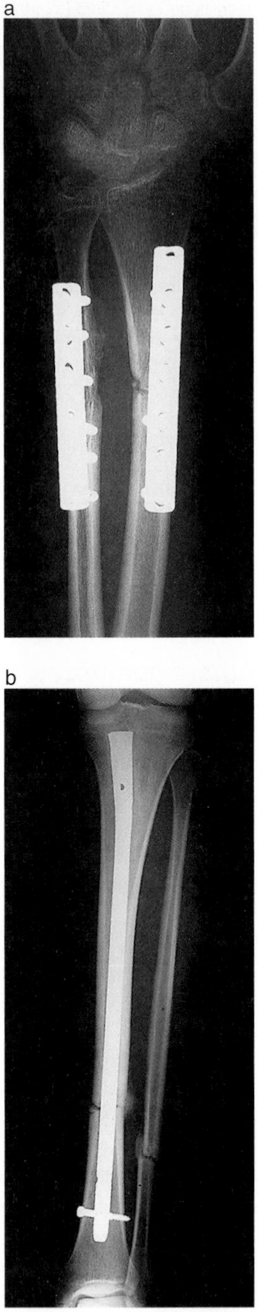

Fig. 35.5 Open reduction and fixation. (a) Plate and screw fixation to the distal third of both radius and ulna. (b) Intramedullary nail fixation of a fracture of the distal third of the tibia.

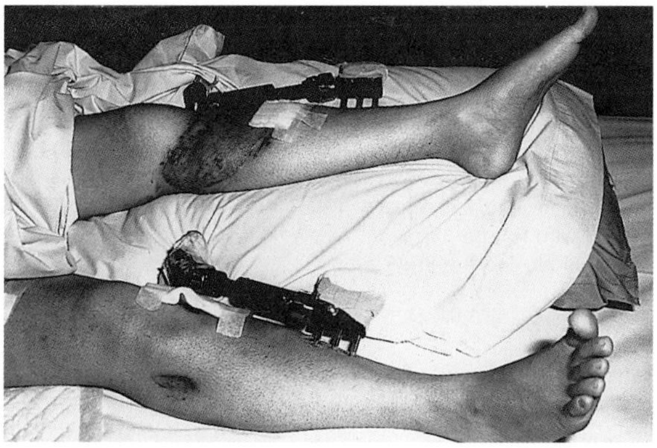

Fig. 35.6 External fixation and management of type III open fracture.

Any of these requires removal of all dressings, external splints and casts so that the fracture site can be inspected and necessary remedial action undertaken.

Active movement and rehabilitation

Rehabilitation starts immediately after treatment. The patient is asked to move the injured part as much as the method of fixation allows. This helps to:

- stimulate union
- decrease disuse osteoporosis
- prevent muscle atrophy
- minimise joint stiffness.

All external splints are removed as soon as there is clinical evidence of union, and the patient is started on a supervised programme of active exercises to restore function (physiotherapy and/or occupational therapy).

Open fractures

The communication of a fracture with the surface is a pathway along which bacteria can contaminate the fracture site and produce infection. Once bone is infected with pyogenic organisms, the inflammation tends to become chronic, especially if foreign material has been carried into the fracture site at the time of injury. Infection delays and may prevent union and, with some virulent infections such as clostridia (Ch. 9), may cause death. Open fractures are surgical emergencies and also represent significant soft-tissue damage where blood supply is also compromised, affecting healing potential.

For first aid in all open injuries of bone, the wound is covered with a sterile dressing soaked in normal saline or aqueous iodine. Parenteral broad-spectrum antibiotic therapy is begun at once and attention paid to tetanus prophylaxis.

In all open fractures, surgical debridement of the wound with removal of all devitalised tissue and foreign material as soon as possible is essential to prevent sepsis. If treatment on these lines is undertaken within 12 hours of injury, the incidence of sepsis is low. Therefore, internal fixation may be done safely by experienced surgeons operating in ideal conditions. In certain type III fractures, external trauma causes extensive skin and muscle damage, often with associated injuries to vessels and nerves. The incidence of sepsis is high, and internal fixation is usually avoided in the first instance. After debridement of the wound, external fixation (Fig. 35.6) and repair of neurovascular structures is usually followed by many staged procedures to achieve skin cover. In the most severe of those injuries (a limb that has been avascular for more than 6 hours or one that has been severely crushed), an amputation both saves life and avoids a long period of invalidity which may have considerable psychological effects.

Box 35.4 Complications of fracture

Early

Local

- Infection
- Haemorrhage
- Injury to other structures – arteries, nerves and viscera
- Skin necrosis
- Deep vein thrombosis
- Compartment syndrome

Systemic

- Hypovolaemic shock
- Fat embolism
- Effects of prolonged immobilisation – chest infection, pressure sores, pulmonary embolism

Late (delayed)

Local

- Malunion
- Delayed union
- Non-union
- Muscle wasting
- Joint stiffness
- Osteoarthritis
- Delayed tendon rupture
- Tardy nerve palsy
- Reflex sympathetic dystrophy
- Myositis ossificans

Systemic

- Osteoporosis
- Changes in lifestyle and psychological state

Complications

In the great majority of fractures union proceeds according to expectation and function is fully restored. Complications do, however, occur and may be considered in two groups: early or delayed. In both, effects may be local or systemic (Box 35.4).

Infection

This can occur in open fractures or in closed fractures treated by operation.

Haemorrhage

Haemorrhage from the bone marrow, periosteum and surrounding soft tissues may not be immediately clinically obvious but can be considerable and cause significant reduction in blood volume. As a general rule, blood loss from adult fractures may be estimated as:

- pelvis: 2–3 L
- femur: 1–2 L
- tibia or humerus: 0.5–1 L.

Patients with open or pathological fractures bleed more profusely. Multiple fractures produce cumulative losses which,

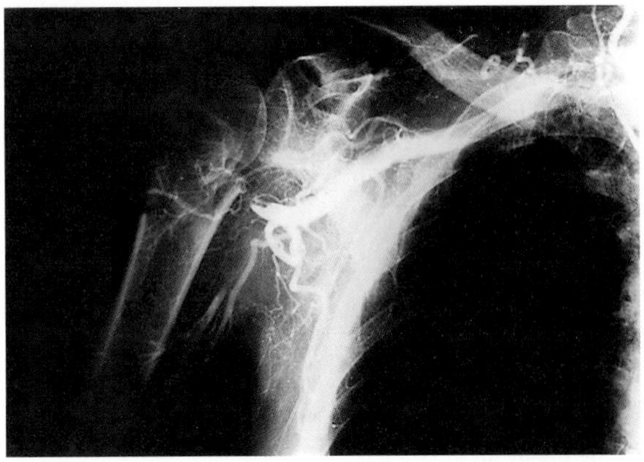

Fig. 35.7 Vascular injury as a consequence of fracture. A fracture of the surgical neck of the humerus has produced a spike that has injured the distal axillary artery, occlusion of which is shown on the arteriogram.

if unrecognised, are sufficient to cause hypovolaemic shock, which is a possible but preventable cause of death.

Arterial and venous injury

This can occur in penetrating injuries such as a gunshot wound or from a spike of bone (Fig. 35.7). All types of injury occur. Some bony injuries are commonly associated with vascular damage – supracondylar fractures of the humerus contuse the brachial artery, and 50% of knee dislocations give rise to an intimal tear in the popliteal artery.

Distal ischaemia may lead to:

- nerve and muscle necrosis
- total limb death with gangrene, necessitating amputation.

The first line of treatment is to reposition the limb so as to correct gross deformity and remove all occlusive dressings. This may solve the problem but, if the signs of ischaemia do not disappear within 15 minutes, surgical intervention is necessary.

Deep venous thrombosis and pulmonary embolism

These are common sequelae to many fractures, particularly in the elderly, and are discussed in Chapter 30.

Nerve damage

Nerve palsies are common after high-energy-transfer (violent) injuries, and nerves are particularly vulnerable in fracture–dislocations. The common associations are given in Table 35.3.

Compartment syndrome

This condition arises because the muscles, vessels and nerves in limbs are held within inelastic osseofascial compartments. Bleeding from a fracture increases the intracompartmental pressure and occludes the venous outflow and hence capillary inflow. The cells first become hypoxic and then swell. There is further rise in intracompartmental pressure and a vicious circle of hypoxia and further swelling ensues. The clinical features are summarised in Box 35.5.

Table 35.3 Nerve injuries frequently associated with fractures and dislocations

Fracture	Nerve injury
Dislocation of the shoulder	Axillary nerve (30%)
Shaft of humerus	Radial (20%)
Injuries around the elbow	Median, ulnar
Dislocation of the hip	Sciatic (20%)
Injuries around the knee	Common peroneal

Box 35.5 Clinical features of compartment syndrome

Early symptoms
- Increasing pain
- Paraesthesia
- Paresis

Early signs
- Pain on passive stretching of the muscle groups in the compartment
- Palpably tense compartment
- Pulses usually normal because arteries traversing the compartment are resistant to a rise in pressure within it

Late symptoms
- Numbness
- Paralysis

Late signs
- Muscle contracture
- Anaesthesia
- Absence of arterial pulses

It is vital that compartment syndrome is detected early, well before the late signs and symptoms occur. Early detection is mainly clinical as seen by pain over and above that which can be explained by the injured part, stretch pain and a tense compartment. An intracompartmental pressure which differs from diastolic pressure by 30 mmHg or less is sufficient to impede capillary inflow, and irreversible damage to nerves and muscles occurs within a matter of 4–6 hours. The skin overlying the compartment is unaffected, but a disabling contracture of the damaged muscles (Volkmann's ischaemic contracture) may result as a late sequelae.

Because of the risks of compartment syndrome, pain relief in fractures by the use of local nerve blocks is not recommended, as this may mask its early features. Vigilance in detection and prompt treatment are both vital. When a compartment syndrome is suspected, any cast and all dressings are removed. If symptoms do not improve immediately, the compartment is surgically decompressed by division of the overlying skin and fascia (open fasciotomy).

Fat embolism

This is more common in patients with multiple fractures but may follow minor trauma. Its cause is not known: either fat from the marrow of the fractured bone enters the circulation and clogs capillaries or some as-yet unidentified factor causes chylomicrons in the bloodstream to aggregate. In either event, large fat globules are present in the bloodstream – on the right side of the heart in the pulmonary circulation and, perhaps aided by a subclinical patent foramen ovale, on the arterial side in the brain and skin. Clinically, a few days after injury the patient becomes increasingly confused, and develops tachypnoea and mild pyrexia. Skin petechiae may be seen, and laboratory investigations usually reveal a reduced PO_2 and thrombocytopenia. Fat globules may be detected in the urine. Maintenance of oxygenation is of paramount importance and may require intubation and ventilatory support.

Pressure sores (decubitus ulcers)

Sores occurring as a result of necrosis of skin over the heel, sacrum, ischium and hips are a real risk in patients confined to bed because of skeletal injury (or for other reasons), especially in the debilitated, the elderly and those with spinal cord injury. Prevention is by good nursing care and early mobilisation.

Malunion

This follows imperfect reduction or redisplacement after satisfactory reduction and leads to cosmetic deformity and loss of function (Fig. 35.8). It is prevented by satisfactory primary management but, if established, may require complex corrective procedures.

Delayed union

Union is said to be delayed if the fracture has not united clinically or radiologically at a time when this would have been expected. The fracture may still continue to heal slowly until it unites and, provided there are not any adverse factors which require correction, a watching policy is adopted while making sure that optimum conditions for continued healing are present.

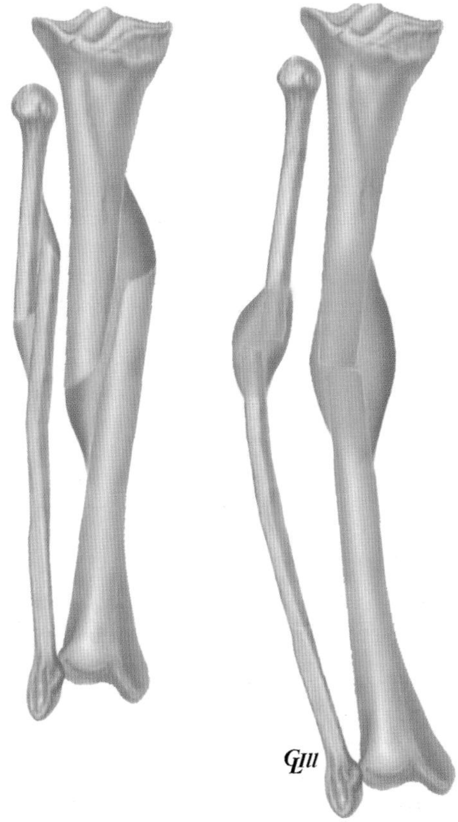

Fig. 35.8 Malunion.

Non-union

This is diagnosed when healing has come to a halt before union has occurred (Fig. 35.9). Two broad types of exist: *hypertrophic non-union* and *atrophic non-union.* In hypertrophic cases the body has tried to heal the fracture but either too much movement is occurring between the bone ends or the bone ends are not in close contact. As a result the callus formed cannot bridge the gap. Radiographs show florid callus formation either side of the fracture but none bridging the gap. In atrophic non-union the body has not attempted to heal the fracture, commonly due to a lack of blood supply or infection. Radiologically the fracture edges have died back and there is little or no evidence of callus formation.

The borderline between delayed union and non-union is often difficult to define, although the differentiation may be important for both the patient and the surgeon. Management is often complex and inevitably requires surgical intervention. In hypertrophic cases, more rigid (usually internal) fixation is required without excessive disturbance of the fracture; in atrophic non-union a direct operation on the fracture site is indicated with removal of sclerotic bone to increase the blood supply, bone grafting and rigid fixation.

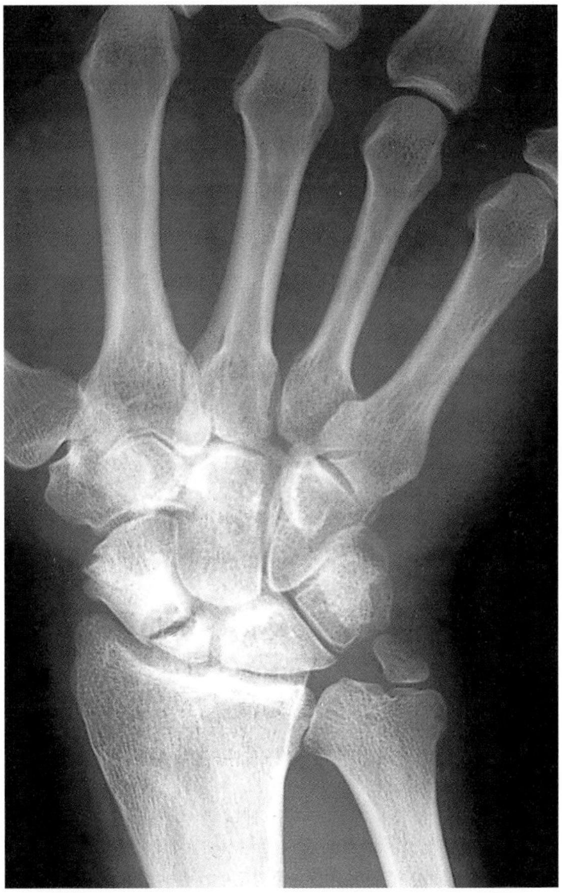

Fig. 35.9 Non-union. This fracture of the scaphoid has failed to unite. There is a radiological gap between the fragments which can be assumed to be filled with fibrous tissue. There is some, although not much, evidence of sclerosis.

Complex regional pain syndrome (CRPS) Type 1

This condition, otherwise known as reflex sympathetic dystrophy or Sudecks's atrophy, presents at intervals of days or weeks after injury as:

- disproportionate pain
- abnormal sensations (dysaesthesia)
- joint stiffness
- thickening of the soft tissues
- abnormal sweating
- loss of hair at the site of injury.

The hand, which is most commonly affected, is characteristically swollen, discoloured, painful, and exquisitely sensitive to touch. Tight plasters, bandages or splints, inactivity and dependence of the limb are common factors. The condition is largely preventable by holding the wrist and the digits in positions of function, by elevation of the part and by early active exercises. Use of the part is essential in treatment. There is a possible role for the post-ganglionic sympathetic efferent fibres in some cases.

Myositis ossificans

This is heterotopic bone forming in the muscles around a fracture or injured joint. Movement is often restricted and painful. The most common site is the elbow, and the cause is possibly too early and too vigorous joint movement.

Fractures which involve articular surfaces

If accurate reduction to obtain congruent surfaces is not achieved and maintained, secondary osteoarthritis can develop. Open reduction and internal rigid fixation are thus indicated. Early joint movement should be encouraged to reduce stiffness and (possibly) to promote the healing of articular cartilage.

Fractures in children

The bones of children are more flexible, and incomplete fractures of the greenstick type (see Fig. 35.1) are common. Turnover of bone is more active in children, so that union occurs in approximately half the time taken in adult fractures.

Remodelling in the plane of movement of the joints after a shaft fracture is usually so perfect that eventually the site is indistinguishable in radiographs (see Fig. 35.3). However, remodelling is incomplete in many situations, such as in varus or valgus deformities of the elbow and in rotational deformities of the forearm, and accurate reduction should be sought in these cases.

Epiphyseal displacement

The growth plate (physis) between the epiphysis and metaphysis provides a relatively weak area which is often involved when forces are concentrated near the ends of the bone. Damage to the growth plate may result in arrest of growth and subsequent deformity. Accurate reduction is necessary.

Non-accidental injury (battering)

This condition is part of child abuse and regrettably common. Suspicious features include a delay to take the child to hospital, inadequate or inappropriate explanation of the injury, multiple bruises of differing ages, non-accidental burns and radiological evidence of previous injuries. A paediatrician should be involved from the outset.

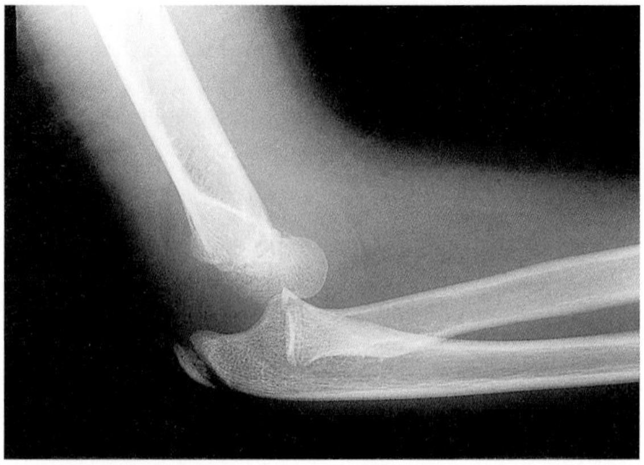

Fig. 35.10 Dislocation of the elbow. There is complete loss of joint apposition.

JOINT INJURIES

In dislocation (luxation) there is complete loss of contact of the articular joint surfaces (Fig. 35.10), and in subluxation there is partial loss of contact. Either may be combined with a fracture.

The clinical features are the same as those of a fracture:

- pain
- deformity
- loss of function.

The diagnosis is confirmed by radiographs in two planes. The integrity of the surrounding nerves and vessels must be assessed clinically because of the relatively high incidence of associated damage. In addition, time factors are important: the risk of avascular necrosis of the femoral head after a traumatic posterior dislocation of the hip is directly proportional to the time interval between dislocation and reduction. Dislocations are therefore surgical emergencies. Treatment is usually by closed reduction; open reduction is rarely required.

SPINAL INJURIES

Damage to the bony and ligamentous structures of the vertebral column as well as to the enclosed neural elements may occur in spinal injuries. During management it is important to prevent further injury, particularly to the spinal cord. For this purpose, spinal injuries are classified into two types:

- **stable** – the vertebral components will not be displaced by normal movements; an undamaged cord is not in danger

- **unstable** – further displacement and damage to the cord may result from movement.

As in long bone fractures, the mechanism of injury may often produce particular injury types. For example, flexion injuries produce a crush fracture to the anterior vertebral body which is usually stable while axial compression may crush the entire vertebral body, often resulting in an unstable fracture. More complex injuries result from combined forces, and may result in fracture–dislocations. Cord injury without either fracture or dislocation may occur in the more elastic tissues of children or in the spondylitic spine of the elderly.

Clinical features

History

Suspicion of instability of the spine may be aroused from the mechanism of injury and, in a conscious patient, by complaints of pain, decreased muscle power and/or sensation and paraesthesiae. An unconscious accident victim should always be assumed to have a spinal injury until proven otherwise.

Physical findings

Injuries to the neurological elements may be complete or incomplete; accurate neurological diagnosis is essential because recovery is more likely if some residual sensation or movement is detectable in the affected area.

Complete neurological lesions

Complete neurological injury, such as a transection of the cord, causes complete permanent motor paralysis below the level of injury, with corresponding loss of sensation. It must be remembered that the level of the bony spinal injury may not correspond with the level of the neurological injury.

Injuries to the lumbar vertebrae will damage only the cauda equina and nerve roots and produce:

- flaccid paralysis and eventual wasting of the leg muscles
- loss of sensation in the lower limbs
- variable effects on the bowel and bladder, including loss of reflexes which initiate micturition and defecation tone.

Complete lesions in the thoracic region result in paraplegia (spastic paralysis of the legs) with:

- reflex spasms
- loss of sensation distal to the lesion
- no voluntary control of bladder, bowel and sexual function, although automatic function is ultimately established.

Injuries to the cervical region lead to quadriplegia with:

- partial or complete involvement of the arms and hands
- similar effects on organ function to paraplegia.

High cervical lesions also lead to:

- phrenic nerve paralysis associated with respiratory failure which may cause immediate or later death
- loss of the potential for an independent life.

Incomplete neurological lesions

These may be the consequence of:

- partial transection
- oedema and bleeding in relation to a spinal fracture or fracture–dislocation.

It is obviously of great importance to recognise that a lesion is incomplete in that efforts to prevent further injury must be rigorous. Although the neurological patterns may be complex, the preservation of any function distal to the established site of injury is an important initial finding; every care must be taken to preserve it. More-detailed neurological analysis can follow later.

Investigation

Accurate imaging is essential. A frequent mistake is not to image the C7/T1 junction clearly, a common site for injury between the mobile cervical and the more-fixed thoracic vertebrae and also a difficult area to show on X-rays. If one fracture is found, the whole spine from the craniocervical junction to the lumbosacral articulation should be examined radiologically, as further fractures occur in 7% of patients.

CT scanning may help visualize specific areas more clearly, demonstrate the extent of injury to the neural arch and the amount of bony neural canal impingement. MRI (Fig. 35.11) outlines the extent of spinal cord compression by bone or intervertebral disc and the type of injury that the cord has sustained, such as oedema or haemorrhage.

Management

Management must start at the scene of the accident and may make the difference between recovery or lifelong paralysis. Paramedical staff are trained to apply rigid spinal support and to move patients only in a way that does not threaten further damage. The same must be the case for the surgical team.

Spinal shock

Immediately after a severe spinal injury, a transient depression of all reflex activity is superimposed on the local neural damage due to cord concussion. There is a flaccid paralysis of all the distally supplied muscles and loss of all reflexes.

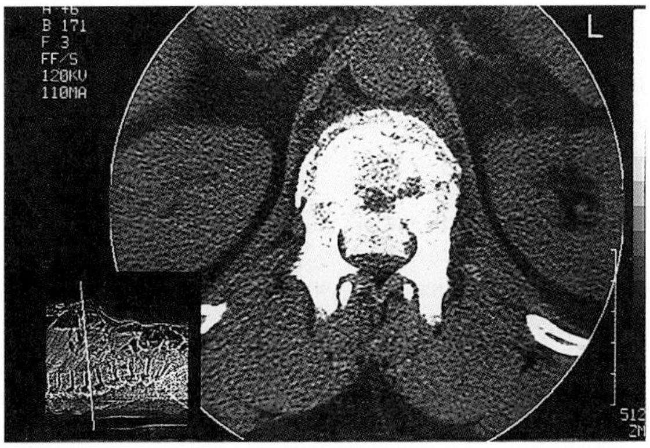

Fig. 35.11 MRI of spinal cord compression. The image is viewed from below, and the posterior aspect of the spine is below. There is a filling defect which is compressing the spinal cord by about a third.

Recovery from spinal shock usually occurs within 24–72 hours and is first evident in men by return of the bulbocavernosus reflex (contraction of the external anal sphincter on stimulation of the glans penis). Identifying the end of spinal shock is important as further improvement in neurological function after this time is minimal.

Neurogenic shock

High thoracic or cervical injuries, resulting in transaction of the sympathetic pathways, may cause systemic vasodilatation, resulting in hypotension and paradoxical bradycardia. This is due to the unopposed parasympathetic action of the vagus nerve. Although hypovolaemic shock is far more common in the trauma situation, the presence of unexplained bradycardia in the shocked patient should be identified, as it may indicate a significant spinal injury and management of the shock will be modified.

Concomitant injuries

Management of other life-threatening conditions, such as head, chest or abdominal trauma, must take precedence over the definitive management of the spinal injury. Reduction of displaced vertebrae is necessary to achieve bony alignment and decrease the distortion of the neural elements and their blood supply and can be achieved either by traction or by operation. Patients with incomplete lesions of the cord and fractures where the bone segments, vertebral disc or a haematoma within the vertebral canal narrow it by more than 50% do better if the canal is surgically decompressed early; the potential for recovery can be significant.

General management

Skin

Rigorous attention must be given to the skin that is anaesthetic in an immobile limb. Alteration of position every 2 hours, cleanliness and avoidance of minor trauma are the best ways of avoiding pressure sores.

Bladder

Initially in spinal shock there is acute retention and this should be relieved as soon as possible. Later, bladder 'training' is by intermittent catheterisation which ultimately results in micturition which can be predicted on the basis of time. A few patients may need a permanent indwelling urethral catheter.

Bowel

Attention to diet and the use of aperients are started as early as possible.

Joint contractures

These must be prevented by regular physiotherapy, and spasms can be controlled by skeletal muscle relaxants such as baclofen.

Mobilisation and fixation

If the injury is confirmed to be stable, early mobilisation with appropriate orthotics is undertaken. Those with unstable injuries can be treated either by 6–12 weeks' bed rest or by rigid fixation of the fracture to facilitate nursing and allow earlier rehabilitation.

Rehabilitation

Return of the patient into society is best carried out by a multidisciplinary team working in a spinal injuries unit, and it is now feasible for most patients to achieve an independent and fulfilling life.

PERIPHERAL NERVE INJURIES

Transection of a major nerve trunk causes severe disability from paralysis, loss of sensation and sometimes pain. If untreated, atrophy and deformity of the injured part follow.

Pathological features

The axons of peripheral nerves are cytoplasmic extensions of cell bodies located in the dorsal root ganglia (sensory) or the ventral horn of the spinal cord (motor). They are composed of axoplasm surrounded by a cell membrane. The axons are themselves enclosed in the sheath formed by Schwann cells and may or may not contain myelin. The peripheral nerves contain motor fibres (to end plates in skeletal muscle), sensory fibres (from organs and endings in skin, muscle, tendon and joint) and autonomic fibres (postganglionic sympathetic fibres) controlling the smooth muscle in blood vessels, sweat glands and in the hair follicles.

Types of injury

Neurotmesis

This is division of a nerve trunk, and it causes well-defined changes both proximally and distally. Proximally, the axons die back for a distance of about 2 cm and the cell body enlarges with increase in RNA and protein. Sprouting of the divided axon at the division may be evident within a day. Distally, Wallerian degeneration occurs with lysis of axoplasm and fragmentation of myelin sheaths. If the nerve is not repaired, no recovery will occur. If the ends of the nerve are apposed, regenerating axons grow into the empty Schwann cell sheath at a rate of approximately 1 mm/day. However, haphazard matching of axonal sprouts with distal sensory receptors and motor units is inevitable. Recovery is therefore almost always incomplete. If the nerve ends are not in contact, the regenerating axons mingle with proliferating Schwann cells and fibroblasts to form a tangled mass – a neuroma – which may be painful.

When the orderly sequence of regrowth into the distal stump is not achieved, with the passage of time the activity of the sprouting neurons diminishes, the distal endoneural tubes narrow and the brain forgets how to use the limb. The diagnosis and repair of nerve injuries are, consequently, a matter of urgency.

Axonotmesis

In this type of injury there is damage to axons but the Schwann cell sheath remains intact. It may, for example, occur from traction on a nerve. Common examples of axonotmesis include many cases of radial palsy after fracture of shaft of humerus. Because the axon is disrupted, Wallerian degeneration occurs, but the potential for recovery is greater than in neurotmesis, as the sprouting neurons do not have to bridge a gap in their sheaths. If the cause is removed, good recovery takes place with time and nerve repair is not required.

Neurapraxia

In this type of injury, there is a physiological block to conduction but the axon is in anatomical continuity. A contusion is one cause – striking the ulnar nerve behind the medial epicondyle to cause the well-known 'funny elbow' is a good example. Function is temporarily absent, but Wallerian degeneration does not take place and, if the cause is removed, recovery is rapid.

The classification given above into neurotmesis, axonotmesis and neurapraxia (described by Seddon) is useful, but it is important to realise that demarcation between different types is not always clear-cut in the individual case.

Clinical features

Early recognition and prompt management of a nerve injury give the patient the best chance of restoring function.

History

After a fracture or dislocation, or any penetrating injury that might conceivably have passed close to a nerve, the history should include specific questions about distal anaesthesia or loss of motor function, because these may not be appreciated by the patient who is more concerned with the bony or soft-tissue injury.

Physical findings

A neurological examination for function of the nerves in the vicinity of all fractures, dislocations and lacerations must be done. The commonest reason for failing to detect a nerve injury is failure to suspect one and make a complete assessment. The critical step is to distinguish between non-degenerative and degenerative lesions.

Non-degenerative lesions (neurapraxia). Some sensation, e.g. for deep pressure, usually persists. Autonomic function – vasomotor and sudomotor control – is also usually intact. The nerve trunk distal to the injury continues to conduct because the axons beyond the injury are still nourished, and this can be established by electrodiagnostic testing. Spontaneous pain is uncommon.

Degenerative lesions. These follow axonotmesis or neurotmesis and cause a complete loss of all nerve function, including vasomotor and sudomotor control. In consequence, the skin innervated by the damaged nerve is red and dry. The nerve trunk distal to the injury conducts impulses only for the first 3 weeks until Wallerian degeneration has occurred.

The difficulty lies in distinguishing between axonotmesis and neurotmesis. Only time or exposure of the nerve will ultimately be diagnostic. Where a fracture or dislocation has been caused by more than a moderate degree of violence and where there has been wide displacement of the skeletal fragments, then absence of function is assumed to be from rupture of the relevant nerve trunk. Similarly, where a laceration is present over the nerve or a surgeon has been operating in the vicinity, loss of function must be assumed to be from division.

Management

It is better to explore too soon (even if the nerve is found to be intact) than too late. However, life-threatening injuries to the head, chest and abdomen take priority over nerve repair.

Nerve repair

The ideal nerve repair should be performed as a primary procedure in an uncontaminated wound by an experienced surgeon and in an operating room with high-quality equipment and lighting. In contaminated wounds, repair is postponed for 3–4 weeks until either the wound is healed or infection has been controlled.

Primary repair is the suture of nerve stumps before a neuroma has had time to form, usually up to 2 weeks after the injury. It gives the best results.

Secondary repair is the later suture of nerve stumps in which a neuroma has formed and requires resection. It is done after any initial wound has healed and oedema and joint stiffness have resolved.

Nerve grafting is required when nerve tissue has been destroyed over a distance that makes direct repair impossible without tension. Nerves commonly used are the sural and the medial cutaneous nerve of the forearm which can be autotransplanted without significant loss of sensation.

Nerve transfer is sometimes indicated. For example, a fascicle from the ulnar nerve may be transferred into the stump of an irreparably damaged musculocutaneous nerve to restore biceps function, and the body learns to use this pathway.

Assessment of recovery

'Tinel's sign' is valuable in the clinical detection of progress. Tinel's sign indicates regenerating axons and it is not present in cases of neurapraxia (conduction block). Percussion along the course of a nerve from distal to proximal elicits painful paraesthesia when the area of regeneration is reached. Tinel's sign is initially at the level of injury and advances distally with time. Rehabilitation should be started while recovery is awaited; the range of joint movement should be preserved and the anaesthetic skin protected.

Prognosis

The outcome of nerve repair depends on:

- age
- delay between injury and repair
- type of lesion – a clean cut has a better prognosis than a crush injury, which in turn is better than a traction injury. Injuries associated with vascular injuries have a very poor prognosis
- nerve type
- size of the gap to be bridged
- surgical skill.

The two most important factors are the violence of injury, which defines the extent of damage to the nerve, and delay between injury and repair.

Table 35.4 Classification of the obstetric brachial plexus palsy[a]

Group	Nerves injured	Extent of paralysis	Natural course
I	C5, C6	Shoulder, elbow flexion	>90% recover completely
II	C5, C6, C7	Shoulder, elbow, wrist extension	70% recover completely
III	C5, C6, C7, C8, T1	Complete	50% recover completely. Residual defects usually affect the shoulder
IV	C5, C6, C7, C8, T1 with Horner's sign	Complete	Few recover completely. 50% regain useful hand function
Over 65% of all cases fall into Groups I and II			

[a]After Narakas.

BRACHIAL PLEXUS INJURIES

Aetiology

Brachial plexus injuries are amongst the most severe of all peripheral nerve lesions. They are usually caused by high-energy-transfer injuries, as in high-speed motorcycle accidents when there is violent distraction of forequarter from the trunk. Open wounds from bullets and other missiles or from knife attacks are increasingly seen. There are about 500 new cases every year in the UK. Life-threatening injuries to head, chest or abdomen are seen in 10%; the spine and spinal cord may be damaged in about 2%; there are fractures or fracture dislocations of long bones in 50%; the subclavian artery is ruptured in about 15%.

Pathological features

The injury to the spinal nerves forming the brachial plexus may be pre-ganglionic or post-ganglionic. In *pre-ganglionic* injury the spinal nerve is separated from the spinal cord, and the level of rupture lies between the dorsal root ganglion and the cord. In *post-ganglionic* rupture the nerve trunk is torn apart, usually above the clavicle but also at varying levels below it.

Clinical features

A severe lesion of the brachial plexus leads to extensive paralysis and loss of sensation. Pain is usually severe and it is characteristic of the pre-ganglionic injury. In one half of cases the injury to the brachial plexus is complete, so that all function in the upper limb is lost. In the remainder, spinal nerves survive, so that there is residual function, usually in the hand. Complete pre-ganglionic injury is seen in about 20% of the whole.

A pre-ganglionic injury is suggested by:

- a high-energy-transfer accident with violent distraction of the forequarter from the trunk
- severe pain – this is characteristic and it usually occurs on the day of injury. There are two patterns of pain. First is a constant, crushing burning bursting or tearing pain which is experienced within the anaesthetic hand. Next are convulsive shoots of 'lightning like' pain which course down the whole of the upper limb within the territory of the damaged nerve. The patient may experience up to 30 or 40 bursts of this convulsive pain every day
- sensory loss above the clavicle
- ipsilateral Bernard–Horner's syndrome
- paralysis of serratus anterior and of the ipsilateral hemidiaphragm.

Management

Other life-threatening injuries take priority in treatment. Plain radiographs of the neck, chest and shoulder, myelography, CT myelography and MR scanning are useful in diagnosis. Nerve conduction studies are valuable in describing the extent of the injury and in distinguishing between pre- and post-ganglionic injury.

Repair of the ruptured nerves is urgently indicated. Pre-ganglionic injuries may be treated by nerve transfer. There is growing interest in the concept of reconnecting the spinal cord to the peripheral nerves by means of interposed grafts in the pre-ganglionic injury.

The process of rehabilitation is lengthy and is directed towards the relief of pain, the restoration of elements of function within the paralysed upper limb, and guiding the patient back to normal life, study and work.

The obstetric brachial plexus palsy (OBPP)

There are approximately 300 new cases in the UK and Ireland every year, an incidence of about 1:2000 live births. There are two patterns (Table 35.4):

- Breech delivery is associated with severe bilateral lesions and paralysis of the phrenic nerves. These babies are small and are often premature. Breech delivery accounts for less than 10% of OBPP cases in the UK.
- In cephalic delivery heavy babies and shorter, heavier mothers are at risk. Shoulder dystocia is recorded in about 60% of these cases.

About 50% of the infants will make a complete spontaneous recovery, and 40% more will recover useful function. Exploration and repair of the brachial plexus may be considered in about 10% of the children. Posterior dislocation of the shoulder is the most significant and common of the secondary deformities in OBPP, occurring in about 25% of all cases. Abnormal posture of the shoulder and restriction of the range of lateral rotation are diagnostic features.

FURTHER READING

Hamblen DL, Simpson HR 2007 Adams's outline of fractures, 12th edn. Churchill Livingstone, Edinburgh

McRae R, Esser M 2008 Practical fracture management, 5th edn. Churchill Livingstone, Edinburgh

O'Brien M 2010 Aids to the examination of the peripheral nervous system, 5th edn. Saunders Edinburgh

Solomon L, Warwick D, Nayagam S (2005) Apley's concise orthopaedics and trauma, 3rd edn. Hodder Arnold, London

36 Principles of paediatric surgery

GENERAL PRINCIPLES

What is paediatric surgery?

Paediatric surgery involves a broad range of bodily systems and is the only surgical specialty defined by the age of the patient as well as the surgical condition. Patients range from children as young as 24 weeks premature weighing only 500 g up to late adolescence.

Assessing the paediatric surgical patient

As with other branches of surgery and medicine the management of a paediatric surgical patient is fundamentally based on the ability to take an accurate history and perform a thorough clinical examination. Challenges lie in our patients who, unlike adults, are often unable and sometimes unwilling to allow such a process. History must often be extracted from those involved in the primary care of the child and examination techniques require skill and carefully applied strategies that develop with experience.

What are the main differences between adult surgery and paediatric surgery?

- Surgical pathology is often related to congenital or inherited disorders as opposed to acquired conditions seen in adults such as atherosclerosis.
- Age-dependent physiological differences such as heart rate and blood pressure must be considered during assessment.
- Individual fluid and drug regimens are necessary as they are weight dependent.
- Children rely on the consent of others, usually parents, for permission to perform surgical procedures that they may require.
- The low incidences of many surgical conditions results in the transfer of many patients to regional centres for specialised anaesthetic and surgical management.

Principles of neonatal and paediatric transfer to a specialist centre

The priorities in care during transfer are:

- temperature control
- nasogastric intubation to keep the stomach empty
- airway protection, e.g. pharyngeal suction for oesophageal atresia (see below) and assisted ventilation via endotracheal tube for respiratory insufficiency
- cardiorespiratory monitoring of pulse rate and oxygen saturation
- intravenous fluids – to provide glucose and sodium; water overload must be avoided; fluid requirements are determined by the infant's age and weight (Table 36.1).

Temperature

Hypothermia is minimised by the use of an incubator and a warming mattress and by an overhead heater in the operating theatre and anaesthetic room. The extremities are wrapped and the infant nursed in warm cotton wool covered by gauze (Gamgee), exposing only the operating field. Covering the abdomen with clear adhesive film decreases convection losses even further. Sick infants may be transferred between hospitals in a transport incubator with other support as detailed below.

Nasogastric intubation

Whenever intestinal obstruction is suspected, a nasogastric tube large enough to keep the stomach empty (8–10 Fr) is essential to minimise the risk of aspiration of gastric contents into the respiratory tract. This should be kept on free drainage and regularly aspirated.

Cardiorespiratory monitoring

Pulse rate and arterial oxygen saturation are sensitive indicators of how the infant is responding to the stresses of illness. Continuous records help to adjust respiratory support and fluid and electrolyte replacement.

Table 36.1 Fluids during first week of life

Day of life	Fluids (mL/kg per day)
Day 1, 2	60
Day 3, 4	90
Day 5, 6	120
Day 7+	150

Table 36.2 Guide to fluid maintenance volume in the infant and child according to weight

3–10 kg	100 mL/kg/d (4 mL/kg/h)
10–20 kg	1000 mL/d + 50 mL/weight in kg less 10/d (40 mL/h + 2 mL/weight in kg less 10/h)
>20 kg	1500 mL/d + 25 mL/weight in kg less 20/d (60 mL/h + 1 mL/weight in kg less 20/h)

Fluid and electrolyte replacement

To avoid hyponatremia this is best given as 0.9% saline with 5–10% glucose with 10 mmol of potassium added to each 500 mL bag. Close monitoring of serum electrolytes allows for volume adjustment. Maintenance fluid of 0.45% saline is acceptable though still hypotonic and must be considered in accordance with the physiological status of the patient. If the child is within the neonatal period (<44 weeks post conception) then a more accurate calculation of daily electrolyte requirement is required according to current serum levels. Any additional losses such as stoma or drain fluid must also be taken into account. Babies who require phototherapy for hyperbilirubinaemia need 20% extra fluid because of increased insensible loss through the skin. The infant and older child's daily fluid requirements must also be calculated according to weight (Table 36.2).

Intravenous nutrition

If enteral feeding is not possible within 7 days of birth, total parenteral nutrition (TPN) is indicated for mature babies but at a younger age for premature and small-for-dates babies as they are born with very low calorie stores of glycogen and fat.

Intravenous fluids can be delivered via peripheral veins but this necessitates frequent re-siting of the cannula. Peripheral administration is not suitable for the hypertonic solutions used in TPN, and central venous catheters are recommended. These may be introduced percutaneously via peripheral veins or surgically via a jugular vein. Central catheters have an increased risk of infection.

Infection in the newborn

Infection is a constant risk for the newborn patient and increases with prematurity. Intensive care and surgical procedures add to that risk and broad-spectrum antibiotic cover is required. Which antibiotic is often determined by the incidence of local resistance. Sepsis may be indicated from temperature instability (high or low), tachycardia or bradycardia as well as high or low white blood cell levels. A rising C-reactive protein (CRP) is often a useful marker and microbiological cultures are routinely taken to assist in therapy.

Prenatal diagnosis and fetal therapy

Evidence for the effectiveness of many fetal surgical interventions is constantly under evaluation. There are currently three methods of surgical access for a prenatally diagnosed anomaly: ultrasound-guided shunt placement into the chest or bladder of an affected fetus; open uterine surgery, which carries a high risk of abortion; and the more minimally invasive fetoscopic approach.

Fetuses with conditions such as congenital diaphragmatic hernia or bladder outflow obstruction secondary to urethral valves, which are considered to have a very poor prognosis, may undergo such interventions. The procedures require a careful evaluation of the risks to the mother and child as well as the potential benefit to the child.

Prenatal diagnosis allows for the appropriate counselling for many surgical conditions and in some cases prompts further investigations such as chromosomal studies to be performed. Some conditions such as gastroschisis have been shown to have survival advantages if the mother is transferred prior to delivery to a centre with paediatric surgery on site.

SURGICAL PATHOLOGY IN CHILDREN

CONDITIONS PRESENTING WITH RESPIRATORY DISTRESS

Oesophageal atresia with tracheo-oesophageal fistula

Oesophageal atresia affects 1 in 3000 births in the UK and is a condition where the upper and lower parts of the oesophagus are not connected. Instead the upper part of the oesophagus is blind ending and the lower part is attached to the trachea and referred to as a tracheo-oesophageal fistula (Fig. 36.1).

There are other presentations with or without the fistula which are less common. Fifty percent of infants born with this condition have other associated defects of the heart renal or skeletal system.

Clinical features

Prenatal polyhydramnios occurs in half of affected infants because the fetus cannot swallow the amniotic fluid. At birth this is seen as an inability to swallow secretions and bubbling at the mouth is common.

Investigation

An inability to pass a nasogastric tube as well as a chest X-ray demonstrating the coiled tube in the upper oesophageal pouch. The presence of a fistula connecting to the stomach can be confirmed if gas is seen in the distal bowel on X-ray.

Echocardiography is usually performed on all these children preoperatively to look for cardiac defects and aortic arch position.

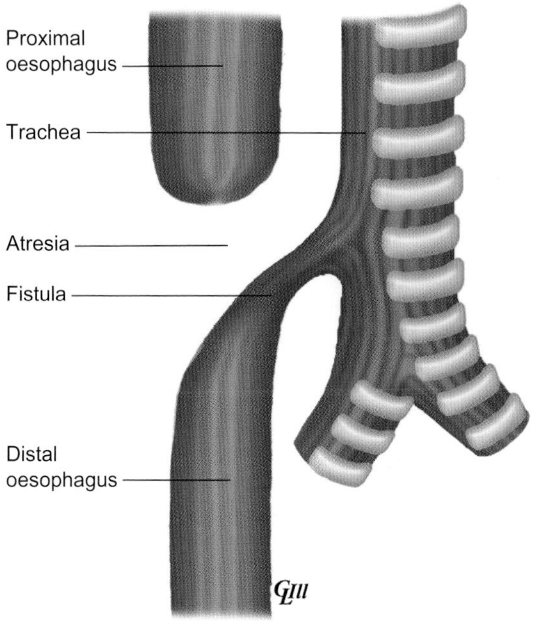

Fig. 36.1 Common variant of oesophageal atresia and tracheo-oesophageal fistula.

Management

Protection of the airway is paramount and achieved by suctioning of the upper pouch. If possible, ventilation is to be avoided. Transfer to a unit with surgical expertise can then occur.

Surgery involves ligation of the fistula and anastomosis to the upper pouch through a thoracotomy. If the gap between the two oesophageal ends is too long then a gastrostomy is sited and a staged procedure occurs. If the gap is still too long for an oesophageal anastomosis then a substitute of either stomach, small bowel or colon is used. A thoracoscopic approach is also possible.

Prognosis

The long-term survival for the majority is excellent. Those born with a low birth weight and cardiac anomalies have a poor prognosis.

Complications commonly encountered are a result of scarring at the anastomosis and up to one-third of patients will require an endoscopic dilatation.

Congenital diaphragmatic hernia

Congenital diaphragmatic hernia occurs in 1 in 2500 births in the UK. The defect usually occurs in the left posterolateral aspect of the diaphragm, though the entire diaphragm may be missing. Bowel within the chest is often seen on the antenatal ultrasound scan. Pulmonary hypoplasia is a common feature as are associated anomalies such as cardiac defects.

Clinical features

The infant often has respiratory distress at birth which requires ventilation.

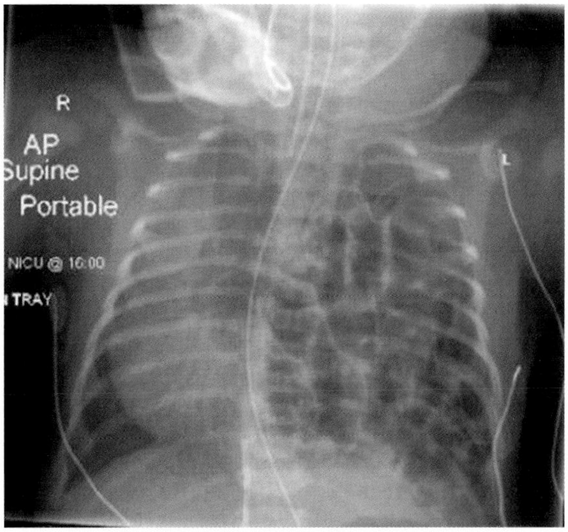

Fig. 36.2 Congenital diaphragmatic hernia.

Patients may also present outside of the neonatal period with recurrent chest infections, intestinal obstruction, or bowel ischaemia or necrosis following intestinal volvulus.

Investigation

A chest and abdominal X-ray usually reveal the condition (Fig. 36.2). Congenital lung cysts are a differential but excluded by the absence of gas on the abdominal X-ray. Gastrointestinal contrast studies can be used for difficult cases.

Management

The pulmonary vascular circulation is under high pressures and stability prior to any surgery is paramount. Extracorporeal membrane oxygenation may be needed in some severe cases.

Once stable the infant's bowel and any other viscera are reduced from the chest via a laparotomy. The defect is repaired using non-absorbable sutures primarily or by using a prosthetic patch. A thoracoscopic approach is increasingly used in many centres worldwide.

Prognosis

Overall survival for this condition is 60% but reduced if a cardiac anomaly is present. Long-term problems are mainly related to gastro-oesophageal reflux disease and reduced pulmonary function, the latter related to the degree of pulmonary hypoplasia.

Future

In utero therapy is reserved for cases where survival is predicted as being poor. Tracheal obstruction using a small endoscopically placed intra-tracheal balloon allows for distension of the pulmonary tree and a reduced hypoplasia at birth. This technique is used in some international centres though efficacy remains unproven.

Cervical cystic lymphangioma

Often referred to as cystic hygroma, this loculated lymphatic lesion can be found anywhere in the body but is often in the left posterior triangle of the neck. If large enough, it can result in tracheal compression and urgent decompression/excision is warranted. Surgery is often complex and success is reported with sclerosing these lesions if they are smaller than 5 cm.

Bilateral choanal atresia

This is a bony or membranous obstruction to the nasal passages at the junction of the hard and soft palates. The newborn is an obligatory nasal breather and can suffocate without the assistance of an oropharyngeal tube to maintain a patent airway.

The diagnosis is confirmed by inability to pass a nasal tube into the pharynx, and a CT scan is helpful in defining the extent of the atresia and planning operative repair, which is undertaken as soon as possible. Under a general anaesthetic, the atresia is resected transnasally using a drill. The resulting nasal airway is stented for a minimum of 6 weeks, and further resection of tissue may be required.

Micrognathia

A hypoplastic mandible causes obstruction of the pharynx by posterior prolapse of the tongue. Combination of this disorder with a cleft palate is known as the Pierre Robin syndrome. The respiratory problem is best relieved by a tracheostomy and the defects repaired at a later date.

THE NEWBORN WITH INTESTINAL OBSTRUCTION

Unlike other surgical specialties the clinical history of any newborn involves two people – the mother and the infant. Important features of the pregnancy such as maternal illness or polyhydramnios provide possible indicators of certain neonatal disorders.

Genetic predisposition to conditions such as Hirschsprung's disease or cystic fibrosis must also be enquired about.

Intestinal obstruction in the newborn commonly presents with either bile-stained vomiting, abdominal distension or a failure to pass stool (meconium) within 24 hours of birth. With the increasing accuracy of prenatal ultrasound many conditions are detected before birth. Chorionic villous sampling or amniocentesis may have been performed to look for associated chromosomal disorders.

Postnatal examination focuses on unusual or dysmorphic facial features which may indicate a chromosomal abnormality or a recognised syndrome, abdominal distension and tenderness as well as normal anatomy such as the presence of a patent anus.

Duodenal atresia/stenosis

One in 5000 newborns has duodenal obstruction with up to one-third having trisomy 21 (Down's syndrome), though the cause remains unknown. Theories include a failure of recanalisation of the duodenum following a solid phase in early fetal life. Prenatally this may present with polyhydramnios and dilated stomach and proximal duodenum on ultrasound.

Clinical features

Dysmorphic features may indicate the presence of trisomy 21. Obstruction may present as persistent vomiting with or without bile depending on the level of obstruction in relation to the ampulla of Vater.

If a stenosis is present (a membrane with a small central opening) then the child may present later with vomiting and failure to thrive.

Investigation

Abdominal X-ray reveals two large gas-filled upper abdominal structures or the 'double bubble' sign and these represent the dilated stomach and duodenum above the obstruction. The rest of the X-ray will be gasless in atresia or normal in stenosis (Fig. 36.3).

Management

Surgery involves a laparotomy to anastomose the proximal with the distal duodenum, care being taken to avoid damage to the ampulla. Laparoscopic repair is also feasible.

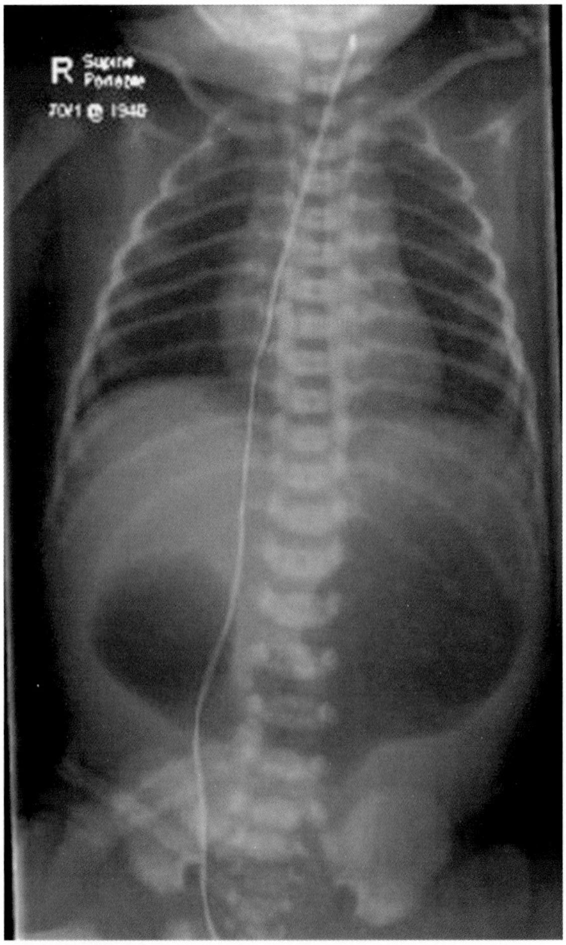

Fig. 36.3 'Double bubble' X-ray.

Prognosis

Feeding can take several weeks to establish in some patients but overall the prognosis is good providing no other anomalies are present.

Atresia of the small and large bowel

More commonly seen in the ileum though can occur anywhere, this interruption of intestinal continuity is thought to be due to mesenteric vascular accidents occurring during fetal life. Dilated bowel maybe seen on a prenatal ultrasound together with polyhydramnios.

Clinical features

Presentation depends on the level of obstruction, with infants being generally well at birth.

Investigation

Plain X-ray may reveal a 'triple bubble' sign in the case of jejunal atresia or multiple dilated bowel loops if the obstruction is more distal. Contrast enema is often performed to delineate the anatomy distal to the atresia prior to any surgical intervention.

Management

Laparotomy is performed with anastomosis of the proximal obstructed bowel to the distal unused segments.

Prognosis

Postoperative outcome depends on the length of bowel anatomically as well as functionally, with malabsorption being a significant problem for many of these children.

Malrotation with volvulus

During fetal life the herniated intestine is rotated clockwise through 270° prior to returning to the abdominal cavity and fixing to the posterior abdominal wall. This process can be halted at any point. Disorders of rotation and fixation present numerous challenges to the paediatric surgeon.

Clinical features

The infant often presents within the first month of life with bile-stained vomiting. The child may have a normal or scaphoid (empty) abdomen on examination. If the intestine has twisted (volvulus) and become ischaemic the presentation is a much more urgent one with a tender distended abdomen in a shocked infant.

Investigation

Malrotation is confirmed with an upper gastrointestinal contrast study to examine the position of the duodenal jejunal flexure. The normal position lies to the left of the midline at the level of the first lumbar vertebrae. If ischaemia is thought likely then an urgent laparotomy is preferred with ongoing resuscitation as ischaemic changes are often irreversible after 6 hours.

Management

Laparotomy is performed to release the abnormal fixating peritoneal bands that can compress and obstruct the duodenum. The bowel is placed into a non-rotated form, thus reducing the risk of the mesentery twisting.

Prognosis

Providing sufficient bowel is maintained, prognosis is good. Long-term intravenous nutrition may be needed in severe cases.

Meconium ileus

This condition occurs as a result of thickened impacted meconium (newborn stool) obstructing the distal ileum. It has a strong association with cystic fibrosis, which is found in up to 95% of affected infants.

Clinical features

The terminal ileum is impacted with firm pellets of meconium, with the colon appearing very narrow and unused and often referred to as a microcolon. Prenatal perforation may take place with a sterile peritonitis and local calcification or pseudocyst formation. The infant presents with bile-stained vomiting and abdominal distension shortly after birth.

Investigation

A plain X-ray confirms distal bowel obstruction, with or without calcification from a sterile perforation. An enema using water-soluble contrast fills the empty colon and may pass through the ileocaecal valve to outline loops of ileum and the impacted meconium.

The underlying cystic fibrosis can be confirmed by the detection of one of the specific defective genes found on chromosome 7 or by the finding of elevated levels of immunoreactive trypsin in the blood.

Management

The high osmolality of the gastrograffin enema may be successful in up to 50% of cases. A hydroscopic effect draws water into the bowel and assists in evacuation.

If unsuccessful then a laparotomy with or without a stoma is used to decompress the ileum. The introduction of feeds postoperatively should include pancreatic enzymes to facilitate the digestion and absorption of fats.

Prognosis

Following initial impaction, further occurrences can take place throughout childhood though usually only if compliance with medication is poor.

Hirschsprung's disease

Congenital aganglionosis of the bowel is referred to as Hirschsprung's disease and occurs in 1 in 5000 births in the UK. Cholinergic ganglia in the myenteric plexus play an important role in the relaxation phase of normal intestinal peristalsis. The failure to relax due to the absence of ganglion cells results in a functional bowel obstruction. The aganglionic segment of bowel extends from the rectum a variable distance proximally. The cause of Hirschsprung's disease is still unclear though is thought to be an arrest of the neural crest cell migration. A genetic role has been identified in several chromosomal disorders.

Clinical features

Abdominal distension and failure to pass meconium within the first 24–48 hours of birth are the most common presenting features. The most frequently affected area is the recto-sigmoid colon which presents as a distal bowel obstruction. Rectal examination may result in an explosive passage of stool. Death can occur if severe inflammation of the proximal bowel or enterocolitis is the presenting feature.

Investigation

Plain abdominal X-ray may reveal multiple dilated large loops of bowel and the diagnosis is confirmed with a rectal biopsy which shows increased staining for anticholinesterase throughout the muscularis mucosa and lamina propria. Contrast enema may further assist in the diagnosis. Failure of relaxation of the internal anal sphincter on manometry is diagnostic.

Management

Therapy begins with administration of broad-spectrum antibiotics and urgent decompression of the obstructed large bowel. Initially this involves regular rectal washouts. If unsuccessful then surgical decompression is indicated in the form of stoma – often in the form of a split sigmoid colostomy (as described by Pena).

Definitive surgery involves using ganglionic bowel to replace the aganglionic segment.

Prognosis

Constipation and soiling can occur in up to one-third of children up to early adolescence but long-term outcome appears good. Early mortality occurs in up to 5–10% and is related to delayed treatment of enterocolitis.

Anorectal anomalies

Perineal inspection at birth is an important aspect of newborn examination. The absence of a patent anus is occasionally overlooked and can result in bowel perforation.

Clinical features

In males this may present as a skin-covered anus or a fistula on the perineum (Fig. 36.4). Higher lesions can result in the rectum connecting to the urethra or bladder. In females, meconium may be seen to exit from the introitus or, more rarely, from the vagina.

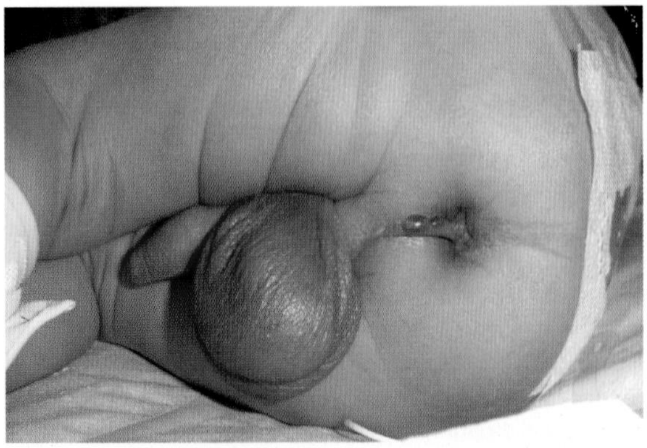

Fig. 36.4 Anorectal anomaly showing closed anus with a perineal fistula (low type).

A more severe form in females is called a cloaca (Greek for sewer) – there is a combined urogenital tract where the urethra, vagina and rectum fuse distally to form a common channel.

Investigation

Ultrasound or prone invertograms (X-ray with infant lying on its abdomen with pelvic elevation) are used by many surgeons to detect the distance of the anal canal from the perineum. Preoperative investigations such as echocardiography may also necessary as this condition may be associated with cardiac and other defects.

Knowledge of the VACTERL (Vertebral, Anorectal, Cardiac, Tracheo-oesophageal, Esophagus, Renal and Limb) complex of associated birth defects assists in the exclusion of other often associated anomalies in these patients.

Management

Surgery involves reconstruction of the anal canal. If a high lesion is present then a staged procedure is performed using a stoma followed by preoperative imaging to determine any possible connection of the anal canal to the lower urinary tract. If the lesion is low then a primary anal reconstruction is often possible.

Prognosis

This depends on the degree of continence and is ultimately related to the level of the initial defect.

Neonatal necrotising enterocolitis (NEC)

Inflammation and necrosis of the intestinal wall or necrotising enterocolitis, affecting the small or large bowel, is the most common neonatal intestinal emergency, affecting 1 in 1000 infants in the UK. The cause is not fully understood but is related to prematurity and feeding.

The risk of developing the condition decreases with increasing gestational age suggesting an immature gut does play a role. Infection is found in up to a third of patients though it is unclear if this is a primary or secondary event.

Clinical features

Systemic infection in neonates is indicated by apnoea, bradycardia, lethargy, fluctuating body temperatures and a low blood sugar together with a failure to absorb gastric feeds. These may also be the initial clinical findings in NEC. Abdominal distension then progresses to tenderness and erythema of the abdominal wall and often a passage of loose stools with blood.

Investigation

Abdominal X-ray often demonstrates dilated loops of bowel with intramural gas (pneumatosis intestinalis) being diagnostic. Free air in the peritoneal cavity indicates a perforation, usually in gangrenous intestine. Gas shadowing over the hepatic shadow is a result of gas-forming organisms in the hepatic portal vein. Serology may reveal a thrombocytopenia and raised inflammatory markers and a metabolic acidosis.

Management

Patients are kept nil by mouth, placed onto nasogastric decompression and antimicrobial therapy commenced for sepsis using broad-spectrum antibiotics. Resuscitation includes intravenous fluids: 10% glucose in 0.18% normal saline to maintain blood sugar, and colloid or blood to expand the circulating volume and to ensure a good urine output of more than 1 mL/kg per hour. Platelet transfusions are also often required. Ventilation may be necessary often when there is respiratory failure secondary to abdominal distension, sepsis or underlying lung disease. With prompt intensive medical treatment, the majority of infants will improve but may require up to 10 days of total parenteral nutrition before reintroduction of gastric feeds. A laparotomy is indicated if:

- a perforation is obvious on X-ray or is clinically suspected
- there is failure to respond to medical management, including persistent acidosis and thrombocytopenia, which are indications of severe necrosis.

Peritoneal drainage is used by some centres as management for very low birth weight infants though randomised controlled trials have failed to show this as a significant advantage to definitive care.

At operation, gangrenous bowel is excised and either a primary anastomosis performed or the two viable ends exteriorised as stomas. If necrosis is found throughout the intestine then either a second-look laparotomy 24–48 hours later could be performed to determine the degree of revascularisation or withdrawal of treatment is undertaken following parental discussion.

Prognosis

Although the mortality rate remains high, some series have reported a 70–80% survival rate in infants surgically treated for NEC.

Longer-term complications in survivors include short-bowel syndrome or malabsorption and fibrotic strictures. With an intact ileocaecal valve, just 20 cm of small bowel can adapt to achieve adequate absorption but, without an ileocaecal valve or ileum, the jejunum has limited ability to compensate. Late strictures present as feeding difficulties or subacute obstruction and can be diagnosed by contrast studies and treated surgically with resection and anastomosis.

CONGENITAL ABDOMINAL WALL DEFECTS

Gastroschisis

Gastro (belly) *schisis* (separation) is the term used to describe an evisceration of intestinal contents through a defect, usually to the right of a normally sited umbilical cord. Intestine returns to the abdominal cavity by week 13 of fetal development and failure to do so results in gastroschisis. The cause is unknown though a vascular event is thought probable as intestinal atresias are associated in 10%. Other anomalies are rare. The incidence also appears to be increasing in many parts of the developed world including the UK.

Investigation

Antenatal ultrasound scanning has a high sensitivity in accurately diagnosing the condition.

Clinical features

The bowel often has a very matted appearance and is seen to eviscerate through a defect in the abdominal wall that is invariably to the right of the umbilical cord.

Management

Vaginal birth is the usual mode of delivery and protection of the bowel with cling film to protect and avoid evaporation together with antibiotics and sufficient fluid resuscitation is required. Delivery of such infants in the surgical centre is preferred. Surgical treatment involves a delayed or primary reduction of the intestinal contents into the abdominal cavity. A silo or intestinal bag may be used to assist a delayed closure (Fig. 36.5).

Prognosis

Patients without atresia have an excellent prognosis, though a prolonged time to reach full feeds is expected. Patients with atresia often require long-term parenteral nutrition.

Exomphalos

Exomphalos differs from gastroschisis in that the intestinal contents are within a sac which involves the umbilical cord. The liver is also often seen in the herniated contents. Other associated defects are common such as cardiac and chromosomal abnormalities. Prenatal detection often includes analysis of cord blood or amniotic fluid for chromosomal analysis to assist in assessing prognosis.

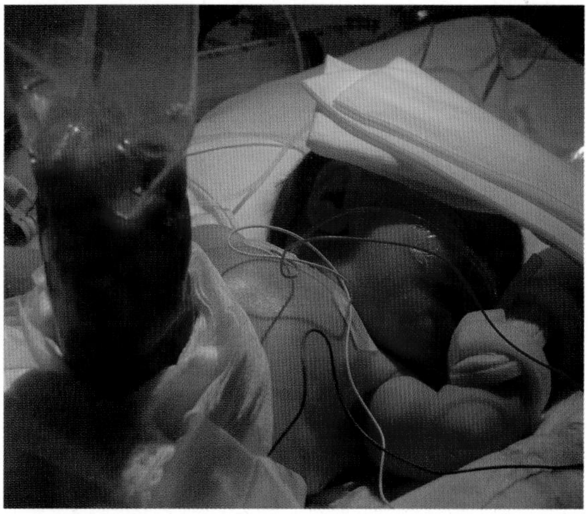

Fig. 36.5 Silo on a newborn with gastroschisis.

Management

As in gastroschisis, primary closure is required and the use of a silo or prosthetic bag may also be needed. If a very large defect is present then the sac is allowed to epithelialise initially and only skin cover is achieved. A definitive muscle closure is performed later in early childhood.

Prognosis

If no other anomalies are present the prognosis is good and mortality low.

Bladder exstrophy

This is a rare anomaly resulting in an exposed bladder affecting boys more frequently than girls (Fig. 36.6).

Investigation

Prenatal ultrasound can detect the lesion which at birth appears as a defect on the lower abdominal wall. The pubic bones are separated and the bladder mucosa is exposed.

Epispadias is when the anterior aspect of the phallus is incomplete and the urethra is exposed. Epispadias is seen alone but is also seen as part of the exstrophy anomaly.

Management

Surgery aims to achieve continence, preserve kidney function and achieve good cosmesis. If untreated for many years the lesion is at risk of adenocarcinoma.

Cloacal exstrophy is a more severe and even rarer condition where the exposed bladder is separated by two intestinal stomas. Most patients also have an associated exomphalos. Defining the gender is often a difficult decision as the penile shaft is very deficient.

DISORDERS OF THE UMBILICUS

The umbilicus is an important part of fetal life. It allows for blood and nutrients to pass initially to and from the yolk sac to the fetus through the vitello-intestinal duct until the placenta continues that function. The umbilicus also allows for a physiological herniation of the gut during early fetal life, allowing for expansion of the fetal abdomen.

The urachus is another fetal structure that passes through the umbilicus and allows the bladder to communicate with the allantois or yolk sac diverticulum. The umbilical ring naturally regresses before birth. Problems during regression may result in a number of clinical conditions.

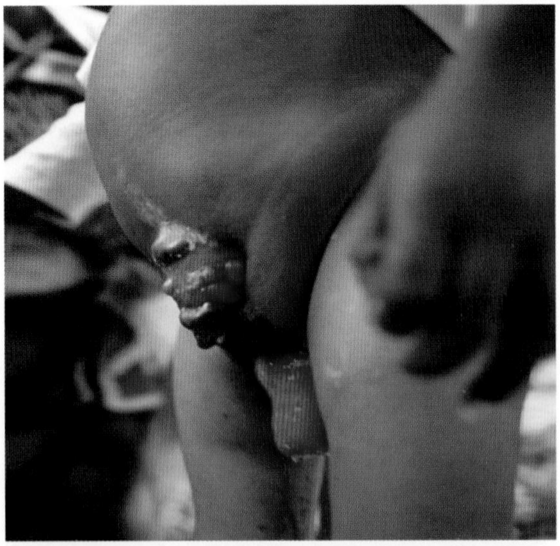

Fig. 36.6 Bladder exstrophy with rectal prolapse in the developing world.

Umbilical hernia

Umbilical hernia appears as a skin-covered protrusion at the umbilicus and is concerning for most parents though rarely causes symptoms. It is more common in Afro-Caribbean children and those with trisomy 21 and 18. Most surgeons would advocate monitoring of small umbilical hernias as surgery is not usually required. Defects of more than 2 cm at 3 years of age are unlikely to resolve spontaneously and are normally repaired. Incarceration is rarely reported.

Umbilical granuloma

Clinical features

Umbilical granuloma presents as a shiny red moist lesion described by parents as never healing following the cord disconnection. It may represent mucosa derived from the fetal intestinal connection or sepsis of the cord remnant.

Occasionally the intestine itself does not regress completely from the umbilicus. This is a patent vitello-intestinal duct and can present with persistent leakage of meconium from the umbilicus.

If the bladder connection with the yolk sac fails to regress this is termed a patent urachus and urine is seen to leak from the umbilicus. Any outflow obstruction to the fetal bladder can result in this condition and therefore renal tract imaging is warranted before surgical closure of the rachis.

Both persistent communications may also develop cysts which present as infected intra-abdominal masses.

Management

A simple granulated lesion can be treated with topical silver nitrate or other form of cauterisation. Abdominal ultrasound may be of use in detecting a patent channel or cyst. Surgical exploration of the umbilicus with disconnection is required for both patent vitello-intestinal duct and patent urachus.

Prune belly syndrome

Absence of the anterior abdominal wall muscles may follow transient but severe prenatal ascites. This is a rare anomaly, seen mostly in boys, and associated with bilateral intra-abdominal testes and an abnormal urinary tract with gross dilatation and poor function. The skin lies in loose wrinkled folds, with the underlying abdominal wall muscles poorly developed and displaced laterally. The management of the urological problems and renal failure is paramount. Staged orchidopexies and surgical repair of the anterior abdominal wall should be considered.

THE INGUINAL REGION

What is the difference between inguinal hydrocele and inguinal hernia?

A hydrocele is a collection of fluid within the processus vaginalis (PV) and results in a swelling in the scrotum occasionally extending into the groin.

An inguinal hernia occurs when abdominal organs protrude into the inguinal canal or scrotum. In children inguinal hernia and hydrocele result from the same defect – failure of closure of the processus vaginalis (Fig. 36.7).

See Box 36.1 for differential diagnoses of swelling in the groin.

Hydrocele

Clinical features

Hydrocele is more common in the first year of life and if still present at the age 2 is unlikely to disappear. Parents report intermittent swelling, worse at the end of the day or when the child has a cough or a cold.

Box 36.1 Differential diagnoses of swelling in the groin

- Inguinal hernia
- Ovary within an inguinal hernia
- Lymph node
- Undescended testicle
- Encysted hydrocele of the cord (outpouching of the patent processus)
- Tumour of spermatic cord (very rare)

On examination the swelling is fluctuant, non-tender and may extend from the scrotum to the inguinal region. It is usually irreducible though a minority may communicate. An ability to get above the swelling differentiates it from hernia. Transillumination is often not a useful tool as hernia may also allow light to shine through as the skin and the bowel wall are so thin.

Management

A ligation of the patent tract or processus is carried out through an inguinal incision. A hydrocele in an adult is different in that surgery is performed through a scrotal approach as the aetiology is different.

Inguinal hernia

This occurs in 1 in 100 male infants and 1 in 500 girls. Hernia is more common in premature infants. Surgery is always required as bowel incarceration can result in intestinal or testicular infarction in up to 10% of obstructed hernia. In girls it is not uncommon for an ovary to be present and be misdiagnosed as a lymph node. Incarceration can lead to ovarian torsion or infarction.

Clinical features

A swelling is seen intermittently in the groin and may extend into the scrotum in a boy. This may be associated with pain or colic and bowel irregularity. Incarceration can present with nausea and vomiting. If obstructed, the swelling may be tender and red in appearance.

Investigation

Clinical examination is usually sufficient though ultrasound is used by some if clinical doubt exists.

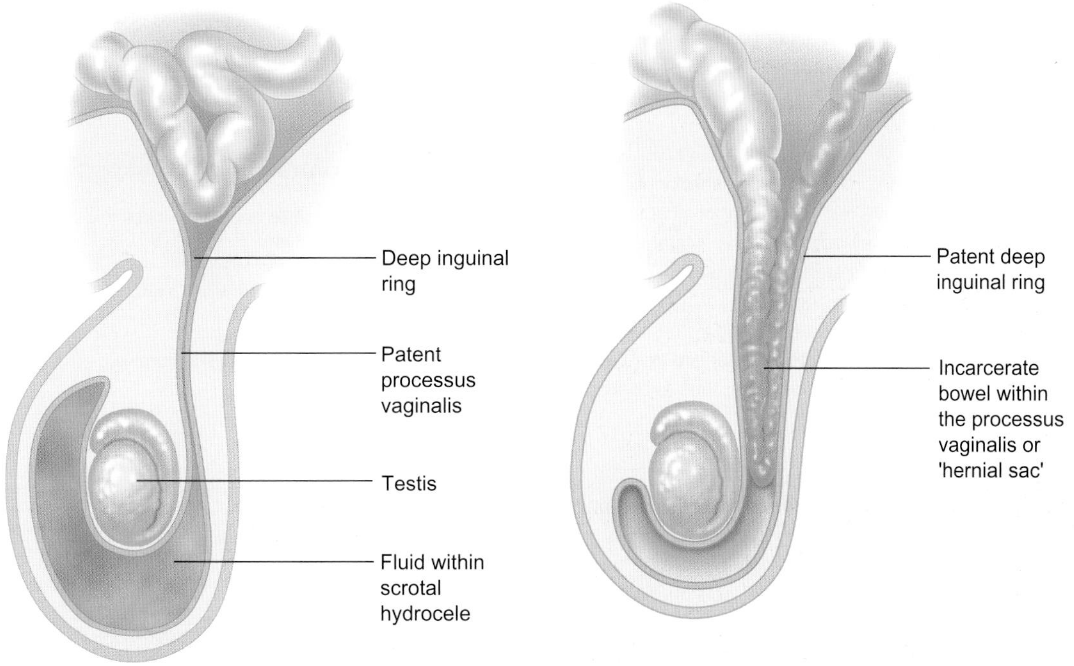

Fig. 36.7 Schematic drawing demonstrating the difference between inguinal hernia and hydrocele.

Management

If possible an attempt should be made to reduce the hernia usually after appropriate analgesia. Once reduced an elective operation can be planned as soon as swelling in the groin has reduced. Most hernias can be reduced by experienced hands but if the hernia remains irreducible, then urgent operative reduction with or without bowel resection will be necessary.

The operation is performed through an inguinal incision with the same technique used in the hydrocele repair. The laparoscopic approach is also now feasible.

1 in 8–10 children will present clinically with a hernia on the opposite side. For this reason laparoscopy through the hernial sac or through the umbilicus is sometimes used to detect contralateral hernias. The recurrence rate is low.

COMMON ABDOMINAL MASSES IN CHILDREN

Pyloric stenosis

Occurs in approximately 1 in 250 children and is more common in white northern Europeans. Gastric outlet obstruction results from hypertrophy of the circular muscle fibres of the pylorus. The cause of this condition is still largely unknown and surgery to the 'tumour' itself has remained unchanged in over a century.

Clinical features

Children commonly present within 3–6 weeks after birth with progressive forceful vomiting and failure to thrive despite appearing hungry.

The condition is more common in males, especially first born, and is seven times more likely if there is a family history. Children are often labelled as suffering from gastro-oesophageal reflux and treated accordingly. On presentation the infant may be below expected weight and may be dehydrated.

Investigation

Diagnosis relies largely on clinical examination but ultrasound is a highly sensitive test to confirm clinical findings.

Blood tests reveal a metabolic alkalosis. Water, hydrogen and chloride ions are all depleted with vomiting. To compensate, ion exchange occurs in the kidney. Water is brought back into the vascular compartment along with sodium and bicarbonate. This renal exchange mechanism results in a further loss of hydrogen ions in the urine, thus exacerbating the alkalosis.

Management

Treatment involves fluid resuscitation and potassium replacement. Once hydrated, metabolically stable and with a good urine output, the operation is commonly performed through a right upper quadrant or supraumbilical incision. The muscle of the pylorus is divided completely to expose the underlying mucosa. The laparoscopic approach is increasingly used in many centres and may have postoperative feeding advantages. The child is fed within hours of the operation or rested overnight and feeds slowly reintroduced. Recurrence is very rare.

Intussusception

Definition and epidemiology

Intussusception is the invagination of one part of the intestine into an adjacent segment. In children this occurs most commonly in the ileocaecal region (80%) (Fig. 36.8) and is secondary to inflammatory enlargement of gut lymphoid tissue following either a respiratory or gastrointestinal tract virus infection.

Intussusuception occurs in 1 in 250–300 children and most commonly occurs in infants between 6 months and 2 years though it can occur at any age. In older children a pathological cause should be considered (Box 36.2 and Box 36.3).

Clinical features

Parental history often reveals a high-pitched inconsolable cry. The child may have intermittent abdominal pain and draws up its legs during such episodes. In between spasms the child may often appear perfectly normal or appear pale

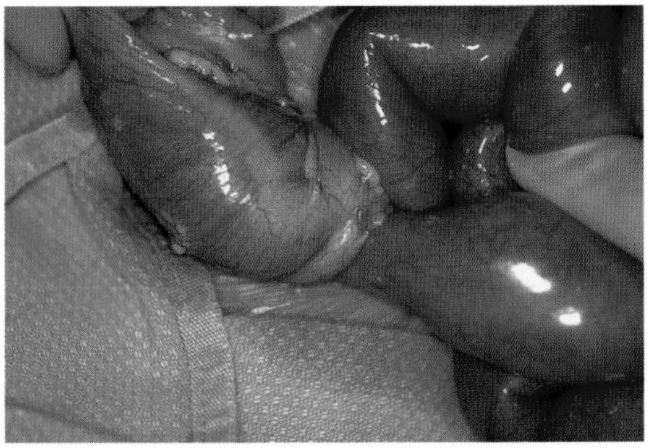

Fig. 36.8 Ileocolic intussusceptions.

Box 36.2 Causes of intussusception in children

- Lymphoid aggregates post viral illness (most common)
- Meckel's diverticulum
- Lymphoma
- Henoch–Schönlein purpura
- Duplication cysts
- Haemangioma of the bowel
- Inspissated meconium in cystic fibrosis
- Intestinal luminal polyp
- Leukaemia
- Nephrotic syndrome

Box 36.3 Diffferential diagnoses of intussusception

- Gastroenteritis
- Appendicitis
- Meckel's diverticulitis
- Malrotation with midgut volvulus
- Incarcerated inguinal hernia

and exhausted. Finally, signs of obstruction and necrosis may result in intermittent vomiting or blood in the nappy, often described as red and jelly-like. The latter represents the intestinal mucosal sloughing as a result of ischaemia.

On examination the child may range from appearing well to signs of hypovolaemic shock. Careful palpation of the abdomen may reveal a right upper quadrant mass or an empty right iliac fossa (Dance's sign) with or without peritonitis. Examination of the nappy or rectal exam may reveal blood and mucus.

Investigation

Ultrasound has a near 100% sensitivity and specificity for diagnosis. Plain abdominal X-ray may reveal bowel obstruction with a paucity of gas in the right lower quadrant. Air or contrast enema is used as a therapeutic rather than a diagnostic aid.

Management

Fluid resuscitation, broad-spectrum antibiotics and, if necessary, analgesia are essential for these patients.

Pneumatic reduction is commonly used but should be performed by experienced radiologists. Operative reduction is reserved for failed air enema (20%) or those patients who are unstable with peritonitis or signs of perforation.

Air is pumped through a rectal catheter around the colon under radiological control until it enters the terminal ileum. If there is progress but incomplete reduction, the air enema can be repeated in a stable patient several hours later.

Operative reduction can be performed either by laparotomy or laparoscopically. One in 10 children will require resection. The intussusception is reduced by gently manipulating the mass back through the bowel it has invaginated. Traction is avoided as perforation may occur. Recurrence following reduction occurs in up to 5% of patients.

Appendix mass

Appendix mass occurs usually following several days illness during which diagnoses other than acute appendicitis were considered. The omentum becomes adherent to the inflamed appendix. If peritonitis does not exist then a trial period of conservative management with intravenous broad-spectrum antibiotics is observed. If symptoms and signs improve then the appendix can be removed electively 6–8 weeks later to prevent recurrent attacks which occur in up to 60% of children.

Hydronephrosis

An obstructed renal pelvis results in a build-up of urine and stagnation which, if untreated, can result in a pyonephrosis. This can lead to hypertension and loss of renal function. Causes are numerous, ranging from strictures within the ureter at the renal pelviureteric junction to external vascular compression.

Clinical features

There may be a history of unexplained fevers or previous renal problems. Older children may show signs of hypertension.

Investigation

Urine testing may reveal infection. Ultrasound can confirm the anatomy and radioisotope studies are used to demonstrate the poor drainage and function of the infected kidney.

Management

Decompression with nephrostomy followed by pyeloplasty if sufficient renal function is present. Nephrectomy is carried out if function is poor and the other kidney is normal.

Faecaloma

A history of constipation would accompany such a clinical finding though often such children report diarrhoeal incontinence. The latter is due to overflow around the mass of liquid stool building up above the rectal faecal mass. If discovered, a rectal enema may be needed to evacuate the rectum. If this is not possible (it is very distressing to many children) then manual evacuation under general anaesthetic may be required.

Careful questioning of early bowel habit is required to eliminate Hirschsprung's disease, and it may be necessary to exclude the condition with a rectal biopsy.

Bladder outflow obstruction

Urinary retention is an often overlooked cause of a tender lower abdominal mass in children. Possible causes include pelvic surgery, constipation or urinary tract infection.

TUMOURS AND THE PAEDIATRIC SURGEON

Nephroblastoma (Wilms' tumour)

This malignant renal tumour most commonly affects children and is rarely seen in adults. Approximately 40 tumours per year are diagnosed in the UK. One in 5 tumours are linked to abnormalities on chromosome 11.

Clinical features

An incidental finding of an abdominal mass in a preschool child is the most common presenting symptom, though 1 in 10 may have painless haematuria. If left sided, a scrotal varicocele may be present caused by obstruction to the left testicular vein.

Investigation

A chest X-ray and CT scan are useful to determine extent of the condition and the latter also examines the opposite kidney.

Treatment

Nephrectomy with chemotherapy with or without radiotherapy depending on the stage.

Prognosis

It is highly responsive to treatment with a greater than 90% 5-year survival rate for localised disease.

Neuroblastoma

This malignant tumour arises from either the adrenal medulla or sympathetic ganglia of the autonomic nervous system. Sites include the retroperitoneum, adrenal gland, thorax and pelvis. Approximately 100 children are diagnosed each year.

Clinical features

Most commonly seen in children under 2 years old, neuroblastoma presents as either intra-abdominal pain with a mass or as a thoracic/cervical tumour resulting in dysphagia or respiratory compromise. A Horner's syndrome (ptosis, miosis, enophthamlos) may result from a cervical mass compressing the cervical sympathetic chain.

Non-metastatic tumour effects include hypertension from circulating cathecholamines and sweating and diarrhoea from vasoactive intestinal polypeptide (VIP) production.

Investigation

High levels of urinary catecholamines are present, MRI is the procedure of choice and can identify intraspinal extension. Radioisotope studies are useful for bone invasion and tissue biopsy helps determine the likely response to different treatment modalities according to the molecular biology of the tumour.

Management

Surgery is indicated in all but the most advanced tumours. Resection may occur later in those children if an adequate response to chemo- and radiotherapy has taken place.

Survival is poor for those with advanced tumours and those diagnosed after the age of 2.

Ovarian tumour

Ovarian tumours are often detected antenatally and observed to decrease in size with increasing postnatal age. They also occur in prepubertal girls.

Clinical features

An abdominal mass may be palpable arising from the pelvis, which often feels firm in adolescents.

Investigation

USS/CT/MRI may show ovarian origin. Features may include calcification or other structures suggestive of multiple cellular origins: e.g. teeth and hair.

Serology should include tumour markers such as alphafetoprotein, beta-HCG and CEA prior to surgery.

Management

Management is by surgical excision either by open laparotomy or laparoscopically assisted if benign nature likely. Malignant ovarian tumours are rare in childhood.

Teratomas

Terato (monstrous) *oma* (swelling) are abnormal developments of germ cells that occur in areas such as the testis, ovary or sacrococcygeum (Fig. 36.9). The tumours contain derivatives of all germ cell layers of endoderm, ectoderm and mesoderm. Most teratomas in children are benign.

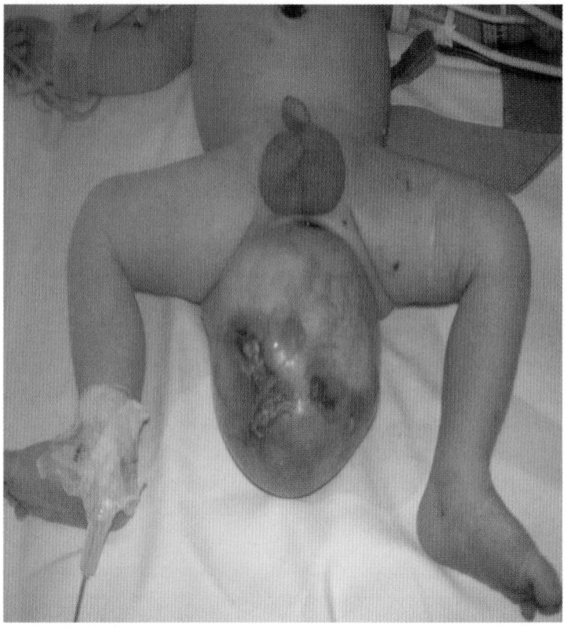

Fig. 36.9 Sacrococcygeal teratoma in a newborn.

Surgery usually takes place within the first few days of life. Long-term management of continence problems is often necessary after excision of sacrococcygeal tumours.

Abdominal tumours often present later in infancy and may be malignant.

DISORDERS OF GENITALIA

Undescended testes

Epidemiology and embryology

One in 30 males have an undescended testis at birth. This rises to nearly 1 in 5 if born prematurely. Descent may occur in the first 3 months in many and at 6 months the incidence overall is considerably reduced.

To understand the testis and why it fails to reach the scrotum, a basic knowledge of embryology is required. In males and females the gonad develops on a ridge on the posterior abdominal wall early in fetal life and descends caudally reaching the inguinal canal by week 32 of fetal life. This occurs under the influence of various hormones. In the second phase of descent the testis passes through the inguinal canal and into the scrotum under the influence of testosterone. The gubernaculum is a structure that elongates distal to the testis, creating a space for the testicle to migrate. Peritoneum elongates with the descent of the testis – referred to as the processus vaginalis. The failure of the gubernaculum to migrate is the probably most common cause of an undescended testis.

Clinical features

Examining a child for the presence of an inguinal testicle can be difficult. It is important to have a warm room and to use distraction techniques. Gentle palpation confirms lack of

Box 36.4 **Problems associated with an undescended testis**

- Abnormal fertility in an undescended testis
- Inability to palpate later in adult life (cancer screening)
- Cosmetic
- Increased risk of torsion
- A 5-fold increased risk of malignancy if undescended at the age of 10

a testicle in the scrotum. Gentle palpation beginning at the lateral point of the inguinal canal and passing medially has the effect of controlling the cremasteric reflex. The other hand can then palpate for the testicle from the scrotum up and laterally along the inguinal canal. If the testicle can be manipulated into the scrotum and remains there momentarily prior to retreating back into the inguinal canal, it is referred to as a retractile testis and does not require surgery. Some patients present at an older age with an impalpable testis, having previously been seen to be in the scrotum. Such patients may represent retractile testes that have 'ascended'. Monitoring on an annual basis is therefore recommended by many surgeons.

Indications for surgery

A testicle that has failed to reach the scrotum by 6 months is unlikely to descend. Surgery is normally performed between 6 and 12 months of age. An undescended testis is associated with a number of potential problems (Box 36.4). It is hoped that operating at an early age will reduce the risk of malignant change.

Investigation

If neither testis is able to be found then a human chorionic gonadotrophin stimulation test should be performed to determine whether testicular tissue is present at all. If testosterone is measured, then laparoscopy is used to identify the intra-abdominal testes. Ultrasound and CT have limited value in location of such intra-abdominal testes.

Surgical management

Orchdio (Greek for testicle) *pexy* (Greek for fixing together) involves a general anaesthetic but can be performed as a day case. The inguinal transverse skin incision allows exposure to the inguinal canal, which is opened and the testicle identified. The gubernaculum is transected to extract the testicle. The spermatic cord, comprising the artery and vein to the testicle, the vas deferens and the processus vaginalis all surrounded by cremasteric muscle, are then carefully mobilised from the inguinal canal. The operation then involves carefully dissecting of the processus vaginalis from the vas and vessels, freeing any adhesions that are preventing the testicle from reaching the scrotum. A tunnel is then created using the surgeon's finger to create a space from the inguinal region to the scrotum. The testicle is then delivered into the scrotum and placed in a pouch created beneath the scrotal skin and may or may not be fixed, depending on the amount of tension. Complications include testicular atrophy (1–2%) and retraction of the testicle back into the groin (1%).

Torsion of the testis and appendix testis

Epidemiology

Testicular torsion can occur at any age, with peak incidences perinatally and between 10 and 20 years of age.

Aetiology

An abnormal horizontal lie of the testis indicates that there is a high attachment of the peritoneal tunica, giving the testis more mobility, and hence a possible predisposition to rotate. This is often referred to as a bell clapper testis. An inguinal testis is more likely to twist than an intrascrotal one for similar reasons.

The appendix testis is a small embryological remnant on the upper pole of the testis. This can also twist and necrose, resulting in a similar clinical picture.

Clinical features

Perinatal torsion presents with a painless blue, often hard swelling in the scrotum, several times larger than the contralateral testis. Occasionally incarcerated inguinal hernia can be mistaken for an acute neonatal testicular torsion.

In later childhood, torsion causes severe pain which is felt in the scrotum and lower abdomen and is usually associated with vomiting and difficulty in walking.

Examination of testicles should be routine in the investigation of abdominal pain, as the pain in the iliac fossa may divert attention from the scrotum and so delay the diagnosis. The history may reveal previous minor episodes indicating intermittent torsion.

Testicular remnant torsion may be distinguishable by the appearance of a blue dot on close examination. Conservative management with analgesics will often suffice; if there is doubt, exploration is warranted.

Investigation

The time taken to diagnose accurately torsion of the testicle only lengthens ischaemia time to the testicle. If suspected, an urgent exploration under general anaesthesia should be performed without further investigation.

Management

Through either a horizontal hemiscrotal or midline incision the testicle is delivered and inspected. The testicle and cord is untwisted, warmed and observed for several minutes to see if colour improves. If operated on within 6 hours a significant number will be saved and can be fixed with 3 non-absorbable sutures to the scrotal fascia. After 24 hours virtually all twisted testes will need removing. Fixation of the opposite side with non-absorbable suture is usually performed to prevent a similar scenario in the future. If a torted remnant or appendix testis is found, this is also removed.

Idiopathic scrotal oedema

This is a form of urticarial angio-oedema of unknown cause.

Clinical features

Bright red oedema of the scrotum or hemiscrotum is observed which often extends posteriorly towards the anus or anteriorly over the inguinal region. The appearance resembles an acute cellulitic infection with some irritation and tenderness. However, fever and pain are not present and antibiotics do not influence the course.

The normal testis is obscured by the intense oedema of the scrotal wall.

Management

The parents are often alarmed and reassurance is necessary. There is resolution over 24–48 hours. Antihistamines and anti-inflammatory medication can speed spontaneous resolution.

Phimosis/paraphimosis and balanoposthitis

Phimosis of the foreskin can be considered as either congenital or acquired; or as physiological or pathological.

Removal of the foreskin or circumcision is the most commonly performed operation in the world and for centuries has been a fundamental rite of passage in many cultures.

A congenital or physiological phimosis is where the foreskin is naturally adherent to the glans penis and does not retract. This can continue to puberty without causing symptoms and up to 3% of males will still be unretractile by the age of 13.

An acquired or pathological phimosis in childhood is usually a result of balanitis xerotica obliterans (sclerotic fibrotic process of the foreskin) or due to chronic balanoposthitis. *Balano* (Greek for acorn) *itis* (inflammation) is inflammation of the glans of the penis, whereas *posthe* (Greek for foreskin) *itis* (inflammation) refers to inflammation of the skin surrounding the glans.

The only absolute indication for circumcision in childhood is a pathological phimosis. Relative indications include recurrent severe posthitis (severe inflammation of the foreskin) and paraphimosis (retraction with a tourniquet effect from the preputial ring).

Circumcision is still performed in up to 60% of males in the United States for cultural and hygienic reasons. The incidence fell dramatically in postwar England and remains at about 2% of the male population.

Recent trials in Africa suggest that circumcising males in a population with minimal use of condoms can reduce infection with HIV.

Clinical features

A physiological foreskin, on gentle examination, will retract to reveal a spout or funnel with healthy mucosa visible. Pathological phimosis will often have a rolled pale edge with white linear radial scars. Both conditions can result in difficulty in urination though it is much more common in a pathological phimosis.

Management

Physiological phimosis requires reassurance as well as advice on careful drying of the foreskin following urination. Drying can help in preventing dermatitis which is secondary to the concentrated ammonia found in urine being in prolonged contact with the foreskin. Topical steroids are used by many clinicians to treat the inflammation.

Circumcision is required for a pathological phimosis to prevent retraction with a tourniquet-like effect as the tight phimotic ring passes over the glans and is unable to be brought forward. This is referred to as a paraphimosis. Gentle retraction with or without a small slit dorsally is required. Circumcision is then usually offered as an elective procedure.

Hypospadias

This refers to a defect in the distal formation of the male urethra as it forms ventrally. The result is a spectrum of abnormally situated urethral openings along the course of the normal urethra. The urethral openings can be situated anywhere from above the coronal sulcus of the glans penis to the perineum in its most extreme form. The latter is often associated with chordae or fibrotic areas on the shaft, resulting in a ventral curvature.

The incidence in the UK is approximately 1 in 250 male births. The cause is thought to be an interruption in the androgenic processes required during ventral urethral formation.

Clinical features

The disorder is usually identified at birth and rarely can be associated with other chromosomal, reproductive or endocrine anomalies. The prepuce is also incomplete and lies dorsally.

Management

Surgery usually takes place in early infancy and involves either a primary or staged procedure to tubularise a new urethra. The incomplete or hooded prepuce is often incorporated into the repair.

PRINCIPLES OF PAEDIATRIC TRAUMA

Trauma is the most common cause of death in children aged over 1 year. Different mechanisms of injury are closely associated with developmental milestones. Head injuries, either as an isolated cause or in association with other injuries, are the most common cause of death.

Thoracic, abdominal and perineal injuries are those most commonly encountered by paediatric general surgeons.

The possibility of non-accidental injury must always be considered, and if any doubt exists the paediatric consultant with responsibility for safeguarding children should be contacted for advice. All staff treating children should undergo child protection training.

Thoracic

This accounts for the second leading cause of death in paediatric trauma with blunt trauma from road traffic accidents being mostly responsible. The paediatric chest wall is more compliant than an adult and thus fractures are less common but pulmonary contusion and pneumothorax are more common. The majority of such injuries can be managed with observation with or without chest drainage. Thoracotomy or thoracoscopy is necessary if more than 20 mL/kg of blood is required in resuscitation or if a drainage rate of >2 mL/kg/h is observed following intercostal drainage of a haemothorax.

Abdominal

If bruising is discovered on a child's abdomen following trauma, then it is likely that significant force has occurred. This may be as a direct blow or from restraint such as the seat or lap belt.

Viscera such as the liver and spleen are less protected in the infant due to nature of rib cage shape and development and a high index of suspicion for visceral injury must be maintained. Splenic injury is common in children, though the majority of intrasplenic lacerations and haemorrhage will resolve if managed conservatively with bed rest and observation for 1–2 weeks.

Deceleration injuries in road traffic accidents can affect hollow viscera such as the duodenum. CT with contrast is the preferred investigation. The mechanism of injury is the sudden visceral compression against the bony spine and shearing forces affecting retroperitoneal structures.

Assessment and management

The Airway Breathing Circulation (ABC) principles of resuscitation apply to children as they do adults. Intravenous fluid and pharmacotherapy, however, is weight based and each child must be considered on an individual basis.

Within the trauma setting the primary concern is the airway together with cervical spine control. Once secured, the breathing is assessed and optimised, followed by support of the circulation. If the child is not breathing and there is no cardiac output, 5 rescue breaths are given prior to cardiac compression. Children require 30 chest compressions for every 2 breaths. Once resuscitation is successful, the neurological status of the patient is then assessed and the patient undergoes a full examination to complete the primary survey. The stabilised child can then undergo the secondary survey to look for additional injuries.

The resuscitation of children in the UK should adhere to the guidelines set out by the advanced paediatric life support (APLS) group and this is mandatory training for all paediatric surgeons.

FURTHER READING

Holcomb GW, Murphy JP 2010 Ashcraft's pediatric surgery, 5th edn. Saunders Elsevier, Philadelphia

Spitz L, Coran A 2008 Operative paediatric surgery. Hodder Arnold, London

Stringer MD, Oldham KT, Mouriquand PDE 2006 Pediatric surgery and urology: long-term outcomes. Cambridge University Press, Cambridge

Thomas DFM, Duffy PG, Rickwood AMK 2008 Essentials of paediatric urology. Informa Healthcare, London

37 Ophthalmology in clinical surgery

The eye is a unique organ because of its specialised function. All ocular structures are transparent to allow the optimal focusing of light; therefore with appropriate instruments the ophthalmologist can examine all structures anterior to and including the retina without resort to special investigations. Moreover, the eye is a window to view the progression of systemic disease.

EVALUATION

The non-ophthalmologist can make an effective assessment of the nature and urgency of a presentation from a detailed history and the use of equipment readily available in any Emergency Department or general practice rooms. Important symptoms and their possible causes are summarised in Table 37.1. Further details are given in the section on common symptoms and signs below. Important features of the examination are in Table 37.2.

Physical findings

The items of equipment needed are:

- a Snellen chart of letters that reduce in size so that, to the eye, a letter from the 6 m line seen at 6 m should have the same size as a letter from the 3 m line seen at 3 m
- bright pen torch
- ophthalmoscope.

Visual acuity

Distance. The Snellen chart at 6 m is most commonly used with the subject wearing full refractive correction and bright ambient illumination. Interpretation of results is in Table 37.3.

Pinhole acuity. If a refractive error is uncorrected, confusion may occur as to whether an intrinsic ocular disorder is responsible for poor vision. A pinhole only allows a central ray of light to pass through, undeviated by the eye's focusing system onto the macula area, and therefore the significance of any refractive error is reduced. Pinhole acuity should be measured whenever the acuity, with or without refractive correction, is worse than 6/9.

Movements of the optic globe

The ability to move both globes is tested by asking the eye to follow the examiner's finger while keeping the head steady. The muscles responsible are illustrated in Figure 37.1.

Visual fields

The confrontation method detects significant neurological field defects:

1. Test distance is approximately 1 m.
2. One eye each of both subject and examiner is occluded, which allows comparison between the visual field of the examiner and that of the subject.
3. The subject is asked to steadily fixate the examiner's eye.
4. Finger counting is carried out in all four quadrants: superotemporal, inferotemporal, inferonasal and superonasal; it is best to present, in a static way, one, two or five fingers.

A hemifield comparison is also made:

1. Similar distance to the confrontation method.
2. Controlled fixation of the subject on the examiner's eye.
3. The examiner holds up both hands on either side of the vertical meridian and the subject is asked to compare their appearance – is one clearer or darker than the other?

Table 37.1 Common symptoms of eye disease

Nature	Type	Causes
Pain	Ocular	Uveitis, acute glaucoma
	Referred	Paranasal sinuses
		Dental
Visual disturbances	Distortion	Disease of the macula
	Photophobia	Uveitis, corneal disease
	Halos	Acute glaucoma
	Flashing lights	Vitreous and retinal disorders, migraines
	Floaters	Vitreous and retinal disorders
	Acute visual loss	Retinal, vascular and neurological disorders
	Chronic visual loss	Media opacities, retinal, vascular and neurological disorders
	Night blindness	Retinal degeneration
Double vision (diplopia)	Monocular	Cataract, refractive errors
	Binocular	Extraocular muscle imbalance
Altered appearance of the eye	Red eye	Conjunctivitis, episcleritis, uveitis, acute glaucoma
	Proptosis	Infection, thyroid eye disease
Lacrimal disturbance	Dry eye	Primary lacrimal failure, Sjögren's syndrome
	Watery eye	Ocular irritation, blocked tear drainage

Table 37.2 Ophthalmic examination

Property examined	Tests and abnormal findings
Visual acuity (normal = 6/6)	At distance
	At near
	Pinhole
Visual field	Confrontation
	Formal perimetry
Ocular motility	Misalignment of visual axis
	Nystagmus
Pupil responses	Unequal size (anisocoria)
	Distortion
	Reaction to light
	Response to accommodation
	Afferent pupil defect
Examination of anterior eye by torch	Redness
	Clarity
	Depth of anterior chamber
Digital tonometry	Subjective hardness of globe
Fundoscopy	Red reflex
	Optic disc
	Macula
	Retinal vessels

Table 37.3 Visual acuity

Snellen acuity	Patient can see	At distance
6/60	60 m line	6 m
6/36	36 m line	6 m
6/24	24 m line	6 m
6/18	18 m line	6 m
6/12	12 m line	6 m
6/9	9 m line	6 m
6/6	6 m line	6 m
6/5	5 m line	6 m
CF	To count fingers	× m
HM	To detect hand movement	× m
PL	To perceive light	

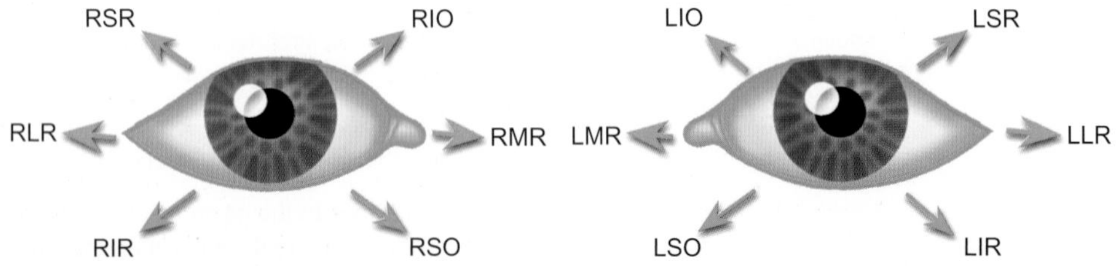

RSR = right superior rectus
RLR = right lateral rectus
RIR = right inferior rectus
RIO = right inferior oblique
RMR = right medial rectus
RSO = right superior oblique

Fig. 37.1 Movements of the optic globe and muscles responsible.

Finally a kinetic field test is done using a white hat-pin with a 5 mm diameter head. The pin is moved in from the periphery, and the point of first detection is recorded.

Simple rules of interpretation of the acuity and field tests

The 'rules of the road' are:

- Lesions anterior to the chiasm affect one eye only.
- Lesions at the chiasm most usually damage the crossing nasal fibres from each eye to give rise to defects in the temporal fields on each side (bitemporal field defect).
- Lesions posterior to the chiasm damage the temporal fibres from one eye plus the nasal fibres from the other eye to cause a homonymous defect (i.e. a defect affecting one visual hemifield).

Pupil responses

Abnormal responses are summarised in Table 37.4.

Anisocoria is a visible difference between the pupil sizes of the two eyes, which may be a normal variation in about 20% of the population.

Light reflex (parasympathetic) and pupillary constriction. If all pathways are intact, a light shone on one eye constricts both pupils at an equal rate and to a similar degree (direct and consensual reflexes).

Pupillary examination

Procedure is described in Clinical Box 37.1.

Ocular motility

The visual acuity must be known, to ensure that the subject can fixate on the targets presented.

- Observe for misalignment of the visual axis in the primary position, which can easily be determined by shining a torch light from 30 cm away and checking that the reflections on the corneas are central.
- Is nystagmus (involuntary oscillations of the eyes) present?
- Ask the subject to follow a target in the six different directions of gaze.
- Is there a complaint of double vision?

Table 37.4 Abnormal responses of the pupil

Abnormality	Common causes
Dilatation	IIIrd nerve lesion Adie pupil (see text) Mydriatic drugs Iris trauma
Constriction	Horner's syndrome Argyll–Robertson pupil Drugs: opiates, cholinergic
Failure of accommodation/ convergence	Extrapyramidal disease (parkinsonism) Pineal tumour
Marcus–Gunn pupil	Damage to the anterior visual pathway up to the lateral geniculate nucleus

Appearance of external eye

Ocular adnexa (eyelids and periocular area):

- skin lesions
- inflammation
- position of the eyelids – ptosis, retraction, entropion (lid margin turning in) or ectropion (lid margin turning out)
- proptosis
- general facial examination.

Redness of the eye and opacities in the cornea can be easily seen with a torch. Fluorescein staining reveals areas of the cornea denuded of epithelium as bright yellow fluorescence when viewed with a blue light.

Digital tonometry

Intraocular pressure is measured most accurately at the slit lamp using a tonometer. An estimate can be made by digital tonometry. The eyes are palpated through the closed lids over the upper outer angle of the orbit where the tarsal plate is thinnest. A hard eye indicates high pressure and, in the presence of a red, painful eye, may indicate acute angle closure glaucoma.

Fundoscopy

The hand-held direct ophthalmoscope provides a magnified (×15) monocular view of the transparent ocular media (cornea, aqueous, lens and vitreous) and the fundus. The field of view is small, especially through an undilated pupil. The technique should be practised until one can reliably see the optic disc through an undilated pupil, as this forms an important part of any neurological examination.

Technical points are described in Clinical Box 37.2.

The examination starts with the ophthalmoscope 30 cm away from the subject and with observation of the red reflex which fills the pupil. It is formed by the reflection of light from the retina and is impaired by any obstruction to that light, e.g. cataract, vitreous haemorrhage. It proceeds

Clinical Box 37.1 Pupillary examination

- Observe the sizes of both pupils in bright and dim illumination.
- Shine a bright torch in one eye and observe the direct and consensual light responses.
- A bright light shone into one eye will cause pupillary constriction in both eyes (direct and consensual light response).
- If there is an afferent defect on one side, e.g. a unilateral optic nerve lesion, then the stimulus to constriction when the light is shone on the affected side will be reduced relative to the response when light is shone on the normal side.
- When the torch is swung quickly across from one eye to the other, dwelling for a second on each, the pupils will dilate when light is shone on the affected side – paradoxical dilatation. The side that dilates is described as having a relative afferent pupillary defect (RAPD). This is a very important sign to elicit in the diagnosis of visual loss.
- Ask for fixation first on a distant target, then present a near target at 15 cm and observe the change in pupillary size as fixation is changed.

Clinical Box 37.2 Fundoscopy

- Use a darkened room, ideally with both pupils dilated – common dilators (mydriatics) in adults are an anticholinergic (tropicamide 1%) and a sympathomimetic (phenylephrine 2.5%).
- Use your right eye to examine the subject's right eye and your left for the subject's left, which allows the instrument to be as close as possible to the subject's pupil.
- The green/red free filter in the ophthalmoscope renders the blood vessels black and easier to view.
- An ophthalmoscope contains a sequential arrangement of lenses of different dioptric power which can be rotated clockwise (plus, convergent or black) to compensate for long sight, and anticlockwise (minus, divergent or red) to compensate for short sight in the subject.
- Refractive errors in the observer which normally require glasses can be dealt with by adjusting the diopter strength in the instrument or by keeping on corrective glasses.

inwards towards the pupil, with one hand on the patient's forehead if necessary to steady the view.

Features to note are the:

- optic disc
- macula
- retinal vessels.

The optic disc. The margin should be sharp and the colour pink. A cup:disc ratio (the cup is the cavity in the centre of the disc) of 0.3 or less is considered normal but a large cup or asymmetry between the two eyes should lead to referral to an ophthalmologist for further investigation.

The macula is the area of central vision which lies approximately 1.5 disc diameters temporal to the optic disc. To examine it, the beam may be directed temporally or the subject asked to look directly at the light. The appearance is of a darker hue than the rest of the retina, with a central glistening area which is the reflection from the fovea – the centre of the macula.

Retinal vessels. Note the following:

- size: arteriolar attenuation (hypertension), venous dilatation (venous obstruction)
- crossing over of the retinal vessels for signs of nipping (hypertension)
- microaneurysms (diabetes).

OPHTHALMIC INJURIES

Fortunately most injuries to the eye seen in the Emergency Department are superficial. The question is if and when an ophthalmologist needs to be involved:

- *Any damage to the lacrimal drainage system which involves the lid margin.* An ophthalmologist repairs the lid margin to avoid notching and also determines any damage to lacrimal drainage.
- *Blunt injuries.* A history of considerable force, e.g. a punch, can cause effects to be transmitted deeper into the eye and should lead to consideration of referral.
- *Blow-out fractures of the orbit.* After a serious blunt injury with or without a fracture to the orbit, a thorough ocular examination is needed. A fracture can cause entrapment of extraocular muscles which can lead to double vision. Sinking of the globe into an enlarged orbital space created by the fracture has the same effect.
- *Suspicion of penetrating injury or possible foreign body.* See below.
- *Chemical injury.* Caustic chemicals, especially alkalis, can penetrate deeply.
- *Contact lenses.* Those with pain, with an acute red eye or with a visible corneal lesion have a high risk of keratitis and must be referred urgently.
- *Recent intraocular procedures.* Trauma may cause breakdown of fragile wounds, and infection may have a delayed presentation.
- *Painful orbital swelling (orbital cellulitis).* Particularly in a child, this is an ocular emergency, as the build-up of orbital pressure may compress the optic nerve.

General approach to ocular injuries

Clinical features

Complaints and history

Special attention should be paid to:

- force applied, including direction and velocity
- what was being done at the time of injury – hammering, other industrial activities
- possible nature of a foreign body.

Physical findings

Be suspicious of an undetected injury, particularly when other and apparently more obvious injuries are present either in the eye or elsewhere; an eyelid laceration can hide a perforated globe, which may in turn hide an intracranial injury.

Investigation

Imaging is most important when a foreign body is suspected: orbital X-ray, CT or (if a non-radio-opaque object is suspected) ultrasound.

General management

In a possible penetrating injury, check anti-tetanus status and bring up to date if necessary. (See below for individual injuries.)

Burns

Aetiology

Thermal injury in civilian practice is usually from molten metal. Rapid, reflex eye closure helps to limit the damage. Ultraviolet damage can arise from arc welding, sunlamps or prolonged exposure to high intensities of natural light (skiing or exploring without wearing sunglasses). Chemical burns are usually alkaline and have the devastating effect of saponifying lipid barriers so that they may penetrate into the anterior chamber.

Clinical features

Extensive oedema in the lids and face after a thermal burn may limit examination and give the false impression of blindness until the swelling subsides. Repeated assessment is necessary.

Management

Involvement of the lids in a thermal burn necessitates referral to an ophthalmologist for lid repair. Ultraviolet burns are usually self-limiting and require reassurance that vision will return, as well as pain relief. Chemical burns need copious irrigation with normal saline until the pH is returned to normal and urgent referral to an ophthalmologist to deal with the potentially serious consequences of corneal melt, glaucoma, cataract and phthisis (opacification and atrophy of the cornea).

Orbital injuries

More than 30% of patients who suffer blunt maxillofacial trauma sustain ocular injuries, of which 3% are blinding. More than 90% of the serious injuries result from midfacial, supraorbital and frontal sinus fractures; 4% of these cause optic nerve damage.

Clinical features

History

The history must include specific questions about:

- diplopia
- decreased vision
- sensory deficits in the skin of the face
- trismus
- rhinorrhoea, which may indicate a compound fracture of the skull.

Physical findings

Assess:

- visual acuity
- pupil and pupil reactions
- specific features – enophthalmos, subcutaneous emphysema, malar flattening and palpable steps in the orbital rim.

All orbital injuries should be examined by an ophthalmologist, and other specialties – maxillofacial and ear, nose and throat – should be involved as appropriate. CT is essential to plan surgical repair.

Blunt ocular trauma

Moderate to severe injury may cause immediate or delayed consequences (Table 37.5). All should be seen by an ophthalmologist.

Table 37.5 Effects of blunt trauma

Structure involved	Immediate injury	Delayed injury
Conjunctiva	Subconjunctival haemorrhage	
Cornea	Abrasion Penetrating laceration	
Iris	Rupture, dialysis hyphaema	Glaucoma
Ciliary body and angle	Recession, dialysis	Hyoptony
Vitreous	Haemorrhage	Macular hole
Retina	Commotio (bruising) Macular haemorrhage or hole Retinal tears/ dialysis	Retinal detachment Subretinal membranes
Choroid	Rupture	Subretinal membranes
Sclera	Rupture	
Optic nerve	Avulsion	Traumatic neuropathy

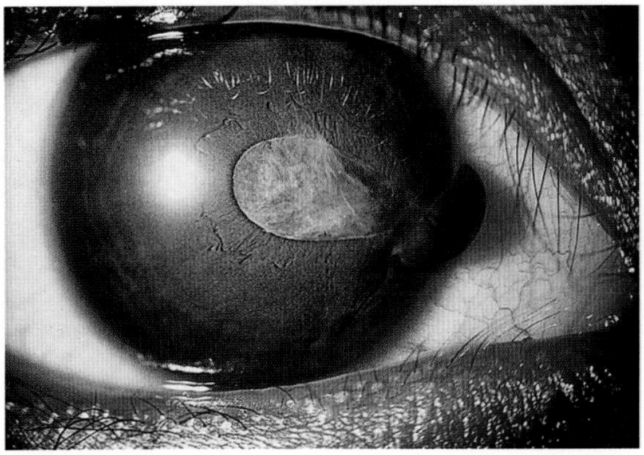

Fig. 37.2 Penetrating injury of the cornea with iris prolapse causing pupillary distortion, and secondary cataract.

Penetrating or perforating ocular injury

A penetrating injury causes cutting or tearing of the walls of the eye. A perforating injury is the same but with the addition of entry and exit wounds.

Clinical features

Suspicious appearances are:

- decreased visual acuity
- soft eye
- distorted iris – a teardrop-shaped pupil points towards the site of the perforation (Fig. 37.2).

Ocular foreign bodies

Most foreign bodies in the eye are either trapped underneath the upper lid (subtarsal) or stuck in the cornea.

Management

Removal is by the steps in Clinical Box 37.3.

Intraocular foreign bodies

Aetiology

These may be the consequence of a penetrating injury and can lodge in any part of the eye. Retrieval of foreign bodies from the eye, especially once they have lodged in the posterior segment, requires complicated vitrectomy techniques, often including lens extraction if a traumatic cataract has formed.

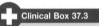

Clinical Box 37.3 Removal of a foreign body

1. Ensure the eye is well anaesthetised with several drops of topical preparation (e.g. tetracaine [amethocaine])
2. Sit the patient at the slit lamp with a warning to keep the forehead firmly against the head rest
3. Instil a drop of fluorescein to stain any corneal abrasions and enhance the presence of subtarsal foreign bodies and errant contact lenses
4. Search systematically with a request to look up, down, right and left; evert the upper eyelid for the same purpose and remove foreign bodies with a sterile cotton bud
5. For a foreign body firmly embedded in the cornea, the ideal instrument is a blunt-tipped burr which can also effectively remove a rust ring which forms around some metallic objects; if this is not available, a green 18-gauge needle can be used with caution to scrape away the affected tissue
6. A 1-week course of topical antibiotic (e.g. chloramphenicol) is prescribed

COMMON SYMPTOMS OF OCULAR DISEASE

Visual loss may be a reduction of visual acuity (blurring) or loss of visual field, either partial or total. Unilateral symptoms are likely to be from lesions of the eye or the optic nerve; bilateral lesions commonly result from defects proximal to the optic chiasm – in the brain. A summary of visual loss is given in Table 37.6.

ACUTE LOSS OF ACUITY

Retinal artery occlusion

Aetiology

Central retinal artery occlusion (CRAO) typically occurs in the optic nerve just behind the visible optic nerve head and is usually the result of thrombosis of atheromatous vessels. Rarer causes include vasculitis. Branch retinal artery occlusions (BRAOs) are embolic – 80% are derived from atheromatous disease of the carotid arteries (Ch. 29). Less commonly, calcified material or cholesterol emboli may be released from other sites (valve vegetations and thrombi of cardiac origin). Emboli may be visualised on fundoscopy as white or yellow particles lodged at the bifurcations of the retinal arterioles.

Clinical features

History

When the central retinal artery is involved, the visual loss is sudden and painless, and the deficit is profound, with acuity usually reduced to counting fingers (CF) or worse, with even a loss of light perception.

Physical findings

There is a relative afferent pupillary defect (impaired direct light response), and fundoscopy shows a pale retina with

Table 37.6 Causes of visual loss

	Painful		
Time course	Red eye	White eye	Painless (white eye)
Acute	Trauma	AION – arteritic	CRAO/ BRAO CRVO/BRVO AION – non–arteritic
Subacute	Uveitis Orbital inflammation Acute glaucoma	Optic neuritis	Wet ARMD Uveitis
Gradual	Uveitis	Optic nerve compression	Wet ARMD Dry ARMD Cataract Optic nerve compression Uveitis Chronic glaucoma
Transient	Migraine AION – arteritic		Migraine TIA (amaurosis fugax) Syncope

AION, anterior ischaemic optic neuropathy; ARMD, age-related macular degeneration; BRAO, branch retinal artery occlusion; BRVO, branch retinal vein occlusion; CRAO, central retinal artery occlusion; CRVO, central retinal vein occlusion; TIA, transient ischaemic attack.

attenuated vessels and a cherry red spot at the macula (Fig. 37.3). In around 20%, the macula receives its blood supply from the choroidal circulation via the cilioretinal artery, and, in these, a small island of central vision with variable retention of visual acuity may remain, but the loss of visual field greatly reduces function.

BRAO affects vision and depends on the location of the vessel affected. A visual field defect (scotoma) results, and, when the macula is involved, there is reduced visual acuity.

CRAO typically occurs in the optic nerve just behind the visible nerve head. The usual cause is atheroma with embolus of a fibrinoplatelet accumulation (Ch. 29) in the carotid bifurcation from atrial fibrillation or myocardial infarction, but vasculitis (including giant cell arteritis) is another possibility. Cardiovascular assessment is required. Emboli can be seen on fundoscopy as white or yellow particles lodged at bifurcations of the retinal arterioles (Fig. 37.4).

Retinal vein occlusion

Aetiology

Diabetes, hypertension and hyperlipidaemia are the major systemic risk factors.

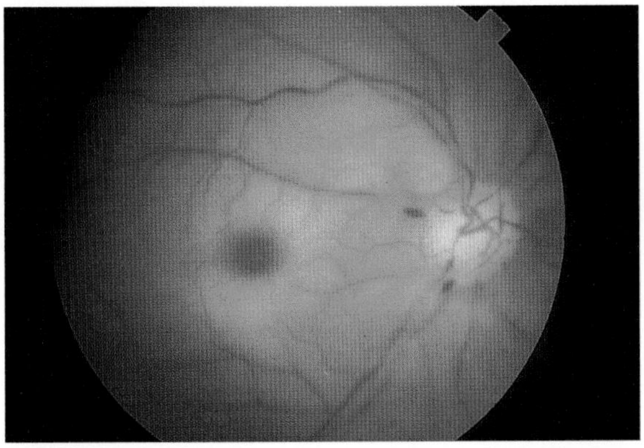

Fig. 37.3 Central retinal artery occlusion with 'cherry red spot'.

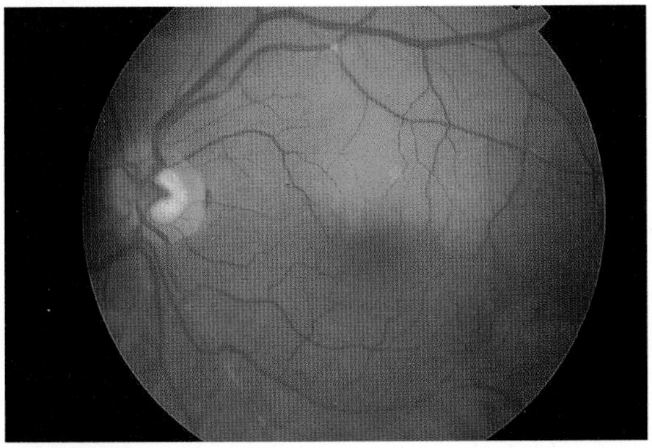

Fig. 37.4 Superior temporal branch retinal artery occlusion (see calcific embolus lodged in bifurcation of retinal arterioles), with cloudy retinal swelling in the distribution of the occluded vessel.

History and findings

Retinal vein occlusion is experienced as a sudden loss of vision of variable severity. Fundoscopy reveals dilated veins, haemorrhages and cotton wool spots in the affected area of retina. It may be localised, as in branch retinal vein occlusions, or involve all four retinal quadrants, often with disc swelling in a case of central retinal vein occlusion.

Anterior ischaemic optic neuropathy (AION)

Aetiology

This is an infarction of the optic nerve head because of closure of the ciliary arteries of supply. Two groups of patients can be identified: 50–60-year-olds and those aged >70 years. Members of the first group are likely to have cardiovascular risk factors such as hypertension and angina caused by thrombosis of atheromatous ciliary vessels. The over-70s may have arteritic AION, usually as a result of giant-cell arteritis.

Clinical features

A sudden visual loss results, which may be total or altitudinal (where the inferior or, less commonly, the superior half of the visual field in one eye is lost). Arteritic AION may be accompanied by symptoms of malaise, weight loss, muscle pains and stiffness, temporal headache and scalp tenderness, and jaw or tongue claudication.

There is a relative afferent pupillary defect, and on fundoscopy a pale, swollen optic disc is seen.

Management

All patients with acute visual loss thought to be of vascular origin should have an urgent ESR and immediate referral to an ophthalmologist if arteritis is suspected, because high-dose systemic steroids may be required to prevent blindness from involvement of the other eye (see also transient visual loss – 'stuttering amaurosis').

SUBACUTE LOSS OF ACUITY

Optic neuritis

Visual loss which develops over a few hours to 2–3 days and which is associated with ocular pain exacerbated by ocular movements is characteristic of optic and retrobulbar neuritis. Loss of acuity is variable but may fall to an absence of perception of light. Colour desaturation (i.e. where colours are seen as being washed out) is a prominent early feature. There is a relative afferent pupillary defect and, if the intraocular optic nerve is affected, a swollen optic disc may be noted (Fig. 37.5). More commonly the inflammation is located in the intraorbital optic nerve and fundoscopy is normal (the patient sees nothing and the doctor sees nothing), and the condition is called retrobulbar neuritis.

The most common cause is multiple sclerosis (MS), and patients tend therefore to be in the 20–40 year age group and are more often female. Enquiry and examination for symptoms or signs of previous neurological disease are essential and, if positive, confirm the diagnosis of multiple sclerosis.

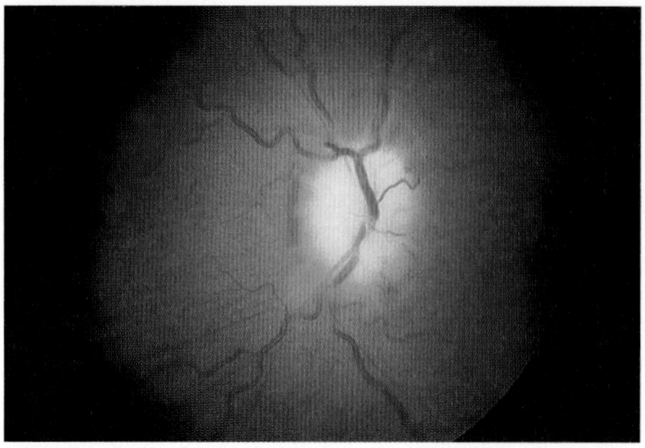

Fig. 37.5 Papilloedema in benign intracranial hypertension.

Referral to an ophthalmologist or neurologist is indicated for confirmation of eye involvement.

Investigation and management

In isolated optic or retrobulbar neuritis, the extent of investigation is controversial; some recommend a full work-up for signs of subclinical lesions elsewhere in order to make the diagnosis of MS; others feel that, because there is as yet no effective intervention, a 'wait and see' attitude should be adopted. Treatment is also controversial; intravenous corticosteroids shorten the acute episode but have no effect on the extent of final visual recovery or the ultimate prognosis.

Prognosis

After visual loss, some degree of recovery always occurs. In most instances, this takes 4–6 weeks and is full or nearly so, although a small residual (subjective) defect is often present. Residual signs include red desaturation, a relative afferent pupillary defect and optic disc pallor, most marked temporally, which develops over a few weeks after an acute episode.

Optic nerve compression

Lesions within the orbit may compress the optic nerve, especially if located posteriorly at the orbital apex where nerves and vessels are crowded together. Many such lesions result in gradual visual loss (see below). Orbital inflammatory disease may, however, be rapidly progressive and is an ophthalmic emergency.

Clinical features

Symptoms
include pain, visual loss and diplopia.

Signs are of:

- reduced acuity
- loss of colour vision
- a relative afferent pupillary defect
- proptosis
- conjunctival chemosis.

Reduction of ocular motility results either from IIIrd, IVth or VIth cranial nerve damage at the orbital apex or from direct mechanical restriction of ocular movement.

Causes to be considered are:

- acute dysthyroid eye disease (Graves' disease, see Ch. 32)
- orbital cellulitis (usually secondary to paranasal sinus disease)
- orbital pseudotumour (idiopathic orbital inflammation which mimics an orbital tumour).

Insidious, unilateral painless visual loss results from compression of the optic nerve by a slowly growing tumour. In children, this is most commonly an optic nerve glioma, sometimes seen as part of type 1 neurofibromatosis. In adults, usually women of 30–50 years, meningioma of the optic nerve sheath or sphenoid wing is most likely.

Fundoscopy shows a pale and sometimes swollen optic disc. Tortuous abnormal vessels on the optic disc (retinochoroidal shunts) are typical of a meningioma.

Management

The patient should be referred to an ophthalmologist who, when the diagnosis is suspected, can confirm it by CT.

Surgical excision often results in damage to the optic nerve. It may be indicated if the sight is already badly damaged and the tumour can be excised whole; otherwise, radiotherapy or observation alone may be preferred.

GRADUAL LOSS OF ACUITY

Gradual diminution of visual acuity is one of the most common complaints encountered in ophthalmology. By contrast, gradual loss of visual field is rarely noticed by the patient – hence the need for screening programmes for chronic glaucoma. Field loss is usually noticed by the patient only when very extensive, because acuity is retained until late in the disease process.

Cataract

A cataract is an opacity of the lens that interferes with vision (Fig. 37.6). Most are of the idiopathic senile type, and the prevalence increases with age. There are many other causes, which include:

- trauma
- uveitis
- metabolic disorders (e.g. diabetes mellitus)
- congenital.

In those regions of the world where therapeutic resources are unavailable, cataract is the most common cause of blindness (visual acuity less than 3/60 in the better eye).

Clinical features

Symptoms include:

- gradual blurring of vision
- change in the prescription for glasses – 'second sight' is the myopic shift induced by nuclear sclerotic cataract that may allow a presbyopic patient to resume reading

Gradual loss of acuity

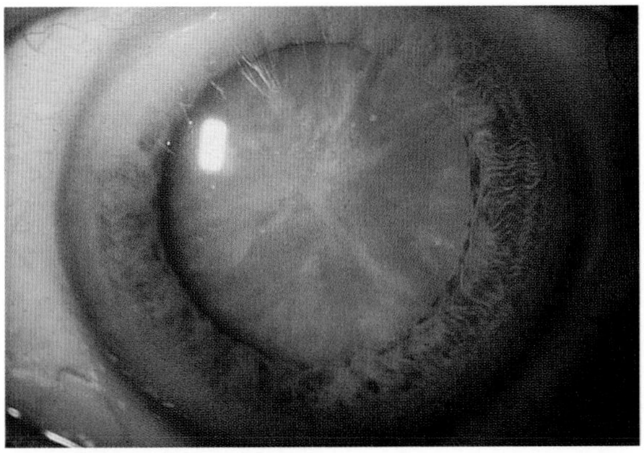

Fig. 37.6 Mature cataract.

without reading glasses after previously having required them

- glare – most marked in bright sunlight or when confronted by oncoming headlights while driving at night; this is typical of a posterior subcapsular cataract.

A cataract is most easily identified as an obstruction of the red reflex during direct ophthalmoscopy.

Management

Treatment is by extraction and insertion of a prosthetic intraocular lens once the reduction of vision is sufficient to interfere with lifestyle. The threshold for an operation is affected by individual visual needs – driving, occupation and hobbies. Cataract surgery is usually performed as a day case under local anaesthesia.

Macular degeneration

Age-related macular degeneration (ARMD) is the most common cause of blindness (visual acuity of less than 3/60 in the better eye) in the developed world. It affects central vision, with reduction of visual acuity and sometimes formation of a central scotoma. There are two types: dry and wet.

Dry ARMD

This is an idiopathic gradual loss of photoreceptors and retinal pigment epithelium in the macular area. Visual loss is gradual, mild to moderate in severity and usually symmetrical. Fundoscopy shows areas of hypo- and hyperpigmentation in the macula. There is no treatment to arrest the process. Management is directed at low-vision optical aids to make the most of what residual function exists. Registration as partially sighted or blind is valuable to increase help from community sources.

Wet ARMD

Wet ARMD is again bilateral, although symptoms usually begin on one side. It tends to occur in a younger age group and results from the development of subretinal neovascular complexes: 'membranes' that leak serum and may bleed into the retina. Presentation is with more-rapid onset of poor vision; central scotomas and visual distortion (see below) are common. Fundoscopy (Fig. 37.7) may reveal dark red blood or grey subretinal elevation (fluid or subretinal membrane) at the macula. Immediate referral to an ophthalmologist is required because treatment with anti-growth factor injected intravitreal can prevent blindness.

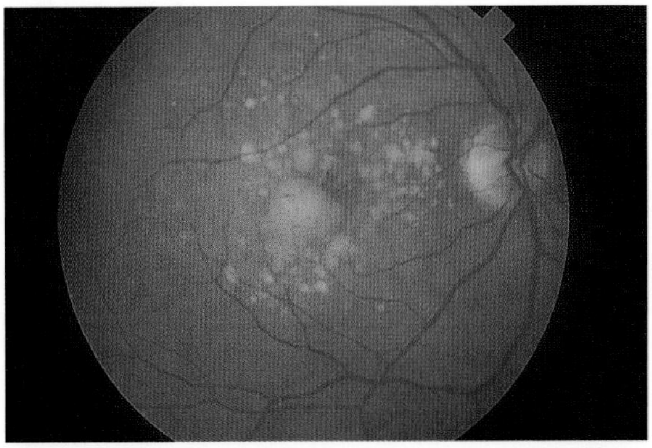

Fig. 37.7 Age-related macular degeneration, with large confluent soft drusen. This eye is at high risk of visual loss from subretinal neovascularisation.

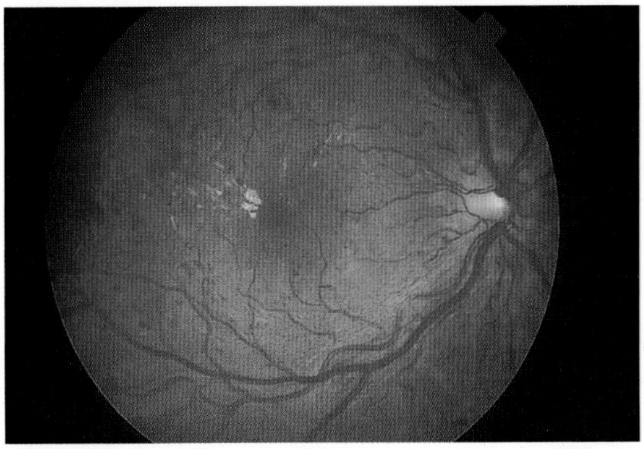

Fig. 37.8 Diabetic maculopathy.

Macular oedema

This is a complication of many ophthalmic disorders rather than a separate entity. It is the major cause of visual loss in diabetic retinopathy (Fig. 37.8) and may be the presenting feature of diabetes in non-insulin-dependent disease. Macular oedema may also be seen in ARMD, in uveitis, in hypertensive retinopathy (Fig. 37.9) and as a complication of intraocular surgery.

Another relatively common cause is central serous retinopathy, an idiopathic condition seen most commonly in men of between 20 and 40 years. Choroidal fluid leaks through the macula to produce a localised serous retinal detachment, which presents with subacute onset of blurring and distortion of the central field characterised by micropsia (objects appear smaller than they actually are). In the great majority, the condition resolves spontaneously, usually within 1–6 months after the onset of symptoms.

Macular hole

This is another degenerative disorder caused by an abnormal vitreoretinal adhesion at the macula which pulls out a circular fragment of retina. The disease is most common in women

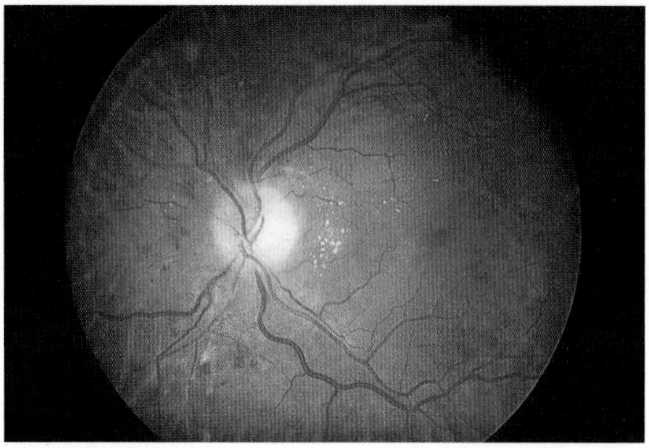

Fig. 37.9 Grade III hypertensive retinopathy. The concentration of exudates and haemorrhages in the peripapillary area is typical.

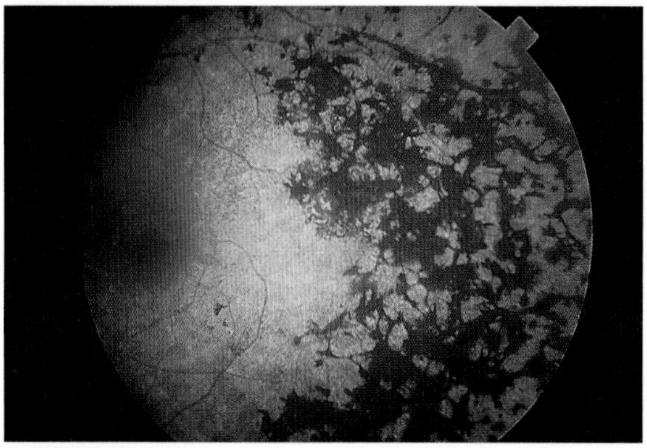

Fig. 37.10 Retinitis pigmentosa with classic bone spicule pigmentation.

in the sixth and seventh decades of life and remains unilateral in 90%.

The presenting features are similar to ARMD: visual distortion, reduced acuity and a central scotoma. On fundoscopy a small (approximately one-third of a disc diameter) red round hole over the fovea may be seen. Referral is indicated because surgical intervention may be possible.

Retinal dystrophies

Gradual visual loss in younger patients is uncommon and always warrants ophthalmic referral. There are a large number of hereditary and sporadic retinal and macular dystrophies that may present with reduced acuity and colour or night blindness. Often the gross ophthalmoscopic appearance is normal. Retinitis pigmentosa is the best known of these conditions, in which case the classic mid-peripheral bone spicule pigmentation may indicate the diagnosis (Fig. 37.10).

Uveitis

Acute uveitis (inflammation of the uvea, i.e. the iris [iritis], ciliary body [iridocyclitis] and choroid [posterior uveitis or choroiditis]) usually presents with a red eye and pain, but chronic uveitis may solely cause visual loss. Chronic anterior uveitis in juvenile rheumatoid arthritis may be asymptomatic until the complications of secondary cataract and (often untreatable) cystoid macular oedema develop. For this reason all children with arthritis must have ophthalmic screening at regular intervals. Intermediate and posterior uveitis may cause gradual or subacute loss of vision, as a result of direct retinal damage, macular oedema or vitritis. The last of these causes a diffuse vitreous haze or floaters (below). All these conditions need specialist assessment. Management is often difficult but may involve periocular or systemic corticosteroids.

TRANSIENT LOSS OF VISION

This is a common symptom. A careful history often allows benign conditions to be separated from more serious disease.

Syncope

A fall in systemic blood pressure from whatever cause (e.g. Stokes–Adams attack, vasovagal response) can result in, initially, the loss of colour vision (grey-out) and subsequently all vision (blackout), as blood flow to the eyes decreases. Symptoms are bilateral and are usually accompanied by faintness, dizziness and palpitations. Provided blood flow is restored (e.g. by falling to a horizontal position), both general recovery and visual recovery are likely to be swift.

Migraine

This is a familial vasospastic disorder that may cause neurological symptoms as a result of intracranial ischaemia, followed in most instances by headache which is thought to be the consequence of compensatory vasodilatation. The most common neurological disturbance is visual, with the appearance of jagged concentric black lines across the visual field (fortification spectra) and a scintillating scotoma. These sensations may last for around 30 minutes and are followed by a severe throbbing ipsilateral hemicranial headache, with debilitation and nausea present for up to several hours, followed by resolution and sleep.

Migraine is, however, protean in its manifestations and should be included in the differential diagnosis of any transient visual disturbance, even without headache, especially in younger patients. If it occurs for the first time after the age of 50, the diagnosis must only be made with caution because an intracranial disorder is possible.

Transient ischaemic attack (TIA)

(See also Ch. 29)

A TIA that involves the central retinal artery circulation has the same cause as a branch retinal arterial occlusion, and those that affect the cerebral hemispheres (embolic disease) usually relate to atheroma of the extracranial carotid arteries. The patient typically describes a grey curtain moving horizontally upwards or downwards across the vision of one eye; it comes on over seconds to minutes and is likely to resolve within a few minutes (amaurosis fugax – fleeting blindness). Fundoscopy is often normal; alternatively, white/yellow refractile emboli may be visible within the retinal arterioles.

Transient loss of vision
Loss of visual field
Retinal detachment
Neurological disease
Visual distortion

The significance of amaurosis fugax is the increased risk of retinal arterial occlusion or stroke. A full assessment is required (Ch. 29). A related symptom is stuttering amaurosis (repeated uniocular episodes of visual loss) which is an occasional precursor of permanent loss of vision in giant-cell arteritis.

LOSS OF VISUAL FIELD

Vascular

All the vascular causes of acute loss of acuity described above can instead present as visual field loss, e.g. with a scotoma in BRAO and BRVO or altitudinal field loss in AION.

RETINAL DETACHMENT

Retinal detachment may be traumatic; however, in the majority of cases it is spontaneous. The condition is more common in myopes.

Pathological and pathophysiological features

Changes in the vitreous gel (posterior vitreous detachment) tear a hole in the retina and allow fluid from the vitreous to enter the subretinal space. The neurosensory retina separates from the underlying retinal pigment epithelium so that the detached area of retina ceases to function. The field defect which results mirrors the site of the detachment. Thus a superior detachment (the most common and rapidly progressive) produces an inferior-field defect, often referred to as a 'shadow in the vision'.

Clinical features

Symptoms

Visual acuity is retained until the macula is involved in the detachment. This is important, because detachment that is surgically repaired when the macula is still on has a much better visual prognosis than when it has come off. Other symptoms include floaters and photopsia.

Physical findings

The index of suspicion must be high – a myopic spectacle correction is easily detected by looking through the spectacle lens, when objects appear smaller. A monocular field defect is usually present. Visual acuity varies depending on the state of the macula. If more than a quarter of the retina has detached, there is a relative afferent pupillary defect. If the detachment is small, fundoscopy may be normal, especially if a direct ophthalmoscope through an undilated pupil is used, because this only affords a small field of view and the detachment starts peripherally. The detachment is seen as an elevated convex area of grey retina which moves with ocular movement and has a wrinkled surface (Fig. 37.11). Therefore, if the history is suggestive but the examination appears to be normal, a referral to an ophthalmologist for more detailed examination is important.

Management

If central vision is retained at the time of diagnosis, detachment is an emergency. Treatment is surgical. It involves either an external approach with the application of a compressive buckle to the outside of the eye, or an internal approach with removal of the vitreous gel and usually internal tamponade with gas or liquid. The aim is to oppose the detached retina and underlying retinal pigment epithelium. Adhesion between the two layers is then achieved by the use of laser or cryoprobe to create inflammation and scarring.

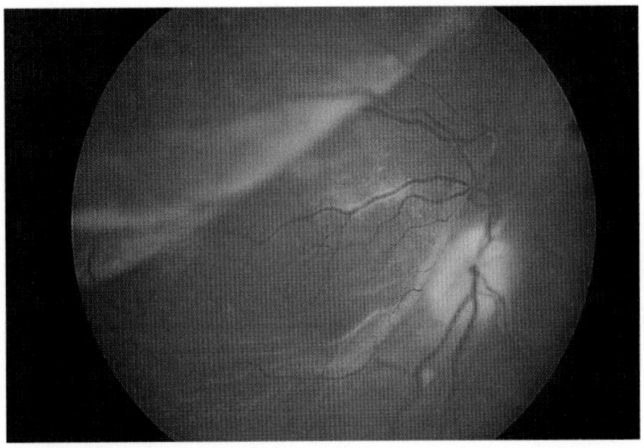

Fig. 37.11 Retinal detachment.

NEUROLOGICAL DISEASE

Lesions of the retrochiasmal optic pathway result in bilateral hemianopic visual field defects that obey the vertical meridian. They can usually be easily detected by confrontation testing and must be specifically sought in all instances of apparently monocular visual loss because a positive finding excludes ocular disease as the cause. In a left homonymous hemianopia, for example, the nasal field defect in the right eye may not be noticed by the patient because it is overlapped by the retained nasal field of the left eye, and it may therefore present as an isolated loss of the left temporal visual field.

Acute-onset hemianopic visual field loss is very likely to be cerebrovascular in origin – 80% of cases are caused by emboli from the extracranial carotid arteries (Ch. 29). Cardiovascular risk factors should therefore be assessed.

Ophthalmic disease in multiple sclerosis is described later in this chapter.

VISUAL DISTORTION

Visual distortion (metamorphopsia) is a symptom restricted to disorders that affect the macula, because it occurs when macular photoreceptors are displaced relative to each other. The result is disruption of macular representation of objects in the central visual field. Altered image size and reduced visual acuity result from the same mechanism.

The formation of a fine membranous scar (epiretinal membrane) may cause metamorphopsia, as may macular oedema from any cause. Detection is easy by asking the patient to examine an Amsler chart, which is a regular grid of black lines on a white background, looked at from a distance of 30 cm. Typically there is distortion and blurring of the grid; the location of worst distortion corresponds to the site of the macular lesion. If an Amsler chart is not available, any straight high-contrast edge will suffice; for example, ask if the edges of a window frame appear straight and regular.

Photopsia

Photopsia refers to the sensation of light arising from non-light stimuli. It may happen when mechanical forces act on the retina: either due to an external force (trauma), which can be transient, or secondary to intraocular disease which is more persistent. The two major intraocular causes are posterior vitreous detachment (see below) and retinal detachment. Mechanical photopsia are unformed visual sensations, as distinct from the structured visual sensations experienced as a result of neurological disease, such as migraine.

Floaters

Floaters are dark spots seen moving in the visual field. They result from opacities within the vitreous gel casting a shadow on the retina, explaining their mobility.

Posterior vitreous detachment

The vitreous gel is increasingly being recognised as a complex structure, rather than simply an amorphous gel, which is reflected in the degenerative changes that are seen in all eyes with increasing age. The gel collapses into itself in places to form denser spots and areas of increased gel mobility, which are of themselves sometimes large enough to be seen as floaters but are not of clinical significance. With further degeneration the volume of the vitreous gel decreases and the retrohyaloid space (the space between the vitreous and retina) is filled with aqueous. Movement of the eye will allow the liquid gel to strip the remaining vitreous away from the retina, to create a posterior vitreous detachment (PVD).

Clinical features

Photopsia may be experienced during the development of a posterior vitreous detachment because of the traction on the retina when the gel collapses. The incidence of PVD increases with age. In the majority, it is annoying but not dangerous. Around 5%, however, sustain damage in the form of a retinal tear as a result of traction. Retinal tears are the major cause of retinal detachments because they allow the liquefied vitreous and/or aqueous to pass through the hole into the subretinal space and detach it from the retinal pigment epithelium.

Retinal tear

Clinical features of a retinal tear include floaters associated with photopsia, and impairment of visual acuity in the case of a larger vitreous haemorrhage. On fundoscopy the PVD and any vitreous blood may be seen as small, mobile, black spots in the red reflex. However, they are difficult to visualise with the direct ophthalmoscope.

Management of suspected PVD or a retinal tear involves same-day referral to an ophthalmologist for thorough dilated indirect ophthalmoscopy. There is no treatment for the PVD, but retinal tears need laser or cryotherapy to seal the tear. Retinal detachments, if present, usually require operation.

Uveitis

Chronic uveitis may lead to organised inflammatory reaction in the vitreous gel which the patient perceives as floaters. The eye is usually painless, and the condition may have been present for some time. Visual loss is common, but in intermediate uveitis/pars planitis, where only the region of the ciliary body is inflamed, visual acuity is usually normal, unless and until cystoid macular oedema supervenes.

Ocular pain

While many disorders of the external eye produce ocular discomfort (e.g. conjunctivitis and blepharitis), ocular pain is less common and may indicate serious disease. It is helpful to elicit whether the pain feels superficial (sharp, scratching) or deep (aching, gnawing), as this sometimes distinguishes corneal from intraocular disease. Headache associated with visual symptoms occurs in migraine and giant-cell arteritis and should not be confused with ocular pain.

Corneal abrasion

Defects in the corneal epithelium expose the underlying plexus of naked nerve terminals, cause severe, sharp pain, worse with lid movement, and excessive lacrimation.

Clinical features

History

There is usually a clear history of trauma to the eye, although sometimes an abrasion results from breakdown of healed epithelium at a site of previous injury. This recurrent corneal erosion syndrome has a characteristic pattern of pain on first opening the eyes in the morning, often preceded by short-lived episodes of pain and redness in the few days before the actual abrasion occurs.

Physical findings

Abrasions are identified with guttae fluorescein 2% stain and cobalt blue light, which shows the abrasion as a fluorescent yellow-green area on the cornea (Fig. 37.12). A blue cover to a penlight torch can be used where a slit lamp is unavailable.

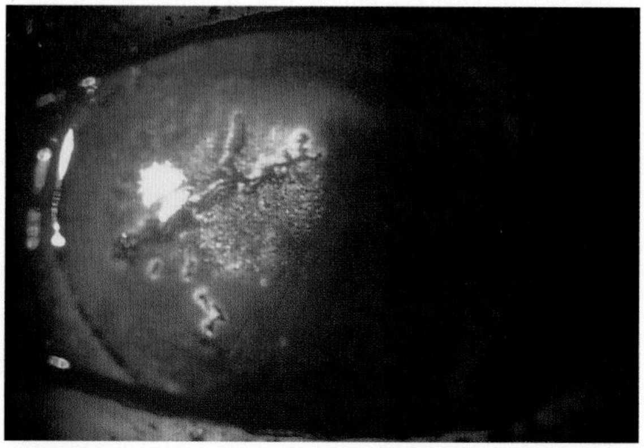

Fig. 37.12 Fluorescein–stained dendritic ulcer (herpes simplex).

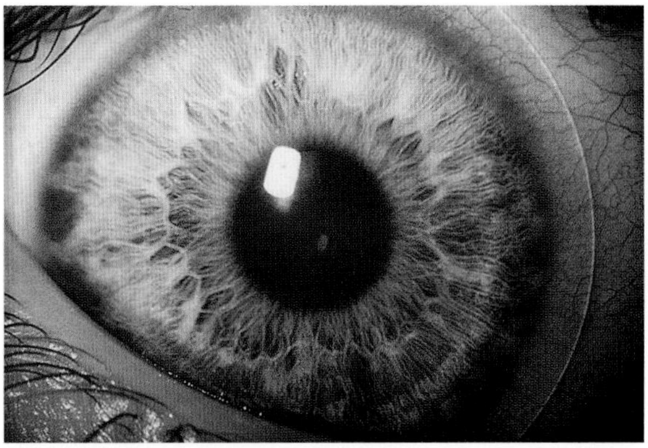

Fig. 37.13 Soft contact lens in situ.

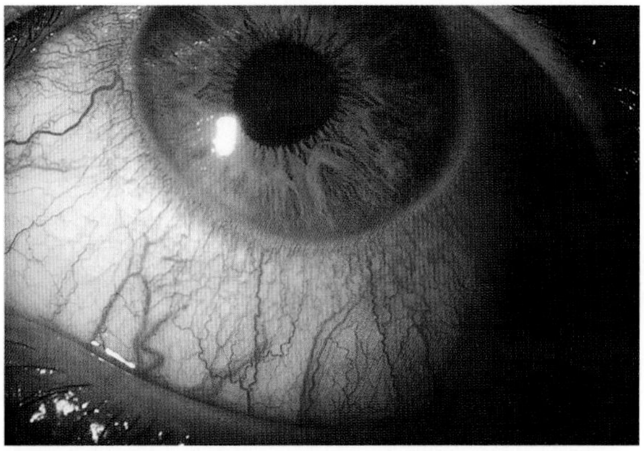

Fig. 37.14 Acute anterior uveitis (iritis) with ciliary flush and a fixed, oval pupil.

Management

Treatment is with broad-spectrum antibiotic eye drops (usually chloramphenicol 0.5% four times a day for 5 days) with cycloplegia and/or an eye patch if the pain is severe. Simple abrasions do not need referral to an ophthalmologist but should be reviewed after 48 hours to confirm a reduction in size.

Keratitis

Inflammation of the cornea is usually infective. Herpes virus infections and related immune keratitis are considered below. Most bacteria require a pre-existing epithelial defect to allow them to breach the cornea, but an important exception is *Neisseria gonorrhoeae*; hence the importance of urgent, aggressive treatment in ophthalmia neonatorum. Predisposing conditions include contact lenses (Fig. 37.13), a dry eye and the long-term use of eye drops that contain corticosteroids. Pain can be severe, partly because of the frequently present secondary uveitis. Suspected keratitis always needs urgent ophthalmic review.

Uveitis

Acute anterior uveitis is inflammation of the iris and/or ciliary body. If only the iris is affected, it may also be called iritis or, if the ciliary body is also involved, iridocyclitis.

Aetiology

There are many possible causes of acute anterior uveitis, including a number of associations with systemic disorders (e.g. HLA B27-positive arthropathies and sarcoidosis). However, in the majority a specific cause is not found.

Clinical features

History

Pain is usually moderate to severe, with photophobia, lacrimation and often reduction of vision.

Physical findings

Redness is most marked around the cornea and typically has a violaceous hue. Miosis is present, and the pupil may also be fixed and irregular because of the formation of adhesions between the iris and the lens – posterior synechiae (Fig. 37.14). In most, the condition is unilateral and should be strongly suspected in the presence of any unilateral, persistently painful red eye.

Management

Uveitis always needs specialist attention, even when the diagnosis appears clear, because the efficacy of treatment and the presence of complications such as glaucoma can only be assessed by slit-lamp examination.

Glaucoma

Glaucoma refers to a group of conditions characterised by retinal nerve fibre damage, resulting in typical optic disc changes (cupping) and visual field loss. There are many subgroups, most importantly acute and chronic glaucoma. Raised intraocular pressure is always a feature of acute glaucoma, and most cases of chronic glaucoma also have raised pressure, but to a lesser degree.

Pain is not a feature of chronic open-angle glaucoma (the most common form). However, in acute angle closure glaucoma, the intraocular pressure rises rapidly and dramatically.

Clinical features of acute glaucoma

The condition is more common with increasing age and is found predominantly in hyperopes (whose glasses magnify images seen through the lens).

The patient is likely to be in distress, with severe pain, blurring of vision and halos around lights. The eye is intensely injected, with clouding of the cornea and a fixed semi-dilated pupil.

Management

Immediate referral is necessary and urgent treatment to lower the pressure is required to alleviate the pain and prevent permanent visual loss due to pressure-induced damage to the retinal nerve fibres as they enter the optic nerve.

Episcleritis and scleritis

Both these conditions present with a red eye and are immune-mediated.

Episcleritis

This is a self-limiting condition characterised by ocular discomfort and diffuse or localised redness. It is rarely associated with underlying disease. If symptoms warrant treatment, a course of oral NSAIDs is usually effective.

Scleritis

This is a much more serious condition that may lead to visual loss. Severe, constant, deep ocular pain is usual. The redness may be localised, diffuse or absent in posterior scleritis. An early ophthalmic opinion should be sought. Scleritis may occur in isolation, but is frequently associated with connective-tissue disorders (systemic lupus erythematosus, rheumatoid arthritis) or vasculitis.

ORBITAL PAIN

It is often very difficult clinically to differentiate between orbital and ocular pain because many describe ocular pain as coming from behind the eye and orbital pain is poorly localised. Orbital inflammatory conditions often lead to secondary scleritis, which adds ocular pain to the clinical picture. Associated features that lead to the suspicion of orbital disease as a cause include proptosis, ophthalmoplegia, ptosis and loss of corneal sensation.

Orbital inflammation

Orbital cellulitis, dysthyroid eye disease and orbital pseudotumour have all been mentioned in the section on visual loss. The severity of pain, inflammatory signs or mass effects varies greatly.

Orbital malignancy

Benign tumours generally present with painless gradual visual loss. Malignant tumours, however, often cause pain as a result of rapid growth or neuronal invasion, which is often associated with proptosis and ophthalmoplegia.

PROPTOSIS

The orbit is bounded by bone on all sides except anteriorly. In consequence, any increase in the volume of the intraorbital contents can only be decompressed by forward displacement of the globe, which causes protrusion of the orbital contents – proptosis. Exophthalmos is a synonymous term but is usually reserved for dysthyroid eye disease (the most common cause of proptosis).

Aetiology

If a lesion is located within the retrobulbar space, bounded by the extraocular muscles (intraconal), the displacement is axial; if extraconal, then non-axial proptosis with mechanical strabismus ensues.

Dysthyroid eye disease and idiopathic orbital inflammation (orbital pseudotumour), orbital cellulitis and other rarer conditions such as tuberculosis and sarcoidosis cause proptosis by increasing the volume of intraorbital fat and connective tissue and also of the extraocular muscles. Tumours of all kinds may cause proptosis, as may vascular disease such as orbital varices and haemorrhagic cysts. Pulsatile proptosis with enlargement and injection of the conjunctival vessels is the hallmark of a carotid-cavernous fistula, in which the orbital venous system becomes arterialised as a result of an abnormal communication between the ophthalmic artery and the cavernous venous sinus.

EPIPHORA

Epiphora (excessive production or running of tears) can be difficult to evaluate. Probably the most important question is: is it constant? Tearing which is only intermittent is unlikely to result from lacrimal duct obstruction. The diagnosis is best approached by considering where the problem may lie:

Lacrimal gland. Primary excessive activity of the gland is very rare but may be seen after injury to the facial nerve with aberrant regeneration (gustatory sweating). Secondary or reflex overactivity is much more common and can result from any painful ocular condition. For chronic epiphora, it is important to examine the lids and ocular surface for irritant lesions such as trichiasis (inturned lashes) and entropion (inturned lid).

Eyelid. Tears are moved across the eye from the superolateral lacrimal gland to the inferomedial drainage system by a combination of gravity and the pumping action of the lids. The mechanism can be upset by ectropion, where the lid margin turns outwards away from the eye; tears spill over the edge and normal apposition of the lacrimal punctum to the pool of tears in the medial canthus is prevented. Even without ectropion, a flaccid orbicularis muscle can impair the pump mechanism and epiphora follows. These changes are commonly involutional in the elderly but may also be seen following VIIth nerve palsy or scarring of the skin of the lower lid.

Lacrimal duct. From the lacrimal punctae, tears drain via the canaliculi to the lacrimal sac and thence to the nasolacrimal duct and the nose. Obstruction at any of these sites causes epiphora. Congenital nasolacrimal duct obstruction affects up to 20% of neonates, but canalisation is completed spontaneously in over 90% by 1 year. When canalisation remains incomplete after this time, probing of the duct usually easily completes the process. In adults, stenosis may be traumatic, infective (e.g. herpes simplex conjunctivitis) or, most commonly, a gradual involutional change. Often a simple explanation of the cause of symptoms is all that is required;

however, some require surgery, which can now often be done under local anaesthesia.

PTOSIS

This is an abnormally low position of the upper eyelid which may be an isolated problem or the presenting feature of serious neurological disease. It should be differentiated from pseudoptosis, which is a relative ptosis because of contralateral lid retraction. Ptosis is best considered initially in relation to age.

Congenital ptosis

Infantile ptosis may be the outcome of any of the causes described under subsequent headings but is most commonly dystrophic with abnormal development of the levator muscle. The condition may be unilateral or bilateral. Any significant ptosis in a young child must be urgently referred because of the risk of occlusion amblyopia. This is a failure of development of the cerebral pathways serving the affected eye due to lack of stimulation during the critical period of development. The eye is physically normal, but processing of visual data from the eye is impaired. In infants, a week of occlusion may be significant; once a child is over around 7 years of age, amblyopia can neither develop nor be treated if present.

Adult

Ptosis in adults of working age may result from a number of causes (Fig. 37.15). Diplopia, rapid muscle fatigue and muscle weakness should be specifically asked for and may indicate myasthenia gravis. The pupil and ocular movements must be examined specifically to look for the down-and-out globe position of a palsy of the IIIrd nerve. In those with diabetes or hypertension, this is commonly a microvascular event; however, the presence of a dilated pupil raises the possibility of an expanding aneurysm of the posterior communicating artery which must be investigated by neuroimaging. Trauma may also cause ptosis, which may not become evident until the initial swelling has died down.

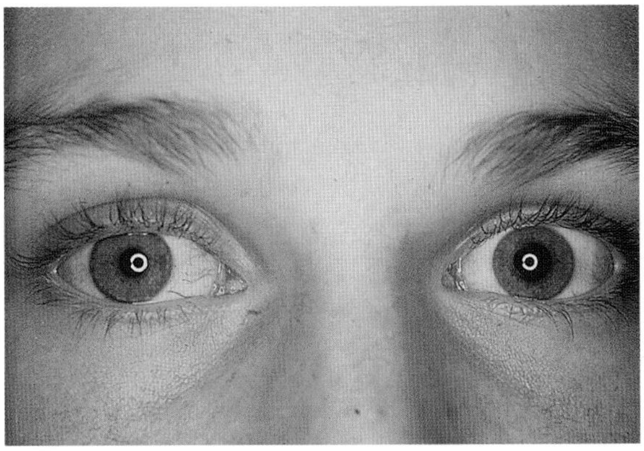

Fig. 37.15 Right Horner's syndrome: pupillary miosis and partial ptosis.

The elderly

The adult causes described above still apply in later life, but the most common cause is degeneration of the attachment of the levator palpebrae superioris aponeurosis to the lid. Five per cent of cataract operations precipitate the condition. There is a drooping upper lid with thin skin, and the horizontal upper lid crease lies high up on the lid. In spontaneous instances, the condition is bilateral but not necessarily symmetrical. Operation to reattach the aponeurosis to the lid tissues can be performed under local anaesthetic.

ANISOCORIA

This is a visible difference in pupil size between the two eyes. It may be a normal variant (seen in 20% of the population at some time; pupillary reactions are normal) or pathological. Pathological causes can be divided into parasympathetic, tonic and sympathetic neurological causes and local (ocular) causes.

Parasympathetic palsy

The innervation of the sphincter pupillae muscle which is responsible for constriction of the pupil (miosis) is by preganglionic parasympathetic axons in the oculomotor nerve with synapses in the ciliary ganglion. The fibres run on the superior border of the nerve within the subarachnoid space where they are vulnerable to compression by intracranial lesions, but their superficial location close to the pial blood vessels spares them from many vascular problems. In consequence, there are two types of lesion: a fixed dilated pupil (surgical) and a pupil-sparing IIIrd (medical).

Tonic (Adie) pupil

This is a dilated pupil with light–near dissociation – the pupil fails to constrict in response to light but does so to accommodation (the near triad of miosis, accommodation and convergence). The lesion is in the ciliary ganglion and is thought to result from viral inflammation. The usual occurrence is in a young woman who presents with blurring of vision because of paresis of accommodation. Regeneration of the nerve results in the return of near vision, but the pupillary responses remain abnormal with a tonic (slow onset and prolonged duration) miosis, initially in response to near vision but which becomes permanent over a few years. The Holmes–Adie syndrome is the association of the tonic pupil with absence of deep tendon reflexes (e.g. knee jerks) which is seen in 60%.

Sympathetic palsy

Horner's syndrome is the triad of partial ptosis, miosis and anhidrosis resulting from a lesion in the sympathetic nervous system. The neuronal pathway originates with pre-ganglionic fibres in the hypothalamus, and then passes through the brainstem and spinal cord to exit in the anterior roots. They ascend in the sympathetic chain and synapse in the superior cervical ganglion. Post-ganglionic fibres pass from the ganglion into the cervical sympathetic chain and perivascular plexi, and thence to the orbit. Ptosis and miosis are seen in all cases, whereas anhidrosis is absent with lesions affecting post-ganglionic fibres.

Horner's syndrome may be transient, as in neuralgic migraine/cluster headache where the neuronal plexus around the carotid artery is affected. Otherwise the lesion may be anywhere along the pathway described, and careful examination supplemented by imaging and pharmacological testing may be required to determine the cause. It is particularly important to examine the root of the neck for evidence of apical lung carcinoma (Pancoast's syndrome).

Local causes

Iris damage may result in an unreactive or poorly reactive pupil. Causes include trauma, uveitis and previous acute glaucoma. Pharmacological mydriasis is the commonest cause of an isolated unreactive pupil; usually the history is apparent, but unprescribed use of eye drops and accidental exposure to mydriatics (e.g. occupational) can also occur. Atropine, the longest-acting mydriatic, has a half-life of around 10 days.

THE RED EYE

Red eye is an initially daunting matter when encountered in primary care or in the Emergency Department. Provided, however, that the main features of pain and visual symptoms are elicited, the most likely cause can be rapidly narrowed down as shown in Table 37.7 or, where features are suggestive of more serious disease, Box 37.1.

Box 37.1 Features of the dangerous red eye

Symptoms
- Severe pain
- Photophobia
- Loss of vision
- Progression of symptoms

Physical features
- Reduced visual acuity
- Unilateral
- Intense injection

High intraocular pressure
- Corneal opacity, epithelial defect
- Proptosis
- Loss of red reflex

At-risk individual
- Neonate
- Immunocompromise
- Contact lenses

Painless red eye with normal vision

This can only be a subconjunctival haemorrhage (SCH), caused by the rupture of an episcleral vein and producing a bright red area over the sclera. Usually it is localised and the remaining conjunctiva can be seen to be normal; sometimes the bleed is more extensive, and swollen conjunctiva can prolapse through the palpebral fissure.

SCHs may be caused by trauma, coughing and straining, clotting disorders or, rarely, hypertension. However, the great majority are spontaneous. Treatment is not required, and the discoloration fades over 1–2 weeks.

Uncomfortable red eye with normal vision

Blepharitis

This is a chronic inflammatory condition that affects the margins of the eyelid. It may be greasy (seborrhoeic) or crusting (staphylococcal), or a combination of both and can be associated with recurrent styes (Fig. 37.16). The complaint is of ocular discomfort, dryness and crusting of the lashes, most noticeable in the mornings. Conjunctival inflammation is mainly inferior from contact with the inflamed lower lid. The cornea may also become involved with a secondary conjunctivitis; more severe cases such as this are often seen in patients with acne rosacea. The main treatment is lid hygiene, with mechanical cleaning of the lid margin using a cotton bud dipped in a dilute solution of baby shampoo or bicarbonate of soda. Artificial tear drops may relieve the symptoms of dryness, and topical antibiotics are also often used initially to eliminate or reduce the load of staphylococci.

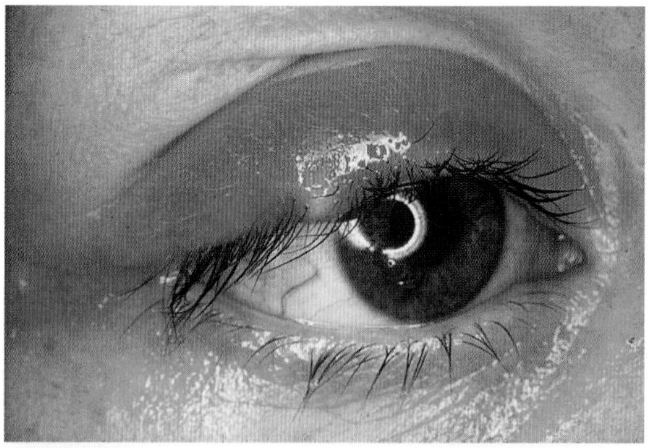

Fig. 37.16 Acute infection of eyelash follicle (stye).

Table 37.7 Causes of red eye

	Painless	Uncomfortable	Painful
Normal vision	Subconjunctival haemorrhage	Blepharitis Conjunctivitis Episcleritis	Anterior uveitis Scleritis Keratitis (peri–peripheral)
Reduced vision	None		Anterior uveitis Posterior scleritis Central keratitis

Conjunctivitis

This is a typical cause of ocular discomfort rather than pain which often begins in one eye but becomes bilateral within a few days. Discharge is an important feature: purulent or mucopurulent is typical in bacterial infection; mucopurulent in chlamydial; mucoid in allergic; and watery in viral (Fig. 37.17). In chlamydial and viral disease, there may be enlarged tender preauricular lymph nodes and conjunctival follicles, visible as small 'rice grains' in the inferior conjunctival fornices.

Bacterial conjunctivitis is commonly caused by Gram-positive cocci, especially *Staphylococcus aureus*. Treatment is with a broad-spectrum topical antibiotic (e.g. chloramphenicol). Swabs are only required if the infection has not resolved within a week of effective treatment or if the condition is initially severe.

Viral conjunctivitis does not need treatment other than explanation and reassurance because the majority are mild and self-limiting. Adenovirus infection may be more severe, and the small proportion that develop keratitis (with visual disturbance and increased pain) require referral for specialist management.

Chlamydial infection is most commonly a sexually transmitted disease in young adults and may be chronic and unilateral. Referral to an ophthalmologist is required for confirmation of the diagnosis. The genitourinary physician is also involved, in order to screen for sexual contacts for *Chlamydia* and other sexually transmitted diseases. Treatment includes topical and systemic tetracyclines.

Episcleritis

See above.

Painful red eyes

Scleritis, keratitis and uveitis are all possible causes of a painful red eye, and they are discussed above in the sections on visual loss, floaters and ocular pain.

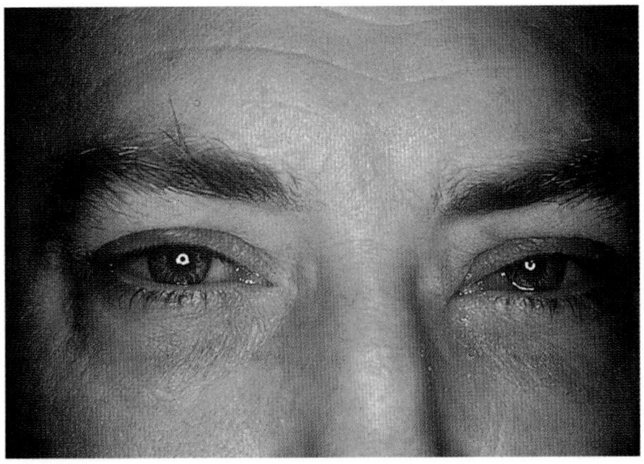

Fig. 37.17 Viral conjunctivitis. The lids are swollen, the eyes are watering, red and uncomfortable.

DISEASES WITH OPHTHALMIC MANIFESTATIONS

Acquired immune deficiency disease (AIDS)

AIDS has a number of ophthalmic manifestations which include primary effects, opportunistic infections and tumours. Only the most important and common are described here. The high incidence of such conditions requires a low threshold for referral for specialist assessment.

Primary effects

The HIV virus has a direct effect on the retinal vasculature, causing cotton wool spots and microaneurysms that are very similar to those seen in background diabetic retinopathy. The lesions are asymptomatic and resolve spontaneously, and treatment is not required.

Secondary infections

Viral infections

Cytomegalovirus is the major sight-threatening disease in HIV infection and is one of the defining illnesses of AIDS, rarely seen when the CD4 T-cell count is greater than 50 cells/μL. It occurs in approximately 30% of those with AIDS. The virus causes retinitis with white areas of retinal necrosis and often extensive retinal haemorrhages (the pizza-pie appearance). Vision is lost as a result of direct retinal destruction, secondary retinal detachment and optic nerve involvement. Treatment initially involves intravenous antiviral agents (ganciclovir is the current first-line agent), with long-term prophylaxis against relapses using intravenous oral or intraocular antivirals.

The recent introduction of protease inhibitors as part of antiretroviral therapy (ART) has allowed lymphocyte counts to rise in some patients such that long-term prophylaxis can be safely stopped.

Herpes simplex and varicella zoster viruses may both cause acute fulminating retinitis with a very high incidence of visual loss.

Bacterial infections

Staphylococcal blepharitis. This is common in those with HIV (see also 'Red eye').

Mycobacteria. Tuberculous choroiditis may occur in isolation or with signs of disease elsewhere.

Syphilis has an increased frequency in AIDS because of both the impaired immunity and the common means of transmission. Uveitis is the most common manifestation.

Fungal infections

Candida albicans causes a severe uveitis. It is seen most often in intravenous drug abusers who use unsterilised needles (see Ch. 9).

Cryptococcus neoformans can cause choroiditis in patients with cryptococcal meningitis.

Protozoal infections

Toxoplasmosis. In the immunocompromised, the condition differs from that in the healthy population by being acquired rather than congenital. Creamy white patches on the retina indicate active retinitis and cause visual loss by direct retinal damage. Systemic anti-protozoals are required to control the initial infection and are continued at a lower maintenance dose for life.

Tumours

Kaposi sarcoma

This is commonly seen on the eyelids or conjunctiva of AIDS patients and is a defining disease. It forms a dark red (or purple) firm mass which may be flat or elevated. In the conjunctiva it may resemble a subconjunctival haemorrhage and must be considered as a possible diagnosis for any such lesion, especially in the young, if persistent for more than 2 weeks.

Rheumatoid arthritis (RA)

Keratoconjunctivitis sicca

This is an example of secondary Sjögren's syndrome, with autoimmune destruction of the lacrimal gland, which leads to dry eye symptoms and corneal damage. The symptoms are distressing and often difficult to control. The mainstay of treatment is ocular lubrication with artificial tears and ointments.

Scleritis and keratitis

Scleritis in rheumatoid arthritis may be acute with a painful red eye and requires urgent referral to an ophthalmologist. More commonly it is chronic, without overt inflammation, eventual scleral thinning and exposure of the underlying uvea (scleromalacia perforans) which renders the eye vulnerable to minor trauma. There is no treatment for scleromalacia.

Keratitis may be painful, with a corneal opacity and conjunctival injection, or a painless non-inflammatory corneal melt which can result in corneal perforation. Again, urgent referral is required.

Iatrogenic disease

Long-term steroid treatment (10 mg/day for more than a year) in rheumatoid arthritis commonly results in cataract.

Systemic lupus erythematosus

Systemic lupus erythematosus (SLE), like RA, may be associated with secondary Sjögren's syndrome. Small-vessel vasculitis may present as scleritis, corneal melt, retinal vasculitis or optic nerve infarction. Involvement of the retina or optic nerve implies central nervous system disease, which is a poor prognostic sign. Specialist management, with close liaison between ophthalmologist and rheumatologist, is required.

Iatrogenic disease

Steroids are commonly used in SLE and, as with RA, may cause cataract. Chloroquine and hydroxychloroquine are used, particularly in the control of skin rashes, and can cause a bull's eye maculopathy which results in irreversible loss of visual acuity. The risk of this complication is much higher with chloroquine than with hydroxychloroquine and is dose-related. Typical dosage regimens of hydroxychloroquine are very unlikely to cause problems within 5 years of beginning the drug. Patients starting on these drugs have a baseline examination by the ophthalmologist and are then warned to stop the drug and seek ophthalmic advice should they subsequently develop visual symptoms or detect a scotoma when viewing an Amsler chart.

Giant-cell arteritis (GCA)

This multisystem disorder results in inflammation of medium-sized arteries with an internal elastic lamina. The terms 'temporal' and 'cranial' arteritis refer to the high incidence of involvement of the arteries of the head; systemic disease results in polymyalgia rheumatica. GCA is a disease of the elderly and is very rarely seen in those less than 50 years old.

Clinical features

Symptoms

The patient experiences temporal headache, scalp tenderness (even necrosis) and jaw and tongue claudication. General malaise is usual, and muscle stiffness and pain may be present. Visual loss is a late event but can be of sudden onset.

Physical findings

There are often no signs to support the diagnosis. Scalp tenderness on the side of the headache may be present. The ipsilateral superficial temporal artery just in front of the ear may be enlarged, tortuous, tender and non-pulsatile.

Investigation

The erythrocyte sedimentation rate must be measured urgently. In GCA it is always elevated. Temporal artery biopsy is usually done to confirm the diagnosis; the histological findings are unaffected by up to a week of steroid treatment, so that treatment of suspected GCA must not be delayed until biopsy can be done.

Management

Hospital admission is usual. Prednisolone 1 mg/kg per day is started orally immediately. If visual loss has occurred or appears imminent ('stuttering amaurosis'), then a loading dose of intravenous hydrocortisone or methylprednisolone may be given. The dose is then gradually reduced according to the clinical response. The majority feel subjectively much better after 48 hours of treatment. Steroid therapy is continued at a low dose for around 2 years depending on ESR results.

Systemic candidiasis

Candida albicans is a yeast-like organism commonly present as a commensal in the healthy gastrointestinal tract. Candidiasis only becomes an ophthalmic problem in immunocompromised patients (e.g. immunosuppressive drugs, haematological malignancy and AIDS) or if the organism is directly introduced into the bloodstream by non-sterile i.v. drug abuse or the presence of indwelling catheters (especially hyperalimentation following bowel surgery).

Clinical features

Blurring of vision and floaters are the main symptoms of candidal endophthalmitis, i.e. infective inflammation of the internal eye, including the vitreous gel. Pain with a red eye is less common.

Vitreous inflammation may obscure the fundus; when it can be seen, there are usually elevated white chorioretinal lesions. The vitritis is frequently organised into localised masses – the string of pearls. In the minority who has associated anterior uveitis, there is ciliary injection and clouding of the anterior chamber.

Investigation and management

Blood cultures for candidaemia and appropriate investigations to assess immunocompromise are required. Ocular investigation involves anterior chamber and vitreous sampling.

Treatment is with vitrectomy and intravitreal and systemic antifungal agents.

Embolic disease

Emboli which affect the visual system are most commonly thromboemboli and arise from the carotid vessels in the neck. Emboli may result in transient visual loss (transient ischaemic attack), sudden permanent visual loss (retinal artery occlusion) or visual field loss (cerebrovascular disease) (see common symptoms above and Ch. 29).

Graves' disease

This is an autoimmune disorder characterised by the production of thyroid-stimulating immunoglobulins (TSIs) that cause thyrotoxicosis (Ch. 32). Orbital inflammation – dysthyroid eye disease or thyroid ophthalmopathy – is associated. The orbital condition may occasionally be seen in those who are both clinically and biochemically euthyroid.

Pathological features

Soft-tissue inflammation in and around the orbits may produce exophthalmos. If severe, the orbital contents, including the optic nerve, may be compressed and vision is lost. After 1–2 years, the acute inflammation tends to subside, leaving residual chronic fibrotic changes in the orbit and ocular muscles.

Clinical features

Symptoms

In the acute phase, sore red eyes are common. A 'staring eyes' appearance may cause self-embarrassment. When the condition is severe, reduced vision may be noted and, rarely, diplopia.

If the condition reaches a chronic phase, diplopia and the poor appearance of exophthalmos and lid retraction are the main complaints.

Physical findings

In acute disease the conjunctiva are injected, particularly over the insertions of the horizontal recti muscles at 3 and 6 o'clock. There may be chemosis and swelling of the lids. Orbital inflammation increases the volume of the orbit which pushes the globes forwards and can lead to exposure of the cornea; downward movement of the upper eyelids may be restricted so that the sclera above the superior limbus becomes visible. This is most obvious in changing from up-gaze to down-gaze – lid lag. Lid retraction contributes to the staring look and to corneal exposure (Fig. 37.18).

Nerve compression may reduce visual acuity, impair colour vision and cause a relative afferent pupillary defect.

In the later stages, inflammation is replaced by fibrosis which restricts ocular movements. Any direction of squint may occur, but most commonly the limitations are in up-gaze and lateral gaze.

Management

Management of the thyroid state is necessary (Ch. 32). In mild thyroid eye disease, treatment may not be needed. Artificial tears may be necessary to ease the ocular discomfort from corneal exposure.

In more severe disease, immunosuppression with systemic corticosteroids or orbital irradiation may be necessary. Surgical interventions include orbital decompression, strabismus correction and methods of lowering the retracted lids.

Multiple sclerosis

This is an autoimmune disorder characterised by demyelinating inflammation within the central nervous system, with recurrent attacks in different locations. Ophthalmic presentations are common and include:

- **Optic and retrobulbar neuritis.** This is the most common ophthalmic complication, with around 70% having evidence of previous attacks. Optic neuritis may occur in isolation, but at least 50% of women and 25% of men with optic neuritis go on to develop MS. The

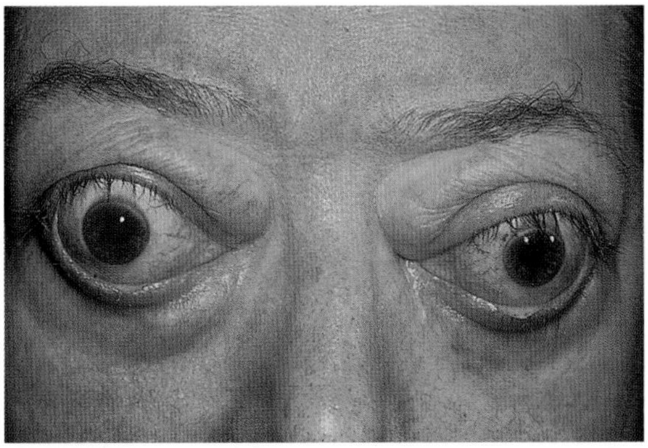

Fig. 37.18 Dysthyroid eye disease, with exophthalmos and strabismus.

clinical features are described under 'Loss of visual acuity'.

- **Ocular motility disorders.** MS may affect individual nerves to cause paretic strabismus. Brainstem lesions of the medial longitudinal fasciculus cause internuclear ophthalmoplegia (INO – commonly bilateral) which affects horizontal gaze away from the side of the lesion so that the eye ipsilateral to the lesion fails to adduct across the midline, while the contralateral eye exhibits nystagmus.
- **Visual field defects.** These are rarely seen but they are the result of a large demyelinating plaque which affects the optic radiations.

Hypertension

Hypertension can cause retinopathy, choroidopathy and optic neuropathy. The changes are most marked in the accelerated hypertension of pre-eclampsia or so-called malignant hypertension. The pathological changes in the eye are usually the consequence of ischaemia with tissue infarction or exudation from a compromised vascular endothelium.

Retinopathy can be graded by the severity and duration of disease. In **chronic disease** (arteriosclerosis):

- Grade 1 – increased arteriolar light reflex
- Grade 2 – deflection of veins at arteriovenous crossings
- Grade 3 – arteriolar narrowing (nipping) at arteriovenous crossings
- Grade 4 – silver wiring of arterioles (increased light reflex and tortuosity of vessels).

In **acute disease:**

- Grade 1 – generalised arteriolar attenuation
- Grade 2 – focal arteriolar attenuation and deflection of veins at arteriovenous crossings
- Grade 3 – hard exudates, flame-shaped haemorrhages and cotton wool spots with arteriolar narrowing (nipping) at arteriovenous crossings
- Grade 4 – grade 3 changes plus silver wiring of arterioles and swelling of the optic disc.

Grade 4 acute retinopathy is usually associated with encephalopathy and requires immediate referral for medical assessment. The fundal changes usually regress after the raised blood pressure has been corrected.

Diabetes

Diabetic retinopathy is a potentially blinding disease and is the leading cause of registration for blindness in the working age population in the UK. It can occur in both Type I and Type II diabetes. Visual loss can occur as a result of macular damage (oedema or ischaemia), vitreous haemorrhage or retinal detachment. The latter two conditions result from proliferative retinopathy (Fig. 37.19) in which retinal ischaemia leads to abnormal neovascularisation. The incidence of retinopathy increases with duration of disease and is reduced by tight control of blood sugar and blood pressure. Argon laser treatment is effective in preventing visual loss from retinopathy, therefore all diabetic patients should be screened for retinopathy. Screening should begin 5 years from diagnosis or at 12 years of age (whichever is the later) in Type I diabetes and at diagnosis in Type II disease. Advanced diabetic eye disease is managed with vitreoretinal surgery and urgent referral is indicated.

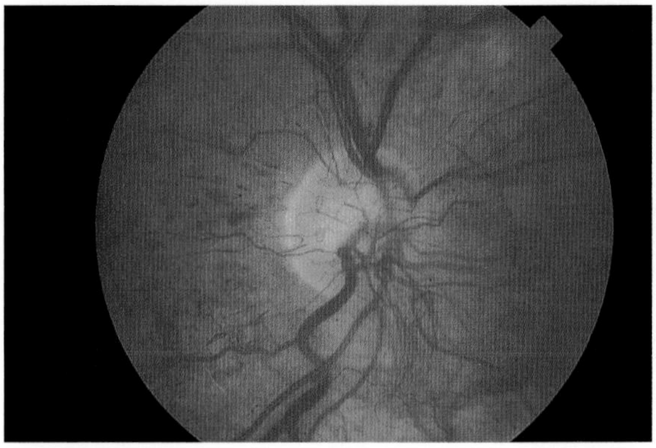

Fig. 37.19 Proliferative diabetic retinopathy, with new vessels growing from the nasal side of the optic disc.

Sarcoidosis

The eye is (after the lungs and lymph nodes) the most common organ to be affected (20–30%) by this condition. Uveitis is the most common manifestation, and granulomatous inflammation can involve the retina and choroid to cause blindness. When this occurs there is a 30% incidence of central nervous system involvement. Granulomas can also affect the eyelid, conjunctiva and the lacrimal gland.

Stevens–Johnson syndrome (erythema multiforme major)

This is an acute, generally self-limiting mucocutaneous vesiculobullous disease which tends to affect young healthy individuals. It involves the conjunctiva in 90%, causing mucopurulent conjunctivitis. Lid scarring may follow and lead to misdirection of the eyelashes with corneal damage. In the acute phase, assessment by an ophthalmologist is necessary. Systemic treatment is generally with steroids.

Sickle cell disease

Eye disease in the sickle haemoglobinopathies occurs in the SC and S-Thal forms but rarely in the SS form. The abnormal red blood cells cause vascular obstruction and infarction. The resulting ischaemia may lead to proliferation of abnormal new blood vessels, which may bleed to cause vitreous and retinal haemorrhages and retinal detachment. Once proliferative retinopathy has developed, there is a 3.4% 8-year incidence of visual loss, although the disease may be self-limiting. Most of the retinal changes occur in the retinal periphery, beyond the field of view of a direct ophthalmoscope. The disease is self-limiting but laser photocoagulation or vitreoretinal surgery is occasionally required.

Wegener's granulomatosis

This disease is characterised by necrotising granulomas of the upper respiratory tract. The eye can be affected by keratoconjunctivitis sicca, scleritis, corneal melt and orbital involvement. Treatment is by systemic immunosuppression, e.g. cyclophosphamide.

FURTHER READING

Kanski J J, Bowling B 2011 Clinical ophthalmology: a systematic approach, 7th edn. Butterworth-Heinemann, Edinburgh

38 Principles of plastic surgery

Derived from the Greek 'plastikos' meaning to mould or to give shape the specialty of plastic surgery is perhaps more accurately described as one of reconstructive surgery. The lay person's perception of plastic surgery is one of cosmetic surgery which represents merely a facet of the specialty, though aesthetic goals along with restoration of form and function underpin the basic principles of the specialty. Unlike other surgical specialties there is no specific territory of the body which is the monopoly of plastic surgery. Although a degree of subspecialisation has developed recently the plastic surgeon might be regarded as the last of the general surgeons in treating a great variety of problems in many sites (although in general, body cavities are excluded) by means of specialised 'plastic surgery techniques'. Some of these techniques have been in use for many years – there are records of reconstructions of the nose with forehead flaps from India dating back 3000 years. The specialty only developed independently in the last 75 years, triggered specifically by mutilations from trench warfare in the First World War, although the increased mechanisation and high-speed travel of the 20th century have maintained the need for soft-tissue reconstruction.

The demands on the specialty have been even greater as a result of the changing behaviour patterns and fashions of society. There has been a dramatic increase in sun-induced skin damage, including skin cancer, as a result of the burgeoning package holiday trade and the belief that a suntan is attractive. With greater emphasis on the merits of an improved physical appearance, the demand for aesthetic plastic surgery has also soared. The definition of plastic surgery from the Union Européenne de Médecins Spécialistes (UEMS) within the EU has therefore recently been modified as 'surgery intended to restore form and function and to promote well being'.

To simplify: the aetiology of defects requiring reconstruction are congenital or acquired, the acquired being either traumatic, degenerative or following tumour excision. Such defects may arise as a result of many different causes in sites all over the body, leading to considerable clinical overlap whereby the plastic surgeon is the member of a team. But while plastic surgery may often be associated with sophisticated reconstructions, the plastic surgeon also manages the commonest tumours of infancy (vascular hamartomata), the commonest form of cancer (skin cancer), the commonest cause of admission to an emergency department (hand and soft-tissue injuries) and the commonest cause of prolonged morbidity in the elderly (chronic wounds and decubitus ulcers).

Examples of types of problems involving the plastic surgeon are shown in Table 38.1.

In practical terms, the commonest reconstruction required is the repair of a breach in the skin or a mucosal surface. However, the defect may extend deeper and involve other structures such as muscle, nerve, tendon and bone, and, where possible, these too will need to be corrected to enable full return of function.

PLASTIC SURGERY TECHNIQUES

There has been an escalation of surgical technology in the last two decades, supported by advances in anaesthetic and monitoring techniques which have allowed a greater range of reconstructive options. Furthermore, development in instrument technology, including fibreoptics and microsurgery, has increased surgical safety and reliability.

However, regardless of the rich choices available, the surgeon should opt for the simplest and safest surgery in the first instance, turning to more complex and potentially more hazardous procedures only when the simpler methods do not meet the reconstructive and occasionally aesthetic requirements. It is therefore helpful to have a mental picture of a ladder of surgical options (Fig. 38.1a), although recent developments have resulted in so many offshoots that the resulting plan resembles more closely a tree (Fig. 38.1b).

Table 38.1 Types of problems involving the plastic surgeon

Aetiology of defect	Example
Congenital abnormality	Cleft lip and palate Congenital hand anomalies
Trauma	Lower limb soft-tissue loss Hand injury
Burns	Extensive skin loss
Neoplasia	Skin cancer Intra-oral cancer excision and reconstruction Breast reconstruction following mastectomy
Degenerative processes	Rheumatoid hand deformities

SPONTANEOUS WOUND HEALING

Wound healing is a natural and spontaneous phenomenon which occurs irrespective of (and sometimes despite) the surgeon. Although the basic events of blood clotting, fibrin deposition, organisation and collagen synthesis have been observed for many years, the factors which initiate and control these processes are incompletely understood. The pattern of wound healing may be affected by sophisticated endocrine, pharmacological and physical manipulation, or simply by surgery, but the most important influence on open wounds is the nature in which they are dressed.

Numerous dressings and topical agents are commercially available, sometimes making extravagant and unproven claims, but there is no evidence that any available dressings accelerate wound healing. They simply provide the optimal environment in which a wound can re-epithelialise. With this in mind, one should select well-tried and tested dressings which should also have the properties of being cheap and painless to apply and remove (Fig. 38.2).

Some wounds will heal completely without surgical intervention. These not only include small wounds but also some large cavernous wounds as might be produced by abscess drainage or excision of a pilonidal sinus. Such wounds may be too heavily contaminated for surgical closure and often contract down surprisingly quickly, particularly if subjected to a negative pressure.

When a wound fails to heal, adverse factors relating to the wound (local factors; Box 8.1) or to the patient (systemic factors; Box 8.2) need to be identified and, if possible, addressed. This is particularly true of chronic wounds if, following thorough debridement, healing is to be achieved.

ADJUNCTS TO SPONTANEOUS WOUND HEALING

Hyperbaric oxygen

Improving tissue oxygen levels by intermittent inhalation of 100% oxygen in a hyperbaric chamber at pressures greater than at sea level (usually 2.2–2.4 atmospheres absolute) can be useful particularly in the treatment of chronic wounds. The positive effects on healing are observed at a cellular level such as enhanced fibroblast proliferation and collagen formation, improved microbial killing and neoangiogenesis.

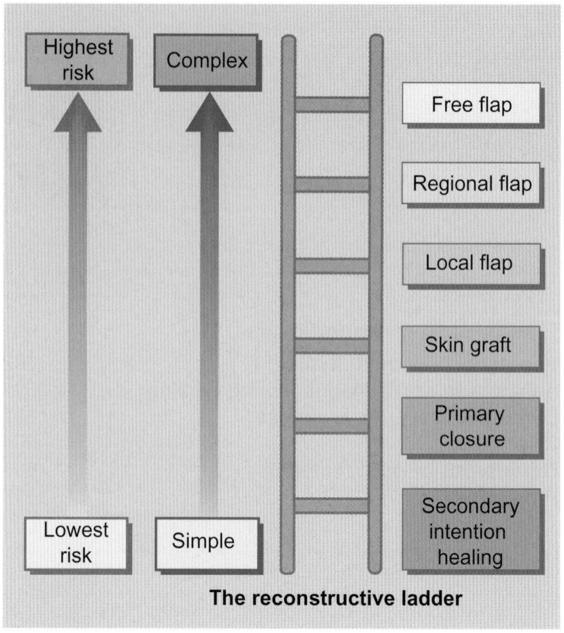

Fig. 38.1a The reconstructive ladder.

The practicalities of such treatment limits its widespread application.

VAC therapy

Vacuum Assisted Closure (VAC®) therapy; KCI USA, San Antonio, TX) involves application of continuous or intermittent negative pressure to a wound through a non-adherent foam dressing via a closed system. Wound healing is assisted by reduction in bacterial load and interstitial fluid with improved angiogenesis and formation of granulation tissue. Suitable for large, deep wounds, it enables improved wound management and can occasionally convert a non-graftable bed into one that will accept a graft.

DIRECT SURGICAL WOUND CLOSURE

The first choice for wound repair is direct closure by suture, a standard and common surgical procedure but one deserving attention to detail to enable the best possible scar. The wound should first be converted to an ellipse whose long axis lies in the same line as the local skin creases and perpendicular to the underlying muscle (failure to do so is likely to produce unsightly dog ears). The wound is sutured so that the edges are exactly matched and slightly everted while reducing any crushing damage of the tissues with the help of fine-toothed forceps or skin hooks. Tension and haematoma must be avoided at all costs by means of meticulous haemostasis and the support of buried intradermal sutures and adhesive tapes. However, the quality of the final scar is determined by the individual's own wound-healing properties.

It is unfortunate that a vigorous scar formation is not in the interests of a good cosmetic result. In some patients the normal equilibrium between collagen synthesis

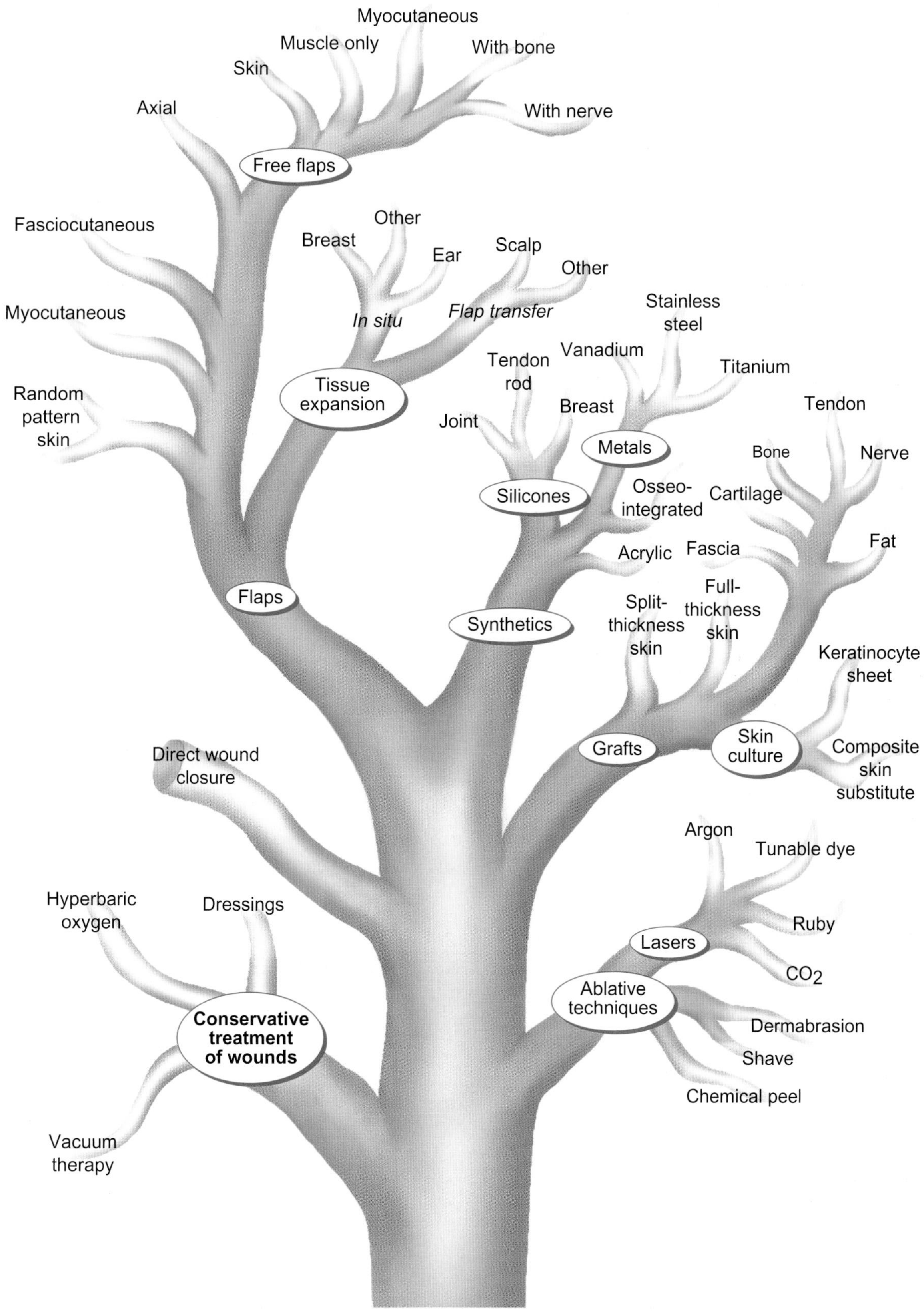

Fig. 38.1b Tree of reconstruction.

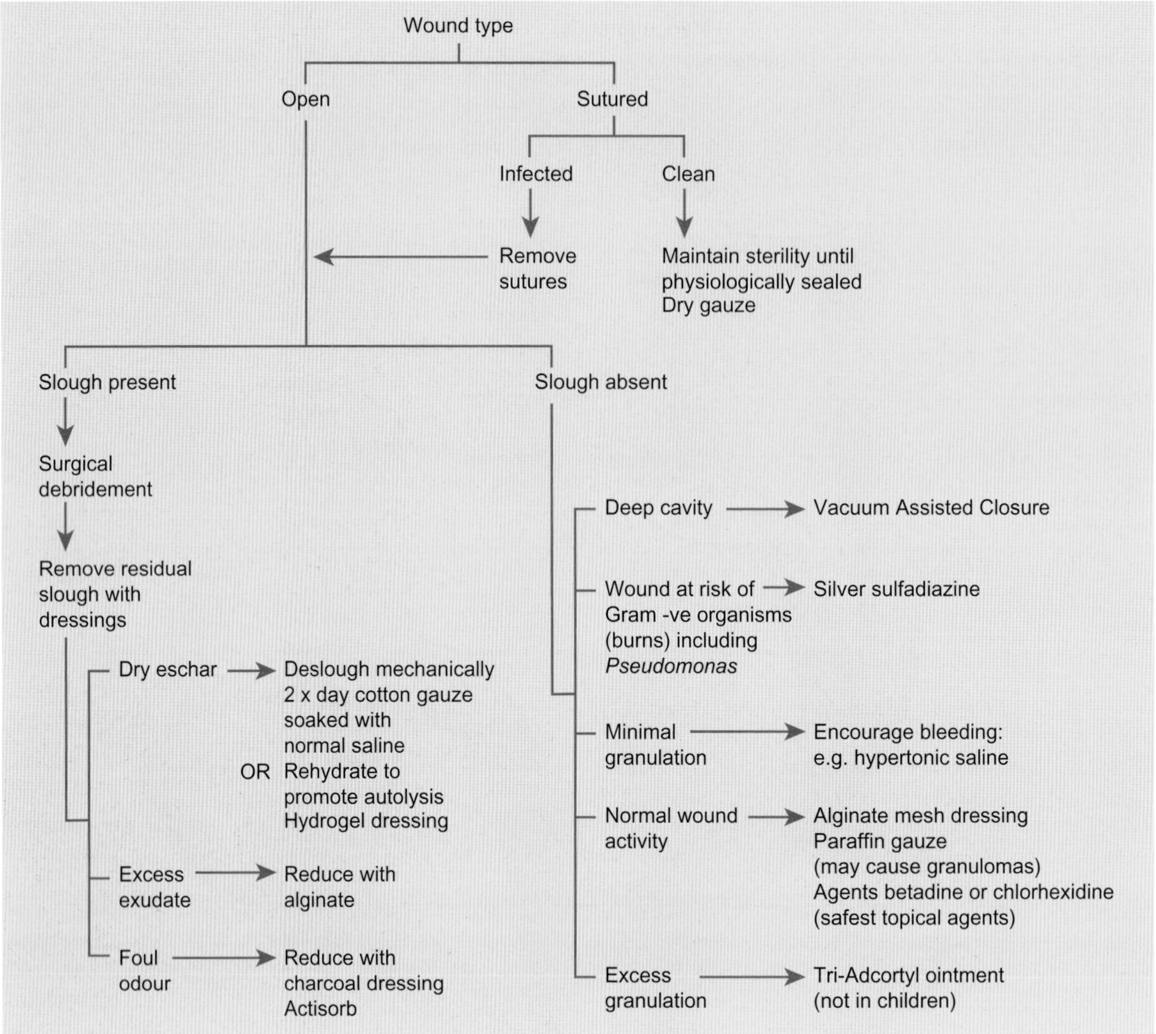

Fig. 38.2 Algorithmic flow chart showing choice and examples of dressings in different situations.

Table 38.2 Treatment of unsatisfactory scars

Treatment	Undesirable features of normal scars	Hypertrophic scars	Keloid scars	Pigmented scars	Stretch scars
Surgical revision	Yes	Yes	Very rarely	Yes	Yes
Topical or intralesional Steroid	Rarely	Yes	Yes	No	No
Dermabrasion	Yes	No	No	Yes	No
Injectable tissue filler	Yes	No	No	No	Yes
External pressure with or without Silastic sheet	No	Yes	Yes	No	No
Low-dose radiotherapy	No	No	Yes	No	No
Cosmetic camouflage	Yes	Yes	No	Yes	Yes

and degradation is disturbed. Instead of scar maturation occurring over a 12-month period, collagen may be produced in excess, resulting in a red, lumpy, hypertrophic scar. If there is extension into surrounding tissues a true keloid will result. The management of abnormal scarring following trauma or surgery is not entirely satisfactory, but the means available are charted (Table 38.2).

SKIN GRAFTS

If a wound is too wide to be closed directly, grafting is the simplest method of repair. A skin graft is a sheet of skin harvested from elsewhere in the body and comprising either its epidermis and superficial dermis (split-thickness graft) or its entire thickness (full-thickness graft). The graft is

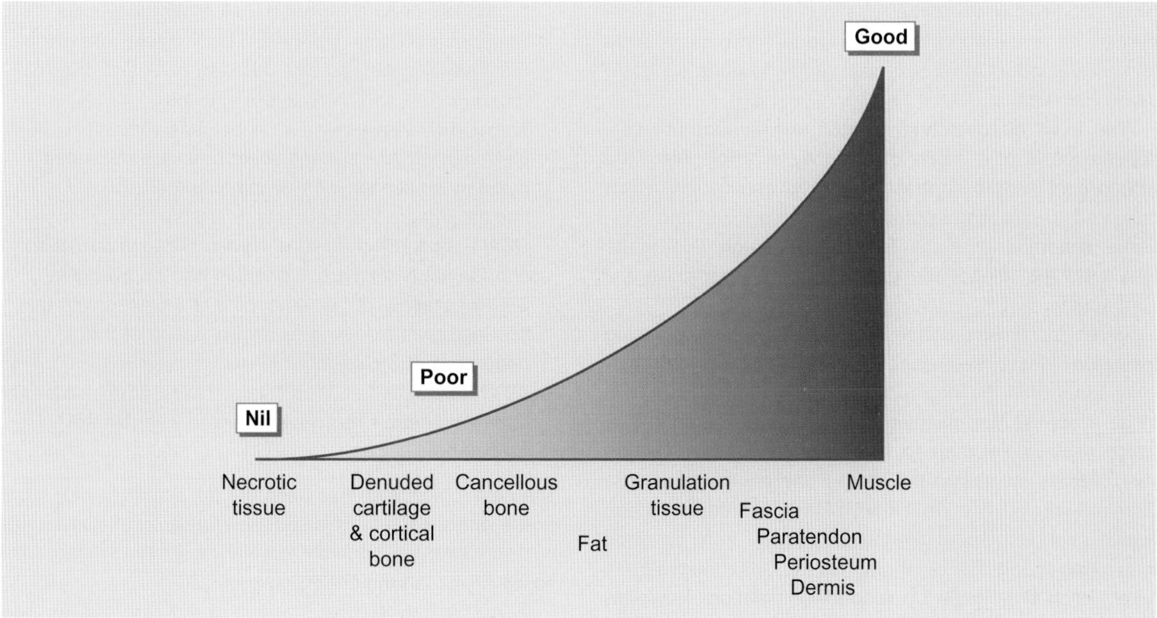

Fig. 38.3 Suitability of tissues to receive split skin grafts.

completely detached from the body and, when applied to the wound, depends entirely on the underlying vascular bed for its nutrition by diffusion of metabolites for a few days before its revascularisation by the ingrowth of blood vessels. A skin graft will therefore only 'take' if applied to wounds which can supply the necessary environment. Graft loss can occur for several reasons: namely, haematoma beneath the graft (minimised by cutting slots [fenestrations] into the graft), infection, inadequate immobilisation of the graft to its bed permitting shear, positioning the graft on an unsuitable bed incapable of nourishing the graft (necrotic tissue, bare endochondral bone [without periosteum]), bare cartilage (without perichondrium), bare tendon (without paratenon), or technical error (placing the graft upside down!) The spectrum of ability of different tissues to receive a graft is shown in Figure 38.3. Most wounds older than 48 hours will be covered by granulation tissue, whose vascularity will be related to that of the underlying tissue.

Split-thickness skin grafts

Split-thickness skin grafts are taken with either hand-held graft knives or by powered dermatomes, both of which cut the superficial layers of the skin 150–300 μm thick (Fig. 38.4). As a large number of epithelial remnants are left behind at the donor site, these will, in the same manner as a bad graze, heal within 2 weeks, provided they are kept free from infection.

'Take' also depends on stability of the graft. Shearing forces which disrupt ingrowing capillary loops must be avoided by immobilising the skin graft with the help of a tie-over dressing or by sutures, staples or cyanoacrylate glue. This dressing is normally left intact for a period of 3–5 days to allow vascular ingrowth of the graft before it is inspected.

Large areas of skin can thus be harvested, but as donor sites often heal with some alteration of pigmentation and occasionally with hypertrophic scars, the sites chosen should be inconspicuous, such as the inner thigh or buttock. In the elderly who may have an attenuated dermis, the healing of these donor sites may be considerably delayed. The most acceptable donor site dressing is an alginate mesh, which should be left undisturbed for at least 10 days. The graft

a

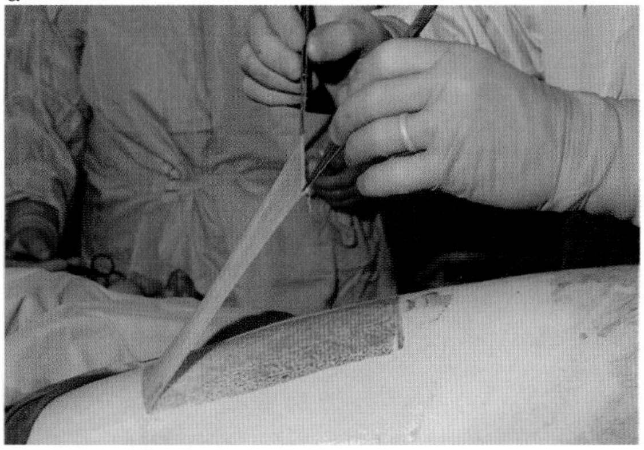

b

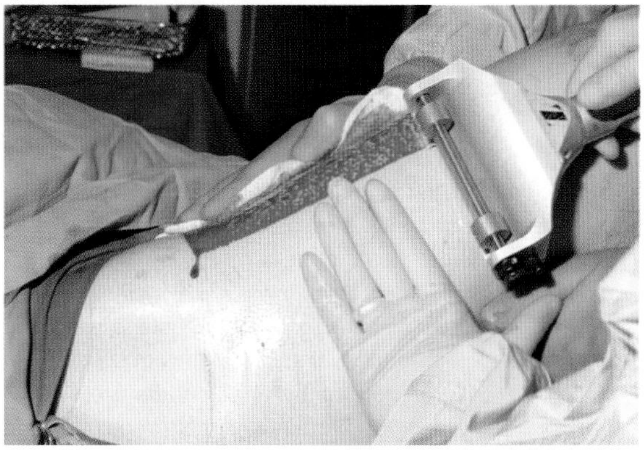

Fig. 38.4 Harvesting a split-thickness skin graft.

donor site heals by re-epithelialisation from remnants of epithelium left in the donor site. The same donor site can be reused to supply further split skin graft providing sufficient dermis remains.

The main disadvantage of split skin is that the final appearance is of a patch of unsightly scarring. Also, the wound continues to contract after graft application, which may lead to disabling contractures across joints and soft-tissue distortion of facial features. Although thin grafts take well, the thinner the graft the more aggressive the contracture.

Given the limited donor sites available for resurfacing extensive defects (like major burns) and the potential morbidity of donor sites, the introduction of the graft mesher proved to be a bonus. The machine cuts slots into the split skin, which enables the graft to be stretched out like a string vest, thereby increasing the area of the original graft. The diamond-shaped slots permit any blood or serum to escape (which might otherwise lift the graft away from its bed), thus reducing the chance of graft failure. Once the graft has taken, each hole heals by secondary intention. However, the disadvantage is that the healed area is like a cobbled surface, implying that it is best suited to inconspicuous recipient beds.

At best, split-thickness grafts must be regarded as 'hole fillers' for the repair of large skin defects.

Full-thickness skin grafts

For smaller wounds in conspicuous areas, over joints or where scar contracture has produced deformity, a full-thickness graft is preferable. Although 'take' of these grafts is less predictable due to the greater volume of tissue requiring nourishment from the graft bed, they retain their original texture with little scarring and contracture, and are particularly suited to the face. However, the colour and texture of the standard postauricular graft is not ideal for all facial areas, and one should consider other donor sites such as redundant upper-eyelid skin, preauricular and supraclavicular skin to achieve optimum facial skin matching.

Cultured skin and skin substitutes

Although not in common usage, there has been considerable clinical experience in the culture of keratinocytes isolated by trypsin from a small split skin graft. These are allowed to proliferate into large sheets of cells on a substrate of fibroblasts. However, such ultrathin layers of cells when applied as a graft are not sufficiently robust to withstand wear and tear and are subject to high infection rates with subsequent graft loss. These cultured epithelial autografts are seldom used alone for coverage. The fundamental problem is that replacement of epidermis alone (e.g. CEA) is insufficient for full-thickness defects and that the complex dermal structure cannot regenerate and be cultured in the same way. This has encouraged development of a wide range of skin substitutes for epidermal and dermal reconstruction that are employed particularly in the burns setting where large areas of skin loss require resurfacing. Some products contain specific growth factors designed to assist healing of chronic wounds:

- Biobrane® (Dow Hickman/Bertek Pharmaceuticals, Sugar Land, Texas, USA) – a Silastic sheet with nylon mesh seeded with porcine collagen and used principally for superficial partial-thickness skin loss.
- Transcyte® (Advanced Tissue Sciences, Inc., La Jolla, California, USA) – silicone sheet on collagen-coated nylon mesh seeded with neonatal fibroblasts.
- Integra (Integra Life Sciences, Plainsboro, New Jersey, USA) – a bilaminar sheet of bovine collagen and shark chondroitin 6-sulphate neodermis with an overlying Silastic sheet which is removed and replaced with thin split autograft following revascularisation of the neodermis at 3 weeks.
- AlloDerm® (LifeCell, Woodlands, Texas, USA) – acellular cadaveric dermis requiring coverage with thin split autograft.

The next logical step has been the development of a composite skin substitute which not only has an epithelial surface but also a tough adherent dermal layer, which raises the possibility of 'off the shelf' banks of skin.

OTHER TYPES OF GRAFT MATERIALS

Other tissues available as free grafts for deep tissue defects, contour defects and functional restoration include bone, cartilage, nerve, tendon and fat. Bone is usually harvested from the ilium or rib and cartilage from the ear concha or the rib. For bridging gaps in nerves, a cutaneous nerve such as the sural nerve may be sacrificed, and for tendon reconstruction vestigial tendons such as palmaris longus and plantaris are used (fascia lata is a reasonable substitute in their absence).

Other tissues such as muscle are used only occasionally as their survival is unpredictable. Fat harvested from any area of abundance can be reinjected to treat small to moderate contour defects. Autografts are preferable (in spite of potential problems at the donor site) on account of their more reliable long-term incorporation. Heterografts and xenografts have the disadvantages of the added expense of denaturing for the sake of reducing antigenicity, while also carrying the higher risk of infection and progressive absorption.

PROSTHESES

Not only has an enormous range of implantable devices been designed in the last 20 years but also improvements in their composition has rendered them safer, with a lower implant failure rate.

Silicone, the most commonly used implant material, is a polymer of silica and oxygen that can take on different physical characteristics from a thin oil to a hard block depending on its degree of polymerisation. It is relatively inert but after implantation, such as in a breast prosthesis or small joint replacement, is characteristically enveloped in a capsule of fibrous tissue of variable thickness lined with smooth mesothelium. An abnormally thick capsule may distort a breast prosthesis and, as yet, this phenomenon is unable to be predicted or prevented.

Other materials used as a bone substitute, either to restore contour such as following loss of the calvarium or for skeletal replacement, include acrylic bone cement and (more commonly) metal such as stainless steel, chrome cobalt and titanium. The recent discovery that bone will produce a very tight bond on a molecular level with titanium even when the latter extends through skin or mucosa has generated 'osseo-integrated' implants as studs on which artificial teeth and, more recently, external facial prostheses, such as a nose or ear, can be securely attached.

FLAPS

Where a skin graft is impossible or a more durable construct is necessary, or indeed when aesthetics dictate, a defect should be resurfaced with a flap. A flap is a block of tissue which retains an attachment to the body, known as a pedicle, through which it receives its blood supply and innervation as required. An encyclopaedia of flaps have been described according to how they are moved, how they are composed and (of far greater importance) how they are vascularised.

The earliest flaps were simply skin and subcutaneous fat designed without appreciation of the underlying blood supply (random pattern flaps), so that their length and mobility were restricted. More reliable and predictable flaps arose from understanding that the skin obtains its blood supply from three main sources: via direct cutaneous arteries, via perforating vessels of underlying muscles and via tributaries of the vascular plexus within the underlying deep fascia and fascial septa. This has led to the development of three different types of flap (Fig. 38.5).

- Axial pattern flaps have a known cutaneous artery which is included by orientating the flap in the same axis as the vessel, thereby enabling a long and versatile flap. The best-known example is the groin flap which has its base over the femoral vessels in the groin and extends laterally following the course of the superficial circumflex iliac artery.
- Fasciocutaneous flaps are similar to skin flaps but also include deep fascia. These are normally used in the limb where there is a very definite layer of well-vascularised deep fascia which permit a surviving length two to three times the length of the corresponding skin flap.
- Muscle flaps usually include a polarised blood supply so that the axis of movement can only be at the site of axial arteriovenous penetration. Muscle flaps alone will require epithelial cover in the form of a skin graft; however, when the muscle is superficial it is possible to include the overlying skin as a 'composite myocutaneous' flap.

Until a flap is incorporated within the defect, it needs to be nourished by an intact pedicle even if it bridges across intact skin. After this time the pedicle may be detached and discarded or returned to its original site. It follows that these flaps can only be transferred locally, although it is possible to transport them to distant sites by a series of staged and unreliable operations involving their inset into a 'carrier' such as the wrist.

Flaps require a warm, tension-free environment until they become well healed. This requires observation to monitor satisfactory perfusion and freedom from haematoma.

FREE TISSUE TRANSFER

As a result of advances in microsurgery, blood vessels as small as 1 mm can be successfully anastomosed. Thus, a new era of single-stage distant flap reconstruction became possible in which the flap is completely detached and its axial vessel is anastomosed to recipient vessels near the defect. Furthermore, this surgical technology obviates the need for multistaged procedures involving long in-patient stays.

These 'free flaps' permit sophisticated reconstructions in either emergency or elective circumstances. The stages are as follows:

1. Elevation of the flap, islanding it on the vascular pedicle.
2. Preparation of the recipient bed and isolation of healthy recipient vessels (ideally performed by a second team of surgeons).

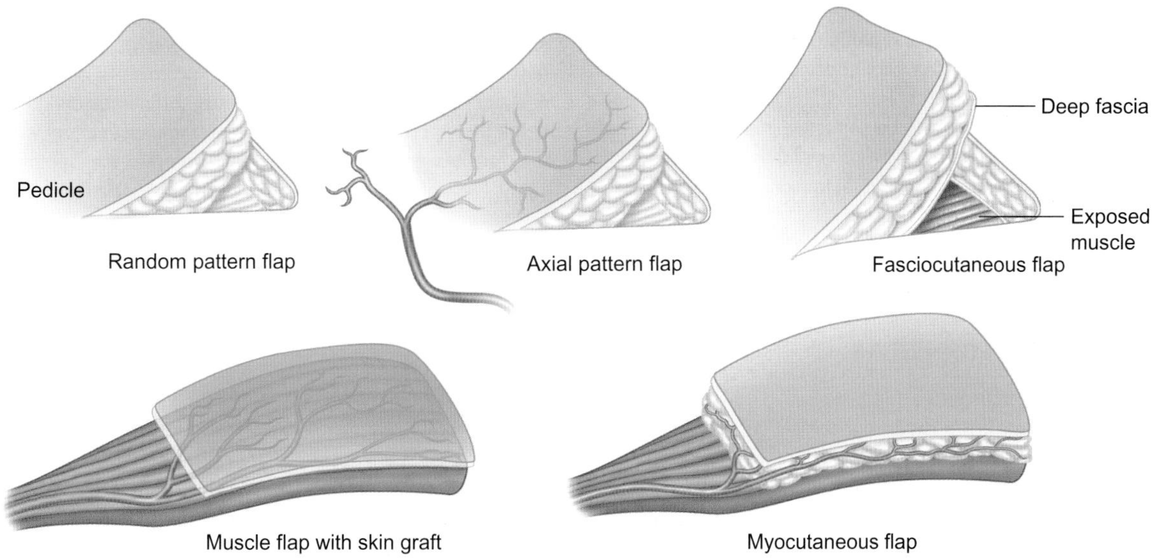

Fig. 38.5 The different types of flap.

3. Detachment of the flap followed by anastomosis of donor to recipient vessels.
4. Inset of flap and closure of donor site.

In the hands of an experienced microsurgeon supported by skilled anaesthesia (controlled, high peripheral perfusion is the key), a patency rate of 95% can be expected. Similar techniques are used in the reattachment of any traumatically amputated parts which must be brought swiftly to hospital, preferably cooled in a plastic bag lying within a second plastic bag filled with ice. If the vessels of the part and the recipient site are sufficiently healthy, one can safely proceed to replantation and revascularisation using an intervening vein graft, if necessary, to avoid any anastomotic tension.

Perforator flaps

In order to limit the adverse effects of flap harvest (donor site morbidity), e.g. loss of one rectus abdominis muscle used in a TRAM (transverse rectus abdominis myocutaneous) flap, recent techniques have focused on sparing muscle by raising a block of tissue supplied by vessel branches that perforate the muscle and dissecting these 'perforators' back to the main pedicle. In the TRAM flap example, one or two perforators from the deep inferior epigastric artery are dissected from the main artery through the rectus abdominis muscle to the overlying abdominal integument (deep inferior epigastric perforator, or DIEP, flap). Many such perforator flaps have been described and their role within reconstructive surgery is becoming clearer.

TISSUE EXPANSION

A tissue expander (which consists of an empty silicone balloon connected by a tube to a filler valve) is implanted subcutaneously adjacent to a defect at an initial operation. Over a period of weeks or months the expander is then inflated by serially injecting saline percutaneously into the filler valve, thereby distending the overlying skin. When enough skin has been generated the expander is removed and the surplus skin used for reconstruction. The great advantage is that the skin adjacent to the defect is most likely to match that of the area to be reconstructed, providing a good aesthetic match. This is particularly important in certain areas where the skin has very specific properties, such as the hair-bearing scalp.

The method appears to be seductive in its simplicity, but in practice there is a 30–40% complication rate including infection, erosion of skin and extrusion. However, tissue expansion still has a place, particularly in breast reconstruction, and it is the treatment of choice in the reconstruction of the hair-bearing scalp (Fig. 38.6).

ABLATIVE TECHNIQUES

In the restoration of normal form, surgical reconstruction may be unnecessary if the lesion concerned can be selectively destroyed. Rhinophyma (a condition characterised by massive hypertrophy of cutaneous sebaceous glands of the nose) is effectively treated by shaving alone. Deep epithelial remnants quickly re-epithelialise the surface of the nose. Dermabrasion is a similar technique in which minor irregularities of the skin such as post-acne scarring can be improved by abrading the superficial epidermo-dermal layers.

However, the laser is the most sophisticated ablative tool. There are many types of medical laser, but those in plastic surgery differ in that they must be very selective in their tissue damage to leave the skin minimally unscarred. The treatment of the intradermal capillary haemangioma (or port wine stain) has been improved initially by an argon laser whose wavelength is similar to that absorbed by haemoglobin, so that abnormal vessels can thus be photocoagulated. However, this has been recently superseded by a tunable dye laser in which a dye is selected which has a wavelength even more specific for haemoglobin. In a similar manner the India ink pigment of amateur tattoos may be vapourised by the ruby laser which emits light of the appropriate wavelength.

OTHER RECONSTRUCTIVE PROBLEMS

Other problems requiring reconstruction can broadly be divided into those of composite tissue loss and loss of function. In composite loss following the deep resection of a tumour, not only skin cover but also loss of mucosal surfaces and intervening tissue including skeletal support must be made good. Here the plastic surgeon is a member of a surgical team either in an excisional role but more commonly in a post-excisional, reconstructive role.

Descriptions of specific reconstruction are beyond the scope of this chapter, but the specific aims of reconstruction will be considered for the major branches of the specialty.

Trauma

Trauma has become a multidisciplinary specialty, and the plastic surgeon who cares for soft-tissue injuries must work as part of a team. Full assessment of the injured patient is essential, as other problems may take priority over the soft tissue.

It is important to assess whether tissues are missing or simply displaced. The viability of remaining tissues is then determined and, if avascular such as amputated parts, their suitability for revascularisation. All debris and devitalised tissue must be removed without compromise to allow subsequent reconstruction. However, it is sometimes difficult to judge the viability of tissues, especially following injury when they are bruised and swollen. For example, the degloving injury, whereby skin is sheared from the underlying deep fascia, is notoriously difficult to accurately diagnose; the devitalisation of other tissues, notably fat, occurs some time after an apparently adequate wound toilet. Thus, if there is any doubt about tissue viability, the patient should be returned to theatre for second and third inspections of the wound with necrectomies and surgical toilet as necessary until a clean wound becomes apparent. It can then be closed with the techniques previously discussed.

Congenital abnormalities

Birth defects result from failure of a variety of development processes, including formation, fusion, separation and

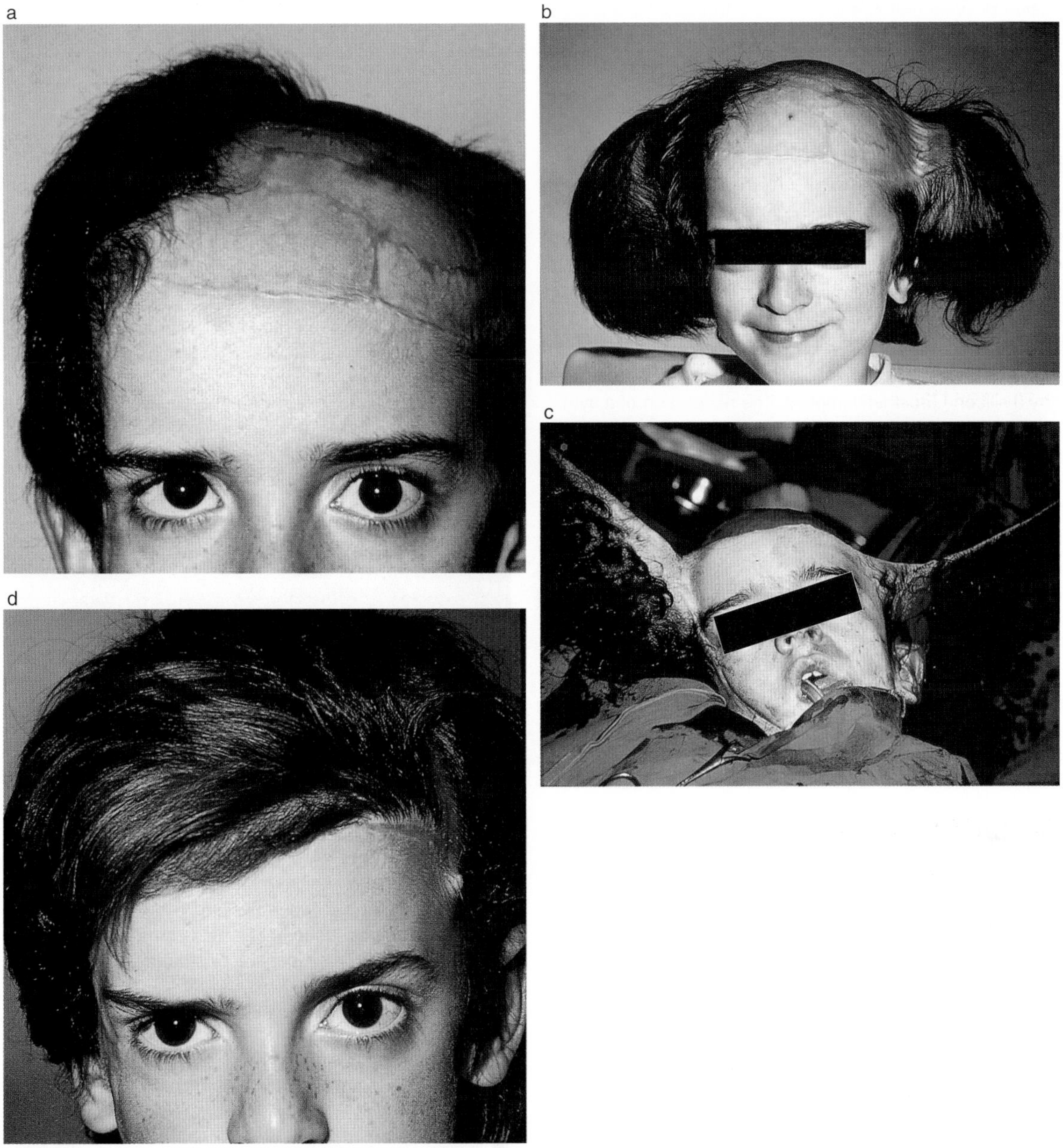

Fig. 38.6 Reconstruction of hair-bearing scalp. (a) Following a compound fracture of the right parietal bone with loss of the overlying scalp, a large scalp flap was used to repair this wound. The skin graft used to cover this flap's donor site has left an obvious area of alopecia. (b) Following insertion and inflation of two tissue expanders. (c) At operation the expanders have been removed and scalp flaps have been raised in the expanded skin prior to excising the skin graft. (d) Six weeks after completion of the reconstruction.

regression of parts. Many abnormalities not only consist of a true shortage of tissues but also of an abnormal anatomy of the adjacent tissues.

The treatment of many of these conditions may be started at a very young age, such as during the first few days of birth in the case of neonatal cleft repair. The essential goal is the restoration of as near normal function and appearance by the time the child starts primary school, and as little interference with schooling as possible by any further intervention. Surgery in infancy may interfere with growth of the operated part: thus while the timing of the procedure and meticulous technique are of obvious importance, there must also be careful follow-up in order to monitor any untoward growth changes.

Developments in anaesthesia, diagnostic imaging and neurosurgery have contributed towards safer and more precise correction of major craniofacial abnormalities. Although these conditions may produce very disfiguring abnormalities, they are not often life threatening, and therefore treatment can only be justified if the morbidity is acceptable. Contrary to other sites in the body, much of the facial skeleton can be mobilised, even if this involves devascularisation, and be expected to survive. Once the skeleton has been rigidly fixed in the correct position, possibly with the addition of bone grafts, it is necessary to consider the correction of soft-tissue abnormalities. Craniofacial surgery has developed into a subspecialty in its own right involving a large team headed by plastic and neurosurgeons.

Breast reconstruction

Despite recent trends towards the conservative management of breast cancer, there are still indications for mastectomy, and there will always be women requesting breast reconstruction. In its simplest terms, breast reconstruction requires the restoration of a skin envelope and the bulk with which to fill it. The former is achieved by a variety of flaps, including tissue expansion, and the latter by the bulk of the flap itself or by a silicone prosthetic implant. The restoration of a symmetrical breast with a natural ptosis and projection is sometimes impossible without surgical compromise involving a mastopexy (uplift) or reduction of the other breast.

Over recent years there has been a trend, when the breast pathology allows, to perform a skin-sparing mastectomy and immediate breast reconstruction utilising the remaining breast skin. Good cosmetic results can be obtained, and this technique is commonly used in cases of ductal carcinoma in situ (Fig 38.7).

Some patients will require a nipple–areolar reconstruction, which can be effected by a variety of local flaps or grafts taken either from the opposite nipple–areolar complex or skin from the upper inner aspect of the thigh.

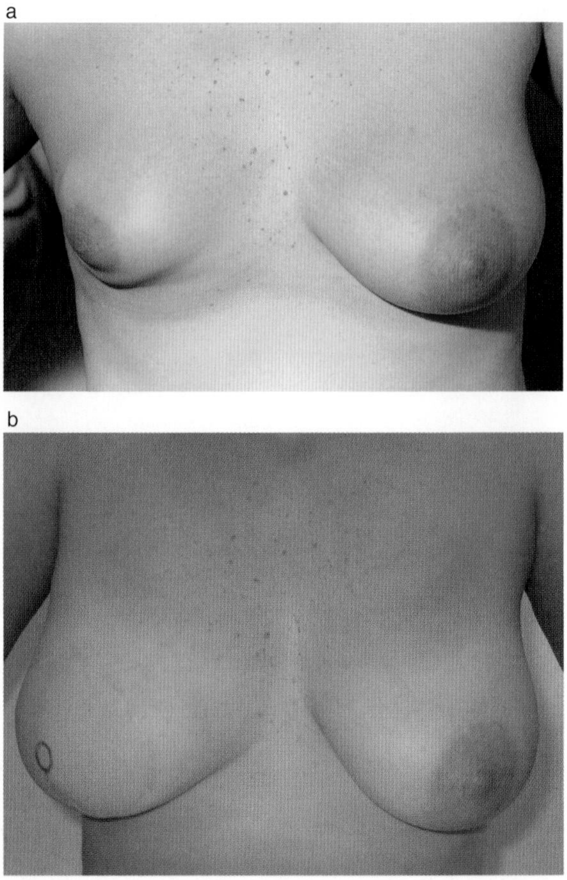

Fig. 38.7 Reconstruction of the right breast with a free TRAM flap following subcutaneous mastectomy. (a) Partial mastectomy defect resulting in asymmetry for volume with distortion of breast contour and nipple–areolar complex and prior to right subcutaneous mastectomy (including nipple–areolar complex) plus reconstruction with a free TRAM flap. (b) Postoperative result of free TRAM reconstruction of right breast (nipple position has been marked for nipple reconstruction using local flaps from TRAM flap skin paddle).

Hand surgery

Although the priority in hand surgery must always be function, the hand, like the face, is never normally covered, and aesthetics must also be borne in mind.

The hand is a sophisticated sensate organ composed of highly specialised and compactly organised moving parts with little wasted space. Thus any surgical intervention should be designed to minimise postoperative oedema and scarring to avoid long-term compromise of function in terms of power, range of movement and sensation.

Surgery of the hand is merely the start of treatment. Without dedicated postoperative treatment by physiotherapists, occupational therapists, orthotists and, in particular, the determination of the patient, even the most skilful surgery may result in an irreversibly stiff hand.

Burns

Although the treatment of burns is performed by a multidisciplinary team the plastic surgeon is normally the main practitioner involved in the treatment of major burns.

As with any major injury a primary survey must be performed and life-saving management begun. In the case of burns the sequence in Clinical Box 38.1 should be followed after first-aid measures to stop the burning process have been taken and the burn wound cooled.

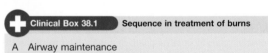

Clinical Box 38.1 Sequence in treatment of burns

- A Airway maintenance
- B Breathing and ventilation
- C Circulation
- D Drip – instigate i.v. fluids
- E Estimate burns size and depth
- F Fluid resuscitation

The initial treatment of patients with major burns is stabilisation by compensating the major fluid loss which will otherwise produce oligaemic shock. The weight of the patient and the extent of the burn, in terms of percentage of body surface area affected, needs to be assessed to determine the expected volume of fluid required to maintain satisfactory perfusion. In adults the rule of nines (see Fig. 10.4) is used to help in this assessment but, as the relative proportions of children differ, specific charts for children are available.

Various formulae for fluid resuscitation have been devised based on the weight and percentage area of burn, using either crystalloid solutions such as Ringer's lactate or colloid solutions such as plasma protein solution (PPS). In the UK for many years colloid resuscitation was favoured, but recently concern has been expressed that capillaries in the area of an extensive burn become so permeable that large molecules such as plasma proteins will pass into the extracellular space. In this situation colloid solutions confer no benefit over crystalloid solutions, and formulae employing the latter have become standard – such as the Parkland formula from Dallas, Texas. This requires a total volume replacement of approximately 4 mL Ringer's lactate (Hartmann's solution) per kg bodyweight per percentage total body surface burnt to be given in the first 24 hours postburn, of which one-half needs to be given within the first 8 hours. It is important to realise that these formulae are guides only and that the patient needs to be repeatedly assessed and the fluid resuscitation matched to clinical parameters such as urine output, haematocrit and blood pressure. The depth of the burn is also assessed to determine which areas are only superficially destroyed (i.e. deeper parts of the dermis are spared, implying spontaneous healing) or whether the damage is deeper and will require surgical excision. Further assessment is needed to determine whether excision should take place in the first few days – reducing the risk of sepsis but increasing the risk of oligaemia – or at a later stage when oligaemia is less likely but septicaemia is a greater risk. In both instances the choice of graft is either whole or mesh split skin, or a combination of the two. In general burns over 15% body surface area in adults and 10% body surface area in children require intravenous resuscitation and would normally in the UK be transferred to regional burns units as soon as possible. The criteria for transfer to a regional burns unit are broad but include any inhalation injury, burns to difficult areas such as hands, perineum, and burns at extremes of age. As a result only small minor burns are managed outside the regional setting. Most deep burns will require intensive nursing care and, in particular, extensive dressings. Physiotherapy will be required to maintain joint mobility – particularly in the hand, which is often best dressed in a plastic bag to avoid the use of restrictive dressings.

Once again, surgery is only the beginning; not infrequently the subsequent disfigurement and deformity from scarring and contracture involve the patient in multiple surgical procedures over many years.

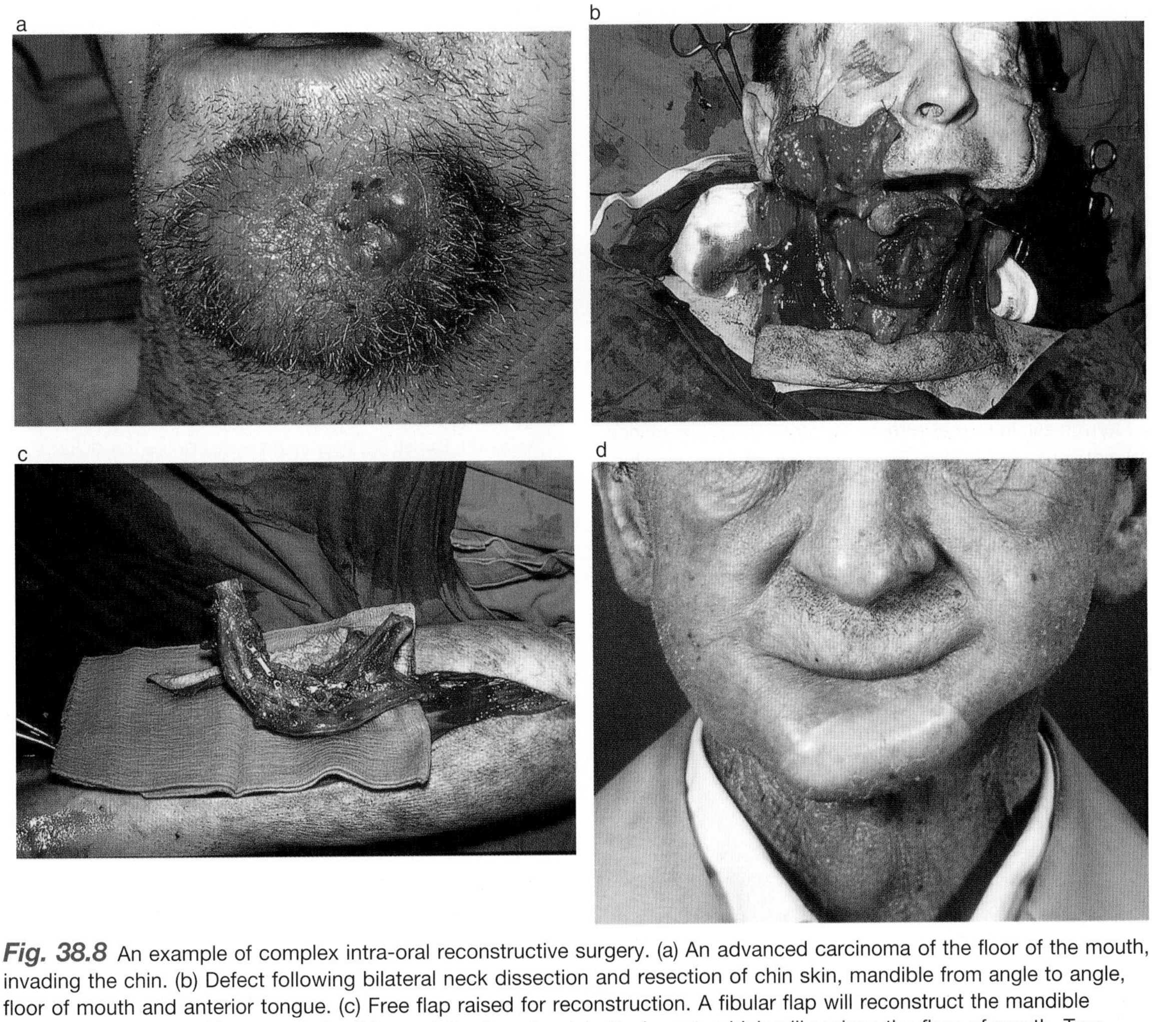

Fig. 38.8 An example of complex intra-oral reconstructive surgery. (a) An advanced carcinoma of the floor of the mouth, invading the chin. (b) Defect following bilateral neck dissection and resection of chin skin, mandible from angle to angle, floor of mouth and anterior tongue. (c) Free flap raised for reconstruction. A fibular flap will reconstruct the mandible with some overlying skin, vascularised through its deep fascial attachment, which will replace the floor of mouth. Two osteotomies have been made in the bone, which has been plated in a design to conform with the resected mandible. (d) Four months following surgery there is good bony union. External skin cover was achieved with an axial skin flap from the upper chest (deltopectoral flap)

Decubitus ulcers

These wounds are caused by pressure necrosis of tissues in an immobilised and often debilitated patient. In those patients who are temporarily incapacitated and subsequently become ambulant, the prognosis is good and the defects can be managed conservatively. The majority of ulcers, however, occur in paraplegic patients in tissues over bony prominences subject to chronic pressure when a combination of poor-quality and insensate tissues, poor general nutrition and, occasionally, poor motivation exacerbate the situation.

Management is directed to improving the nutritional status with the help of a dietician and excluding coexistent vascular disease. Continued pressure must be alleviated by regular turning of the patient, with mechanical assistance such as the low-air-loss bed. These patients are demanding of nursing time and require frequent dressings and repeated necrectomy. Eventually some of these wounds may heal spontaneously, though in many the resulting defect is of a size that can only be closed with a local flap. The surgery of decubitus ulcers can be expensive and time consuming and is inadvisable if measures cannot subsequently be taken to prevent any recurrence.

Head and neck surgery

Reconstruction in the head and neck demands the highest possible standards and encapsulates all the principles of restoration of form, appearance and function. In the face the cosmetic result is all important and, with this in mind, the surgeon may well opt for a more complicated method of repair. However, prostheses are indicated when the defect may be beyond the scope of surgical reconstruction or the patient too frail for extensive surgery. The materials of the prosthesis together with the secure fixation with osseointegration or the new biological adhesives has initiated a new era in prosthetic rehabilitation.

Conversely, intra-oral surgery demands the maintenance and restoration of function. Failure to adequately replace lost mucosal surfaces will produce tethering within the mouth, which is disastrous when it involves the tongue, resulting in interference with speech and swallowing. Thin and pliable flaps are ideal, as they drape the contours of the oral cavity. In many flaps it is possible to include vascularised bone, which permits single-stage mandibular reconstruction. If part of the lip is resected, dynamic reconstitution of the oral sphincter should be achieved to prevent oral incontinence. An example of complex reconstruction in this region is shown in Figure 38.8.

AESTHETIC PLASTIC OR COSMETIC SURGERY

In cosmetic surgery there is no obvious surgical pathology. The source of distress may either be variants of normal appearance or the aftermath of normal ageing processes, often out of proportion to the degree of physical abnormality as perceived by others. It is therefore essential that the surgeon does not trivialise cosmetic surgery or impart his prejudices on patients, many of whom enjoy a dramatic improvement in the quality of their lives following appropriate treatment. Meticulous patient selection and detailed discussion of the treatment options are paramount, so that the potential benefits and harms can be fully understood. In no other form of surgery is the implementation of fully informed consent more important. In no other form of surgery is there such a thin line between success and failure; between a happy grateful patient and an unhappy, resentful and potentially litigious patient.

FURTHER READING

Barret-Nerin J, Hemdon DN 2004 Principles and practice of burn surgery. Informa Healthcare, New York

McGregor AD, McGregor IA 2000 Fundamental techniques of plastic surgery: and their surgical applications, 10th edn. Churchill Livingstone, London

Settle JAD 1996 Principles and practice of burns management. Churchill Livingstone, Edinburgh

Thorne CH, Bartlett SP, Beasley RW, Aston SJ, Gurtner GC 2006 Grabb and Smith's plastic surgery, 6th edn. Lippincott Williams & Wilkins, Boston

Warwick D, Dunn R, Melikyan E, Vadher J 2009 Oxford specialist handbooks in surgery – hand surgery. OUP, Oxford

39 Skin disorders

INTRODUCTION

The most useful tool for diagnosing a skin complaint is skilful history-taking. The skin should be examined using the naked eye: the characteristics of the individual lesion(s) and their distribution are key to making the diagnosis. The whole skin surface must be examined even if the patient presents with an apparently solitary lesion, and careful consideration should be made of the need to examine the mucous membranes and the skin appendages, including nails and hair. It is also important to examine the regional lymph nodes draining the area of involvement, particularly in suspected neoplastic conditions.

Most skin conditions examined in surgical practice are benign or malignant tumours. Other conditions encountered include inflammatory rashes, perhaps triggered by drugs or a physical stress such as surgery, so a broader understanding of dermatological conditions is essential.

Embryology and anatomy

There are three layers to the skin (Fig. 39.1):

- epidermis
- dermis
- subcutis.

Epidermis

The epidermis originates from the embryonic ectoderm, in contrast to the other two deeper layers which are of mesodermal origin. Some epidermal structures – the pilosebaceous unit and nail matrix (see below) – migrate inwards during development and are anatomically located in the dermis. Similarly, some cells of mesodermal origin, such as melanocytes which are of neural crest origin, migrate outwards to the epidermis and are located within the basal cell layer.

The interface between the epidermis and dermis is convoluted – the dermal projection of the epidermis is a rete peg and the upwardly projecting portion of the dermis is the papillary dermis (Fig. 39.2). Between the epidermis and dermis there is a basement membrane zone which is traversed by anchoring fibrils, which are important in adherence of the two structures.

Epidermal cells

The *keratinocyte* is the predominant cell of the epidermis. The epidermis is made up of stratified keratinising squamous epithelium the layers of which can be identified histologically and represent stages of the maturation of cell division of the keratinocytes. The cells mature progressively as they migrate from the basal layer towards the surface. Initially, in the basal-layer keratinocytes, keratin filaments appear in the cytoplasm. As the cells mature further, the cytoplasm becomes progressively replaced by keratin – a structural protein which is surrounded by a phospholipid envelope that was the original cell membrane. As the cells with each division migrate towards the surface they flatten and by the time they reach the surface they form a laminated structure – the stratum corneum (Fig. 39.1) which serves as a physiological barrier to chemical and microbiological invasion from without, as well as fluid and salt loss from within. The epidermal transit time from the basal layer to stratum corneum is about 28 days. Disruption of this smooth transition occurs in inflammatory conditions of the epidermis such as psoriasis, and also as a result of actinic (sun-induced) damage to the basal cell – a process known as dyskeratosis which makes the affected epidermis unstable.

Melanocytes are cells of neural crest origin which produce the ultraviolet (UV) radiation-absorbing pigment melanin.

They are located along the basement membrane between the basal keratinocytes and have a dendritic shape with multiple root-like projections. Different racial groups have the same number of melanocytes, but there is a difference in the amount and type of melanin produced: Celtic races, for example, produce predominantly phaeomelanin, a yellow-red pigment which gives poorer UV protection than brown-black eumelanin. Increased melanin production can be stimulated by UV light and the cytokines released by inflammatory processes. Melanocytes distribute their melanin granules to the surrounding basal cells through their dendrites. Once these granules are taken up by the basal cells, they are dispersed through the cytoplasm to absorb UV radiation, which protects the nuclei as well as deeper cells from UV damage. Thus melanin has a key role in preventing malignant change to basal cells and photodamage to the underlying collagen: individuals who produce phaeomelanin which is less photoprotective will burn rather than tan and are more vulnerable to developing UV-induced skin tumours and wrinkling.

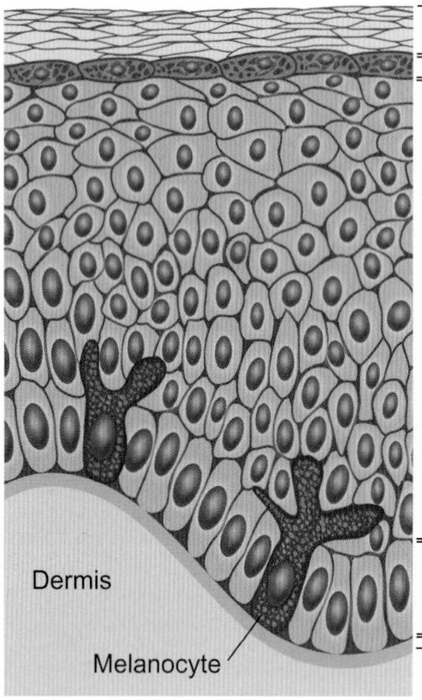

Fig. 39.1 Structure of normal epidermis.

Immunocompetent cells are of a number of classes: *Langerhans cells* are derived from bone marrow and are closely related to the macrophage. They are located just above the basal layer of keratinocytes in the so-called suprabasal layer. They express HLA receptors on their surface and are central to the presentation of antigens to other immunocompetent cells. They also, in their own right, release cytokines such as interleukin-2. Their prime importance is in immunosurveillance of the skin and mediation of the cutaneous immune response.

Lymphocytes are present in small numbers in the normal epidermis – mainly T lymphocytes of both CD4 and CD8 subsets. The T lymphocytes are derived from the thymus, which also like the epidermis is of ectodermal origin, and it is believed that they migrate through the epidermis as part of their surveillance of immune function. The interaction between Langerhans cells and lymphocytes makes the epidermis an important component of the body's immune system. This can be disturbed in some inflammatory conditions of the epidermis which are T-cell mediated: e.g.

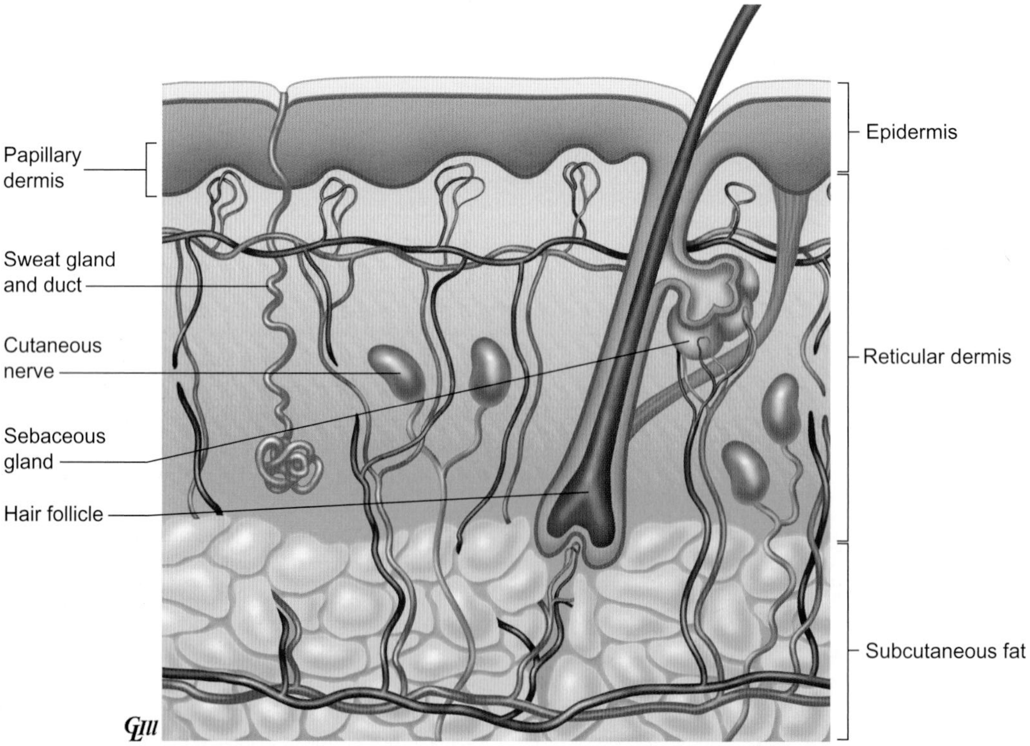

Fig. 39.2 Structure of normal skin.

psoriasis in which T lymphocytes release lymphokines into the epidermis, resulting in keratinocyte proliferation. In the cell-mediated (type IV) reaction, such as that seen to adhesives used in wound dressings, the colophony allergen is presented by an antigen-presenting cell, such as a Langerhans cell, to a T lymphocyte, setting off the cascade of events which result in allergic contact eczema.

The epidermal immune system may be suppressed in various ways. UV light can suppress type IV reactions in the skin. Some skin diseases such as atopic eczema are associated with local immunodeficiency and patients are prone to cutaneous infections with *Staphylococcus aureus*. The cutaneous immune system may also be suppressed during systemic diseases such as diabetes mellitus, HIV and leukaemia.

Merkel cells These, like melanocytes, are of mesodermal origin derived from the neural crest. They function as mechanoreceptors to help sense touch, and so are found particularly on the digital pads of the fingers.

Dermis

The major component of the dermis is connective tissue composed mainly of collagen fibres within an amorphous ground substance. The papillary dermis is the uppermost layer of the dermis, intertwined with the rete ridges of the epidermis. Below this, the reticular dermis is less cellular and contains more densely packed collagen and elastic fibres (Fig. 39.2). The dermis contains blood vessels which derive from a deep vascular plexus, sweat glands, nerves, lymphatics, and muscle fibres associated with a pilosebaceous unit (see below).

Dermal collagen is produced by fibroblasts which lie between the collagen bundles. It forms a mesh-like network which provides a supportive framework for skin structures, and gives the skin strength and elasticity. Changes in collagen occur with ageing and from UV light, both of which make collagen less flexible and less able to provide support for other structures. Wrinkles result, and purpura may also follow from the increased fragility of blood vessels.

Dermal blood vessels arise from a deep arterial plexus which then subdivides and finally a capillary loop which supplies the dermal papillae. Blood then drains through a papillary venous network and back into the subcutaneous vessels.

Lymphatic channels can be recognised within the dermis. Their obstruction or failure causes cutaneous lymphoedema.

Dermal nerve fibres are:

- afferent for cutaneous sensation
- efferent vasomotor and also to the sweat glands, both of which help regulate body temperature; there is also a supply to the erector pili muscle.

Sweat glands are of two types:

- eccrine glands are present throughout all skin and secrete an aqueous fluid
- apocrine glands occur in the intertriginous areas of the axillae and groin and also the scalp – their secretion is greasy.

Pilosebaceous units are a combination of a hair shaft, hair follicle and a sebaceous gland. Attached to the hair shaft are muscle fibres of the pili erector muscle. The keratin of the hair shaft is derived from a germinal layer of the hair bulb which lies deep in the dermis. The hair follicle is richly supplied by nerves and blood vessels. The sebaceous gland produces an oily secretion, sebum, which is discharged into the hair follicle via the pilosebaceous duct.

Nail matrix produces the specialised keratin of the nail plate which grows out beneath the proximal nail fold (Fig. 39.3). The plate is closely adherent to the underlying nail bed. Melanocytes can be present in the nail matrix, causing linear pigmented striae within the nails, as well as providing a starting place for melanoma (see Fig. 39.23). On either side of the nail plate are the lateral nail folds. The nail plate can grow into the soft nail fold, giving rise to an ingrowing nail; if the nail folds become infected, this is termed paronychia (Fig. 39.4).

Subcutis

The subcutis, which predominantly contains loose adipose tissue and elastin, serves to attach the skin to underlying muscle and bone as well as supplying it with blood vessels and nerves.

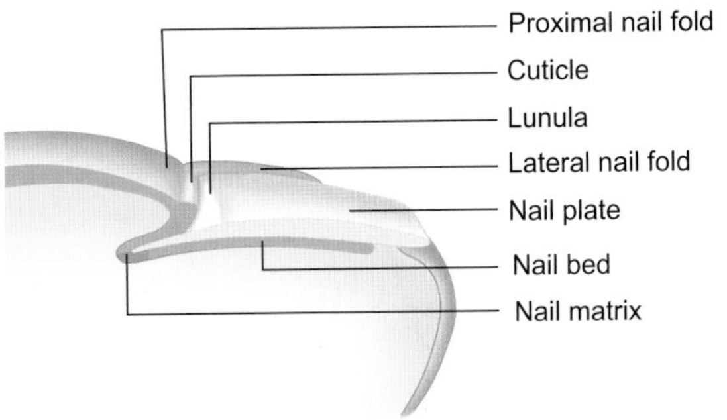

Fig. 39.3 Sagittal view of the nail anatomy.

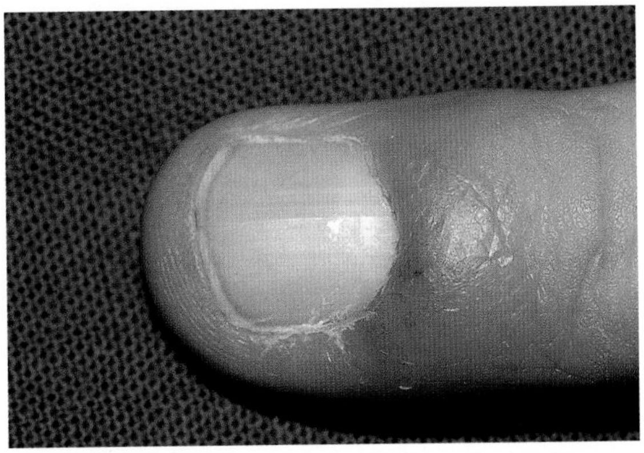

Fig. 39.4 Paronychia, showing loss of cuticle and swelling of nail fold.

Principles of investigation: the biopsy

Histological examination is required to confirm diagnosis, especially where there is doubt on clinical grounds. Small lesions may be completely excised (an excisional biopsy), larger ones may be removed initially in part (an incisional biopsy) before definitive therapy is decided on. When biopsying a rash, a relatively fresh representative lesion should be biopsied, and the biopsy should be taken across the edge of a lesion. It is important to provide adequate material for histological interpretation, which usually means a full-thickness biopsy including epidermis, dermis and a small amount of subcutis. Skin surgery is usually performed under local anaesthetic.

Full-thickness skin biopsies

Any incision into collagen (i.e. through the dermis) leaves a scar on healing, and this inevitable consequence must be explained to the patient beforehand. Hypertrophic and keloid scarring is always a possibility, especially for surgery on the upper trunk and shoulders, and the risk is higher in patients with black skin tone. Full-thickness skin biopsies may be incisional or excisional, and a variety of techniques can be used including:

- **Punch biopsy** (Fig. 39.5). A small sharp tool, not dissimilar to an apple-corer is used to obtain a cylindrical sample of full-thickness skin. This technique is often used to obtain an incisional biopsy for diagnostic purposes. Very small punch biopsies can heal well by secondary intention; otherwise, primary closure is achieved with sutures.
- **Ellipse biopsy** (Fig. 39.6). Using a scalpel an ellipse-shaped full-thickness biopsy is obtained of the skin. This technique is often used to perform excisional biopsies, e.g. of a melanoma, or when good-sized samples of the subcutis as well as the more superficial skin is required, e.g. in investigating inflammation of the fat. The wound is closed with sutures which are left in situ for 5–20 days dependent upon the site of the surgery and other wound-healing factors.

For larger wound defects a variety of techniques are used to close wounds, including skin grafts and rotation flaps (Ch. 38).

Principles of therapy

Neoplastic lesions must be excised without primary regard for the cosmetic outcome, and the sample submitted for histological examination to confirm the diagnosis and to check that the margins taken were adequate. For benign lesions, however, cosmesis must be given consideration.

A variety of therapeutic surgical techniques may be used: punch and ellipse biopsies as above, and also these methods below which in experienced hands have the advantage of removing superficial skin lesions without damaging collagen.

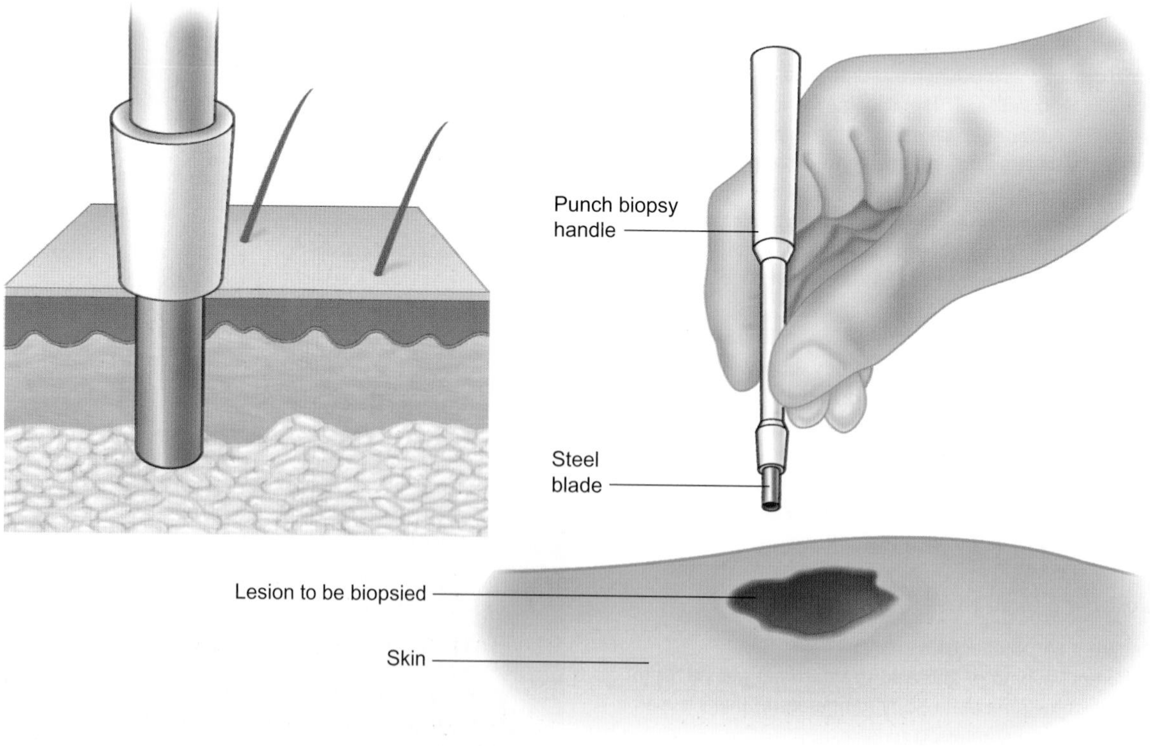

Fig. 39.5 Punch biopsy technique: the sharp instrument is driven into the skin to obtain a cylindrical section of skin. Inset: the sample obtained is of full-thickness skin down to subcutis.

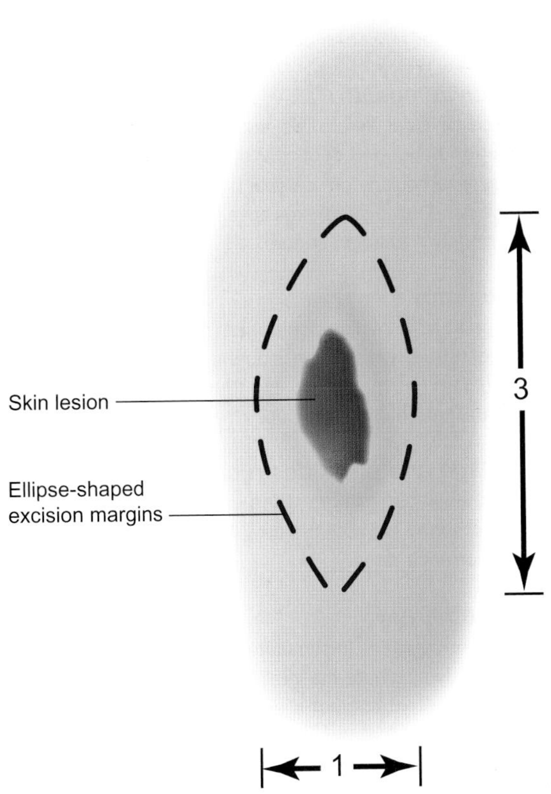

Fig. 39.6 Ellipse biopsy of skin showing the planned excision margins for a pigmented lesion, with the 3:1 ratio typically used to ensure a thin linear scar after suturing.

Curettage. A ring or spoon-shaped curette is used to remove the epidermal lesion, by drawing the curette with pressure over the lesion, e.g. seborrhoeic keratoses.

Shave biopsy. A scalpel or razor blade is used to remove a superficial skin lesion in a single piece of unfragmented tissue, e.g. a benign intradermal melanocytic naevus which catches on clothing.

Snip excision. Sterile scissors are used to remove pedunculated skin lesions, e.g. skin tags. Haemostasis is then achieved to the resultant erosion using cautery, hyfrecation or chemically using topical aluminium chloride solution.

Cryosurgery can also be used to treat superficial lesions such as viral warts (see below) satisfactorily. Patients should be warned of the likelihood of pain and blistering after this treatment, and, especially in patients with pigmented skin types, of the risk of pigmentary changes. Injudicious use of this method may result in deeper tissue injuries, such as digital nerve or extensor tendon damage when used on the dorsal aspects of the fingers.

Lasers can be used to treat benign vascular and pigmented lesions. The emission wavelength of the laser can be matched to the absorption spectrum of the pigment present, e.g. haemoglobin or melanin. Carbon dioxide lasers are more destructive, but give immediate haemostasis and vaporise a lesion; they have a role in ablative therapy especially.

DISORDERS OF THE SKIN

The skin is the body's largest organ – by weight, up to 15% of body mass. It is, along with the mucosal surface of the gastrointestinal tract, with which it is continuous, the interface between the external and internal environment and has a number of important functions in protection and in the maintenance of homeostasis. It is extensively exposed to agents which are actually or potentially noxious, including chemicals, carcinogens and pathogenic organisms. Also, it is at constant risk of physical trauma and subject to a large number of endogenous diseases such as eczema, lichen planus and psoriasis and may be involved in systemic problems such as vasculitis and granulomatous diseases (e.g. sarcoidosis). The prevalence of skin disorders is summarised in Box 39.1.

Box 39.1 Prevalence of skin disorders in the UK

- Skin disease affects between 25% and 33% of the population at any given time
- Skin disorders account for 15% of all consultations in general practice
- The commonest skin disorders seen in general practice are eczema, acne, infections and psoriasis
- Skin cancer accounts for 50% of the skin problem referrals from general practice to secondary care

INFECTIONS

The skin is constantly exposed to infectious agents. Protection is afforded by the physical barrier of the stratum corneum and the very effective immunological barrier of the epidermis.

Host defences may be breached as a result of:

- Physical injury, e.g. trauma or surgery to the skin
- Endogenous skin diseases, e.g. eczema or venous ulceration
- Immunosuppression, e.g. HIV or leukaemia
- Pathogenic organisms that are able to penetrate the normal skin defence mechanisms, e.g. fungal and candidal infection.

VIRAL INFECTIONS

Human papillomaviruses

These are a group of RNA viruses, and more than a hundred subtypes have been identified so far. The skin manifestation is a wart.

Epidemiology and aetiology

Warts are common, and most people suffer infection at some stage. They are mostly prevalent in children, where they are probably acquired from direct contact or from communal recreational facilities such as swimming pools. Genital (including perianal) warts are usually found in adults, and are most commonly, though not exclusively, acquired as a result of sexual intercourse so that they may coexist with other sexually transmitted infections.

History

Cutaneous warts may present suddenly with rapid growth or more gradually creep up on their hosts over many weeks, even years. Itching may be a feature. Larger lesions can become painful, especially if they are on pressure points such as the heel or ball of the foot. Lesions can be of cosmetic concern when on exposed sites such as the hands or face.

Clinicopathological features

The virus infects the basal keratinocytes of the epidermis, resulting in increased proliferation of these cells. In stratified squamous epithelium this gives rise to hyperkeratosis and a hard wart is seen. The characteristics of a wart are loss of the normal dermatoglyphics of the skin and thrombosed capillaries that are seen as small black dots which bleed if the overlying hard skin is pared away (Fig. 39.7). On mucosal surfaces the wart is softer – a fleshy papilloma.

Management

Prevention

Vaccines have been produced against HPV subtypes 16 and 18, which together are associated with 70% of cervical cancers, and are also associated with many cases of anal cancer. Routine HPV immunisation of girls aged 9–14 years has been introduced in the UK and other countries. One currently available vaccine also protects against HPV types 6 and 11, which cause 90% of genital warts. These developments open up the future possibility of a vaccine against the HPV types (e.g. 1 and 2) more typically involved in cutaneous warts on the hands and feet.

Natural history

Spontaneous resolution is the rule once natural immunity has developed, but this takes longer in adults than in children, so that infection can last for many years. The multiplicity of treatment options for management of viral warts reflects the relatively poor efficacies of these individual treatments.

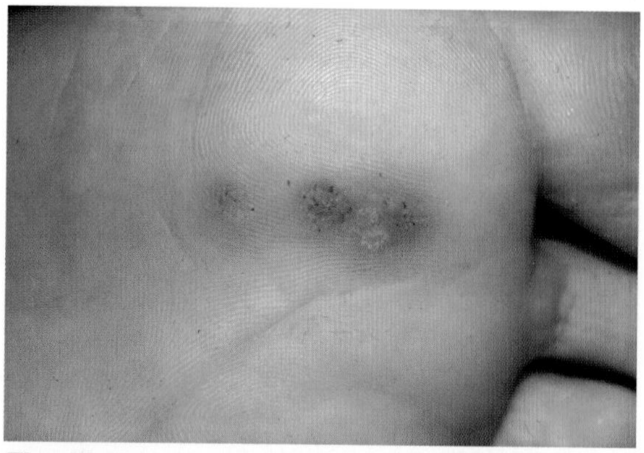

Fig. 39.7 Viral warts (verrucae) on the sole, demonstrating thrombosed capillaries which clinically appear as 'black dots'.

Keratolytic agents

The use of local keratolytic agents such as salicylic acid paints for hand and foot warts remains the mainstay of therapy, particularly in children. Even when cure is not achieved the removal of excessive keratin helps to limit discomfort until resolution occurs.

Cryotherapy

The application of liquid nitrogen can destroy the virus-infected tissue, which then sloughs off. Early resolution in individual lesions may follow, but there is a high rate of recurrence and treatment is painful.

Curettage and other destructive measures

Physical ablation of larger warts can be achieved by curettage, diathermy or laser therapy, but they also have significant recurrence rates.

Immunotherapy

Immunotherapy aims to stimulate the body's immune system to effectively eliminate the virally infected cells, e.g. diphencyprone, a potent contact allergen which in expert hands is used to induce localised eczema associated with clearance of the warts; and imiquimod, a topical immune modulator which binds to cell-surface toll-like receptors resulting in the secretion of numerous pro-inflammatory cytokines including interferon-α, resulting in clearance of the warts.

Cytotoxic agents

Podophyllin (a compound preparation which contains the agent podophyllotoxin) is particularly helpful in treating genital warts. Its application must be closely monitored, however, because it causes soreness and is teratogenic and therefore must not be used during pregnancy. Bleomycin has also been successfully used by injecting intralesionally.

Special problems with genital warts (syn. condylomata acuminatum)

It is important when assessing a patient with genital warts to ensure that they have not also acquired any other sexually transmitted disease. In addition to podophyllin and imiquimod, these warts may be treated with physical destruction or excision under general anaesthesia. Excision has the benefit of providing histology as dysplasia and even squamous cell carcinoma may be present especially in immunocompromised patients.

Molluscum contagiosum

Aetiology and pathological features

This is caused by a pox virus. The individual lesions are smooth and dome-shaped, they have a characteristic central depression or umbilication and, if squeezed, a central white core can be expressed called the molluscum body. Florid molluscum contagiosum may occur in immunosuppressed patients, particularly those with HIV infection. When patients acquire immununity to the virus the lesions disappear.

Management

Early resolution of individual lesions can be induced by minor trauma such as cryotherapy or superficial diathermy; imiquimod has also been used to good effect.

Herpes viruses

There are two types of infection:

- Herpes simplex due to a number of subtypes of herpes simplex viruses (HSV)
- Herpes zoster due to varicella-zoster virus (VZV).

The distinction is summarised in Box 39.2.

Herpes simplex

This condition can affect any area of the skin, however it is most commonly seen close to the mucous membranes of the lips in HSV type 1 and the genitalia in HSV type 2. The patient notices a prodromal tingling of the skin followed by the eruption of clusters of small vesicles. The active lesions are infectious, and surgeons need to take care to avoid direct contact, as this can result in a herpetic whitlow on a finger.

Herpes zoster

This is caused by VZV; the primary widespread infection is chickenpox. The virus then lies dormant in the dorsal root ganglia of the CNS and is reactivated along peripheral nerves to produce vesicles and pustules in a dermatomal distribution, known as shingles or herpes zoster. Its relevance for surgeons is that herpes zoster can be triggered by stresses such as surgery. Additionally the prodromal phase, before the development of vesicles, gives rise to pain in the skin of the affected dermatome which may cause diagnostic difficulties by mimicking other nerve lesions such as sciatica, or an acute abdomen. Treatment with aciclovir or valaciclovir shortens attacks.

Box 39.2 Herpes simplex and zoster

Herpes simplex
- Subtype 1 – onset in childhood and usually orofacial
- Subtype 2 – onset in adults and usually genital
- Attacks may be precipitated by UV light, or an intercurrent illness, e.g. upper respiratory infection

Herpes zoster
- Caused by activation of dormant varicella-zoster (chickenpox) virus
- Distribution is characteristically dermatomal and unilateral – more widespread infection suggests immunosuppression, e.g. HIV infection
- Can present with unilateral abdominal pain before skin lesions appear
- Rarely recurs but may be complicated in the long term by severe post-herpetic neuralgia
- Antiviral drugs reduce the acute pain and duration of herpes zoster and should always be given

BACTERIAL INFECTIONS

Staphylococcal infections

Aetiology, pathological features and management

Staphylococcus aureus (SA) can cause primary skin infections such as impetigo, furunculosis and acute paronychia. Diabetic patients are particularly susceptible. Since the 1950s the majority of strains of *S. aureus* have been resistant to many commonly used antibiotics such as penicillin; from the mid-1990s there has been an increasing incidence of methicillin-resistant SA or MRSA such that it is now endemic in British hospitals. Community acquired MRSA infections are also increasingly seen. Panton–Valentine leukocidin (PVL) is a toxic substance produced by some strains of *S. aureus* which is associated with an increased ability to cause disease. This PVL SA remains relatively uncommon in the UK.

Impetigo

This condition mainly affects the face and is much more common in children than in adults: presentation is as flaccid blisters underneath the stratum corneum which rupture early on, so giving rise to a raw eroded base. Impetigo is contagious, and infected children should be kept away from school. Swabs are taken to determine the antibiotic sensitivities of the organism. Both staphylococcal and streptococcal bacteria may cause the condition. If the lesions are localised, topical antibiotics such as fucidic acid or mupirocin are effective, dependent on sensitivities. If lesions are more widespread, they are treated with systemic flucloxacillin.

Furunculosis

This term describes a group of conditions characterised by staphylococcal infection of the hair follicles. Staphylococcal folliculitis is a pyoderma localised to the hair follicle and can be either superficial or deep. A furuncle (boil) is a deep-seated inflammatory nodule which develops around a hair follicle from a preceding, more superficial folliculitis. A carbuncle is a more-extensive and even deeper infiltrating inflammation which occurs in thick and inelastic skin – commonly on the back of the neck.

The acute lesions of furunculosis are characterised by pain and tenderness of the infected area and soft tissue. Localisation of pus gives rise to abscesses. The natural history of the lesions is for the pus to discharge and this to be followed by resolution. Treatment of the early soft-tissue phase is with systemic antibiotics. If a deep abscess forms, then surgical drainage is indicated. Carbuncles and ecthyma represent infective gangrene of the deep tissues. The subcutaneous tissues become painful and indurated and drain to the surface through sinuses. Surgical debridement may be necessary, in addition to a course of antibiotics.

Paronychia

This is the term given to inflammation of the nail fold. Infection is usually acquired through loss of the cuticle of the proximal nail fold, sometimes the consequence of a self-inflicted injury at manicure. Paronychia may be acute when caused by *S. aureus* infection, or chronic when the result of

Candida infection whose acquisition is difficult to determine (Fig. 39.4). Treatment is by surgical debridement – which may have to include the nail – under local anaesthetic.

Streptococcal infections

Streptococcus pyogenes (beta-haemolytic streptococcus Lancefield group A) causes dermal infections of two types:

- erysipelas – infection in the deep dermis but not the subcutaneous tissues
- cellulitis – full-thickness infection of the skin with involvement of the subcutaneous tissues.

The presentation of both may be that of the systemic features of severe sepsis, with rigor and fever but without initial overt evidence of skin involvement. The earliest cutaneous sign is erythema. The leg and face are most commonly affected, although any site may be involved. The infection spreads through the tissue by the release of toxins, giving rise to a brawny erythema spreading across the skin with a sharp well-demarcated edge (Fig. 39.8). If left untreated, the infection will eventually resolve, but there is a significant mortality from overwhelming toxaemia and septicaemia.

The treatment of choice for streptococcal cellulitis is bed rest with intravenous antibiotics. The majority of streptococci are sensitive to penicillin, and this is the agent of choice. The fever usually settles within 24–48 hours, and the erythema and swelling subside slowly. Streptococcal cellulitis can complicate chronic skin conditions such as venous leg ulceration (Ch. 30) and lymphoedema (Ch. 30). When this occurs, treatment with antibiotics may have to be prolonged to prevent early relapse.

Necrotising fasciitis

Necrotising fasciitis is an acute and potentially life-threatening infection. It occurs in healthy individuals, often after mild trauma, usually on the leg. It may be caused by a single bacterium or a synergistic combination of different bacteria. The organisms commonly cultured include group A streptococcus, *S. aureus* (including MRSA), *Vibrio vulnificus*, *Clostridium perfringens* and *Bacteroides fragilis*. An ill-defined erythema develops which rapidly becomes necrotic. The patient complains of severe pain and is found to have a high fever and the other features of systemic inflammatory response out of proportion to the local skin findings. The infection spreads quickly in the fascial plane and involves both skin and subcutaneous tissues. Urgent CT or ultrasound scanning may confirm the diagnosis and help to define the extent of the disease, but these should not delay definitive surgical treatment. Urgent surgical wide debridement of the affected tissues is required together with intravenous antibiotics (e.g. linezolid with meropenem or piperacillin/tazobactam). Antibiotic treatment may be modified once bacteriological culture results are available. Repeat operation is often performed within a few hours in case further tissue excision is required. Transfer to a plastic surgical unit for reconstructive surgery is usually required once the patient's condition has improved.

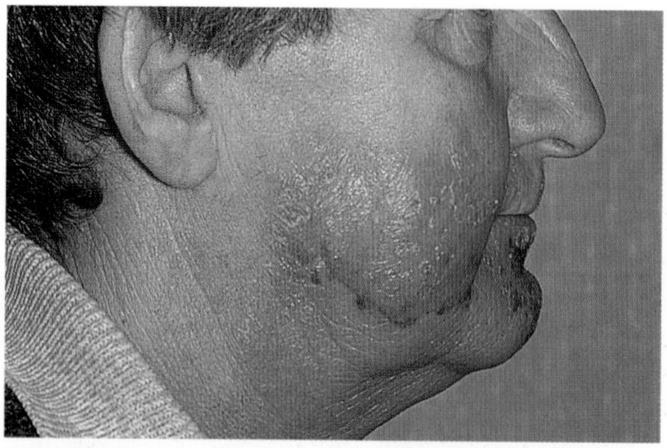

Fig. 39.8 Erysipelas, showing indurated red plaque spreading across face.

Venous ulceration

Ulceration in the gaiter area of the leg is common in patients with post-thrombotic venous hypertension and is also seen with advanced varicose veins. These ulcers may become secondarily infected and cause surrounding cellulitis. The condition and its treatment are described in detail in Chapter 30.

FUNGAL INFECTIONS

Superficial mycoses

These infections are due to fungi that can only invade fully keratinised tissues. The clinical appearance depends on the severity of the inflammatory reaction to the fungi. When mild, the lesions are red and scaly; when severe, boggy areas of inflammation may arise; when present on the scalp or beard this is known as a kerion (Fig. 39.9). It is important to recognise this to prevent inappropriate surgical intervention as these lesions can best be treated medically with appropriate systemic antifungals. Mycological examination of the tissue

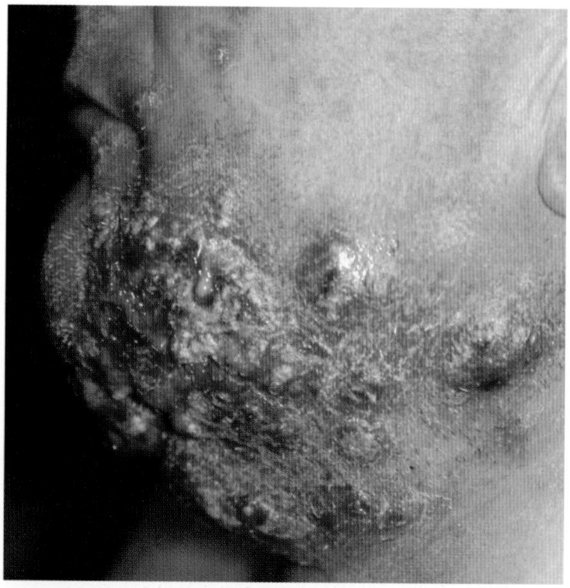

Fig. 39.9 Kerion in the beard area due to *Trichophyton verrucosum*. Treatment is with systemic antifungal therapy: this lesion resolved without scarring after treatment with oral terbinafine.

Fungal infections
Tumours
Benign tumours of the epidermis

conducted by direct microscopy is used to confirm the diagnosis.

TUMOURS

The skin is exposed to chronic irritation and carcinogens. Tumours of the skin, as with any other tissue, can be benign or malignant. The latter may be primary or secondary.

A number of premalignant conditions can be identified and are discussed below. Tumours that derive from the epidermis (ectodermal) have different clinical features from those of the dermis (mesodermal).

BENIGN TUMOURS OF THE EPIDERMIS

Seborrhoeic keratosis/wart (*syn*. basal cell papilloma)

These lesions are common in the elderly.

Clinical features

History

These are rough lesions which may catch on clothing; this or other trauma may cause minor bleeding. The appearance is unattractive, and cosmetic distaste is a common reason for presentation.

Physical findings

Raised, well-circumscribed lesions may occur anywhere on the body, although the trunk is the most common site. They are initially flat with varying amounts of pigmentation. The surface is waxy with superficial clefting and fissuring (Fig. 39.10).

Management

The differential diagnosis of deeply pigmented papillomas from malignant melanoma can be difficult; if there is doubt, excision biopsy is indicated.

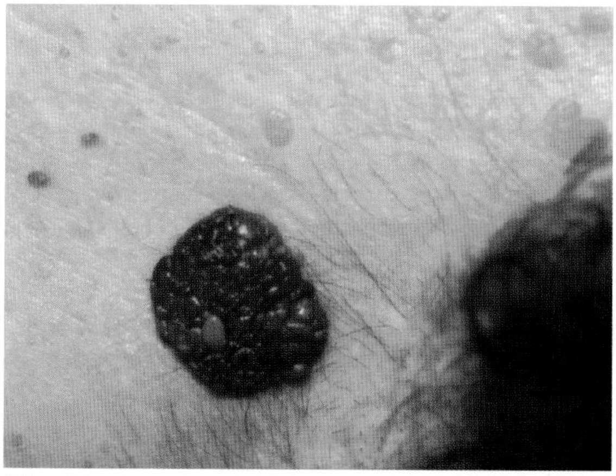

Fig. 39.10 Large, deeply pigmented seborrhoeic keratosis with greasy, ceribriform surface. Close by, several smaller skin-coloured seborrhoeic keratoses may also be seen.

However, if the diagnosis is certain, shaving back the lesion or curettage and cautery give a satisfactory cosmetic result with the additional benefit of providing a specimen for histological confirmation of the diagnosis.

Skin tags

These lesions are usually found in sites where skin surfaces rub together and the skin is therefore chronically irritated. There is a loose connective tissue core covered by epidermis which is variably pigmented.

Skin tags are irritated by clothing and bleed as well as causing local symptoms in areas such as the skin surrounding the anus. Patients often present to request removal. The diagnosis is obvious to the naked eye.

Management is by snip excision and cautery carried out under local anaesthetic.

Solar (actinic) keratoses

These scaling red macular (flat) lesions occur on sun-exposed areas of the skin, often on a background of collagen damage known as solar elastosis. The basal epidermal cells are dysplastic: clinically this results in the skin surface changing from smooth to scaly with excessive keratin. Induration or pain can occurs if the lesion becomes invasive; progression to a squamous cell carcinoma may take place, although this is rare.

Management

Isolated superficial lesions are dealt with by cryotherapy. If there is any induration, curettage and cautery are used and the fragments sent for histological examination. Where there is a high suspicion of squamous cell carcinoma lesions should be excised to avoid ambiguous histology. Close follow-up is indicated when the histological diagnosis is uncertain.

Extensive areas of sun damage with multiple solar keratoses are better managed topically with application of cytotoxic creams such as 5-fluorouracil or immunomodulators such as imiquimod to stabilise the epithelium; this has to be done under close supervision.

Keratoacanthoma

This lesion arises from squamous epithelium. It is most common on exposed areas of the body and is thought to result from minor trauma. As its name suggests, it has a central keratin plug with a surrounding collar of acanthotic thickened epidermis (Fig. 39.11).

Clinical features

The lesion is characterised by rapid onset and growth. It then enters a static phase, which may last 3–4 months before spontaneous resolution. The appearance of the lesion by itself can be very difficult to distinguish from a squamous cell carcinoma (see below), although the latter usually grows progressively but less rapidly. The same difficulty also occurs on histological examination, but carcinoma always invades the deeper dermis. Treatment is by excision with a margin of

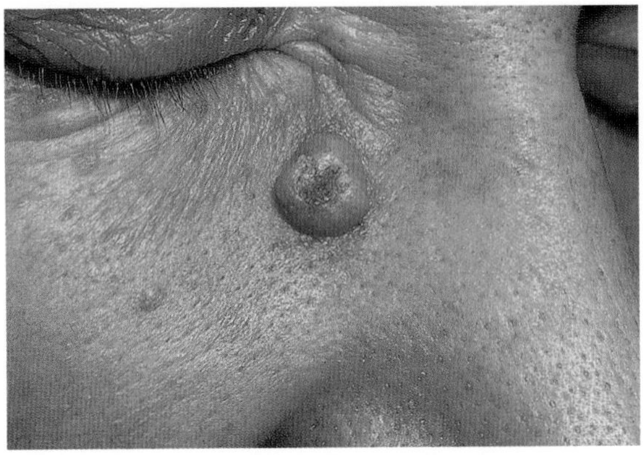

Fig. 39.11 Keratoacanthoma on cheek, showing central keratin plug with surrounding acanthotic collar.

surrounding skin; if there is any remaining doubt about the diagnosis, careful follow-up is indicated.

OTHER BENIGN SKIN TUMOURS

Benign pigmented skin lesions

Freckles (*syn.*ephelides)

Freckles are areas of the epidermis where melanocytes produce more melanin, usually in response to ultraviolet light. The number of melanocytes is normal, and they are quite stable.

Lentigo (plural lentigines)

Lentigines are areas of the epidermis where the number of melanocytes is increased and melanin production is excessive. They are found in areas of chronic sun exposure and hence are most common on the face, hands and shoulders. If seen in young patients, they are the sites of solar damage, and the patient should be advised against unnecessary exposure to the sun.

Melanocytic pigmented naevus (plural naevi): 'moles'

The term naevus is not necessarily confined to melanocytic skin lesions; it may equally refer to blood vessels (vascular naevi). The more correct generic term is a hamartoma. Essentially there is an abnormal collection of a normal skin constituent: in this case, melanocytes. Congenital melanocytic naevi are rare, often darkly pigmented and may be hairy or papillary. Melanocytic naevi may occur anywhere on the skin – including the nail bed, where they give rise to a linear pigmented stria. According to the clinical and histological features, melanocytic naevi can be subdivided into five types:

- junctional – at the dermo–epidermal interface (clinically brown and flat)
- intradermal – entirely within the dermis (clinically skin-coloured and raised)
- compound – features of both junctional and intradermal (clinically brown and raised)
- blue – deep dermal with considerable pigmentation which gives rise to their colour (blue-black and flat)
- Spitz naevus – reddish brown in colour, usually on the face or limbs of children and young adults; they are benign (but see below).

Most moles which are not present at birth will develop in the second or third decade. A Spitz naevus may undergo rapid growth and for this reason is often removed to exclude malignancy. Histological examination shows large cells which are pleomorphic and can be very difficult to distinguish from those of malignant melanoma. Skilled histological assessment is necessary.

Dermatofibroma

This is a tumour (often multiple) of dermal connective tissue which contains histiocytes and is of unknown cause. There have been suggestions that they arise from insect bites as the lower leg is the most commonly affected site, and they are more common in women than in men. A small intradermal nodule is present. Pigmentation is usual, and the overlying epidermis is tethered to the lesion, giving a puckered appearance if the lesion is squeezed.

As the lesion matures it changes from red-brown to pale, although often with a retained surrounding halo of pigmentation. A slow increase in size may occur, and excision may be necessary especially with the darker lesions, to exclude melanoma and establish the diagnosis with certainty.

Benign abnormalities of the blood vessels

Haemangiomas are distinguished by the size of the blood vessel that is involved.

Pathological features

Capillary haemangiomas are common and may give rise to salmon pink discoloration on the surface of the skin. The back of the neck is a common site. Other variants include the port wine stain on the face, which may be associated with ipsilateral intracranial haemangiomata, giving rise to epilepsy (Sturge–Weber syndrome). Strawberry naevi may appear in infancy and grow with age before resolving spontaneously by the early teens. Campbell de Morgan spots appear as small cherry papules on the trunk, are very common and of no significance, although they can become increasingly numerous with age and give rise to cosmetic embarrassment. Pyogenic granulomas are exuberant granulation tissue, an exaggerated healing response to minor trauma, and are usually found on the finger or the lip (Fig. 39.12). In spite of their name, the lesions are not infective in cause. They are friable and bleed readily. Glomus tumours appear as small vascular blebs on the skin. They have a generous nerve supply and are tender, especially if they occur within a confined space such as the nail bed.

Neurofibromas

These are benign tumours of the fibroblasts of the nerve sheath. The usual presentation is a solitary lesion in the area of a peripheral nerve. On clinical examination they are soft and fleshy (Fig. 39.13).

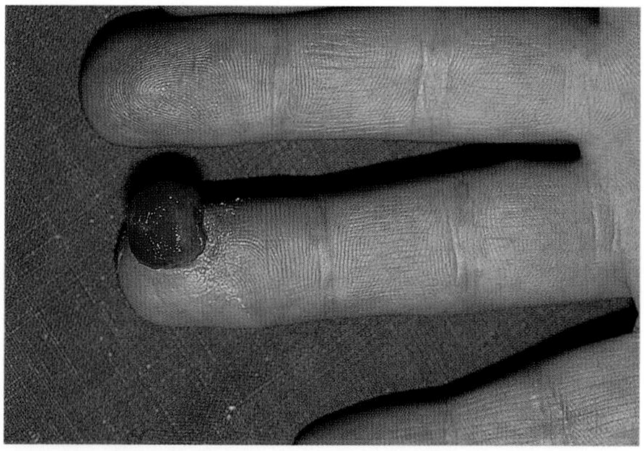

Fig. 39.12 Pyogenic granuloma on finger, showing friable vascular tumour.

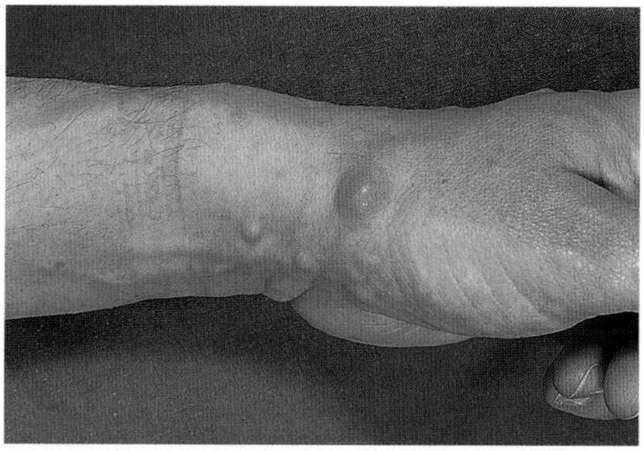

Fig. 39.13 Neurofibroma on wrist, showing soft fleshy swelling.

Schwannomas are benign tumours arising from the Schwann cells around the peripheral nerves, are much firmer nodules than neurofibromas and are closely tethered to an identifiable nerve. Pressure on the tumour may cause pain in the area of distribution of the nerve, and excision has to be performed with great care.

Some patients have multiple neurofibromas, which form part of the syndrome of neurofibromatosis with associated cafe-au-lait spots and axillary freckling. There are sometimes schwannomas of the larger cranial nerves and phaeochromocytoma. Two types of neurofibromatosis exist with identified mutations on chromosome 17q (neurofibromin protein, type 1) and 22q (merlin protein, type 2). They are both autosomal dominant, although there is a high spontaneous mutation rate seen in approximately 50% patients.

Benign appendage tumours

Skin appendages, such as sweat glands and hair follicles, are a source of benign tumours. Non-specific tumours such as syringomata or trichofolliculomas are not usually diagnosed clinically but only retrospectively following excision of a nondescript skin nodule. A cylindroma is of hair follicle origin and gives rise to a fleshy nodule. They usually occur on the scalp and may become very large, giving rise to what in the past was labelled a turban tumour.

Cysts

A cyst is an epithelium-lined cavity usually filled with thick products of epithelial secretion or of cell breakdown which have undergone degeneration. The most common type originates from the hair follicle.

Epidermoid and pilar cysts

These are sometimes incorrectly termed sebaceous cysts. Epidermoid cysts have walls derived from the follicular infundibular epithelium, so they are found anywhere on the body where hair follicles occur. Many are solitary but multiple lesions occur. They range in size from a few millimetres to several centimetres. The cyst is located in the deep dermis but is connected to the superficial epithelium through the pilosebaceous duct. A blocked duct may be visible on the surface as a central black punctum. Clinically, they are soft and are mobile over deeper structures. Pilar cysts have walls derived from the outer root sheath of the hair follicle, and are almost invariably found on the scalp.

Epidermoid and pilar cysts are not usually painful unless they are injured with disruption of the contents into the surrounding dermis, where they cause an intense inflammatory reaction. When this occurs, the area swells and becomes tender.

Uninflamed cysts are excised; care must be taken that all abnormal epithelial elements are removed, or recurrence is likely. If the cyst has become inflamed, then the contents are best drained and the inflammation allowed to subside, at which point the whole cyst can be excised.

Dermoid cysts

Congenital

These are rare and arise from abnormalities of development where epithelial remnants occur. They are found in lines of embryological fusion; the midline of the neck, the scalp and the face are common sites. The contents of the cysts include ectodermal structures of hair and sebaceous glands in addition to keratin.

Implantation dermoids

In this condition, a usually insignificant injury drives a fragment of dermis into the subdermal layer from where its secretions cannot escape. The fingertip is the commonest site (e.g. rose gardeners), although they may occur at any site of injury.

Lipomas

This is strictly a growth of fat deep to the skin proper. The overlying skin is normal, and the lump can be moved in relation to it. Fluctuation can be elicited, although the lesion is not cystic. The histological appearance is of a mass of adipose tissue with thin fibroid septa. The size varies, and penetration into muscles can occur. Treatment is by excision, particularly if the lipoma increases in size or becomes tender.

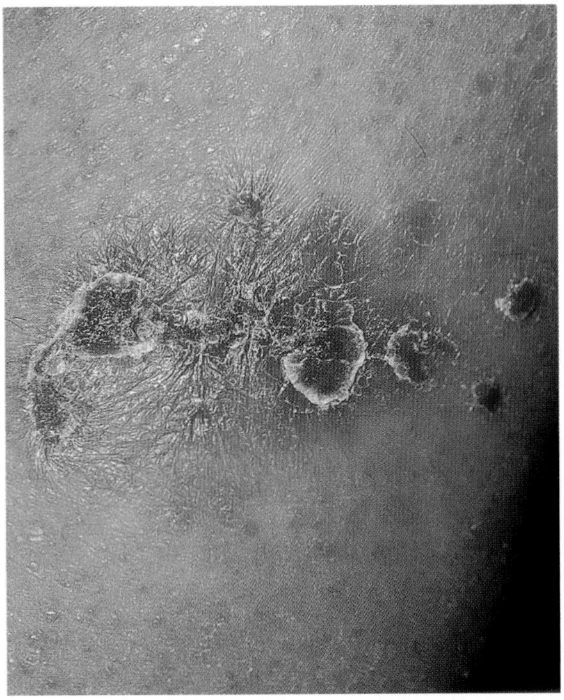

Fig. 39.14 Bowen's disease on leg, showing psoriasiform plaque.

PREMALIGNANT CONDITIONS OF THE EPIDERMIS

Bowen's disease

This is characterised by a well-circumscribed scaly plaque (Fig. 39.14) most commonly on the lower legs although it can occur anywhere on the body including at the anus. The clinical appearance is similar to a solitary patch of psoriasis. Histological examination shows full-thickness epidermal dysplasia sometimes amounting to carcinoma in situ. The condition is potentially malignant although progression is slow.

Management

A variety of methods can be used to treat the condition, including curettage and cautery, the use of topical cytotoxic drugs, excision, cryotherapy, and sometimes superficial radiotherapy. The choice depends on the size of the lesion, its site and the age of the patient.

Leucoplakia

In this condition, a fixed white plaque is seen on mucous membranes. The differential diagnosis is from lichen planus – a common inflammatory condition of the skin and mucous membranes – which has a more lace-like appearance, and *Candida* where the white plaques can be brushed off from the surface mucosa. Oral candidiasis usually occurs in immunocompromised patients, in diabetics or in those on systemic corticosteroid therapy. If there is any doubt, the plaque should be biopsied to exclude dysplasia and, if positive, the area ablated by cryotherapy or laser.

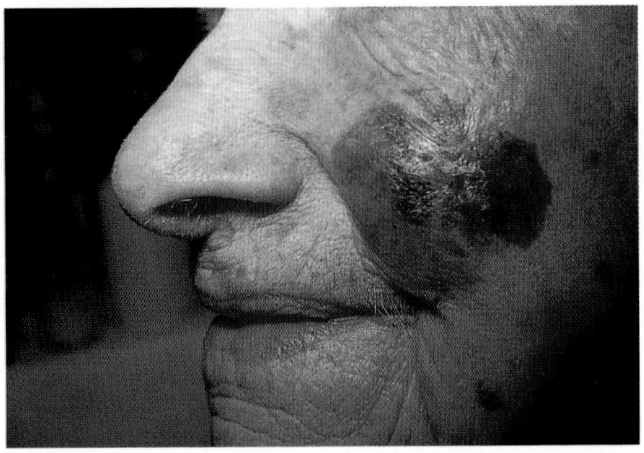

Fig. 39.15 Lentigo maligna on cheek, showing plaque with variation in pigmentation.

Paget's disease of the nipple

This is discussed in detail in Chapter 28.

Lentigo maligna

This is a rare plaque-like condition which tends to develop in late middle age, most commonly on the cheek, and increases slowly in size with time. Initially the plaque is uniformly pigmented, but as the lesion develops, irregular pigmentation occurs which is the early superficial spreading phase of a malignant melanoma (Fig. 39.15). If left untreated, the melanoma advances and enters a deep invasive phase with the same risk of metastases as melanoma elsewhere.

Management

Smaller lesions should be excised. There is a problem here with lesions that occupy a large surface area, and excision is not usually possible without grafting. A graft is unsightly, and the condition may be managed expectantly by close and regular follow-up. Action is taken if there is a change in appearance.

NON-MELANOMA SKIN CANCER

Classification

There are two commoner clinical types of carcinoma, both of which arise from keratinocytes:

- basal cell carcinoma
- squamous cell carcinoma.

A variety of factors predispose the epidermis towards these malignancies:

- exposure to the sun
- immunosuppression, e.g. from therapy to prevent rejection of organs
- hereditary disorders, e.g. xeroderma pigmentosum, a condition of failure of DNA repair

The annual incidence of non-melanoma skin cancer is increasing, and basal cell carcinoma is the more common.

Basal cell carcinoma

This generally arises in sites exposed to the sun. Ninety percent of lesions are on the face.

Classification

There are four clinical types:

- nodulocystic – the most common
- pigmented
- superficial spreading
- morphoeic or sclerotic.

Pathological features

Basal cell carcinomas cause local invasion and destruction of surrounding tissues. They penetrate into subcutaneous tissue and can erode into vital structures such as the orbit and brain. Histologically, the tumour cells have strongly basophilic nuclei and little cytoplasm. Cells at the periphery of the tumour give rise to a palisade pattern reminiscent of normal basal cells. Metastases are extremely rare.

Clinical features

A **nodulocystic** lesion has fluid-filled spaces and initially presents as a small translucent or pearly nodule which eventually breaks down, usually as the result of minor trauma, to produce an ulcer – a rodent ulcer characterised by a rolled pearly edge with surface telangiectasia (Fig. 39.16).

A **pigmented form** has characteristic pearly nodules around the edge (Fig. 39.17).

Superficial spreading carcinoma is a scaly plaque, usually on the trunk, with epidermal atrophy; pearly translucent nodules can usually be seen around the periphery of the lesion (Fig. 39.18).

Morphoeic or **sclerotic lesions** heal by fibrosis and scarring and may be multifocal; they do not look at all like cystic basal cell carcinomas, do not have pearly nodules but appear as a rather depressed plaque of sclerotic skin (Fig. 39.19).

Management

It is important that the tumour is treated adequately on the first occasion to render recurrence unlikely. Treatment depends on the site and size of the lesions at the time of

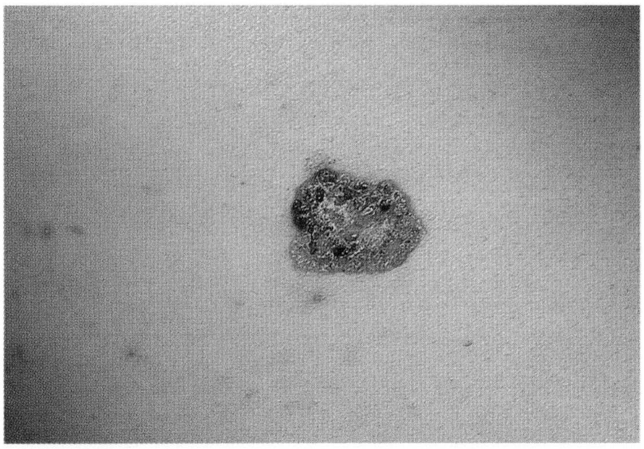

Fig. 39.17 Pigmented basal cell carcinoma showing pigmentation of lesion.

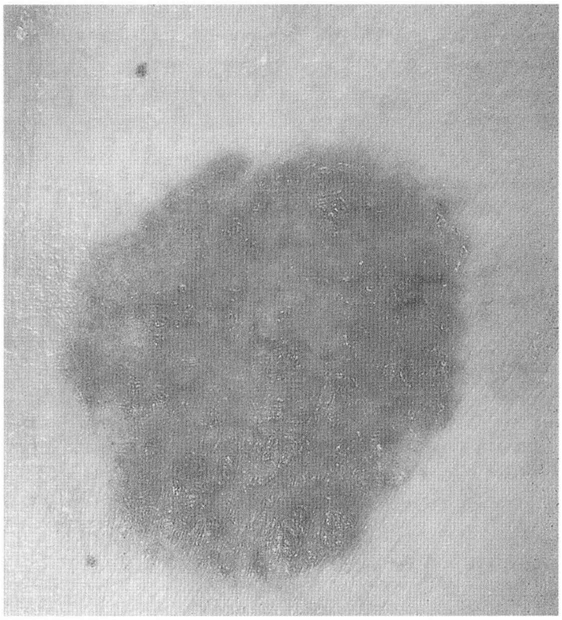

Fig. 39.18 Superficial basal cell carcinoma on back, showing spreading flat, red plaque.

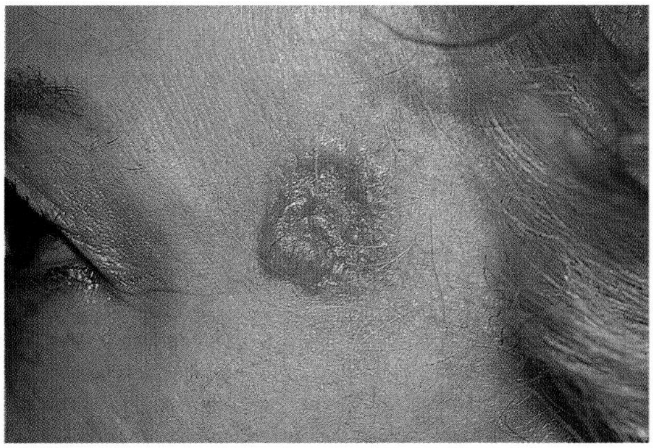

Fig. 39.16 Cystic basal cell carcinoma on temple, showing central breakdown and ulceration.

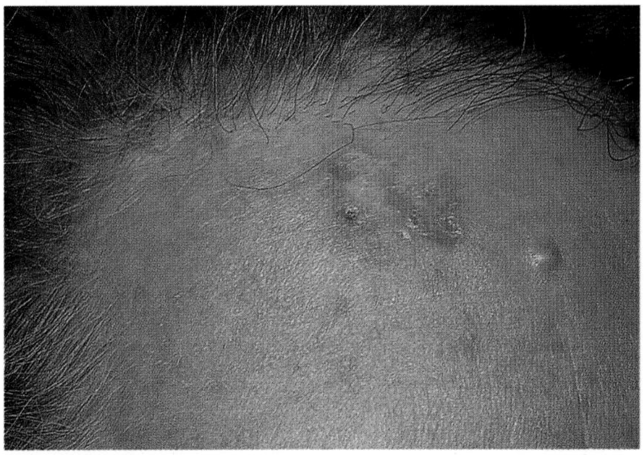

Fig. 39.19 Sclerotic basal cell carcinoma on forehead showing depressed white plaque.

diagnosis. Small lesions can be dealt with by curettage and cautery, although local excision is usually preferred to ensure there is a margin of clearance around the tumour. Larger lesions may require extensive reconstructive surgery or be treated by radiotherapy. Superficial lesions can be treated with topical immunomodulators such as imiquimod, topical chemotherapeutic agents such as 5-fluorouracil, photodynamic therapy or cryotherapy.

Squamous cell carcinoma

Aetiology and pathological features

Older age groups than those with basal cell carcinoma are usually affected and lesions are also most commonly found on skin repeatedly exposed to ultraviolet light. Industrial carcinogens are also important in their development (ionising radiation, arsenic and chronic exposure to coal tar and mineral oils). They can also arise as a consequence of chronic inflammation, e.g. within chronic leg ulcers. Smokers are prone to squamous cell carcinomas of the lip. The origin of the tumour is within the epidermis, and the cells show some degree of maturation towards keratin formation. Occurrence may be de novo or in pre-existing skin lesions such as active solar keratoses, leucoplakia or Bowen's disease. Squamous cell carcinoma invades the dermis and deeper tissues such as bone and cartilage. Metastasis to distant sites via both the lymphatics and the bloodstream takes place, although the second is usually a late and uncommon complication of the disease. Lesions of the lip (Fig. 39.20) and ear are prone to spread early.

Clinical features

The usual presentation is with either an enlarging painless ulcer with a rolled indurated margin or a papillomatous appearance with areas of ulceration, bleeding or serous exudation from secondary infection on the surface. An unexplained area of ulceration or thickening of the lip must be biopsied at once to establish a diagnosis.

Management

Although metastases from squamous cell carcinoma of the skin are rare, there is a need for adequate local treatment to eradicate the tumour. Most lesions are small, and local excision suffices. Problems can occur with larger lesions, where reconstruction by grafting or flap procedures (Ch. 38) may be necessary. Where extensive surgery seems likely, radiotherapy can be considered, although long-term sequelae include radiodermatitis, and an unattractive white, avascular scar may make this choice inappropriate for exposed areas such as the face. Tumours on the lip and ear must be treated vigorously from the outset.

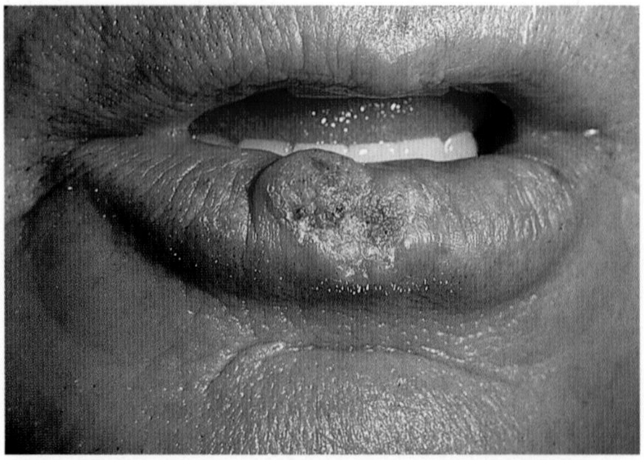

Fig. 39.20 Squamous cell carcinoma on lower lip showing infiltrated keratinised lesion with ulceration.

MALIGNANT MELANOMA (*SYN.* MELANOMA)

This is a highly malignant tumour derived from melanocytes (Box 39.3).

Epidemiology and aetiology

Malignant melanoma can arise de novo or from a pre-existing melanocytic naevus, especially a large congenital or atypical melanocytic naevus. Melanomas are rare in dark-skinned races and most common in fair-skinned people of Celtic origin. The highest incidence in the world is in northern and western Australia, perhaps because of the exposure of Northern hemisphere migrant ethnic groups to UV light for which their past genetic experience has not prepared them.

The incidence of melanoma has been rising, because of the fashion of sun exposure for its perceived enhancement of lifestyle. In young adults its incidence is increasing more rapidly than for any other cancer, and for this age group it represents the second most common cancer (when non-melanoma skin cancer is excluded). Over the last 40 years or so mortality rates for melanoma in Britain for men have continuously risen from around 1.2 to 3.1 per 100 000 of the population. In women, rates have also risen but less so: from 1.4 to 2.2 per 100 000. These figures reflect the rising melanoma incidence seen but are much less pronounced than the incidence figures would suggest, and this is thought to be due to more patients presenting at an earlier stage, with thinner melanomas.

Box 39.3 Malignant melanoma

- UK incidence 19/100 000 per year
- Incidence has increased fourfold over the last 30 years – it is the most rapidly increasing malignancy in young adults
- Risk factors include:
  - a family history of melanoma
  - previous melanoma
  - presence of a large number of moles (>100)
  - presence of atypical moles
  - significant ultraviolet exposure and burning
  - skin type I
  - affluence[a]
- Prognosis of malignant melanoma is related to tumour thickness at the time of excision (Breslow thickness)
- Adequate excision of primary tumour is most important aspect of surgical management

[a]Public awareness of significance of changes in moles is important to allow early detection and treatment.

Malignant melanoma (*syn.* melanoma)

Pathological features

All skin areas are vulnerable, although the most commonly affected sites are the lower extremities in women and the trunk) in men. Tumours may also arise in the choroid of the eye and in the oral mucosa. The classification of spread is dealt with below under 'Management'. However, the pathways are:

- direct extension into the underlying dermis and thence to the subcutaneous tissues
- satellite nodules – around the lesion and perhaps caused by tumour deposits lodging in the draining lymphatics
- to regional lymph nodes
- blood-borne to distant organs.

Clinical classification

There are five clinical types of malignant melanoma:

- lentigo maligna
- superficial spreading melanoma (Fig. 39.21)
- nodular melanoma (Fig. 39.22)
- acral lentiginous melanoma (Fig. 39.23)
- amelanotic melanoma (Fig. 39.24) – a lesion where the malignant melanocytes are not producing melanin; this is uncommon.

Clinical features that suggest a melanoma

Most patients present with a new skin lesion or a change in the character of a pre-existing naevus. The features are summarised in Box 39.4.

Other presentations

Malignant melanoma can also present with metastases – localised lymph node enlargement or distant spread such as cerebral deposits.

Prophylaxis

Public awareness campaigns are an important part of the management of the disease. Patients should be persuaded to check their skin regularly for moles that change and should

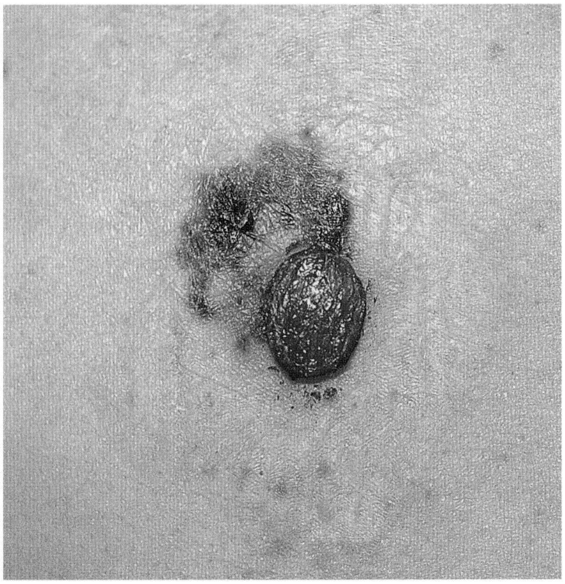

Fig. 39.21 Superficial spreading malignant melanoma showing asymmetry, irregular border and variation in colour with raised nodule developing.

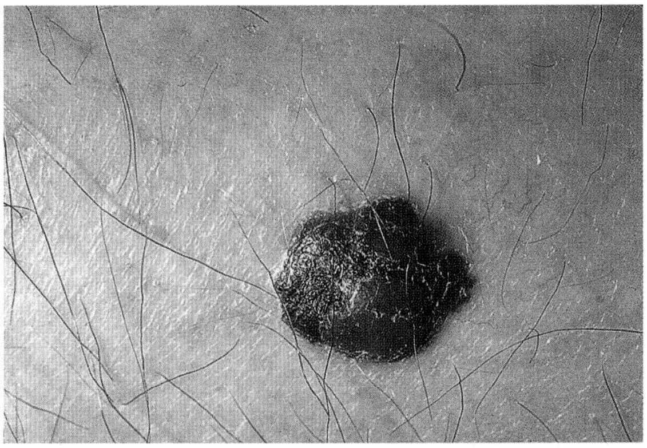

Fig. 39.22 Nodular malignant melanoma showing raised, deeply pigmented tumour.

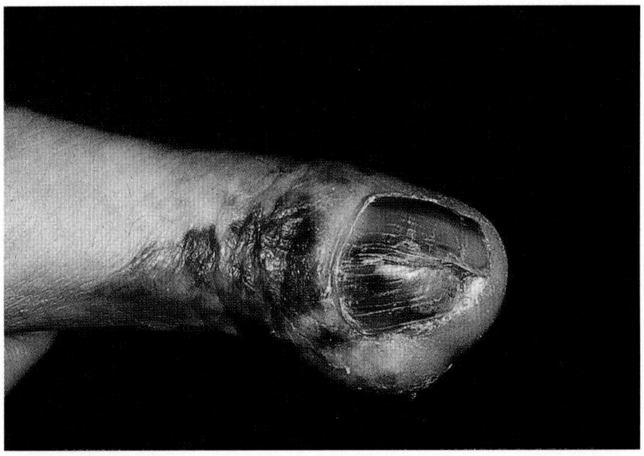

Fig. 39.23 Acral melanoma spreading under nail.

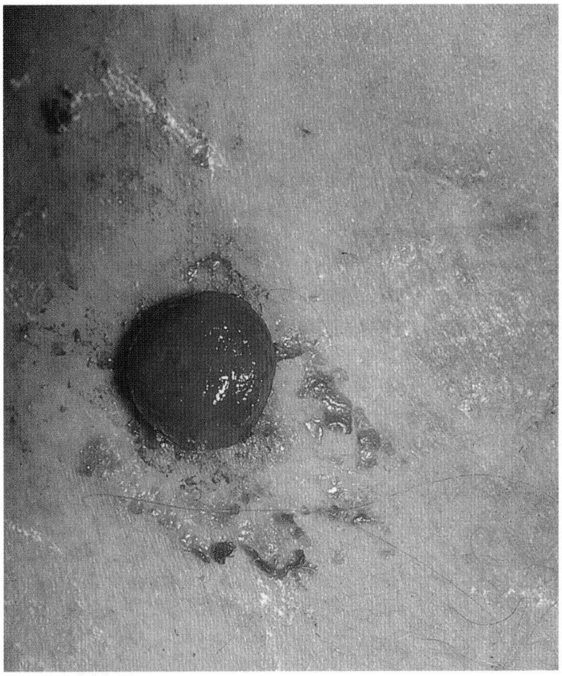

Fig. 39.24 Amelanotic malignant melanoma on neck, showing raised, non-pigmented tumour.

Box 39.4 Changes in pigmented lesions indicative of malignant melanoma

American Cancer Society checklist

A Asymmetry of lesion
B Irregular border
C Irregular colour
D Diameter >6 mm

Glasgow seven-point checklist

	Major features		Minor features
1	Change in size	4	Diameter of lesion >7 mm
2	Change in shape	5	Inflammation around lesion
3	Change in colour	6	Bleeding of lesion
		7	Itch/altered sensation

One major feature indicates removal of lesion

A feature of both checklists is the presence of a changing lesion which identifies it as being different from other pigmented lesions on the patient.

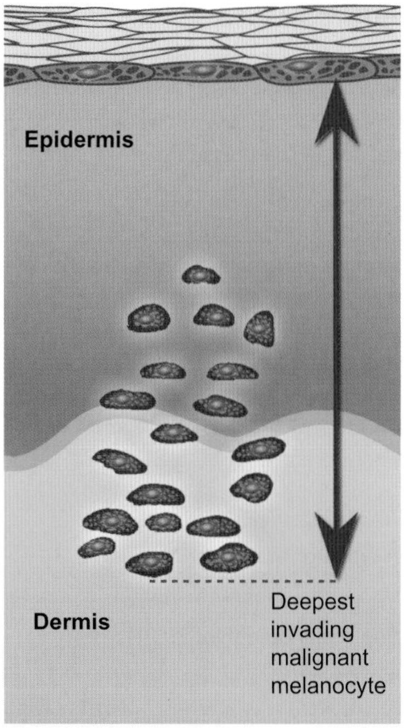

Fig. 39.25 Breslow classification. The pathologist measures the thickness of the tumour in millimetres as the distance from the granular cell layer of the epidermis to the deepest invading melanoma cell.

then come early to their doctor if there is concern. Avoidance of unnecessary exposure to the sun by the use of hats, clothing and effective barrier creams is an important message to communicate to the public and should, in the long term, reduce the incidence of both malignant melanoma and other epidermal cancers.

Patients with a greatly increased risk of melanoma are those with a giant (20 cm or more) congenital pigmented naevus and those with a strong family history of melanoma. Patients who have had a previous primary melanoma or who have >100 typical moles or >2 atypical moles have a moderately increased chance of developing melanoma. Individuals with fair skin and poor tanning ability or freckling should also be advised to take great care with sun avoidance and protection.

Management and prognosis

Suspicious lesions

Any questionable lesion on either history or physical examination must always be completely excised down to subcutis and sent for histological examination. A more difficult decision is when a patient presents with multiple naevi which are showing variation in the evenness of pigmentation within lesions and between lesions. Patients with this so-called 'atypical naevus syndrome' have a higher than normal risk of developing melanoma. They should be managed by careful photography of the lesions to act as a yardstick for future change. Any suspicious lesions should be excised and examined microscopically.

Establishing the diagnosis

Initial management is by local full thickness skin excision. It is essential to have a clear peripheral and deep margin. The specimen is then assessed histologically to confirm the diagnosis and to assess depth of invasion.

Histological classification is in two ways:

- Breslow thickness (which has become the widely adopted best criterion for assessment) – measurement of penetration of malignant cells in millimetres from the granular cell layer of the epidermis through to the deepest invading melanocyte (Fig. 39.25). Tumours less than 0.76 mm at the time of primary excision carry an excellent prognosis, but those that have penetrated further have a poorer prognosis proportionate to depth. Although the inverse relationship between thickness and survival is generally linear, there are occasional melanomas that do not follow the rule. Tumour thickness is the most important prognostic factor but others such as age, sex and size of lesion, metabolic rate, and tumour-infiltrating lymphocytes need to be considered.
- Clark's classification – grades the tumour on the depth within the dermis of malignant invasion (Table 39.1)

Table 39.1 Clark's classification of levels of malignant melanoma

Level	Definition
I	Lesion confined to epidermis (melanoma in situ)
II	Invasion into upper (papillary) dermis
III	Occupation and expansion of papillary dermis by melanoma cells
IV	Invasion into deeper (reticular) dermis
V	Invasion into subcutaneous fat

Five-year survival figures fall steadily with deeper layers.

TMN classification is also based on tumour thickness but includes other variables such as ulceration and mitotic rate (Table 39.2).

Further excision can then be planned. Until recently, very wide excision with a skin graft was the normal practice, although recent experience suggests that this does not

Table 39.2 TNM staging of melanoma

T stage	
T0	No evidence of primary tumor
Tis	Melanoma in situ (the tumor remains in the epidermis)
T1a	The melanoma is less than or equal to 1.0 mm thick, without ulceration and without any dermal mitoses (a mitotic rate of $0/mm^2$)
T1b	The melanoma is less than or equal to 1.0 mm thick. It is ulcerated and/or there is one or more dermal mitoses (a mitotic rate is equal to or greater than $1/mm^2$)
T2a	The melanoma is between 1.01 and 2.0 mm thick without ulceration
T2b	The melanoma is between 1.01 and 2.0 mm thick with ulceration
T3a	The melanoma is between 2.01 and 4.0 mm thick without ulceration
T3b	The melanoma is between 2.01 and 4.0 mm thick with ulceration
T4a	The melanoma is thicker than 4.0 mm without ulceration
T4b	The melanoma is thicker than 4.0 mm with ulceration
N stage	
N0	No spread to nearby lymph nodes
N1	Spread to 1 nearby lymph node
N2	Spread to 2 or 3 nearby lymph nodes, or spread of melanoma to nearby skin or toward a nearby lymph node area (without reaching the lymph nodes)
N3	Spread to 4 or more lymph nodes, or spread to lymph nodes that are clumped together, or spread of melanoma to nearby skin or toward a lymph node area and into the lymph node(s)
M stage	
M0	No distant metastasis
M1a	Distant metastases to skin or subcutaneous (below the skin) tissue or distant lymph nodes
M1b	Metastases to lung
M1c	Metastases to other organs

improve the prognosis. Current practice for thin tumours is to excise with a 1 cm margin for each millimetre depth of invasion. Sentinel node biopsy is an important part of staging the tumour and is used in specialised melanoma centres for clinical trial work.

It must be emphasised that malignant melanoma is a curable disease if treated early.

Thicker melanoma/metastases

The prognosis is worse in patients with tumours of greater Breslow thickness. There is currently no standard additional treatment after surgical excision for patients whose tumour was of Breslow thickness 2 mm or more, or with surface ulceration. Such patients should be considered for clinical trials or given palliative treatment as appropriate.

Extensive local tumour

Treatment is by wide excision including subcutaneous tissue down to the deep fascia. Evidence that this enhances survival is not established.

Satellite limb lesions

Clinical control can be achieved by either chemotherapy (see below) or isolated limb perfusion of chemotherapy.

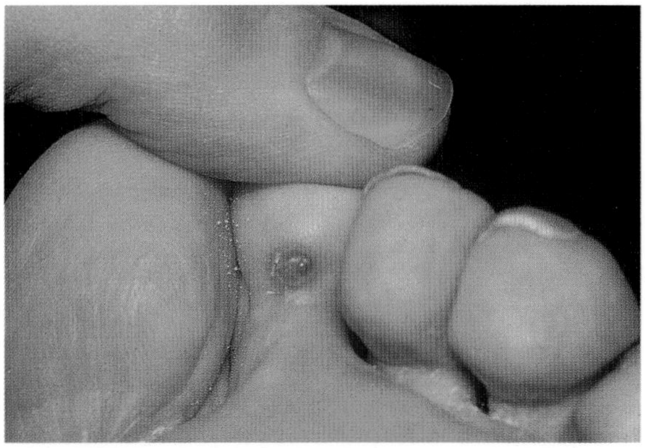

Fig. 39.26 Kaposi sarcoma showing purple nodule.

Lymph node involvement

Sentinel node biopsy, by which the local draining node is identified by injection of dye or radioisotope at the time of wide excision of the primary tumour and then removed for histological analysis, is helpful in assessing local node involvement. If positive, block dissection of the regional nodes is commonly performed. This helps prevent local recurrence and gives valuable prognostic information but its contribution to survival is unproven and it may cause lymphoedema in the limb with significant morbidity.

Chemotherapy and immunotherapy

Local excision, without lymph node dissection but combined with cytotoxic agents (such as dacarbazene), has been used to lengthen the period to tumour relapse.

Although some studies have shown that high-dose interferon can lengthen the recurrence-free period in a subset of patients with high-risk melanoma, other have not, and there is no evidence that it improves overall survival. Additionally the drug is associated with significant side-effects.

B-RAF is a protein kinase involved in cell proliferation signalling. The gene which encodes this is commonly mutated in melanoma, resulting in the kinase becoming continuously active, leading to increasing cell proliferation and the development of cancer. Inhibitors of B-RAF kinase (and similarly targeted drugs) are currently in the research phase of development and offer hope for melanoma therapy in the future.

MALIGNANT TUMOURS OF THE DERMIS

These are rare. The dermis is of mesodermal origin, and therefore malignant tumours are classified as sarcomas. They initially present as small nodules which increase in size and may become tender.

Kaposi sarcoma

This is a type of haemangiosarcoma which used to be a relatively rare disease and was found most commonly as a small purple nodule usually on a lymphoedematous leg either of an elderly person of central European Jewish extraction or in sub-Saharan Africa. More recently, however, it has become recognised as an opportunistic tumour in immunosuppressed patients, especially those with HIV infections, in association with herpes simplex virus type 8 infection. In this context there are a variety of clinical presentations. The most usual is that of a small purple nodule (Fig. 39.26), but a dusky purple plaque or with mucosal involvement is not uncommon. The treatment is usually surgical excision for small discrete lesions and radiotherapy for larger ones.

OTHER MALIGNANCIES OF THE SKIN

Lymphoma

Most cutaneous lymphomas are T cell in origin and as they present with diffuse scaly plaques which may look like a cutaneous fungal infection (hence they are also known as mycosis fungoides) they rarely present to surgeons. B-cell lymphomas, however, may present with a solitary nodule or cluster of nodules, and the diagnosis is made on biopsy.

Secondary carcinoma

The skin may be the site of distant spread of internal carcinoma. Sometimes solitary nodules arise in the skin that are the result of blood-borne metastases or direct involvement through the lymphatics. Biopsy of the lesion usually provides a clue to the site of the primary disorder. Solitary nodules may occur in cancers that are known to spread with single metastases such as thyroid and renal carcinoma.

Cutaneous signs of internal malignancy

The skin is well recognised as a marker for non-metastatic signs of internal malignancy:

- pruritus may be a presenting feature of myeloproliferative malignancies, particularly in young people – polycythaemia vera, lymphoma
- deep jaundice from obstruction of the bile duct – carcinoma of the head of the pancreas
- increased pigmentation – ACTH secretion in carcinoma of the bronchus
- finger clubbing – colonic/bronchial carcinoma
- unusual annular erythemas such as erythema gyratum repens – carcinoma of the bronchus
- tylosis (diffuse keratinous thickening) with palmar plantar hyperkeratosis – carcinoma of the oesophagus
- acanthosis nigricans (a velvety papillomatous appearance in the intertriginous areas of the axillae and groin and around the neck) – upper gastrointestinal tumours
- acquired ichthyosis – any internal malignancy.

FURTHER READING

Bolognia JL, Jorizzo JL, Rapini RP 2007 Dermatology, 2nd edn. Mosby Elsevier, St Louis

Burns T, Breathnach S, Cox N, Griffiths CEM (eds) 2010 Rook's textbook of dermatology, 8th edn. Wiley-Blackwell, Oxford

Buxton PK, Morris-Jones R 2009 ABC of dermatology (ABC series), 5th edn. BMJ Books, London

Calonje JE, Brenn T, Lazar AJ, McKee PH 2011 Pathology of the skin: with clinical correlations, 4th edn. Mosby Elsevier, Philadelphia

Du Vivier A 2002 Atlas of clinical dermatology, 3rd edn. Churchill Livingstone, Edinburgh

Wolff K, Johnson RA 2009 Fitzpatrick's color atlas and synopsis of clinical dermatology, 6th edn. McGraw-Hill Medical, New York

40 Surgery in the developing world

INTRODUCTION

Whilst there are some excellent surgical centres, the provision of healthcare in many developing countries is often rudimentary, with available expenditure greatly skewed towards the largest conurbations. For many isolated rural communities, secondary care is frequently non-existent (Box 40.1). While preventative medicine and primary care (e.g. mass immunisation programmes) are often supported by international organisations, secondary care (hospital-based) receives less attention. Millions of people do not have access to even basic surgical care.

Against this backdrop, the impact of appropriately delivered primary surgery can be huge. For example, the impact of simple repair of an obstructed inguinal hernia, or the elective repair of a vesicovaginal fistula, can far exceed the value for money in quality life years delivered (including return to communal life and work) that is commonly assumed to accompany primary medical care.

However, investment into the provision of surgical care in resource-poor nations lags unacceptably behind other domains of healthcare – notable the 'big three' well-resourced conditions of TB, HIV and malaria. There are signs that this discrepancy is now being recognised, but data describing the prevalence of surgically remediable disease and dysfunction is scarce, and good research urgently required.

Perspective for surgical visitors from developed countries

A considerable challenge for the surgical visitor is the relevance of experience gained in highly technical surgical settings to resource-poor environments. Twenty-first-century developed surgery is highly technical and managed within narrow sub-specialties. In contrast, surgery in poor rural communities is usually delivered by the highly diverse skills of a generalist working with little technical support. Surgeons are often called upon to undertake emergency obstetric and elective gynaecological operations in addition to general surgical procedures. In isolated areas they need experience in urology, orthopaedics, paediatric surgery, plastic procedures, neurosurgery and thoracic surgery.

Many experienced surgical teams working in developing countries attest to the overwhelming importance of training and capacity-building in developing surgical resources for sustainable development in the longer term. Thus the ideal model for support from wealthier groups is to develop partnerships built on mutual respect, two-way learning from poor to rich and vice versa, with capacity-building a prime goal. The most valuable partnerships between developed and developing countries are multiprofessional. Long-term relationships flourish in contrast to short, one-off, visits, and longer-term exchanges of professionals are extremely beneficial. When such support does extend to short-term visits, such visitors must be prepared to empathise with local challenges faced by national colleagues working in developing countries, respect cultural differences, make an effort with the language and readily accept that they will probably receive more than they can give both professionally and personally.

Not surprisingly, therefore, many surgeons from developed economies will attest to the impact of a surgical elective – undertaken whilst a medical student – on their career choice. Further into their career, surgeons may have opportunities to return to a developing country for varied periods of time. In the past the focus of these trips has been surgical service provision. In recent years, the focus of partnerships has shifted towards teaching and training, and the model of all forms of partnership between surgeons, surgical departments and institutions is now encouraged.

It is beyond the remit of this chapter to discuss the specific management of all diseases that present to the surgeon. In fact, many of the diseases encountered are found in developed countries and have been discussed in previous chapters. The focus of this chapter will be on:

- understanding the multifactorial reasons for late and advanced surgical presentations
- the difference in management of surgical disease
- surgical presentations rarely seen in developed countries.

GENERAL CHALLENGES OF THE ENVIRONMENT

Although there are many centres of excellence providing surgical care in the poorer developing nations, the overall provision of surgical care is low. This is a direct consequence of the many challenges faced by the population and healthcare workers, as set out in Box 40.2. At first glance these may not appear to be surgically relevant, but in fact they have a profound impact on surgical delivery.

Box 40.1 Statistics on surgery in the developing countries

- Only 10% of all major surgery required is actually performed
- Only 2% of all minor surgery required is actually performed
- 10% of surgery requires specialist surgical training
- 40% of surgery requires postgraduate surgical training
- 50% of surgery requires minimal training

Poverty and low literacy rates

Two indicators for health include the life expectancy at birth and the infant mortality rate (IMR). These indicators are influenced by the gross domestic product (GDP) and the percentage of GDP spent on health. Figure 40.1 shows the correlation between GDP per capita and infant mortality rates.

In developing countries the percentage of GDP spent on education mirrors that spent on health, and adult literacy rates are consequently low. This impacts on public health awareness and health itself.

Lack of clean water and basic sanitation

This relates directly to poverty but deserves a separate mention, as its impact on health is so profound. Over two-thirds of the population in the poorest countries are still without access to clean drinking water. Approximately 40% of the world's population lack even basic sanitation. The

Box 40.2 Challenges to patients and healthcare workers in developing countries

- Poverty and low literacy rates
- Lack of clean water and basic sanitation
- Poor infrastructure, civil unrest, military conflict, distance from health centres and lack of patient transport
- Cultural practices and beliefs
- Poor health facilities and limited trained human resources
- Infectious diseases, malnutrition and the immunocompromised patient
- Problems in perioperative management

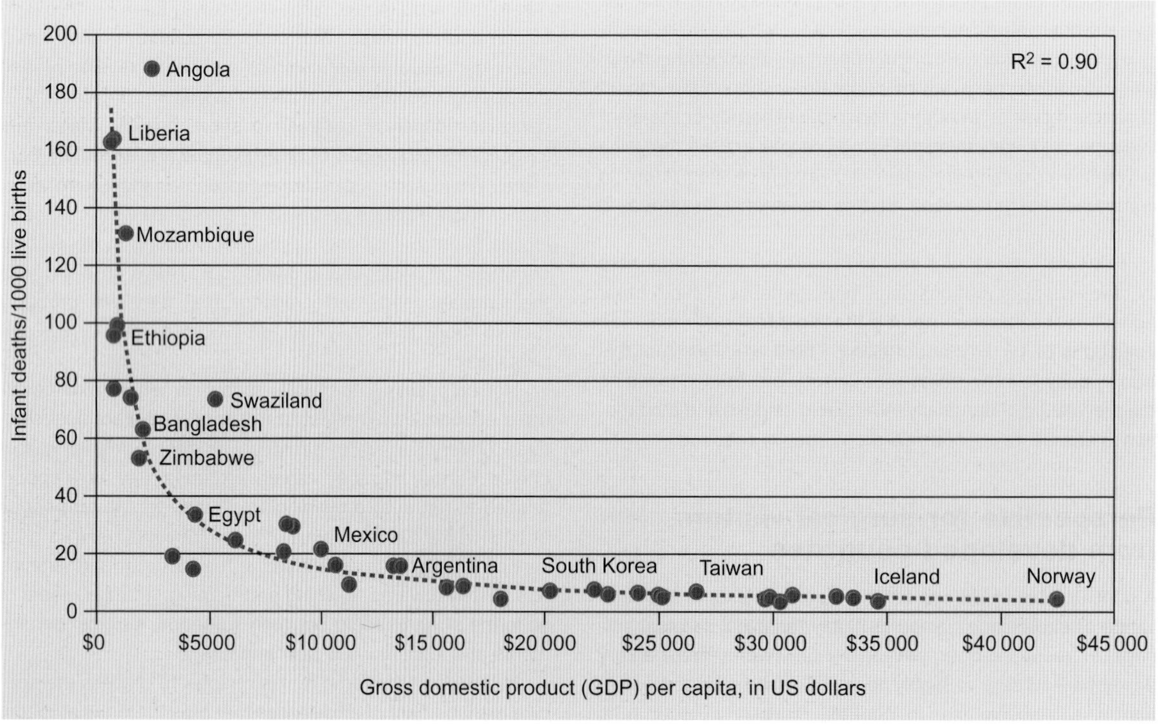

Fig. 40.1 Infant mortality and GDP per capita (CIA Worldfactbook 2006).

combination of poor hygiene, contaminated water and poor sanitation results in a heavy burden of infectious disease. The impact of this for surgeons will be discussed below. Water-borne diseases, spread by the faeco-oral route, are responsible for patients occupying half of the world's hospital beds. Clean running water is frequently sporadic even within hospitals, adding further to the difficulties of providing a surgical service.

Poor infrastructure, civil unrest, military conflict, distance from health centres and lack of patient transport

Public health in any nation is a function not only of the system of delivery of basic healthcare services but also of the general state of the nation's infrastructure. The developing world continues to struggle with inadequate delivery systems and poor infrastructure.

Subsistence farmers who make up the rural poor may have some access to the limited service of a local health centre but this limited access might be completely confounded by inability to get transport to urban hospitals. Travel to health facilities incurs time away from their land (and therefore food supply as well as livelihood), and the financial obstacle may be insurmountable to a family. Travel by foot, bicycle, cart, bus or car may be impossible during rainy seasons when roads are impassable. Civil unrest and military conflict add to these difficulties by disrupting health service provision, destroying infrastructure and adding gross trauma to the burden of disease. Patients able to travel are frequently accompanied by relatives who need to remain with the patient to provide supportive care including food for themselves and the patient (Fig. 40.2).

Inadequate health facilities and limited trained human resources

Not only are there limited numbers of health facilities in poor nations but also they may be poorly distributed within the country. In Nigeria, three-quarters of health facilities are in urban areas, where only 30% of the population live. Where hospitals do exist, standards may be poor. A survey undertaken by the World Bank revealed that of 15 publicly operated hospitals in Kenya, 40% of the buildings were in 'poor and unsatisfactory condition'. Without reliable mains electricity, hospitals require additional expensive equipment in order to function effectively (e.g. kerosene or solar fridges for maintaining the cold chain for vaccines). This is often unavailable. Phone and internet services may be non-existent or unreliable, reducing access to current literature and recent advances, second opinions/telemedical support and ongoing medical education – all of which improve isolated services.

Surgeons frequently cope with only basic equipment (Fig. 40.3). Resources such as infusion lines, intravenous fluids, drugs and antibiotics are scarce. Surgical instruments are often old or of poor quality, demanding greater expertise from the isolated surgeon. Improvisation of instrumentation and dressings, together with and reuse of all materials, is an invaluable asset. Suture material is expensive and supplies may be erratic. As a result surgeons may have to compromise either with the type of needle or suture material they are using or by modifying their techniques. For instance, reusable needles may be preferred and knots tied with instruments rather than hands to save suture material.

In the developed world, aspects of care managed by a clinical nurse specialist (CNS) are increasing to include many roles traditionally carried out by doctors (including surgical assistants). In many countries, nurses have carried out such extended surgical roles for many years. The ratio of medical staff to the general population is much lower than in developed nations; however, the spectrum of health workers carrying out surgical procedures is broader. Those involved in the care of surgical patients include:

- traditional healers
- health officers in rural health clinics
- nurses and doctors in hospitals (district, regional and specialist)
- visiting teams (e.g. Flying Eye Doctor).

Provision of a surgical service is by no means limited to skills delivered by trained clinical staff. Limited human resources affect non-medical essential staff as well (e.g. store keeping, maintenance and accountancy). Inadequate staffing in these areas has a considerable impact on the general running of a hospital and especially affects the provision of specialist services. By way of example, a physician with no pharmacy might still run an out-patient clinic and give the patient a

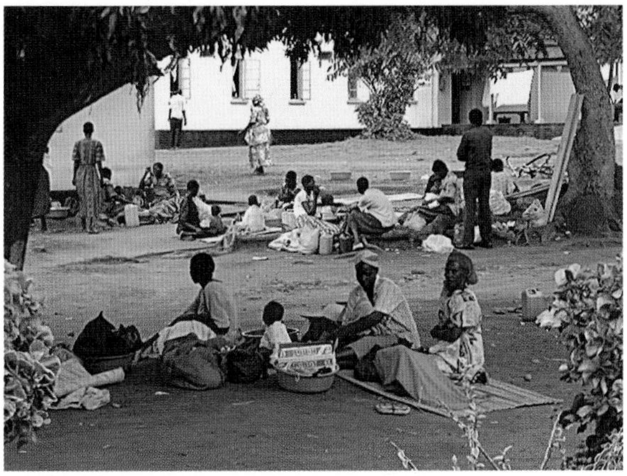

Fig. 40.2 Patients, relatives and essentials!

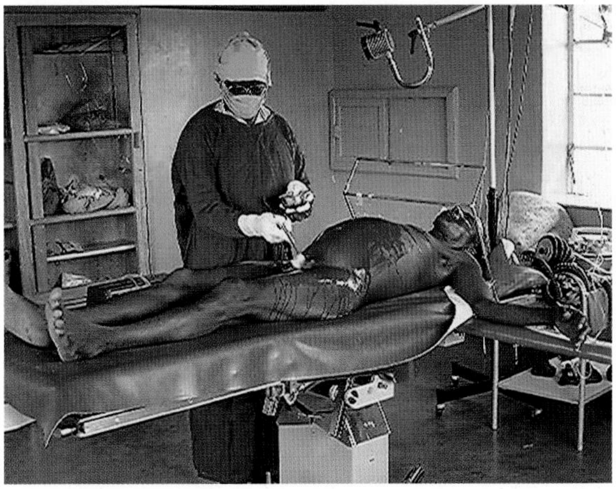

Fig. 40.3 A theatre in East Africa.

script to buy medicine elsewhere, but a surgeon can do little without at least basic facilities.

Cultural practices and beliefs

All societies have their fair share of diverse cultural, religious and personal beliefs, and some established attitudes can prevent individuals seeking medical intervention. These can result in increased morbidity and mortality and, not infreqently, the hospital is the last place for patients to seek help. Advice might be sought from traditional healers, which often leads to late presentation of established pathology. Surgeons are thus more likely to encounter patients *in extremis* with advanced disease. Figure 40.4 shows a patient who presented with surgical disease but had previously been 'branded' on the abdominal wall in order to exorcise the 'evil spirits'. In sub-Saharan Africa female genital mutilation is still widely practised despite a growing effort to stop the practice. It is a cause of increased risk of morbidity during childbirth and also increases the risk of a stillbirth up to fourfold. Traditional herbal medicines are known to mimic surgical disease, for example by inducing an ileus complicating post-operative recovery.

Infectious disease, malnutrition and the immunocompromised patient

Of those patients who do present to the surgical team, many are malnourished and as a result have a degree of immunocompromise. Such a condition may also result from parasitic infestation and infectious disease such as HIV, tuberculosis and malaria. Specific surgical presentations relating to infections will be covered later.

HIV. The epidemic of HIV in developing countries is taking its toll on life and resources. In the last 10 years the estimated number of people living with HIV/AIDS has almost tripled, with Africa being the hardest hit region. About 28 million people are thought to be infected in sub-Saharan Africa alone, and 18 million deaths occur in the same region each year. The second most affected area is South and South-East Asia. Pathology resulting from HIV infection is common. Figure 40.5 illustrates a patient with Kaposi sarcoma, a manifestation of advanced HIV. Challenges for the surgical team include:

- immunocompromised patients
- surgical presentations related to HIV
- risks to staff from needlestick injury and mucous membrane contact
- lack of antiretroviral prophylaxis after exposure.

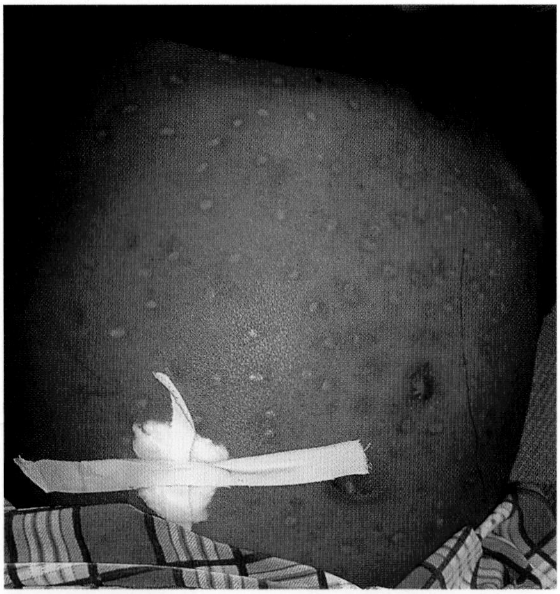

Fig. 40.4 Patient whose abdominal wall has been branded to exorcise 'evil spirits'.

Malaria kills 3000 children in Africa a day, as well as draining billions of dollars from the continent's economy each year from lost work time and burden of care. Increasing drug resistance is a serious problem. Chronic malaria is a cause of massive splenomegaly that is associated with its own complications such as traumatic rupture and sepsis.

Tuberculosis remains a major global cause of death due to an infectious agent. Nearly one-third of the world population is infected with tuberculosis. Resurgence of the disease has occurred because of the increasing prevalence of immunocompromised patients, mainly with HIV. Drug-resistant strains have contributed to the problem.

Malnutrition can result from lack of calorific intake, protein, vitamins and/or trace elements. All these in the context of surgery predispose to higher risk of infection, slower healing, wound breakdown and wound dehiscence. Surgical patients who are malnourished need supplemental nutrition to aid healing. Perioperative nutrition (enteral and parenteral) in developed countries is often managed by specialist teams working in conjunction with the surgical team. Sustaining an adequate nutritional status can be a difficult (if not an impossible) task without the skill, knowledge and technological support usually associated with such team-based care.

Problems within perioperative management

Regional or local anaesthesia is often preferred to general anaesthesia for safely and management logistic reasons. The only drugs available for such techniques are usually lidocaine and bupivacaine. Oxygen supplies are often poor and piped oxygen scarce, making postoperative ventilation

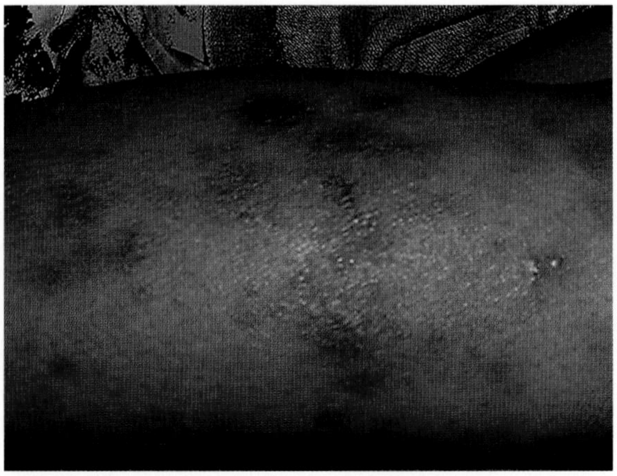

Fig. 40.5 Kaposi sarcoma in a surgical patient.

impossible. Opiates may be in scarce supply, and perioperative analgesia inadequate. Ketamine anaesthesia has been highly refined within poor settings, and good courses now exist to train in appropriate and relevant anaesthetic techniques (www.nda.ox.ac.uk/announcements/anaesthesia-in-developing-countries). However, much investment is required for safer anaesthesia to become the norm in developing countries (Walker & Wilson, 2008). The 'Lifebox' safer surgery initiative aims, amongst a package of care for surgery, to ensure that pulse oximetry is available during every general anaesthetic. It is a new initiative that all surgeons in developing nations should be aware of (www.lifebox.org).

Caring for critically ill surgical patients is a daunting task in the absence of specialised high-dependency and intensive-care units. Basic pathology tests measuring postoperative electrolytes may not be available, necessitating a different approach to patient care. Blood products are scarce, and their safety is often questioned. Other services including histology may be unavailable, with reliance on one or other of the extraordinarily valuable postal pathology services. The patient in Figure 40.6a underwent excision of a submandibular tumour (Fig. 40.6b), but unfortunately no histological diagnosis was possible. Figure 40.7 illustrates the lack of oncological and palliative care for a woman with local recurrence of breast carcinoma following a previous mastectomy. Stoma therapy in rural areas may not be possible, thus restricting surgical options.

Late presentation and advanced pathology

As a result of these many challenges patients present in the elective and emergency setting with late and advanced pathology (Fig 40.8). The reasons for this are multifactorial and illustrated in Box 40.3.

Decision-making and advanced pathology

Decision-making and good judgement are essential capabilities of surgeons worldwide. In developing countries, there may be added challenges often involving ethical dilemmas of when and when not to intervene because absent or inadequate resources might make the attendant risks of surgery greater. Managing advanced pathology in such areas with limited resources presents difficult questions. Elective surgery may be appropriately restricted in favour of life- or limb-saving surgery. Often a 'wait-and-watch' or conservative method of treatment can be preferable when the pathology is primarily of cosmetic significance only. It is imperative for surgeons to recognise that not all instances of grossly enlarged pathology require surgical resection. Very substantial salivary gland lumps are a classic example of this, and the morbidity attendant on unnecessary resection is the responsibility of the surgeon, who may wield considerable influence over the informed consent of a poorly educated patient. Rationalisation is important when deciding which pathology deserves scarce operative resources. A good example might be when dealing with a patient presenting with a goitre. A smaller goitre may, initially, appear innocent compared with an obvious larger thyroid mass. However, the smaller one may extend retrosternally, with risk of the tracheal or oesophageal compression. This is illustrated in Figure 40.9, where only one patient was symptomatic.

a
b
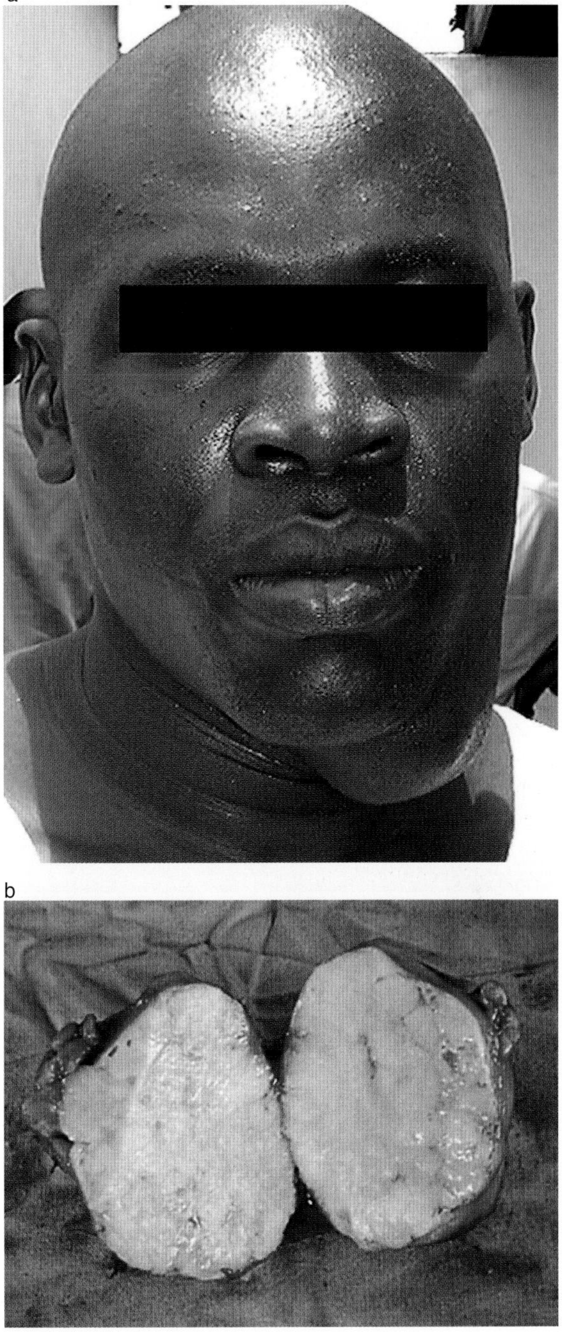

Fig. 40.6 (a) Submandibular tumour. (b) Resected specimen of the tumour.

The social pressure to operate on gross paediatric pathology such as a large AV malformation (Fig. 40.10) may be hard to resist. Indeed, operative intervention may be appropriate after full consent, provided the attendant risks of surgery are fully acknowledged and understood by both patient and surgeon. However, such lesions are notoriously prone to unexpected clinical presentation, and wise judgement might advocate referral to whatever regional centre is available (despite what might be great waits or cost).

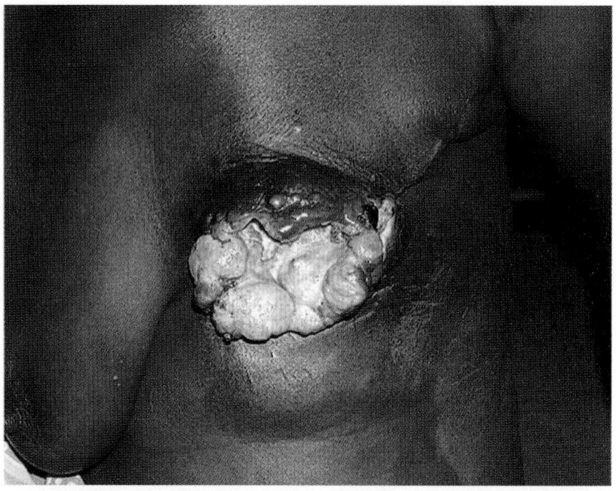

Fig. 40.7 Recurrent breast carcinoma.

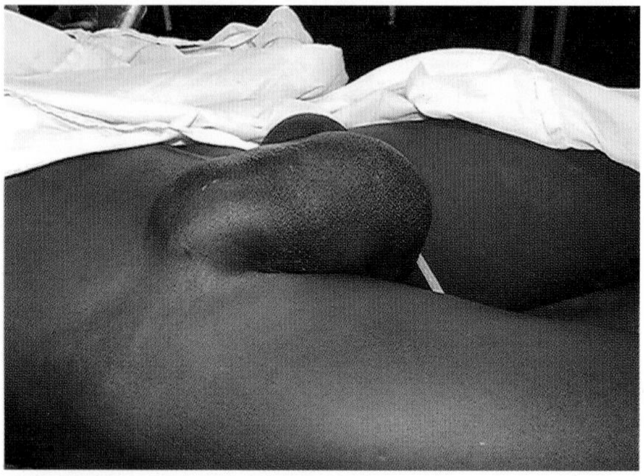

Fig. 40.8 Obstructed inguinal hernia.

Box 40.3 Emergency presentation of an obstructed inguinal hernia

- Inguinal hernia develops
- Absence of surgical care at the primary level, economic factors and social taboos lead to pathology being ignored
- Obstruction and surgical emergency (Fig. 40.8)
- Prolonged travel to surgical care leads to development of haemodynamic compromise, strangulation and sepsis
- Lack of trained surgical staff, technical equipment and nursing ability to look after critically ill surgical patient
- Multi-organ failure associated with preventable morbidity and mortality

Congenital and acquired orthopaedic pathology frequently present late, and patients may have significant disability. The fundamental question for the general surgeon outside a specialist centre to address is whether the functional outcome for the patient can and should be improved. This is sometimes much more important than cosmesis, which (as in the case of facial clefting) is likely to be far better addressed in the long term by waiting for specialist provision by referral or visiting team. Figure 40.11 illustrates a patient with chronic dislocation of the right hip and significant disability. Local resources were good, and operative intervention was undertaken. Conversely, Figure 40.12 illustrates a child with gross talipes equinovarus but remarkably good function despite appearance. Conservative management was followed. The management of congenital talipes has, in

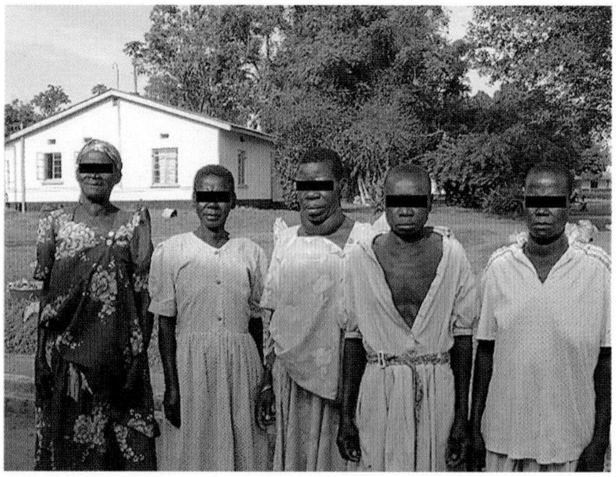

Fig. 40.9 Only one (second from right) among these patients with goitres was symptomatic.

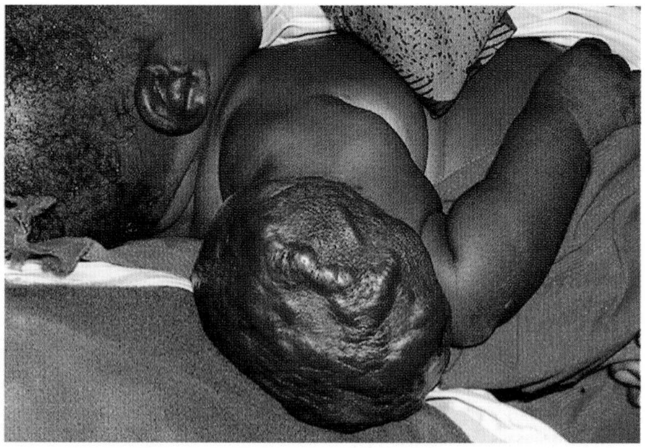

Fig. 40.10 Large arteriovenous malformation.

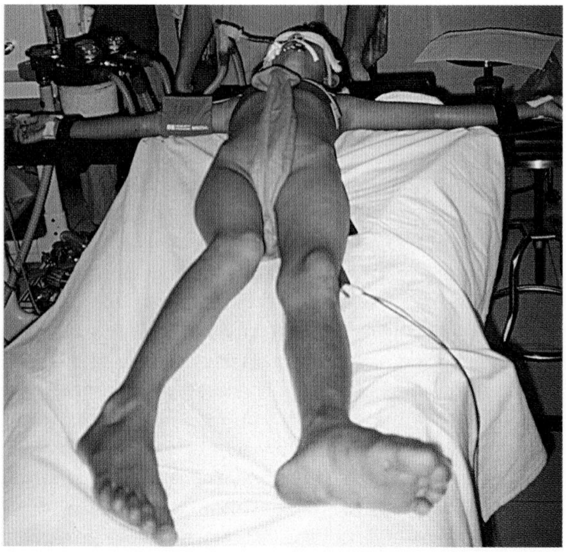

Fig. 40.11 Chronic dislocated right hip. (By courtesy of Mr D Rajan, King's College Hospital, London.)

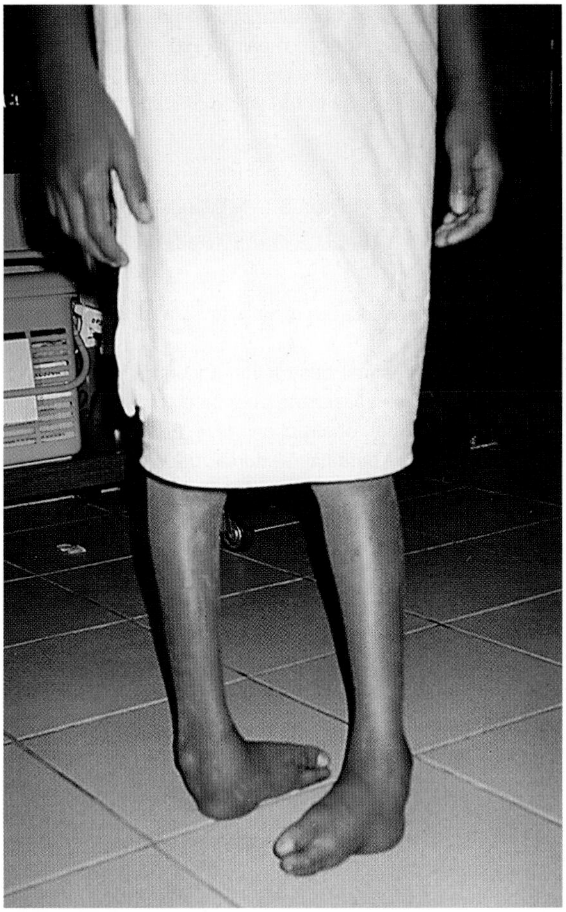

Fig. 40.12 Gross talipes equinovarus. (By courtesy of Mr D Rajan, King's College Hospital, London.)

the great majority of cases, been radically transformed in recent years by the introduction of the Ponsetti method of conservative splinting and manipulation.

Surgery of the poor

The example of obstetric fistulae

There is probably no surgical pathology more illustrative of the plight of the isolated rural poor than the development of obstetric fistula from vagina to bladder and bowel in young women. Patients are often in their early teens, with cephalopelvic disproportion, and may have suffered an obstructed labour lasting many days, far from any medical help. Many women die in childbirth under these circumstances. If the mother survives and passes a macerated fetus, she may be left with a vesicovaginal fistula (VVF) and sometimes a rectovaginal fistula (RVF).

Prolonged compression of the anterior vaginal wall, base of the bladder and urethra between the fetal head and the posterior surface of the pubis results in pressure necrosis and the development of a VVF. A similar process compressing the posterior vaginal wall and rectum between the fetal head and sacral promontory results in further necrosis and the development of an RVF. These women suffer constant incontinence of urine and/or faeces, leaving them wet, smelly, leading to social and psychological isolation (Fig. 40.13a). The complexity of the fistula repair varies

a

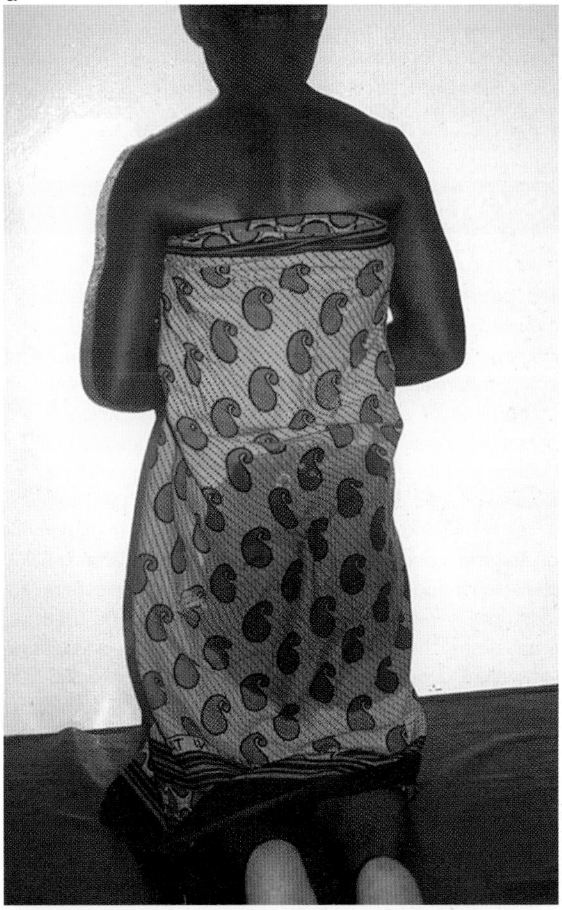

b

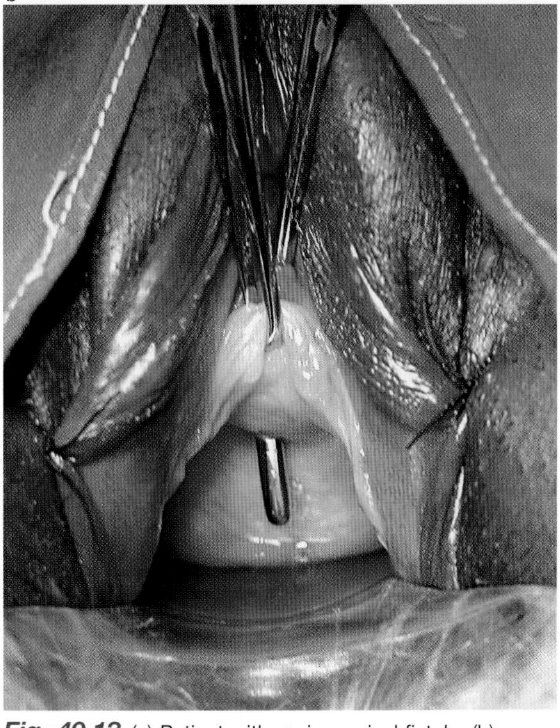

Fig. 40.13 (a) Patient with vesicovaginal fistula. (b) Simple vesicovaginal fistula. (By courtesy of Mr B Hancock, Manchester.)

enormously. A simple mid-vaginal VVF (Fig. 40.13) can be simply repaired in two layers (occasionally interposing a transposed local fat flap) through the vagina. Other cases associated with far more extensive injuries and resultant scarring require complex dissection and reconstruction. The overall success rate for repair in experienced hands is about 90%, and successful closure is one of the most life-transforming procedures in the whole of surgery.

SYSTEMS REVIEW

The pattern of surgical disease presentation varies enormously between the developed and less developed world. For example, appendicitis – although a common cause of acute abdominal pain in the West – is a rarer differential in many parts of sub-Saharan Africa. Inconsistencies in the prevalence of surgical diseases also occur between neighbouring countries. Hence, familiarity with the distribution of disease presentation to the local area is important.

As mentioned previously, the diagnosis and management of surgical conditions presents the surgeon with specific challenges. Indeed, the lack of hospital and community resources available to diagnose and manage patients emphasises the importance of clinical skills and sound judgement. Described below are some of the conditions commonly encountered by surgeons practising in developing countries. The emphasis throughout this chapter is on the challenges that these pathologies present to the surgeon and on aspects of management that differ from those delivered in wealthier healthcare systems.

GENERAL SURGERY

THE ACUTE ABDOMEN

The most common procedure for the general surgeon is the drainage of abscesses. These are a consequence of inadequate hygiene, immunosuppression and malnutrition. Infections are frequently neglected, and abscesses of significant size and chronicity consequently have to be dealt with. In rural areas elective abdominal surgery is rarely performed; however, patients frequently present with acute abdominal pain. The initial management of patients with acute abdominal pain commences with resuscitation. It comprises: intravenous rehydration, correction of metabolic disorder, nasogastric aspiration, antibiotic treatment for sepsis and provision of analgesia. In contrast to the Western world, however, accurate preoperative diagnosis is often impossible in a developing country.

In the absence of a definitive diagnosis, subsequent clinical management requires a pragmatic approach. In the first instance the surgeon must decide whether operative intervention is required. The general indications for operative intervention include conditions where a diagnosis has been made, e.g. perforated peptic ulcer that requires an operation. In addition, laparotomy is indicated in some circumstances when a diagnosis has not been secured and clinical improvement has not occurred despite resuscitation. In contrast, operations should be avoided for diagnosed abdominal conditions where surgery is not indicated and also for undiagnosed abdominal pain where the patient is improving.

In Uganda intestinal obstruction accounts for over 90% of all presentations with acute abdominal pain. The general causes of intestinal obstruction have been described in Chapter 24. The cardinal features of vomiting, colicky abdominal pain, distension and constipation should alert the surgeon to the likely diagnosis of obstruction. The generic diagnosis of obstruction, and the differentiation between small- and large-bowel obstruction, can generally be made with ease. The specific cause of obstruction can usually be identified from the history (e.g. adhesions if previous laparotomy). In other instances, a physical sign denotes the cause (e.g. an incarcerated hernia). The surgeon must be alert to physical signs that may represent pathology endemic to the area but not frequently seen in developed countries. For instance, in the obstructed patient, a mass in the right iliac fossa might represent ileocaecal tuberculosis rather than an appendix mass, the probable diagnosis in a Western country.

In cases of simple obstruction, fluid and electrolyte resuscitation takes precedence over an operation. When closed-loop or strangulated obstruction has occurred, aggressive rehydration is required as well as prompt operative intervention. Some causes of simple obstruction that resolve spontaneously on conservative treatment include:

- post-surgical adhesions
- a localised inflammatory mass (e.g. appendix mass or pyosalpinx)
- a mass due to *Ascaris* worms.

Non-operative management of obstruction should never be maintained if strangulation supervenes.

SPECIFIC CAUSES OF INTESTINAL OBSTRUCTION COMMONLY SEEN IN DEVELOPING COUNTRIES

Sigmoid volvulus

Aetiology and epidemiology

The high-fibre diet consumed in underdeveloped countries produces a large residue in the colon. This results in colonic distension and also impacts on motility, facilitating volvulus formation. In contrast, this condition is relatively uncommon in the West, where diseases of a low-fibre diet, such as diverticular disease, predominate. In parts of East Africa, sigmoid volvulus commonly occurs in adult males.

Clinical features

The condition may present acutely, but in many instances a history of subacute episodes can be elicited.

The clinical features of large-bowel volvulus generally commence with constipation (for flatus), followed by increasing abdominal distension. The abdomen can distend to huge proportions, but often little pain is experienced and tenderness is minimal. This disparity between the patients' apparent comfort and the abdominal signs is often striking. When available, abdominal radiography will classically display the 'coffee-bean' appearance of a sigmoid volvulus.

Management

Management of sigmoid volvulus depends largely on the type of volvulus that presents. In most instances, the volvulus is subacute and there is no impairment of intestinal blood supply. The aim should be to treat this group non-operatively if possible. In acute cases, however, the mesenteric blood supply to the large bowel is impaired and septic shock can occur rapidly. These cases will require aggressive resuscitation as well as prompt intervention. In the first instance, decompression can be attempted with a sigmoidoscope and flatus tube. This technique is successful in 75% of cases. When successful, a flatus tube can be placed into the sigmoid colon to aid decompression and prevent recurrence. When successful decompression has been achieved an elective sigmoid colectomy should be considered as the incidence of recurrence is high. If, however, in the acute setting, the sigmoid decompression fails or there are signs of strangulation and gangrene, a laparotomy will be required. At operation, if the affected large bowel is viable, as in Figure 40.14, it requires untwisting with insertion of a rectal tube and/or suturing the colon to the abdominal wall to prevent further attacks. If the volvulus has strangulated, however, resection will be required. The surgical options depend largely on the condition of the patient and the technical ability of the surgeon. Much consideration is required prior to creating a stoma. Poverty and lack of specialist nursing staff makes successful stoma management unlikely. In this instance, however, when a sigmoid colon has required acute resection either a defunctioning transverse loop, end (Hartmann's) or double-barrelled colostomy will be required.

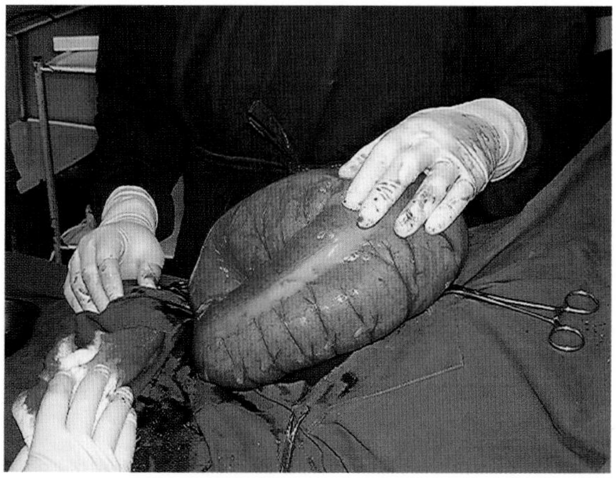

Fig. 40.14 Sigmoid volvulus.

Caecal volvulus

Caecal volvulus is rare in developed countries. In some instances the caecum, ascending colon and ileum are all free to rotate and undergo volvulus. The clinical presentation of this condition is much the same as that of an acute sigmoid volvulus. Plain abdominal radiographs may demonstrate a large gas shadow placed centrally with a suspicious absence of gas in the right lower quadrant.

Management

Caecal volvulus in the absence of access to colonoscopy will almost always require a laparotomy. If the caecal volvulus can be untwisted and appears viable at operation a caecopexy procedure may be performed to anchor the caecum to the anterior abdominal wall. Alternatively a caecostomy with a Foley catheter passed through the anterior abdominal wall is fashioned. If, however, the bowel is not viable a right hemicolectomy will be required.

Small-bowel volvulus

Aetiology

Volvulus of the small gut is encountered rarely in the developed world. When it does occur it is usually seen in infants as a result of intestinal malrotation or another congenital anomaly. In adults this condition is extremely rare and usually results from a 'twist' that has occurred around a fixed post-surgical adhesion. In contrast, however, small-bowel volvulus is seen frequently in developing countries in all age groups. The aetiology commonly arises from a congenital band which tethers the bowel from the posterior abdominal wall to a point a few centimetres proximal to the ileocaecal valve. In other cases post-surgical adhesions are to blame.

Clinical features and management

The characteristic clinical features of small-bowel volvulus include the sudden onset of colicky abdominal pain, distension and vomiting. The impact of rapid cessation of blood flow to the bowel is profound. Over a short period of time haemodynamic instability supervenes secondary to hypovolaemia and sepsis. For this reason these patients require aggressive resuscitation with intravenous fluid and antibiotics. In theory, treatment is easy if the condition is detected early. In these cases 'untwisting' of the affected gut can be performed at laparotomy if irreversible bowel wall strangulation has not already occurred. In many cases small-bowel resection will be necessary, however. At the time of surgery, care must be taken not to rupture the affected bowel loop. Under these circumstances overall mortality rises to approximately 30%.

Adhesion obstruction

Postoperative adhesions can cause intestinal obstruction many years following previous abdominal surgery. Management of obstruction that occurs secondary to adhesions virtually always affects the small bowel. Treatment for this form of obstruction is usually non-operative. Replacement of fluid and electrolyte losses as well as nasogastric decompression (drip and suck) forms the basis of management. The indications to discontinue non-operative treatment include signs of peritonism or sepsis. Under these circumstances the surgeon must suspect that bowel infarction has supervened.

Intussusception

Epidemiology and aetiology

Intussusception is rarely seen in adults in the developed world. In the developing world, however, it is encountered more frequently, although the condition still predominates in infants and young children. Telescoping of the ileum into the caecum (ileocaecal intussusception) is the type most commonly seen. In addition, adult caeco-colic, colo-colic and ileo-ileal intussusceptions are seen in parts of Nigeria and Uganda. Sometimes intussusception occurs secondary to a polyp or tumour acting as a lead-point but in many cases no specific cause is identifiable.

Clinical features

The combination of colicky abdominal pain, bloody diarrhoea and an abdominal mass should alert the surgeon to the possibility of intussusception.

Management

In children an intussusception will sometimes resolve spontaneously. This is not the case in adults. In developed countries it is sometimes possible to achieve reduction of an intussusception hydrostatically using contrast media. This is rarely possible in developing countries and should not be attempted without adequate access to surgical services. When an operation is required an attempt at manual reduction of the intussusception should be afforded. This is successful in approximately 80% of cases. When reduction is not possible, or the intussuscepted segment has strangulated, resection or exteriorisation of the affected bowel segment will be necessary.

Obstruction due to tuberculosis

See below.

Obstruction due to *Ascaris* worms

Aetiology

Ingested *Ascaris* ova grow into worms within the gut lumen. *Ascaris* infestation is generally an indication of poor sanitation and consequently is seen frequently where poverty prevails. Only rarely is intestinal contamination so heavy that bowel obstruction occurs. Indeed, obstruction often follows an attempt at decontamination, as paralysis of the worms may result in a bolus and predispose towards complete blockage.

Clinical features

A diagnosis of ascaris bowel obstruction may be considered when a child presents with a history of having passed worms rectally or having vomited them. In some cases an irregular mobile abdominal mass can be palpated.

Management

When ascaris obstruction has been diagnosed, and there are no features of peritoneal irritation, conservative management should be instituted. This involves the administration of intravenous fluids and nasogastric decompression. Deworming with mebendazole should not be attempted until the obstruction has resolved, as there is a risk of aggravating the condition. In most instances non-operative treatment is successful and surgery is not required. In some cases, however, when the obstruction has failed to resolve, or perforation has occurred, a laparotomy is indicated. When surgery is required for uncomplicated obstruction, every attempt should be made to avoid enterotomy, and instead attempts should be made to break up the mass and milk the worms into the caecum from where they can be passed safely.

HERNIA

A comprehensive account of the presentation, complications and management of inguinal hernias has been given in Chapter 27. Although inguinal hernias are commonly seen throughout the world, the presentation and management of this condition varies widely between developed and developing countries.

Hernias often reach a gigantic size before treatment is sought. Size, in itself, is seldom the determinant for presentation; rather it is the negative impact of pain on work and earning capacity. Indeed, presentation is often delayed until complications such as incarceration or strangulation have supervened.

Management

Standard treatment of inguinal hernias includes excision of the hernial sac (herniotomy) and repair of the abdominal wall defect (herniorrhaphy). The latter is achieved for inguinal hernia in developed countries by using a mesh which is fixed to the posterior wall of the inguinal canal. In developing countries, the technique generally requires modification. Certainly for large inguinoscrotal hernias, excision of the sac may require extensive dissection into the scrotum. Under these circumstances the sac can be divided once the contents have been reduced into the abdomen. The distal portion of the sac remains in situ in the scrotum. As a sterile mesh is expensive, repair of the posterior wall is usually achieved with the conventional *Bassini* or *Shouldice* procedures.

PLASTIC SURGERY

Plastic surgery, or the surgery of reconstruction, is frequently neglected in the provision of comprehensive surgical care in developing countries. This is unfortunate, since at least 20% of the surgical case load of a hospital in rural Africa is likely to require plastic surgical methods as part or all of the management (Box 40.4). Plastic surgery frequently requires no more than basic surgical resources, with little of the specialised equipment that can be associated with other surgical disciplines. Its primary role is in restoring tissues to their

Box 40.4 Main areas of plastic surgery in developing countries

Post trauma
- Face
- Hands
- Lower limb, especially compound fractures
- Urogenital
- Skin, especially burns and degloving or crush

Congenital anomaly
- Face, especially clefting
- Hands
- Urogenital
- Skin, especially lymphatic, vascular, tumours

Cancer and sequelae
- Skin
- Facial
- Sarcomas
- Advanced cancers of many forms

Soft-tissue infection
- Hand infections
- Necrotising fasciitis
- Neglected infections, which may include bone

'Difficult' wounds
- Overlying 'privileged' areas, or in diabetics, immunosuppressed patients, or following irradiation

normal form and function, thereby enabling the patient to feel more confident and function socially.

Plastic surgery methodology (see Ch. 38) includes careful discipline for tissue handling, the use of grafts of all tissue types (which are transferred without their blood supply) and a wide repertoire of flaps (which are transferred with a nutrient blood supply). Basic principles include dealing adequately with the underlying pathology before reconstruction (which may follow immediately or be delayed) and not expecting grafted material to 'take' on sites which have exposed, dried bone or are otherwise denuded of nutrient supply for wound healing. Tissues which are raised for transfer must be mobilised with a clear understanding of the underlying blood supply, and put into the new position without tension, underlying blood or exudates, and with careful handling to avoid early damage or loss.

BURN INJURY

It is outside the scope of this chapter to give a detailed account of burn management (see Ch. 10). Burn injury is one of the most commonly seen conditions in hospitals in the developing world, and is frequently neglected. Common causes include childhood scalds and falls into open fires used for cooking. Burns from petrol, electric shock and house fires are also remarkably common, and have been joined in many countries recently by conflict-related burns and acid burns following domestic violence. Burn injury is naturally more common where public health measures to control the use of volatile liquids and acids are less well organised. Likewise, poverty restricts cooking to open fires, and a reduction in severe burn injury usually follows significant periods of economic prosperity.

The severity of a burn relates to its site and depth, and the mortality of given types increases with early childhood and also old age. Scalds treated rapidly with cold water may remain superficial depending upon the initial fluid temperature, and also whether secondary infection follows. They are usually treated locally, sometimes with traditional remedies, and do not constitute the main problem in developing-world hospitals.

Most burns following flame injury, untreated scald, electrical injury and acid/alkali are full thickness, and should be assumed so unless proven otherwise. Minor burns do not require hospital admission, although relatively small-surface-area burns of important areas (such as the hands or eyelids) should be given urgent priority because of the severe consequences of neglected treatment.

Clinical Box 40.1 First aid in burns cases

- Manage airway/ventilation if inhalational element is present
- Insert intravenous access line if burn >10% in adults, >6% in children
- Divide any circumferential full-thickness constricting burn immediately – so-called 'escharotomy', does not require anaesthetic
- Give appropriate analgesia
- Give fluids according to a regimen with which you are familiar – take great care *not* to fluid overload, especially in children
- Give tetanus prophylaxis

Immediate care

Many burns cases in rural areas present late. In urban areas, however, they may arrive early, and require first aid. Initial assessment should include the following:

- Is there evidence of inhalational (smoke or toxic fume) injury?
  - singed nasal hairs
  - soot visible in back of throat
  - dyspnoea
- What is the approximate body surface area of the burn?
  - 'rule of nines' in adults (see Ch.10); palm = 1%; children, the head and trunk have a higher proportion of surface area
- What is the depth of the burn?
  - full thickness is insensate
  - superficial burns blister
  - history
- Are any of the extremities circumferentially burnt, causing distal ischaemia?
  - tight leather-like band of burn, with blue or white hand/foot.

First aid

See Clinical Box 40.1.

Burn management

Consider early excision of full-thickness burns, before they become infected and can be grafted 'cleanly'. Hand burns are usually best managed in plastic bags with some antiseptic fluid, in order to maintain mobility. Eyelid burns must be managed urgently to prevent exposure of the corneas.

Many hospitals in the developing world do not operate early on severe burns, because of the lack of facilities to undertake safe surgical excision with the inevitable fluid loss. This is unfortunate, since many of the later consequences of burn contracture and infection could be avoided if this were possible.

If burns are to be dressed, areas which might be expected to heal should be dressed early with non-stick dressings and left intact for 4–5-day periods to prevent secondary contamination. Deeper burns are ideally dressed daily with silver sulfadiazine (Flamazine) or a hypertonic agent such as pure honey. There is no role for topical antibiotics. Facial burns can be covered with simple liquid paraffin for comfort and washed regularly. Regular washing with clean water is a cheap, comfortable and often life-saving action which reduces the overall bacterial concentration in the wound colonisation, thereby reducing the incidence of invasive cellulitis (which is the first cause of septicaemia in burns).

Areas of up to 15% of body surface area burn can be excised and split skin grafted at one session, depending upon anaesthetic and postoperative support. Areas which often require more than a split skin graft include eyelids, exposed skuil, tendons and nerves, and the neck. These may be best treated with flap cover or full-thickness grafting (difficult technique for large areas).

Longer-term management and contracture prevention

The paramount importance of splintage and mobilisation following burn injury cannot be overemphasised. Simple plastic rings fashioned from strips of suction tubing connected together and placed around the neck can prevent severe neck flexion contracture developing. Hands, which are not being used, must be splinted, usually with wrist extended, metacarpophalangeal joints flexed, and fingers straight.

The social needs of badly burnt patients must also be addressed. Significant scarring and loss of function may often be unavoidable, and it is vital to begin to help the victim and their family early on in coming to terms with this, as well as planning for future occupation, and social reintegration.

Burn contracture

Burn contractures present one of the most common and enduring images of disabling injury in the developing world (Fig. 40.15). The loss of function of limbs, and hands in particular, is all the more devastating to lives where physical function is an essential component in personal or family survival. These disabilities also influence future marriage prospects and social integration.

Contracture release requires careful planning, and a certain amount of overall skin loss can be compensated for by mobilising adjacent tissue (such as in the versatile 'Y to V plasty' for dense linear flexion contractures). However, many contractures when released require the defect to be covered with additional skin, usually in the form of split graft. Thicker grafts are more difficult to get to 'take', and they leave poorly healing donor sites, but are most successful in preventing contracture relapse. Grafted areas must be splinted postoperatively until the joint has healed fully and is actively mobile.

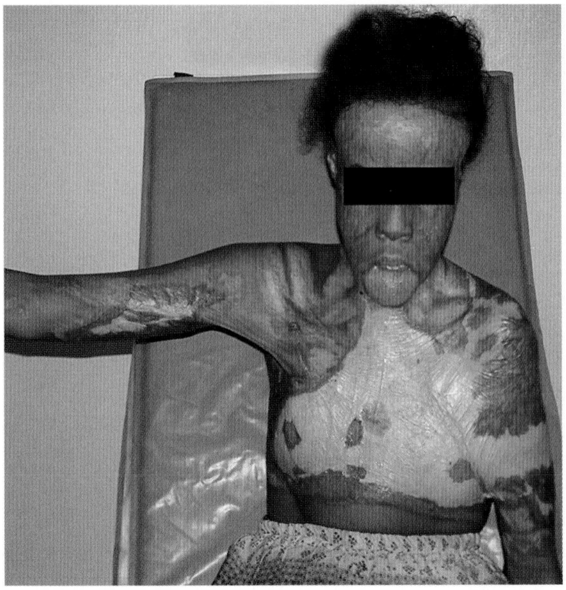

Fig. 40.15 Burn contracture.

When contracture release exposes major nerves, joints, or tendons, it is wise to attempt to cover these with local flaps of full-thickness tissue, and use split graft for the remaining areas. Contractures may often benefit from multiple operative releases and grafts, and the wise surgeon will anticipate this in taking care of available donor sites and careful attention to detail. Blood and exudates must be prevented from accumulating beneath the grafts, and this is usually best done by tying over dressings onto the graft in the early days.

OTHER INJURIES

Facial injuries

Facial injuries are usually predominantly either bony or soft-tissue, although severe road accidents and conflict injuries are inevitably combined. The most severe mid-facial bony fracture (classified as the Le Fort III, or 'craniofacial disjunction') can compromise the airway, and first aid involves pulling the upper jaw firmly forward to disimpact the fracture and clear the airway. Most other fractures fall into well-described patterns and can be corrected electively.

Soft-tissue facial injury in the developing world frequently involves loss of a major part, from animal or human bites, avulsion or weapon. It is not possible to describe all possible reconstructions, but two principles are essential:

- First, tissues such as the lip and nasal margin, the eyelid or the ear, are all irreplaceable, and therefore should be preserved if at all possible and only sacrificed if utterly destroyed or irredeemably damaged. Limited amounts of such remaining tissue should even be replaced, often contrary to the accepted teaching of surgical practice on wound debridement and toilet.
- Second, most secondary, elective, reconstruction will involve flap mobilisation, with little role for 'simple' grafts or flaps. Such surgery is not complicated, but is usually best reserved for those with previous experience

rather than risking the production of additional scars in unfavourable places which is often seen following poor reconstruction.

Hand injuries

Hand injuries require early wound care and washing, with preservation of all possible vital structures. The difficulties encountered with using dynamic splints following tendon repair in poor rural communities mean that tendon injuries are usually best given an attempt at primary repair and protected mobilisation (if fine instruments and suture materials are available). Flexor tendon injuries can have major long-lasting adverse effects on livelihood, and should always be managed with the best attention available for physiotherapy post surgery. Failing such a level of facilities, is the option of leaving the wound closed and treated with elective secondary tendon grafting at a later date (as was the case in major hand units up to about 30 years ago in developed health centres). Most bone injuries of the hand sustained in hot climates are best managed as conservatively as possible, using Kirchner wire fixation and pinning when necessary. There is an urgent need for many more dedicated hand injury treatment centres to be developed throughout poor countries, since this aspect of healthcare is ideally suited to management by skilled healthcare assistants and therapists (as has been shown clearly in India). It is also of greatest importance when livelihoods might be adversely affected by loss of hand function in manual labourers. The goal of all hand surgery is upgrading the injured or deformed hand to the best possible functional level.

Lower-limb injuries

Compound injuries of the lower limb can cause major disability, and are often treated with immediate below-knee amputation. In recent years, this amputation rate has been reduced by the introduction of a range of local, pedicled and distantly transferred ('free') flaps, which can be used to cover a carefully debrided and stabilised fracture site. Even complex injuries thus covered can subsequently be built up with cancellous bone grafting so long as an adequately vascularised soft-tissue 'envelope' has been created. The value of such lower-limb conservation has been challenged by some trauma authorities. However, the value of maintaining a viable limb without lifelong prosthetic requirements, to the rural communities of the developing world, cannot be overestimated.

Such reconstructions are rarely indicated for the mangled and heavily contaminated landmine injury, and any major neurovascular loss (the so-called 'Gustilo Grade 3c injury') is usually an absolute indication for amputation in the developing world.

ADVANCED CANCER

Much cancer in the developing world presents in an advanced stage. Clearly this may be terminal if metastatic disease is also present, but many tumours do not progress rapidly to such a stage before there has been advanced local tissue destruction. Neglected tumours (rarely seen in developed health centres) may be painful, smelly and debilitating, with blood loss and suppuration. Such tumours may be of the breast, skin, thyroid, oropharynx, bladder, or other rarer conditions. In rural areas, other treatments, such as radiotherapy, chemotherapy and opiate analgesia are usually not available or a scarce resource. Surgical excision may often be the only reasonable option both for potential cure and for palliation if there is no hope of successful eradication.

Major fungating cancers can present the surgeon with formidable problems in how to manage the resulting defect. Plastic surgery techniques are often able to deal with such tissue loss during the same operation, and can render cases operable which would otherwise be deemed not so. A common example is the use of the latissimus dorsi myocutaneous flap to cover massive anterior chest wall defects (including rib and pleural loss) following breast cancer excision.

CONGENITAL DEFORMITY

Common congenital deformities which can be successfully reconstructed include facial clefts (approx 1 in 350 births in Asia, 1 in 650 births in Europe, 1 in 800 births in Africa), some urogenital defects (1 in 300 births) (Fig. 40.16) and hand anomalies. Cleft lip and palate in particular carries various stigmata: for example the speech disorder associated with unrepaired cleft palate is often thought to indicate mental deficiency (which it clearly does not). Since cleft repair is a method that is easily taught, but can produce very poor results in untrained hands, it should be confined to those with the relevant expertise. Most parts of the world now have either their own highly trained group of surgeons or are visited by one of the teams of volunteers who undertake such work.

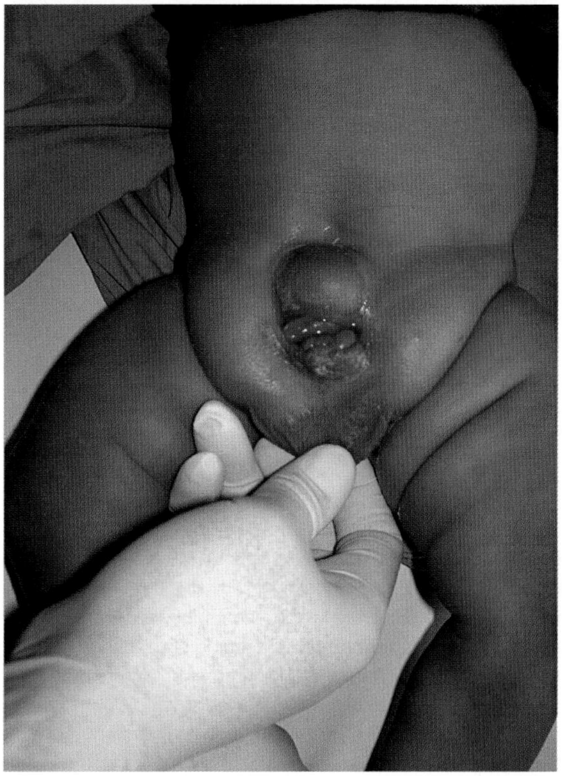

Fig. 40.16 Ectopia vesicae.

CONCLUSION

Plastic techniques are versatile and overlap with many other disciplines. Thus, complex and difficult wounds encountered by trauma surgeons, gynaecologists, ENT, eye and neurosurgeons might all benefit from access to surgeons trained in reconstructive methodology. Such a repertoire does not have to be comprehensive, and there is a real role for the training of healthcare assistants with skills confined to wound care, simple grafting and local flap management. The numbers of people throughout the poor world with untreated wounds and injuries (especially in war-torn areas) is simply massive and is one of the most pressing public health needs in the world today.

INFECTIONS

Many infections are disease entities that the visiting surgeon will not usually have encountered in regular practice. Unlike most surgery in developed countries which involves degenerative, malignant and traumatic conditions, surgery of sepsis and infection is proportionately much greater in developing nations. A description of common infections that often require surgical intervention follows.

Typhoid fever

Pathophysiology

During the second or third week of a typhoid illness, heavy gut contamination occurs through bilious excretion and bacteraemic spread. Typhoid (*Salmonella typhi*) colonises the lymphoid tissue of the jejunum, caecum, appendix and ascending colon. This leads to oedema and hyperplasia of the lymphoid follicles and may progress to ulceration and perforation.

Diagnosis

The diagnosis of an intestinal typhoid perforation is often suggested by the clinical features of peritonitis in a region where the disease is known to be endemic. Blood cultures are positive in 80% of patients in the second week. At this time, stool and urine cultures also become positive in those that have not received antimicrobial treatment.

Management

The surgical management of an intestinal perforation due to typhoid involves resuscitation and early laparotomy along with antimicrobial treatment. The perforation is usually found on the antimesenteric bowel border. Small perforations can be closed simply, but resection may be required for larger defects. The acutely ill patient with multiple perforations found at laparotomy might be best managed by simple 'exteriorisation' of the perforated area(s) and stabilisation of systemic disorder (with antimicrobial treatment) before definitive care of the bowel lesions as a delayed procedure.

Acute cholecystitis due to typhoid infection is rare. Chronic cholecystitis due to *Salmonella typhi* can however perpetuate a carrier state where patients continue to excrete microbes in the stool despite antimicrobial treatment. Cholecystectomy may be indicated for this group.

Abdominal tuberculosis

Abdominal tuberculosis (TB) refers to mycobacterial infection of the gastrointestinal tract, mesenteric lymph nodes, peritoneum and omentum, as well as the liver and spleen. A recent resurgence of TB has occurred both in the West as well as the developing world as a result of the proliferation of HIV.

Pathophysiology

Primary gastrointestinal infection occurs by ingestion of the bovine strain of *Mycobacterium tuberculosis* in milk. Secondary intestinal disease occurs from swallowing sputum infected with the bacteria. The terminal ileum and caecum are the most susceptible parts of the GI tract. The tubercle initially localises in the mucosal glands and, from there, spreads to Peyer's patches, where ulceration, inflammation and/or sclerosis occur. The disease may extend to involve the peritoneum, producing widespread tuberculous deposits. The usual presentation involves a history of insidious ill health, abdominal pain and weight loss. In addition, an acute abdomen may result from peritonitis or obstruction depending on whether the ulcerative or inflammatory process has predominated.

Management

Surgical treatment of intestinal TB is only indicated if gut complications, such as obstruction or peritonitis, have occurred. Otherwise, antituberculous chemotherapy is the mainstay of management.

Amoebiasis and amoebic liver abscess

Pathophysiology

Amoebiasis is caused by infestation with *Entamoeba histolytica* – a protozoal parasite. Approximately 10% of the world population have been infected, but many carriers remain asymptomatic. The active trophozoite subsists in the colon and, consequently, the disease is spread via the faeco-oral route. Amoebiasis exists in two forms: intestinal and extraintestinal. The intestinal form affects the large bowel, sparing the terminal ileum. The extraintestinal form affects the liver, lung, skin and brain.

Clinical features

Clinical presentation may be insidious, but patients often present acutely with high fever, tenesmus and colicky abdominal pain associated with bloody diarrhoea (amoebic dysentery or colitis). Colonic perforation is accompanied by signs of peritonitis and shock. Operative treatment is not usually required but is indicated when perforation or severe bleeding has supervened.

Liver abscess

Liver abscess is a potential complication of amoebic colitis (see Ch.19). The organ is affected by the portal spread of protozoa. Rupture of this abscess into the abdominal cavity or into the pleural space is a life-threatening complication. Surgery is rarely needed for the treatment of amoebic liver abscesses, as most can be managed with metronidazole with or without needle aspiration.

Hydatid disease

Pathophysiology and clinical features

The liver is the commonest site of involvement for the tapeworm *Echinococcus granulosus* (see Ch. 19), although any organ can be affected. Ova are generally passed in the faeces of affected animal hosts, usually dogs, and consequently pass to humans via the faeco-oral route. The *Echinococcus* ova penetrate the intestine to pass into the portal circulation and thence to the liver. In the liver the ova develop into cysts and enlarge insidiously. Symptomatic patients may present with a history of vague abdominal pain, hepatomegaly, jaundice and fever.

Management

Surgical management remains the mainstay of treatment for hepatic hydatid disease. Spillage of contents of the cyst should be avoided to prevent seeding. Surgical emergencies occur when rupture of the cyst occurs following trauma to an enlarged diseased liver. Medical treatment with albendazole is recommended perioperatively and for patients with disseminated disease.

Schistosomiasis (bilharzia)

Three schistosomes produce human disease: *Schistosoma haematobium*, *S. mansoni* and *S. japonicum*. The latter is prevalent in the Far East, whereas the other species cause infection mostly in Africa and South America (see also Ch. 33).

Pathophysiology

Cercaria represent the infective form of the parasite to humans. Snails act as vectors for the parasite. Human infection occurs following penetration of the skin by cercaria. The parasites then migrate to the liver and lungs via the venous system as schistosomules. Once mature, pairs of worms migrate to the mesenteric venules via the portal vein or to the bladder submucosa, where they replicate. The eggs can then leave the body in the faeces or urine by penetrating the intestinal or bladder wall. The larvae (miracidia) hatch once they enter fresh water, where they then infect host snails to perpetuate the cycle.

Clinical features

The clinical features of schistosomal infection are widespread. Acute infection is generally heralded by an acute inflammatory response at the site of the invading cercaria. This is often termed 'swimmers' or 'bathers' itch. Within a few days of infection an acute febrile illness generally supervenes. The clinical features of acute infection include fever, myalgia, urticaria, eosinophilia, diarrhoea and cough. The clinical features of chronic schistosomal infestation depend mostly on the type of the schistosome involved.

S. mansoni is the most prevalent schistosome in Africa and Latin America. It usually affects the colon, where it causes erythema, ulceration and inflammatory pseudopolyps. In its progressive form, fibrosis and stricture formation supervene. Granulomatous hepatitis followed by portal hypertension can give rise to hepatosplenomegaly and oesophageal varices. Pulmonary schistosomiasis occurs as the schistosomules pass to the lungs. Chronic pulmonary infection leads to pulmonary hypertension and cor pulmonale.

S. haematobium predominantly affects the urinary tract. It is most prevalent in Egypt and Middle Eastern countries. The presence of *S. haematobium* ova in 3000-year-old Egyptian mummies suggests that this disease was also prevalent in ancient times. Dysuria, haematuria and frequency result from the chronic inflammatory process that affects the urological system. In the latter stages, obstructive uropathy and chronic pyelonephritis supervene. Epidemiological studies suggest that schistosomal infection of the bladder is associated with both squamous cell and transitional cell cancer.

Diagnosis and management

The diagnosis of schistosomal infection is often made on clinical grounds alone. Ova can, however, be detected in the stools and urine as well as on rectal biopsy. Antischistosomal chemotherapeutic agents include praziquantel and oxamniquine. In endemic areas reinfection occurs rapidly following treatment.

Tropical ulcer

Tropical ulcer is common throughout the village communities in the tropics and subtropics.

Acute tropical ulcer

Pathophysiology

Acute tropical ulcer results from a cutaneous synergistic bacterial infection usually following trivial injury to the leg below the knee. A combination of anaerobes and facultative aerobes have been implicated in the pathogenesis (*Fusobacterium fusiforme* and *Borrelia vincentii*). Necrotising infection spreads within a few days until an area of demarcation is reached. Blistering of the skin with an area of central gangrene is usually surrounded by an area of cellulitis. Slough separation occurs early to reveal a bed of healthy granulation tissue surrounded by normal skin.

Differential diagnosis

There are numerous causes of severe ulceration in tropical environments. In recent years, the widespread incidence of deeply necrosing ulcers from *Mycobacterium ulcerans* infection – the 'Burulli ulcer' – has been identified, and is the subject of a WHO Global Initiative to raise awareness and direct best practice in management (www.who.int/buruli/en/). Antimycotic therapy is essential first-line treatment for such ulcers, with surgery having a major role in debriding dead tissue, effecting viable cover for exposed vital structures, and managing contractures and disabling functional loss.

Other causes of ulceration include other mycobacteria, cutaneous leishmaniasis (oriental sore), TB, leprosy, cutaneous anthrax, syphilitic gumma, and naturally causes such as venous stasis, and diabetic ulceration which are ubiquitous in presentation.

Management

Treatment of acute tropical ulcer might require prompt administration of intravenous systemic antibiotics with broad-spectrum cover. Unfortunately, most patients present at a later stage when skin necrosis is established. These patients may require antimicrobial treatment if persistent surrounding cellulitis is still present, as well as surgical debridement to remove non-viable tissue. Frequent washing with clean water and regular dressing changes then form the basis of local infection control. Small clean ulcers will heal spontaneously by epithelialisation from the ulcer edges. Larger ulcers (greater than 1–2 cm) can be encouraged to heal more rapidly with a split skin graft (meshed or perforated to encourage 'take' and allow exudate to escape).

Chronic tropical ulcer

Pathophysiology and differential diagnosis

When acute tropical ulcers fail to heal they become chronic. The strict definition of a chronic tropical ulcer is an acute lesion that has become chronic; however, numerous disease processes produce identical lower-limb ulceration. These differential diagnoses (Box 40.5 – not exhaustive) can be difficult to distinguish from chronic tropical ulceration on clinical grounds alone. The chronic ulcer has a pale and scarred appearance and the ulcer base is usually adjacent to the tibial periosteum. Over an extended period, repeated fibrosis can lead to severe contracture formation. Most ulcers remain indolent over many years, with malnutrition often influencing adequate wound healing. Any significant change in ulcer size or associated pain may signal squamous cell malignant change (the development of a so-called 'Marjolin's ulcer').

Management

Treatment of chronic tropical ulceration comprises local infection control (usually by removal of dead tissue, copious washing and provision of skin cover). The latter is usually best achieved by shaving the ulcer down to a healthy bed, and covering with a split skin graft that has been perforated or meshed. The graft should be immobilised with a firm dressing while it 'takes' over 10–14 days, and supported with an external pressure dressing (such as Tubigrip) for several months after surgery.

Box 40.5 Differential diagnosis for chronic tropical ulceration

- Syphilitic infection
- Yaws infection
- Mycobacterial ulceration
- Burulli ulcer
  - Tuberculosis
  - Leprosy
- Venous ulceration
- Arterial disease
- Diabetic ulceration
- Trauma

SOME OTHER SPECIALTIES

Obstetrics and gynaecology

Obstetricians and gynaecologists perform operations, yet in the developed world the specialty is a separate entity from other surgical disciplines. In developing countries, with obstetric specialists scarce, general surgeons are often called upon to perform emergency obstetric procedures and even elective gynaecological operations. Common O&G surgical procedures include:

- obstetric
  - caesarean section or symphysiotomy for obstructed labour, or in cases of pre-eclampsia/eclampsia
  - emergency hysterectomy or uterine repair for uterine rupture
- gynaecological
  - bilateral tubal ligation
  - hysterectomy – abdominal and vaginal
  - ovarian cystectomy
  - vesicovaginal fistula repair.

Trauma and orthopaedics

The most common cause of disability worldwide is trauma following road traffic injury (22.8%). War and civil unrest also results in a high volume of patients needing urgent treatment and thus stretching already scarce resources – with war and violence accounting for another 14.4 % of global injury. Disability as a long-term outcome of such injury is common, especially amongst those in poor countries where few have access to surgery, artificial limbs and rehabilitation.

Recent global initiatives have attempted to address this urgent need. Primary Trauma Care is a comprehensive programme of appropriate methods and support for trauma delivery in resource-poor nations (www.nda.ox.ac.uk/ptc/)

Provision of orthopaedic treatment in rural centres can be basic and is sometimes provided by a general surgeon. The most appropriate methods for fracture management might not be the more widely used internal fixation techniques adopted in developed hospitals with ultra-clean environments. The closed management of fractures using balanced traction and other well-established methods (Charnley 2007) may be. Serious complications of fractures such as malunion, delayed and non-union are common. This is illustrated in Figure 40.17, where a young man with non-union required hospital care for about 18 months. Immobilisation with such injury for long periods results in muscle atrophy, joint stiffness and possible further debilitation from pressure sore formation.

Orthopaedic surgical procedures undertaken in poor environments are associated with a high incidence of complications, especially postoperative sepsis. Osteomyelitis (either primary or secondarily following compound fracture) is common and is difficult to erradicate without access to radical surgical excision, reconstruction (including soft-tissue transfer) and prolonged therapy with multiple antibiotics.

Ophthalmology

It is estimated that blindness affects 37 million people worldwide (Table 40.1). Approximately three-quarters of all cases

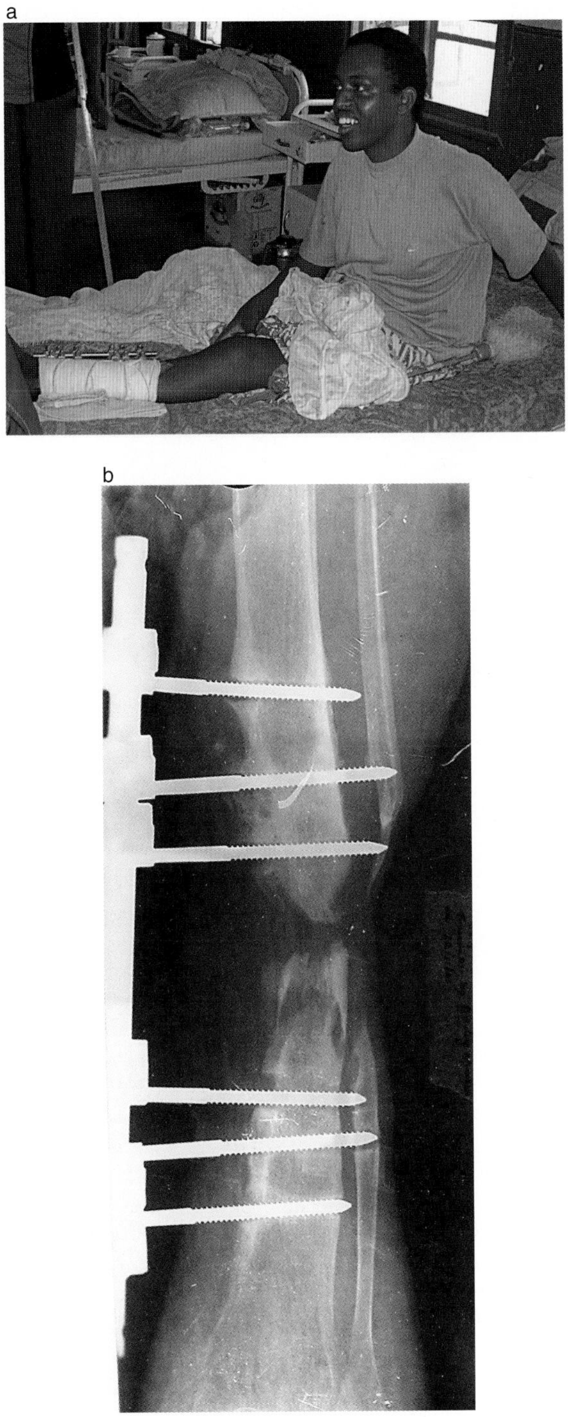

Fig. 40.17 (a) Young patient with non-union of lower-limb fracture. (b) X-ray of non-union.

Table 40.1 WHO estimates of prevalence of blindness for different regions (2002)

Region	Prevalence of blindness
European region	2.7 million
Americas	2.4 million
SE Asia	11.6 million
Africa	6.7 million
Western Pacific region	9.3 million
Eastern Mediterranean region	4.0 million
World total	36.7 million

Table 40.2 Estimated causes of blindness worldwide (WHO 2010)

Cause	%
Cataract	48
Glaucoma	12
Macular degeneration	9
Diabetic retinopathy	5
Corneal opacities	5
Childhood blindness	4
Trachoma	4
Onchocerciasis	1
Others	12

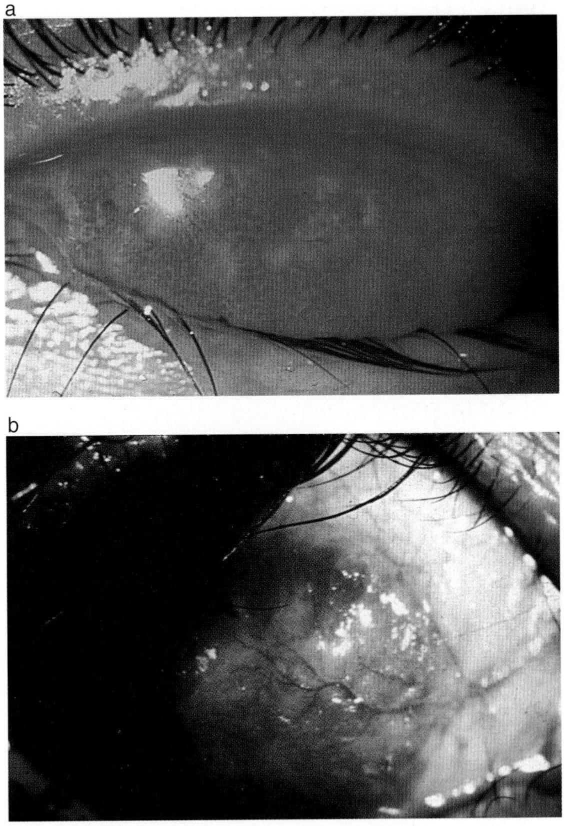

Fig. 40.18 Trachoma: (a) subtarsal scarring in stage III; (b) corneal neovascularisation and scarring. (By courtesy of Mr D McHugh, King's College Hospital, London.)

of blindness are preventable or amenable to cure. Data on the worldwide causes of visual loss are given in Table 40.2. Trachoma is present in epidemic proportions in many developing countries and accounts for a high proportion of preventable blindness. Figure 40.18a shows typical subtarsal scarring seen in stage III trachoma, and Figure 40.18b illustrates corneal neovascularisation and scarring.

FURTHER READING

Charnley J 2007 The closed treatment of common fractures. Golden Jubilee edn. Cambridge University Press, Cambridge

Walker IA, Wilson IH 2008 Anaesthesia in developing countries – a risk for patients. The Lancet 371: 968–969

Warrell DA, Cox TM, Firth JD (eds) 2010 Oxford textbook of medicine, 5th edn. Oxford University Press, Oxford

World Health Organisation 2002 World Health Report, WHO, Geneva. Available online. Accessed 18 January 2011 www.who.int/violence_injury_prevention/publications/road_traffic/world_report/

Index

Page numbers followed by "f" indicate figures, "t" indicate tables, and "b" indicate boxes.

A

C

F

G

H

I

J

K

N

O

T

U

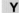

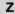